The American Psychiatric Publishing

Textbook of Substance Abuse Treatment

Third Edition

The American Psychiatric Publishing

Textbook of Substance Abuse Treatment

Third Edition

Edited by

Marc Galanter, M.D.
Herbert D. Kleber, M.D.

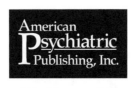

American Psychiatric Publishing, Inc.

Washington, DC
London, England

Manufactured in the United States of America on acid-free paper
08 07 06 05 04   5 4 3 2 1
Third Edition

Typeset in Adobe's New Baskerville and Futura Book

American Psychiatric Publishing, Inc.
1000 Wilson Boulevard
Arlington, VA 22209-3901
www.appi.org

Library of Congress Cataloging-in-Publication Data
The American Psychiatric Publishing textbook of substance abuse treatment / edited by Marc Galanter,
    Herbert D. Kleber.—3rd ed.
        p. ; cm.
    Rev. ed. of: The American Psychiatric Press textbook of substance abuse treatment. 2nd ed. c1999.
    Includes bibliographical references and index.
    ISBN 1-58562-099-8 (alk. paper)
    1. Substance abuse—Treatment. I. Galanter, Marc. II. Kleber, Herbert D. III. American Psychiatric Press
textbook of substance abuse treatment. IV. Title: Textbook of substance abuse treatment.
    [DNLM: 1. Substance-Related Disorders—therapy. WM 270 A5108 2004]
    RC564.A526 2004
    616.86'06—dc22
                                                                                                2003058354

British Library Cataloguing in Publication Data
A CIP record is available from the British Library.

Contents

PART

I

The Nature of Addiction

PART

IV

Treatment Approaches

PART

V

Special Approaches and Treatment Programs

PART
VI
Special Populations

Contributors

James C. Anthony, Ph.D.
Professor and Chairman, Department of Epidemiology, Medical School, Michigan State University, East Lansing, Michigan

Samuel A. Ball, Ph.D.
Associate Professor of Psychiatry, Yale University School of Medicine, New Haven, Connecticut

Steven L. Batki, M.D.
Professor and Director of Research, Department of Psychiatry, State University of New York Upstate Medical University, Syracuse, New York

Terry C. Blum, Ph.D.
Dean and Tedd Munchak Professor of Management, DuPree College of Management, Georgia Institute of Technology, Atlanta, Georgia

Sheila B. Blume, M.D.
Clinical Professor of Psychiatry, State University of New York at Stony Brook, Stony Brook, New York; Former Medical Director, Addiction Services, South Oaks Hospital, Amityville, New York

Lisa Borg, M.D.
Senior Research Associate and Associate Physician, Laboratory of the Biology of Addictive Diseases, Rockefeller University; Clinical Assistant Professor of Psychiatry, Weill Medical College of Cornell University, New York, New York

Kathleen T. Brady, M.D., Ph.D.
Professor of Psychiatry and Behavioral Sciences, Medical University of South Carolina, Charleston, South Carolina

David W. Brook, M.D.
Professor of Community and Preventive Medicine, Mount Sinai School of Medicine, New York, New York

Kirk J. Brower, M.D.
Associate Professor of Psychiatry, University of Michigan Department of Psychiatry and Addiction Research Center, Ann Arbor, Michigan

Kathleen M. Carroll, Ph.D.
Professor of Psychiatry, Division of Substance Abuse, Yale University School of Medicine, New Haven; VA Connecticut Healthcare System, West Haven, Connecticut

Chuan Yu Chen, Ph.D.
Postdoctoral Fellow, Johns Hopkins Bloomberg School of Public Health, Baltimore, Maryland

C. Robert Cloninger, M.D.
Wallace Renard Professor of Psychiatry and Genetics, Department of Psychiatry, Washington University School of Medicine, St. Louis, Missouri

Eric D. Collins, M.D.
Assistant Professor of Clinical Psychiatry, Department of Psychiatry, Columbia University College of Physicians and Surgeons, New York, New York

J. Douglas Crowder, M.D.
Associate Professor of Psychiatry, University of Texas Southwestern Medical Center, Dallas, Texas

Thomas J. Crowley, M.D.
Professor and Director, Division of Substance Dependence, Department of Psychiatry, University of Colorado School of Medicine; Attending Physician, University of Colorado Hospital, Denver, Colorado

George De Leon, Ph.D.
Director, Center for Therapeutic Community Research at National Development and Research Institutes; Clinical Professor of Psychiatry, New York University School of Medicine, New York, New York

Robert L. DuPont, M.D.
President, Institute for Behavior and Health, Inc., Rockville, Maryland; Clinical Professor of Psychiatry, Georgetown University School of Medicine, Washington, D.C.

Chad D. Emrick, Ph.D.
Assistant Clinical Professor of Clinical Psychology in Psychiatry, University of Colorado Health Sciences Center; Director, Substance Abuse Treatment Program, Denver Veterans Affairs Medical Center, Denver, Colorado

Loretta P. Finnegan, M.D.
Professor of Pediatrics, Psychiatry, and Human Behavior (Adjunct), Jefferson Medical College of Thomas Jefferson University, Philadelphia, Pennsylvania

Richard J. Frances, M.D.
Director of Public and Professional Education, Silver Hill Hospital, New Canaan, Connecticut; Clinical Professor of Psychiatry, New York University, New York, New York; Adjunct Professor of Psychiatry, University of Medicine and Dentistry of New Jersey, Newark, New Jersey

John E. Franklin, M.D.
Associate Professor of Psychiatry and Director, Division of Addiction Psychiatry, Feinberg School of Medicine, Northwestern University, Chicago, Illinois

Kimberly Frost-Pineda, M.P.H.
Coordinator for Public Health Research Group, Department of Psychiatry, Division of Addiction Medicine, University of Florida, Gainesville, Florida

Marc Galanter, M.D.
Professor of Psychiatry and Director of the Division of Alcoholism and Drug Abuse, New York University Medical Center, New York, New York

David R. Gastfriend, M.D.
Director, Addiction Research Program, Department of Psychiatry, Massachusetts General Hospital and Harvard Medical School, Boston, Massachusetts

Dean R. Gerstein, Ph.D.
Senior Vice President, National Opinion Research Center at the University of Chicago, Washington Office, Washington, D.C.

Richard A. Glennon, Ph.D.
Professor of Medicinal Chemistry, Department of Medicinal Chemistry, School of Pharmacy, Medical College of Virginia, Virginia Commonwealth University, Richmond, Virginia

Mark S. Gold, M.D.
Distinguished Professor, Departments of Psychiatry, Neuroscience, Community Health, and Family Medicine; Chief, Division of Addiction Medicine, University of Florida McKnight Brain Institute, Gainesville, Florida

Sarah J. Golden-Schulman, Ph.D.
Clinical Psychologist, Tucson, Arizona

Edith S. Lisansky Gomberg, Ph.D.
Professor Emerita, Department of Psychiatry, University of Michigan, Ann Arbor, Michigan

Shelly F. Greenfield, M.D., M.P.H.
Assistant Professor of Psychiatry, Harvard Medical School, Boston, Massachusetts; Medical Director of Alcohol and Drug Abuse Ambulatory Treatment Program, McLean Hospital, Belmont, Massachusetts

Erik W. Gunderson, M.D.
Assistant Clinical Professor of Medicine in Psychiatry, Columbia University College of Physicians and Surgeons and New York State Psychiatric Institute, New York, New York

Margaret Haney, Ph.D.
Associate Professor of Clinical Neuroscience, Department of Psychiatry, College of Physicians and Surgeons of Columbia University and New York State Psychiatric Institute, New York, New York

Sarah H. Heil, Ph.D.
Research Assistant Professor, Department of Psychiatry, University of Vermont, Burlington, Vermont

Grace Hennessy, M.D.
Assistant Professor of Clinical Psychiatry, Columbia University; Assistant Medical Director, Substance Treatment and Research Service, New York State Psychiatric Institute, New York, New York

Reid K. Hester, Ph.D.
Director, Research Division, Behavior Therapy Associates LLP, Albuquerque, New Mexico

Stephen T. Higgins, Ph.D.
Professor, Departments of Psychiatry and Psychology, University of Vermont, Burlington, Vermont

Paula L. Hoffman, Ph.D.
Professor, University of Colorado Health Sciences Center, Department of Pharmacology, Denver, Colorado

Harold D. Holder, Ph.D.
Senior Scientist, Prevention Research Center, Pacific Institute for Research and Evaluation, Berkeley, California

William S. Jacobs, M.D.
Assistant Professor, Department of Psychiatry, University of Florida College of Medicine, Gainesville, Florida; Medical Director, Gateway Community Services, Jacksonville, Florida

Ari B. Jaffe, M.D.
Associate Clinical Director, Mental Illness Research and Clinical Center, VISN3, Veterans Affairs Medical Center, Bronx, New York

Jerome H. Jaffe, M.D.
Clinical Professor, Department of Psychiatry, Division of Alcohol and Drug Abuse, University of Maryland School of Medicine, Baltimore, Maryland; Adjunct Professor, Department of Mental Hygiene, Johns Hopkins University School of Public Health, Baltimore, Maryland

Yifrah Kaminer, M.D.
Professor of Psychiatry, Alcohol Research Center, Department of Psychiatry, University of Connecticut Health Center, Farmington, Connecticut

Kyle M. Kampman, M.D.
Associate Professor of Psychiatry, University of Pennsylvania and Philadelphia Veterans Affairs Medical Center, Philadelphia, Pennsylvania

Stephen R. Kandall, M.D.
Professor of Pediatrics (Retired), Albert Einstein College of Medicine, Bronx, New York

Edward Kaufman, M.D.
Clinical Professor of Psychiatry, Department of Psychiatry and Human Behavior, University of California at Irvine, College of Medicine, Irvine, California

Edward J. Khantzian, M.D.
Clinical Professor of Psychiatry, Harvard Medical School at the Cambridge Hospital, Cambridge, Massachusetts; Associate Chief of Psychiatry, Tewksbury Hospital, Tewksbury, Massachusetts

Gregory L. Kirk, M.D.
Chief of Psychiatry for Hospital and Consultation Services, Kaiser-Permanente, Colorado Region, Denver, Colorado

Herbert D. Kleber, M.D.
Professor of Psychiatry and Director of the Division on Substance Abuse, Columbia University College of Physicians and Surgeons and New York State Psychiatric Institute, New York, New York

Thomas R. Kosten, M.D.
Professor and Deputy Chief of Psychiatry, Yale University School of Medicine, VA Connecticut Healthcare System, Department of Psychiatry, West Haven, Connecticut

Sari Kutch, M.S.W.
Ackerman Institute for the Family, New York, New York

Frances Rudnick Levin, M.D.
Q.J. Kennedy Associate Professor of Clinical Psychiatry, Columbia University College of Physicians and Surgeons and New York State Psychiatric Institute, New York, New York

Petros Levounis, M.D.
Assistant Professor of Clinical Psychiatry, Columbia University College of Physicians and Surgeons; Director, Smithers Alcoholism Treatment and Training Center, New York, New York

Lester Luborsky, Ph.D.
Professor of Psychology in Psychiatry, Department of Psychiatry, University of Pennsylvania, Philadelphia, Pennsylvania

Avram H. Mack, M.D.
Physician, Bellevue Hospital Center, New York, New York

Robert J. Malcolm, M.D.
Professor of Psychiatry and Behavioral Sciences, Medical University of South Carolina, Charleston, South Carolina

Peter A. Mansky, M.D.
Clinical Associate Professor, Department of Psychiatry, and Adjunct Associate Professor, Department of Pharmacology and Toxicology, Albany Medical College of Union University, Albany, New York; Medical Director, Committee for Physicians' Health (Physicians' Health Program), Medical Society of the State of New York

Billy R. Martin, Ph.D.
Louis and Ruth Harris Professor and Chair, Department of Pharmacology and Toxicology, Virginia Commonwealth University School of Medicine, Richmond, Virginia

Steve Martino, Ph.D.
Associate Professor of Psychiatry, Yale University School of Medicine, New Haven, Connecticut

William E. McAuliffe, Ph.D.
Director, North Charles Research and Planning Group, Cambridge; and Associate Professor, Department of Psychiatry, Harvard Medical School, Boston, Massachusetts

David M. McDowell, M.D.
Director, Buprenorphine Program, and Senior Medical Advisor, Substance Abuse Research and Treatment Service, Columbia University College of Physicians and Surgeons, New York State Psychiatric Institute Division on Substance Abuse, New York, New York

Delinda Mercer, Ph.D.
Staff Psychologist, Partners in Behavioral Health at Region West Medical Center, Scottsbluff, Nebraska

Edgar P. Nace, M.D.
Clinical Professor of Psychiatry, University of Texas Southwestern Medical Center, Dallas, Texas

Kalpana I. Nathan, M.D.
Adjunct Clinical Assistant Professor of Psychiatry, Stanford University School of Medicine, Stanford, California; Program Director, New Horizons, Palo Alto Veterans Affairs Health Care System, Menlo Park, California

Charles P. O'Brien, M.D., Ph.D.
Kenneth E. Appel Professor and Vice Chair of Psychiatry, University of Pennsylvania and Philadelphia Veterans Affairs Medical Center Mental Illness Research, Education and Clinical Center, Philadelphia, Pennsylvania

Judith K. Ockene, Ph.D., M.Ed.
Professor of Medicine, Division of Preventive and Behavioral Medicine, University of Massachusetts Medical School, Worcester, Massachusetts

Lori Pbert, Ph.D.
Associate Professor of Medicine, Division of Preventive and Behavioral Medicine, University of Massachusetts Medical School, Worcester, Massachusetts

Robert N. Pechnick, Ph.D.
Associate Director of Research, Department of Psychiatry, Cedars-Sinai Medical Center; Professor of Psychiatry, Department of Psychiatry and Biobehavioral Sciences, David Geffen School of Medicine at UCLA, Los Angeles, California

Sandrine Pirard, M.D.
Clinical Research Fellow, Addiction Research Program, Department of Psychiatry, Massachusetts General Hospital and Harvard Medical School, Boston, Massachusetts

Harrison G. Pope Jr., M.D.
Professor of Psychiatry, Harvard Medical School and Director, Biological Psychiatry Laboratory, McLean Hospital/Harvard Medical School, Belmont, Massachusetts

Jennifer Sharpe Potter, Ph.D., M.P.H.
Research Director, Alcohol and Drug Abuse Treatment Program, McLean Hospital, Belmont, Massachusetts; Instructor in Psychology, Department of Psychiatry, Harvard Medical School, Boston, Massachusetts

Sarah Reiff-Hekking, Ph.D.
Assistant Professor of Medicine, Division of Preventive and Behavioral Medicine, University of Massachusetts Medical School, Worcester, Massachusetts

Jonathan I. Ritvo, M.D.
Clinical Associate Professor of Psychiatry and Training Director, Addiction Psychiatry Program, Denver Health Medical Center, University of Colorado School of Medicine, Denver, Colorado

Paul M. Roman, Ph.D.
Distinguished Research Professor of Sociology and Director, Center for Research on Behavioral Health and Human Service Delivery, Institute for Behavioral Research and Department of Sociology, University of Georgia, Athens, Georgia

Joseph T. Sakai, M.D.
Instructor/Fellow, Department of Psychiatry, University of Colorado Health Sciences Center, Denver, Colorado

Sidney H. Schnoll, M.D., Ph.D.
Clinical Professor of Internal Medicine and Psychiatry, Medical College of Virginia, Virginia Commonwealth University, Richmond, Virginia

Richard Steven Schottenfeld, M.D.
Professor of Psychiatry, Department of Psychiatry, Substance Abuse Treatment Unit, Yale University School of Medicine, New Haven, Connecticut

Marc A. Schuckit, M.D.
Professor of Psychiatry, University of California at San Diego School of Medicine, and San Diego Veterans Hospitals, San Diego, California

Carl M. Selavka, Ph.D.
Director, Massachusetts State Police Crime Laboratory, Sudbury, Massachusetts

David E. Smith, M.D.
Founder and Medical Director, Haight-Ashbury Free Clinics; Professor, University of California, San Francisco; San Francisco, California

Mehmet Sofuoglu, M.D., Ph.D.
Associate Professor of Psychiatry, Yale University School of Medicine, VA Connecticut Healthcare System, Department of Psychiatry, West Haven, Connecticut

Daniel D. Squires, M.S., M.P.H.
Psychology Intern, Brown University School of Medicine, Providence, Rhode Island

Peter Steinglass, M.D.
Executive Director, Ackerman Institute for the Family; Clinical Professor of Psychiatry, Weill Medical College of Cornell University, New York, New York

Barry Stimmel, M.D.
Katherine and Clifford Goldsmith Professor of Medicine and Professor of Medical Education, Mount Sinai School of Medicine, New York, New York

Boris Tabakoff, Ph.D.
Professor and Chair, University of Colorado Health Sciences Center, Department of Pharmacology, Denver, Colorado

Susan Tapert, Ph.D.
Assistant Professor of Psychiatry, University of California at San Diego, San Diego, California

Ralph E. Tarter, Ph.D.
Professor, School of Pharmacology, University of Pittsburgh, Pittsburgh, Pennsylvania

J. Scott Tonigan, Ph.D.
Co-Director, Center on Alcoholism, Substance Abuse, and Addictions, University of New Mexico, Albuquerque, New Mexico

J. Thomas Ungerleider, M.D.
Professor Emeritus of Psychiatry, Department of Psychiatry and Biobehavioral Sciences, David Geffen School of Medicine at UCLA, Los Angeles, California

Michael F. Weaver, M.D.
Assistant Professor of Internal Medicine and Psychiatry, Medical College of Virginia, Virginia Commonwealth University, Richmond, Virginia

Roger D. Weiss, M.D.
Clinical Director, Alcohol and Drug Abuse Treatment Program, McLean Hospital, Belmont, Massachusetts; Associate Professor of Psychiatry, Harvard Medical School, Boston, Massachusetts

Donald R. Wesson, M.D.
Consultant, CNS Medications Development, Oakland, California

Joseph Westermeyer, M.D., M.P.H., Ph.D.
Chief, Psychiatry Services, Minneapolis Veteran Affairs Medical Center and St. Cloud Veteran Affairs Medical Center; Professor of Psychiatry and Adjunct Professor of Anthropology, University of Minnesota, Minneapolis, Minnesota

George E. Woody, M.D.
Behavioral Health Service, Philadelphia Veterans Affairs Medical Center; Professor, Department of Psychiatry, University of Pennsylvania, Philadelphia, Pennsylvania

Monica L. Zilberman, M.D., Ph.D.
Psychiatrist and Fellow, Institute of Psychiatry, University of São Paulo, São Paulo, Brazil

Preface

Substance abuse, a worldwide problem of major dimensions, was identified in a 2001 report to the Robert Wood Johnson Foundation as the number one health problem in the United States. The estimated annual U.S. economic cost of substance abuse is more than $414 billion. In the United States, 18% of the population experiences a substance use disorder at some point in life. Furthermore, an average of 20% of patients in general medical facilities and 35% in general psychiatric units present with substance use disorders—and in some settings, the percentage is much higher. Although the sequelae of addiction, such as cirrhosis, psychopathology, trauma, and infection, generally receive proper medical attention, patients' primary addictive problems often go untreated.

Nonetheless, we stand on the threshold of important opportunities in the addiction field. In recent years many advances have emerged in receptor mechanisms, membrane chemistry, and patterns of genetic transmission. Public awareness of the need for greater research and treatment resources has been aroused as well, and substance abusers now seek help earlier, at a point when treatment can be administered more effectively. Furthermore, the health community has been alerted to the need for early diagnosis and comprehensive care. New treatment concepts, both pharmacological and psychosocial, have made recovery a possibility for most alcohol- and drug-abusing patients.

The first edition of this volume emerged from a growing commitment of psychiatry to address the problem of substance abuse. In 1982, the American Psychiatric Association (APA) established its Task Force on Treatment of Psychiatric Disorders, consisting of 26 panels. The editors of this textbook served as chairpersons of the panels on psychoactive substance use disorders, alcohol, and other drugs. In response to this APA initiative, we brought together a group of experts who could provide a carefully drawn perspective on addiction treatment, perhaps the most comprehensive one to date. After several years' work, our panels developed reports for the Task Force that were published by the APA in 1989 in the four-volume set *Treatments of Psychiatric Disorders.*

Soon after the appearance of these volumes, we decided that it was important to update and amplify the substance abuse treatment information. In addition, we wanted to focus on the most recent developments in biological and psychosocial therapies and the problems of specific populations. The resulting volume, the first edition of this textbook, appeared in 1994, and the second edition followed in 1999. We are now pleased to present a fully updated version of this textbook, tailored to represent the most current basic and clinical perspectives on the substance abuse field.

Most important to the development of the current edition was the maturation of the substance abuse field itself. As recently as the mid-1980s, American departments of psychiatry, as well as academic programs for other health professionals, paid little heed to the importance of training for substance use treatment. Although the medical addiction community had been vocal over the previous two decades about the need for better care, investment in addiction training was relatively small and had only a limited association with academic teaching centers. This situation has changed dramatically in recent years. Substance abuse training is now an integral part of undergraduate curricula in most medical schools and is a one-month full-time equivalent component of psychiatry residency training programs. Courses about substance abuse are also regularly taught in graduate psychology and social work programs. The federal institutes on drug and alcohol abuse are fully aware of the need for research training and are working closely with organizations in the addiction field to promote growth in clinical teaching as well.

The approval of the American Board of Psychiatry and Neurology for an Added Qualification in Addiction Psychiatry was of major importance in establishing addiction as a medical subspecialty. The American Board of Medical Specialties, under its guidelines for establishing subspecialties, sanctioned this process. The first certifying examination was given in 1993, and certification is now given by APBN on the basis of an examination and a minimum of one year of associated training in an accredited residency. The Accreditation Council for Graduate Medical Education reviews the curricula of these respective training programs, and completion of such a program is required by candidates to sit for the subspecialty examination. In 1996 the first PGY V and PGY V–VI addiction psychiatry residencies were approved, and certified programs are now listed in the Graduate Medical Education Directory.

As of this printing, more than 1,800 psychiatrists are certified in Addiction Psychiatry. These subspecialists will meet a variety of clinical and academic needs, and the range of training experiences provided by the addiction residency programs has been designed to prepare them for this. These residents spend about half their time on patient care and devote the rest of their time to research, teaching, and their own learning. Postresidency fellowships in addiction psychiatry now number more than 40. These programs are showing great vitality and are playing an influential role in ensuring quality treatment for the future. Unfortunately, less than half of the population in need of substance abuse treatment actually receives it—a function both of the reluctance of private and public payors to adequately fund treatment and of the reluctance of the affected population to seek it.

We have designed this volume to serve clinicians in practice and researchers concerned with addiction as well as trainees in psychiatry, general medicine, and other health professions. We therefore hope that this book will serve as a valuable treatment resource for any health care professional concerned with the problems posed by the issue of substance abuse.

Marc Galanter, M.D.
Herbert D. Kleber, M.D.

The Nature of Addiction

Neurobiology of Alcohol

Boris Tabakoff, Ph.D.
Paula L. Hoffman, Ph.D.

Ethanol, or beverage alcohol, is an organic molecule composed of two carbon atoms, six hydrogen atoms, and one oxygen atom. This molecule seemingly carries little chemical information in its structure but generates myriad effects in the central nervous system (CNS) and in peripheral organs of mammals and other organisms. The chronic ingestion of ethanol can result in the alterations of CNS function observed in the alcohol dependence syndrome (American Psychiatric Association 2000; World Health Organization 1992). The diagnosis of alcohol dependence in the United States is usually based on DSM-IV-TR (American Psychiatric Association 2000).

Alcohol dependence can be considered a pharmacogenetic disease in which the "disease"-causing agent (alcohol) interacts with the genetic background of the "host" organism (human) to produce the manifestations of the "disease." It is also generally acknowledged that not only genetic but environmental factors influence both the level of alcohol intake by an individual and the propensity to develop dependence on alcohol.

A clear demonstration of the interaction of genetics and environment is an animal behavior study in which responses to ethanol (incoordination, anxiolysis, anesthesia) were tested in the same panel of inbred strains of mice (which are genetically identical) in several different laboratories (Crabbe et al. 1999). In spite of the genetic homogeneity of the animals and concerted efforts to control certain environmental influences, significant differences in behavioral responses to ethanol occurred between laboratories. These types of studies underscore the importance of realizing that even a discussion of ethanol's actions at a cellular or molecular level should not ignore the influence of genotype or environment (e.g., the culture conditions for neuronal primary cultures) on the mechanisms by which ethanol produces acute intoxication and/or dependence.

Another important issue sometimes overlooked in discussions of ethanol's cellular action is the dose-response relationship of the effects of ethanol on particular receptors, signal transduction systems, and

The authors' work is supported by the National Institute on Alcohol Abuse and Alcoholism and the Banbury Fund.

neurotransmitter networks. As the concentration of ethanol in brain is increased, the actions of ethanol spread from a limited number of targets to involve multiple molecular sites of action. This occurrence differentiates ethanol from drugs (e.g., morphine) that are limited in their spectrum of action by specific interaction with only certain families of receptors (e.g., the opiate μ, δ, κ receptors) for both their analgesic and reinforcing effects and high-dose toxicologic actions. When discussing the neurobiology of alcohol's actions, we limit ourselves to effects primarily noted at concentrations compatible with survival in humans (i.e., 5–100 mM or 23–460 mg/100 mL). The LD_{50} dose for ethanol in humans is approximately 600 mg/100 mL).

Molecular Interactions That Mediate the Effects of Ethanol

Historically, the acute actions of ethanol in the CNS were believed to be mediated through a disordering of neuronal membrane bulk lipids (Goldstein et al. 1982; Meyer 1901). However, a careful examination of the concentrations of ethanol needed to produce a generalized perturbation of the neuronal lipid bilayer (100–1,000 mM) indicated that the lipid-disordering effect of ethanol could not be reconciled with many of ethanol's nonanesthetic effects in the CNS. That is not to say that lipids or hydrophobic interactions have nothing to do with ethanol's actions. The conformation and proper localization of a cellular (neuronal membrane) protein, which often is a prerequisite for a protein's action, is dependent on the protein's interaction with lipid domains and on protein-protein interactions. It is currently acknowledged that ethanol's biophysical (amphipathic) properties may well affect protein-lipid and protein-protein interactions, in the context of either multisubunit receptor/effector systems or disruption of scaffold systems devoted to bringing together protein complexes (e.g., protein kinases and their substrates; Pawson and Scott 1997).

There is also beginning to be significant evidence that ethanol may interact with specific domains of single proteins per se ("alcohol-sensitive pockets"). For example, ethanol has been shown to increase the action of the inhibitory neurotransmitter γ-aminobutyric acid (GABA) at the $GABA_A$ receptor (Mihic 1999). Mutations of certain amino acid residues in the α or β

subunits of the $GABA_A$ receptor altered the ability of ethanol to potentiate GABA responses (Ueno et al. 2001), even though the mutant proteins were expressed in the identical cells used for studies of the wild-type (i.e., normal) protein. These data implicated the primary as well as the tertiary and quaternary structure of the multisubunit $GABA_A$ receptor protein complex in mediating certain effects of ethanol. Similar studies were performed with glycine receptor proteins with modified subunit primary structures produced by mutagenic techniques (Mihic et al. 1997). A modification of one amino acid (the substitution of isoleucine for a serine at amino acid 267 of the glycine receptor $α_1$ subunit) produced a receptor complex that was completely resistant to the effects of ethanol. Ethanol significantly potentiated the function of the wild-type glycine receptor; and the mutation, although it eliminated the glycine receptor's response to ethanol, did not significantly alter the characteristics of the mutant glycine receptor response to the classic agonists or antagonists of this receptor. The importance of such studies rests not only in the insight provided into the mechanism of ethanol's action but also in the demonstration that a mutational (genetic) difference that changes the sequence of a protein by only one amino acid can drastically alter a protein's (and possibly a human's) response to ethanol.

Most of the ethanol-sensitive systems described in this chapter are either multisubunit systems—for example, the $GABA_A$ receptor system, the N-methyl-D-aspartate (NMDA) receptor system, the 5-hydroxytryptamine (serotonin) type 3 (5-HT_3) receptor, and the nicotinic cholinergic receptor system—or multicomponent systems, such as the receptor-coupled adenylyl cyclase system, which consists of various neurotransmitter receptors (e.g., dopamine receptors) coupled through the guanine nucleotide–binding proteins (G proteins) to the catalytic unit of adenylyl cyclase. The effect of ethanol in these systems can depend on the components (subunit composition) of the system. Much evidence has accumulated that the subunit composition of receptor-gated ion channels such as the $GABA_A$, NMDA, and nicotinic cholinergic receptors varies in an anatomically and neuronally specific manner in brain. It would therefore be expected that ethanol would also act in an anatomically selective manner, dependent on the distribution of the particularly ethanol-sensitive complexes. For example, low concentrations of ethanol generally enhance responses of nicotinic cholinergic receptors, but certain receptors in brain (depending on their subunit composition) are insensitive to ethanol (Covernton and Connolly 1997; Yu et al. 1996; Zuo et al. 2002).

GABA Receptor System

GABA is the major inhibitory neurotransmitter in brain tissue. For many years, the CNS-depressant actions of ethanol were hypothesized to result primarily from ethanol's interactions with GABA-mediated neurotransmission. Benzodiazepines and barbiturates can potentiate the actions of GABA at the GABA$_A$ receptor by their interactions with receptor sites for these compounds on the GABA$_A$ receptor complex (Whiting et al. 1999). It was suggested that the sedative, anticonvulsant, anxiolytic, and incoordinating effects of ethanol could be explained by ethanol's interactions with the GABA$_A$ receptor because the spectrum of effects produced by the benzodiazepines and barbiturates resembled the spectrum of ethanol's actions (Suzdak et al. 1986).

Molecular biological and electrophysiological studies have further implicated the GABA$_A$ receptor system in certain actions of ethanol and have brought a greater understanding of the variables that contribute to ethanol's interactions with the GABA$_A$ receptor. Electrophysiological assessment of the interactions of ethanol and GABA on single neurons has uncovered a discordance in observation (for reviews, see Mihic and Harris 1996; Tabakoff and Hoffman 1996b). For example, with the use of whole cell patch-clamp recording, ethanol was reported to enhance the response of neurons of the dorsal root ganglion to GABA in one study but not in another (Nakahiro et al. 1991; White et al. 1990). In studies using slices of hippocampus, ethanol had little or no effect on GABA actions, but when the levels of adenosine triphosphate (ATP) were more carefully preserved in the cells of the hippocampal slices, ethanol significantly potentiated GABA's effects (Weiner et al. 1994). In the cerebellum, ethanol had little effect on GABA's actions on cerebellar Purkinje cells unless cyclic adenosine monophosphate (cyclic AMP; cAMP) levels in these cells were increased simultaneously with the administration of ethanol (Lin et al. 1991, 1993). Systemic administration of ethanol, coupled with iontophoretic administration of GABA, demonstrated that ethanol could potentiate GABA inhibition of cell firing in the medial septal area of the brain but not in the lateral septum (Givens and Breese 1990; Simson et al. 1991). The studies mentioned here demonstrated that neurons in different brain areas and under different metabolic conditions respond differentially to ethanol with regard to ethanol's interactions with GABA at the GABA$_A$ receptor.

The GABA$_A$ receptor is composed of a pentameric array of subunits. The subunits composing this array have been classified into groups based on similarities in the primary structure of these proteins. Six types of α subunits (α_1–α_6), three β subunits (β_1–β_3), three γ subunits (γ_1–γ_3), and δ, ε, π, and θ subunits have been identified (Whiting et al. 1999). The native GABA$_A$ receptor can be composed of different combinations of these subunits, and the pharmacological profile (i.e., the response of the receptor to various compounds) depends on the receptor's subunit composition (Whiting et al. 1999). The GABA$_A$ receptor's subunit composition in various areas of mammalian brain differs in a defined manner and contributes to region-specific sensitivity to particular drugs, including ethanol. For example, zolpidem's actions seem to be concentrated on brain areas possessing GABA$_A$ receptors containing α_1 subunits. Zolpidem is more a sedative than an anxiolytic medication, and thus the α_1 subunit has been considered important for sedation (McKernan et al. 2000). Studies of regional sensitivity of the GABA$_A$ receptor to ethanol seem to indicate that ethanol sensitivity also follows the brain distribution of the GABA$_A$ receptor α_1 subunit (Criswell et al. 1993). With regard to another subunit, GABA$_A$ receptor δ subunit knockout mice were behaviorally and physiologically evaluated and showed a reduced anticonvulsant response to ethanol, as well as reduced ethanol withdrawal (convulsions) and reduced ethanol consumption (Mihalek et al. 2001). Interestingly, these mice demonstrated normal sedative (hypnotic) and anxiolytic responses to ethanol (Mihalek et al. 2001). Electrophysiological analysis of recombinant GABA$_A$ receptor subunit combinations expressed in *Xenopus* oocytes demonstrated that combinations containing the δ subunit ($\alpha_4\beta_2\delta$) responded to ethanol concentrations as low as 3 mM with an increase in chloride current through this receptor (Sundstrom-Poromaa et al. 2002). Such demonstrations, and other examples of receptor subunit changes that alter GABA$_A$ receptor sensitivity to ethanol and alter only a subset of ethanol effects, speak to the fact that the full spectrum of ethanol's actions is dependent on a variety of receptor systems and on the subtypes of receptors as defined by subunit composition.

It was also reported that the δ subunit knockout mice demonstrated upregulation of the γ_2 GABA$_A$ receptor subunit in brain (Tretter et al. 2001). One always has to be careful when ascribing behavioral changes in a knockout animal definitively to the gene which was disrupted. However, mice with a targeted disruption of the γ_2 [γ_{2L}] gene did not show altered acute behavioral or electrophysiological responses to ethanol (Homanics et al. 1999).

An influence of the γ_2 subunit of the GABA$_A$ receptor on certain acute and chronic effects of ethanol and neuroadaptive phenomena cannot, however, be totally discounted. A polymorphism in the gene encoding the γ_2 subunit of the GABA$_A$ receptor, which resulted in a variation in amino acid sequence—either a threonine or an alanine residue at position 11 of the protein—was found to be associated with significant differences in ethanol withdrawal, ethanol-conditioned taste aversion, motor incoordination, and ethanol-induced hypothermia (Hood and Buck 2000).

Recent studies have also supported the concept that GABA$_A$ receptor subunit phosphorylation is an important factor in mediating the response of the GABA$_A$ receptor to ethanol. Studies with mice in which the brain-specific γ isoform of protein kinase C (PKC) was knocked out showed that the mice deficient in PKCγ were resistant to the hypnotic effects of ethanol and that their GABA$_A$ receptor function was also less sensitive to ethanol compared with wild-type mice (Harris et al. 1995). Mice lacking PKCγ also showed decreased anxiety and a decreased anxiolytic response to ethanol in comparison with wild-type mice (Bowers et al. 2000, 2001). The knockout of another isoform of PKC, PKCε, produced mice that were *more* sensitive to several behavioral effects of ethanol (i.e., locomotor stimulation by low doses of ethanol, sedative effect of ethanol). The GABA$_A$ receptors in the PKCε knockout mice were also more sensitive to activation by ethanol and benzodiazepines. Interestingly, these mice voluntarily consumed less alcohol than did wild-type mice (Hodge et al. 1999; Olive et al. 2000). These results are consistent with the idea that PKC can modulate the response of the GABA$_A$ receptor to ethanol, but the exact mechanism of this effect (i.e., phosphorylation of subunits of the receptor or associated proteins), as well as the importance of different PKC isoforms and the brain localization of the relevant GABA$_A$ receptor complexes, remains to be determined.

The sensitivity of the GABA$_A$ receptor to ethanol in certain brain areas is also controlled by the activity of adenylyl cyclase, cAMP, and protein kinase A (PKA). Purkinje cell GABA$_A$ receptors are insensitive to etha-

nol unless adenylyl cyclase is activated concomitantly with the administration of ethanol (Lin et al. 1993). The lack of evidence for such interactions in other parts of the brain may be a result of the particular subunit composition of the GABA$_A$ receptors in the cerebellum (Whiting et al. 1999) and of the presence of an ethanol-sensitive adenylyl cyclase in cerebellar Purkinje cells (Mons et al. 1998; Yoshimura and Tabakoff 1995). In Purkinje cells, ethanol can act in a feedforward manner by activating the ethanol-sensitive adenylyl cyclase, which generates cAMP and activates PKA. The activated PKA can then phosphorylate Purkinje cell GABA$_A$ receptors to increase their sensitivity to ethanol.

NMDA Receptor System

The NMDA subtype of glutamate receptor has structural similarities to the GABA$_A$ receptor. It is a multisubunit, receptor-gated ion channel that has binding sites for several psychoactive drugs. The glutamatergic system is the major excitatory system of the brain, and activation of the NMDA receptor by glutamate and its coagonist glycine produces neuronal membrane depolarization by increasing the permeability of the membrane to sodium, potassium, and calcium ions. The entry of calcium into the neuron through the activated NMDA receptor not only adds to membrane depolarization but also contributes to significant alterations in the intracellular homeostasis of the neuron (i.e., calcium acts as an intracellular second messenger and activator of several important signaling cascades within the neuron). The NMDA receptor has an important role in the initial stages of memory formation, in neural excitability and seizures, in excitotoxic brain damage, and in neural development (Choi 1992; Collingridge and Lester 1989).

Ethanol is a potent inhibitor of NMDA receptor function when the receptor is acutely exposed to ethanol at concentrations as low as 10 mM (approximately 50 mg/100 mL) (for reviews, see Tabakoff and Hoffman 1996a, 1996c; Woodward 2000). The effect of ethanol, in the presence of saturating levels of the neurotransmitter glutamate, is selective for the NMDA receptor in comparison with the other subtypes of ionotropic or metabotropic glutamate receptors. At lower concentrations of glutamate, however, ethanol also has effects on the kainate/α-amino-3-hydroxy-5-methyl-4-isoxazole propionate (AMPA) subtypes of glutamate receptors. The ionotropic NMDA and AMPA glutamate receptors are heteromultimeric proteins. The AMPA receptor consists of GluR1–4 subunits, and the NMDA receptor consists of a required NR1 subunit in combination with one or more NR2 subunits (NR2A, B, C, or D). NR1 is distributed throughout the brain, whereas the NR2 subunits show more discrete localization (Hollmann and Heinemann 1994). A more recently identified NR3 subunit has a modulatory effect on receptor function and is expressed primarily during nervous system development.

Ethanol's actions on the NMDA receptor seem to be less dependent on the subunit composition of this receptor than are ethanol's actions on the GABA$_A$ receptor, but phosphorylation of the NMDA receptor subunits may play an important role in determining the receptor's activity and sensitivity to ethanol. In cerebellar granule cells, phorbol esters, which activate PKC, inhibited NMDA receptor function in a manner similar to that of the inhibition produced by ethanol, and inhibitors of PKC blocked the inhibition of the NMDA receptor produced by phorbol esters and the inhibition produced by ethanol (Popp et al. 1999; Snell et al. 1994). However, in other brain areas, such as hippocampus, activation of PKC, which may lead to serine/ threonine phosphorylation or tyrosine phosphorylation of the receptor or receptor-associated proteins, was found to increase NMDA receptor activity (Lu et al. 1999). When hippocampal slices were exposed to ethanol, ethanol inhibition of NMDA receptor function was associated with decreased tyrosine phosphorylation of the NMDA receptor. It was suggested that ethanol increased phosphatase activity in the hippocampus, leading to receptor dephosphorylation and inhibition of function (Alvestad et al. 2003).

The converse of this proposal is that phosphorylation of the NMDA receptor would counter the effect of ethanol, leading to a decreased sensitivity of the receptor to ethanol-induced inhibition. Results to support this hypothesis were found when the effect of ethanol on NMDA receptors in the ventral midbrain region of the brain (nucleus accumbens [NAc]) was studied. In this brain region, activation of a PKA-mediated pathway led to increased phosphorylation of the NR1 subunit of the receptor and decreased ethanol inhibition (Maldve et al. 2002). Tyrosine kinase–mediated phosphorylation of the NR2B subunit has also been implicated in the action of ethanol on the NMDA receptor. The role of the tyrosine kinase Fyn was investigated by comparing knockout mice deficient in Fyn (Fyn-negative mice) and mice in which Fyn was functional (Fyn-

positive mice) (Miyakawa et al. 1997). In the presence of ethanol, phosphorylation of the NMDA receptor (NR2B subunit) in the hippocampus of the Fyn-positive mice was increased, whereas no such ethanol-associated increase in phosphorylation was evident in the Fyn-negative mice. The Fyn-negative mice were also significantly more sensitive to the hypnotic actions of ethanol and did not acquire the acute tolerance to ethanol that the Fyn-positive mice acquired. These findings suggest 1) that ethanol inhibition of NMDA receptor function in this brain area may initially reflect dephosphorylation of the receptor and 2) that a subsequent rephosphorylation of the receptor by the tyrosine kinase Fyn results in an adaptive response (acute tolerance) that decreases the effect of ethanol on the receptor.

Work on ethanol's acute actions on the NMDA and GABA$_A$ receptors indicates that certain of the sedative, incoordinating, amnestic, and anxiolytic effects of ethanol may be mediated by ethanol's inhibition of the NMDA receptor system and by ethanol's potentiation of activation of the GABA$_A$ receptor. Thus ethanol can be considered an inhibitor of a component of the major excitatory system in the brain (i.e., the glutamate transmitter system) and an enhancer of the major inhibitory system in the brain (i.e., the GABA$_A$ transmitter system). In both cases, ethanol's actions seem to be dependent on receptor subunit composition and/or phosphorylation events influencing these receptors.

Serotonin$_3$ Receptors and Nicotinic Cholinergic Receptors

Ethanol also modulates the activity of two other receptor-gated ion channels. Concentrations of ethanol that produce moderate intoxication (i.e., 25 mM) potentiate the effects of serotonin (5-HT) at the 5-HT$_3$ subtype of the 5-HT receptor. The 5-HT$_3$ receptor is the only 5-HT receptor subtype that is a receptor-gated ion channel. Interestingly, ethanol has direct actions at only this subtype of 5-HT receptor, although other 5-HT receptor subtypes (the G protein–coupled subtypes) may be affected secondarily by ethanol-induced increases in brain 5-HT release and turnover (for review, see Tabakoff and Hoffman 1996b). The structure of the 5-HT$_3$ receptor was originally thought to be a pentameric configuration of a single subunit, but more recent evidence suggests that the 5-HT$_3$ receptor subunit may interact with subunit proteins thought to be part of the nicotinic acetylcholine receptors (Lovinger

1999). Ethanol potentiation of 5-HT$_3$ receptor function seems to be mediated by an increased probability of channel opening (Lovinger et al. 2000) at lower concentrations of 5-HT. In other words, ethanol increases the effectiveness of 5-HT to activate the 5-HT$_3$ receptor. The finding that ethanol can enhance the function of the 5-HT$_3$ receptor in the CNS (Sung et al. 2000) lends credence to the possible role of this receptor in the reinforcing and/or intoxicating effect of ethanol (see below).

Investigations of ethanol's actions on nicotinic cholinergic receptors were promoted by the observation of extensive concomitant use of tobacco and alcohol by many individuals. The effects of subunit composition of the nicotinic cholinergic receptors on the manifestation of ethanol's action are as profound as the effects of subunit composition noted for the GABA$_A$ receptor system. In brain, nicotinic cholinergic receptors are predominantly composed of α (α_2–α_{10}) and β (β_2–β_4) subunits. A major subtype of brain nicotinic receptor consists of $\alpha_4\beta_2$ subunits, and other receptor subtypes ($\alpha_3\beta_4$, $\alpha_3\beta_2$) are prominent in certain brain areas (Perry et al. 2002). The α_7 subunit is another component of the nicotinic cholinergic receptors in brain and in fact is specifically localized to brain (e.g., cortex and hippocampus). When ethanol (5–100 mM) was applied to cells in which different subunit combinations of the nicotinic cholinergic receptor were expressed, the acetylcholine receptor–gated channels consisting of $\alpha_3\beta_4$ subunit combinations could be significantly potentiated *or* inhibited by these ethanol concentrations (Covernton and Connolly 1997). Receptors consisting of $\alpha_4\beta_2$ or $\alpha_3\beta_2$ subunits were generally insensitive to ethanol, whereas α_7 subunit–containing nicotinic receptors were inhibited by ethanol (Yu et al. 1996; Zuo et al. 2002).

These studies not only restate the importance of the subunit composition of multisubunit receptor systems in ethanol's action but also bring attention to the fact that even receptors of a particular subunit composition (e.g., $\alpha_3\beta_4$) may show differential responses to ethanol (potentiation or inhibition), depending on the state of the receptor within a cell—for example, whether the receptor is in a phosphorylated form. The nicotinic cholinergic receptors can be phosphorylated by PKA, PKC, other Ca^{2+}-regulated kinases, and protein tyrosine kinases. Both serine/threonine and tyrosine phosphorylation were demonstrated to regulate desensitization of nicotinic receptors (Swope et al. 1999).

Role of Receptor-Gated Ion Channels and Certain G Protein–Coupled Receptors in the Reinforcing Properties of Ethanol

Although the pleasurable and reinforcing properties of ethanol are part of a spectrum of ethanol's actions in many animals, not all humans or other mammals experience the drug's reinforcing properties. Selective breeding studies with rats have demonstrated that ethanol's reinforcing properties and other actions may be under genetic control to a significant extent (Li et al. 1993). The dopaminergic neuron systems that project from the brain stem to the NAc, frontal cortex, and other limbic areas (i.e., the mesolimbic dopamine systems) are activated by administered or ingested ethanol in experimental animals (Di Chiara and Imperato 1988; Gessa et al. 1985), and this action of ethanol may be more efficacious in animals selectively bred for alcohol preference (Li and McBride 1995).

Similar activation of the mesolimbic dopamine system is evident with administration of cocaine, morphine, nicotine, and other drugs (Di Chiara and Imperato 1988). Di Chiara (1995) reported that the increased firing of the mesolimbic dopamine neurons produced by ethanol led to increased release of dopamine in the NAc, an event associated with the presence of several other motivational stimuli. The molecular process by which ethanol activates the mesolimbic dopamine system is still poorly understood. Ethanol was reported to excite dopamine-containing ventral tegmental neurons directly, in the absence of input from neighboring neurons (Brodie et al. 1999). Activation of these dopamine neurons would lead to dopamine release in the NAc. Evidence was also reported for a more indirect action of ethanol: ethanol's actions at the NMDA, nicotinic cholinergic, and 5-HT$_3$ receptor systems may be initiating ethanol's activation of the mesolimbic dopamine system (Di Chiara et al. 1994; Wozniak et al. 1990). Nicotine is known to increase dopamine release in the NAc (Di Chiara and Imperato 1988) through activation of nicotinic acetylcholine receptors on dopamine cell bodies in the ventral tegmental area. There is a heterogeneous population of nicotinic cholinergic receptors on dopamine neurons in the ventral tegmental area, and the ability of ethanol to enhance the action of acetylcholine at particular subtypes of nicotinic acetylcholine receptors (discussed above) is likely to contribute to the finding that ethanol and nicotine produce additive effects on dopamine release in the NAc (Tizabi et al. 2002). A significant pharmacological consequence of this interaction is suggested by the finding that mecamylamine, a nicotinic cholinergic receptor antagonist, decreased the rewarding effect of ethanol in humans (Blomqvist et al. 2002).

The 5-HT$_3$ receptor antagonist tropisetron (ICS 205-930) also blocks the ethanol-induced enhancement of dopamine release in the NAc; and NMDA antagonists, which, like ethanol, *inhibit* NMDA receptor function, can *increase* the release of dopamine in the NAc. Both 5-HT$_3$ receptor antagonists and various NMDA receptor antagonists can reduce ethanol consumption in humans and ethanol self-administration in animals (e.g., Rassnick et al. 1992; Rodd-Henricks et al. 2000; Sellers et al. 1994). However, the mechanism of this reduced intake may differ. The 5-HT$_3$ antagonists, by blocking ethanol-induced dopamine release, may reduce ethanol's reinforcing effect, and extinction of ethanol-ingestive behavior would occur. On the other hand, the NMDA receptor antagonists, by increasing dopamine release, could substitute for the effect of ethanol. Because of this substitution, the animal would no longer "need" the ethanol in order to increase dopamine release. Not only do the 5-HT$_3$ antagonists and NMDA receptor blockers antagonize or mimic ethanol's action on dopaminergic neurotransmission and reduce ethanol consumption, they also influence the discriminative stimulus properties of ethanol. In animals trained to distinguish ethanol from other fluids, 5-HT$_3$ receptor antagonists blocked ethanol's discriminative stimulus properties (Grant 1995). In contrast, NMDA receptor antagonists were able to generalize to the ethanol cue (Grant and Colombo 1993). The trained animals' response to NMDA receptor antagonists indicates that the animals perceived the NMDA receptor antagonists to be, in certain respects, like ethanol.

Other receptors (G protein–coupled receptors) may synergize with 5-HT$_3$, nicotinic cholinergic, and NMDA receptors in mediating ethanol's actions on the mesolimbic dopamine neurons. Low to moderate (≤ 50 mM) concentrations of ethanol promoted the binding of opioid agonists to μ opioid receptors (Tabakoff and Hoffman 1983). The μ opioid receptors are present on the cell bodies of the dopaminergic neurons in the ventral tegmental area, and activation of these receptors promotes the firing of dopaminergic neurons and the release of dopamine in the NAc. Thus, it is of some interest that the opioid receptor antagonist naltrexone was able to reverse the dopamine-

releasing effects of ethanol in rats and that, when administered to human ethanol-dependent subjects, naltrexone reduced relapse (O'Brien et al. 1996). The limited effectiveness of naltrexone in human patients with alcoholism (Volpicelli et al. 1995) may indicate that actions of ethanol at receptors other than the opioid receptors (e.g., NMDA, 5-HT$_3$) contribute significantly to the positive reinforcing effects of ethanol.

The Stimulus for Neuroadaptation

The cAMP-generating system is a signaling system that is intimately involved in neural adaptation and that also impinges on the short-term excitability of neurons; cAMP plays a major role in the control of intracellular energy metabolism, in the functional control of ion channels, and in the control of transcriptional events. Many of the actions of cAMP are mediated through the activation and translocation of the serine/threonine kinase PKA. The enzyme adenylyl cyclase produces cAMP. There are nine characterized forms of this enzyme, which are all products of individual genes (Hanoune and Defer 2001). With respect to ethanol's action, type VII adenylyl cyclase (AC7) is two to three times more sensitive to ethanol than are other adenylyl cyclase isoforms (Yoshimura and Tabakoff 1995). Work with AC7-transfected cells in culture has demonstrated that concentrations of ethanol in the range of 10–25 mM can significantly activate AC7 and that this activation occurs only with the simultaneous activation of the G$_s$ proteins. In other words, ethanol (at low to moderate levels) potentiates the action of G$_s$-coupled receptors, but only if these receptors are specifically linked to AC7.

A number of laboratories have demonstrated the activation of PKA (Yoshimura and Tabakoff 1999) and translocation of PKA upon exposure of cells containing AC7 to ethanol. Gordon and colleagues (Constantinescu et al. 1999; Dohrman et al. 2002) found that a 30-minute exposure of NG 108–15 cells to ethanol resulted in the translocation of PKA from a neuronal membrane location to the cytosol and cell nucleus. Such events represent a prelude to activation of transcriptional machinery. One of the most direct pathways for cAMP to affect gene transcription is through the PKA-mediated phosphorylation of the cAMP response element binding protein (CREB). The phosphorylation of CREB enhances its binding to cAMP response element (CRE) promoter regions in the 5' sequences of particular genes, and given the proper steady state of other promoter/repressor elements, the phosphorylated CREB would enhance transcription. Ethanol-induced increases in CREB phosphorylation have been shown to occur in cultured cells and in brains of animals treated with ethanol (Asher et al. 2002; Constantinescu et al. 1999; Yang et al. 1996). Therefore, the acute actions of ethanol on cAMP-mediated cell signaling, via activation of AC7, can result in the initiation of neuroadaptive events that are dependent on gene transcription, as well as more proximate effects in time and space to modulate the sensitivity of certain receptor systems to ethanol.

The effect of ethanol on the NMDA receptor system, which gates calcium, can also be thought of as a signal for neuronal adaptation. Calcium is an important intracellular signal that modulates the activity of a number of protein kinases, including PKC and calmodulin (CaM) kinase isoforms. The phosphorylation state of many proteins determines their cellular localization and action, and the state of phosphorylation is determined by a balance of kinase and phosphatase activities. Thus, one can surmise that the inhibition of calcium fluxes through the NMDA receptor ion channel by acute administration of ethanol would lead to a shift in the balance of kinase and phosphatase activities. This shift would in turn lead to changes in the phosphorylation state of proteins, changes in phosphoprotein activity, and possibly changes in a protein's continued sensitivity to ethanol (acute tolerance or sensitization), as well as instigation of longer-term changes in cellular physiology generated through activation or suppression of transcriptional events.

Neuroadaptive Phenomena Associated With Alcohol Consumption

Tolerance and Dependence

The neurochemistry of short- and long-term memory was modeled in an invertebrate system by Kandel and colleagues (Kandel 1997), who identified phosphorylation events as critical mediators of short-term changes associated with learning. For example, phosphorylation of an ion channel or receptor can lead to changes in its activity that mediate the adaptation associated with short-term memory. Tolerance, like learning, can be considered an adaptation of the brain to an external stimulus. In the case of ethanol, as discussed above, phosphorylation of the NMDA receptor led to decreased sensitivity to the effects of ethanol or acute tolerance (Miyakawa et al. 1997).

Some evidence suggests that adaptation to chronic ethanol exposure may proceed in two stages. The first stage involves a more rapid or profound development of acute (within-session) tolerance or dependence. A later, second phase of adaptation, which lasts from one drinking session to another, may be likened to the adaptations that underlie long-term memory.

It has been suggested that these secondary changes involve transcription of new proteins and anatomical reorganizations (Kandel 1997). The second phase of adaptation to ethanol may also involve changes in processes such as gene transcription, or translation or stabilization of proteins, as well as the formation of new synaptic connections. An example is the finding that chronic exposure of cultured neuronal (PC12) cells to ethanol produces an increase in the number of voltage-sensitive Ca^{2+} channels (VSCCs) (implicated in ethanol withdrawal signs in chronically ethanol-treated animals; Watson and Little 2002) by a mechanism involving PKC (McMahon et al. 2000). Thus, the activity of PKC, which can rapidly affect the sensitivity of ligand-gated ion channels to ethanol, also causes a long-term neuroadaptation to ethanol in the form of synthesis of VSCCs. It was also noted that chronic ethanol exposure and withdrawal caused increases in the expression of transcription factors known as *immediate early genes* (Beckmann et al. 1997; Dave et al. 1990), which are regulated by phosphorylation. Chronic ethanol exposure was also shown to change the architecture of PC12 cells by inducing neurite outgrowth by means of a PKC-dependent mechanism (Roivainen et al. 1995). These examples suggest that the rapid and reversible changes associated with acute intoxication and rapid adaptation to ethanol (e.g., phosphorylation) can also lead, over time, to more stable adaptations involving transcriptional, translational, or morphologic events.

Transcriptional or other long-term changes that are involved in chronic neuroadaptation to ethanol are often related to changes generated in the proteins involved in the acute effects of ethanol. For example, the chronic administration of ethanol to animals for periods sufficient to produce functional tolerance and signs of physical dependence results in changes in the subunit characteristics and functions of the $GABA_A$ and NMDA receptor systems in the brain (for review, see Hoffman et al. 2000). Neuroadaptive changes in VSCCs, exemplified by increases in the binding of nitrendipine, an L-type VSCC blocker, are also evident (Watson and Little 1999). Although changes in the quantities of several $GABA_A$ receptor subunits have been observed in the brains of ethanol-dependent animals (i.e., increases in β and α_6 subunits, decreases in α_2 subunits), the most consistent changes have been significant decreases in α_1 subunits (Hoffman et al. 2000). As noted earlier, $GABA_A$ receptors with a particular subunit composition (i.e., those containing the α_1 subunits; Criswell et al. 1993) may be selectively sensitive to ethanol, and investigations of brain synaptoneurosomes obtained from chronically alcohol-treated animals demonstrated a reduced effect of ethanol in potentiating GABA-mediated chloride flux through the $GABA_A$ receptor channel complex (i.e., the system had become tolerant to ethanol's actions).

Substantial evidence also indicates upregulation of the NMDA receptor complex in the brains of humans and experimental animals after chronic ethanol ingestion. This upregulation is observed as an increase in the binding of ligands specific for the NMDA receptor and an increase in NMDA receptor–mediated influx of calcium into neurons that have been chronically exposed to ethanol. Tabakoff and Hoffman (1996a) suggested that the increase in NMDA receptor number and function may lead to neuronal hyperexcitability, which is responsible for some signs and symptoms of ethanol withdrawal (e.g., seizures, sleep disturbances, anxiety). NMDA receptor–induced neuronal excitability during ethanol withdrawal also predisposes neurons to glutamate-induced excitotoxicity and neuronal death (for review, see Hoffman et al. 2000). NMDA receptor antagonists, although not available for use in humans, effectively alleviate alcohol withdrawal signs in animals.

The benzodiazepines, acting as potentiators of GABA effects at the $GABA_A$ receptor, are also effective in the treatment of alcohol withdrawal signs and may protect brain from excitotoxic damage. However, the more severe withdrawal signs (seizures, convulsions) may not be the result of $GABA_A$ receptor changes observed after chronic ethanol ingestion. Electrophysiological studies of brain slices from ethanol-dependent animals suggested that ethanol withdrawal seizures result from a synergistic effect of increased NMDA recep-

tor and VSCC function rather than from changes in the function of $GABA_A$ receptors (Ripley et al. 1996). The effectiveness of high doses of benzodiazepines in controlling alcohol withdrawal seizures and convulsions may be the result of general anticonvulsant properties of the benzodiazepines rather than specific actions of benzodiazepines on the molecular systems that initiate withdrawal-induced neuronal hyperexcitability.

Neuroadaptations Leading to Craving for Alcohol

The termination of alcohol consumption by an alcohol-dependent individual usually generates a state of anhedonia and initiates the withdrawal hyperexcitability mentioned earlier. Withdrawal from ethanol also generates a decrease in the firing of dopaminergic neurons in the ventral tegmental area of the brain and a decrease in the release of dopamine from these neurons (Bailey et al. 1998; Rossetti et al. 1991). This phenomenon is opposite to the increased dopaminergic activity observed after acute administration of ethanol to animals. NMDA receptors may exert a tonic inhibitory control over the firing of the mesolimbic dopamine neurons (Rossetti et al. 1992). The upregulated NMDA receptor system, which has been noted in alcohol-dependent animals, could thus generate an increase in this tonic inhibitory control. The increased inhibitory control would result in the decreased dopaminergic neuron activity and decreased dopamine release observed after alcohol withdrawal (Rossetti et al. 1991).

Congruent with the proposal of NMDA receptor–mediated inhibitory control of dopaminergic neurons is the observation that an NMDA receptor antagonist reversed the decreased dopamine release associated with alcohol withdrawal (Rossetti et al. 1991). Systemic administration of alcohol also reversed the decreased release of dopamine in the NAc of alcohol-withdrawn animals (Diana et al. 1993), and alcohol-withdrawn animals were found to ingest alcohol in quantities that returned dopamine release to control levels (Weiss et al. 2001). It was also found that, following chronic ethanol exposure and withdrawal, dopamine neurons were more sensitive to excitatory effects of ethanol (Brodie 2002). Because the decreased mesolimbic dopaminergic transmission is believed to be an important contributor to the negative affect associated with alcohol and other drug withdrawal, the increased

NMDA receptor function noted during withdrawal could underlie an affective state that increases the compulsion to drink alcohol. A study using an animal model that mimics the craving for ethanol following chronic ethanol consumption and withdrawal provided evidence that an NMDA receptor antagonist can reduce this craving (Holter et al. 2000). Furthermore, acamprosate (Ca^{2+}-homotaurine), which is being used in humans to reduce craving for alcohol (Stromberg et al. 2001), exerts its actions at least partially on the NMDA receptor (e.g., al Qatari et al. 2001).

In addition to the alterations in glutamate receptors, decreased activity of opiate systems and decreases in opiate receptor number (Khatami et al. 1987; Sim-Selley et al. 2002) following chronic ethanol exposure could contribute to decreased function of dopaminergic neurons. It must again be emphasized, however, that several neuronal systems, including the $GABA_A$ receptor system, interact with dopaminergic neurotransmission to generate control or loss of control over alcohol intake. As noted, alcohol-dependent rats increased their responding to ethanol during a period of alcohol withdrawal, but the injection of the $GABA_A$ receptor agonist muscimol into the amygdala of these animals attenuated their increased ethanol intake (Roberts et al. 1996). Experiments in which muscimol was administered into the NAc further demonstrated that the postsynaptic $GABA_A$ receptor in certain anatomically distinct areas of brain may be intimately involved in the early termination of alcohol self-administration, whereas the presynaptic dopaminergic systems projecting to the NAc and amygdala were more focused on the initiation or maintenance of alcohol-reinforced responding in animals (Hodge et al. 1995). In essence, if one has decreased $GABA_A$ receptor function in the appropriate brain areas, as well as changes in NMDA and opiate receptors that alter dopaminergic neuron function, chronic ethanol ingestion and withdrawal produce a state of the CNS in which initiation and maintenance of ethanol intake is promoted and termination of intake is impaired.

Although much attention has focused on possible changes in the neuronal systems that directly mediate ethanol reinforcement as a basis for craving for alcohol in alcohol-dependent individuals, the factors that contribute to such craving may be more diffuse. Some individuals display a protracted withdrawal syndrome following the resolution of the acute withdrawal syndrome. The slowly resolving symptomatology (sometimes lasting more than 1 year after cessation of alcohol intake) includes changes in sleep latency and frequency of awakening, variations in autonomic function, spontaneous anxiety, and depressive episodes (Gallant 1999). A number of systems that are altered by chronic ethanol exposure could directly or indirectly contribute to the signs and symptoms of the protracted withdrawal syndrome. In addition to decreases in the activity of mesolimbic dopamine neurons described above (which have been shown to remain for up to several months following ethanol withdrawal; Bailey et al. 2000), ethanol withdrawal was reported to be associated with decreased activity of 5-HT neurons and 5-HT release in the NAc (Weiss et al. 2001). In persons with chronic alcoholism, deficits in 5-HT neuron activity and 5-HT receptors were also reported (Weiss et al. 2001). Decreased activity of the 5-HT systems may contribute to sleep disturbances as well as depression. Neuroendocrine systems are also altered during ethanol withdrawal. In particular, corticotropin-releasing factor (CRF), which regulates pituitary secretion of adrenocorticotropic hormone but is also thought to be a "stress hormone" in other brain areas, is elevated in the amygdala during withdrawal. The amygdala is a brain area that regulates anxiety, and elevated CRF in this area may contribute to anxiety and stresslike symptoms that occur in the protracted withdrawal syndrome (Valdez et al. 2002). Interestingly, CRF in the amygdala was found to increase progressively during a 6-week period following cessation of ethanol intake by rats (Weiss et al. 2001). It is likely that physiologic and affective symptoms and long-term neurochemical and neuroanatomic changes ("addictive" memory) may promote relapse to alcohol use.

Conclusion

Overall, the selective potency of ethanol's actions on receptor-gated ion channels and cAMP-generating systems may contribute significantly to the acute and chronic neurobiological effects of ethanol. The ethanol ingestion–associated phosphorylation of the receptor-gated ion channels, as observed with the NMDA, nicotinic cholinergic, and $GABA_A$ receptors and adenylyl cyclase, appears to alter the channels' sensitivity to ethanol and may explain such phenomena as acute tolerance and/or sensitization. The longer-term (e.g., transcriptional) changes initiated by ethanol's actions on cAMP signaling cascades and other kinases and/or phosphatases generate neuroadaptive events leading to the development of chronic alcohol tolerance and physical dependence. Long-term neuroadaptations also play an integral role in the compulsion to drink alcohol in the alcohol-dependent individual.

References

al Qatari M, Khan S, Harris B, et al: Acamprosate is neuroprotective against glutamate-induced excitotoxicity when enhanced by ethanol withdrawal in neocortical cultures of fetal rat brain. Alcohol Clin Exp Res 25:1276–1283, 2001

Alvestad RM, Grosshans DR, Coultrap MD, et al: Tyrosine dephosphorylation and ethanol inhibition of N-methyl-D-aspartate receptor function. J Biol Chem 278:11020–11025, 2003

American Psychiatric Association: Diagnostic and Statistical Manual of Mental Disorders, 4th Edition, Text Revision. Washington, DC, American Psychiatric Association, 2000

Asher O, Cunningham TD, Yao L, et al: Ethanol stimulates cAMP-responsive element (CRE)-mediated transcription via CRE-binding protein and cAMP-dependent protein kinase. J Pharmacol Exp Ther 301:66–70, 2002

Bailey CP, Manley SJ, Watson WP, et al: Chronic ethanol administration alters activity in ventral tegmental area neurons after cessation of withdrawal hyperexcitability. Brain Res 803:144–152, 1998

Bailey CP, Andrews N, McKnight AT, et al: Prolonged changes in neurochemistry of dopamine neurones after chronic ethanol consumption. Pharmacol Biochem Behav 66:153–161, 2000

Beckmann AM, Matsumoto I, Wilce PA: AP-1 and Egr DNA-binding activities are increased in rat brain during ethanol withdrawal. J Neurochem 69:306–314, 1997

Blomqvist O, Hernandez-Avila CA, Van Kirk J, et al: Mecamylamine modifies the pharmacokinetics and reinforcing effects of alcohol. Alcohol Clin Exp Res 26:326–331 2002

Bowers BJ, Collins AC, Tritto T, et al: Mice lacking PKC gamma exhibit decreased anxiety. Behav Genet 30:111–121, 2000

Bowers BJ, Elliott KJ, Wehner JM: Differential sensitivity to the anxiolytic effects of ethanol and flunitrazepam in PKCgamma null mutant mice. Pharmacol Biochem Behav 69:99–110, 2001

Brodie MS: Increased ethanol excitation of dopaminergic neurons of the ventral tegmental area after chronic ethanol treatment. Alcohol Clin Exp Res 26:1024–1030, 2002

Brodie MS, Pesold C, Appel SB: Ethanol directly excites dopaminergic ventral tegmental area reward neurons. Alcohol Clin Exp Res 23:1848–1852, 1999

Choi DW: Excitotoxic cell death. J Neurobiol 23:1261–1276, 1992

Collingridge GL, Lester RA: Excitatory amino acid receptors in the vertebrate central nervous system. Pharmacol Rev 41:143–210, 1989

Constantinescu A, Diamond I, Gordon AS: Ethanol-induced translocation of cAMP-dependent protein kinase to the nucleus: mechanism and functional consequences. J Biol Chem 274:26985–26991, 1999

Covernton PJ, Connolly JG: Differential modulation of rat neuronal nicotinic receptor subtypes by acute application of ethanol. Br J Pharmacol 122:1661–1668, 1997

Crabbe JC, Wahlsten D, Dudek BC: Genetics of mouse behavior: interactions with laboratory environment. Science 284:1670–1672, 1999

Criswell HE, Simson PE, Duncan GE, et al: Molecular basis for regionally specific action of ethanol on gamma-aminobutyric acid$_A$ receptors: generalization to other ligand-gated ion channels. J Pharmacol Exp Ther 267:522–537, 1993

Dave JR, Tabakoff B, Hoffman PL: Ethanol withdrawal seizures produce increased c-fos mRNA in mouse brain. Mol Pharmacol 37:367–371, 1990

Diana M, Pistis M, Carboni S, et al: Profound decrement of mesolimbic dopaminergic neuronal activity during ethanol withdrawal syndrome in rats: electrophysiological and biochemical evidence. Proc Natl Acad Sci U S A 90:7966–7969, 1993

Di Chiara G: The role of dopamine in drug abuse viewed from the perspective of its role in motivation. Drug Alcohol Depend 38:95–137, 1995

Di Chiara G, Imperato A: Drugs abused by humans preferentially increase synaptic dopamine concentrations in the mesolimbic system of freely moving rats. Proc Natl Acad Sci U S A 85:5274–5278, 1988

Di Chiara G, Morelli M, Consolo S: Modulatory functions of neurotransmitters in the striatum: ACh/dopamine/NMDA interactions. Trends Neurosci 17:228–233, 1994

Dohrman DP, Chen HM, Gordon AS, et al: Ethanol-induced translocation of protein kinase A occurs in two phases: control by different molecular mechanisms. Alcohol Clin Exp Res 26:407–415, 2002

Gallant D: Alcohol, in The American Psychiatric Press Textbook of Substance Abuse Treatment, 2nd Edition. Edited by Galanter M, Kleber HD. Washington, DC, American Psychiatric Press, 1999, pp 151–164

Gessa GL, Muntoni F, Collu M, et al: Low doses of ethanol activate dopaminergic neurons in the ventral tegmental area. Brain Res 348:201–203, 1985

Givens BS, Breese GR: Site-specific enhancement of gamma-aminobutyric acid–mediated inhibition of neural activity by ethanol in the rat medial septal area. J Pharmacol Exp Ther 254:528–538, 1990

Goldstein DB, Chin JH, Lyon RC: Ethanol disordering of spin-labeled mouse brain membranes: correlation with genetically determined ethanol sensitivity of mice. Proc Natl Acad Sci U S A 79:4231–4233, 1982

Grant KA: The role of 5-HT$_3$ receptors in drug dependence. Drug Alcohol Depend 38:155–171, 1995

Grant KA, Colombo G: Discriminative stimulus effects of ethanol: effect of training dose on the substitution of N-methyl-D-aspartate antagonists. J Pharmacol Exp Ther 264:1241–1247, 1993

Hanoune J, Defer N: Regulation and role of adenylyl cyclase isoforms. Annu Rev Pharmacol Toxicol 41:145–174, 2001

Harris RA, McQuilkin SJ, Paylor R, et al: Mutant mice lacking the gamma isoform of protein kinase C show decreased behavioral actions of ethanol and altered function of gamma-aminobutyrate type A receptors. Proc Natl Acad Sci U S A 92:3658–3662, 1995

Hodge CW, Chappelle AM, Samson HH: GABAergic transmission in the nucleus accumbens is involved in the termination of ethanol self-administration in rats. Alcohol Clin Exp Res 19:1486–1493, 1995

Hodge CW, Mehmert KK, Kelley SP, et al: Supersensitivity to allosteric GABA(A) receptor modulators and alcohol in mice lacking PKCepsilon. Nat Neurosci 2:997–1002, 1999

Hoffman PL, Morrow AL, Phillips TJ, et al: Neuroadaptation to ethanol at the molecular and cellular levels, in Review of NIAAA's Neuroscience and Behavioral Research Portfolio. Edited by Noronha A, Eckardt M, Warren K (NIAAA Research Monograph No 34). Rockville, MD, National Institute on Alcohol Abuse and Alcoholism, 2000, pp 85–188

Hollmann M, Heinemann S: Cloned glutamate receptors. Annu Rev Neurosci 17:31–108, 1994

Holter SM, Danysz W, Spanagel R: Novel uncompetitive N-methyl-D-aspartate (NMDA)-receptor antagonist MRZ 2/579 suppresses ethanol intake in long-term ethanol-experienced rats and generalizes to ethanol cue in drug discrimination procedure. J Pharmacol Exp Ther 292:545–552, 2000

Homanics GE, Harrison NL, Quinlan JJ, et al: Normal electrophysiological and behavioral responses to ethanol in mice lacking the long splice variant of the gamma$_2$ subunit of the gamma-aminobutyrate type A receptor. Neuropharmacology 38:253–265, 1999

Hood HM, Buck KJ: Allelic variation in the GABA A receptor gamma$_2$ subunit is associated with genetic susceptibility to ethanol-induced motor incoordination and hypothermia, conditioned taste aversion, and withdrawal in BXD/Ty recombinant inbred mice. Alcohol Clin Exp Res 24:1327–1334, 2000

Kandel ER: Genes, synapses, and long-term memory. J Cell Physiol 173:124–125, 1997

Khatami S, Hoffman PL, Shibuya T, et al: Selective effects of ethanol on opiate receptor subtypes in brain. Neuropharmacology 26:1503–1507, 1987

Li T-K, McBride WJ: Pharmacogenetic models of alcoholism. Clin Neurosci 3:182–188, 1995

Li T-K, Lumeng L, Doolittle DP: Selective breeding for alcohol preference and associated responses. Behav Genet 23:163–170, 1993

Lin AM, Freund RK, Palmer MR: Ethanol potentiation of GABA-induced electrophysiological responses in cerebellum: requirement for catecholamine modulation. Neurosci Lett 122:154–158, 1991

Lin AM, Freund RK, Palmer MR: Sensitization of γ-aminobutyric acid-induced depressions of cerebellar Purkinje neurons to the potentiative effects of ethanol by beta adrenergic mechanisms in rat brain. J Pharmacol Exp Ther 265:426–432, 1993

Lovinger DM: 5-HT$_3$ receptors and the neural actions of alcohols: an increasingly exciting topic. Neurochem Int 35:125–130, 1999

Lovinger DM, Sung KW, Zhou Q: Ethanol and trichloroethanol alter gating of 5-HT$_3$ receptor-channels in NCB-20 neuroblastoma cells. Neuropharmacology 39:561–570, 2000

Lu WY, Xiong ZG, Lei S, et al: G-protein-coupled receptors act via protein kinase C and Src to regulate NMDA receptors. Nat Neurosci 2:331–338, 1999

Maldve RE, Zhang TA, Ferrani-Kile K, et al: DARPP-32 and regulation of the ethanol sensitivity of NMDA receptors in the nucleus accumbens. Nat Neurosci 5:641–648, 2002

McKernan RM, Rosahl TW, Reynolds DS, et al: Sedative but not anxiolytic properties of benzodiazepines are mediated by the GABA(A) receptor alpha1 subtype. Nat Neurosci 3:587–592, 2000

McMahon T, Andersen R, Metten P, et al: Protein kinase C epsilon mediates up-regulation of N-type calcium channels by ethanol. Mol Pharmacol 57:53–58, 2000

Meyer HZTdA: Der einfuss wechselnder temperatur auf wirkungsstarke und theilungscoefficient der narcotina. Naunyn Schmiedebergs Arch Exp Pathol Pharmakol 46:338–346, 1901

Mihalek RM, Bowers BJ, Wehner JM, et al: GABA(A)-receptor delta subunit knockout mice have multiple defects in behavioral responses to ethanol. Alcohol Clin Exp Res 25:1708–1718, 2001

Mihic SJ: Acute effects of ethanol on GABA$_A$ and glycine receptor function. Neurochem Int 35:115–123, 1999

Mihic SJ, Harris RA: Alcohol actions at the GABA$_A$ receptor/chloride channel complex, in Pharmacological Effects of Ethanol on the Nervous System. Edited by Deitrich RA, Erwin VG. Boca Raton, FL, CRC Press, 1996, pp 51–72

Mihic SJ, Ye Q, Wick MJ, et al: Sites of alcohol and volatile anaesthetic action on GABA$_A$ and glycine receptors. Nature 389:385–389, 1997

Miyakawa T, Yagi T, Kitazawa H, et al: Fyn-kinase as a determinant of ethanol sensitivity: relation to NMDA-receptor function. Science 278:698–701, 1997

Mons N, Yoshimura M, Ikeda H, et al: Immunological assessment of the distribution of type VII adenylyl cyclase in brain. Brain Res 788:251–261, 1998

Nakahiro M, Arakawa O, Narahashi T: Modulation of gamma-aminobutyric acid receptor-channel complex by alcohols. J Pharmacol Exp Ther 259:235–240, 1991

O'Brien CP, Volpicelli LA, Volpicelli JR: Naltrexone in the treatment of alcoholism: a clinical review. Alcohol 13:35–39, 1996

Olive MF, Mehmert KK, Messing R, et al: Reduced operant ethanol self-administration and in vivo mesolimbic dopamine responses to ethanol in PKCepsilon-deficient mice. Eur J Neurosci 12:4131–4140, 2000

Pawson T, Scott JD: Signaling through scaffold, anchoring, and adaptor proteins. Science 278:2075–2080, 1997

Perry DC, Xiao Y, Nguyen HN, et al: Measuring nicotinic receptors with characteristics of alpha4beta2, alpha3beta2 and alpha3beta4 subtypes in rat tissues by autoradiography. J Neurochem 82:468–481, 2002

Popp RL, Lickteig RL, Lovinger DM: Factors that enhance ethanol inhibition of N-methyl-D-aspartate receptors in cerebellar granule cells. J Pharmacol Exp Ther 289:1564–1574, 1999

Rassnick S, Pulvirenti L, Koob GF: Oral ethanol self-administration in rats is reduced by the administration of dopamine and glutamate receptor antagonists into the nucleus accumbens. Psychopharmacology (Berl) 109:92–98, 1992

Ripley TL, Whittington MA, Butterworth AR, et al: Ethanol withdrawal hyperexcitability in vivo and in isolated mouse hippocampal slices. Alcohol Alcohol 31:347–357, 1996

Roberts AJ, Cole M, Koob GF: Intra-amygdala muscimol decreases operant ethanol self-administration in dependent rats. Alcohol Clin Exp Res 20:1289–1298, 1996

Rodd-Henricks ZA, McKinzie DL, Edmundson VE, et al: Effects of 5-HT(3) receptor antagonists on daily alcohol intake under acquisition, maintenance, and relapse conditions in alcohol-preferring (P) rats. Alcohol 21:73–85, 2000

Roivainen R, Hundle B, Messing RO: Ethanol enhances growth factor activation of mitogen-activated protein kinases by a protein kinase C-dependent mechanism. Proc Natl Acad Sci U S A 92:1891–1895, 1995

Rossetti ZL, Melis F, Carboni S, et al: Marked decrease of extraneuronal dopamine after alcohol withdrawal in rats: reversal by MK-801. Eur J Pharmacol 200:371–372, 1991

Rossetti ZL, Hmaidan Y, Gessa GL: Marked inhibition of mesolimbic dopamine release: a common feature of ethanol, morphine, cocaine and amphetamine abstinence in rats. Eur J Pharmacol 221:227–234, 1992

Sellers EM, Toneatto T, Romach MK, et al: Clinical efficacy of the 5-HT$_3$ antagonist ondansetron in alcohol abuse and dependence. Alcohol Clin Exp Res 18:879–885, 1994

Sim-Selley LJ, Sharpe AL, Vogt LJ, et al: Effect of ethanol self-administration on mu- and delta-opioid receptor-mediated G-protein activity. Alcohol Clin Exp Res 26:688–694, 2002

Simson PE, Criswell HE, Breese GR: Ethanol potentiates gamma-aminobutyric acid–mediated inhibition in the inferior colliculus: evidence for local ethanol/gamma-aminobutyric acid interactions. J Pharmacol Exp Ther 259:1288–1293, 1991

Snell LD, Iorio KR, Tabakoff B, et al: Protein kinase C activation attenuates N-methyl-D-aspartate-induced increases in intracellular calcium in cerebellar granule cells. J Neurochem 62:1783–1789, 1994

Stromberg MF, Mackler SA, Volpicelli JR, et al: Effect of acamprosate and naltrexone, alone or in combination, on ethanol consumption. Alcohol 23:109–116, 2001

Sundstrom-Poromaa I, Smith DH, Gong QH, et al: Hormonally regulated alpha(4)beta(2)delta GABA(A) receptors are a target for alcohol. Nat Neurosci 5:721–722, 2002

Sung KW, Engel SR, Allan AM, et al: 5-HT(3) receptor function and potentiation by alcohols in frontal cortex neurons from transgenic mice overexpressing the receptor. Neuropharmacology 39:2346–2351, 2000

Suzdak PD, Glowa JR, Crawley JN, et al: A selective imidazobenzodiazepine antagonist of ethanol in the rat. Science 234:1243–1247, 1986

Swope SL, Moss SI, Raymond LA, et al: Regulation of ligand-gated ion channels by protein phosphorylation. Adv Second Messenger Phosphoprotein Res 33:49–78, 1999

Tabakoff B, Hoffman PL: Alcohol interactions with brain opiate receptors. Life Sci 32:197–204, 1983

Tabakoff B, Hoffman PL: Alcohol addiction: an enigma among us. Neuron 16:909–912, 1996a

Tabakoff B, Hoffman PL: Effect of alcohol on neurotransmitters and their receptors and enzymes, in The Pharmacology of Alcohol and Alcohol Dependence. Edited by Begleiter H, Kissin B. New York, Oxford University Press, 1996b, pp 356–430

Tabakoff B, Hoffman PL: Ethanol and glutamate receptors, in Pharmacological Effects of Ethanol on the Nervous System. Edited by Deitrich RA, Erwin VG. Boca Raton, FL, CRC Press, 1996c, pp 73–93

Tizabi Y, Copeland RL Jr, Louis VA, et al: Effects of combined systemic alcohol and central nicotine administration into ventral tegmental area on dopamine release in the nucleus accumbens. Alcohol Clin Exp Res 26:394–399, 2002

Tretter V, Hauer B, Nusser Z, et al: Targeted disruption of the GABA(A) receptor delta subunit gene leads to an up-regulation of gamma 2 subunit-containing receptors in cerebellar granule cells. J Biol Chem 276:10532–10538, 2001

Ueno S, Harris RA, Messing RO, et al: Alcohol actions on GABA(A) receptors: from protein structure to mouse behavior. Alcohol Clin Exp Res 25:76S–81S, 2001

Valdez GR, Roberts AJ, Chan K, et al: Increased ethanol self-administration and anxiety-like behavior during acute ethanol withdrawal and protracted abstinence: regulation by corticotropin-releasing factor. Alcohol Clin Exp Res 26:1494–1501, 2002

Volpicelli JR, Volpicelli LA, O'Brien CP: Medical management of alcohol dependence: clinical use and limitations of naltrexone treatment. Alcohol Alcohol 30:789–798, 1995

Watson WP, Little HJ: Correlation between increases in dihydropyridine binding in vivo and behavioural signs of ethanol withdrawal in mice. Alcohol Alcohol 34:35–42, 1999

Watson WP, Little HJ: Selectivity of the protective effects of dihydropyridine calcium channel antagonists against the ethanol withdrawal syndrome. Brain Res 930:111–122, 2002

Weiner JL, Zhang L, Carlen PL: Potentiation of GABA$_A$-mediated synaptic current by ethanol in hippocampal CA1 neurons: possible role of protein kinase C. J Pharmacol Exp Ther 268:1388–1395, 1994

Weiss F, Ciccocioppo R, Parsons LH, et al: Compulsive drug-seeking behavior and relapse: neuroadaptation, stress, and conditioning factors. Ann N Y Acad Sci 937:1–26, 2001

White G, Lovinger DM, Weight FF: Ethanol inhibits NMDA-activated current but does not alter GABA-activated current in an isolated adult mammalian neuron. Brain Res 507:332–336, 1990

Whiting PJ, Bonnert TP, McKernan RM, et al: Molecular and functional diversity of the expanding GABA-A receptor gene family. Ann N Y Acad Sci 868:645–653, 1999

Woodward JJ: Ethanol and NMDA receptor signaling. Crit Rev Neurobiol 14:69–89, 2000

World Health Organization: International Statistical Classification of Diseases and Related Health Problems, 10th Revision. Geneva, World Health Organization, 1992

Wozniak KM, Pert A, Linnoila M: Antagonism of 5-HT$_3$ receptors attenuates the effects of ethanol on extracellular dopamine. Eur J Pharmacol 187:287–289, 1990

Yang X, Diehl AM, Wand GS: Ethanol exposure alters the phosphorylation of cyclic AMP responsive element binding protein and cyclic AMP responsive element binding activity in rat cerebellum. J Pharmacol Exp Ther 278:338–346, 1996

Yoshimura M, Tabakoff B: Selective effects of ethanol on the generation of cAMP by particular members of the adenylyl cyclase family. Alcohol Clin Exp Res 19:1435–1440, 1995

Yoshimura M, Tabakoff B: Ethanol's actions on cAMP-mediated signaling in cells transfected with type VII adenylyl cyclase. Alcohol Clin Exp Res 23:1457–1461, 1999

Yu D, Zhang L, Eisele JL, et al: Ethanol inhibition of nicotinic acetylcholine type alpha 7 receptors involves the amino-terminal domain of the receptor. Mol Pharmacol 50:1010–1016, 1996

Zuo Y, Kuryatov A, Lindstrom JM, et al: Alcohol modulation of neuronal nicotinic acetylcholine receptors is alpha subunit dependent. Alcohol Clin Exp Res 26:779–784, 2002

Neurobiology of Opioids

Jerome H. Jaffe, M.D.
Ari B. Jaffe, M.D.

The euphorigenic, mood-altering, and dependence-producing properties of the opioids have been known for at least 300 years. Nonmedical opioid use and opioid dependence is a worldwide problem. This chapter, intended for the psychiatrist or physician who specializes in treating problems of drug abuse, summarizes current knowledge about the biological basis of opioid actions and the process by which initial use can develop into the syndrome of opioid dependence.

Opioid Actions

Opioid drugs act by binding to specific receptors on neurons distributed throughout the central nervous system (CNS), the peripheral nervous system, and tissues of the immune system. Several types of opioid receptors exist. Drugs that bind to these receptor types can act as agonists, partial agonists, or antagonists. These opioid receptors are the binding sites for several families of endogenous peptides that play important roles in modulating responses to stress and pain; in regulating temperature, respiration, endocrine and

gastrointestinal activity, and mood and motivation; and in other functions (Gutstein and Akil 2001; Vaccarino and Kastin 2001). When opioid receptors are activated by an agonist (either endogenous or exogenous), a cascade of intracellular changes involving second and third messenger systems is set in motion. These changes not only produce immediate changes in the responsiveness of the opioid receptor–bearing neurons but also lead to adaptive changes in other neural systems that interact with them. Intracellular adaptive changes include alterations to intracellular messenger systems and to protein phosphorylation and changes in gene expression. Some of these intracellular changes are related to the development of tolerance (decreased responsiveness to the same concentration of the opioid at the receptor) and altered excitability (withdrawal) when the agonist is removed after a period of receptor occupancy. Other intracellular changes are related to sensitization. In the intact organism, the opioid withdrawal syndrome represents changes within the opioid receptor–bearing neurons themselves and altered activity in other neuronal systems affected indirectly by opioid actions in the CNS (Koob and Le Moal 2001; Nestler 1997, 2001).

Opioid Receptors

Four major types of opioid or opioid-like receptors have been identified thus far: μ, κ, δ, and OFQ/N (defined later in this section). All these receptors belong to a larger superfamily of receptors that have seven transmembrane α helices and are coupled to guanine nucleotide–binding proteins (G proteins).

Selective antagonists for each of the four receptor types have also been developed. Each of the major receptor types has a distinct distribution in the CNS and the peripheral nervous system. Activation of the μ and δ receptors produces generally similar actions that are quite distinct from those resulting from κ receptor activation. Agonist activation of OFQ/N receptors can produce either analgesic or pronociceptive actions, depending on the site of administration (Gutstein and Akil 2001).

On the basis of binding-affinity studies in neural material that use very specific agonists and antagonists, responses in knockout mice, and antisense techniques, researchers have proposed additional receptor subtypes of the major types of opioid receptors. Some work in mice suggested that there are subtypes of the μ receptor and that heroin, morphine 6-β glucuronide, and certain other opioids exert their actions at a μ receptor subtype that is distinct from the one at which morphine acts. The existence of μ receptor subtypes could help to explain why there is less than complete cross-tolerance among μ agonists (Pasternak 2001). However, studies in monkeys suggest that morphine, heroin, and 6-acetylmorphine act at pharmacologically similar μ opioid receptors (Negus et al. 2003). Evidence points to interactions among opioid receptor types. Such apparent interactions may represent complexes or dimerizations among distinct receptor types, and such complexes may be an alternative explanation for the data suggesting the existence of distinct receptor subtypes (Jordan et al. 2000).

There are probably significant differences among individuals in levels of expression of the μ receptors. Studies of knockout mice with all, some, or no μ receptors expressed suggest that the different neural systems regulated by μ receptor agonists have very different levels of receptor reserve. Differences in expression between individuals, as well as intraindividual differences within neural systems, may explain some of the variability in response to opioids (Sora et al. 2001).

Single-nucleotide polymorphisms have been identified in the human μ, δ, and κ opioid receptor genes and in the genes coding for pro-opiomelanocortin (POMC), enkephalin, and dynorphin. Although some differences of borderline significance have been found between opioid-dependent subjects and control subjects, and sometimes between alcoholic subjects and control subjects, these differences have not been robust. Some receptor variants have been associated with changes in the binding or potency of exogenous and endogenous opioid ligands (LaForge et al. 2000).

The OFQ/N receptor, identified in cloning studies, exhibits a high degree of homology to the three original opioid receptors (μ, κ, δ). Because none of the exogenous or endogenous ligands of the original three exhibit significant affinity for the OFQ/N receptor, the receptor was initially designated *orphan opioid-like receptor (ORL-1)*. Subsequently, an endogenous peptide ligand for this orphan receptor was identified and designated *orphanin FQ* by one group of researchers and *nociceptin* by another. The ligand is now commonly designated *orphanin FQ/nociceptin* (OFQ/N), or N/OFQ, and the ORL-1 receptor is now often named after the ligand. Researchers now consider the OFQ/N (ORL-1) receptor and its ligands to belong within an extended opioid receptor family and have recommended terminology in which the μ, κ, δ, and OFQ/N receptors are designated as MOP_1, KOP_1, DOP_1, and NOP_1 (Gutstein and Akil 2001).

Endogenous Opioid Peptides

Several genetically distinct families of endogenous opioid peptides have been defined thus far: the pro-enkephalin, prodynorphin, pro-opiomelanocortin (POMC), pro-OFQ/N, and endomorphin peptide families. The precursor proteins for most of these peptides can be processed to produce a number of active peptides with varying affinities for the major types of opioid receptors. Although the endogenous peptide ligands and the currently available exogenous opioids bind preferentially to one or more subtypes of receptor, they are often not as highly selective in their binding characteristics as are some recently developed synthetic ligands.

As a generalization, the enkephalin peptides prefer the δ receptor, the dynorphin principal peptides prefer the κ receptor, the endorphins show about comparable affinity for the μ and the δ receptors, the endomorphins bind preferentially to µ receptors, and OFQ/N binds to OFQ/N (ORL-1 [NOP1]) receptors (Akil et al. 1997, 1998; Gutstein and Akil 2001; Mogil and Pasternak 2001; Zadina 2002).

Posttranslational processing of the endogenous opioid peptides can substantially alter their receptor affinities and preferences. For example, met-enkephalin binds preferentially to δ receptors, whereas two of the other proenkephalin peptides bind equally or preferentially to κ receptors. Most of the prodynorphin peptides bind preferentially to κ receptors, but dynorphin 1-6 also shows roughly equivalent binding at µ and δ. Some smaller dynorphin peptides can have nonopioid actions. Furthermore, some processing produces peptides that still have affinity for the opioid receptors but act functionally as antagonists. For example, although β-endorphin 1-31 is a potent agonist at µ and δ receptors, β-endorphin 1-27 has one-tenth the activity and can antagonize the actions of β-endorphin 1-31, and fragments of OFQ/N can antagonize the actions of the full 17–amino acid peptide (Mogil and Pasternak 2001). Some of the precursor proteins that yield opioid peptides also contain peptides that act on other systems. Thus, POMC also yields adrenocorticotropic hormone (ACTH) and melanocyte-stimulating hormone (MSH) (Akil et al. 1997, 1998); pro-OFQ/N yields several OFQ/N peptides and also a peptide, nocistatin, that antagonizes the pronociceptive effects of OFQ/N and appears to act at a distinct receptor.

Opioid Drugs: Agonists, Partial Antagonists, Antagonists, Mixed Agonist/Antagonists

More than 20 clinically available drugs exert actions at opioid receptors. Most of these drugs, such as morphine, are prototypical µ agonists: they produce analgesia, altered mood (often euphoria), decreased anxiety, respiratory depression, inhibition of certain spinal polysynaptic reflexes, inhibition of gastrointestinal motility, suppression of cough, suppression of corticotropin-releasing factor and adrenocorticotropic hormone release, and miosis (pinpoint pupils); they can also produce pruritus, nausea, and vomiting. When brain levels rise rapidly, which occurs when opioid drugs are injected intravenously or inhaled, users may experience a brief, intense, usually pleasurable sensation called a *rush* or *thrill*. This sensation is followed by a longer-lasting period of altered feeling state—the *high*. Most of the µ agonists are full agonists, able to produce maximal responses in opioid-responsive systems. In clinical dosages, few of the available agonists have any significant actions at the δ or κ receptors. When any µ agonist is used chronically, tolerance and physical dependence develop (see below).

Several opioid antagonists (e.g., naloxone, naltrexone, nalmefene) are now available for clinical use. These drugs bind primarily to the µ receptor, but in higher dosages they can bind to δ and κ receptors. Also available are several drugs that are often described as mixed agonist/antagonists. They bind to several receptor types, usually acting as antagonists or partial agonists at the µ receptor; some have agonist actions at the κ receptor. Drugs in this group include pentazocine, nalbuphine, butorphanol, and dezocine (Gutstein and Akil 2001).

The drug buprenorphine is best described as a partial µ agonist, although in animals it also has κ antagonist activity. Buprenorphine produces typical µ agonist effects; however, as the dosage is increased, the response intensity plateaus, reaching a ceiling comparable to about 20–30 mg of morphine parenterally. Thus buprenorphine is far less likely to produce the severe respiratory depression observed with high dosages of full µ agonists. Like other µ agonists, buprenorphine produces tolerance and physical dependence, but withdrawal is less intense because of the ceiling effect and possibly because buprenorphine binds quite tightly to the receptor. Higher doses of antagonists such as naloxone are required in order to reverse the actions of buprenorphine once it has bound to its receptors. Buprenorphine is now approved for use in the treatment of opioid dependence as both a detoxification and a maintenance agent (see "Opioids: Antagonists and Partial Agonists," Chapter 25 in this volume).

Virtually all the opioids that are abused are prototypical µ agonists. Diacetylmorphine, or heroin, is the most widely used illicit opioid. Heroin is, in part, a prodrug, metabolized within minutes to 6-monoacetylmorphine and to morphine. However, heroin is more lipid soluble than morphine, passing more rapidly into the brain.

The likelihood of a µ agonist drug being misused (abused) depends in part on its pharmacokinetics and the route by which it is administered. Drugs with short half-lives that are used intravenously (e.g., heroin, morphine, hydromorphone, fentanyl) produce behavioral syndromes characterized by a brief period of intoxication (the high) followed within hours by a period of relative withdrawal, drug-seeking behavior, or the administration of more drug. Drugs with long half-lives—for example, methadone or L-α-acetylmethadol (LAAM)—given orally, can allow a relatively stable pattern of behavior; once tolerance has developed, there is minimal or no impairment of mood, judgment, and psychomotor performance (see "Opioids: Maintenance Treatment," Chapter 24 in this volume).

There are sporadic cases of abuse and dependence involving mixed agonist/antagonists, but there is virtually no abuse of κ agonists. Although they can produce analgesia, κ agonists also typically produce dysphoria and a distinct form of physical dependence. There is no cross-dependence between μ and κ agonists.

Neurobiological Models of Opioid Use and Dependence

Drug dependence is characterized by continued, repetitive use of a substance, despite risk to personal health and well-being. Drugs of abuse typically (at least initially) produce subjective feelings of pleasure and are reinforcing in animal models. Neurobiological models of opioids of abuse and dependence typically focus on three phenomena: 1) the euphorigenicity of drugs, 2) their capacity to positively reinforce drug-seeking behavior, and 3) the avoidance of aversive feelings, including but not limited to those associated with drug withdrawal (i.e., negative reinforcement).

Dopamine, Positive Reinforcement, and Hedonic Regulation

The two brain regions most often identified as mediating the pleasurable and positively reinforcing properties of drugs are the ventral tegmental area (VTA) and the nucleus accumbens (NAc). Dopaminergic neurons projecting from the VTA to the NAc form the central pathway of the mesocorticolimbic dopamine system. In animal models, direct stimulation of the NAc and microinjection of dopamine agonists into the region are reinforcing (Koob 2000; Robinson and Berridge 2000).

The limbic projection areas of this circuit include the amygdala and the hippocampus, which are in-

volved in the memory of emotionally charged stimuli. The cortical projection areas of this circuit include prefrontal, anterior cingulate, and frontal cortices, which are involved in drug expectation, stimulus salience, and craving (Goldstein and Volkow 2002). These regions are also central to organizing goal-directed behavior toward naturally pleasurable stimuli, such as food or sex, and such stimuli (as well as anticipation of such stimuli) are associated with dopamine efflux.

However, despite the fact that the action of dopamine in the NAc and related structures plays a critical role in the reinforcing effects of many psychoactive drugs, some argument does exist about exactly how dopamine release engenders drug-seeking behavior. Does dopamine release act as a signal of potential reward, or as the mechanism of the reward itself? Much evidence suggests that the rise in dopamine levels in the NAc produces an effect experienced as pleasure or intense euphoria (Koob and Le Moal 2001; Wise 1998). Other interpreters of the evidence, such as Robinson and Berridge (2000), emphasize dopamine's role not as merely a "pleasure signal" but as a "salience signal," which focuses an organism's attention toward potentially rewarding stimuli and motivates behavior toward obtaining those stimuli. Proponents of this view (called the incentive-sensitization hypothesis) note that dopamine-releasing agents can sensitize dopaminergic motor systems, and these researchers hypothesize that a similar phenomenon occurs in parallel dopaminergic motivational systems. The result is that organisms that experience repeated exposure to drugs of abuse may experience a behavioral sensitization for the wanting of or craving for the drug (Robinson and Berridge 2000).

Although it is common to consider the euphorigenic (hedonic) effects of drugs such as opioids or cocaine to be equivalent to their rewarding or reinforcing effects (effects that increase the likelihood of drug-using behavior), these two phenomena are actually separable ones. For example, in human subjects, some drugs of abuse can engender drug-taking behavior at doses too low to produce subjective hedonic effects. Robinson and Berridge (2000) argue that not only are liking and wanting dissociable, but they are also subserved by partially distinct neural systems. In making a distinction between *wanting* or *craving* and *liking*, the authors argue further that sensitization of neural systems responsible for attributing salience to stimuli can produce goal-directed (drug-seeking) behavior—wanting even in the absence of conscious awareness of wanting. The authors also note that there is great individual variation in susceptibility to sensitization and that there are powerful environmental influences on the development of sensitization. Because, in animals, sensitization of the locomotor system can persist for prolonged periods after the cessation of drug administration, the authors postulate that, in parallel fashion in humans, the salience of drug-related stimuli that elicit craving can also persist for very long periods. Thus far, however, the evidence is correlational, with no proven causal relationship between sensitization and relapse vulnerability in humans (Shalev et al. 2002).

Another perspective that also emphasizes the increased salience of drug-related stimuli is that of Goldstein and Volkow (2002). They note the role of the frontal cortex in inhibition of the amygdala (which is involved in memories of drug effects) and the evidence that in animal models and several brain imaging studies in abstinent addicts there are decreases in frontal lobe volume. The authors postulate that a deficit in frontal lobe function leads to impaired response inhibition to drug-related stimuli such as craving, and they conceptualize addiction as "a syndrome of impaired response inhibition and salience attribution" (Goldstein and Volkow 2002, p. 1643).

A central feature of all current efforts to explain addictive behavior is the critical role of learning. The effects of drugs and external stimuli associated with their use (implements, packaging, etc.) can become linked through learning so that these stimuli can become cues of drug availability or can trigger memories of positive drug effects and can elicit drug craving (Childress et al. 1999; Goldstein and Volkow 2002). Similarly, drug withdrawal can become conditioned to the external environmental stimuli that are present when withdrawal occurs so that these stimuli alone can elicit a sense of withdrawal distress. Learning can also link internal stimuli such as stress, anger, and depression to the drugs that have been used to control these states, and consequently these affective states can elicit craving for the drug (O'Brien et al. 1992).

Opioid Influences on Dopaminergic Reward Systems

The μ and δ opioid agonists increase the activity of dopaminergic neurons originating in the VTA by inhibiting the γ-aminobutyric acid (GABA)–ergic interneurons that normally exert a tonic inhibitory effect on the dopaminergic neurons. These VTA dopamine neurons project fibers to the NAc. Neurons in the NAc itself express at least three types of opioid receptors. Actions at these receptors are probably responsible for direct reinforcing actions of μ and δ agonists in the NAc that do not depend on dopamine (Koob and Le Moal 2001; Nestler 1997, 2001). Some neurons in the NAc have recurrent fibers expressing dynorphin that synapse on κ receptor–bearing dopaminergic neurons projecting from VTA to the NAc (see Figure 2–1).

Activation of these κ receptors is inhibitory to this population of neurons. That arrangement results in a negative feedback loop in which activation of the dynorphin-containing neurons in the NAc results in feedback inhibition of dopaminergic activity. Consistent with this model, currently available κ agonists decrease the activity of VTA dopaminergic neurons and produce aversive effects (presumably mediated by decreased efflux of dopamine at the terminals of these neurons in the NAc) (Akil et al. 1997; Di Chiara and Imperato 1988).

Negative Reinforcement and the Maintenance of Opioid Dependence

Although positive reinforcement, behavioral sensitization, and pleasure probably play important roles in the initiation of opioid abuse, many observers believe that negative reinforcement (the avoidance of aversive internal stimuli) gradually assumes a dominant role in *maintenance* of opioid dependence (although the recurrent search for subjective pleasure continues to be a motive for many, if not all, users). Koob and Le Moal (2001) conceptualized the addicted state as one in which the neurotransmitter systems responsible for positive affective states are hypofunctional, whereas those responsible for aversive affective states are overactive. This situation provides a motivation to seek to end the aversive affective states by further use of a drug. These authors hypothesized that recurrent opioid use may interfere with reward systems by affecting levels of neurotransmitters, such as dynorphin, neuropeptide FF, and OFQ/N, which are believed to dampen the activity of reward systems.

More broadly, Koob and Le Moal (2001) see addiction as an example of *allostasis*, a process in which a perturbed physiological system, rather than maintaining its normal homeostatic balance, instead shifts to a state in which an abnormal set point is maintained.

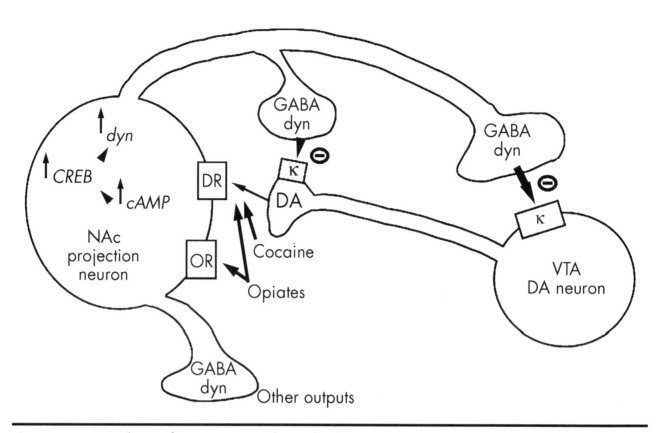

Figure 2–1. Regulation of cAMP response element binding protein (CREB) by drugs of abuse.

A ventral tegmental area (VTA) dopamine (DA) neuron innervating a class of nucleus accumbens (NAc) GABAergic projection neuron that expresses dynorphin (dyn). Dynorphin serves a negative feedback mechanism in this circuit: dynorphin, released from terminals of the NAc neurons, acts on κ opioid receptors (OR) located on nerve terminals and cell bodies of the DA neurons to inhibit their functioning. Chronic exposure to cocaine or opiates upregulates the activity of this negative feedback loop via upregulation of the cyclic adenosine monophosphate (cAMP) pathway, activation of CREB, and induction of dynorphin. GABA=γ-aminobutyric acid. DR=dopamine receptor.

Source. Reprinted from Nestler EJ: "Molecular Neurobiology of Addiction." *American Journal on Addictions* 10:201–217, 2001. Used with permission.

Specifically, the model postulates an imbalance between brain reward systems and stress response systems, resulting in abnormally low sensitivity of the former and abnormally high sensitivity of the latter and requiring multiple neurotransmitter and hormonal systems to be activated in order to maintain normal reward functions.

Environmental stress has long been known to increase likelihood of relapse in drug abuse. In animal models, stress (or the administration of corticosteroids) can sensitize animals to the effects of drugs and increase their tendency to self-administer. Stress can also trigger reinitiation of drug self-administration in animals after a period of extinction. A number of brain systems have been implicated in mediating this stress response. For example, stress has been associated with the activation of excitatory projections from

the prefrontal cortex to the VTA. There, the dopamine projections from the VTA to the NAc are activated, and drug self-administration is stimulated by release of dopamine in the NAc, as described earlier in the chapter (Koob and Le Moal 2001).

Further evidence implicating the brain's stress response system comes from studies of the effects of corticotropin-releasing factor (CRF) on drug-related behaviors. CRF is the hormone responsible for the release of ACTH from the pituitary, but research has shown that it also has actions at other sites in the CNS and may act as a key neurotransmitter in mediating the brain's response to environmental stress. Administration of exogenous CRF stimulates heroin-seeking behavior in dependent animals, and intracerebral injections of CRF antagonists can partially reduce stress-induced relapse. The exact mechanism by which CRF exerts this effect is not clear. Some effects may be mediated directly by CRF acting as a neurotransmitter. Other effects may be mediated by CRF activation of the hypothalamic-pituitary-adrenal (HPA) axis. Glucocorticoid receptors are known to be located on dopamine neurons in the VTA, and corticosteroids appear to increase the sensitivity of these neurons to excitatory inputs, potentiating the stress-induced release of dopamine in the NAc. Blocking the glucocorticoid response to stress eliminates the enhanced behavioral sensitivity to morphine and amphetamine that is induced by stress (Koob and Le Moal 2001; Self and Nestler 1998).

Clinical evidence also supports the notion that the brain's stress system, and specifically the HPA axis, is deranged in opioid-addicted individuals. HPA axis function also appears to be abnormal in abstinent heroin users (although it is normal in patients stably maintained on methadone) (Kreek and Koob 1998). HPA axis activation can be induced by exposure to doses of opioid antagonists too small to result in the appearance of subjective withdrawal. Consistent with this finding are the high levels of glucocorticoids exhibited by opioid addicts during withdrawal and the rises in ACTH (and β-endorphin, also a gene product of POMC) that precede the onset of other signs and symptoms of opioid withdrawal. Heroin addicts demonstrate abnormally high releases of POMC gene products in response to stress chemically induced by metyrapone, a blocker of cortisol synthesis that causes feedback inhibition of brain CRF, ACTH, and β-endorphin. This hyperresponsiveness to stress may be related to relapse. In stabilized methadone-maintained patients, it was possible to elicit classical signs of opioid withdrawal by the administration of metyrapone, suggesting that the activation of the HPA axis (e.g., through increases in CRF and ACTH) may serve as an internal cue of opioid withdrawal (Kreek 1997; Kreek and Koob 1998).

Tolerance, Physical Dependence, and Long-Lasting Neural Adaptation

The Phenomena in Brief

With repeated use, tolerance develops to most of the actions of μ agonist drugs, but it does not develop with equal rapidity in all systems. For example, tolerance develops to the drugs' miotic and constipating effects far more slowly than to their euphoriant and respira-

tory depressant effects. Patients stably maintained on methadone for years may continue to complain of constipation and excessive sweating (Kreek 1997). Generally, there is a considerable degree of cross-tolerance among agonists that act at the same receptor but no cross-tolerance between agonists acting at distinct receptors.

Some level of physical dependence on near-clinical dosages of μ agonist drugs develops quite rapidly, and some symptoms of withdrawal (e.g., yawning, rhinorrhea, dysphoria, nausea) can be elicited by administration of a large dose of naloxone 12–24 hours after a single dose of morphine (Heishman et al. 1989). The μ agonist withdrawal syndrome consists of a number of physiological disturbances that can be thought of as rebound hyperactivity in the biological systems that the agonists suppressed. Thus, instead of analgesia, euphoria, tranquillity, dampened sympathetic activity, miosis, depressed spinal reflexes, and decreased gastrointestinal motility, individuals experience hyperalgesia, dysphoria, anxiety, muscle aches and bone pain, spinal reflex hyperactivity that causes kicking movements ("kicking the habit"), dilated pupils, cramps, and diarrhea. They also experience yawning, sweating, and rhinorrhea. The intensity of the syndrome is generally proportional to the opioid dosage and duration of use.

The onset and duration of the syndrome are closely correlated with the rate at which the drug is cleared from the receptors. With short-acting drugs such as heroin, the onset of early visible symptoms occurs at about 8 hours, and the peak of the syndrome at about 48–72 hours, after the last dose is taken. Once significant physical dependence has developed, the effort to avoid withdrawal becomes a powerful new motive for continued drug taking. With longer-acting opioids such as methadone and LAAM, 24–72 hours may elapse before the onset of withdrawal; peak intensity, which is typically not as severe as with short-acting drugs, may not be reached until the fifth or sixth day. Although, at its peak, withdrawal from longer-acting opioids may be less severe than from comparable doses of short-acting drugs, the prolonged discomfort and hypophoria may be experienced as less tolerable. The acute withdrawal syndrome with short-acting drugs such as morphine or heroin largely subsides within 5–7 days, but with drugs such as methadone it may persist in milder form for 14–21 days. In both situations, the acute phase of withdrawal may be followed by a longer-lasting period characterized by decreased self-esteem, unstable mood, and dysphoria (Martin et al. 1973). The instability of the HPA axis is also part of this longer-lasting syndrome. The dysphoria or hypophoria may be one aspect of the dysregulation of hedonic tone mentioned previously. It is not always clear whether protracted abstinence syndromes represent a later manifestation of opioid-induced biological changes or the emergence of one of several varieties of mood disorders that commonly co-occur among heroin addicts (Brooner et al. 1997).

The general principle that intense opioid withdrawal is relatively brief and that in slower withdrawal the symptoms are less intense but more protracted led to efforts to shorten the duration of withdrawal by using small doses of antagonists to precipitate withdrawal. Benzodiazepines and, later, benzodiazepines plus clonidine were used to make the experience more tolerable. That technique has now been extended to using large doses of antagonists to induce opioid withdrawal during anesthesia. In this way the duration of the acute phase can be shortened to 24–48 hours, although some withdrawal discomfort may persist for several more days (Brewer 1997). (A more complete description of the opioid withdrawal syndrome is found in Chapter 23, "Opioids: Detoxification," in this volume.)

Mechanisms of Tolerance, Dependence, and Long-Lasting Neural Adaptations

Tolerance to opioids involves several mechanisms. Acutely, agonists at all types of opioid receptor (μ, κ, δ, and OFQ/N) produce an inhibition of adenylyl cyclase and a decrease in intracellular cyclic adenosine monophosphate (cAMP) levels. There are also G_i and/or G_o protein–mediated changes in conductance of an inhibitory K^+ ion channel that do not involve cAMP (Figure 2–2).

A type of acute tolerance that develops over minutes may be mediated by protein kinase C (PKC) phosphorylation of the μ and δ receptors (Akil et al. 1997). The tolerance that develops more gradually with chronic drug exposure involves a compensatory upregulation of the cAMP pathway, probably by upregulation of several forms of adenylyl cyclase, an internalization of μ and δ opioid receptors, and adaptive changes in other neural systems that interact with those directly influenced by the opioids. Still another mechanism might involve a decrease in the abundance of the G proteins that couple the opioid receptors to

the second messengers and ion channels (Akil et al. 1997, 1998; Nestler 1997, 2001; Nestler and Aghajanian 1997).

The upregulation of adenylyl cyclase is mediated by the transcription factor cAMP response element binding protein (CREB). CREB is activated when it is phosphorylated by protein kinase A (PKA) or other protein kinases. Opioid inhibition of cAMP initially reduces PKA activity, lowering active CREB, but this process results in more transcription of CREB, which in turn increases expression of adenylyl cyclase (Nestler 2001).

Upregulation of the cAMP pathway occurs in a number of neural systems affected by opioids, including the locus coeruleus (LC), the NAc, the VTA, and the periaqueductal gray (PAG). When the opioids are removed, there is a sharp rise (overshoot) in cAMP levels. Some of the phenomena seen during opioid withdrawal could be explained by the upregulation of cAMP in the VTA and PAG regions, particularly within the GABAergic neurons that innervate these regions. For example, increased activity in GABAergic neurons that normally inhibit dopaminergic neurons in the VTA would result in reduced dopamine release at the NAc—an action consistent with the states of dysphoria, depression, and anhedonia observed during clinical withdrawal and sometimes for long periods following withdrawal (Koob and Bloom 1988; Koob and Le Moal 2001; Nestler 1997, 2001).

Upregulation of the cAMP systems in NAc cells themselves may contribute to tolerance to neural inputs that mediate reward. As evidence for this possibility, activators of PKA (a cAMP-dependent protein kinase) injected into the NAc decrease the rewarding effects of opioids, and inhibitors of PKA increase the rewarding effects (Nestler 2001).

Other withdrawal effects are consistent with rebound hyperactivity of the LC. The LC has the largest concentration of noradrenergic neurons in the brain, with extensive connections to other brain structures. Activity of these neurons generates feelings of anxiety and many of the autonomic symptoms (e.g., increased blood pressure, nausea, sweating, gastrointestinal distress) that emerge during opioid withdrawal. The role of LC hyperactivity during opioid withdrawal is of some clinical relevance because LC neurons express not only receptors for μ and δ opioids but also α_2-adrenergic receptors. The α_2-adrenergic agonists, such as clonidine and lofexidine, can suppress some of the symptoms of opioid withdrawal but apparently not

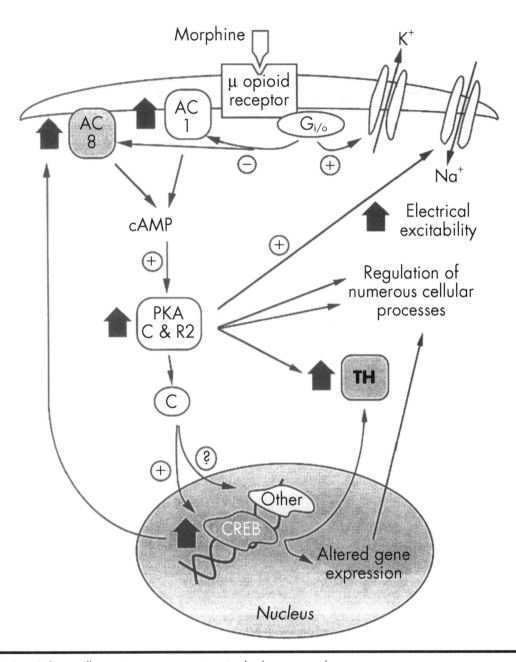

Figure 2–2. Scheme illustrating opiate actions in the locus coeruleus.

Opiates acutely inhibit locus coeruleus neurons by increasing the conductance of an inwardly rectifying K^+ channel via coupling with subtypes of $G_{i/o}$ proteins and by decreasing a Na^+-dependent inward current via coupling with $G_{i/o}$ and the consequent inhibition of adenylyl cyclase (AC). Reduced levels of cyclic adenosine monophosphate (cAMP) decrease protein kinase A (PKA) activity and the phosphorylation of the responsible channel or pump. Inhibition of the cAMP pathway also decreases phosphorylation of numerous other proteins and thereby affects many additional processes in the neuron. For example, it reduces the phosphorylation state of cAMP response element binding protein (CREB), which may initiate some of the longer-term changes in locus coeruleus function. Upward bold arrows summarize effects of chronic morphine in the locus coeruleus. Chronic morphine increases levels of AC types 1 (AC1) and 8 (AC8), PKA catalytic (C) and regulatory type 2 (R2) subunits, and several phosphoproteins, including CREB and tyrosine hydroxylase (TH), the rate-limiting enzyme in norepinephrine biosynthesis. These changes contribute to the altered phenotype for the drug-addicted state. For example, the intrinsic excitability of LC neurons is increased by enhanced activity of the cAMP pathway and Na^+-dependent inward current, which contributes to the tolerance, dependence, and withdrawal exhibited by these neurons. Upregulation of AC8 and TH is mediated via CREB, whereas upregulation of AC1 and of the PKA subunits appears to occur via a CREB-independent mechanism not yet identified.

Source.   Reprinted from Nestler EJ: "Molecular Neurobiology of Addiction." *American Journal on Addictions* 10:201–217, 2001. Used with permission.

the craving, dysphoria, or muscle cramps (Gowing et al. 2002).

Additional mechanisms besides rebound increases in cAMP in opioid receptor–bearing neurons are probably involved in withdrawal. In the LC, for example, the increased activity results also from increased excitatory glutaminergic inputs (Nestler and Aghajanian 1997). Similarly, multiple changes in the VTA could account for dysphoria during acute withdrawal and perhaps for hypophoria during protracted withdrawal.

Chronic opioid use reduces neurofilament proteins and the average size of dopamine neurons in the VTA—changes that may be associated with functional hypoactivity following a period of exposure (Nestler 1997, 2001). Such structural changes could underlie long-lasting changes in drug sensitivity. Alterations in the NAc may also contribute to dysphoric states. During withdrawal, increased activity in a subset of NAc neurons expressing dynorphin can further dampen dopamine release by actions at presynaptic κ receptors of neurons projecting to the nucleus accumbens (Nestler 2001) (see Figure 2–1).

Drug-induced changes in the endogenous opioid systems might also be relevant to postwithdrawal functioning, protracted abstinence, and relapse. Studies of the effects of chronic exposure to μ and κ agonists and μ antagonists on levels of endogenous peptides or on transcription of opioid precursor genes, manifested as changes in messenger RNA (mRNA), have not produced consistent results. However, chronic treatment with μ opioid antagonists has been shown to lead to an upregulation of μ receptor density (Vaccarino and Kastin 2001). In rodents, this upregulation of μ opioid receptors appears to contribute to a hyperresponsiveness to μ opioid agonists when antagonist administration is stopped. These findings in animal models have raised some concern that patients who relapse to opioid use following a period of treatment with antagonists might be more vulnerable to opioid toxicity (Daws and White 1999). Some studies have found decreased affinity and density of opioid receptors, and others have found no significant change in the number of opioid receptors, after chronic exposure to opioid agonists. Some of the inconsistency may be explained by differences in the capacity of different μ opioids to produce μ receptor downregulation.

Some neurons expressing opioid receptors also express receptors for one or more glutamatergic receptors, and evidence indicates that these glutamatergic receptors play a role in the development of opioid tol-erance and dependence. Activation of the *N*-methyl-D-aspartate (NMDA) receptor by glutamate leads to calcium and calmodulin–mediated activation of nitric oxide synthase, resulting in increased levels of nitric oxide. The development of opioid tolerance and dependence can be influenced by agents that act at various points in the pathway from the NMDA receptor to the rise in nitric oxide. In rodents, agents that block the NMDA receptor or inhibit nitric oxide synthase activity can attenuate or prevent the development of opioid tolerance and dependence. Such agents include MK801, phencyclidine (PCP), memantine, and dextrorphan (a metabolite of the widely used antitussive agent dextromethorphan) (Inturrisi 1997; Vaccarino and Kastin 2001). Glutamate also appears to be involved in sensitization to the actions of other psychoactive drugs such as cocaine, and glutamate blockers prevent the development of this sensitization (Wolf 2002).

Acute administration of several varieties of drugs results in production of several members of the Fos family of transcription factors, many of which are unstable. With repeated drug administration, isoforms of Fos proteins (such as ΔFosB) that are more stable begin to accumulate and can persist in various brain regions. (CREB, which, as noted above, increases with chronic opioid exposure, probably plays a role in this process.) In the NAc, ΔFosB seems to accumulate in dynorphin-containing neurons. This increase in ΔFosB results in an increased sensitization to both the rewarding and the locomotor effects of opioids (and cocaine). A suggested mechanism for the sensitization is ΔFosB-induced changes in subunits of AMPA glutamate receptors. Nestler (2001) suggested that the accumulation of ΔFosB "is both a necessary and sufficient mechanism" (p. 210) that could account for long-lasting sensitization to cocaine and opioids and could thereby contribute to relapse. Other drug-induced perturbations that could have long-lasting effects are alterations in the function of neurotrophic factors, such as brain-derived neurotrophic factor (BDNF) and glial cell line–derived neurotrophic factor (GDNF) (Nestler 2001).

Relapse

A prominent feature of addictive disorders is the tendency to relapse to drug use weeks or months after cessation and the disappearance of measurable withdrawal phenomena. Entire systems of treatment are built on teaching patients how to avoid situations likely to lead to drug use and relapse. Those situations include exposure to stimuli associated with drug use (e.g., people who use drugs or implements for using drugs). Formerly dependent subjects exposed to drug-related stimuli expressed increased craving and increased brain activity in the amygdala, orbitofrontal cortex, and lateral prefrontal cortex and related areas, as shown by positron emission tomography scans and magnetic resonance imaging (Bonson et al. 2002; Childress et al. 1999; Daglish et al. 2001; Goldstein and Volkow 2002; Wang et al. 1999). Stress, anger, and depression are the emotional states most frequently reported to trigger craving for drug use. It is almost axiomatic that any use of an individual's drug of addiction can lead to an increase in craving and may lead to further use. Goldstein and Volkow postulated that frontal lobe deficits might impair the individual's capacity to inhibit responses to stimuli previously associated with drug use.

The long-lasting behavioral changes that are induced by repeated drug exposure imply altered synaptic plasticity. There is now evidence that repeated administration of morphine, amphetamine, or cocaine can alter the density of dendritic spines of certain neurons in the NAc and the caudate-putamen. The changes are found on the distal, but not the proximal, dendrites of medium spiny neurons, structures at the specific site of convergence of dopaminergic and glutamatergic signaling on medium spiny neurons. These changes could provide a structural basis for long-lasting sensitization to drugs and vulnerability to relapse (Li et al. 2003).

An area of intensive inquiry is the neurobiology of relapse and the situations that reinstate the behavior. An animal model of relapse is the return to drug self-administration following a period of extinction. This area was reviewed by Shalev et al. (2002). Three distinct conditions can reliably induce such a return to drug use: 1) stress, induced by foot shock or hunger, 2) exposure to conditioned drug cues, and 3) a priming dose of the previously self-administered drug or one that has similar effects. The neural systems involved in these three methods of inducing reinstatement (relapse) are somewhat distinct. For example, μ opioid antagonists and dopamine antagonists can block drug seeking induced by a priming dose of heroin, but they have no effect on reinstatement induced by foot shock. Antagonists of CRF that can block rein-

statement induced by foot shock have no effect on reinstatement induced by priming doses. Shalev et al. (2002) concluded that the neural systems subserving drug-induced reinstatement of drug use are pharmacologically separable from those that mediate drug reinforcement.

Vulnerability Factors and Genetics

Not everyone who tries opioids continues to use them or does so to the point at which dependence develops. In the National Comorbidity Survey, only 7.5% of respondents who had ever tried any opioid for nonmedical purposes developed opioid dependence. Of those who had used heroin, 23% had a lifetime history of opioid dependence, whereas 16.7% of those who had ever used cocaine became cocaine dependent (Anthony et al. 1994). What is known about vulnerability factors for opioid dependence is based on clinical, epidemiological, and animal studies. There appear to be significant differences in the way μ agonists such as morphine are experienced: former addicts generally report euphoria, whereas nonaddicted subjects are more likely to report mental clouding and dysphoria.

There is evidence that genetic factors play a role in vulnerability to opioid dependence. Animal studies show that marked differences exist between strains of rodents in the rapidity and enthusiasm with which they learn to self-administer opioid drugs and in their sensitivity to them. In a study population of Vietnam era veterans, monozygotic twins were more likely than dizygotic twins to be concordant for heroin dependence. Multivariate biometric modeling showed that there were common vulnerability factors underlying the abuse of a variety of drugs (influenced by genetic and environmental factors), as well as genetic influences that appear to be substance specific. Heroin abuse had a greater specific genetic influence than marijuana, stimulants, or sedatives (Tsuang et al. 1998). Other twin studies have found both genetic and shared environmental effects on risks for substance abuse/dependence, but the genetic effects were not substance specific (Kendler et al. 2003). Certain behavioral syndromes in childhood (e.g., conduct disorder) and certain psychiatric disorders in adulthood (especially antisocial personality disorder) also increase the likelihood of drug use and dependence, including opioid dependence. These syndromes have both biological and environmental roots (Lyons et al. 1995).

Opioid Toxicity

Opioids given by mouth in therapeutic doses are relatively nontoxic, and drugs such as methadone have been used over prolonged periods with little or no major organ damage (see Chapter 24, "Opioids: Maintenance Treatment," in this volume). However, a number of toxic effects have been associated with the self-administration of injected or inhaled opioids. The etiology of the toxic effects is not always apparent.

The most dramatic of the toxic effects are acute opioid overdoses characterized by stupor or coma, depressed respiration, and typically extreme miosis. Pulmonary edema may also occur. If respiratory depression persists, anoxia may lead to hypotension and dilated pupils. Overdoses with a more gradual onset but a similar clinical picture have been observed in nontolerant opioid users who are given methadone. Although the use of antagonists increases the likelihood of survival, there may still be subtle or occasionally serious sequelae of anoxia. Whether such insults account for the cognitive deficits observed in some studies among opioid-dependent patients is not clear (Mintzer and Stitzer 2002).

Injection use of illicit opioids has also been associated with neurological lesions, such as necrosis of spinal gray matter and degeneration of globus pallidus (found at autopsy), transverse myelitis, amblyopia, and plexitis. Inhaled opioids have also been associated with neurological damage such as spongiform encephalopathy (Strang et al. 1997). The role of contaminants in these syndromes is not clear; the reported cases of toxicity associated with inhaled opioids typically involved inhaling vapors from a mixture heated on aluminum foil. A known contaminant in the illicit manufacture of meperidine, 1-methyl-4-phenyl-1,2,3,6-tetrahydropyridine (MPTP), causes destruction of dopaminergic neurons and is responsible for several cases of severe parkinsonism seen among drug users. Intramuscular injection of meperidine and certain other opioids, such as pentazocine, can produce long-lasting induration and sclerosis of muscle tissues. Some infectious disorders (e.g., human immunodeficiency virus [HIV], hepatitis, subacute bacterial endocarditis, skin ulcers) are found in opioid users who do not use sterile techniques or who share injection equipment.

There are a few exceptions to the general rule about the safety of opioids. Some opioids can affect heart rhythm by prolonging the QT interval, an effect that is not unique to the opioids. In extreme cases, lengthening the QT, which is caused by the blocking of a specific K^+ channel, can result in serious cardiac arrhythmias, such as torsades de pointes. Opioid agonists differ in their potency in exerting this effect. An in vitro study using human cells transfected with the gene for that K^+ channel concluded that morphine and codeine had the widest safety margins and that LAAM and methadone had the lowest (Katchman et al. 2002).

Some opioids have toxic metabolites. For example, normeperidine, a metabolite of meperidine, can produce seizures and confused delirium. Normeperidine accumulates if it is given frequently in high dosages (as may be seen in physician addicts), in ordinary dosages when renal function is impaired, and as a consequence of certain drug interactions.

References

Akil H, Meng F, Devine DP, et al: Molecular and neuroanatomical properties of the endogenous opioid system: implications for treatment of opiate addiction. Seminars in Neuroscience 9:70–83, 1997

Akil H, Owens C, Gutstein H, et al: Endogenous opioids: overview and current issues. Drug Alcohol Depend 51:127–140, 1998

Anthony JC, Warner LA, Kessler RC: Comparative epidemiology of dependence on tobacco, alcohol, controlled substances, and inhalants: basic findings from the National Comorbidity Survey. Exp Clin Psychopharmacol 2:244–268, 1994

Bonson KR, Grant SJ, Contoreggi CS, et al: Neural systems and cue-induced craving. Neuropsychopharmacology 26:376–386, 2002

Brewer C: Ultra-rapid, antagonist-precipitated opiate detoxification under general anaesthesia or sedation. Addict Biol 2:291–302, 1997

Brooner RK, King VL, Kidorf M, et al: Psychiatric and substance use comorbidity among treatment-seeking opioid abusers. Arch Gen Psychiatry 54:71–80, 1997

Childress AR, Mozley PD, McElgin W, et al: Limbic activation during cue-induced cocaine craving. Am J Psychiatry 156:11–18, 1999

Daglish MR, Weinstein A, Malizia AL, et al: Changes in regional cerebral blood flow elicited by craving memories in abstinent opiate-dependent subjects. Am J Psychiatry 158:1680–1686, 2001

Daws LC, White JM: Regulation of opioid receptors by opioid antagonists: implications for rapid opioid detoxification. Addict Biol 4:391–397, 1999

Di Chiara G, Imperato A: Opposite effects of mu and kappa opiate agonists on dopamine release in the nucleus accumbens and in the dorsal caudate of freely moving rats. J Pharmacol Exp Ther 244:1067–1080, 1988

Goldstein RZ, Volkow ND: Drug addiction and its underlying neurobiological basis: neuroimaging evidence for the involvement of the frontal cortex. Am J Psychiatry 159:1642–1652, 2002

Gowing LR, Farrell M, Ali RL, et al: α_2-Adrenergic agonists in opioid withdrawal. Addiction 97:49–58, 2002

Gutstein HB, Akil H: Opioid analgesics, in Goodman and Gilman's The Pharmacological Basis of Therapeutics, 10th Edition. Edited by Hardman JG, Limbird LE. New York, McGraw-Hill, 2001, pp 569–620

Heishman SJ, Stitzer ML, Bigelow GE, et al: Acute opioid physical dependence in humans: effect of varying the morphine-naloxone interval, I. J Pharmacol Exp Ther 250:485–491, 1989

Inturrisi CE: Preclinical evidence for a role of glutamatergic systems in opioid tolerance and dependence. Seminars in Neuroscience 9:110–119, 1997

Jordan BA, Cvejic S, Devi LA: Opioids and their complicated receptor complexes. Neuropsychopharmacology 23 (4 suppl):S5–S18, 2000

Katchman AN, McGroary KA, Kilborn MJ, et al: Influence of opioid agonists on cardiac human ether-a-go-go-related gene K^+ currents. J Pharmacol Exp Ther 303: 688–694, 2002

Kendler KS, Karkowski LM, Neale MC, et al: Illicit psychoactive substance use, heavy use, abuse and dependence in a US population-based sample of male twins. Arch Gen Psychiatry 57:261–269, 2000

Kendler KS, Jacobson KC, Prescott CA, et al: Specificity of genetic and environmental risk factors for use and abuse/dependence of cannabis, cocaine, hallucinogens, sedatives, stimulants, and opiates in male twins. Am J Psychiatry 160:687–695, 2003

Koob GF: Neurobiology of addiction: toward the development of new therapies. Ann N Y Acad Sci 909:170–185, 2000

Koob GF, Bloom FE: Cellular and molecular mechanisms of drug dependence. Science 242:715–723, 1988

Koob GF, Le Moal M: Drug addiction, dysregulation of reward, and allostasis. Neuropsychopharmacology 24:97–129, 2001

Kreek MJ: Clinical update of opioid agonists and partial agonist medications for the maintenance treatment of opioid addiction. Seminars in Neuroscience 9:140–157, 1997

Kreek MJ, Koob GF: Drug dependence: stress and dysregulation of brain reward pathways. Drug Alcohol Depend 51:23–47, 1998

LaForge KS, Yuferov V, Kreek MJ: Opioid receptor and peptide gene polymorphisms: potential implications for addictions. Eur J Pharmacol 410:249–268, 2000

Li Y, Kolb B, Robinson TE: The location of persistent amphetamine-induced changes in the density of dendritic spines on medium spiny neurons in the nucleus accumbens and caudate-putamen. Neuropsychopharmacology 28:1082–1085, 2003

Lyons MJ, True WR, Eisen SA, et al: Differential heritability of adult and juvenile antisocial traits. Arch Gen Psychiatry 52:906–915, 1995

Martin WR, Jasinski DR, Haertzen CA, et al: Methadone—a reevaluation. Arch Gen Psychiatry 28:286–295, 1973

Mintzer MZ, Stitzer ML: Cognitive impairment in methadone maintenance patients. Drug Alcohol Depend 67:41–51, 2002

Mogil JS, Pasternak GW: The molecular and behavioral pharmacology of the orphanin FQ/nociceptin peptide and receptor family. Pharmacol Rev 53:381–415, 2001

Negus SS, Brandt MR, Gatch MB, et al: Effects of heroin and its metabolites on schedule-controlled responding and thermal nociception in rhesus monkeys: sensitivity to antagonism by quadazocine, naltrindole and beta-funaltrexamine. Drug Alcohol Depend 70:17–27, 2003

Nestler EJ: Molecular mechanisms underlying opiate addiction: implications for medications development. Seminars in Neuroscience 9:84–93, 1997

Nestler EJ: Molecular neurobiology of addiction. Am J Addictions 10:201–217, 2001

Nestler EJ, Aghajanian GK: Molecular and cellular basis of addiction. Science 278:58–63, 1997

O'Brien CP, Childress AR, McLellan AT, et al: Classical conditioning in drug-dependent humans. Ann N Y Acad Sci 654:400–415, 1992

Pasternak GW: The pharmacology of mu analgesics: from patients to genes. Neuroscientist 7:110–231, 2001

Robinson TE, Berridge KC: The psychology and neurobiology of addiction: an incentive sensitization view. Addiction 95 (suppl 2):S91–S117, 2000

Self DW, Nestler EJ: Relapse to drug-seeking: neural and molecular mechanisms. Drug Alcohol Depend 51:49–60, 1998

Shalev U, Grimm JW, Shaham Y: Neurobiology of relapse to heroin and cocaine seeking: a review. Pharmacol Rev 54:1–42, 2002

Sora I, Elmer G, Funada M, et al: Mu opiate receptor gene dose effects on different morphine actions: evidence for differential in vivo mu receptor reserve. Neuropsychopharmacology 25:41–54, 2001

Strang J, Griffiths P, Gossop M: Heroin smoking by "chasing the dragon": origins and history. Addiction 92:673–683, 1997

Tsuang MT, Lyons MJ, Meyer JM, et al: Co-occurrence of abuse of different drugs in men. Arch Gen Psychiatry 55:967–972, 1998

Vaccarino AL, Kastin AJ: Endogenous opiates: 2000. Peptides 22:2257–2328, 2001

Wang GJ, Volkow ND, Fowler JS, et al; Regional brain metabolic activation during craving elicited by recall of previous drug experiences. Life Sci 64:775–784, 1999

Wise R: Drug-activation of brain reward pathways. Drug Alcohol Depend 51:13–22, 1998

Wolf ME: Addiction: Making the connection between behavioral changes and neuronal plasticity in specific pathways. Molecular Interventions 2:146–157, 2002

Zadina JE: Isolation and distribution of endomorphins in the central nervous system. Jpn J Pharmacol 89:203–208, 2002

Neurobiology of Stimulants

Margaret Haney, Ph.D.

Cycles of amphetamine and cocaine abuse have occurred throughout the world for more than 100 years. In the United States, use of methamphetamine, which is the primary form of amphetamine abused, has dramatically increased. The number of individuals entering treatment for methamphetamine has also increased in recent years. Between 1993 and 1999, treatment admissions for methamphetamine increased by 100%–250% in the western United States (Substance Abuse and Mental Health Services Administration 2001). By comparison, cocaine use has declined relative to its extremely widespread use in the 1980s to early 1990s. Nonetheless, cocaine arrest statistics, drug treatment records, and emergency room mentions demonstrate that cocaine remains a major public health issue (U.S. Office of National Drug Control Policy 2001). Currently, there are no medications available to treat stimulant abuse. Continued progress in our understanding of the behavioral, cellular, and molecular consequences of chronic cocaine and amphetamine use will be important in the development of effective treatment medications.

Mechanism of Action

Cocaine's behavioral effects are mediated primarily by its binding to the dopamine transporter and inhibiting the reuptake of synaptic dopamine (Ritz et al. 1987). Given that reuptake is the primary mechanism of terminating dopamine transmission, cocaine administration results in dose-dependent increases in extracellular levels of dopamine (e.g., Wise et al. 1995). Cocaine also blocks the reuptake of norepinephrine and serotonin. In fact, the affinity of cocaine for serotonin-binding sites is greater than its affinity for dopamine-binding sites (Koe 1976).

Amphetamine has a more complex mechanism of action than cocaine; amphetamine both decreases dopamine reuptake and promotes dopamine release via the dopamine transporter (e.g., Saunders et al. 2000). Another important difference between amphetamines and cocaine is the duration of action: cocaine is rapidly metabolized, whereas amphetamine metabolism is relatively slow, with effects lasting several hours longer than those of cocaine.

Although methamphetamine is the primary type of amphetamine that is abused, laboratory studies have often used dextroamphetamine (*d*-amphetamine), which has behavioral and dopaminergic effects similar to that of methamphetamine but a different pattern of effects on serotonin and norepinephrine, particularly following repeated administration (Kuczenski et al. 1995). Thus we present data on methamphetamine when available.

Subjective and Discriminative Stimulus Effects

Among the most important behavioral effects of cocaine and methamphetamine are their mood-altering properties (Johanson and Fischman 1989). Both cocaine and amphetamine dose-dependently increase subjective-effects measures considered to describe euphoria and decrease such measures considered to describe sedative-like effects. Behavioral methods have been developed to obtain information from laboratory animals on the discriminative stimuli of drugs of abuse that are thought to model subjective drug effects in humans. In a typical drug discrimination experiment, laboratory animals are trained to make a particular behavioral response when they receive an active dose of a drug and to make another behavioral response when they receive a placebo. Specifically, after receiving a training dose of a drug, making a drug-appropriate behavioral response results in reinforcer delivery (e.g., food), whereas making a placebo-appropriate response does not result in reinforcer delivery.

Once animals have been trained, drugs from the same or different pharmacological classes can be administered, and the behavioral response the animal makes provides information about how similar or different the test drug is from the training drug. These procedures indicate that the discriminative stimulus effects of cocaine and amphetamine are similar. That is, if trained to discriminate cocaine from saline, animals respond on the cocaine-appropriate lever when given amphetamine, and vice versa.

Reinforcing Effects

Stimuli that maintain behavior leading to their administration are classified as reinforcers. The most salient feature of drug addiction is repeated, compulsive drug use, indicating that drugs of abuse are reinforcers. A great deal of research has focused on the reinforcing effects of stimulant drugs because of their substantial abuse. The primary method used to determine whether a drug functions as a reinforcer is the self-administration paradigm, in which the drug is delivered after a specific behavioral response is emitted. The robust reinforcing effects of cocaine and amphetamine are thought to result from their effects on the mesolimbic/mesocortical dopaminergic neuronal systems, including the ventral tegmental area (VTA), nucleus accumbens, ventral pallidum, and medial prefrontal cortex. The following data support the hypothesis that dopamine has a primary role in the reinforcing effects of psychostimulant drugs (Fischman and Johanson 1996):

- Dopamine receptor antagonists decrease the reinforcing effects of cocaine and amphetamine in laboratory animals.
- A depletion of dopamine produced by the injection of neurotoxin into these dopaminergic pathways attenuates cocaine and amphetamine self-administration by laboratory animals.
- The amount of cocaine self-administered is correlated positively with extracellular dopamine levels in the nucleus accumbens (Pettit and Justice 1991).
- The magnitude of the self-reported "high" in humans correlates with the occupancy of the dopamine transporter by cocaine, and the time course for these ratings parallels cocaine concentrations in the striatum (Volkow et al. 1997).

Neither norepinephrine nor serotonin appears to specifically mediate the reinforcing effects of cocaine or amphetamine. Serotonin modulates dopamine in the ventral striatum, but the relationship is complex. In laboratory animals, increasing serotonin levels has been shown to decrease cocaine's effects on extracellular dopamine levels and to decrease cocaine self-administration, yet responding for food may decrease as well, suggesting that the effects are not specific. In human laboratory studies, maintenance on fluoxetine, a serotonin reuptake inhibitor, reduced the subjective effects of low doses of cocaine but did not improve treatment outcome in clinical trials of cocaine abusers (Czoty et al. 2002; Walsh and Cunningham 1997). It may be that selective modulation of one or more of the 14 subtypes for the serotonin receptor will prove useful therapeutically, but currently there are few specific compounds available to test in humans. Thus, further work is needed to clarify if selective serotonergic agonists or antagonists will prove useful as potential pharmacotherapies for cocaine and amphetamine abuse.

Other neurotransmitter systems may also influence cocaine or amphetamine self-administration by modulating dopamine. For instance, glutamate projects to dopaminergic neurons in the nucleus accumbens, and injections of selective N-methyl-D-aspartate (NMDA) receptor antagonists into the nucleus accumbens block both the dopaminergic effects of psychostimulants and their reinforcing effects in laboratory animals (Pap and Bradberry 1995; Schenk et al. 1993b). The inhibitory neurotransmitter γ-aminobutyric acid (GABA) also interacts with dopamine neurons in the nucleus accumbens and the VTA, and pharmacological manipulation of GABA alters both dopamine activity and cocaine self-administration (e.g., Roberts et al. 1996). A number of preclinical human studies currently under way are investigating the effects of NMDA antagonists and GABA agonists for the treatment of psychostimulant abuse.

These data demonstrate that dopamine plays a primary role in mediating the reinforcing effects of cocaine and amphetamine. However, because of the intricate interactions between dopamine and other neurotransmitters, cocaine and amphetamine use can be modulated by medications acting on a range of neurochemical sites.

Consequences of Repeated Stimulant Exposure

Stimulant drugs are generally abused in repeated dose bouts, called binge-crash cycles, which impinge on the reward pathway with a longevity and intensity that do not occur with natural rewards. Repeated, frequent drug use produces disruptions in homeostatic mechanisms and leads to enduring neuroadaptations that may provide the neurobiological basis for consequences such as addiction or the compulsive use of cocaine and amphetamine following repeated self-administration. The consequences of repeated stimulant exposure depend on the pattern of use. Intermittent exposure increases the motor-activating effect of stimulant drugs in laboratory animals, and in humans such exposure can lower the threshold for developing stimulant psychosis. Chronic stimulant exposure can result in tolerance, or a decrease in the effects of stimulant drugs, and may result in neurotoxicity; and cessation of chronic stimulant use may result in symptoms of withdrawal.

Sensitization

Sensitization is defined as a leftward shift in the dose-response curve, meaning that smaller doses produce an effect that once was obtained only at higher doses. Repeated, intermittent administration of cocaine or amphetamine to laboratory animals results in sensitization to the motoric and convulsant effects of these drugs. There are data suggesting that the reinforcing effects of cocaine and amphetamine also become sensitized. In laboratory animals, doses of these drugs that were subthreshold for maintaining self-administration maintained the behavior if the animals were preexposed to these doses (e.g., Lorrain et al. 2000; Piazza et al. 1989). However, nonhuman primates show remarkably stable patterns of cocaine self-administration over periods of months without indication of changes in sensitivity to cocaine's reinforcing effects (Wilson et al. 1971). Thus, the notion of sensitization to reinforcing effects is unclear.

Sensitization to the reinforcing or subjective effects of stimulants has not been demonstrated in humans, and the role played by sensitization in cocaine or amphetamine addiction is unknown. Sensitization, however, does appear to affect the development of behavioral pathology in humans. At its most extreme, this pathology can include psychosis, characterized by paranoia, impaired reality testing, and vivid visual, auditory, and tactile hallucinations that are virtually indistinguishable from schizophrenia (Post and Kopanda 1976). Methamphetamine-related psychosis may last as long as several days or weeks, whereas cocaine-related psychosis tends to have a briefer duration (Jackson 1989). Chronic stimulant abusers who have experienced drug-induced psychosis report that this state readily recurs with readministration of even a small dose of the drug, and laboratory investigations support these findings: amphetamine psychosis has been replicated reliably in drug-free volunteers who were given small but frequent doses of the drug over the course of several days (Griffith et al. 1972). Thus, sensitization appears to play a role in the behaviorally toxic consequences of psychostimulant abuse.

Neurochemical Basis

Drugs that are capable of inducing behavioral sensitization stimulate dopamine transmission either directly or indirectly. The neuroanatomical loci mediating the initiation of sensitization are distinct from those mediating the expression of sensitization. It appears that the initiation of sensitization to both cocaine and amphetamine occurs in the VTA, where dopamine cell bodies that project to the nucleus accumbens are located, whereas the expression of sensitization is mediated in the nucleus accumbens. Dopamine receptors are classified as D_1 or D_2 receptors. In the initial phases of sensitization, the firing rate of dopamine neurons originating in the VTA increases because of a decrease in sensitivity of the inhibitory, impulse-regulating D_2 autoreceptors. This subsensitivity in the D_2 autoreceptors is not maintained for long, and therefore it is not the mechanism by which sensitization is maintained. Sensitization is expressed in the nucleus accumbens, where D_1 receptors become supersensitive to the effects of extracellular dopamine (Henry and White 1992). Thus, sensitization in part reflects decreased sensitivity of D_2 autoreceptors in the VTA, resulting in increased dopamine release, and increased sensitivity of postsynaptic D_1 receptors in the nucleus accumbens.

Glutamate also plays an important role in the initiation of stimulant sensitization. Repeated administration of stimulants results in an enhanced response to glutamate's excitatory effects on dopaminergic neurons in the VTA; this enhanced response is not present 14 days later (Zhang et al. 1997). The coadministration of NMDA-receptor antagonists with cocaine or methamphetamine prevents the development of sensitization to the locomotor and reinforcing effects of these drugs (e.g., Schenk et al. 1993a). NMDA antagonists coadministered with amphetamine also block D_2 autoreceptor subsensitivity in the VTA and postsynaptic D_1 receptor supersensitivity in the nucleus accumbens (Wolf et al. 1994). These studies demonstrate that glutamatergic synapses in the VTA are critical to the initiation of sensitization.

The mechanisms of amphetamine and cocaine sensitization are not identical. Inhibitors of nitric oxide (NO) (which is produced following NMDA receptor activation), coadministered with cocaine, prevented the development of sensitization; in contrast, the same NO inhibitors coadministered with methamphetamine attenuated but did not abolish the development of sensitization (Itzhak 1997).

Other neurotransmitters and neuromodulators also influence the development and expression of stimulant sensitization, often through their effects on dopamine. For example, cocaine produces a larger inhibition of serotonin firing rate in the dorsal raphe nucleus in sensitized rats than in drug-naive rats. Because serotonin inhibits dopamine neurotransmission, a decrease in serotonin release in areas such as the VTA and the nucleus accumbens results in increased dopamine neurotransmission (Cunningham et al. 1992). Furthermore, coadministering serotonin antagonists

with cocaine blocks the development of sensitization (King et al. 1997). Antagonists at the nicotinic receptor (Schoffelmeer et al. 2002), and at the μ, κ, σ, or δ opioid receptor (e.g., Ujike et al. 1996) also block the initiation of methamphetamine or cocaine sensitization. Thus, it is clear that the mechanisms underlying sensitization are complex and involve interactions among a variety of neurochemical pathways within the central nervous system.

Addiction

Addiction can be defined as compulsive drug seeking and drug taking, with a loss of control over drug use. Part of this loss of control not only includes an inability to regulate drug intake but also an inability to maintain abstinence. Addiction is considered a chronic relapsing disorder. Most individuals addicted to cocaine or amphetamine, for example, relapse within 1 year of initiating abstinence. One factor believed to increase the likelihood of relapse is exposure to the sensory cues associated with drug taking, often producing an overwhelming desire for the drug. Associations between these cues and drug use, often formed over hundreds of occasions, can profoundly influence the motivation to use drugs even after years of drug abstinence.

Neurochemical Basis

Brain structures such as the basolateral amygdala and the hippocampus, which mediate the association between environmental stimuli and drug effects, are essential to the influence of drug-related cues on drug seeking. In laboratory animals, presentation of the cues associated with cocaine or amphetamine increase dopamine levels in the nucleus accumbens and amygdala, and, more importantly, increase drug-seeking behavior; D_1 antagonists at the level of the amygdala block drug seeking following cue presentation (Everitt and Wolf 2002). In humans, functional imaging studies show that cocaine-related cues are associated with increased activity in the basolateral amygdala, the cingulate cortex, and the orbitofrontal cortex (London et al. 1999). Thus, one mechanism by which environmental cues trigger cocaine or amphetamine seeking appears to involve projections from limbic cortical structures to the nucleus accumbens.

The persistence of drug addiction may reflect altered patterns of synaptic connectivity, as occurs during normal memory foundation. Conventional reinforcers, such as palatable food, increase dopamine in the nucleus accumbens and in other areas of the extended amygdala; this process helps form the association between the reinforcer and the stimuli associated with the reinforcer. With repeated exposure to the palatable food, the dopamine response habituates. Stimulants however, elicit a prolonged increase in dopamine that does not habituate. This lack of habituation may be one reason why drug-related stimuli gain excessive control over behavior (Di Chiara 1998). That is, stimulants, by enhancing dopamine action to a greater extent than nondrug reinforcers, may lead to *excessive* strengthening of the behaviors associated with drug use, perhaps explaining the powerful influence of drug-related cues on drug use.

Another consequence (or precursor) of chronic cocaine or amphetamine use may be impaired impulse control. Frontal cortical structures mediating decision making and impulse inhibition, which are closely linked with the nucleus accumbens, the amygdala, and the VTA, appear to be affected by chronic stimulant exposure (Jentsch and Taylor 1999). As compared with nondrug users, both cocaine and methamphetamine users have alterations in dopamine D_2 receptors and metabolic activity in the frontal cortex that persist for months after detoxification (Volkow and Fowler 2000). In general, damage within the frontal cortex leads to a preferential response for small reinforcers over larger, delayed reinforcers, as well as perseveration in responding, even in the absence of reinforcement. The similarity between these behaviors and the compulsive use of cocaine and amphetamine at the expense of other behaviors implicates the frontal cortex in the mediation of addictive behaviors.

Given the role of dopamine in the neurobiology of addiction, a number of preclinical human studies have tested dopaminergic agonists and antagonists as potential treatment medications, much as opioid agonists and antagonists have been used in the treatment of opioid abuse. Kosten and Sofuoglu (Chapter 16 of this volume) provide a more detailed explanation of the treatment of stimulant abuse; therefore the discussion in this chapter is largely limited to preclinical studies. The discussion is also limited to cocaine because few studies, other than preliminary investigations using oral *d*-amphetamine to treat amphetamine abuse (e.g., Shearer et al. 2001), have investigated potential medications for methamphetamine abuse.

In terms of an agonist approach to stimulant treatment, dopamine D_1 receptor agonists show more promise than those acting at the D_2 receptor. Acute pretreatment with the D_1 agonist ABT-431 produced dose-dependent decreases in the effects of smoked cocaine, such as ratings of the high obtained and ratings of the quality and potency of cocaine (Haney et al. 1999). These data support the theory that D_1 agonists may have utility as medications for treating cocaine abuse. D_2 receptor agonists, by contrast, were not promising in laboratory studies (e.g., Haney et al. 1998) or in the clinic (e.g., Malcolm et al. 2000).

In terms of dopaminergic antagonists, in laboratory studies, maintenance on the D_1/D_2 receptor antagonist flupenthixol did not alter the pattern of cocaine self-administration, and flupenthixol at higher doses was associated with extrapyramidal side effects (Evans et al. 2001). Acute administration of the D_1 antagonist ecopipam decreased the euphoric effects of cocaine in a laboratory setting (Romach et al. 1999), yet maintenance on ecopipam actually *enhanced* cocaine's reinforcing and subjective effects compared with placebo (e.g., Haney et al. 2001a). These data emphasize the importance of studying the chronic administration of potential treatment medications, because chronic and acute drug administration often produce different effects.

Tolerance

Tolerance is defined as a rightward shift in the dose-response curve, meaning that larger doses are needed to produce an effect that previously was obtained at a lower dose. In humans, acute tolerance to many of cocaine's effects develops during a single episode of cocaine use. That is, the first dose administration produces larger cardiovascular and subjective effects than do subsequent doses, despite sustained elevations in cocaine plasma levels (Foltin and Fischman 1991). During a binge, cocaine users often use large amounts of cocaine to attempt to achieve the effect obtained by the first dose.

There is little evidence in nonhuman or human laboratory studies to support longer-term tolerance to cocaine's or amphetamine's reinforcing effects (e.g., Ward et al. 1997; Wilson et al. 1971). That is, there is little indication that experienced stimulant abusers are less sensitive to the reinforcing effects of cocaine or amphetamine than are those who have less experience using stimulants. Thus, although tolerance to certain stimulant effects, such as anorexia, has been clearly demonstrated, long-term tolerance to the reinforcing effects of cocaine or amphetamine does not appear to occur.

Neurochemical Basis

Although there are numerous neurochemical consequences of repeated cocaine and amphetamine use, it is difficult to definitively ascribe acute tolerance to any of these changes.

Dependence

Dependence is defined as the presence of withdrawal symptoms on termination of drug use. Psychostimulants, unlike opiates or alcohol, do not produce adaptations in areas mediating somatic and autonomic function and therefore are not associated with physical withdrawal symptoms. However, both clinical observations (e.g., Weddington et al. 1990) and controlled laboratory studies (e.g., Foltin and Fischman 1997) demonstrate that abstinence following the repeated use of intravenous or smoked cocaine is associated with increased depression, anxiety, and irritability. Thus, stimulant withdrawal is primarily characterized by disorders in mood.

Neurochemical Basis

In laboratory animals, abstinence following unlimited stimulant self-administration coincides with decreased extracellular dopamine and serotonin and increased dynorphin in the nucleus accumbens, which are hypothesized to contribute to mood symptoms during stimulant withdrawal (Koob et al. 1997).

In humans, the effects of chronic stimulant use on serotonin and dopamine pathways are difficult to study directly. Yet there is indirect evidence supporting alterations in serotonin pathways during cocaine withdrawal. Serotonin stimulates prolactin and cortisol release; therefore, one method of assessing central serotonergic function is to measure plasma prolactin and corticosterone following administration of the serotonin releaser and reuptake inhibitor d-fenfluramine. Cocaine users who self-administered a controlled amount of crack cocaine in the laboratory had a blunted neuroendocrine response to d-fenfluramine that lasted for at least 2 weeks of cocaine abstinence as compared with control subjects who did not abuse drugs. By contrast, there was no disruption in the hormonal response to the D_2 agonist bromocriptine during cocaine abstinence, even shortly after a controlled cocaine "binge" (Haney et al. 2001b). A deficit of central serotonin transmission during stimulant withdrawal is consistent with the hypothesized etiology of clinical depression. Thus, the long-lasting and selective disruption in serotonin pathways that follows chronic cocaine use may provide a neurochemical basis for the changes in mood commonly reported during cocaine withdrawal.

Neurotoxicity

An additional consequence of chronic exposure to psychostimulants, particularly amphetamine, may be neurotoxicity. In laboratory animals, repeated administration of large doses of d-amphetamine or methamphetamine is associated with decreased tissue concentrations of dopamine and serotonin, decreases in dopamine uptake sites, and an inhibition of tyrosine hydroxylase and tryptophan hydroxylase (Seiden and Sabol 1996). In humans, postmortem analyses of methamphetamine abusers revealed decreased neural levels of striatal dopamine, tyrosine hydroxylase, and dopamine transporters compared with those of control subjects (Wilson et al. 1996). Brain imaging studies in detoxified methamphetamine abusers also showed decreased dopamine transporters in the caudate and putamen that appeared to last at least several months after the last drug use (e.g., Volkow et al. 2001). Although it is possible that the results reflect neuroadaptations rather than dopamine terminal degeneration, the persistence of these effects suggests that dopamine transporter levels were not simply downregulated. Nonetheless, there is evidence in rats (Cass and Manning 1999) and in nonhuman primates (Melega et al. 1997) that dopamine functioning recovers over time. Thus, there is a need for more studies on the precise behavioral and physiological consequences of methamphetamine's long-term effects on dopamine and serotonin. Also needed are studies that approximate the doses and patterns of human methamphetamine abuse. Most laboratory animal studies demonstrating neurotoxicity used higher doses and more frequent dose administrations than used by humans (e.g., Villemagne et al. 1998); therefore, the relevance of these studies to human methamphetamine abuse remains to be determined.

Cocaine has not been shown to produce the same degree of dopaminergic neurotoxicity as methamphetamine. In laboratory animal studies comparing doses of cocaine and *d*-amphetamine that produced comparable levels of weight loss, behavioral activation, and lethality, amphetamine resulted in axonal degeneration in the neostriatum and frontal cortex, but cocaine did not (Ryan et al. 1988). There was also little evidence of toxicity to dopaminergic nerve terminals in human cocaine-overdose patients compared with drug-free age-matched control subjects (Staley et al. 1997). Cocaine may have neurotoxic effects outside dopamine pathways. Chronic cocaine administration has been shown to produce axonal degeneration in the lateral habenula. Furthermore, cocaine abusers (who often abuse other drugs as well) also tend to show deficits in cerebral blood perfusion and cerebral glucose metabolism that persist after detoxification from cocaine. These abnormalities, which mimic certain neurological disorders, may play a role in cocaine's behavioral toxicity (Majewska 1996).

Neurochemical Basis

Depending on the dose and route of administration of methamphetamine, the dopamine whose release is thus induced may be auto-oxidized to 6-hydroxydopamine, which results in neurodegeneration. In fact, the magnitude of dopamine release correlates with the amount of neurotoxicity. Thus, the destruction of both serotonin and dopamine neurons has been shown to be reduced or prevented in laboratory animals if one of the following steps is taken before methamphetamine administration: 1) dopamine reuptake blockers are administered, 2) dopamine synthesis inhibitors or antagonists are administered, or 3) brain dopamine levels are depleted (Seiden and Sabol 1996). Antioxidants protect dopamine from damage induced by methamphetamine, suggesting that treating methamphetamine abusers during early withdrawal with antioxidants may attenuate potential pathology.

Neurotoxicity with repeated methamphetamine abuse may also be partly the result of increased glutamate release, which underlies the neuron-damaging effects of a range of central nervous system insults. Toxic doses of methamphetamine increase glutamate efflux in the striatum, where neurotoxicity occurs, but not in the nucleus accumbens, where neurotoxicity does not occur (Abekawa et al. 1994). NMDA antagonists prevent both dopaminergic and serotonergic neurotoxicity (e.g., Johnson et al. 1989), suggesting that these medications also have potential for decreasing methamphetamine's toxic effects.

Conclusion

Cocaine and amphetamine share a number of important features. Acutely administered, these drugs have similar subjective, reinforcing, and discriminative stimulus effects, and repeated exposure results in sensitization or tolerance to certain effects, depending on the dosage and patterning of drug administration. Some important distinctions between cocaine and amphetamine exist. First, cocaine's effects are relatively short lasting, resulting in a pattern of more frequent self-administration over a shorter period of time than with amphetamine. Second, the neurochemical effects of cocaine and amphetamine are distinct, which may explain differences in their neurotoxic effects. Cocaine inhibits the reuptake of dopamine, whereas amphetamine both inhibits dopamine reuptake and promotes dopamine release. This finding means that amphetamine is more neurotoxic to dopaminergic neurons than is cocaine.

There can be a range of consequences to repeated psychostimulant self-administration, including sensitization, tolerance, dependence, and addiction. The mechanisms for these adaptations are distinct, and therefore each has a distinct time course and etiology. The substantial advances in understanding of the complex neuroadaptations that follow cocaine or amphetamine abuse have formed the basis for studies attempting to reverse or treat the consequences of chronic drug use with medications. The far-reaching effects of psychostimulant abuse on a range of neurochemical systems illustrate the difficulty of this task, because finding a compound that acts specifically is difficult. In addition, the development of treatment medications becomes further complicated if the normal mechanisms of experience-dependent learning and memory formation are usurped by chronic drug exposure. Pharmacotherapeutic interventions will probably not cure a chronic, relapsing disorder such as stimulant abuse, but such interventions may decrease craving, initiate or prolong abstinence, or block the acute stimulant effects of the drug being abused. These effects may provide a window of opportunity during which behavioral and psychosocial interventions can be applied (Johanson and Fischman 1989). I believe that continued efforts at the basic preclinical level, combined with human laboratory investigations aimed at detailing the mechanisms of action of prospective medications, will lead to effective pharmacological adjuncts for the treatment of cocaine and methamphetamine abuse.

References

Abekawa T, Ohmori T, Koyama T: Effects of repeated administration of a high dose of methamphetamine on dopamine and glutamate release in rat striatum and n. accumbens. Brain Res 643:276–281, 1994

Cass WA, Manning MW: Recovery of presynaptic dopaminergic functioning in rats treated with neurotoxic doses of methamphetamine. J Neurosci 19:7653–7660, 1999

Cunningham KA, Paris JM, Goeders NE: Serotonin neurotransmission in cocaine sensitization. Ann N Y Acad Sci 654:117–127, 1992

Czoty PW, Ginsburg BC, Howell LL: Serotonergic attenuation of the reinforcing and neurochemical effects of cocaine in squirrel monkeys. J Pharmacol Exp Ther 300:831–837, 2002

Di Chiara G: A motivational learning hypothesis of the role of mesolimbic dopamine in compulsive drug use. J Psychopharmacol 12:54–67, 1998

Evans SM, Walsh SL, Levin FR, et al: Effect of flupenthixol on subjective and cardiovascular responses to intravenous cocaine in humans. Drug Alcohol Depend 64:271–283, 2001

Everitt BJ, Wolf ME: Psychomotor stimulant addiction: a neural systems perspective. J Neurosci 22:3312–3320, 2002

Fischman MW, Johanson CE: Toward an integrated neurobehavioral approach, in Pharmacological Aspects of Drug Dependence: Toward an Integrated Neurobehavioral Approach (Handbook of Experimental Pharmacology, Vol 118). Edited by Schuster CR, Kuhar MJ. New York, Springer-Verlag, 1996, pp 159–195

Foltin RW, Fischman MW: Smoked and intravenous cocaine in humans: acute tolerance, cardiovascular and subjective effects. J Pharmacol Exp Ther 257:247–261, 1991

Foltin RW, Fischman MW: A laboratory model of cocaine withdrawal in humans: intravenous cocaine. Exp Clin Psychopharmacol 5:404–411, 1997

Griffith JD, Cavanaugh J, Held J, et al: Dextro-amphetamine: evaluation of psychotomimetic properties in man. Arch Gen Psychiatry 26:97–100, 1972

Haney M, Fischman MW, Foltin RW: Effects of pergolide on cocaine self-administration in men and women. Psychopharmacology (Berl) 137:15–24, 1998

Haney M, Collins ED, Ward AS, et al: Effects of a selective dopamine D₁ agonist (ABT-431) on smoked cocaine self-administration in humans. Psychopharmacology (Berl) 143:102–110, 1999

Haney M, Ward AS, Foltin RW: Effects of ecopipam, a selective dopamine D1 antagonist, on smoked cocaine self-administration by humans. Psychopharmacology (Berl) 155:330–337, 2001a

Haney M, Ward AS, Gerra G, et al: Neuroendocrine effects of d-fenfluramine and bromocriptine following repeated smoked cocaine in humans. Drug Alcohol Depend 64:63–73, 2001b

Henry DJ, White FJ: Electrophysiological correlates of psychomotor stimulant-induced sensitization, in The Neurobiology of Drug and Alcohol Addiction. Edited by Kalivas PW, Samson HH. New York, New York Academy of Sciences, 1992, pp 47–59

Itzhak Y: Modulation of cocaine- and methamphetamine-induced behavioral sensitization by inhibition of brain nitric oxide synthase. J Pharmacol Exp Ther 282:521–527, 1997

Jackson JG: Hazards of smokable methamphetamine (letter). N Engl J Med 321:907, 1989

Jentsch JD, Taylor JR: Impulsivity resulting from frontostriatal dysfunction in drug abuse: implications for the control of behavior by reward-related stimuli. Psychopharmacology (Berl) 146:373–390, 1999

Johanson CE, Fischman MW: The pharmacology of cocaine related to its abuse. Pharmacol Rev 41:3–52, 1989

Johnson M, Hanson GR, Gibb JW: Effect of MK-801 on decrease in tryptophan hydroxylase induced by methamphetamine and its methylenedioxy analog. Eur J Pharmacol 165:315–318, 1989

King GR, Xiong Z, Ellinwood EH Jr: Blockade of cocaine sensitization and tolerance by the co-administration of ondansetron, a 5-HT₃ receptor antagonist, and cocaine. Psychopharmacology (Berl) 130:159–165, 1997

Koe BK: Molecular geometry of inhibitors of the uptake of catecholamines and serotonin in synaptosomal preparations of rat brain. J Pharmacol Exp Ther 199:649–661, 1976

Koob GF, Caine SB, Parsons L, et al: Opponent process model and psychostimulant addiction. Pharmacol Biochem Behav 57:513–521, 1997

Kuczenski R, Segal DS, Cho AK, et al: Hippocampus norepinephrine, caudate dopamine and serotonin, and behavioral responses to the stereoisomers of amphetamine and methamphetamine. Neuroscience 15:1308–1317, 1995

London ED, Bonson KR, Ernst M, et al: Brain imaging studies of cocaine abuse: implications for medication development. Crit Rev Neurobiol 13:227–242, 1999

Lorrain DS, Arnold GM, Vezina P: Previous exposure to amphetamine increases incentive to obtain drug: long-lasting effects revealed by progressive ratio schedules. Behav Brain Res 107:9–19, 2000

Majewska MD: Cocaine as a neurological disorder: implications for treatment, in Neurotoxicity and Neuropathology Associated With Cocaine Abuse (NIDA Research Monograph 163). Edited by Majewska MD. Rockville, MD, National Institute on Drug Abuse, 1996, pp 1–26

Malcolm R, Kajdasz DK, Herron J, et al: A double-blind, placebo-controlled outpatient trial of pergolide for cocaine dependence. Drug Alcohol Depend 60:161–168, 2000

Melega WP, Raleigh MJ, Stout DB, et al: Recovery of striatal dopamine function after acute amphetamine- and methamphetamine-induced neurotoxicity in the vervet monkey. Brain Res 766:113–120, 1997

Pap A, Bradberry CW: Excitatory amino acid antagonists attenuate the effects of cocaine on extracellular dopamine in the nucleus accumbens. J Pharmacol Exp Ther 274:127–133, 1995

Pettit HO, Justice JB Jr: Effect of dose on cocaine self-administration behavior and dopamine levels in the nucleus accumbens. Brain Res 539:94–102, 1991

Piazza PV, Deminiere JM, Le Moal M, et al: Factors that predict individual vulnerability to amphetamine self-administration. Science 245:1511–1513, 1989

Post RM, Kopanda RT: Cocaine, kindling and psychosis. Am J Psychiatry 133:627–634, 1976

Ritz MC, Lamb RJ, Goldberg SR, et al: Cocaine receptors on dopamine transporters are related to self-administration of cocaine. Science 237:1219–1223, 1987

Roberts DCS, Andrews MM, Vickers GJ: Baclofen attenuates the reinforcing effects of cocaine in rats. Neuropsychopharmacology 15:417–423, 1996

Romach MK, Glue P, Kampmann K, et al: Attenuation of the euphoric effects of cocaine by the dopamine D_1/D_5 antagonist ecopipam (SCH 39166). Arch Gen Psychiatry 56:1101–1106, 1999

Ryan LJ, Martone ME, Linder JC, et al: Cocaine, in contrast to D-amphetamine, does not cause axonal degeneration in neostriatum and agranular frontal cortex of Long-Evans rats. Life Sci 43:1403–1409, 1988

Saunders C, Ferrer JV, Shi L, et al: Amphetamine-induced loss of human dopamine transporter activity: an internalization-dependent and cocaine-sensitive mechanism. Proc Natl Acad Sci U S A 97:6850–6855, 2000

Schenk S, Valadez A, McNamara C, et al: Development and expression of sensitization to cocaine's reinforcing properties: role of NMDA receptors. Psychopharmacology (Berl) 111:332–338, 1993a

Schenk S, Valadez A, Worley CM, et al: Blockade of the acquisition of cocaine self-administration by the NMDA antagonist MK-801 (dizocilpine). Behav Pharmacol 4:652–659, 1993b

Schoffelmeer ANM, De Vries JT, Wardeh G, et al: Pyschostimulant-induced behavioral sensitization depends on nicotinic receptor activation. J Neurosci 22:3269–3276, 2002

Seiden LS, Sabol KE: Methamphetamine and methylenedioxymethamphetamine neurotoxicity: possible mechanisms of cell destruction, in Neurotoxicity and Neuropathology Associated With Cocaine Abuse (NIDA Research Monograph 163). Edited by Majewska MD. Rockville, MD, National Institute on Drug Abuse, 1996, pp 251–276

Shearer J, Wodak A, Mattick RP, et al: Pilot randomized controlled study of dexamphetamine substitution for amphetamine dependence. Addiction 96:1289–1298, 2001

Staley JK, Talbot JZ, Ciliax J, et al: Radioligand binding and immunoautoradiographic evidence for a lack of toxicity to dopaminergic nerve terminals in human cocaine overdose victims. Brain Res 747:219–229, 1997

Substance Abuse and Mental Health Services Administration: Amphetamine treatment admissions increase: 1993–1999. The Dasis Report, November 16, 2001. Rockville, MD, Substance Abuse and Mental Health Services Administration, 2001

U.S. Office of National Drug Control Policy: National Drug Control Strategy: 2001 Annual Report. Washington, DC, U.S. Government Printing Office, 2001

Ujike H, Kuroda S, Otsuki S: σ Receptor antagonists block the development of sensitization to cocaine. Eur J Pharmacol 296:123–128, 1996

Villemagne V, Yuan J, Wong DF, et al: Brain dopamine neurotoxicity in baboons treated with doses of methamphetamine comparable to those recreationally abused by humans: evidence from [^{11}C]WIN-35,428 positron emission tomography studies and direct in vitro determinations. J Neurosci 18:419–427, 1998

Volkow ND, Fowler JS: Addiction, a disease of compulsion and drive: involvement of the orbitofrontal cortex. Cereb Cortex 10:318–325, 2000

Volkow ND, Wang GJ, Fischman MW, et al: Relationship between subjective effects of cocaine and dopamine transporter occupancy. Nature 386:827–839, 1997

Volkow ND, Chang L, Wang G-J, et al: Association of dopamine transporter reduction with psychomotor impairment in methamphetamine abusers. Am J Psychiatry 158:377–382, 2001

Walsh SL, Cunningham KA: Serotonergic mechanisms involved in the discriminative stimulus, reinforcing and subjective effects of cocaine. Psychopharmacology (Berl) 130:41–58, 1997

Ward AS, Haney M, Fischman MW, et al: Binge cocaine self-administration in humans: intravenous cocaine. Psychopharmacology (Berl) 132:375–381, 1997

Weddington WW, Brown BS, Haertzen CA, et al: Changes in mood, craving and sleep during short-term abstinence reported by male cocaine addicts. Arch Gen Psychiatry 47:861–868, 1990

Wilson JM, Kalasinsky KS, Levey AI, et al: Striatal dopamine nerve terminal markers in human, chronic methamphetamine users. Nat Med 2:699–703, 1996

Wilson MC, Hitomi M, Schuster CR: Psychomotor stimulant self-administration as a function of dosage per injection in the rhesus monkey. Psychopharmacologia 22:271–281, 1971

Wise RA, Newton P, Leeb K, et al: Fluctuations in nucleus accumbens dopamine concentration during intravenous cocaine self-administration in rats. Psychopharmacology (Berl) 120:10–20, 1995

Wolf ME, White FJ, Hu XT: MK-801 prevents alterations in the mesoaccumbens dopamine system associated with behavioral sensitization to amphetamine. J Neurosci 14:1735–1745, 1994

Zhang XF, Hu XT, White FJ, et al: Increased responsiveness of ventral tegmental area dopamine neurons to glutamate after repeated administration of cocaine or amphetamine is transient and selectively involves AMPA receptors. J Pharmacol Exp Ther 281:699–706, 1997

Neurobiology of Hallucinogens

Richard A. Glennon, Ph.D.

Hallucinogenic agents represent an old and very large class of drugs. Nearly every major civilization throughout history has had a preferred drug of abuse, or mind-altering substance, and in many instances these agents have been hallucinogens or hallucinogen-related agents or plant products. What constitutes a hallucinogen? Various agents can produce hallucinogenic episodes, and terms used to describe such agents include, for example, *hallucinogens, psychotomimetics, psychedelics, inebriants,* and *intoxicants.* Many agents have been included in this general class of psychoactive agents. Do agents as structurally diverse as (+)lysergic acid diethylamide [(+)LSD], phencyclidine (PCP, angel dust), tetrahydrocannabinol (THC; a constituent of marijuana), amphetamine, and mescaline all produce the same (or a common) effect? Do they all work by means of a common pharmacological mechanism? Studies over the past several decades suggest that they do not. Hollister (1968) wrote that "one can scarcely get any agreement upon the term used to describe this class of drugs" (p. 18). How, then, do we define *hallucinogen?* Hollister (1968) attempted to define these agents on the basis of their pharmacological effects:

- In proportion to other effects, changes in thought, perception, and mood should predominate.

- Intellectual or memory impairment should be minimal at dosages that produce the effects listed above.
- Stupor, narcosis, or excessive stimulation should not be an integral effect.
- Autonomic nervous system side effects should be neither disabling nor severely disconcerting.
- Addictive craving should be minimal.

Although these criteria allowed the classification of certain agents by a process of elimination, they still allowed inclusion of a rather wide variety of pharmacologically distinct agents. Hallucinogenic agents do not appear to represent a behaviorally homogeneous class of agents. Evidence indicates that agents once included in the single general category of hallucinogenic/psychotomimetic agents should be further subclassified. For example, psychotomimetic PCP-related agents probably produce many of their actions through interaction at PCP receptors, cannabinoid receptors may account for some of the actions of various cannabinoids, and hallucinogenic episodes associated with amphetamine psychosis probably involve a dopaminergic mechanism. Many agents remain, and none of the previously mentioned categories would accommodate hallucinogens such as LSD or mescaline. The term *classical hallucinogen* has evolved to account for some of these agents (Glennon 1999; Lin and Glennon 1994).

Classical Hallucinogens: Classification

The best working definition of *classical hallucinogen* is an agent that meets the Hollister criteria and that 1) binds at serotonin type 2 (5-HT$_2$) receptors and 2) is recognized by animals trained to discriminate 1-(2,5-dimethoxy-4-methylphenyl)-2-aminopropane (DOM) from nondrug, or vehicle, in tests of stimulus generalization (Glennon 1996, 2003). These criteria may account for many of the remaining agents.

Although a significant amount of human data is available (Brimblecombe and Pinder 1975; Hoffer and Osmond 1967; Jacob and Shulgin 1994; Lin and Glennon 1994; Shulgin and Shulgin 1991; Siva Sankar 1975), many putative hallucinogens have been poorly investigated, if at all, in humans. There are some results from animal studies; however, no reliable animal model of hallucinogenic activity has been developed (Glennon 1992). As a result, animal data must be interpreted cautiously.

Nevertheless, a procedure that has become widely accepted for classifying centrally acting agents is the *drug discrimination paradigm*, usually performed with rats, pigeons, or monkeys as test subjects (Glennon 1994). Using a typical two-lever operant behavioral paradigm, animals can be trained to respond in one manner (e.g., to press one of two levers) under a given set of conditions and to respond in a different manner (e.g., to press the opposite of the two levers) under a different set of conditions. Thus, animals can be reliably trained to discriminate administration of a centrally acting agent from vehicle. Typically, the drug stimulus is reliable and robust, and results are replicable from laboratory to laboratory.

Once animals are trained to discriminate a given training drug from vehicle, several types of studies can be conducted. Two of the most useful and widely used studies are tests of stimulus generalization and tests of stimulus antagonism. In the former, challenge drugs are administered intermittently to the trained animals to determine whether the agents produce stimulus effects similar to those of the training drug. Results are both qualitative and quantitative; that is, the method

allows classification of the type of action produced and also provides information about the potency of the challenge drugs relative to the training drug. In tests of stimulus antagonism, the training drug's mechanism of action can be explored by attempting to antagonize the stimulus effects of the drug with various neurotransmitter antagonists. Although such studies are not limited to the investigation of hallucinogens and have been used more for the investigation of nonhallucinogens, they have provided a wealth of information regarding the classification and mechanism of action of hallucinogenic agents. Furthermore, results obtained from such studies can be compared with results of human studies in which data are available to corroborate the findings.

The strength of the drug discrimination paradigm is that stimulus generalization does not occur between agents that do not produce common stimulus effects. For example, animals trained to discriminate (+)LSD do not recognize PCP or THC, animals trained to discriminate (+)amphetamine do not recognize mescaline, and so on. Using this procedure, several classical hallucinogens have been used as training drugs, including (+)LSD, DOM, mescaline, and 5-methoxy-*N,N*-dimethyltryptamine (Glennon 1996). Moreover, animals trained to one of these agents recognize each of the other agents, further attesting to the similarity of their stimulus effects. Several hundred agents have been examined in rats trained to discriminate DOM from vehicle, and this research has aided the classification of the agents. Table 4–1 shows categories and examples of classical hallucinogens, and Figure 4–1 shows chemical structures of selected examples. The agents in Table 4–1 seem to share a common component of action in that they are recognized by DOM-trained animals.

Classical Hallucinogens: Mechanism of Action

Tests of stimulus antagonism have been conducted with various neurotransmitter antagonists, and serotonin antagonists can antagonize the effects of hallucinogens. Ketanserin, pirenperone, and other antagonists with an affinity for a particular population of serotonin receptors (i.e., 5-HT$_2$ receptors) are the most effective in blocking the stimulus effects of the classical hallucinogens, leading to the concept that

Table 4–1. Categories and examples of classical hallucinogens

Category	Subcategory	Examples
Indolealkylamines	Tryptamines	N,N-Dimethyltryptamine (DMT)
		N,N-Diethyltryptamine (DET)
		4-Hydroxy-DMT (psilocin)
		5-Methoxy-DMT
	α-Alkyltryptamines	α-Methyltryptamine (α-MeT)
		5-Methoxy-α-MeT
	Lysergamides	Lysergic acid diethylamide (LSD)
	β-Carbolines[a]	Harmaline
Phenylalkylamines	Phenylethylamines	Mescaline
		2-(4-Bromo-2,5-dimethoxyphenyl)-1-aminoethane (Nexus)
	Phenylisopropylamines	α-Methylmescaline (3,4,5-TMA)
		1-(2,5-Dimethoxy-4-methylphenyl)-2-aminopropane (DOM)
		1-(4-Bromo-2,5-dimethoxyphenyl)-2-aminopropane (DOB)
		1-(2,5-Dimethoxy-4-iodophenyl)-2-aminopropane (DOI)
		1-(3,4-Methylenedioxyphenyl)-2-aminopropane (MDA; love drug)

[a] Categorization as classical hallucinogens is tentative. Although certain β-carbolines bind at serotonin type 2A (5-HT$_{2A}$) receptors and are recognized by DOM-trained animals, none has been shown to produce a 5-HT$_{2A}$-mediated agonist effect (e.g., phosphatidylinositol [PI] hydrolysis).

classical hallucinogens act as 5-HT$_2$ agonists. Subsequently, the 5-HT$_2$ receptor affinities of various hallucinogens were measured, and a significant correlation was found between any two of the following parameters: 1) drug discrimination–derived potencies, 2) human hallucinogenic potencies, and 3) 5-HT$_2$ receptor affinities. It would appear, then, that hallucinogens act as 5-HT$_2$ receptor agonists. This theory has become known as the *5-HT$_2$ hypothesis of classical hallucinogen action* (Glennon 1994), and this class of agents has been alternatively referred to as *serotonergic hallucinogens* (Glennon 2003). This hypothesis does not preclude a role for other populations of receptors in the actions of hallucinogens. Indeed, individual hallucinogens can display widely varying binding profiles. Nevertheless, 5-HT$_2$ receptor affinity is the one feature that all classical hallucinogens have in common. In the first clinical study of its kind, the actions of the indolealkylamine hallucinogen psilocybin, the phosphate ester of psilocin, was recently shown to be antagonized in humans by the 5-HT$_2$ antagonist ketanserin (Vollenweider et al. 1998).

Three populations of 5-HT$_2$ receptors (5-HT$_{2A}$, 5-HT$_{2B}$, and 5-HT$_{2C}$) have been identified since the 5-HT$_2$ hypothesis was proposed. Although hallucinogens bind at all three subpopulations (Nelson et al. 1994), work from several laboratories indicates that hallucinogens may act primarily via a 5-HT$_{2A}$ mechanism (Fiorella et al. 1995; Ismaiel et al. 1993; Schreiber et al. 1994).

Hallucinogen-Related Designer Drugs

Designer drugs, or controlled substance analogues, are structural variants of known drugs of abuse. For example, the designer drug "Nexus" (2-CB; see Table 4–1) is a mescaline-like analogue of the phenylisopropylamine (PIA) hallucinogen 1-(4-bromo-2,5-dimethoxyphenyl)-2-aminopropane (DOB) and is a hallucinogen. The PIAs represent one of the largest categories of hallucinogens, and a wealth of human data is available on them (Shulgin and Shulgin 1991). Not all PIA designer drugs are hallucinogenic. Amphetamine (Figure 4–2), a nonhallucinogen central stimulant that can produce hallucinations (called *amphetamine psychosis*) upon chronic administration of high dosages, is also a PIA; amphetamine and some related PIAs are amphetamine-like central stimulants rather than hallucinogens. Methcathinone ("cat") is an example of a designer drug with stimulant activity. Other PIAs produce empathogenic effects (i.e., increased empathy, talkativeness, openness, and feelings of well-being); an agent with this activity is the *N*-methyl ana-

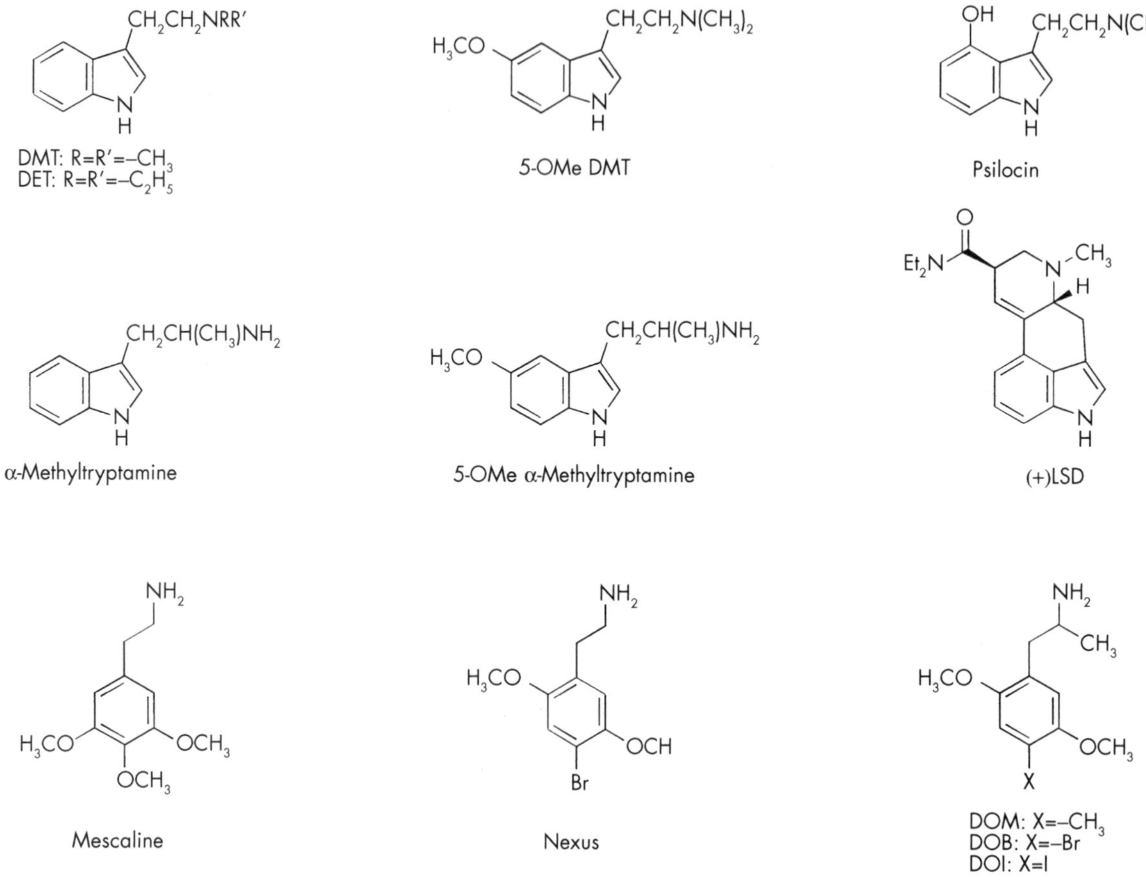

Figure 4–1. Structures of some of the examples of hallucinogenic agents listed in Table 4–1.

DET=*N,N*-diethyltryptamine; DMT=*N,N*-dimethyltryptamine; DOB=1-(4-bromo-2,5-dimethoxyphenyl)-2-aminopropane; DOI=1-(2,5-dimethoxy-4-iodophenyl)-2-aminopropane; DOM=1-(2,5-dimethoxy-4-methylphenyl)-2-aminopropane; (+)LSD=(+)lysergic acid diethylamide.

logue of 1-(3,4-methylenedioxyphenyl)-2-aminopropane (MDA) (i.e., MDMA; "XTC," "Ecstasy," "X," "e") (Nichols and Oberlender 1989). Yet another type of PIA is typified by the designer drug *N*-methyl-1-(4-methoxyphenyl)-2-aminopropane (PMMA), a nonhallucinogen nonstimulant. Thus, minor structural alterations in a PIA can result in agents with central stimulant, hallucinogenic, or other actions (see Figure 4–3). A PIA might have more than one such action, depending on its specific chemical structure. Unlike stimulant PIAs, hallucinogenic PIAs are not typically self-administered by animals; however, the multiplicity of effect of PIAs may explain why certain PIA hallucinogens are self-administered, whereas most are not.

By use of the new classification scheme (Figure 4–3), Nexus can be classified as a DOM-like hallucinogen, and methcathinone as an amphetamine-like stimulant. MDMA is best characterized as an S/P-type agent

in that it produces both amphetamine-like and PMMA-like effects. On the other hand, *N*-methyl-1-(3,4-methylenedioxyphenyl)-2-aminobutane (MBDB; "Eden," "Methyl-J"), a homolog of MDMA that lacks stimulant character (Nichols and Oberlender 1989), is defined as a PMMA-like agent (Rangisetty et al. 2001). Racemic MDA represents the common intersect because it produces all three actions; however, its individual optical isomers R(-)MDA and S(+)MDA are classified as H/P- and S/P-type agents, respectively (Glennon and Young 2002). PMMA and 1-(4-methoxyphenyl)-2-aminopropane (PMA; "white death," "chicken powder") have been used to adulterate MDMA or have been represented on the street as MDMA; PMA produces PMMA-like effects. An example of a new PMMA-like agent is 1-(4-methylthiophenyl)-2-aminopropane (4-MTA; "flatliners"). Such a classification scheme has also been extended to indolealkylamine hallucinogens such as

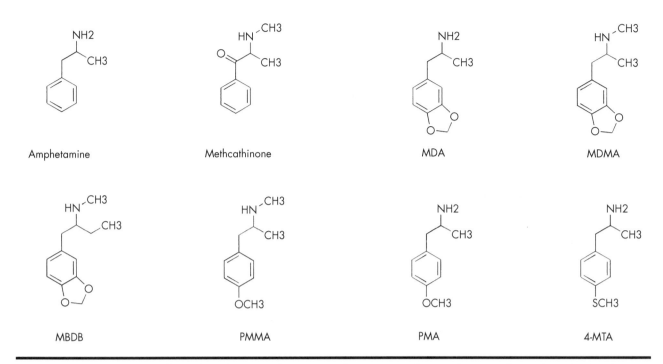

Figure 4-2. Structures of the phenylisopropylamine amphetamine and some designer drugs described in the text.

MBDB=N-methyl-1-(3,4-methylenedioxyphenyl)-2-aminobutane; MDA=1-(3,4-methylenedioxyphenyl)-2-aminopropane; MDMA=methyl-1-(3,4-methylenedioxyphenyl)-2-aminobutane; 4-MTA=1-(4-methylthiophenyl)-2-aminopropane; PMA=1-(4-methox-yphenyl)-2-aminopropane; PMMA=N-methyl-1-(4-methoxyphenyl)-2-aminopropane.

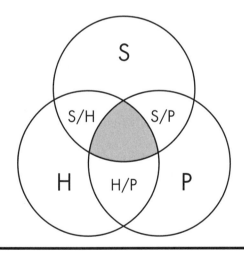

Figure 4-3. Venn diagram representing possible overlapping activities or behavioral similarities among the psychoactive phenylisopropylamines.

H=hallucinogenic, typified by 1-(2,5-dimethoxy-4-methylphe-nyl)-2-aminopropane (DOM); **S**=central stimulant, typified by (+)amphetamine; **P**=other activity, typified by N-methyl-1-(4-methoxyphenyl)-2-aminopropane (PMMA). The agent 1-(3,4-methylenedioxyphenyl)-2-aminopropane [(±)MDA] seems to represent the common (shaded) intersect in that it produces all three actions. See Glennon et al. (1997) and Glen-non and Young (2002) for further discussion.

α-ethyltryptamine (α-ET; "ET"). The specific mix of actions of certain agents may contribute to their attrac-tiveness as drugs of abuse and also may explain the dif-ficulty of classifying various PIAs with respect to their observed clinical effects (Glennon et al. 1997). Various new agents are appearing on the street; little is known about their actions and mechanisms of action. These agents (including their metabolites and synthetic by-products) require further investigation.

Conclusion

Hallucinogens/psychotomimetics represent a diverse group of agents that are perhaps best understood by subdividing them into several categories (e.g., PCP-like psychotomimetics, cannabinoids, cholinergic hal-lucinogens). The agents that generally come to mind when one hears the term *hallucinogen,* such as LSD and mescaline, are termed *classical hallucinogens.* Although the agents in this latter class do not necessarily pro-duce identical effects, they do seem to produce a com-mon effect that may represent the activation of 5-HT$_{2A}$ receptors in the brain. Structural modification of these agents modulates their potency and action. That is, certain designer drugs may produce hallucinogenic, central stimulant, and/or other actions, and these effects may need to be considered when addressing or treating hallucinogen abuse.

References

Brimblecombe RW, Pinder RM: Hallucinogenic Agents. Bristol, England, Wright-Scientechnica, 1975

Fiorella D, Rabin RA, Winter JC: The role of 5-HT$_{2A}$ and 5-HT$_{2C}$ receptors in the stimulus effects of hallucinogenic drugs, I: antagonist correlation analysis. Psychopharmacology (Berl) 121:347–356, 1995

Glennon RA: Animal models for assessing classical hallucinogens, in Animal Models for the Assessment of Psychoactive Drugs. Edited by Boulton AA, Baker GB, Wu PH. Clifton, NJ, Humana Press, 1992, pp 345–381

Glennon RA: Classical hallucinogens: an introductory overview, in Hallucinogens: An Update (NIDA Research Monograph 146). Edited by Lin GC, Glennon RA. Rockville, MD, National Institute on Drug Abuse, 1994, pp 4–32

Glennon RA: Classical hallucinogens, in Pharmacological Aspects of Drug Dependence (Handbook of Experimental Pharmacology, Vol 118). Edited by Schuster CR, Kuhar MJ. Berlin, Springer, 1996, pp 343–372

Glennon RA: Arylalkylamine drugs of abuse: an overview of drug discrimination studies. Pharmacol Biochem Behav 64:251–256, 1999

Glennon RA: The pharmacology of serotonergic hallucinogens and "designer drugs," in Principles of Addiction Medicine, 3rd Edition. Edited by Graham AW, Schultz TK, Mayo-Smith M, et al. Chevy Chase, MD, American Society of Addiction Medicine, 2003, pp 271–285

Glennon RA, Young R: Effect of 1-(3,4-methylenedioxyphenyl)-2-aminopropane and its optical isomers in PMMA-trained rats. Pharmacol Biochem Behav 72:307–311, 2002

Glennon RA, Young R, Dukat M, et al: Initial characterization of PMMA as a discriminative stimulus. Pharmacol Biochem Behav 57:151–158, 1997

Hoffer A, Osmond H: The Hallucinogens. New York, Academic Press, 1967

Hollister LE: Chemical Psychoses. Springfield, IL, Charles C Thomas, 1968

Ismaiel AM, De Los Angeles J, Teitler M, et al: Antagonism of the 1-(2,5-dimethoxy-4-methylphenyl)-2-aminopropane stimulus with a newly identified 5-HT$_2$- versus 5-HT$_{1C}$-selective antagonist. J Med Chem 36:2519–2525, 1993

Jacob P III, Shulgin AT: Structure-activity relationships of the classical hallucinogens and their analogs, in Hallucinogens: An Update. Edited by Lin GC, Glennon RA. Washington, DC, U.S. Department of Health and Human Services, 1994, pp 74–91

Lin GC, Glennon RA (eds): Hallucinogens: An Update. Washington, DC, U.S. Department of Health and Human Services, 1994

Nelson DL, Lucaites VL, Wainscott DB, et al: Comparisons of hallucinogenic phenylisopropylamine binding affinities at cloned human 5-HT$_{2A}$, 5-HT$_{2B}$, and 5-HT$_{2C}$ receptors. Naunyn Schmiedebergs Arch Pharmacol 359:1–6, 1999

Nichols DE, Oberlender R: Structure-activity relationships of MDMA-like substances, in Pharmacology and Toxicology of Amphetamine and Related Designer Drugs (NIDA Research Monograph 94). Edited by Ashgar K, De Souza EB. Rockville, MD, National Institute on Drug Abuse, 1989, pp 1–29

Rangisetty JB, Bondarev ML, Chang-Fong J, et al: PMMA-stimulus generalization to the optical isomers of MBDB and 3,4-DMA. Pharmacol Biochem Behav 69:261–267, 2001

Schreiber R, Brocco M, Millan MJ: Blockade of the discriminative stimulus effects of DOI by MDL 100,907, and the atypical antipsychotics clozapine and risperidone. Eur J Pharmacol 264:99–102, 1994

Shulgin A, Shulgin A: Pihkal. Berkeley, CA, Transform Press, 1991

Siva Sankar DV: LSD: A Total Study. Westbury, NY, PJD Publications, 1975

Vollenweider FX, Vollenweider-Scherpenhuyzen MF, Babler A, et al: Psilocybin induces schizophrenia-like psychosis in humans via a serotonin-2 agonist action. Neuroreport 9:3897–3902, 1998

Neurobiology of Marijuana

Billy R. Martin, Ph.D.

Marijuana (the common name for the plant *Cannabis sativa*) is the most widely used illicit drug today. It has been used for centuries for its therapeutic and mood-altering properties. The magnitude of health consequences from recreational use of marijuana and the medical efficacy of this plant remain highly controversial. The sudden emergence, in the early 1970s, of marijuana as a major substance of abuse was accompanied by intense interest in understanding how the drug produces its centrally mediated effects and, more important, the biological consequences of acute and chronic use. Marijuana has prominent effects on the central nervous system and has numerous peripheral effects as well. Acutely, marijuana produces an altered state of consciousness characterized by mild euphoria, relaxation, perceptual alterations including time distortion, and enhancement of ordinary sensory experiences (Hall et al. 1994). Cognitive effects such as impairment of short-term memory are also marked. Motor skills and reaction time are also impaired, with the result that various types of skilled activities are frequently disrupted (Hall et al. 1994). In early studies, the cannabinoids appeared to have numerous potential therapeutic uses, given their effects in laboratory animal models, but the biological actions of cannabinoids remained elusive.

The identification of Δ^9-tetrahydrocannabinol (THC) as the psychoactive constituent in marijuana was the first significant step in establishing the pharmacological properties of the drug. However, elucidating the neurobiology of cannabinoids proceeded more slowly, for several reasons. First, few cannabinoids were available as investigational probes. The high water-insolubility of cannabinoids made it difficult to conduct in vivo and in vitro experiments. It became apparent that high concentrations of THC were effective in altering numerous biochemical processes in vitro (Martin 1986). The difficulty arose when attempts were made to establish the pharmacological relevance of these findings. Because THC affects a wide range of biochemical processes, from enzymatic activity to neurotransmitter uptake, and because relatively high concentrations of THC were required, researchers continued to speculate that cannabinoids produced at least some of their actions through nonselective perturbation of membranes. However, recent progress has clarified the existence of an endogenous cannabinoid system that includes specific receptors, signal transduction systems, and endogenous ligands. More important, the roles of this endogenous system in normal physiological processes and in disease states are beginning to emerge.

Receptors

Often, one of the first indications of receptor involvement in drug action is enantioselectivity and/or structure-activity relationships. Even the earliest research provided strong indications of structural requirements for cannabinoid activity. Extensive structure-activity relationship studies strongly suggested that cannabinoids act through a receptor mechanism (Razdan 1986). The subsequent development of novel synthetic analogues of THC ultimately played a major role in the characterization and cloning of the cannabinoid CB_1 receptor. One of these analogues was CP 55,940, a highly potent cannabinoid receptor agonist that was radiolabeled and used to characterize cannabinoid binding sites in the brain (Devane et al. 1988). These sites exhibit high affinity for cannabinoids but not for other centrally active compounds. These binding sites are also present in high quantities and are distributed widely throughout the brain (Herkenham et al. 1990). Receptor cloning proved the existence of this CB_1 receptor. The CB_1 receptor complementary DNA was isolated from a rat brain library by a homology screen for guanine nucleotide–binding protein (G protein)–coupled receptors, and its identity was confirmed by transfecting the clone into Chinese hamster ovary (CHO) cells and demonstrating cannabinoid-mediated inhibition of adenylyl cyclase (Matsuda et al. 1990). The CB_1 receptor is a seven-transmembrane protein with characteristics similar to those of G protein–coupled receptors. The rat and human CB_1 receptors are highly conserved, with 93% identity at the nucleic acid level and 97% at the amino acid level.

A second cannabinoid receptor clone, CB_2 (which has a different sequence but a similar binding profile, compared with the CB_1 receptor clone), was discovered by a polymerase chain reaction–based strategy designed to isolate G protein–coupled receptors in differentiated myeloid cells (Munro et al. 1993). The CB_2 receptor, which has been found in the spleen and in the cells of the immune system, has 44% amino acid identity with the CB_1 receptor and thus represents a receptor subtype. CB_2 receptors have been detected in B lymphocytes, macrophages, mast cells, microglia, natural killer cells, peripheral mononuclear cells, CD4 lymphocytes, CD8 lymphocytes, lymph nodes, Peyer's patches, and the spleen (Howlett et al. 2002). There is no evidence of their presence in neuronal membranes.

THC binds equally well to these two receptor subtypes, whereas endogenous ligands (discussed in their own section later in the chapter) have somewhat higher affinity for CB_1 receptors. Efforts to develop highly selective ligands for these two receptor subtypes have been successful. Removal of the phenolic hydroxyl of THC-like compounds led to the first selective CB_2 receptor agonist (Huffman et al. 1996), and improvements followed (Howlett et al. 2002). Several selective CB_1 receptor agonists were developed on the basis of the preference of endogenous ligands for this receptor. The development of antagonists has proved to be critical for verifying a role of these receptors in cannabinoid actions. Furthermore, the synthesis of selective receptor antagonists has made possible the distinction between CB_1 and CB_2 receptor function. The selective CB_1 receptor antagonist SR 141716A effectively blocks CB_1 receptor–mediated effects both in vitro and in vivo (Dutta et al. 1995; Rinaldi-Carmona et al. 1994). The selective CB_2 receptor antagonist SR 144528 was developed later (Rinaldi-Carmona et al. 1998) and blocks immunoinhibitory and anti-inflammatory effects of THC.

CB_1 Receptor Distribution in the Brain

The distribution of the cannabinoid receptor was carefully mapped in rat brain (Herkenham et al. 1990). The highest densities were found in the basal ganglia (substantia nigra pars reticularis, globus pallidus, entopeduncular nucleus, and lateral caudate putamen) and in the molecular layer of the cerebellum. Receptor localization in these regions most likely explains cannabinoid interference with movement. Intermediate levels of binding were found in the pyramidal cell layers of the hippocampus, the dentate gyrus, and layers I and VI of the cortex—observations consistent with THC disruption of short-term memory in humans. The presence of cannabinoid receptors in regions associated with brain reward (e.g., ventromedial striatum and nucleus accumbens) suggests an association with dopamine neurons. Sparse receptor levels were detected in the brain stem, hypothalamus, corpus callosum, and deep cerebellum nuclei. Low levels of receptors in brain stem areas controlling cardiovascular and respiratory functions are also consistent with the lack of lethality of marijuana. As for cellular distribution, high densities of CB_1 receptors are found on axonal fibers, especially at the terminals. CB_1 receptors are found almost entirely on presynaptic terminals in the hippocampus, whereas there is a broader distribution in the striatum (Howlett et al. 2002).

Signal Transduction

Cannabinoid agonists inhibit adenylyl cyclase in brain tissue and neuronal cells containing CB_1 receptors and in immune cells expressing CB_2 receptors (Howlett and Mukhopadhyay 2000). CB_1 receptors also regulate potassium and calcium channels. CB_1 and CB_2 receptor–mediated inhibition of adenylyl cyclase activity is pertussis toxin–sensitive, and thus implicates coupling to $G_{i/o}$ proteins (Howlett et al. 2002). Activation of the CB_1 receptor can also stimulate adenylyl cyclase via coupling to G_s proteins. These proteins activate potassium channels and inhibit voltage-gated L, N, P, and Q calcium channels via a $G_{i/o}$ mechanism. Investigations of tertiary messenger systems for the cannabinoids have also been described. When administered to rats, the cannabinoid receptor agonist CP 55,940 induced expression of the immediate early gene *krox*-24 in striosomes. Stimulation of the CB_1 receptor also induced expression of Krox-24 in human astrocytoma cells, an effect that is blocked by the cannabinoid receptor antagonist SR 141716A. In addition, *jun*-B and *krox*-20 are also induced by cannabinoids, but c-*fos* is not. The induction of *krox*-24 expression is mediated by a pertussis toxin–sensitive G protein but probably not via cyclic adenosine monophosphate. The CB_1 receptor is functionally linked to the mitogen-activated protein kinase cascade. This pathway provides a critical link between the CB_1 receptor and regulation of *krox*-24. The signaling pathway associated with stimulation of the CB_2 receptor involves mitogen-activated protein kinase and induction of *krox*-24 expression.

Endogenous Ligands

Definitive evidence of a cannabinoid receptor led to identification of endogenous ligands. Anandamide (arachidonylethanolamide) was isolated from porcine brain and was shown to bind to the cannabinoid receptor and produce THC-like effects (Devane et al. 1992). Anandamide produces many of the same pharmacological effects as the classical cannabinoid ligands, including hypomotility, antinociception, catalepsy, and hypothermia (Fride and Mechoulam 1993). However, it is 4- to 20-fold less potent than THC in producing these effects, and it has a shorter duration of action. In addition, rats trained to discriminate between THC and vehicle identified anandamide as THC-like (Wiley et al. 1995). Synthetic and degradative pathways for anandamide have also been described. It is thought that anandamide is incorporated in the membrane lipid backbone with the transfer of arachidonic acid from diarachidonylphosphatidylcholine to phosphatidylethanolamine in a calcium-dependent process. Anandamide is then released by a phosphodiesterase-mediated cleavage of *N*-arachidonylphosphatidylethanolamine (Howlett et al. 2002).

Anandamide is highly susceptible to enzymatic hydrolysis and is therefore difficult to study either in vivo or in vitro. Structure-activity relationship studies led to development of metabolically stable and potent analogues that have helped clarify anandamide's pharmacological properties. Hydrolytic cleavage of anandamide forms arachidonic acid and ethanolamine, a process blocked by enzyme inhibitors such as phenylmethylsulfonyl fluoride. This hydrolytic enzyme, termed *fatty acid amidohydrolase,* has been fully characterized and cloned (Cravatt et al. 1996). It represents the major metabolic pathway for anandamide and is located in neurons. Anandamide may also be inactivated through a putative active reuptake mechanism, although less is known about this process.

Anandamide may only be representative of a family of endogenous compounds because fatty acid amides are prevalent in neural tissue. Another arachidonic acid derivative (2-arachidonylglycerol) was identified as an endogenous cannabinoid (Mechoulam et al. 1995). This ligand is found in high concentrations in brain and produces THC-like effects. This derivative binds to both CB_1 and CB_2 receptors. Although synthetic and metabolic pathways for 2-arachidonylglycerol have not been characterized, it can be assumed that they will differ from those for anandamide because of the structural differences between these two ligands. A glyceryl ether of arachidonic acid (noladin) was recently identified as an endogenous cannabinoid (Hanus et al. 2001). Little is known about this compound.

Plasticity of the Endogenous Cannabinoid System

After a period of chronic exposure, laboratory animals readily develop tolerance to most pharmacological effects of THC, including anticonvulsant activity, catalepsy, sedation, hypothermia, hypotension, immunosuppression, and motor incoordination (Compton et al. 1990). Humans develop tolerance to THC's effects on cardiovascular and autonomic functions, sleep, and mood. For behavioral tolerance to be achieved, high doses of cannabinoids are required for a sustained period. If doses are sufficiently small and infrequent, little behavioral tolerance seems to develop. The fact that cannabinoid tolerance develops in the absence of appreciable pharmacokinetic changes implies that biochemical and/or cellular changes are responsible for this adaptation. Indeed, most studies have shown that chronic administration of cannabinoids leads to downregulation of the CB_1 receptor. There is also a concomitant reduction in functionality, despite considerable cannabinoid receptor reserve (Sim-Selley and Martin 2002). Although the consequences of changes in receptor function that result from chronic drug exposure have not been fully defined, they likely contribute to the development of dependence. In addition, other changes in the endogenous cannabinoid system may well contribute to the development of dependence.

Functional Significance of the Endogenous Cannabinoid System

It is now thought that most of the effects of THC are mediated through the endogenous cannabinoid system. THC's central effects are blocked by the CB_1 receptor antagonist and are eliminated in CB_1 receptor knockout mice. There is now abundant evidence that the endogenous cannabinoid system plays a role in diverse physiological processes through direct or indirect actions. Dysfunction of the endogenous cannabinoid system may well contribute to several pathophysiological conditions, because it is quite evident that cannabinoids modulate several neuronal pathways that may either contribute to or alleviate abnormal neuronal function. Although it is not possible to review all the putative roles of the endogenous cannabinoid system, a few will be discussed here.

Regulation of Neurotransmission

The neuroanatomical distribution of the CB_1 receptor provides a framework for identifying brain regions and neural circuits as sites of cannabinoid actions. At the neuronal level, there is evidence of localization of CB_1 receptors both pre- and postsynaptically. However, the predominant action of cannabinoids appears to be inhibition of neurotransmitter release through activation of CB_1 receptors located presynaptically (Elphick and Egertova 2001; Howlett et al. 2002). Cannabinoids are known to activate potassium channels (thereby shortening presynaptic action potential) and to inhibit calcium ion channels, either of which actions could account for decreased neurotransmitter release. Additionally, anandamide acts as a retrograde signaling molecule through postsynaptic release. After synthesis and release from a postsynaptic cell, anandamide diffuses presynaptically to activate CB_1 receptors and attenuate neurotransmitter release (Elphick and Egertova 2001). Although cannabinoids directly inhibit neurotransmitter release, this action may well lead to disinhibition of other neuronal systems and increased neurotransmitter release.

Several lines of evidence support an interrelationship between cannabinoid and dopamine receptors. Studies in which unilateral 6-hydroxydopamine lesions were associated with an increase in CB_1 receptor messenger RNA (mRNA) levels in the ipsilateral side suggested a negative dopaminergic influence on cannabinoid receptor 1 gene expression. Furthermore, treatment with dopamine receptor antagonists also increased CB_1 receptor mRNA levels. Previous experiments had documented the disappearance of CB_1 receptors after ibotenic acid lesioning of the striatum but not after 6-hydroxydopamine lesioning, indicating that cannabinoid receptors are not co-localized with dopamine-containing neurons but are probably on axonal terminals of striatal intrinsic neurons (Elphick and Egertova 2001). Glutamatergic regulation of CB_1 receptor mRNA levels in the striatum has also been reported. Unilateral cerebral decortication and treatment with the N-methyl-D-aspartate (NMDA) receptor antagonist MK-801 resulted in decreases in CB_1 receptor mRNA levels, suggesting that NMDA receptor activation increases or maintains CB_1 receptor mRNA levels.

Cognition

The well-established observation that marijuana impairs cognitive function in both humans and laboratory animals has stimulated considerable interest in the role of the endogenous cannabinoid system in memory and learning processes (Lichtman et al. 2002). Cannabinoids exert greater influence on short-term or working memory than on long-term or reference memory. Direct injection of cannabinoids into the hippocampus disrupts performance in laboratory animal models of working memory. At the neuronal level, CB_1 receptors are expressed in γ-aminobutyric acid (GABA)–ergic interneurons, in pyramidal cells in the hippocampus, and on axonal inputs from the entorhinal cortex and the medial septal complex, the latter of which releases acetylcholine that can be blocked by cannabinoids (Elphick and Egertova 2001). Cannabinoids also inhibit glutamate release in the hippocampus; long-term potentiation and long-term depression of glutamate release is thought to be essential for memory formation. The fact that cannabinoids also inhibit GABA release, which presumably leads to disinhibition of pyramidal cells and increased long-term potentiation, is not easily understood. It is assumed that the actions on glutamate predominate, because cannabinoid agonists suppress long-term potentiation and impair memory. In this context, the possibility of an endogenous system for "forgetting" is intriguing. Attempts to attenuate the endogenous tone of this system with the CB_1 receptor antagonist SR 141716A have resulted in memory enhancement in some but not all studies.

Pain Perception

Cannabinoid agonists are effective in blocking nociception in most animal models of pain, and they are analgesics in humans (Martin and Lichtman 1998). Several lines of evidence implicate the endogenous cannabinoid system in pain perception. Cannabinoid antinociceptive effects are blocked by the CB_1 receptor antagonist SR 141716A and are blunted in CB_1 receptor knockout mice. Moreover, endogenous cannabinoid ligands have antinociceptive properties. SR 141716A produced hyperalgesia in some studies, which suggests cannabinoid basal tone. However, other studies failed to demonstrate SR 141716A–induced hyperalgesia. Knocking out fatty acid amidohydrolase, the enzyme that inactivates anandamide, leads to in-

creased levels of this endogenous ligand and an increase in pain threshold (Cravatt et al. 2001). In brain areas controlling descending and ascending pain pathways, there are abundant CB_1 receptors. Electrical stimulation of the periaqueductal gray induces CB_1-mediated analgesia while leading to the release of anandamide from this region of the brain stem. Also, injection of formalin into a paw induces a nociceptive response with a concomitant release of anandamide in the periaqueductal gray area. There is evidence that both CB_1 and CB_2 receptors are involved in perception of peripheral pain. CB_1 receptors are present in peripheral sensory afferents in the skin and appear to be involved in the control of inflammatory pain.

There has also been considerable interest in determining what role cannabinoids play in opioid-induced antinociception. Numerous animal studies have shown that cannabinoids can potentiate morphine analgesia. However, potentiation most likely involves second messenger systems, in that opioid antagonists are not very effective in blocking cannabinoid analgesia and cannabinoid antagonists fail to block opioid analgesia. Cannabinoids stimulate release of endogenous opioids, which most likely contributes to cannabinoid potentiation of opioid analgesia. In addition, the rostral ventromedial medulla that contributes to the pain-suppressing effects of morphine is also required for the analgesic effects of cannabinoids. Endogenous cannabinoids tonically regulate pain thresholds, in part through modulation of rostral ventromedial medulla neuronal activity. Although cannabinoids and opioids act at similar brain stem circuitry for regulation of pain, cannabinoids are centrally acting analgesics with a distinct mechanism of action.

Drug Dependence

It is well known that cessation of chronic marijuana use does not result in severe withdrawal symptoms like those reported for several other classes of drugs. The withdrawal syndrome is more likely to be described as flulike symptoms. The predominant characteristic of marijuana dependence is an inability to reduce or stop use despite adverse health or legal consequences. The highest risk for initiating marijuana use occurs at age 18 years, and the time for meeting criteria for marijuana dependence is age 17–18 years (Wagner and Anthony 2002). Eight percent of marijuana users become dependent within 10 years of initial use. In numerous cases, marijuana is the primary cause of individuals seeking treatment for dependence. The risk of marijuana dependence is probably similar to that of alcohol dependence, and daily use over a period of weeks to months results in the greatest risk of dependence (Hall et al. 1994). It has been reported that the majority of marijuana users seeking treatment for marijuana dependence have experienced symptoms consistent with either moderate or severe dependence. These patients typically complain of being unable to stop or decrease their use despite experiencing sleepiness, depression, an inability to concentrate, and memorization difficulties, all of which symptoms they directly attribute to marijuana exposure (Budney et al. 1998). A comparison of marijuana- and cocaine-dependent patients revealed comparable histories of substance use and a range of impairments in both groups. Although marijuana-dependent patients show less severe dependence, they are more ambivalent and less confident about stopping their marijuana use than cocaine users are about stopping cocaine use. Therefore, treatment-seeking, marijuana-dependent individuals exhibit substantial problems that require effective treatment (Budney et al. 1998).

The development of the cannabinoid antagonist, SR 141716A, made it possible to develop a model of physical withdrawal syndrome for cannabinoids in several animal species (Lichtman and Martin 2002). The implication of these findings is that the endogenous cannabinoid system undergoes changes during chronic exposure to exogenous cannabinoids, and these changes are most readily observed when agonist effects are abruptly interrupted, such as by antagonist challenge. The cannabinoid withdrawal syndrome was very similar to the opioid withdrawal syndrome in rodents. Moreover, morphine self-administration and dependence are attenuated in mice lacking the CB_1 receptor and cannabinoid dependence is reduced in mice lacking the opioid receptor. Recent studies have also shown that the cannabinoid antagonist influences self-administration of both alcohol and cocaine. Therefore, it is possible that the endogenous cannabinoid system plays a role in drug dependence generally, rather than in cannabinoid dependence alone. It is clear in humans, THC is an essential reinforcing component in marijuana. Contrary to the majority of drugs abused by humans, it has been quite difficult to train animals to self-administer cannabinoids. Although the physical characteristics of cannabinoids probably contributed to this difficulty, the general opinion persisted that cannabinoids lack rewarding effects and therefore are devoid of dependence liability. However, it has now been shown that rats will self-administer THC under proper experimental conditions (Tanda et al. 2000).

Immune Modulation

Cannabinoids are immunosuppressive in a wide range of animal models and cell culture systems. The endogenous ligands and the two receptor systems are also present in most immune cells. Endogenous cannabinoids and THC have been shown to be anti-inflammatory, possibly through the inhibition of the production and action of tumor necrosis factor α and other acute-phase cytokines (Klein et al. 2000). Other cytokines suppressed by cannabinoids include granulocyte-macrophage colony-stimulating factor, interleukin (IL)–6, interferon γ, and IL-12, whereas levels of interleukins such as IL-1, IL-4, IL-10, and IL-6 may be increased. Unfortunately, the immunomodulatory effects of cannabinoids are often conflicting, which makes interpretation difficult. However, sufficient information exists to conclude that the endogenous cannabinoid system exerts a significant influence on the immune system. The cannabinoid receptors are involved in some, but not all, of these actions.

Appetite and Reward

Cannabinoid agonists stimulate appetite. The presence of CB_1 receptors in the arcuate nucleus and the medial preoptic area of the hypothalamus, the presence of endocannabinoids and their biosynthetic precursors in the hypothalamus and the pituitary, and the effect of endocannabinoids on body temperature, food intake, and pituitary hormone release suggest that endocannabinoids play a role in the control of hypothalamic functions, and in particular, in the control of appetite. There is also evidence that hormonal control of appetite involves the endogenous cannabinoid system (Di Marzo et al. 2001). A major action of leptin is to decrease food intake. The observations that leptin also decreases anandamide levels and that anandamide levels increase when leptin is absent suggest that anandamide plays a role in the regulation of appetite (Di Marzo et al. 2001). Furthermore, SR 141716A inhibits food intake in rodents, a finding that is consistent with the idea of a modulatory role for the endogenous cannabinoid system.

Another brain region possibly involved in the control of appetite and craving is the limbic forebrain—more particularly, the nucleus accumbens. In this brain area, cannabinoids enhance the release of dopamine from dopaminergic terminals originating in the ventral tegmental area, and therefore cannabinoids may participate in the regulation of feelings of craving and reward. It is possible that dopamine released in the nucleus accumbens in the context of chronic treatment with THC triggers anandamide release, as previously shown for other brain regions. Conversely, dopamine may be released in this region after activation of CB_1 receptors by anandamide, thereby participating in the regulation of reward, craving, and pleasure. There are indications that withdrawal after chronic cannabinoid administration is associated with reduced dopaminergic transmission in the limbic system, similar to that observed with other addictive drugs—a finding consistent with the concept that dopamine plays a role in drug craving and relapse into drug addiction or a role in the reinforcing effects of drugs of abuse.

Conclusion

The major challenge facing researchers is to elucidate the physiological role of the endogenous cannabinoid system. An understanding of this system may provide insight into the mechanism by which cannabinoids produce their unique behavioral effects. Through the use of selective agonists and antagonists, along with CB_1 and CB_2 receptor knockout mice, a better understanding of the system's role is emerging. The presence of cannabinoid presynaptically on both inhibitory and excitatory neurons indicates an important modulatory role for the endogenous cannabinoid system. Although the direct action of cannabinoids is to inhibit neurotransmitter release, they can also stimulate neurotransmitter release through disinhibition or retrograde signaling. There is evidence that the endocannabinoids are directly involved in cognitive processes, pain pathways, reward mechanisms, and appetite circuitry and movement. The greatest challenge remains—namely, to elucidate the physiological control of synthesis, degradation, storage, and release of endocannabinoids. Only then will an understanding of the pathological consequences of a dysfunctional cannabinoid system emerge.

References

Budney AJ, Radonovich KJ, Higgins ST, et al: Adults seeking treatment for marijuana dependence: a comparison with cocaine-dependent treatment seekers. Exp Clin Psychopharmacol 6:419–426, 1998

Compton DR, Dewey WL, Martin BR: Cannabis dependence and tolerance production, in Addiction Potential of Abused Drugs and Drug Classes. Edited by Erickson CK, Javors MA, Morgan WW. Binghamton, NY, Hayworth, 1990, pp 129–147

Cravatt BF, Giang DK, Mayfield SP, et al: Molecular characterization of an enzyme that degrades neuromodulatory fatty-acid amides. Nature 384:83–87, 1996

Cravatt BF, Demarest K, Patricelli MP, et al: Supersensitivity to anandamide and enhanced endogenous cannabinoid signaling in mice lacking fatty acid amide hydrolase. Proc Natl Acad Sci U S A 98:9371–9376, 2001

Devane WA, Dysarz FA, Johnson MR, et al: Determination and characterization of a cannabinoid receptor in rat brain. Mol Pharmacol 34:605–613, 1988

Devane WA, Hanus L, Breuer A, et al: Isolation and structure of a brain constituent that binds to the cannabinoid receptor. Science 258:1946–1949, 1992

Di Marzo V, Goparaju SK, Wang L, et al: Leptin-regulated endocannabinoids are involved in maintaining food intake. Nature 410:822–825, 2001

Dutta A, Sard H, Ryan W, et al: The synthesis and pharmacological evaluation of the cannabinoid antagonist SR 141716A. Medicinal Chemistry Research 5:54–62, 1995

Elphick MR, Egertova M: The neurobiology and evolution of cannabinoid signalling. Philos Trans R Soc Lond B Biol Sci 356:381–408, 2001

Fride E, Mechoulam R: Pharmacological activity of the cannabinoid receptor agonist, anandamide, a brain constituent. Eur J Pharmacol 231:313–314, 1993

Hall W, Solowij N, Lemon J: The health and psychological consequences of cannabis use (National Drug Strategy Monograph Series, no 25). Canberra, Australian Government Publication Service, 1994

Hanus L, Abu-Lafi S, Fride E, et al: 2-Arachidonyl glyceryl ether, an endogenous agonist of the cannabinoid CB_1 receptor. Proc Natl Acad Sci U S A 98:3662–3665, 2001

Herkenham M, Lynn AB, Little MD, et al: Cannabinoid receptor localization in the brain. Proc Natl Acad Sci U S A 87:1932–1936, 1990

Howlett AC, Mukhopadhyay S: Cellular signal transduction by anandamide and 2-arachidonoylglycerol. Chem Phys Lipids 108:53–70, 2000

Howlett AC, Barth F, Bonner TI, et al: International Union of Pharmacology. XXVII. Classification of cannabinoid receptors. Pharmacol Rev 54:161–202, 2002

Huffman JW, Yu S, Showalter V, et al: Synthesis and pharmacology of a very potent cannabinoid lacking a phenolic hydroxyl with high affinity for the CB_2 receptor. J Med Chem 39:3875–3877, 1996

Klein TW, Lane B, Newton CA, et al: The cannabinoid system and cytokine network. Proc Soc Exp Biol Med 225:1–8, 2000

Lichtman AH, Martin BR: Marijuana withdrawal syndrome in the animal model. J Clin Pharmacol 42 (11 suppl):20S–27S, 2002

Lichtman AH, Varvel SA, Martin BR: Endocannabinoids in cognition and dependence. Prostaglandins Leukot Essent Fatty Acids 66:269–285, 2002

Martin BR: Cellular effects of cannabinoids. Pharmacol Rev 38:45–74, 1986

Martin BR, Lichtman AH: Cannabinoid transmission and pain perception. Neurobiol Dis 5:447–461, 1998

Matsuda LA, Lolait SJ, Brownstein MJ, et al: Structure of a cannabinoid receptor and functional expression of the cloned cDNA. Nature 346:561–564, 1990

Mechoulam R, Ben-Shabat S, Hanus L, et al: Identification of an endogenous 2-monoglyceride, present in canine gut, that binds to cannabinoid receptors. Biochem Pharmacol 50:83–90, 1995

Munro S, Thomas KL, Abu-Shaar M: Molecular characterization of a peripheral receptor for cannabinoids. Nature 365:61–64, 1993

Razdan RK: Structure-activity relationships in cannabinoids. Pharmacol Rev 38:75–149, 1986

Rinaldi-Carmona M, Barth F, Héaulme M, et al: SR141716A, a potent and selective antagonist of the brain cannabinoid receptor. FEBS Lett 350:240–244, 1994

Rinaldi-Carmona M, Barth F, Millan J, et al: SR 144528, the first potent and selective antagonist of the CB_2 cannabinoid receptor. J Pharmacol Exp Ther 284:644–650, 1998

Sim-Selley LJ, Martin BR: Effect of chronic administration of R-(+)-[2,3-dihydro-5-methyl-3-[(morpholinyl)methyl]pyrrolo[1,2,3-de]-1,4-benzoxazinyl]-(1-naphthalenyl)methanone mesylate (WIN55,212–2) or delta(9)-tetrahydrocannabinol on cannabinoid receptor adaptation in mice. J Pharmacol Exp Ther 303:36–44, 2002

Tanda G, Munzar P, Goldberg SR: Self-administration behavior is maintained by the psychoactive ingredient of marijuana in squirrel monkeys. Nat Neurosci 3:1073–1074, 2000

Wagner FA, Anthony JC: From first drug use to drug dependence; developmental periods of risk for dependence upon marijuana, cocaine, and alcohol. Neuropsychopharmacology 26:479–488, 2002

Wiley J, Balster R, Martin B: Discriminative stimulus effects of anandamide in rats. Eur J Pharmacol 276:49–54, 1995

Epidemiology of Drug Dependence

James C. Anthony, Ph.D.
Chuan Yu Chen, Ph.D.

In drug dependence epidemiology, as in all main branches of epidemiology in public health, the main point of departure is a clinical concept of disease, disorder, or syndrome. Epidemiologists now can orient their work with respect to a reasonably well measured concept of drug dependence as a clinically meaningful biobehavioral syndrome (i.e., a syndrome with observable clinical features that run together and cohere to a degree beyond that of chance co-occurrence).

Practitioners who treat drug dependence in clinical settings can use epidemiology as a lens to look beyond the clinic's threshold, out toward the population from which drug-dependent patients surface. Epidemiologists have grown fond of depicting the ratio of treated cases to untreated cases in terms of an iceberg (see Figure 6–1). Epidemiological field survey estimates have long shown that for every treated case of drug dependence, there are at least three untreated cases with similar clinical features (Anthony and Helzer 1991; Grant 1997a). Recent estimates suggest that about 90% of young people with current problems related to use of illegal drugs have received no treatment (Substance Abuse and Mental Health Services Administration 2002b).

This chapter, mainly a revision of the chapter prepared for the second edition of this book, originates from more detailed discussions published elsewhere by Anthony (2002), Anthony and Forman (2003), Anthony and Helzer (1995, 2002), and Anthony and Van Etten (1998). In this chapter, we apply the concept of drug use that was introduced by Anthony et al. (1994) and that encompasses a range of drug-taking behaviors: tobacco smoking or use of other nicotine products; consumption of alcoholic beverages; use of illegal drugs; medically unauthorized but not necessarily illegal use of prescription drugs such as morphine or secobarbital (e.g., use of a larger dose than is authorized on the doctor's prescription); use of prescribed medicines, over-the-counter medicines, or other legally available products for purposes other than those intended by the manufacturer (e.g., toluene sniffing or consumption of prescribed or over-the-counter cough medicine to get high); and use of legal products marketed for the sole purpose of intoxication (e.g., Ek-Sta-Sis, Ex-1, Bliss Extra, Space Cadets, and Druids Fantasy).

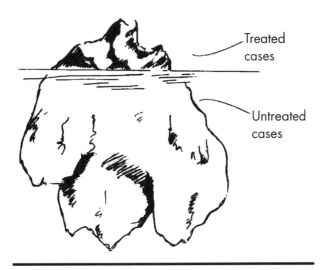

Figure 6–1. The "iceberg" phenomenon of treated and untreated cases.

Graphics: Patricia J. Anthony, 1998, for this publication.

Public health leaders charged with responsibility for the health of a population must pay attention to both treated and untreated cases. This public health work is especially difficult and complex when the goal is to increase the number of treated cases relative to the number of untreated cases and to reduce total occurrence of cases in a population. The work becomes even more complex when one case begets others, as in contagious, person-to-person spread or diffusion. Some drug users inadvertently or deliberately introduce others to drug-taking practices, whereas individuals whose drug dependence has been treated effectively tend not to do so. Hence, population-oriented or public health–oriented initiatives to prevent drug dependence rely on effective intervention programs to reach individuals with untreated drug dependence and individuals or groups responsible for person-to-person spread of drug taking.

Epidemiology also has another, more ambitious agenda. It seeks basic evidence for the purpose of forming a solid foundation for comprehensive prevention and intervention programming. In this search for evidence, five main rubrics are applied, expressed in the following questions:

1. In the community at large, how many people are affected by drug dependence?
2. Where are the affected people more likely to be found?
3. Why do some people in the community become drug dependent while others do not?

4. What linkages of states and processes influence who becomes and who remains drug dependent?
5. What can be done to prevent and intervene in drug dependence?

Anthony and Van Etten (1998) provided a detailed review of these rubrics for psychiatric epidemiology, and the literature now includes several rubric-oriented reviews on cannabis dependence, drug dependence in general, and topics such as the relationship between drugs and crime (Anthony 2002; Anthony and Forman 2003; Anthony and Helzer 2002). In this chapter, we introduce these rubrics using selected examples and evidence from epidemiological studies of dependence on alcohol and/or internationally regulated controlled drugs such marijuana and cocaine. We also present selected estimates concerning tobacco and caffeine dependence.

A Question of Quantity

In the Community at Large, How Many People Are Affected by Drug Dependence?

The quest to estimate the frequency and occurrence of mental and behavioral disturbances in the U.S. population began more than 150 years ago, as part of national censuses and local field surveys. For example, in the 1840 United States census, local census-takers were instructed to count every citizen and resident, free or enslaved. Census procedures eventually involved asking knowledgeable informants within each household and area about residents who might be characterized as "insane" or "idiots." Later in the nineteenth century, the scope of this census inquiry was enlarged to encompass chronic inebriety (Anthony and Van Etten 1998; Wines 1888).

For the 1880 United States census, nearly 100,000 doctors in all parts of the country were contacted, furnished with blank forms, and asked to report to the Census Office all so-called idiots and mentally disordered persons "within the sphere of their personal knowledge" (Wines 1888). In several local area surveys concerning habitual use of opium-containing preparations of that era, druggists and apothecaries were asked to provide information about citizens' drugstore purchases.

A more formal and rigorous approach to epidemiological field surveys of drug dependence and psychiatric disturbances emerged early in the twentieth century (Rosanoff 1917). By 1980, it had become customary to adopt a set of diagnostic criteria, such as those published in DSM-III (American Psychiatric Association 1980), and to translate these criteria into interview measurements for standardized field surveys of general population samples, as was done for the Epidemiologic Catchment Area (ECA) surveys. Because of surveys of this type, completed since 1979, epidemiologists have more complete evidence about the frequency and occurrence of drug dependence in the population. The prevalence estimates reported in this chapter are based on diagnostic criteria presented in DSM-III, DSM-III-R (American Psychiatric Association 1987), or DSM-IV (American Psychiatric Association 1994), and these estimates were derived from the ECA surveys (Anthony and Helzer 1991, 1995, 2002), the National Comorbidity Survey (NCS) (Anthony et al. 1994; Kessler et al. 1994; Warner et al. 1995), the National Longitudinal Alcohol Epidemiologic Survey (NLAES) (Grant 1995, 1997b), and other surveys (Substance Abuse and Mental Health Services Administration 2000a, 2000b, 2002a, 2002b, 2002c, 2002d). Prevalence estimates for DSM conditions were derived from Diagnostic Interview Schedule assessments made by lay interviewers in the ECA surveys—or from adaptations or refinements of the Diagnostic Interview Schedule approach in the cases of the NCS, NLAES, and Substance Abuse and Mental Health Services Administration Office of Applied Studies surveys. Standardized clinical examinations conducted for the ECA surveys by board-eligible psychiatrists yielded slightly higher estimates of DSM-III alcohol or drug use disorders, perhaps because clinicians cross-examined individuals to detect recent evidence of alcohol or drug use disorders (Anthony et al. 1985).

Even with lay interviewing, some variation in observed survey estimates can be traced to differences in diagnostic criteria and methods of assessment, but in many instances, observed study-to-study variation depends on the age composition of survey populations. For example, the NCS focused on 15- to 54-year-olds, whereas the National Household Surveys on Drug Abuse (conducted by the Office of Applied Studies) are focused on all household residents age 12 years or older. Hence, NCS-derived estimates of dependence on alcohol or other drugs are generally higher than estimates derived from Office of Applied Studies surveys, because the NCS focused on the age range in which dependence syndromes are more common, and the population surveyed by the Office of Applied Studies included the youngest adolescents (12–14 years old) and the oldest adults (age 55 years or older). Compared with 15- to 54-year-olds, 12- to 14-year-olds and those age 55 years or older have substantially lower rates of alcohol and other drug dependence (Anthony and Helzer 2002; Wagner and Anthony 2002a). Some of the survey similarities and differences are presented in Table 6–1.

Lifetime Prevalence

According to community surveys conducted in the United States, with case ascertainment based on modern diagnostic criteria and standardized methods, roughly 6%–14% of Americans are dependent on alcohol. Lower values are obtained when DSM-III criteria are used, and higher values are obtained when DSM-IV criteria are used and when the youngest adolescents and the oldest adults are excluded from survey samples. With respect to dependence on marijuana, cocaine, or other controlled drugs, lifetime prevalence estimates are 3%–4% when DSM-III criteria are used, with estimates being modestly higher when DSM-IV criteria are used.

Annual Incidence

Virtually all retrospectively oriented population surveys can produce cumulative occurrence (lifetime prevalence) estimates of how many individuals have become affected by drug dependence. Completing a prospective or longitudinal study, a much more difficult task, is necessary to produce a direct estimate of the risk of developing dependence for the first time in one's life. The first-time risk of developing dependence is conventionally estimated during a 1-year interval, giving the annual incidence rate. According to the ECA surveys, the most recently completed prospective investigation of drug dependence in an adult household population sample in the United States, the estimated annual incidence (based on DSM-III criteria) of alcohol dependence and/or abuse is 1.8%; the estimated annual incidence of controlled-drug dependence and/or abuse is 1.1%. That is, the risk of developing adult-onset alcohol abuse and/or dependence during a 1-year follow-up interval is about 1 in 55 when the information across all ages, from young adulthood (age 18 years) through late life (age 90 years and older),

Table 6–1. Estimated prevalence of recent alcohol and drug use disorders[a]

Survey	Survey years	Diagnostic criteria	Assessment tool	Study population	Survey estimates	Alcohol	Other drugs[b]
ECA (*n*=20,291) New Haven, CT; St. Louis, MO; Baltimore, MD; Los Angeles, CA; Raleigh-Durham, NC	1979–1984	DSM-III	DIS	18-year-olds to oldest adults; residents of households, group quarters, and institutional living quarters	Lifetime prevalence (cumulative occurrence), interval prevalence (12 months and 1 month), annual incidence	7.0%	2%–3%
NCS (*n*=8,098) 48 contiguous states	1990–1992	DSM-III-R	UM-CIDI[c]	15- to 54-year-olds; noninstitutional (mainly household) residents	Lifetime prevalence (cumulative occurrence), interval prevalence (12 months and 1 month)	9.7%	3.6%
NLAES (*n*=42,862) United States	1991–1992	DSM-III-R, DSM-IV	AUDADIS	18-year-olds to oldest adults; noninstitutional (mainly household) residents	Lifetime prevalence (cumulative occurrence), interval prevalence (12 months and 1 month)	7.4%	1.5%
NHSDA[d] (*n* varies by year; *n*≈69,000 in 2001) All 50 states and Washington, DC	Now yearly	DSM-IV	Abbreviated scale based on DIS and CIDI-like items	12-year-olds to oldest adults; noninstitutional (mainly household) residents	Lifetime prevalence (cumulative occurrence), interval prevalence (12 months)	5.9%	2.5%

Note. AUDADIS=Alcohol Use Disorders and Associated Disabilities Interview Schedule; CIDI=Composite International Diagnostic Interview; DIS=Diagnostic Interview Schedule; ECA=Epidemiologic Catchment Area; NCS=National Comorbidity Survey; NHSDA=National Household Survey on Drug Abuse; NLAES=National Longitudinal Alcohol Epidemiologic Survey; UM-CIDI=University of Michigan version of the Composite International Diagnostic Interview.
[a]Includes both dependence and abuse.
[b]Not including tobacco.
[c]Includes coverage of inhalant drugs.
[d]Conducted by the Office of Applied Studies, Substance Abuse and Mental Health Services Administration, and now known as the National Survey on Drug Use and Health.

is summarized. The corresponding 1-year risk estimate for controlled drugs is about 1 in 90 (Eaton et al. 1989). To date, there are no prospectively determined estimates—based on DSM-III-R, DSM-IV, or DSM-IV-TR criteria—of annual incidence or the risk of developing alcohol or other drug dependence for comparison with these DSM-III criteria–based estimates. Prospective studies applying DSM-IV criteria are under way.

Prevalence of Recently Active Drug Dependence

The standard lifetime prevalence proportion reflects the probability of developing a particular condition (i.e., becoming an active case) during one's lifetime, among those who survive to be assessed, up to and including the date of assessment. The standard incidence rate reflects the probability of developing a particular condition for the first time during some fixed interval, such as 1 year (as in an annual incidence rate).

In contrast with incidence rates (which convey the probability of becoming something, or changing in state, per unit of time), all prevalence estimates are proportions, assessed as of some point in time. In standard form, these proportions reflect the probability of developing a particular condition after some point in time, with at least one active clinical feature during some fixed prior interval of time. For example, in a 1-year prevalence proportion, the numerator includes not only first-time cases but also cases with clinical features that became manifest during the year before cross-sectional assessment.

In ECA surveys based on DSM-III criteria, the prevalence of recently active alcohol dependence in the United States was estimated to be about 4%. An additional 3% of individuals had recently active DSM-III alcohol abuse but did not have alcohol dependence. As shown in Table 6–1, more recent estimates derived from national surveys (the NCS, NLAES, and National Household Surveys on Drug Abuse) are not too distant from these ECA values.

With respect to marijuana and other controlled drugs, the ECA surveys based on DSM-III criteria found that an estimated 1%–2% of American adults have recently active drug dependence; an additional 1% have recently active DSM-III drug abuse but not dependence. Lower DSM estimates were found in the NLAES (0.5% and close to 1%, respectively). Estimates derived from the recent National Household Surveys on Drug Abuse are more congruent with estimates ob-

tained through the ECA surveys, and the NCS estimates are somewhat higher (see Table 6–1).

To place these estimates of alcohol and controlled drug use into perspective, according to the NCS, which also used lay interview methods, an estimated one in four 15- to 54-year-old United States residents (24%) has met DSM-III-R criteria for tobacco dependence (Anthony et al. 1994). The majority of active smokers smoke cigarettes daily (Substance Abuse and Mental Health Services Administration 2002b). An estimated one in five to six American adults (15%–20%) drinks at least five cups of coffee per day (Anthony and Arria 1999).

A Question of Location

Where Are the Affected People More Likely to Be Found?

It is a short step from the first rubric of epidemiology to the second rubric, location. Here, *location* refers to placement of cases in time and geography (e.g., as reflected in time trends, space-time clustering, or variation across geopolitical boundaries). *Location* also refers to personal characteristics (i.e., age, gender, and race or ethnicity).

One striking finding of the ECA surveys of psychiatric disturbances in the United States was that drug dependence and most other DSM-III psychiatric disorders were more likely to occur in persons ages 18–54 years. Except for cognitive impairments, these disorders were quite infrequent among persons age 55 years or older. This was true for both incidence and prevalence estimates (Anthony and Helzer 1991; Eaton et al. 1989).

The foundation of evidence from coordinated ECA surveys in five U.S. metropolitan areas made it possible to argue persuasively for a nationally representative probability sample survey of U.S. community residents ages 15–54 years. The resulting survey, the NCS, has provided a sharper focus on the prevalence of drug dependence in the United States, specific for individual categories of psychoactive drugs and specific for age.

According to findings of the NCS, an estimated 92% of 15- to 54-year-old United States residents have consumed alcoholic beverages. Among these drinkers, about 15% have become alcohol dependent. The resulting estimated lifetime prevalence of alcohol dependence in the population is close to 14%. Males were more likely than females to have become alcohol dependent (Anthony et al. 1994).

Fewer 15- to 54-year-old United States residents have smoked tobacco than have consumed alcoholic beverages, but the estimated prevalence of dependence among users is greater for tobacco than for any of the other drugs studied. For example, an estimated 32% of tobacco smokers have developed tobacco dependence. In comparison, an estimated 9% of marijuana smokers ages 15–54 have developed marijuana dependence, and an estimated 16%–17% of cocaine users have developed cocaine dependence (Anthony et al. 1994).

When limited to studying locations of cases in the population, epidemiologists do not seek to draw causal inferences. Rather, they attempt to discern patterned occurrences of health conditions within and between populations. The detection of these disease patterns might have a pragmatic implication for the delivery of prevention or intervention services. These patterns also are important guides to more probing causal research.

To illustrate, as noted earlier in this section, evidence highlights a general tendency for a male excess in the frequency and occurrence of drug dependence for many (but not all) drug categories (e.g., alcohol). These descriptive estimates do not address the causes of the male excess, but they confirm a need for treatment services and outreach for both men and women who have become drug dependent. Furthermore, these estimates highlight the importance of a policy debate about existing outreach and treatment programs. Given that women are underrepresented in drug dependence treatment, should outreach and treatment services for women be expanded until the male-to-female ratio of treated cases is approximately equivalent to the ratio noted in epidemiological studies?

When epidemiologists investigate the location of cases in the population, they define *location* broadly to encompass geographic differences and variation over time. For example, Figures 6–2 and 6–3 depict geographic variation in prevalence of recently active dependence on alcohol and illegal drugs, based on state-by-state estimates derived from recent Office of Applied Studies surveys as described in Table 6–1. Analysts sought to determine geographic variation but were not able to explain the evidence, including an interesting observation that higher prevalence values tend to occur in states of west of Minnesota, Iowa, Mis-

souri, and Arkansas (Substance Abuse and Mental Health Services Administration 2002a, 2002b, 2002c, 2002d).

Cross-national comparisons also are of interest. For example, comparisons of drug dependence between the United States and the United Kingdom have been made possible through calibration of measurements and case definitions used in nationally representative sample surveys in the United States and the United Kingdom. Before calibration, the U.K. prevalence estimate for recently active drug dependence was 2.2% (Meltzer et al. 1995), somewhat higher than corresponding values obtained through U.S. surveys in similar years. However, after calibration of measurements and case definitions, the U.K. prevalence estimate was found to be not too distant from the U.S. prevalence estimate, and it may well be lower than the U.S. prevalence estimate once urban-rural differences are taken into account (Furr-Holden and Anthony 2003).

These considerations do not undercut the value of epidemiological surveys that serve a mainly descriptive function in disclosing variations in frequency and occurrence of drug dependence within and across populations and time periods. Studies of the location of cases represent an important scientific step toward studies of causes, causal mechanisms, prevention, and intervention (as demonstrated in the history of psychiatric epidemiology and epidemiology generally) (Anthony and Van Etten 1998).

A Question of Causes

Why Do Some People in the Community Become Drug Dependent While Others Do Not?

Twin studies have played an important role in research on the genetics of alcohol and drug dependence (see Chapter 7, "Genetics of Substance Abuse," in this volume). Some of these studies were clinically oriented, in that recruitment of twin pairs began with identification of treated index patients or probands, with later follow-back to untreated siblings. Other studies are more epidemiological, in that sampling and recruitment are from population registries of twin pairs and are not influenced by treatment status of a proband.

Twin studies have provided the strongest evidence that experiential conditions play an important role and that environmental conditions and processes in-

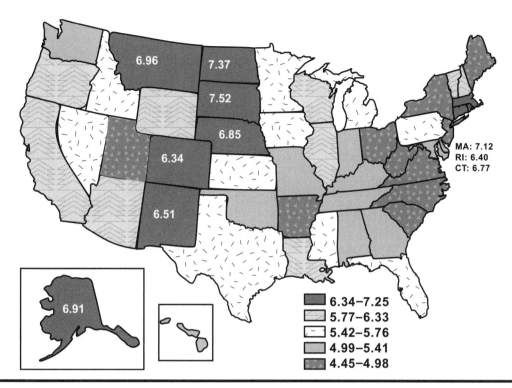

Figure 6–2. Estimated state-specific prevalence (%) of recently active alcohol use disorders (DSM dependence or abuse) among persons age 12 years or older in 2000.

Source. U.S. Substance Abuse and Mental Health Services Administration. Public domain. Posted at: http://www.samhsa.gov/oas.htm.

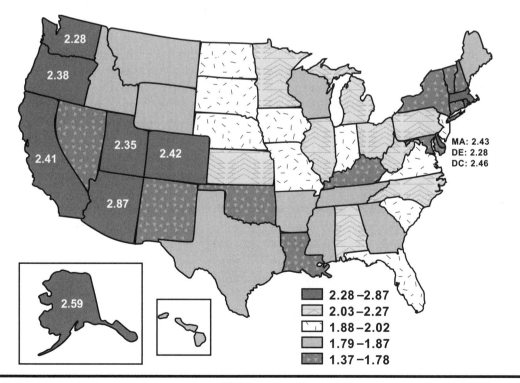

Figure 6–3. Estimated state-specific prevalence (%) of recently active illegal drug use disorders (DSM dependence or abuse) among persons age 12 years or older in 2000.

Source. U.S. Substance Abuse and Mental Health Services Administration. Public domain. Posted at: http://www.samhsa.gov/oas.htm.

fluence the risk of developing dependence on alcohol and other drugs. Estimates of heritability for alcohol dependence and other drug dependence have tended to fall between 25% and 65%, depending on the sex of the twins under study, ascertainment methods, and other factors. Many twin studies yield heritability estimates on the higher end of this range, especially when the transition from drug use to drug dependence is ignored. Nevertheless, these estimates leave considerable room for the influence of noninherited characteristics in the etiology of drug dependence. Looking across a broad array of twin studies, one can see attempts to partition individual-specific environmental causation from shared family environmental causation, independent of family genetic effects and gene-environment interactions. In these analyses, against the backdrop of substantial heritability values in the aforementioned range, the estimated contribution of nongenetic familial transmission of drug dependence often tends to be notably smaller than the estimated contribution from individual-specific (nonshared) environmental causes. Future studies involving monozygotic twins discordant for age at onset of drug dependence will disclose features of nonshared environments that may be causing drug dependence to occur later rather than earlier, and these findings will aid prevention research.

Recognition of experiential and environmental conditions in drug dependence often starts with an appreciation that drug dependence cannot develop until effective contact has occurred between the drug and a vulnerable individual. Effective contact can be measured by using a biomarker such as immune response to the drug-antigen or, as is more typical in epidemiological studies, by administering a survey questionnaire or conducting an interview.

Processes governing effective contact are central in the epidemiological study of drug dependence, including contagious person-to-person diffusion of drug-taking practices and variations in availability of drugs. For example, estimates of heritability in twin studies generally do not take into account that one twin might be a source of drugs for the other twin. Given that monozygotic twins are more likely than dizygotic twins to share drugs with each other, heritability estimates for drug dependence will be inflated unless opportunities to use drugs are measured and controlled in the analysis.

Natural experiments of variation in drug availability are critical in the epidemiological study of expe-

riences and environments that promote risk of drug dependence. An example of epidemiological research in this tradition is a Vietnam veteran study in which almost 20% of veterans in an epidemiological sample had become dependent on heroin and other opioid drugs while in Vietnam, a high-availability zone for these compounds in the early 1970s (Helzer 1985). When the subjects were reassessed within a few years after their return to the United States from Vietnam, fewer than 5% remained opioid dependent or had returned to opioid dependence. Adding to this natural experiment, the researchers found that the probability of returning to opioid dependence was associated with living in a metropolitan area. That is, veterans who returned from Vietnam to lower-availability nonmetropolitan areas were at extremely low risk for becoming readdicted after detoxification; the relative risk of readdiction was greater among veterans who returned to higher-availability areas (Helzer 1985; O'Brien et al. 1980).

In attempting to understand why metropolitan area residents might be more likely to become or remain opioid dependent, one may entertain both social causation and social selection hypotheses. That is, greater drug availability and other conditions of city life might promote drug dependence, if only by heightening the risk of effective contact and drug exposure (see Anthony and Helzer 2002 and Van Etten and Anthony 1999). Alternatively, individuals vulnerable to drug involvement or dependence might be selective in their choice of residence and might migrate to metropolitan areas with greater occurrence and perhaps greater neighborhood clustering of drug involvement in order to gain more ready access to drugs of choice (Petronis and Anthony 2003).

The contending hypotheses of social selection and social causation cannot be investigated with randomized experiments. Instead, epidemiologists must turn to specialized research tactics, typically learned in doctoral or postgraduate research training. For example, in a formal experiment, randomization can be used to control potentially distorting variables. Randomization helps balance the array of potentially distorting influences that might otherwise complicate causal inferences. If randomization cannot or does not balance these distorting influences, alternative tactics must be used during or after sampling of subjects for an epidemiological study. To augment matching and stratification, statistical modeling can be used to constrain potentially distorting influences during data analysis.

A study that involved Sephardic and Ashkenazi sub-samples of Jewish-heritage residents living in Israel illustrates how nonexperimental tactics can probe social causation versus social selection processes (Dohrenwend et al. 1992). The researchers worked from a premise that the Sephardic subjects' heritage would confer a greater social disadvantage because of their prominent African family background, physical appearance, and ethnicity. Assessing the Sephardic and Ashkenazi subjects' lifetime histories of psychiatric disorders, the research team plotted frequency and occurrence of drug dependence and other disorders in relation to the research subjects' levels of education. Using a mix of stratification and statistical modeling, the team expressed occurrence of different types of psychiatric disorders in the two groups as a function of acquired education and social status. The result was a pattern of association consistent with a more prominent influence of social selection in relation to disorders such as schizophrenia and a pattern of association more consistent with a prominent influence of social causation in relation to disorders such as dependence on alcohol and other drugs. This study shows how epidemiological studies can shed light on important issues of cause-effect relationships that are difficult, if not impossible, to examine in randomized controlled trials.

The Human Envirome Project

Using tactics such as matching, stratification, and statistical modeling, epidemiological investigators have searched for an array of life experiences and environmental conditions and processes that might promote or reduce an individual's risk of drug dependence. This search is a central mission of psychiatric epidemiology and drug dependence epidemiology. In brief, epidemiology now is responsible for a longer-term Human Envirome Project, running parallel with the more rapidly evolving Human Genome Project and the recently initiated HapMap project, an elaboration of the Human Genome Project. The Human Genome Project and HapMap are completing maps of the total ensemble of human genes, with a special focus on genes and haplotypes that impinge on human health, and the Human Envirome Project likewise seeks to map the total ensemble of experiential or environmental conditions and processes that affect human health, including gene-environment interactions provoking drug dependence (Anthony 2001; Anthony et al. 1995).

Candidate conditions within the Human Envirome Project can be specified along a timeline from conception to death. For example, one might suppose that maternal exposure to tobacco smoking yields an increased risk of teen smoking or nicotine dependence (given effective contact) among genetically vulnerable offspring (or an increased risk of nicotine-associated depressed mood or conduct disorder), but there is limited epidemiological support for these inferences (Kandel and Udry 1999). A more substantial argument based on epidemiological evidence can be made for a childhood environment of especially inept parental supervision or monitoring of children. For example, deficient parental monitoring in the home seems to influence the risk of early-onset drug taking (Chilcoat and Anthony 1996; Duncan et al. 1998), which is linked to a later increased risk of drug problems associated with drug dependence (Anthony and Petronis 1995).

Youths' affiliation with misbehaving and deviant peers seems to increase the risk of drug use and drug dependence in childhood, adolescence, and adulthood. Affiliation with deviant peers might promote deviant attitudes and otherwise enhance pharmacologically based reinforcing functions of drug taking (D. W. Brook et al. 2002; J. S. Brook et al. 1998, 2001; Newcomb and Bentler 1988). Youthful affiliation with misbehaving and drug-using peers has been found to depend on prior levels of parental supervision and monitoring (Lloyd and Anthony 2003). Moreover, recent research involving nonhuman primates suggests that early maternal-peer socialization experiences and within-peer-group social stratification experiences may be determinants of later drug-taking and reinforcing functions served by drugs such as cocaine and alcohol (Fahlke et al. 2000; Morgan et al. 2002).

Affiliation with misbehaving peers in adolescence is important but is not the only characteristic that must be considered in relation to the risk of drug taking. For example, LSD ingestion and other psychedelic drug use peak sharply in the late teen years and in the early 20s (Chilcoat and Schutz 1996). This location of psychedelic drug use in relation to the personal characteristic of age (in years) does not settle the issue of causation, but it points strongly toward linkages between late high school and early college experiences and the critical social environments that may promote initiation and persistence of use of these drugs.

It would be a mistake to conclude that environmental conditions and processes do not affect the risk of drug dependence after adolescence. Muntaner et al. (1995) and Crum et al. (1995) identified conditions in the psychosocial work environment that seem to enhance the risk of adult-onset drug and alcohol dependence syndromes. The strongest evidence obtained by Muntaner and colleagues (1995) implicated risk-increasing aspects of physically hazardous work environments that allow little room for decision making. Crum et al. (1995) found that the risk of alcohol dependence syndromes also varies in relation to aspects of job strain in the work environment. The connection between the risk of drug use and drug dependence and the conditions of work, family, and community life during adulthood is an underinvestigated aspect of the Human Envirome Project.

An important research tactic, called an encouragement design or randomized incentive design, may be especially helpful in the Human Envirome Project because it permits researchers to address social selection processes that limit inferences about conditions and interventions affecting drug dependence. The randomized incentive design involves randomization of levels of incentive to participate in epidemiological, prevention, or treatment research, and the purpose of such randomization is to gain experimental control over selection processes that otherwise distort estimates of relative risk, efficacy, and effectiveness (Barnard et al. 2003). Inference from findings of most experimental intervention research on drug dependence is compromised by selection processes that influence who will or will not consent to the intervention (Committee on Data and Research for Policy on Illegal Drugs 2001). Researchers can gauge the effect of the intervention on those who are willing, but it is more difficult to project what the intervention effect might be in a less selected context (e.g., if treatment resources were expanded for coverage of all drug-dependent persons in need of treatment). These selection processes have become more prominent within epidemiological research in general. For example, four or five decades ago, response rates to community surveys in the United States were 97%–99%, whereas in recent years, response rates have been 69%–73% or lower (Substance Abuse and Mental Health Services Administration 2002a, 2002d).

Use of encouragement or randomized incentive designs in epidemiological, prevention, and treatment research permits experimental control over selection processes that influence consent to participate. Monetary or other tangible incentives are ranked within an acceptable range (i.e., from no incentive to the maximum incentive allowable with regard to feasibility, ethics, and protection of subjects). Before recruitment and the consent process, the prospective participant is assigned probabilistically to one of the levels of incentive. This incentive is stated when the research is introduced, and the incentive is clarified during the formal study description, disclosure, and consent process before enrollment. If the incentives have been ranked wisely, there will be some degree of experimental control over the selection process, yielding a gradient of participation levels in relation to the graded ranking of incentive levels, with resulting information to aid inference about relative risk, efficacy, and effectiveness levels when a study aim is to generalize beyond the constraints of the observed sample. Application of the randomized incentive design in National Institute on Drug Abuse–supported epidemiological and intervention research is being guided by prior applications in health economics and in experimental research on the use of school vouchers (Barnard et al. 2003). Research reports with the key words *encouragement designs* and *randomized incentive* should begin to appear in the near future.

Of course, when randomized incentive designs are used in drug dependence research, investigators must recognize that drug-dependent individuals may have different characters of response to incentives. The different character may reflect individual-level susceptibility traits present before effective contact with any drug (e.g., long-standing personality traits such as novelty seeking, openness to experience, or reward dependence). In addition, drug involvement may elicit characteristics that are expressed along with drug taking, possibly seen in levels of receptor density or other underlying neuroadaptive substrates, as in primate laboratory research by Morgan et al. (2002), or in behavioral phenomena such as delay discounting, as described by Bickel and Marsch (2001). These possibilities mean that in drug dependence research, the randomized incentive design must be an adaptation of the design used in health economics and school voucher research.

Individual Vulnerabilities and Their Consequences

Although epidemiological studies tend to concentrate on more malleable experiential and environmental conditions and processes leading to drug-taking behavior and drug dependence, important findings are being obtained regarding the individual temperament, personality, and constitutional characteristics that might influence an individual's risk of drug dependence. When more fixed characteristics such as specific candidate genes, haplotypes, or an early-established trait are brought into focus, the tendency in epidemiology is to search for experiential or environmental conditions under which these predispositions are expressed or not expressed (Anthony et al. 2000; Zandi et al. 2002).

Perhaps as early manifestations of gene expression and gene-environment interactions (e.g., altered gene expression after first-trimester fetal exposure to cocaine), individual vulnerabilities in the form of temperament, personality, and behavior are among the suspected causal determinants of drug involvement. For example, prenatal and perinatal obstetric complications such as hypoxia might be associated with later reduced risk of drug involvement, perhaps as a result of greater parental vigilance and more careful supervision of vulnerable youths (Buka et al. 1993). During the next decade, as "crack babies" and other infants exposed to cocaine become adolescents, it will become possible to answer important epidemiological research questions about biologically plausible interactions that involve candidate genes underlying individual-level susceptibility with persistence of maternal cocaine use during pregnancy (e.g., markers on chromosome 11, discussed by Uhl et al. [2002]) that might be modulated by cocaine or other fetal exposures in the earliest weeks or months after conception. To date, investigations involving cocaine-exposed infants have yielded fairly convincing evidence of excess prenatal mortality, reduced gestational age and fetal growth, and modest to moderate neurobehavioral and neuropsychological adversities (Bandstra et al. 2001; Morrow et al. 2001), but follow-up of the children into and through adolescence will be required to obtain evidence about their possibly excess drug involvement. Excess drug involvement might be seen early, in the form of earlier and more frequent drug exposure opportunities. Evidence of gene-environment interactions (e.g., involving genetic susceptibility markers and levels of fetal cocaine exposure) may be more prominent in fetally exposed adolescents' responses to a first chance to try drugs such as tobacco, alcohol, or cocaine—possibly in the form of excess risk of transitions from first opportunity to first drug use, but even more plausibly in excess risk of transitions from first

drug use to the prodromal clinical features of drug dependence (Wagner and Anthony 2002a).

There are a number of leads for epidemiological research on individual-level vulnerabilities and their consequences, including observations by Kellam et al. (1980) with respect to early misbehavior in primary school and a mixture of early shyness or socially withdrawn behavior with aggressiveness or early acting out. Studying youths in relation to a hypothesized drug dependence liability trait, Tarter and colleagues determined that early irritability and "difficult temperament" may be early traits that account for excess adolescent drug involvement (Blackson et al. 1994).

Later in life, an individual's social attachment to parents and bonding to conventional social institutions such as school have theoretically compelling links to reduced risk of drug involvement (D.W. Brook et al. 2002; J.S. Brook et al. 1990, 2001). Similarly, poor school performance also has been associated with both reduced and excess risk of teen drug involvement (Boyle et al. 1993; Duncan et al. 1998; Fleming et al. 1982), and definitive evidence on this facet of individual vulnerability is still lacking. The increased risk sometimes observed in relation to precocious school readiness might be associated with personality traits such as novelty seeking or openness to experience. Elsewhere, these characteristics have been investigated as modulators of vulnerability to drug use and drug dependence, but results are mixed and evidence is still nondefinitive (Laviola et al. 1999; Wills et al. 1994).

Dropping out of high school or college has been studied both as a consequence of earlier drug taking and as a suspected cause of later drug dependence. Experimental trials, with randomized assignment of subjects to interventions promoting school retention, will likely be needed to sort out this network of relationships (Crum et al. 1993; Kasen et al. 1998).

Some of the most robust indicators of risk of serious drug involvement by middle adolescence or later, at least for boys, are early deviance or conduct problems in childhood, unconventionality in adolescence, and antisocial personality traits later in life (D.W. Brook et al. 2002; J.S. Brook et al. 1998; Kellam et al. 1980; Robins 1966). To some extent, these characteristics reflect lower degrees of social bonding and attachment to parents and to conventional social norms. Among males, this suspected causal linkage is supported by prospective and longitudinal studies and by experimental trials in which primary school interventions have been used to modify levels of early misbehavior in school (Kellam and Anthony 1998; O'Donnell et al. 1995; Storr et al. 2002).

A Question of Mechanisms

What Linkages of States and Processes Influence Who Becomes and Who Remains Drug Dependent?

The study of mechanisms in drug dependence epidemiology encompasses research on the natural history of these syndromes as they develop without early intervention or treatment, their clinical courses during and after interventions, and precursor and prodromal processes. Researchers taking this approach have gained insights through conducting longitudinal research and through making daily contacts or "rounds" with untreated drug users and drug-dependent individuals in the community (Schick et al. 1978). Topics investigated include stepping-stone and gateway hypotheses about linked progressions from one drug to the next in a developmental sequence (Chen and Kandel 1995). Many investigators have presumed that public health interventions at each stage in the developmental sequence might yield reduced prevalence of serious drug involvement (Wagner and Anthony 2002a, 2002b). However, several lines of investigation suggest that underlying individual-level predispositions might account for observed covariation of tobacco, alcohol, and illegal drug involvement in this sequence. If this is correct, then different predispositions may have different implications for drug policy and public health interventions (Anthony 2002; Lynskey et al. 1998; Morral et al. 2002).

In natural history studies generally, clinicians observe the progress of signs and symptoms during eras of no effective treatments. Although noteworthy contributions have been made by a handful of clinical investigators (Van Etten et al. 1998; Warner-Smith et al. 2001; Wilsnack et al. 1997), much of the natural history of drug dependence has been learned by anthropologists and ethnographers who have looked into the population for drug users who never have had contact with treatment services (Kaplan and Lambert 1995) and by epidemiologists and behavioral scientists who have had no intimate contact with drug-using participants in their large studies (J. S. Brook et al. 1998; Kandel et al. 1999; Robins 1966; Rosenberg and Anthony 2001; Wagner and Anthony 2002a, 2002b). Many valuable observations made in this population research (conducted by nonclinicians) on natural history, mechanisms, and early stages of drug dependence have been integrated into professional practice in the form of outreach, treatment, and prevention programs (Agar 1997; Carlson et al. 1995).

The history of epidemiology has also illustrated that firm knowledge of causes and causal mechanisms is unnecessary for effective prevention and intervention. Many current methods of preventing and treating disease were discovered decades before anyone had sorted out the causal mechanisms. Of course, the knowledge base for effective prevention and intervention will be improved when more is learned about causal mechanisms. Each firmly identified mechanism highlights new targets for intervention (Anthony and Van Etten 1998).

At a very simplistic level, the process or causal mechanism for becoming drug dependent can be decomposed into a linked sequence of stages or transitions, with intermediate dimensional progressions within these stages. On the way toward drug dependence, the earliest stage of drug involvement occurs before drug taking begins. The start can be marked by the first age or discretely observable time at which an individual has an opportunity to try a given drug such as marijuana, although some observers might prefer to begin with a process that is more difficult to measure—namely, contemplation in anticipation of the first drug exposure opportunity. The next stage occurs when drug taking begins—another discrete event that can be linked to a particular date or age. A subsequent stage occurs when drug dependence has developed (Anthony and Helzer 1995). The four parts of Figure 6–4 are based on epidemiological data related to the use of marijuana, cocaine, psychedelic drugs (e.g., LSD, Ecstasy), and heroin. The figure shows the estimated proportions of the United States population (at various age ranges) that had an opportunity to try the drugs (opportunity to use), the proportions that tried them (history of use), and the proportions that developed dependence (history of dependence).

From this figure, one can discern that a possible mechanism underlying generally lower risk of drug dependence among older adults is the formerly lower probability of having an opportunity to try these drugs. Similarly, if the experience of late adolescents during the 1990s rings true with that of their older brothers and sisters, the observed data suggest an increased prevalence of drug dependence in the first decades of

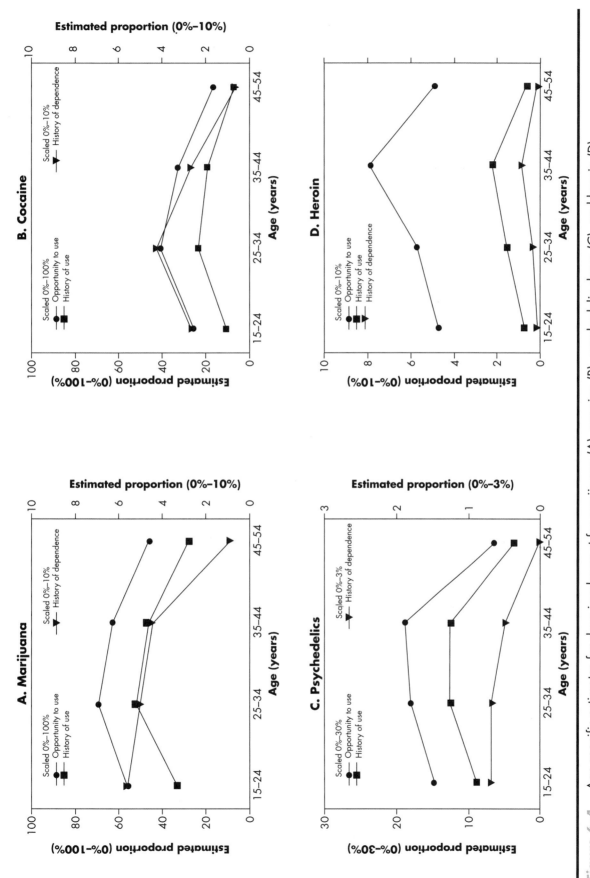

Figure 6–4. Age-specific estimates for drug involvement for marijuana (A), cocaine (B), psychedelic drugs (C), and heroin (D).

Opportunity to use data are from the National Household Surveys on Drug Abuse; *history of use* and *history of dependence* data are from the National Comorbidity Survey, United States, 1990–1992.

Source. Anthony et al. 1994; Van Etten and Anthony 2002. (Graphics: Scott Hubbard, 1998, for this publication.)

the twenty-first century (due to greater opportunities for young people to try these drugs in the waning years of the twentieth century).

There are more challenging examples of how causal mechanisms are being examined in epidemiological field studies, and the resulting observations have implications for prevention and public health action. For example, Duncan et al. (1998) described the Oregon Social Learning Center model for antisocial behavior and adapted it to drug taking:

> According to this model, parental mismanagement of early oppositional and aggressive behavior shapes further aggressive behavior which leads to a pattern of coercive interactions and conflict between parents and children. Parental attempts at discipline are inconsistent and [are] met with the child's aggression. Seeking to avoid these aversive interactions, parents become increasingly inconsistent in their parenting practices and become less involved with their children. The child's aggressive behavior and noncompliance then become well-established.... [T]his pattern of non-compliance and aggressive behavior is extended to the school environment and often places the child on a trajectory that includes rejection by normal peers and academic failure in the classroom. These outcomes contribute to a drift toward other rejected, aggressive peers by early adolescence, where further problematic behavior is shaped and reinforced. Continued association with this deviant peer group places the child at high risk for developing a consistent pattern of antisocial and delinquent behavior. Thus, this model accounts for delinquent and antisocial behavior in adolescents through proximal peer influence, but suggests that poor family management practices (especially conflict and poor parental monitoring) explain the adolescent's engagement with deviant peers. (Duncan et al. 1998, p. 58)

This type of developmental causal model, and its many intermediate pathways and mechanisms, can be tested only with epidemiological sampling of children early in life and with multiple longitudinal observations through the years of schooling and beyond. To the extent that these hypothesized mechanisms are confirmed, they become targets for preventive interventions with respect to early-onset drug taking and later risk of drug dependence. In some of our research group's recent work, mechanisms of drug exposure opportunity and drug purchase opportunity were integrated within these developmental models, and resulting observations indicate that parental supervision and monitoring between middle childhood and middle adolescence can influence the child's affiliation

with deviant peer groups, independent of the child's prior and sustained levels of antisocial behavior (Lloyd and Anthony 2003). Furthermore, it is possible that effective parental supervision and monitoring can reduce or delay a child's first drug exposure opportunities, reduce early-onset drug taking, and prevent or delay more serious forms of drug involvement (Wagner and Anthony 2002b).

To date, elements of cognitive science and behavioral economics have not been prominent in these theories of causal mechanisms that lead to serious drug involvement and drug dependence. However, the integration of these elements into epidemiological field studies is under way, concurrent with a renaissance of cognitive sciences in the late twentieth century and parallel developments in behavioral economics. Longitudinal studies now under way should yield definitive epidemiological evidence on the roles played by deficits in general executive functions (direction, planning, and behavioral control) and by more specific executive functions such as delay discounting. For example, little is currently known about executive dysfunctions, the process of affiliation with drug-using peer groups, and subsequent disaffiliations. Research on these processes is especially complex because executive functions and discounting decisions can influence whether, when, and how much drug taking occurs, but in addition, impairments in these executive functions and discounting decisions can be induced by drug taking. Randomized trials can help sort out steps in these processes, but longitudinal studies involving children and adolescents, after epidemiological sampling, will be important if these steps are to be placed in context with social stratification and peer clustering processes (Link and Phelan 1996; Oetting and Donnermeyer 1998; Szapocznik and Coatsworth 1999).

A Question of Prevention and Intervention

What Can Be Done to Prevent and Intervene in Drug Dependence?

The search for a solid foundation of evidence has led many epidemiologists to conduct randomized controlled intervention and prevention trials. Our research group has undertaken several long-term randomized prevention trials to test the previously mentioned hypotheses about causal mechanisms linking early childhood aggression and later risk of early-onset drug taking (Kellam and Anthony 1998; Storr et al. 2002).

The search for a solid foundation of evidence for prevention and intervention has also led epidemiologists to use the randomized incentive design (discussed in an earlier section, "The Human Envirome Project"). Designs of this type, nested within epidemiological studies, will be needed to answer questions about the effects of interventions on the many drug users who do not come into contact with treatment specialists or who would not ordinarily agree to receive help for their problems. More definitive answers to these questions are crucial if public policy questions are to be answered about the value of investing resources in supply reduction versus demand reduction, treatment, and prevention (Committee on Data and Research for Policy on Illegal Drugs 2001).

Hence, the fifth main rubric for drug dependence epidemiology is expressed in relation to prevention and intervention. When successful, randomized prevention trials not only clarify which programs merit widespread dissemination and which do not, they also marshal important evidence about causal hypotheses and suspected causal mechanisms. Prevention is examined in more detail in Chapter 49, "Prevention of Alcohol-Related Problems," in this volume.

Prospects for the Future

Ongoing epidemiological field studies have been expanding. In the United States, national surveys on drug use and health now involve larger samples, and there is a new prospective follow-up component of the ECA survey and the NCS. In addition, more than 25 other countries—including China, Japan, South Africa, Ukraine, Belgium, and Brazil—are the sites of mental health surveys on drug dependence and other psychiatric disorders meeting DSM-IV and ICD-10 (World Health Organization 1992) criteria (Kessler 1999).

More exciting new evidence in drug dependence epidemiology is likely to come when the Human Genome Project and the HapMap project intersect with the Human Envirome Project in a deliberate effort to find gene-environment interactions that influence the risk of drug dependence in adolescence and early adulthood. In the short run, some of the most promising research on these gene-environment interactions will arise from genome scans within current twin and affected sibling research projects, in tandem with studies involving monozygotic twins and siblings who are discordant for age of transition from one stage of drug involvement to the next (e.g., opportunity, history of use, history of dependence). In addition, there is good reason to include genome scans and investigations of gene-environment interactions in ongoing prospective and longitudinal studies involving adolescents whose mothers took cocaine during pregnancy. Where there are opportunities for genome scans of these mothers, their cocaine-exposed children, and the full or half siblings of these children, there will be opportunities for research on gene-environment interactions, especially in the transition from first drug use by the cocaine-exposed children and subsequent risk of drug dependence.

Epidemiological studies of this type should lead to an increased understanding of the causes and causal mechanisms underlying drug involvement and the stages and processes that lead toward drug dependence and related hazards of drug use. In this fashion will be forged a new generation of experimental intervention and prevention trials with epidemiological samples of sufficient size and generality to yield definitive evidence—as is now the case with large-sample trials in cancer and cardiovascular disease epidemiology.

References

Agar MH: Ethnography: an overview. Subst Use Misuse 32:1155–1173, 1997

American Psychiatric Association: Diagnostic and Statistical Manual of Mental Disorders, 3rd Edition. Washington, DC, American Psychiatric Association, 1980

American Psychiatric Association: Diagnostic and Statistical Manual of Mental Disorders, 3rd Edition, Revised. Washington, DC, American Psychiatric Association, 1987

American Psychiatric Association: Diagnostic and Statistical Manual of Mental Disorders, 4th Edition. Washington, DC, American Psychiatric Association, 1994

Anthony JC: The promise of psychiatric enviromics. Br J Psychiatry Suppl 40:S8–S11, 2001

Anthony JC: Death of the "stepping-stone" hypothesis and the "gateway" model? Comments on Morral et al. Addiction 97:1505–1507, 2002

Anthony JC: Epidemiology of drug dependence, in Neuropsychopharmacology: The Fifth Generation of Progress. Edited by Davis KL, Charney D, Coyle JT, et al. Philadelphia, PA, Lippincott Williams & Wilkins, 2002, pp 1557–1574

Anthony JC: The epidemiology of cannabis dependence, in Cannabis Dependence: Its Nature, Consequences, Treatment. Edited by Roffman RA, Stephens RS. New York, Cambridge University Press (in press)

Anthony JC, Arria AM: Epidemiology of psychoactive drug dependence in adulthood, in Sourcebook on Substance Abuse: Etiology, Epidemiology, Assessment, and Treatment. Edited by Ott PJ, Tarter RE, Ammerman RT. Needham Heights, MA, Allyn & Bacon, 1999, pp 32–48

Anthony JC, Forman V: At the intersection of public health and criminal justice research on drugs and crime, in Toward a Drugs and Crime Research Agenda for the 21st Century. Special Report No 194616. Edited by Hart SV. Washington, DC, National Institute of Justice, 2003. Available at: http://www.ojp.usdoj.gov/nij. Accessed August 4, 2003

Anthony JC, Helzer JE: Syndromes of drug abuse and dependence, in Psychiatric Disorders in America: The Epidemiologic Catchment Area Study. Edited by Robins LN, Regier DA. New York, Free Press, 1991, pp 116–154

Anthony JC, Helzer JE: Epidemiology of drug dependence, in Textbook in Psychiatric Epidemiology. Edited by Tsuang MT, Tohen M, Zachner GEP. New York, Wiley-Liss, 1995, pp 361–406

Anthony JC, Helzer JE: Epidemiology of drug dependence, in Textbook in Psychiatric Epidemiology, 2nd Edition. Edited by Tsuang MT, Tohen M. New York, Wiley-Liss, 2002, pp 479–561

Anthony JC, Petronis KR: Early onset drug use and risk of later drug problems. Drug Alcohol Depend 40:9–15, 1995

Anthony JC, Van Etten ML: Epidemiology and its rubrics, in Comprehensive Clinical Psychology. Edited by Bellack A, Hersen M. Oxford, UK, Elsevier Science, 1998, pp 355–390

Anthony JC, Folstein M, Romanoski AJ, et al: Comparison of the lay Diagnostic Interview Schedule and a standardized psychiatric diagnosis: experience in eastern Baltimore. Arch Gen Psychiatry 42:667–675, 1985

Anthony JC, Warner LA, Kessler RC: Comparative epidemiology of dependence on tobacco, alcohol, controlled substances, and inhalants: basic findings from the National Comorbidity Survey. Exp Clin Psychopharmacol 2:244–268, 1994

Anthony JC, Eaton WW, Henderson AS: Looking to the future in psychiatric epidemiology. Epidemiol Rev 17:240–242, 1995

Anthony JC, Breitner JC, Zandi PP, et al: Reduced prevalence of AD in users of NSAIDs and H_2 receptor antagonists: the Cache County study. Neurology 54:2066–2071, 2000

Bandstra ES, Morrow CE, Anthony JC, et al: Intrauterine growth of full-term infants: impact of prenatal cocaine exposure. Pediatrics 108:1309–1319, 2001

Barnard J, Frangakis CE, Hill JL, et al: A principal stratification approach to broken randomized experiments: a case study of School Choice vouchers in New York City. Journal of the American Statistical Association (with discussion) 98:299–323, 2003

Bickel WK, Marsch LA: Toward a behavioral economic understanding of drug dependence: delay discounting processes. Addiction 96:73–86, 2001

Blackson TC, Tarter RE, Martin CS, et al: Temperament-induced father-son family dysfunction: etiological implications for child behavior problems and substance abuse. Am J Orthopsychiatry 64:280–292, 1994

Boyle MH, Offord DR, Racine YA, et al: Predicting substance use in early adolescence based on parent and teacher assessments of childhood psychiatric disorder: results from the Ontario Child Health Study follow-up. J Child Psychol Psychiatry 34:535–544, 1993

Brook DW, Brook JS, Rosen Z, et al: Correlates of marijuana use in Colombian adolescents: a focus on the impact of the ecological/cultural domain. J Adolesc Health 31:286–298, 2002

Brook JS, Brook DW, Gordon AS, et al: The psychosocial etiology of adolescent drug use: a family interactional approach. Genet Soc Gen Psychol Monogr 116:111–267, 1990

Brook JS, Brook DW, De La Rosa M, et al: Pathways to marijuana use among adolescents: cultural/ecological, family, peer, and personality influences. J Am Acad Child Adolesc Psychiatry 37:759–766, 1998

Brook JS, Brook DW, Arencibia-Mireles O, et al: Risk factors for adolescent marijuana use across cultures and across time. J Genet Psychol 162:357–374, 2001

Buka SL, Tsuang MT, Lipsitt LP: Pregnancy/delivery complications and psychiatric diagnosis: a prospective study. Arch Gen Psychiatry 50:151–156, 1993

Carlson RG, Siegal HA, Falck RS: Qualitative research methods in drug abuse and AIDS prevention research: an overview. NIDA Res Monogr 157:6–26, 1995

Chen K, Kandel DB: The natural history of drug use from adolescence to the mid-thirties in a general population sample. Am J Public Health 85:41–47, 1995

Chilcoat HD, Anthony JC: Impact of parent monitoring on initiation of drug use through late childhood. J Am Acad Child Adolesc Psychiatry 35:91–100, 1996

Chilcoat HD, Schutz CG: Age-specific patterns of hallucinogen use in the US population: an analysis using generalized additive models. Drug Alcohol Depend 43:143–153, 1996

Committee on Data and Research for Policy on Illegal Drugs: Informing America's Policy on Illegal Drugs: What We Don't Know Keeps Hurting Us. Edited by Manski CF, Pepper JV, Petrie CV. Washington, DC, National Academy Press, 2001

Crum RM, Helzer JE, Anthony JC: Level of education and alcohol abuse and dependence in adulthood: a further inquiry. Am J Public Health 83:830–837, 1993

Crum RM, Muntaner C, Eaton WW, et al: Occupational stress and the risk of alcohol abuse and dependence. Alcohol Clin Exp Res 19:647–655, 1995

Dohrenwend BP, Levav I, Shrout PE, et al: Socioeconomic status and psychiatric disorders: the causation-selection issue. Science 255:946–952, 1992

Duncan SC, Duncan TE, Biglan A, et al: Contributions of the social context to the development of adolescent substance use: a multivariate latent growth modeling approach. Drug Alcohol Depend 50:57–71, 1998

Eaton WW, Kramer M, Anthony JC, et al: The incidence of specific DIS/DSM-III mental disorders: data from the NIMH Epidemiologic Catchment Area Program. Acta Psychiatr Scand 79:163–178, 1989

Fahlke C, Lorenz JG, Long J, et al: Rearing experiences and stress-induced plasma cortisol as early risk factors for excessive alcohol consumption in nonhuman primates. Alcohol Clin Exp Res 24:644–650, 2000

Fleming JP, Kellam SG, Brown CH: Early predictors of age at first use of alcohol, marijuana, and cigarettes. Drug Alcohol Depend 9:285–303, 1982

Furr-Holden CDM, Anthony JC: Epidemiologic differences in drug dependence: a U.S.-U.K. cross-national comparison. Soc Psychiatry Psychiatr Epidemiol 38:165–172, 2003

Grant BF: Comorbidity between DSM-IV drug use disorders and major depression: results of a national survey of adults. J Subst Abuse 7:481–497, 1995

Grant BF: Barriers to alcoholism treatment: reasons for not seeking treatment in a general population sample. J Stud Alcohol 58:365–371, 1997a

Grant BF: Prevalence and correlates of alcohol use and DSM-IV alcohol dependence in the United States: results of the National Longitudinal Alcohol Epidemiologic Survey. J Stud Alcohol 58:464–473, 1997b

Helzer JE: Specification of predictors of narcotic use versus addiction, in Studying Drug Abuse. Edited by Robins LN. New Brunswick, NJ, Rutgers University Press, 1985, pp 173–197

Kandel DB, Udry JR: Prenatal effects of maternal smoking on daughters' smoking: nicotine or testosterone exposure? Am J Public Health 89:1377–1383, 1999

Kandel DB, Johnson JG, Bird HR, et al: Psychiatric comorbidity among adolescents with substance use disorders: findings from the MECA Study. J Am Acad Child Adolesc Psychiatry 38:693–699, 1999

Kaplan CD, Lambert EY: The daily life of heroin-addicted persons: the biography of specific methodology. NIDA Res Monogr 157:100–116, 1995

Kasen S, Cohen P, Brook JS: Adolescent school experiences and dropout, adolescent pregnancy, and young adult deviant behavior. J Adolesc Res 13:49–72, 1998

Kellam SG, Anthony JC: Targeting early antecedents to prevent tobacco smoking: findings from an epidemiologically based randomized field trial. Am J Public Health 88:1490–1495, 1998

Kellam SG, Ensminger ME, Simon MB: Mental health in first grade and teenage drug, alcohol, and cigarette use. Drug Alcohol Depend 5:273–304, 1980

Kessler RC: The World Health Organization International Consortium in Psychiatric Epidemiology (ICPE): initial work and future directions—the NAPE Lecture 1998. Nordic Association for Psychiatric Epidemiology. Acta Psychiatr Scand 99:2–9, 1999

Kessler RC, McGonagle KA, Zhao S, et al: Lifetime and 12-month prevalence of DSM-III-R psychiatric disorders in the United States: results from the National Comorbidity Survey. Arch Gen Psychiatry 51:8–19, 1994

Laviola G, Adriani W, Terranova ML, et al: Psychobiological risk factors for vulnerability to psychostimulants in human adolescents and animal models. Neurosci Biobehav Rev 23:993–1010, 1999

Link BG, Phelan JC: Understanding sociodemographic differences in health: the role of fundamental social causes. Am J Public Health 86:471–472, 1996

Lloyd JJ, Anthony JC: Hanging out with the wrong crowd: how much difference can parents make in an urban environment? J Urban Health 80:383–399, 2003

Lynskey MT, Fergusson DM, Horwood LJ: The origins of the correlations between tobacco, alcohol, and cannabis use during adolescence. J Child Psychol Psychiatry 39:995–1005, 1998

Meltzer H, Gill B, Petticrew M, et al: The Prevalence of Psychiatric Morbidity Among Adults Living in Private Households (OPCS Surveys of Psychiatric Morbidity in Great Britain, Report 1). London, H.M.S.O., 1995

Morgan D, Grant KA, Gage HD, et al: Social dominance in monkeys: dopamine D_2 receptors and cocaine self-administration. Nat Neurosci 5:169–174, 2002

Morral AR, McCaffrey DF, Paddock SM: Reassessing the marijuana gateway effect. Addiction 97:1500–1500, 2002

Morrow CE, Bandstra ES, Anthony JC, et al: Influence of prenatal cocaine exposure on full-term infant neurobehavioral functioning. Neurotoxicol Teratol 23:533–544, 2001

Muntaner C, Anthony JC, Crum RM, et al: Psychosocial dimensions of work and the risk of drug dependence among adults. Am J Epidemiol 142:183–190, 1995

Newcomb MD, Bentler PM: Impact of adolescent drug use and social support on problems of young adults: a longitudinal study. J Abnorm Psychol 97:64–75, 1988

O'Brien CP, Nace EP, Mintz J, et al: Follow-up of Vietnam veterans, I: relapse to drug use after Vietnam service. Drug Alcohol Depend 5:333–340, 1980

O'Donnell J, Hawkins JD, Catalano RF, et al: Preventing school failure, drug use, and delinquency among low-income children: long-term intervention in elementary schools. Am J Orthopsychiatry 65:87–100, 1995

Oetting ER, Donnermeyer JF: Primary socialization theory: the etiology of drug use and deviance, I. Subst Use Misuse 33:995–1026, 1998

Petronis KR, Anthony JC: Perceived risk of cocaine use and experience with cocaine: do they cluster within US neighborhoods and cities? Drug Alcohol Depend 57:183–192, 2000

Petronis KR, Anthony JC: A different kind of contextual effect: geographic clustering of cocaine incidence in the US. J Epidemiol Community Health 57:893–900, 2003

Robins LN: Deviant Children Grown Up: A Sociological and Psychiatric Study of Sociopathic Personality. Baltimore, MD, Williams & Wilkins, 1966

Rosanoff AJ: Survey of mental disorders: in Nassau County, New York; July–Oct, 1916. Psychiatr Bull 2:1–73, 1917

Rosenberg MF, Anthony JC: Early clinical manifestations of cannabis dependence in a community sample. Drug Alcohol Depend 64:123–131, 2001

Schick JF, Dorus W, Hughes PH: Adolescent drug using groups in Chicago parks. Drug Alcohol Depend 3:199–210, 1978

Storr CL, Ialongo NS, Kellam SG, et al: A randomized controlled trial of two primary school intervention strategies to prevent early onset tobacco smoking. Drug Alcohol Depend 66:51–60, 2002

Substance Abuse and Mental Health Services Administration: National Household Survey on Drug Abuse: Main Findings 1998 (DHHS Publ No SMA 00-3381). Rockville, MD, Substance Abuse and Mental Health Services Administration, Office of Applied Studies, 2000a

Substance Abuse and Mental Health Services Administration: Summary of Findings From the 1999 National Household Survey on Drug Abuse (DHHS Publ No SMA 00-3466). Rockville, MD, Substance Abuse and Mental Health Services Administration, Office of Applied Studies, 2000b

Substance Abuse and Mental Health Services Administration: Detailed Tables for 1999 and 2000 National Household Survey on Drug Abuse (DHHS Publ No SMA 02-3760). Rockville, MD, Substance Abuse and Mental Health Services Administration, Office of Applied Studies, 2002a

Substance Abuse and Mental Health Services Administration: National and State Estimates of the Drug Abuse Treatment Gap: 2000 National Household Survey on Drug Abuse (DHHS Publ No SMA 02-3640). Rockville, MD, Substance Abuse and Mental Health Services Administration, Office of Applied Studies, 2002b

Substance Abuse and Mental Health Services Administration: Results From the 2001 National Household Survey on Drug Abuse, Vol I: Summary of National Findings (DHHS Publ No SMA 02-3758). Rockville, MD, Substance Abuse and Mental Health Services Administration, Office of Applied Studies, 2002c

Substance Abuse and Mental Health Services Administration: Results From the 2001 National Household Survey on Drug Abuse, Vol II: Technical Appendices and Selected Data Tables (DHHS Publ No SMA 02-3759). Rockville, MD, Substance Abuse and Mental Health Services Administration, Office of Applied Studies, 2002d

Szapocznik J, Coatsworth JD: An ecodevelopmental framework for organizing risk and protection for drug abuse: a developmental model of risk and protection, in Drug Abuse: Origins & Interventions. Edited by Glantz MD, Hartel CR. Washington, DC, American Psychological Association, 1999, pp 331–336

Uhl GR, Liu QR, Naiman D: Substance abuse vulnerability loci: converging genome scanning data. Trends Genet 18:420–425, 2002

Van Etten ML, Anthony JC: Comparative epidemiology of initial drug opportunities and transitions to first use: marijuana, cocaine, hallucinogens and heroin. Drug Alcohol Depend 54:117–125, 1999

Van Etten ML, Higgins ST, Budney AJ, et al: Comparison of the frequency and enjoyability of pleasant events in cocaine abusers vs. non-abusers using a standardized behavioral inventory. Addiction 93:1669–1680, 1998

Wagner FA, Anthony JC: From first drug use to drug dependence; developmental periods of risk for dependence upon marijuana, cocaine, and alcohol. Neuropsychopharmacology 26:479–488, 2002a

Wagner FA, Anthony JC: Into the world of illegal drug use: exposure opportunity and other mechanisms linking the use of alcohol, tobacco, marijuana, and cocaine. Am J Epidemiol 155:918–925, 2002b

Warner LA, Kessler RC, Hughes M, et al: Prevalence and correlates of drug use and dependence in the United States: results from the National Comorbidity Survey. Arch Gen Psychiatry 52:219–229, 1995

Warner-Smith M, Darke S, Lynskey M, et al: Heroin overdose: causes and consequences. Addiction 96:1113–1125, 2001

Wills TA, Vaccaro D, McNamara G: Novelty seeking, risk taking, and related constructs as predictors of adolescent substance use: an application of Cloninger's theory. J Subst Abuse 6:1–20, 1994

Wilsnack SC, Vogeltanz ND, Klassen AD, et al: Childhood sexual abuse and women's substance abuse: national survey findings. J Stud Alcohol 58:264–271, 1997

Wines FH: Report on the Defective, Dependent, and Delinquent Class of the Population of the United States at the Tenth Census (June 1, 1880). Washington, DC, U.S. Government Printing Office, 1888

World Health Organization: International Statistical Classification of Diseases and Related Health Problems, 10th Revision. Geneva, World Health Organization, 1992

Zandi PP, Anthony JC, Hayden KM, et al: Reduced incidence of AD with NSAID but not H_2 receptor antagonists: the Cache County Study. Neurology 59:880–886, 2002

Genetics of Substance Abuse

C. Robert Cloninger, M.D.

Twin and adoption studies have recently distinguished the effects of genes that influence initiation of drug use from the effects of genes that influence the transition from use to abuse or dependence (Tsuang et al. 1999). The genes that influence initiation of drug use are related to antisocial personality traits—in particular, high novelty seeking. The same genes have a strong influence on initiation of use of a wide variety of substances, including stimulants, opiates, psychedelics, sedatives, marijuana, alcohol, and nicotine. In contrast, the transition from drug use to abuse or dependence is weakly influenced by heritable traits, such as low self-directedness and low P300 amplitude. However, the transition to abuse is largely influenced by factors unique to each individual. Linkage and association studies have identified several chromosomal regions and specific genes that influence initiation of substance use and transitions to abuse and dependence. For example, several genes influencing dopaminergic and serotonergic neurotransmission have been implicated in initiation of drug abuse. These genes include genetic polymorphisms influencing the activity of the dopamine and serotonin transporters, the dopamine D_4 receptor (*DRD4*) and the serotonin 1B (5-HT_{1B}) receptor. The greater influence of genes on initiation of drug abuse than on transition to abuse or dependence suggests that treatment should facilitate development of self-efficacy and acceptance of responsibility for one's choice to abuse drugs.

Genetic Epidemiology of Substance Abuse

Family, twin, and adoption studies have consistently confirmed that genetics influences the risk of substance abuse. However, clinicians observed that the same individual often abused several classes of substances, and that different individuals in the same family sometimes abused different substances despite similar opportunities for drug use. A variety of explanations were offered for such polysubstance abuse and individ-

Supported in part by National Institutes of Health grants AA08403, MH31302, MH60879, and MH62130.

ual differences in drug preferences. For example, some investigators hypothesized that use of readily available substances, such as marijuana and cigarettes, is a gateway that may or may not lead to use of drugs that are less often used, such as stimulants, opiates, and psychedelics. Others suggested that vulnerability to each drug has specific genetic antecedents but that environmental influences common to siblings (such as availability in particular neighborhoods) favor use of the same drugs by members of a family.

However, data from twins and adoptees indicate that neither the gateway hypothesis nor the common-environment hypothesis can explain the heritability of polysubstance abuse (Tsuang et al. 1998). Recent findings clearly show that the strongest genetic influences on the risk of drug abuse are the genes that influence initiation of drug use. The genes that influence initiation of use have a strong effect on the ultimate risk of abuse, and they are largely nonspecific for the class of drug. For example, heritable personality traits, such as high novelty seeking, increase the risk of experimentation with a wide variety of drugs (Cloninger et al. 1988; Comings et al. 2000; Howard et al. 1997). The level of availability largely dictates what drugs are used if any experimentation occurs. Once an opportunity to use a drug exists, the genetic factors for initiation of use are largely the same for all classes of drugs except opiates (see Figure 7–1).

The genes uniquely involved in use of specific drugs are unknown. Even the alcohol dehydrogenase 3 (*ADH3*) and μ opioid receptor genes appear to influence susceptibility to polysubstance abuse (Uhl et al. 2001). This nonspecificity of gene effects is not explained by indiscriminant drug use due to intoxication, because cigarette smoking, which is not intoxicating, shares most of its genetic variance with alcoholism (True et al. 1999) and hence with other forms of substance abuse.

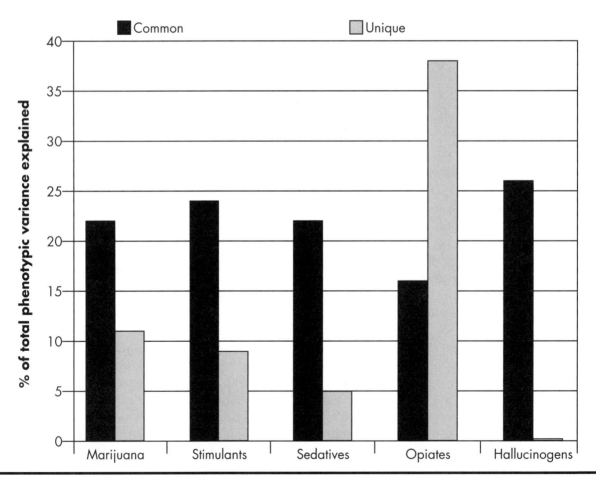

Figure 7–1. Common and unique genetic variance in Vietnam Era Twin Registry subjects, by drug or drug class.
Source. Adapted from Tsuang et al. 1998.

Genes that influence the transition from use to abuse or dependence are not the same genes as those that influence initiation (Kendler et al. 1999, 2000; Sigvardsson et al. 1996; Tsuang et al. 1999). Furthermore, once drug use is initiated, the factors that influence the transition from initiation to repeated use, abuse, or dependence are largely nongenetic factors unique to each individual (see Figure 7–2). In other words, the heritability of transition from use to abuse is weak. The heritability of initiation is compared with the heritability of the transition to abuse in Figure 7–3.

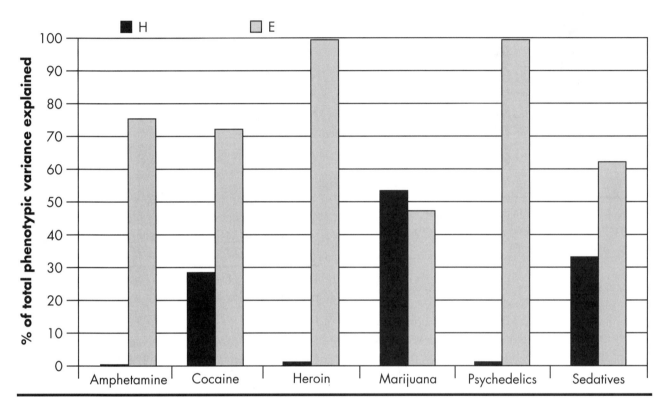

Figure 7–2. Genetic (H) and unique environmental (E) influences on the transition (in Vietnam Era Twin Registry subjects) from initiation of drug use to use of the drug five or more times, by drug or drug class.

Source. Adapted from Tsuang et al. 1999.

Personality Antecedents of Substance Abuse

Antisocial personality traits in a person's biological parents predict an increased risk of early-onset alcoholism and substance abuse (Cadoret et al. 1995). This is true even if children are adopted away from their biological parents at an early age (Cadoret et al. 1995; Cloninger 1987; Sigvardsson et al. 1996). Adopted men whose biological fathers had early-onset alcoholism and were antisocial had a ninefold-increased risk of type 2 alcoholism compared with those without such genetic predisposition (18% vs. 2%), regardless of the quality of the adoptee's home placement (Cloninger 1987). In contrast, severe type 1 alcohol dependence was only weakly heritable in the absence of environmental influences that encouraged heavy drinking. These adoption findings are consistent with the recent twin findings of strong heritability of initiation of substance abuse (as seen in type 2 alcoholism) in contrast to the weak heritability of transition from drug use to abuse or dependence (as seen in severe type 1 alcoholism).

Likewise, antisocial personality traits in a person's own childhood and adolescence predict early onset of substance abuse. The only prospective study focused on the onset of alcoholism before age 28 years (Cloninger et al. 1988). Personality was rated at age 11 years, before any substance use. High novelty seeking (impulsive-aggressive traits) and low harm-avoidance

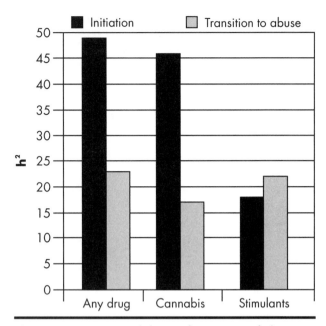

Figure 7–3. Heritabilities of initiation of drug use and transition to drug abuse in female twins in Virginia.

Source. Adapted from Kendler et al. 1999.

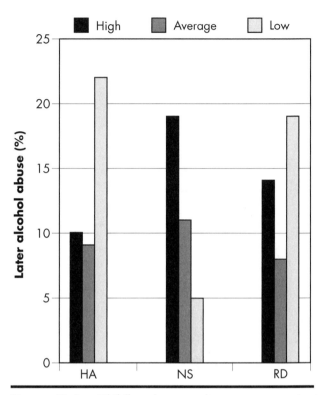

Figure 7–4. Childhood personality as a prospective predictor of alcoholism.

Personality traits were measured in 233 Swedish boys at age 11 years, and alcohol abuse was rated independently in the same group at age 28 years. The triad of antisocial characteristics—low harm-avoidance (HA), high novelty seeking (NS), low reward dependence (RD)—predicted alcoholism.

Source. Adapted from Cloninger et al. 1988.

(risk taking) were most strongly predictive of early-onset alcohol abuse, as shown in Figure 7–4. These two childhood variables distinguished boys who had nearly 20-fold differences in their risk of alcohol abuse: the risk of alcohol abuse varied from 4% to 75%, depending on childhood personality. Likewise, reviews of the personality correlates of substance abusers confirm that novelty seeking, as measured by reliable personality inventories, predicts early-onset alcoholism, other substance abuse, and criminality (Howard et al. 1997).

In addition to being associated with novelty seeking, severe alcohol dependence (meeting ICD-10 [World Health Organization 1992] criteria) is also strongly correlated with the personality trait of low self-directedness and with low P300 amplitude in evoked potential studies. Self-directedness and P300 amplitude are themselves moderately correlated. The effect sizes (as determined in the Collaborative Study on the Genetics of Alcoholism) of personality traits distinguishing subjects with severe alcohol dependence from those with no alcohol dependence are shown in Figure 7–5. Individuals with low self-directedness are described as irresponsible, goalless, helpless, and undisciplined. They have difficulty controlling their emotional impulses in order to accomplish long-term goals such as sobriety. Individuals with low cooperativeness are described as prejudiced, selfish, hostile, revenge-

ful, and unprincipled. In other words, individuals with high novelty seeking, low self-directedness, and low cooperativeness have impulsive (cluster B) personality disorders, which carry a high risk of comorbid substance abuse. These individuals most frequently receive diagnoses of antisocial or borderline personality disorders. These persons are characterized by an inability to delay gratification, leading to both early initiation of drug experimentation and frequent transition to substance abuse or dependence.

Genome Scans for Detecting Linkage and Association

Four large-scale genome scans have been carried out to identify chromosomal regions containing susceptibility genes for substance dependence (see review by Uhl et al. [2001]) and personality traits related to sub-

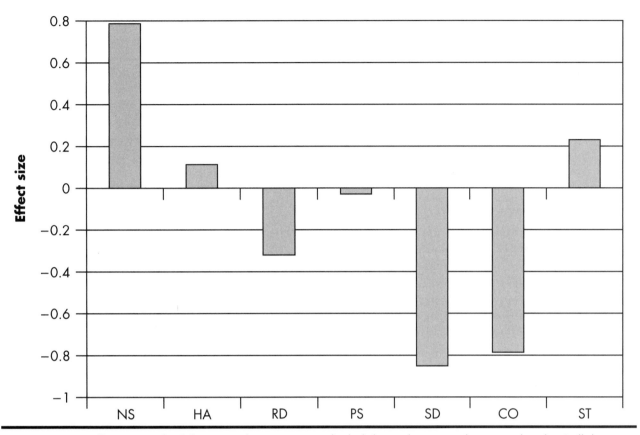

Figure 7–5. Effect sizes of adult personality on severe alcohol dependence, as determined in the Collaborative Study on the Genetics of Alcoholism.

NS=novelty seeking; HA=harm avoidance; RD=reward dependence; PS=persistence; SD=self-directedness; CO=cooperativeness; ST=self-transcendence.

stance dependence (Cloninger et al. 1998). Despite the difficulty of replicating linkage findings for complex phenotypes such as substance dependence, some findings about linkage to alcohol dependence have been replicated in independent samples (Foroud et al. 2000) (see Table 7–1). For example, there is evidence that a region on chromosome 4, near the *ADH3* locus, has a protective effect against development of alcoholism in Americans of European or African descent. This is consistent with evidence that the high-activity isoforms of alcohol dehydrogenase 2 and *ADH3,* as well as low-activity isoforms of acetaldehyde dehydrogenase 2, protect against alcoholism in East Asians (Chen et al. 1999). These variant enzymes lead to high levels of acetaldehyde, which cause unpleasant flushing and decrease the risk of alcohol dependence.

A gene for the 5-HT$_{1B}$ receptor has been linked to type 2 alcoholism in two independent samples. In further work, this gene was associated with harm-avoidance, which mediated its effect on alcohol dependence.

Table 7–1. Multipoint linkage findings of genome scans for alcoholism-related traits

Trait	Linkage
Low risk of any abuse (protective effect)	LOD 2.5, chromosome 4, near *ADH3* locus
High risk of mild dependence	Replicated LOD 2.6, chromosome 1
High risk of severe dependence	Replicated LOD 2.9, chromosome 7
P300 amplitude	LOD>3, chromosomes 2 and 6

Note. Data were obtained in the Collaborative Study on the Genetics of Alcoholism. *ADH3*=alcohol dehydrogenase 3 gene; LOD=logarithm of odds.

According to twin studies, alcohol and nicotine dependence share most of their genetic variance, but little overlap in specific chromosomal regions was identified in two preliminary genome scans of cigarette smokers (Bierut et al. [in press]; Straub et al. 1999)

Table 7–2. Findings of genome scans of cigarette smokers

Suggestive evidence of linkage to habitual smoking:

On chromosomes 2, 4, 10, 16, 17, and 18
(Virginia results independently supported in New Zealand) (Straub et al. 1999)

On chromosomes 5, 9, 11, and 21
(Initial results of Collaborative Study o78
n the Genetics of Alcoholism only modestly supported in replication sample) (Bierut et al., in press)

(see Table 7–2). However, a polymorphism of the dopamine transporter is associated with individual differences in initiation and continuation of cigarette smoking, an association that is mediated by the joint relationship of cigarette smoking and the dopamine transporter with novelty seeking (Sabol et al. 1999).

A genome scan of 667 substance abusers and 327 control subjects, using 1,494 single nucleotide polymorphisms, identified 42 associations with substance abuse that were replicated in blacks and whites (Uhl et al. 2001) (see Table 7–3). Nine loci were also replicated in the four prior genome scans of substance abusers (Uhl et al. 2001) (see Table 7–4). These nine replicated loci included the chromosome 4 region near the *ADH3* locus and the locus for brain-derived neurotrophic factor, which is known to regulate dopamine and serotonin neurotransmitters strongly associated with substance dependence.

Researchers have investigated genetic factors that influence the risk of specific end-organ complications, particularly in the context of alcoholic liver disease. The risk of liver disease in alcoholic persons depends on individual differences in genes regulating specific cellular processes involving cytokines and cytochromes (Grove et al. 2000; Reed et al. 1996; Savolainen et al. 1997).

These replicated findings are encouraging. However, it is not possible to identify specific genes that are necessary or sufficient for development of substance dependence. In substance abuse and other complex behaviors with multifactorial etiologies, the effects of individual genes are small and dependent on nonlinear interactions with other genes and environmental events. For example, the 7-repeat allele of the *DRD4* exon 3 has been associated with high novelty seeking and increased risk of opiate dependence (Kotler et al. 1997). However, high novelty seeking has also been reported to be associated with the 10-repeat allele of the dopamine transporter gene (*DAT1*), but only when the

---

Table 7–3. Genome scan–identified associations with polysubstance abuse

---

42 associations replicated in blacks and whites
9 associations also replicated in other genome scans
6 associations common to alcoholism:
Chromosomes 3, 4, 9, 11, 12, and 13
2 associations common to nicotine dependence:
Chromosomes 10 and X
1 association common to both alcoholism and nicotine dependence:
Chromosome 16

Note.   Genome scan of 1,004 subjects, using 1,494 nucleotide polymorphisms (Uhl et al. 2001).

Table 7–4. Convergent associations with polysubstance abuse

Chromosome	Locus
Chromosome 3	*D3S3053* (drugs, alcohol)
Chromosome 4	*ADH3* locus (drugs, alcohol)
Chromosome 9	*D9S319* (drugs, alcohol)
Chromosome 10	*D10S2469* (drugs, nicotine)
Chromosome 11	BDNF locus (drugs, alcohol)
Chromosome 12	*D12S1045* (drugs, alcohol)
Chromosome 13	*D13S762* (drugs, alcohol)
Chromosome 16	*D16S675* (drugs, alcohol, nicotine)
Chromosome X	*DXS8061* (drugs, nicotine)

Note.   ADH3=alcohol dehydrogenase 3 gene; BDNF=brain-derived neurotrophic factor.
Source.   Uhl et al. 2001.

DRD4 7-repeat allele is absent (Van Gestel et al. 2002). Consequently, it may be necessary to identify and evaluate sets of several genes simultaneously to predict risk of a complex behavior such as substance use or abuse in a particular individual (Comings et al. 2000).

Implications for Treatment of Substance Abuse

Insufficient knowledge exists to individualize treatment according to a person's genetic profile. However, as more specific molecular targets are identified, therapies can be developed to influence susceptibility and thereby prevent abuse or relapse into abuse.

The transition from substance use to abuse is largely influenced by nongenetic events unique to each individual. Likewise, military veterans who developed physiological dependence during wartime have been found to give up abuse on returning home (Robins et al. 1975). These findings indicate that individual self-efficacy, not genetic predisposition or physiological dependence, is the most important determinant of successful cessation of substance abuse. Accordingly, rather than blame the substance abuser's genetic predisposition or external influences that determine substance availability, the therapist must encourage the patient to accept responsibility for his or her abuse.

References

Bierut LJ, Rice JP, Goate A, et al: A genomic scan for habitual smoking in families of alcoholics. Am J Med Genet (in press)

Cadoret RJ, Yates WR, Troughton E, et al: Adoption study demonstrating two genetic pathways to drug abuse. Arch Gen Psychiatry 52:42–52, 1995

Chen CC, Lu RB, Chen YC, et al: Interaction between the functional polymorphisms of the alcohol-metabolism genes in protection against alcoholism. Am J Hum Genet 65:795–807, 1999

Cloninger CR: Neurogenetic adaptive mechanisms in alcoholism. Science 236:410–416, 1987

Cloninger CR, Sigvardsson S, Bohman M: Childhood personality predicts alcohol abuse in young adults. Alcohol Clin Exp Res 12:494–504, 1988

Cloninger CR, Van Eerdewegh P, Goate A, et al: Anxiety proneness linked to epistatic loci in genome scan of human personality traits. Am J Med Genet 81:313–317, 1998

Comings DE, Gade-Andavolu R, Gonzalez N, et al: A multivariate analysis of 59 candidate genes in personality traits: the temperament and character inventory. Clin Genet 58:375–385, 2000

Foroud T, Edenberg HJ, Goate A, et al: Alcoholism susceptibility loci: confirmation studies in a replicate sample and further mapping. Alcohol Clin Exp Res 24:933–945, 2000

Grove J, Daly AK, Bassendine MF, et al: Interleukin 10 promoter region polymorphisms and susceptibility to advanced alcoholic liver disease. Gut 46:540–545, 2000

Howard MO, Kivlahan D, Walker RD: Cloninger's tridimensional theory of personality and psychopathology: applications to substance use disorders. J Stud Alcohol 58:48–66, 1997

Kendler KS, Karkowski LM, Corey LA, et al: Genetic and environmental risk factors in the aetiology of illicit drug initiation and subsequent misuse in women. Br J Psychiatry 175:351–356, 1999

Kendler KS, Karkowski LM, Neale MC, et al: Illicit psychoactive substance use, heavy use, abuse, and dependence in a US population–based sample of male twins. Arch Gen Psychiatry 57:261–269, 2000

Kotler M, Cohen H, Segman R, et al: Excess dopamine D$_4$ receptor (*D4DR*) exon III seven repeat allele in opioid-dependent subjects. Mol Psychiatry 2:251–254, 1997

Reed T, Page WF, Viken RJ, et al: Genetic predisposition to organ-specific endpoints of alcoholism. Alcohol Clin Exp Res 20:1528–1533, 1996

Robins LN, Helzer JE, Davis DH: Narcotic use in southeast Asia and afterward: an interview study of 898 Vietnam returnees. Arch Gen Psychiatry 32:955–961, 1975

Sabol SZ, Nelson ML, Fisher C, et al: A genetic association for cigarette smoking behavior. Health Psychol 18:7–13, 1999

Savolainen VT, Pajarinen J, Perola M, et al: Polymorphism in the cytochrome P450 2E1 gene and the risk of alcoholic liver disease. J Hepatol 26:55–61, 1997

Sigvardsson S, Bohman M, Cloninger CR: Replication of the Stockholm Adoption Study of Alcoholism: confirmatory cross-fostering analysis. Arch Gen Psychiatry 53:681–687, 1996

Straub RE, Sullivan PF, Ma Y, et al: Susceptibility genes for nicotine dependence: a genome scan and followup in an independent sample suggest that regions on chromosomes 2, 4, 10, 16, 17 and 18 merit further study. Mol Psychiatry 4:129–144, 1999

True WR, Xian H, Scherrer JF, et al: Common genetic vulnerability for nicotine and alcohol dependence in men. Arch Gen Psychiatry 56:655–661, 1999

Tsuang MT, Lyons MJ, Meyer JM, et al: Co-occurrence of abuse of different drugs in men: the role of drug-specific and shared vulnerabilities. Arch Gen Psychiatry 55:967–972, 1998

Tsuang MT, Lyons MJ, Harley RM, et al: Genetic and environmental influences on transitions in drug use. Behav Genet 29:473–479, 1999

Uhl GR, Liu QR, Walther D, et al: Polysubstance abuse–vulnerability genes: genome scans for association, using 1,004 subjects and 1,494 single-nucleotide polymorphisms. Am J Hum Genet 69:1290–1300, 2001

Van Gestel S, Forsgren T, Claes S, et al: Epistatic effect of genes from the dopamine and serotonin systems on the temperament traits of novelty seeking and harm avoidance (letter). Mol Psychiatry 7:448–450, 2002

World Health Organization: International Statistical Classification of Diseases and Related Health Problems, 10th Revision. Geneva, World Health Organization, 1992

Principles of Learning in the Study and Treatment of Substance Abuse

Stephen T. Higgins, Ph.D.
Sarah H. Heil, Ph.D.

This chapter is an overview of experimental and clinical psychology research demonstrating that drugs promote repeated drug use for nonmedical purposes, in part through operant and respondent conditioning and social learning processes. This knowledge has led to a valuable and widely used set of theoretical concepts and experimental methods for studying substance use disorders in preclinical and clinical settings. Perhaps most important, this work has elucidated underlying behavioral processes involved in substance abuse (e.g., reinforcement, stimulus control) that have significant treatment implications. This information has been well integrated into basic science and clinical research practices in the area of substance use disorders but has been less well integrated into community treatment and policy arenas. For example, books on the treatment of substance use disorders sometimes fail to mention the reinforcing effects of abused drugs, and clinicians or policy makers sometimes discuss substance use disorders exclusively in terms of physical dependence and withdrawal or underlying psychopathology. Although those processes and concepts are an important part of a comprehensive account of substance use disorders, they do not completely explain them. Conditioning and social learning make fundamental contributions to the genesis and maintenance of substance use disorders and to their treatment. In this chapter, we attempt to illustrate how a broader appreciation of the importance of these learning processes can improve efforts to reduce substance use disorders.

Preparation of this chapter was supported in part by National Institute on Drug Abuse research grants R01-DA09378 and R01-DA08076 and training grant DA07242.

Drugs as Reinforcers

In the 1940s, experimental psychologists began developing methods for studying voluntary self-administration of drugs in laboratory animals (Spragg 1940). Initial studies used animals that were first made physically dependent on drugs through experimenter-administered drug exposure (e.g., Thompson and Schuster 1964). The animals learned an arbitrary response that resulted in delivery of a drug injection. These studies were important because of the methodology they introduced, but the effects observed were easily integrated with extant theories that posited that substance use disorders were driven by physical dependence and withdrawal. Shortly thereafter, however, studies using this new methodology showed that rats and monkeys that were not physically dependent would similarly learn to self-administer commonly abused drugs such as morphine, amphetamine, or cocaine (e.g., Deneau et al. 1969). Experimental variations of parameters such as the scheduled relationship between the learned response and drug administration influenced behavior in the same manner as when comparable manipulations were made using food, sex, or other unconditioned reinforcers as behavioral consequences. These findings provided an empirical foundation for the conclusion that abused drugs could function as unconditioned positive reinforcers (just as food, water, and sex could) and that drug seeking and use conformed to the principles of operant conditioning.

Operant conditioning is a basic form of learning in which the probability of voluntary behavior is influenced by its consequences. Several decades of experimental research have conclusively demonstrated that drug self-administration conforms to the principles of operant conditioning and that laboratory animals voluntarily consume most of the same drugs that humans abuse (Griffiths et al. 1980). Psychomotor stimulants, ethanol, nicotine, opioids, and sedatives function as reinforcers and promote voluntary self-administration of drugs in a variety of species. Physical dependence, tolerance, and withdrawal influence patterns of drug consumption in these self-administration arrangements, but the evidence shows that those are consequences of repeated drug use and not necessary conditions for drug self-administration to be established and maintained. When given unconstrained access to drugs of abuse such as cocaine and opiates, laboratory animals sometimes consumed lethal doses of the drugs

or engaged in repeated drug use to the exclusion of basic sustenance (Aigner and Balster 1978; Deneau et al. 1969). Such findings demonstrated that even these most extreme characteristics of substance abuse are not exclusively human phenomena.

Respondent conditioning, another basic form of learning, occurs when an environmental stimulus (a person, place, or thing) reliably predicts presentation of an unconditioned stimulus (e.g., drug delivery). Previously neutral environmental stimuli that reliably predict drug reinforcement often acquire conditioned stimulus effects through this conditioning process. For example, environmental stimuli become discriminative stimuli, or occasion setters, for urges to use drugs as well as for drug seeking and use. Such effects have been well documented in humans and nonhumans and are related to activation of limbic and other brain regions (Childress et al. 1999; Robinson and Berridge 1993). Environmental stimuli that are paired with drug use also acquire conditioned reinforcing effects, which work in concert with the unconditioned reinforcing effects of abused drugs to sustain the often extraordinary efforts of drug abusers to obtain and use drugs (Schindler et al. 2002).

Social Learning Factors

A complementary body of research on drug dependence as learned behavior addressed the fundamentally important influence of social factors on the behavioral action of drugs in humans. An important advance in this area applied the social learning concepts of modeling and imitation to human drug use. For example, alcoholic individuals imitate the rates and patterns of alcohol ingestion modeled by others drinking in their presence (Caudill and Lipscomb 1980).

In another set of experimental studies, prototypical drugs of abuse shared the effect of facilitating social interaction. For example, when under the acute influence of alcohol or other abused drugs, individuals would forgo opportunities to earn money, preferring to interact socially with other research volunteers (Higgins et al. 1989). These studies illustrated that in addition to the conditioned and unconditioned reinforcing effects of abused drugs, repeated drug use might also be supported through drug-produced enhancement of reinforcement derived from social interaction.

Another series of rigorous experimental studies demonstrated that drinking by alcoholic persons was sensitive to social consequences (Griffiths et al. 1978). For example, drinking decreased significantly when hospitalized alcoholic patients had to forgo—as a consequence of drinking—either social interaction with other alcoholic patients on the ward or visitation privileges with a romantic partner.

In a series of studies, the behavioral effects of drugs were influenced significantly by what drug users were told or believed about the drugs they consumed, as opposed to the pharmacological effects of the substances per se. Instructing subjects that the substance they consumed was an active drug was a more important determinant of outcome than the pharmacological content of the substance. For example, whether social drinkers or nonabstinent alcoholic individuals consumed relatively large amounts of a beverage in a taste-testing procedure was determined by whether they were told that the beverage contained alcohol, rather than by the alcohol content of the drink (Marlatt et al. 1973). Alcohol doses were typically on the low side in these studies (0.5 g/kg), and there seems to be little doubt that use of higher doses would reveal a greater influence of pharmacological factors. That point notwithstanding, these findings illustrated a striking influence of nonpharmacological factors on behavioral effects of ethanol that theretofore had been attributed to the direct pharmacological effects of the drug. Such interactions are not unique to alcohol or to humans. A recent study involving nonhuman primates, for example, demonstrated a striking interaction between social context, neurobiology, and the reinforcing effects of cocaine (Morgan et al. 2002).

Theoretical Implications

Such advances regarding the role of learning in drug use and its behavioral consequences have had important theoretical implications. First, theories on substance use disorders couched exclusively in terms of physiological and pharmacological processes of tolerance and withdrawal (Jellinek 1960), even theories including conditioned tolerance and withdrawal (Wikler 1980), are recognized to be incomplete. This advance in the conceptual understanding of substance use disorders is discernible across consecutive editions of DSM. In DSM-III (American Psychiatric Association 1980), the psychoactive substance use disorders were defined exclusively in terms of tolerance and withdrawal. In DSM-III-R (American Psychiatric Association

1987), tolerance and withdrawal made up four of the nine symptoms, and the remaining five were behavioral symptoms. In DSM-IV (American Psychiatric Association 1994) and DSM-IV-TR (American Psychiatric Association 2000), tolerance and withdrawal were retained and in some ways were made more prominent than in DSM-III-R, but they represent only two of the seven symptoms and are explicitly noted to be neither necessary nor sufficient for a diagnosis of dependence.

Second, this body of scientific evidence contradicts self-medication theories in which personality disorders or other psychiatric disturbances are necessary conditions for substance use disorders. The literature on drug self-administration provides compelling scientific evidence that repeated substance use is a product of normal learning processes that are an integral part of the evolutionary history of humans and other species. Thus, any healthy individual is deemed to possess the neurobiological systems necessary to experience drug-produced reinforcement and hence has the potential to develop a substance use disorder, given appropriate opportunity and supporting environmental circumstances. In brief, psychopathology can significantly increase the probability that a substance use disorder will develop (Regier et al. 1990) but the presence of psychopathology is not necessary for such a disorder to emerge.

Third, studies on instructions and beliefs as determinants of the behavioral actions of alcohol have provided the impetus for current theoretical and clinical interests in cognitive and expectancy factors in substance use disorders (see Chapter 29, "Cognitive, Behavioral, and Motivational Therapies," in this volume). Humans bring complex histories to drug-using situations—histories often involving years of direct and vicarious experience with drug use and years of assimilating peer influence and other cultural views about reasons for and consequences of substance use. These rich histories influence substance consumption practices and the consequences of substance use, and they provide therapeutic targets for treatment interventions.

A Learning-Based Conceptual Framework

This learning-based approach raises an important question: If all biologically intact humans possess the basic prerequisites for a substance use disorder, and drug use for recreational purposes is quite prevalent, why is the prevalence of these disorders not higher? A complete answer to this question is not available, but several decades of behavioral research have revealed a number of determinants of substance use, abuse, and dependence that have important clinical and policy implications.

First, cost is an important determinant of substance use by recreational users and dependent individuals (Chaloupka et al. 1999). *Cost* is used broadly here to subsume 1) monetary price; 2) the effort required to search out and obtain substances; 3) adverse events encountered while obtaining and using substances and while recovering from substance use; and 4) what is forfeited by choosing to allocate time to substance consumption.

Second, environmental context is an important determinant of substance use. Contexts lacking alternative sources of nonpharmacological reinforcement, for example, can promote acquisition of drugs and maintenance of drug use (Higgins 1997). Similarly, individuals lacking skills or resources necessary to locate available sources of alternative reinforcement are likely to be at greater risk for substance use disorders. Such skill deficits likely contribute to the higher prevalence rates of these disorders among individuals with severe mental illness, those with lower educational achievement, and those who are unemployed (Drake et al. 2002; Substance Abuse and Mental Health Services Administration 2002). Also, as noted above in the section on social learning factors, social or peer influence can modulate the risk of substance use disorders, likely through modeling of abusive or risky consumption patterns and through social reinforcement of deviant behavior (Guo et al. 2002). Family context also influences the risk of substance use disorders, not only through the substance use practices and views of the parents but also through family behavior-management practices, interpersonal conflict, and the degree of parent monitoring of child behavior. Finally, neighborhoods and other settings can influence risk, through substance-using opportunities afforded to youths and probably through other social-learning processes (see Chapter 6, "Epidemiology of Drug Dependence," in this volume).

Third, individual differences must be considered. Genetics significantly influence the risk of smoking, alcoholism, and other substance use disorders (see Chapter 7, "Genetics of Substance Abuse," in this volume). How such genetic differences in risk are expressed is not well understood. Twin and adoption studies show an association between impulsive personality characteristics and the risk of severe forms of early-onset polysubstance abuse (see Chapter 7). Variations in individual sensitivity to drug-produced reinforcement and to related learning factors discussed in this chapter have been well demonstrated in preclinical studies and offer a reasonable possibility that is being pursued by researchers in behavioral genetics (Elmer et al. 1998).

Consistent with the association between impulsivity and risk of substance abuse, noted in twin and adoption studies, recent research has documented a potentially important association between discounting of delayed reinforcement and substance abuse (Bickel and Johnson 2003; Bickel et al. 1999). In this area of research, *impulsive behavior* is defined as choosing a smaller, more immediate reinforcer over a larger, more delayed reinforcer. Individual preference for immediate versus delayed reinforcement is assessed by having subjects make a series of choices between different amounts of money or drugs or between other reinforcing events, with all described as being available after different temporal delays. A typical question might be "Would you prefer $100 today or $200 a month from now?" Cigarette smokers, opioid abusers, problem drinkers, and heterogeneous samples of substance abusers have been demonstrated to exhibit greater preference for smaller, more immediate reinforcement than for larger, more delayed reinforcement, compared with samples of nonabusers matched for relevant sociodemographic characteristics (Bickel and Johnson 2003). Interestingly, former abusers have been shown to score between current abusers and nonabusers (Bickel et al. 1999). Women with family histories positive for alcohol dependence have been shown to be distinguishable from those with negative histories through the former's greater preference for smaller, more immediate reinforcement, but men with differing family histories were not distinguishable on that basis (Petry et al. 2002). Although it is a relatively new area of research in terms of application to substance abuse, delay discounting may provide insights into differences in risk of substance abuse between individuals and within individuals over time.

Clinical Practices

Knowledge regarding the role of conditioning and social learning processes in substance use disorders has contributed to the development of a number of efficacious treatments for substance abuse. Some key examples are briefly described here.

Contingency Management

Much of the information in this chapter underscores the operant nature of drug abuse (i.e., behavior influenced by its consequences). It follows logically that the probability that patients will abstain from drug use should be modifiable through frequent, systematic delivery of reinforcing consequences for abstinence. Interventions designed to provide such systematic reinforcement are termed *contingency-management interventions* and are typically used as adjuncts to more broadly focused therapies. In controlled trials, contingency-management interventions have reduced most forms of substance use, especially illicit drug abuse (Higgins and Silverman 1999).

The most thoroughly researched of the contingency-management interventions used to achieve drug abstinence is an approach that involves vouchers exchangeable for retail items, the earning of which is contingent on drug abstinence (Higgins et al. 2002). This approach was originally developed to improve retention and increase cocaine abstinence among cocaine-dependent outpatients (Budney and Higgins 1998). The efficacy of the use of vouchers for the purpose of outpatient treatment of cocaine dependence is now well established (Higgins et al. 2002), and plans are under way to move the intervention into effectiveness testing in community clinics. Vouchers are also now used in the treatment of dependence on alcohol (Petry et al. 2000), marijuana (Budney et al. 2000), nicotine (Donatelle et al. 2000), and opioids (Bickel et al. 1997). Use of vouchers holds promise as an efficacious intervention for special populations of substance abusers, including pregnant and recently-postpartum women (Donatelle et al. 2000), adolescents (Corby et al. 2000), and patients with serious mental illness (Sigmon et al. 2000). Overall, voucher-based incentives hold promise as an innovative intervention for a wide range of substance abuse problems and populations.

Skills Training

The skill levels of many substance abusers are limited to an extent sufficient to make managing challenges of everyday life stressful and to preclude participation in important activities that could function as alternatives to substance abuse. Efficacious skills-training interventions, developed by learning-based therapists, reduce those deficits and improve substance abuse treatment outcomes; these interventions include social-skills and coping-skills training (Monti et al. 1995), relapse prevention training (see Chapter 29, "Cognitive, Behavioral, and Motivational Therapies," in this volume), and behavioral marital therapy involving communication skills (O'Farrell 1995).

Community Reinforcement Approach

Participation in communities that reinforce a healthy lifestyle is considered by many experts in substance abuse to be important to successful recovery. Learning-based therapists have developed interventions designed to systematically rearrange significant aspects of local communities to differentially support an abstinent lifestyle. For example, the community reinforcement approach attempts to increase alternatives to a substance-abusing lifestyle through improved family and marital relations and through vocational, social, and recreational activities. To the extent possible, participation in these alternatives is contingent on abstinence from substance abuse. In a series of controlled trials, the community reinforcement approach produced impressive treatment outcomes in severely and less impaired alcoholic individuals (Meyers and Smith 1995), in homeless alcoholic persons (Smith et al. 1998), and, when used in combination with voucher-based incentives, in cocaine-dependent and opioid-dependent outpatients (Bickel et al. 1997; Higgins et al. 2000).

Brief Interventions

Learning-based therapists have been leaders in the development of efficacious, cost-effective, brief interventions that can be delivered in primary care and other medical settings and through community agencies (Fiore 2000; Heather 2002). These interventions are most commonly used to treat problem drinkers (usually at an early point) and cigarette smokers. Treatment content and duration vary depending on the population, setting, and other factors, but treatment typically involves problem identification and assessment, a specific recommendation for reducing or discontinuing problematic substance use, and follow-up visits to assess change, with treatment sessions as short as 10–15 minutes. Despite these relatively modest characteristics, brief interventions have achieved impressive reductions in substance abuse and related problems. The likely mechanism of action of these interventions is a socially significant individual's (e.g., a physician's) verbal mediation of a contingency between continuing substance abuse and a serious adverse consequence (e.g., liver disease).

Learning-Based Treatments and Comorbidity

There is growing recognition of the importance of offering integrated substance abuse and mental health services to patients with comorbid substance abuse and other mental illness (Drake et al. 2002). Learning-based interventions for substance use disorders are conceptually consistent and thus easily integrated with many efficacious treatments for other psychiatric disorders. For example, behavioral treatments for anxiety disorders, depression, and insomnia are included as components of the community reinforcement approach used for cocaine dependence (Budney and Higgins 1998). Combining pharmacotherapies with learning-based treatments for substance use disorders is common, and it is likely to be associated with fewer philosophical objections to psychopharmacology than is sometimes the case with more traditional treatments for substance abuse.

Conclusion

Substance use disorders result from a complex interplay of many factors. Operant and respondent conditioning and social learning are important psychological factors that contribute to the genesis and maintenance of and recovery from these disorders. These psychological factors and their related methods are not a magic bullet to alleviate substance use disorders. Rather, they represent a thoroughly researched set of scientific concepts, principles, and practices that, if better disseminated and applied, can improve efforts to reduce substance use disorders. Persons trained in the health sciences are probably the best source for the dissemination of such scientific information into community settings and practices.

References

Aigner TG, Balster RL: Choice behavior in rhesus monkeys: cocaine versus food. Science 201:534–535, 1978

American Psychiatric Association: Diagnostic and Statistical Manual of Mental Disorders, 3rd Edition. Washington, DC, American Psychiatric Association, 1980

American Psychiatric Association: Diagnostic and Statistical Manual of Mental Disorders, 3rd Edition, Revised. Washington, DC, American Psychiatric Association, 1987

American Psychiatric Association: Diagnostic and Statistical Manual of Mental Disorders, 4th Edition. Washington, DC, American Psychiatric Association, 1994

American Psychiatric Association: Diagnostic and Statistical Manual of Mental Disorders, 4th Edition, Text Revision. Washington, DC, American Psychiatric Association, 2000

Bickel WK, Johnson MW: Delay discounting: a fundamental behavioral process in drug dependence, in Time and Decision: Economic and Psychological Perspectives on Intertemporal Choice. Edited by Loewenstein G, Reed D, Baumeister R. New York, Russell Sage, 2003, pp 419–440

Bickel WK, Amass L, Higgins ST, et al: Effects of adding behavioral treatment to opioid detoxification with buprenorphine. J Consult Clin Psychol 65:803–810, 1997

Bickel WK, Odum AL, Madden GL: Impulsivity and cigarette smoking: delay discounting in current, never, and ex-smokers. Psychopharmacology (Berl) 146:447–454, 1999

Budney AJ, Higgins ST: Treating Cocaine Dependence: A Community Reinforcement Plus Vouchers Approach. Rockville, MD, National Institute on Drug Abuse, 1998

Budney AJ, Higgins ST, Radonovich KJ, et al: Adding voucher-based incentives to coping skills and motivational enhancement improves outcomes during treatment for marijuana dependence. J Consult Clin Psychol 68:1051–1061, 2000

Caudill BD, Lipscomb TR: Modeling influences on alcoholics' rates of alcohol consumption. J Appl Behav Anal 13:355–365, 1980

Chaloupka FJ, Grossman M, Bickel WK, et al (eds): The Economic Analysis of Substance Use and Abuse: An Integration of Econometric and Behavioral Economic Research. Chicago, IL, University of Chicago Press, 1999

Childress AR, Mozley PD, McElgin W, et al: Limbic activation during cue-induced cocaine craving. Am J Psychiatry 156:11–18, 1999

Corby EA, Roll JR, Ledgerwood DW, et al: Contingency management interventions for treating the substance abuse of adolescents: a feasibility study. Exp Clin Psychopharmacol 8:371–376, 2000

Deneau G, Yanagita T, Seevers MH: Self-administration of psychoactive substances by the monkey. Psychopharmacologia 16:30–48, 1969

Donatelle RJ, Prows SL, Champeau D, et al: Randomised controlled trial using social and financial incentives for high risk pregnant smokers: significant other supporter (SOS) program. Tob Control 9 (suppl 3):III67–III69, 2000

Drake RE, Wallach MA, Alverson HS, et al: Psychosocial aspects of substance abuse by clients with severe mental illness. J Nerv Ment Dis 190:100–106, 2002

Elmer GI, Miner LL, Pickens RW: The contributions of genetic factors in cocaine and other drug abuse, in Cocaine Abuse Research: Behavior, Pharmacology, and Clinical Applications. Edited by Higgins ST, Katz JL. San Diego, CA, Academic Press, 1998, pp 289–311

Fiore MC: US public health service clinical practice guideline: treating tobacco use and dependence. Respir Care 45:1200–1262, 2000

Griffiths RR, Bigelow GE, Liebson IA: Relationship of social factors to ethanol self-administration in alcoholics, in Alcoholism: New Directions in Behavioral Research and Treatment. Edited by Nathan PE, Marlatt GA, Loberg TT. New York, Plenum, 1978, pp 351–379

Griffiths RR, Bigelow GE, Henningfield JE: Similarities in animal and human drug taking behavior, in Advances in Substance Abuse: Behavioral and Biological Research. Edited by Mello NK. Greenwich, CT, JAI Press, 1980, pp 1–90

Guo J, Hill KG, Hawkins JD, et al: A developmental analysis of sociodemographic, family, and peer effects on adolescent illicit drug initiation. J Am Acad Child Adolesc Psychiatry 41:838–845, 2002

Heather N: Effectiveness of brief interventions proved beyond reasonable doubt. Addiction 97:293–294, 2002

Higgins ST: The influence of alternative reinforcers on cocaine use and abuse: a brief review. Pharmacol Biochem Behav 57:419–427, 1997

Higgins ST, Silverman K (eds): Motivating Behavior Change Among Illicit Drug Abusers: Research on Contingency Management Interventions. Washington, DC, American Psychological Association, 1999

Higgins ST, Hughes JR, Bickel WK: Effects of d-amphetamine on choice of social versus monetary reinforcement: a discrete-trial test. Pharmacol Biochem Behav 34:297–301, 1989

Higgins ST, Wong CJ, Badger GJ, et al: Contingent reinforcement increases cocaine abstinence during outpatient treatment and one year of follow-up. J Consult Clin Psychol 68:64–72, 2000

Higgins ST, Alessi SM, Dantona RL: Voucher-based incentives: a substance abuse treatment innovation. Addict Behav 27:887–910, 2002

Jellinek EM: The Disease Concept of Alcoholism. New Brunswick, NJ, Hillhouse, 1960

Marlatt GA, Deming B, Reid J: Loss of control drinking in alcoholics. J Abnorm Psychol 81:233–241, 1973

Meyers RJ, Smith JE: Clinical Guide to Alcohol Treatment: The Community Reinforcement Approach. New York, Guilford, 1995

Monti PM, Rohsenow DJ, Colby SM, et al: Coping and social skills training, in Handbook of Alcoholism Treatment Approaches: Effective Alternatives, 2nd Edition. Edited by Hester RK, Miller WR. Boston, MA, Allyn & Bacon, 1995, pp 221–241

Morgan D, Grant KA, Gage HD, et al: Social dominance in monkeys: dopamine D_2 receptors and cocaine self-administration. Nat Neurosci 5:169–174, 2002

O'Farrell TJ: Marital and family therapy, in Handbook of Alcoholism Treatment Approaches: Effective Alternatives, 2nd Edition. Edited by Hester RK, Miller WR. Boston, MA, Allyn & Bacon, 1995, pp 195–220

Petry NM, Martin B, Cooney JL, et al: Give them prizes, and they will come: contingency management for treatment of alcohol dependence. J Consult Clin Psychol 68:250–257, 2000

Petry NM, Kirby KN, Kranzler HR: Effects of gender and family history of alcohol dependence on a behavioral task of impulsivity in healthy subjects. J Stud Alcohol 63:83–90, 2002

Regier DA, Farmer ME, Rae DS, et al: Comorbidity of mental disorders with alcohol and other drug abuse. JAMA 264:2511–2518, 1990

Robinson TE, Berridge KC: The neural basis of drug craving: an incentive-sensitization theory of addiction. Brain Res Brain Res Rev 18:247–291, 1993

Schindler CW, Panlilio LV, Goldberg SR: Second-order schedules of drug self-administration in animals. Psychopharmacology (Berl) 163:327–344, 2002

Sigmon SC, Steingard S, Badger GJ, et al: Contingent reinforcement of marijuana abstinence among individuals with serious mental illness: a feasibility study. Exp Clin Psychopharmacol 8:509–517, 2000

Smith JE, Meyers RJ, Delaney HD: The community reinforcement approach with homeless alcohol-dependent individuals. J Consult Clin Psychol 66:541–548, 1998

Spragg SDS: Morphine Addiction in Chimpanzees (Comparative Psychology Monographs, Vol 15). Baltimore, MD, Johns Hopkins University Press, 1940

Substance Abuse and Mental Health Services Administration: 2001 National Household Survey on Drug Abuse. Rockville, MD, Substance Abuse and Mental Health Services Administration, Office of Applied Studies, 2002

Thompson T, Schuster CR: Morphine self-administration, food-reinforced, and avoidance behaviors in rhesus monkeys. Psychopharmacologia 71:87–94, 1964

Wikler A: Opioid Dependence. New York, Plenum, 1980

Cross-Cultural Aspects of Substance Abuse

Joseph Westermeyer, M.D., M.P.H., Ph.D.

The term *culture* refers to the sum total of a group's life ways, including the group's material culture, worldview, social organization, symbols, status, child raising, language, technology, and citizenship. The term *ethnicity,* as used in multiethnic societies, applies to peoples from diverse cultural backgrounds who share a common national culture. Distinctive characteristics include identity with a national origin, religious practice, language besides English spoken in the home or neighborhood, dress, diet, nonnational holidays or ceremonial events, traditional family rituals, and use of disposable income and free time (Keyes 1976). *Subculture* refers to groups within a culture that have distinctive cultural characteristics but that cannot exist independent of the group. Substance use, abuse, or commerce can foster highly cohesive and distinctive subcultures, such as tavern culture, cocktail lounge culture, opium den culture, and crack house culture (Bourgois 1989; Dumont 1967; Westermeyer 1974a). *Cross-cultural* can refer to the comparison of psychosocial characteristics across two or more culture groups or, in the medical context, to treatment in which the clinician and the patient belong to different cultures (Comas-Diaz and Griffith 1988). Comparisons across cultures are often termed *etic,* whereas noncomparable, culture-specific elements or patterns are termed *emic* (Lefley and Pedersen 1986).

Prehistory

The development of psychoactive substances began millennia before written records (Westermeyer 1988). People of Africa, Asia, and Europe prepared beverage alcohol from fruits, grains, tubers, and mammalian milk. They also grew opium, cannabis, and some plants with stimulant properties, such as khat (also spelled *chat, kat,* and *qat*) in the Red Sea area, kola in other parts of Africa, kratom in Southeast Asia, and betel across South Asia to Oceania (Burton-Bradley 1977; Getahun and Krikorias 1973).

The champions of psychoactive substance invention were the peoples of the Americas. Before A.D. 1500, they developed several hundred stimulant or hallucinogenic compounds, including tobacco, cocaine, coffee, and peyote (DuToit 1977). American Aztecs and Papago prepared beverage alcohol from cactus and other plants—methods still used commercially today (Anawalt and Berdan 1992; Waddell 1976).

Routes of Administration

People in Africa, Asia, and Europe consumed psychoactive substances primarily by ingesting them. They also chewed some substances—for example, betel nut and khat (Getahun and Krikorias 1973). Again, the peoples of the Americas before A.D. 1500 were foremost in developing innovative means for consuming drugs. They discovered several other routes of administration besides eating, drinking, and chewing (Negrete 1978)—namely snuffing, smoking, and rectal clysis (Furst and Coe 1977). Chewing, smoking, snuffing, and clysis avoided first-pass metabolism in the liver and accelerated onset of drug effect.

Social Controls

Laws regarding substance use and abuse appeared in the earliest codes of law (Anawalt and Berdan 1992). The Aztecs had laws governing when and how much alcohol could be imbibed, and these laws took into account one's social status, role, and age; the punishments for breaking the laws ranged up to and included death (Anawalt and Berdan 1992). Typical patterns of informal social control have included the following:

- Substance use restricted to ceremonies or holidays
- Substance use restricted to large group or extended family events
- Proscription of taboo substances by certain groups (e.g., prohibition of alcohol use by some Christians, Hindus, and Muslims)

History

Before A.D. 1500, sporadic cases of alcoholism and addiction were recognized over hundreds of years. Wine, tobacco, and probably other substances were traded within localized commercial regions. However, no known dramatic changes in substance use or abuse accompanied these early empires and localized commercial routes (Westermeyer 1988).

Around A.D. 1500, improved methods of shipbuilding and new navigation technology led to safer and less-expensive commerce. These changes resulted in the exchange of psychoactive substances across thousands of miles. The post–A.D. 1500 world produced two momentous substance abuse epidemics, one associated with opium in Asia and one associated with alcohol in Europe. It could be argued that alcohol and volatile inhalant abuse among the aboriginal peoples of the Americas and Australia is a third epidemic (Brady 1992; Eastwell 1979; Manson et al. 1992).

Tobacco smoking, which spread rapidly around the world during the 1500s, may have set the stage for the subsequent Asian opium epidemic. Tobacco smoking reached the China Sea within decades of its discovery by Europeans in North America. Asian smokers consumed it in tobacco houses, the meeting places of the day. Tobacco houses subsequently became associated with political sedition and were outlawed in many Asian countries. Tobacco raising and smoking went underground and continued. Around the same time, opium—previously known as an herbal medication—began to be smoked in social settings. By the 1600s, the Asian opium epidemic was well under way, dwarfing the tobacco smoking habit that preceded it. Commercial interests, huge profits, and international politics fueled the epidemic, which was also fostered by local corruption and an absence of cultural strictures against opium use (Fields and Tararin 1970; Merrill 1942; Terry and Pellens 1928).

Attempts at addressing the opium epidemic included enactment of anti-opium laws, establishment of government ministries charged with eliminating opium production and commerce, and formation of private anti-opium societies that aided addicted people trying to quit using opium and that warned the general public about opium. By the mid-1900s, an estimated 18 million Chinese were addicted to opium. Democratic, leftist, and rightist governments in China, Japan, both Koreas, and Taiwan also reversed their opium endemics around the same time (i.e., the 1950s and 1960s). The opiate endemic continues in Thailand, Laos, Burma, Malaysia, Bangladesh, Pakistan, India, Afghanistan, and several countries in the Middle East.

The gin epidemic began in England around the 1600s and continued for almost two centuries, with some vestiges remaining in the 1900s. It involved rum and gin from the Caribbean, where it could be purchased cheaply (because of slave labor) and then used as ballast in ships returning from commercial voyages. Although mead had been drunk traditionally in England, the population had limited experience with distilled beverage alcohol. During the development of the gin epidemic, the Industrial Revolution was also under way, with a massive shift of the population from farms and small towns to industrial towns of various sizes. Because a calorie of alcohol cost less than a calorie of carbohydrate in bread, potent economic forces favored the use of gin and rum as food. Because workers were thought to perform better after moderate drinking, taverns were open briefly in the morning and again at noon so that workers could imbibe before and during work (Rodin 1981).

Public and private efforts gradually brought the gin epidemic under control in the seventeenth, eighteenth, and nineteenth centuries. An import duty on beverages reduced economic incentives to drink. Eight-page booklets detailed the family, health, and social consequences of excessive drinking. Around this time, abstinence-oriented Christian denominations developed, leading eventually to the founding of Alcoholics Anonymous in the twentieth century (Aaron and Musto 1981).

The first pandemic of youthful drug abuse began in the mid-1900s and involved all continents (Cameron 1968). During World War II, tens of millions of young men were transported long distances from home and exposed to years of combat. This tremendous undertaking affected not only the combatants but also many civilian populations in Asia. Combatants were exposed to beverage alcohol, amphetamines, opiates, and other drugs not known in their native lands. Returning home to high unemployment, lost youth, and devastated countries, many combatants used nontraditional forms of psychoactive substances. A *youth culture* with its own nontraditional dress, music, mores, morals, and drugs appeared in many countries during the latter half of the twentieth century (Deutsch 1975; Gfroerer and De La Rosa 1993; Maddahian et al. 1986). The resurgence of fundamentalist (and abstinence-oriented) Buddhist, Christian, and Islamic sects across the globe may have its roots in societal responses to youth culture, including youthful drug use and abuse, just as widespread drug use may have been a response to fundamentalist religiosity (Galanter and Buckley 1978; Galanter and Westermeyer 1980; Westermeyer and Walzer 1975).

From Cottage Industry to High-Tech Industry

Before the 1800s, much of the production and distribution of drugs of abuse depended on high-labor, low-tech methods. Substances such as opium and alcohol were produced in agricultural settings, using human and animal power. Rapid, efficient intercontinental sailing ships and navigation technology had stimulated intercontinental trade in substances, but local distribution depended largely on human and animal transport. Because the technology of the day was widely known and available to virtually anyone, alcohol and drugs were produced and distributed mostly on a small scale to meet local needs. Distribution was effected through local barter and shopkeepers. Until the opium and gin epidemics, few producers, shippers, or retailers depended solely on alcohol or drugs for their livelihoods. As cottage industry techniques gave way to myriad technological advances, new substance-focused occupations and even industries evolved. New social and health problems also appeared (Westermeyer 1988).

Since the early 1800s, advancing technology has resulted in more efficient and rapid means of drug administration. The development of the syringe and hollow needle permitted the user to avoid the first-pass effect of the liver and consume the entire drug dose. Cigarette production fostered all-day tobacco smoking and dependence. Some drugs can be administered via skin patches. These new methods of administration have resulted in new medical and public health challenges (Davoli et al. 1997). Parenteral drug administration has produced epidemics of drug-related maladies (e.g., AIDS, hepatitis B and C), which have led to increased drug smoking and snuffing in recent years (Perez-Jimenez and Robert 1997).

Concentration of Traditional Substances

Alcohol distillation and the preparation of hashish oil were early inventions to increase potency. During the 1800s, chemical concentrates of opium (morphine and heroin) and coca leaves (cocaine) were developed. These concentrates facilitated the use of these substances by snorting, smoking, and parenteral injection. Whereas crude plant compounds had limited shelf lives and were bulky, odoriferous, and easily detected, heroin and cocaine had long shelf lives and were highly compact and much less odoriferous. These concentrated compounds lent themselves to prolonged storage, smuggling, and secretive retail commerce. In addition, some new compounds (such as heroin) crossed the blood-brain barrier more rapidly than traditional mixtures and therefore came to be in greater demand (Westermeyer 1982).

Synthetic Psychoactive Substances

In the 1800s, synthetic psychoactive substances began to be produced. Soon after the development of the gaseous anesthetics nitrous oxide, chloroform, and ether, recreational users began using them. Early abusers were principally medical and pharmaceutical workers. Development of the petroleum industry during the later 1800s and early 1900s led to inexpensive, readily available industrial, cleaning, and fuel compounds that could produce relaxation or an altered state of consciousness. Abusers of petroleum chemicals have included industrial workers, gas station workers, mechanics, unemployed individuals, children and adolescents, alcoholic and addicted prisoners, aboriginal peoples, and military inductees in basic training or on bivouac (Beauvais et al. 1985; Westermeyer 1987).

In the early 1900s, invention of synthetic sedatives and stimulants brought the newly developing pharmaceutical industry into the picture as a producer of addictive drugs. By the 1930s, barbiturate addiction was appearing in industrialized countries. Sporadic cases of amphetamine abuse were seen before World War II, but the use of these drugs by the military catapulted them into widespread use in some countries, producing the first amphetamine epidemics after the war (Tamura 1989). In preparation for World War II, various pharmaceutical houses developed synthetic opioid drugs, anticipating that raw opium might not be available during conflict. This process led to the development of many synthetic opioids with various durations of action—from methadone at one extreme to the short-acting drug fentanyl at the other. In the later 1900s, "outlaw" chemists synthesized new compounds with psychoactive properties, the so-called designer drugs that were supposed to have specific desirable effects.

Smuggling and Distribution of Illicit Substances

Smuggling involves actions by individuals sophisticated in operating illegally at one or more national boundaries. World War II, which displaced millions of people, created a huge reservoir of such persons in many countries around the world, and refugee movements since that time have done the same. Although the vast majority of these people are law-abiding, a sufficient number are drawn by the drug trade, keeping it

not only viable but also active and largely successful. Small airplanes, cigarette boats, and extensive ship, boat, and truck traffic have enabled the transportation of illicit substances over great distances with relative ease (Simmons and Gold 1973).

Community-level retail distribution of illicit substances remains a cottage industry around the world. Its features include the following:

- Low capital investment for starting up (e.g., a storefront or car, a gun, a day's or week's supply of drugs)
- A relationship and/or shared identity between buyer and seller
- Multiple distribution and sales points (so that inactivation of one point does not eliminate the trade)
- High profits relative to investment
- Reduced risk through corruption of police and elected officials

Ethnic Identity and Substance Use

Culturally prescribed use, in which an individual must use a psychoactive substance under certain cultural circumstances, exists among many ethnic groups in the United States. Examples include consumption of wine at Jewish Passover seders and at Catholic masses and peyote chewing at ceremonies of the Native American Church (La Barre 1964). Prescribed use subserves religious and social ends. Duration of use and dosages are also prescribed. Failure to use the substance can be considered unfriendly.

Forbidden use or *taboo* for some substances exists in all societies. Use of certain substances is forbidden under any circumstances. Examples include heroin in the United States, alcohol in Saudi Arabia, and caffeine among Mormons. Taboo tends to work well as long as the individual remains affiliated with the ethnic group proscribing the use; separation from the group tends to erode the taboo. Because no society can enculturate its members into the safe, healthful use of all available substances, most psychoactive substances are forbidden or available only under specific circumstances (e.g., through medical prescriptions).

Substances have taken on symbolic meaning in some instances. Psychoactive substances have come to represent certain values, attitudes, identities, or characteristics. One form of substance-related symbolism involves ethnic identity (Carstairs 1954). For example, among many Jewish people, drunkenness or alcoholism is seen as non-Jewish. Many Muslims consider any use of alcohol to be sinful (Chafetz 1964). Throughout history, substances have at times possessed political symbolism. For example, the Irish long distilled the illicit whiskey poteen in order to avoid English taxation and English-manufactured beverage alcohol (Connell 1961). In recent decades, cannabis has been a symbol of rebellion against established order (Cameron 1968).

Substance use has also been a social bridge. In parts of Latin America, drinking establishments have served as meeting places for persons of differing class and ethnic backgrounds (Heath 1971). Likewise, in parts of Africa, beer gardens have served as egalitarian social venues for people of different races and tribes (Wolcott 1974).

Cultural Risk Factors

Lack of prescription or proscription, in which the culture or ethnic group neither requires nor forbids use of a substance, leaves the decision to the individual (Baasher 1981). This in-between state most predisposes individuals to substance abuse and dependence, especially abuse of and dependence on highly addictive substances such as alcohol, cocaine, opiates, and tobacco.

Norm conflict occurs when ideal norms and behavioral norms differ within a culture. One ideal norm may be that substance use does not occur, whereas behavioral norms may imply that such use is expected. As the gap between ideal and behavioral norms increases, the presumed conflict increases. Norm conflicts occur because individuals rather than entire societies make the choices regarding substance use (Westermeyer 1999).

Pathogenic use patterns can occur as a behavioral norm, especially in groups with norm conflict regarding substance use. An example of such a pathogenic use pattern is bingeing on alcohol. This pattern exists among some northern European groups, some Native American tribes, some island communities in the Pacific, and many American college students. It is likely to lead to pathological use of alcohol among vulnerable persons; in some groups, lifetime risk of alcohol abuse can occur in up to half of the men and a quarter of the women (Boehnlein et al. 1992–1993; Robin et al. 1998).

Technological changes can render a traditional use pattern unsafe. Particularly at risk are societies that formerly accepted very heavy intoxication at ceremonial times or that permitted alcohol or drug use during certain types of work. For example, a heavy drinker riding home in an oxcart from a New Year celebration may be relatively safe and is unlikely to harm others. The same person riding a bicycle or a motorcycle, or driving a car or a truck, is at serious risk of harming himself or herself and others. Intoxicated mariners today risk the lives of hundreds of people (e.g., in the case of a ferryboat) or risk damaging an entire ecosystem (e.g., in the case of an oil tanker). Even low blood levels of psychoactive substances can impede certain highly complex tasks, such as landing an airplane.

Inadequate *ensocialization* occurs if the prescriptions and proscriptions regarding substances are not taught to children. Teaching occurs initially by role modeling and later through supervised use in ritual settings. To be effective, this aspect of culture must be taught in a consistent fashion during infancy, childhood, and adolescence. Some ethnic groups do an excellent job of ensocializing their children into appropriate prescriptions and proscriptions regarding substances (Bennett and Ames 1985). Individuals who leave their ethnic groups of origin are at risk for substance abuse if they migrate to groups that foster pathogenic substance use (Eaton and Weil 1955).

Disenfranchised groups can play major roles in the drug trade. Examples of these groups include the Chiu Chao minority in Hong Kong, Hmong and Iu Mien minorities in Laos and Thailand, Corsicans and Sicilians in Europe, and Middle Eastern refugees and immigrants in parts of Latin America. Funds raised by such groups through the drug trade have supported revolutionary and nationalistic movements, guerilla wars, and terrorism (Westermeyer 1982).

Generational change can influence the forms of psychoactive substance use within a given culture (Keaulana and Whitney 1990). Such change often involves the replacement of traditional cottage industry substances (e.g., locally grown tobacco, locally produced beer or wine) with industry-produced substances (e.g., manufactured cigarettes, imported beer or spirits). In some situations, young people have used substances unfamiliar to earlier generations. Secular use then replaces ritual or ceremonial use, individual choice replaces group decision making, and untried patterns replace patterns that evolved over centuries.

Anomie, loss of a positive ethnic identity, is apt to occur among traditional peoples whose technological culture has been rapidly and extensively undermined by the sudden influx of foreign influences. Rapid and fundamental changes in technological bases of a culture can provoke tremendous changes in social organization, family relationships, cultural symbols, and other aspects of culture that affect psychoactive use patterns (Caetano et al. 1983). Conquest by a foreign power with dramatically different values and mores can also precipitate cultural tumult and subsequent substance abuse epidemics (Wallace 1970). Examples of substance abuse accompanying anomie include an amphetamine epidemic in postwar Japan (Tamura 1989) and abuse of alcohol and inhalants by aboriginal peoples of the Americas, Australia, and Oceania (Kahn et al. 1990; Walker et al. 1985).

Factors Affecting Ethnic Distribution of Substance Use

Smuggled drugs, such as cocaine and heroin, tend to prevail in border, coastal, and commercial areas. By dint of *geographic location,* various ethnic groups become associated with the drug trade. Mafia members, Hispanic refugees and immigrants, and urban African Americans have been highly identified with the coastal, urban-centered heroin and cocaine drug trade in recent decades.

Smuggling can thrive under the following community circumstances:

- A national boundary that lends itself to secret movement (e.g., a remote seacoast, roadless mountains or deserts, a crowded seaport)
- Occupation of the boundary region by a group that is economically disadvantaged relative to fellow citizens
- Boundary occupation by a distinct ethnic group that is sociopolitically disenfranchised
- Differing national laws or economics across the boundary, so that smuggling pays handsome profits

For smuggling to be successful and stable, there must be social support. The local people must accept it morally—as a necessary evil if not as an honorable trade. Those who engage in smuggling as an occupation typically have other seasonal occupations, such as farming, fishing, trading, or crafting (Westermeyer 1982).

Locally grown drugs, especially cannabis, hold much greater sway in the middle of the United States.

Cannabis cash crops have become a key source of income in the Carolinas, Tennessee, Kentucky, Arkansas, Missouri, eastern Oklahoma, Kansas, and some of the western states. In these ecological niches, community leaders may be accepting—even supportive—of the drug trade, considering it a necessary evil that brings jobs and wealth into the community. Successful drug trade requires a *shadow government,* whose key members may share ethnic identity, kinship, and community affiliation. Security to conduct the trade, retribution in the event of nonpayment or theft, and allocation of retail franchises are key to a thriving drug trade.

Status conflict may affect the decision to choose an occupation in the illicit drug trade. The distance between a person's aspired status and his or her actual status in the community constitutes the individual's status conflict. Status conflict can be a source of motivation, driving the individual to work or strive harder. An overwhelming degree of status conflict, with no possible resolution, may motivate an individual to accept the inherent risks of an illicit trade.

Availability, access, and acceptance of illicit drugs are central features of an active drug trade within a small neighborhood or community. An illicit drug may be geographically available in a community, but all ethnic groups may not have equal access to the drug. Access involves factors such as knowing when and where drugs can be purchased, from whom they can be purchased, and how to effect a purchase. At the retail level, safety in conducting illicit sales lies in knowing one's clientele. Unfamiliar customers pose a risk. Selling only to identifiable members of one's own ethnic group may reduce this risk. Thus, to gain access to an illicit substance, the potential buyer must be accepted by the retailer. This same analogy holds in gaining access to the wholesale trade. As one gains access to higher levels of wholesale trade, the profits mount and the severity of the punishments (although not necessarily the risk of punishment) may also increase. In addition, the risk of theft, robbery, or violent takeover of a lucrative trade also exists. Trust can develop across cultures and ethnicities, but it is more difficult to achieve.

Effects of Addiction on Ethnic Affiliation

A decline in ethnic affiliation among addicted individuals accompanies reduced participation in activities that reinforce ethnic identity and support ethnic organizations. Examples include declining participation in extended family gatherings, religious rituals, ethnic celebrations, and other community activities. Disposable income goes to alcohol or drugs rather than to institutions representing community development. Addicted individuals who are parents contribute to anomie by not acculturating their children to the norms and values of their ethnic groups.

Social role conflicts ensue when addicted individuals do not fulfill social expectations and responsibilities (e.g., parenting, working, otherwise meeting community obligations). Inability to discharge the responsibilities of a social role leads to social role conflict, with reduced social status.

Alienation and isolation from an ethnic group can be either a cause or an effect of addiction. Some alienated or isolated people seek solace in substance abuse. Alternatively, an addicted individual may become alienated from his or her family, social network, and community (Holmgren et al. 1983). The effect of increasing social distance may be a reduction in the universal taboo against harming one's family or ethnic group. Thus, addicted individuals may steal from relatives and former friends, or they may use resources meant for the family to purchase drugs or alcohol. Alienation from the family produces a downward spiral into further substance abuse, because of the diminished family support in dealing with loss or stress. During recovery, the regaining of trust among family and former friends always takes at least many months and may require years (Godlaski et al. 1997).

Ethnicity and Treatment

Treatment access, like access to drugs, requires more than availability in the community. Kane (1981) found that a particular ethnic group did not seek alcohol or drug treatment from a local program because the program staff did not include any members of the ethnic group. Because of this lack in staffing, the program was not sensitive to the social aspects of addiction in that ethnic group. An element of acceptance lies in a staff's appreciating and perhaps employing the models of healing and changing preferred by a particular ethnic group (Keene and Raynor 1993). Many examples of ethnic-sensitive or ethnic-specific programs have been described in the literature (Argeriou 1978; Johnson and Westermeyer 2000; J. Red Horse 1982; Y. Red Horse 1982; Shore and Von Fumetti 1972).

Cultural recovery involves regaining a viable ethnic identity; acquiring a functional social network committed to the person's recovery; making a religious, spiritual, or moral recommitment; reengaging in recreational or avocational activities; and gaining a social role in the recovering community, society at large, or both (Westermeyer 1992). Individuals who fail to make a satisfactory cultural recovery are at risk for readdiction. Most recovering people return to their culture of origin (or ethnic group of origin). Old conflicts, aversions, and rejections related to the culture of origin may make recovery in that culture impossible. Some people are able to recover in another cultural, ethnic, or religious group besides their own (Porter 2002). Recovering as an adult in a foreign culture or ethnic group is not a simple or brief task, because individuals are best acculturated into a culture during infancy, childhood, or adolescence. Some persons who recover outside their ethnic group later provide support to their ethnic peers by helping others get treatment, by serving as a sponsor, or by hiring a recovering person.

Recovery subcultures are substitute social groups and networks that can foster early recovery (Lieberman and Borman 1976). Such subcultures may have their own jargon, values, customs, symbols, status markers, and social organizations. A subculture of therapists, therapy groups, and self-help groups can guide the individual toward health and stability. These recovery subcultures can provide support as needed, can confront or challenge the recovering person according to the situation, and can help the person avoid dangerous situations that might precipitate relapse. The recovering person's family and friends may not be able to do this.

In some cases, the recovery group may attempt to dominate the recovering person and keep him or her away from outside influences, even when the person is ready to cope with such influences. Likewise, people who begin recovery in religious cults may find their further progress stifled by isolation in the group. Or some individuals may not be able to recover sufficiently to cope with the world as it is. Consequently, some recovering people remain tied to the recovery group.

Cultural reentry occurs when the recovering person reaches a point at which further progress involves branching out from the recovery subculture. Reentry may grow out of a desire for additional education, a new occupation, or a new avocation. This movement into new groups involves risks (e.g., exposure to alcohol or drugs, failure at a new enterprise, rejection by those biased against former alcoholic or addicted individuals). If the recovery subculture has done its work well, the recovering person should be prepared for this step (Westermeyer 1989).

Specific Populations

Ethnic Minority Patients

Recovery among ethnic minority patients may require dealing with identity issues. For these patients, substance abuse may have been a means of coping psychologically and socially with their feelings about minority status or the majority society (Lampkin 1971). During recovery, such people may find themselves consumed with ethnic issues (Westermeyer 1990). One type of problem is a negative ethnic self-identity. Another problem is an overwhelming hostility toward the majority society. Ideally, early attempts at resolving these ethnic issues should take place with a therapist or peers from the same ethnic group as the recovering person. After recovery is well under way, work with therapists or peers of other ethnic groups may not be a problem; it may even provide a means for working on cross-ethnic issues involving trust, projection, demonization of the other, and so forth. Work at a legitimate occupation can enhance the individual's self-esteem and increase his or her chances of recovery (Stead et al. 1990).

Travelers, Foreign Students, Immigrants, and Refugees

"Going geographic," long recognized in substance abuse subcultures, consists of an addicted person's using travel or relocation to cope with a problem, when alcohol or drugs no longer effect such coping. This tactic is generally seen as a symptom of substance abuse rather than a means of dealing with it (Kimura et al. 1975). In some cases, however, relocation may be used to promote early recovery efforts. Maddux and Desmond (1981) first described the utility of this method among individuals whose repeated returns to the same family, friends, work, or neighborhood precipitated relapses into substance abuse. Relocation to a different school, neighborhood, or even town can have a salutary effect, especially if accompanied by treatment, including family counseling. When returning home, the recovering person should plan carefully, considering alternatives and support systems, reentry into treatment, and other protective measures.

Victimized Persons

Refugees, combat veterans, and individuals who have been raped may find that substance abuse temporarily stifles posttraumatic stress symptoms. In some cases, the symptoms may progress to posttraumatic stress disorder, which can complicate recovery. Substance abuse at the time of victimization or loss may also predispose individuals to posttraumatic stress disorder, by compromising their ability to adapt to victimization, integrate the experience, and recover from it (Green et al. 1992). Studying refugees in Australia, Krupinski et al. (1973) noted a window in time—several years to a decade after relocation—when refugees are at greatest risk of developing substance abuse.

Prevention

Prevention of substance abuse lies in creating communities safe from licit and illicit drugs. Creating such a community is a difficult, lengthy, expensive task if substance abuse is already established. The community must be able to assume responsibility for itself, to develop leadership that can establish and ensure responsible use of licit substances and eradicate illicit substances. This complex task involves close and active collaboration among public and private leaders, including those responsible for the public's health, education, and security. An approach that relies on outside agencies (e.g., the state or national government) or on members of any one profession (e.g., clinicians, police, teachers) or any one sector of the population (e.g., parents, youths, workers) is doomed to failure. Moreover, once members of a community have been made safe from substance abuse, relapse to widespread substance abuse is still a risk if vigilance is suspended. Local eradication of highly prevalent substance abuse has occurred in Asian villages (Kato 1990), Native American communities (J. Red Horse 1982; Y. Red Horse 1982), and elsewhere (Smart et al. 1988). National prevention is also feasible but is not easily, rapidly, or cheaply accomplished (Smart et al. 1988). Passing antiaddiction legislation without undertaking intensive and extensive health, education, law enforcement, and social programs can exacerbate rather than reduce substance-related problems (Westermeyer 1974b).

References

Aaron P, Musto D: Temperance and prohibition in America: a historical overview, in Alcohol and Public Policy: Beyond the Shadow of Prohibition. Edited by Moore M, Gerstein D. Washington, DC, National Academy Press, 1981, pp 127–181

Anawalt PR, Berdan FF: The Codex Mendoza. Sci Am 266 (6, June):70–79, 1992

Argeriou M: Reaching problem-drinking blacks: the unheralded potential of the drinking driver programs. Int J Addict 13:443–459, 1978

Baasher T: The use of drugs in the Islamic world. Br J Addiction 76:233–243, 1981

Beauvais F, Oetting ER, Edward RW: Trends in the use of inhalants among American Indian adolescents living on reservations: 1975–1983. Am J Drug Alcohol Abuse 11:209–229, 1985

Bennett LA, Ames GM: The American Experience With Alcohol: Contrasting Cultural Perspectives. New York, Plenum, 1985

Boehnlein JK, Kinzei JD, Leung PK, et al: The natural history of medical and psychiatric disorders in an American Indian community. Cult Med Psychiatry 16:543–554, 1992–1993

Bourgois P: In search of Horatio Alger: culture and ideology in the crack community. Contemporary Drug Problems 15:619–649, 1989

Brady M: Ethnography and understandings of Aborigine drinking. Journal of Drug Issues 22:699–712, 1992

Burton-Bradley BG: Some implications of betel chewing. Med J Aust 2:744–746, 1977

Caetano R, Suzman RM, Rosen DG, et al: The Shetland Islands: longitudinal changes in alcohol consumption in a changing environment. Br J Addict 78:21–36, 1983

Cameron DC: Youth and drugs: a world view. JAMA 206:1267–1271, 1968

Carstairs GM: Daru and bhang: cultural factors in the choice of intoxicant. Q J Stud Alcohol 15:220–237, 1954

Chafetz ME: Consumption of alcohol in the Far and Middle East. N Engl J Med 271:297–301, 1964

Comas-Diaz L, Griffith EEH (eds): Clinical Guidelines in Cross-Cultural Mental Health. New York, Wiley, 1988

Connell KH: Illicit distillation: an Irish peasant industry. Historical Studies of Ireland 3:58–91, 1961

Davoli M, Perucci CA, Rapiti E, et al: A persistent rise in mortality among injection drug users in Rome, 1980 through 1992. Am J Public Health 87:851–853, 1997

Deutsch A: Observations of a sidewalk ashram. Arch Gen Psychiatry 32:166–175, 1975

Dumont M: Tavern culture: the sustenance of homeless men. Am J Orthopsychiatry 37:938–945, 1967

DuToit BM: Drugs, Rituals and Altered States of Consciousness. Rotterdam, The Netherlands, Balkema, 1977

Eastwell HD: Petrol-inhalation in aboriginal towns—its remedy: the homelands movement. Med J Aust 2:221–224, 1979

Eaton JW, Weil RJ: Culture and Mental Disorders. Glencoe, IL, Free Press, 1955

Fields A, Tararin PA: Opium in China. Br J Addict 64:371–382, 1970

Furst PT, Coe MD: Ritual enemas. Natural History 86:88–91, 1977

Galanter M, Buckley P: Evangelical religion and meditation: psychotherapeutic effects. J Nerv Ment Dis 166:685–691, 1978

Galanter M, Westermeyer J: Charismatic religious experience and large-group psychology. Am J Psychiatry 137:1550–1552, 1980

Getahun A, Krikorias AD: Chat: coffee's rival from Hirar, Ethiopia. Economic Botany 27:353–389, 1973

Gfroerer J, De La Rosa M: Protective and risk factors associated with drug use among Hispanic youth. J Addict Dis 12:87–107, 1993

Godlaski TM, Leukefeld C, Cloud R: Recovery: with and without self-help. Subst Use Misuse 32:621–627, 1997

Green BL, Lindy JD, Grace MC, et al: Chronic posttraumatic stress disorder and diagnostic comorbidity in a disaster sample. J Nerv Ment Dis 180:760–766, 1992

Heath D: Peasants, revolution, and drinking: interethnic drinking patterns in two Bolivian communities. Human Organization 30:179–186, 1971

Holmgren C, Fitzgerald BJ, Carmen RS: Alienation and alcohol use by American Indian and Caucasian high school students. Journal of School Psychology 120:139–140, 1983

Johnson DR, Westermeyer J: Psychiatric therapies influenced by religious movements, in Psychiatry and Religion: The Convergence of Mind and Spirit. Edited by Boehnlein JK. Washington, DC, American Psychiatric Press, 2000, pp 87–108

Kahn MW, Hunter E, Heather N, et al: Australian aborigines and alcohol: a review. Drug and Alcohol Review 10:351–366, 1990

Kane GP: Inner-City Alcoholism: An Ecological Analysis and Cross-Cultural Study. New York, Human Sciences Press, 1981

Kato M: Brief history of control, prevention and treatment of drug dependence in Japan. Drug Alcohol Depend 25:213–214, 1990

Keaulana KA, Whitney S: Ka wai kau mai o Maleka (water from America): the intoxication of the Hawai'ian people. Contemporary Drug Problems 17:161–194, 1990

Keene J, Raynor P: Addiction as a "soul sickness": the influence of client and therapist beliefs. Addiction Research 1:77–87, 1993

Keyes CF: Towards a new formulation of the concept of ethnic group. Ethnicity 3:202–212, 1976

Kimura SD, Mikolashek PI, Kirk SA: Madness in paradise: psychiatric crises among newcomers in Honolulu. Hawaii Med J 34:275–278, 1975

Krupinski J, Stoller A, Wallace L: Psychiatric disorders in Eastern European refugees now in Australia. Soc Sci Med 7:31–45, 1973

La Barre W: The Peyote Cult. Hamden, CT, Shoe String Press, 1964

Lampkin LC: Alienation as a coping mechanism, in Crises of Family Disorganization; Programs to Soften Their Impact on Children. Edited by Pavenstedt E, Bernard VW. New York, Behavioral Publications, 1971

Lefley HP, Pedersen PB: Cross-Cultural Training for Mental Health Professionals. Springfield, IL, Charles C Thomas, 1986

Lieberman MA, Borman LD: Self-help groups. The Journal of Applied Behavioral Science 12:261–303, 1976

Maddahian E, Newcomb MD, Bentler PM: Adolescents' substance use: impact of ethnicity, income, and availability. Adv Alcohol Subst Abuse 5:63–78, 1986

Maddux JF, Desmond DP: Careers of Opioid Users. New York, Praeger, 1981

Manson SM, Shore JH, Baron AE, et al: Alcohol abuse and dependence among American Indians, in Alcoholism in North America, Europe, and Asia. Edited by Helzer JE, Canino GJ. New York, Oxford University Press, 1992, pp 113–130

Merrill TF: Japan and the Opium Menace. New York, Institute of Pacific Relations, 1942

Negrete JC: Coca leaf chewing: a public health assessment. Br J Addict 73:283–290, 1978

Perez-Jimenez JP, Robert MS: Transitions in the route of heroin use. Addiction Research 3:93–98, 1997

Porter E: Protestant faiths appeal to Hispanics and win many over. Wall Street Journal, July 2, 2002, pp A1, A6

Red Horse J: American Indian community mental health: a primary prevention strategy, in New Directions in Prevention Among American Indian and Alaska Native Communities. Edited by Manson SM. Portland, Oregon Health Sciences University, 1982, pp 217–230

Red Horse Y: A cultural network model: perspectives for adolescent services and para-professional training, in New Directions in Prevention Among American Indian and Alaska Native Communities. Edited by Manson SM. Portland, Oregon Health Sciences University, 1982, pp 173–184

Robin RW, Long JC, Rasmussen JK, et al: Relationship of binge drinking to alcohol dependence, other psychiatric disorders, and behavioral problems in an American Indian tribe. Alcohol Clin Exp Res 22:518–523, 1998

Rodin AE: Infants and gin mania in 18th century London. JAMA 245:1237–1239, 1981

Shore JH, Von Fumetti B: Three alcohol programs for American Indians. Am J Psychiatry 128:1450–1454, 1972

Simmons LRS, Gold MB: The myth of international control: American foreign policy and the heroin traffic. Int J Addict 8:779–800, 1973

Smart R, Murray GF, Arif A: Drug abuse and prevention programs in 29 countries. Int J Addict 23:1–17, 1988

Stead P, Rozynko V, Berman S: The SHARP carwash: a community-oriented work program for substance abuse patients. Soc Work 35:79–80, 1990

Tamura M: Japan: stimulant epidemics past and present. United Nations Bulletin of Narcotics 41:81–93, 1989

Terry CE, Pellens M: The Opium Problem. Montclair, NJ, Patterson Smith, 1928

Waddell J: The place of the cactus wine ritual in the Papago Indian ecosystem, in Realm of the Extra-Human: Ideas and Actions. Edited by Bharati A. The Hague, Mouton, 1976, pp 213–228

Walker RD, Benjamin GA, Kivlahan D, et al: American Indian alcohol misuse and treatment outcome, in Alcohol Use Among U.S. Ethnic Minorities (NIAAA Research Monograph no 18; DHHS Publ No [ADM] 89-1435). Edited by Spiegler DL, Tate DA, Aitken SS, et al. Rockville, MD, National Institute on Alcohol abusse and Alcoholism, 1985, pp 301–311

Wallace AFC: The Death and Rebirth of the Seneca. New York, Knopf, 1970

Westermeyer J: Opium dens: a social resource for addicts in Laos. Arch Gen Psychiatry 31:237–240, 1974a

Westermeyer J: The pro-heroin effects of anti-opium laws in Asia. Arch Gen Psychiatry 33:1135–1139, 1974b

Westermeyer J: Poppies, Pipes and People: Opium and Its Use in Laos. Berkeley, University of California Press, 1982

Westermeyer J: The psychiatrist and solvent-inhalant abuse: recognition, assessment, and treatment. Am J Psychiatry 144:903–907, 1987

Westermeyer J: The pursuit of intoxication: our 100 century-old romance with psychoactive substances. Am J Drug Alcohol Abuse 14:175–187, 1988

Westermeyer J: Monitoring recovery from substance abuse: rationales, methods and challenges. Adv Alcohol Subst Abuse 8:93–106, 1989

Westermeyer J: Treatment for psychoactive substance use disorder in special populations: issues in strategic planning. Adv Alcohol Subst Abuse 8:1–8, 1990

Westermeyer J: The sociocultural environment in the genesis and amelioration of opium dependence, in Anthropological Research: Process and Application. Edited by Pogge J. New York, State University of New York Press, 1992, pp 115–132

Westermeyer J: The role of cultural and social factors in the cause of addictive disorders. Psychiatr Clin North Am 22:253–273, 1999

Westermeyer J, Walzer V: Drug usage: an alternative to religion? Dis Nerv Syst 36:492–495, 1975

Wolcott HF: The African Beer Gardens of Bulawayo: Integrated Drinking in a Segregated Society. New Brunswick, NJ, Publications Division, Rutgers Center of Alcohol Studies, 1974

Overview of
Treatment

Assessment of the Patient

Shelly F. Greenfield, M.D., M.P.H.
Grace Hennessy, M.D.

Clinicians encounter patients with substance use disorders in all clinical settings. In 1995, health care spending associated with alcohol, tobacco, and drug abuse was estimated to be more than $114 billion (Horgan 2001). In 2000, there were 601,776 drug-related emergency room episodes, representing an increase of 62% in total drug-related emergency room visits since 1990 (Substance Abuse and Mental Health Services Administration 2001). As much as 40% of medical inpatient admissions are related to the complications of alcohol dependence (Horgan 1993), and on any given day more than 900,000 individuals receive alcohol or drug treatment in specialized treatment programs, with most of these receiving treatment as outpatients (Horgan 2001). However, despite the prevalence of these disorders in both general and treatment-seeking populations, substance use disorders are often undetected and undiagnosed in a variety of clinical settings (Deitz et al. 1994).

A thorough and accurate substance use history should therefore be a part of any medical or psychiat-

ric interview. A number of factors influence the accurate identification, assessment, and diagnosis of substance use disorders among patients presenting for treatment. These include the clinical setting; the style of interviewing; the attitude of the clinician; and patient characteristics such as the patient's motivation and stage of readiness to change, the presence of another co-occurring medical or psychiatric disorder, and the stage of use or abuse of the substance (e.g., current intoxication, current withdrawal, early abstinence, sustained abstinence, or recent relapse).

Successful treatment of substance use disorders depends on a careful, accurate assessment and diagnosis. The goals of assessment of patients with substance use disorders are 1) identifying the presence of substance abuse or dependence as well as identifying signs and symptoms of harmful or hazardous substance use so that prevention and early intervention might take place, 2) making an accurate diagnosis and relating this to any other co-occurring medical or psychiatric

Work for this chapter was supported in part by grant DA00407-02 from the National Institute on Drug Abuse (Dr. Greenfield) and from the Dr. Ralph and Marion Falk Medical Research Trust (Drs. Greenfield and Hennessy).

disorder, 3) formulating and helping to initiate appropriate interventions and treatment, and 4) enhancing the patient's motivation for change. In this chapter we review principles of eliciting the history of substance abuse, key elements of the history, formulation of an accurate diagnosis, the use of biological tests and interviews with significant others, the use of screening instruments and structured interviews, and the enhancement of motivation through the interview.

Eliciting the Substance Abuse History

The interview and elicitation of the substance abuse history are essential to making an accurate diagnosis. The setting of the interview, the clinician's style of interviewing, and patient factors can influence the accuracy of the history.

Setting

Accurate assessment is facilitated by interview settings that provide privacy and patient confidentiality and that permit adequate time to ask key questions, to follow up on positive patient responses, and to give feedback to the patient. It is important to address patients' concerns about confidentiality (Senay 1997). Patients may be concerned about whether their history will be transmitted to parents, spouses, employers, licensing boards, the courts, or other parties. The laws governing patient confidentiality—especially with respect to substance abuse in minors—may vary according to state or federal jurisdiction or with respect to the class of drug involved (e.g., narcotic treatment supported by federal funds has strict safeguards for confidentiality). It is important for the clinician to be aware of these particular laws and to communicate them to the patient (Senay 1997). A statement that gives the patient accurate information regarding confidentiality can be critical in the patient's willingness to provide a valid self-report. Similarly, privacy in the interview setting can also allow the patient to feel comfortable providing an accurate history. Research studies have shown that patients give valid self-reports when honest self-reporting is encouraged (Weiss et al. 1998) and when they perceive few negative consequences. The time allotted should be sufficient to accomplish the essential tasks of the interview. For example, it is helpful to give

the patient several minutes to freely describe his or her problem. The clinician can then move toward a more active style of gathering the history through specific questions. After completion of the history taking, there must be sufficient time for the clinician to provide the patient with a summary of what he or she has heard from the patient, to provide feedback about possible diagnoses and treatment options or recommendations, and to address the patient's specific questions.

Interviewing Style

The clinician's attitude and style of history taking can also facilitate a thorough and accurate assessment. One key to accurate assessment of individuals with substance use disorders is to be mindful of the great heterogeneity of these patients. Patients with substance use disorders may be of any ethnic background, socioeconomic circumstance, age, gender, marital or partner status, and level of employment. The epidemiology of substance use disorders (Robins and Regier 1991) reveals that there is no "typical" person with substance abuse or dependence. The first possible mistake in an accurate assessment is not asking the appropriate questions to elicit the substance use history because the patient does not fit a particular profile that the clinician has in mind. A substance use history should therefore be obtained from all patients presenting for treatment.

Patients with substance use disorders often exhibit certain typical defenses including denial, minimization, rationalization, projection, and externalization (Schottenfeld and Pantalon 1999). It is important to recognize these defenses and note that they can present obstacles to obtaining an accurate history. A number of interview strategies and approaches can help to circumvent these obstacles. It is often useful to begin the interview by asking an open-ended question such as "How can I help you?" or "What brought you here to see me today?" Allowing the patient to begin this way can help the clinician understand how the patient defines the problem, and this can set the direction for the rest of the interview. At the start of the interview, the clinician can permit the patient to take several minutes to further elaborate his or her understanding of the nature of the problem before moving into a more active and detailed mode of history taking. This also allows the clinician to get to know the patient more fully before obtaining a detailed substance abuse history. For example, it is helpful to ask the patient about other areas of his or her life history that might be less threatening, including work, family, or relationships. This helps develop rapport with the patient and can help the patient feel more at ease.

Patients with substance use disorders may vary in their insight into the nature of the problem, their readiness to change, their feelings of shame, or their own explanations for what has caused their problem. For this reason, as in most psychiatric interviewing, asking questions in a simple and straightforward manner and maintaining a nonjudgmental stance is most helpful. This may be demonstrated by the phrasing of specific questions. For example, the clinician can ask, "How has cocaine caused you problems?" rather than "How has your use of cocaine been a problem?" Instead of asking "Why did you drink alcohol then?" the clinician might ask "How were you feeling before you drank?" or "Do you think there were any specific circumstances or triggers to drinking at that time?" Another approach to diminishing shame can be to phrase questions in a manner such as "Some people with alcohol problems experience blackouts (or other negative consequence or behavior). I am wondering if you have ever had that experience?" This technique can be used to convey to the patient a range of experiences that others with similar problems have had and can show that the clinician is knowledgeable about these experiences and is able to hear what the patient might have to say. It can thereby serve to reduce shame. Finally, clinicians can avoid using labels; instead, they can ask patients to describe their pattern of use without labeling it. For example, if the patient says, "I just drink socially but I am not an alcoholic," the clinician can explain, "It would be most helpful for me to be able to understand the pattern of your drinking, so if we look at this past week/month/etc., tell me about your drinking."

Patient Characteristics

The interview can also be influenced by a number of patient characteristics that can affect the clinical presentation of a substance use disorder. Bearing in mind this matrix of patient characteristics can help the clinician adjust the interview to most effectively facilitate an accurate history. These patient factors include

1. Age, gender, partner or marital status, legal and employment status, and ethnicity
2. Degree of insight into and explanation for the nature of his or her problem

3. Medical or psychiatric comorbidity
4. Stage in the course of the illness (e.g., recovery, recent relapse, first treatment)
5. Current phase of use (e.g., intoxicated, withdrawing, interepisode)
6. Stage of readiness for change and motivation

A number of patient characteristics can influence the approach to the interview. For example, an interview with an adolescent who is dependent on marijuana is likely to require a different interview style than an interview with an elderly widow who has developed a drinking problem in the several years following her husband's death. Women may be more likely than men to explain their presenting problem as mood or anxiety and may see their drinking or substance use as a consequence of these difficulties and not the primary problem (Greenfield and O'Leary 2002). Cultural norms may differ regarding the quantity or frequency of use of a substance and may affect the social acceptability and the patient's description of his or her use (Westermeyer 1997). A patient's marital or partner status and employment status may also influence his or her presentation; individuals may present themselves for evaluation because of the urging or demand of significant others or because of work or legal complications of their substance use.

The clinical presentation may also vary depending on whether the patient presents for treatment early in the course of the illness or at a more advanced phase. For example, a patient who has intermittent binge alcohol use may present for treatment after a recent legal charge of driving while intoxicated. The patient's alcohol use may not yet qualify for a diagnosis of an alcohol use disorder. However, this interview may allow for identification of an alcohol problem early in its evolution and may provide an opportunity for early intervention. This interview will likely differ in scope and focus, for example, from that with a patient with a 15-year history of alcohol dependence presenting for a second admission for detoxification.

The current phase of drug use will also influence the clinical presentation and interview. Patients may present in different clinical settings in a state of intoxication, withdrawal, remission, slip, relapse, or maintenance. The clinician is unlikely to elicit a valid history from a patient who is acutely intoxicated (Babor et al. 1987). If possible, during intoxication the interview may be confined to ascertainment of acute medical conditions in need of intervention (e.g., respiratory depression, pancreatitis, gastrointestinal bleeding). The complete history is best deferred to a time when the patient is no longer intoxicated. Similarly, ascertainment of the medical need for detoxification and the prevention of withdrawal complications (e.g., seizures, delirium tremens) are the most important goals of the interview for patients in an acute withdrawal state.

A patient may also present in full, sustained remission from a substance use disorder but may report symptoms of another medical or psychiatric illness or a new onset of urges and cravings. It is important in this instance to find out the supports the patient has used to maintain abstinence and recovery, to examine how any other illness, whether it is chronic or of new onset, may be affecting the patient's ongoing recovery, and to ascertain what types of treatments or interventions may help support the patient's ongoing recovery. Similarly, the interview with a patient who presents with a recent slip or relapse to substance use may be directed toward understanding the triggers to the recent drug use as well as an effort to identify strategies that will help circumscribe the relapse and help the patient get back on the recovery track.

The patient's current stage of motivation for change will also affect the interview (Prochaska et al. 1992). The interview with a patient who is precontemplative will usually require more probing to elicit the history. Interview strategies that focus on establishing a pattern of use and that then elicit "advantages" and "disadvantages" of such use may be helpful. To establish a pattern of use, the clinician might say to the patient, "It would be helpful for me to understand the pattern of your alcohol/cocaine/marijuana/etc. use. As you know, people's use of alcohol/cocaine/marijuana/etc. varies greatly, and it would help me to understand the usual pattern for you." The clinician might then proceed to use a calendar method of ascertaining days of use in the past week, month, or year (Sobell and Sobell 1992). The application of this calendar method in clinical settings would be to ask the patient to describe his or her pattern of use over the past week, month, 3 months, 6 months, and year. For the more recent time periods, the clinician can ask for patterns of use (type of substance, quantity, frequency, time of day, etc.) for each day of the past week or month. For the more distant time periods, it is helpful to anchor the questions in seasonal events or events important to the patient. So, for example, the clinician might ask whether the patient's use was the same during the previous winter holidays as it is currently. Alternatively, the clinician might ask the patient to compare the past week's or month's use of a substance to previous 6-month time intervals, such as "Would you say the current pattern of use that you just described is the same pattern you have had for the last 6 months? What about the previous 6 months? Was there ever a period when you were using more heavily? When was that?" A similar style of interviewing can be used to obtain the lifetime substance abuse history, with the clinician asking for patterns of use during successive developmental periods, such as, "Tell me about your first use. Your use in high school? College? Your twenties? After you were married?" until the clinician is satisfied that he or she has understood the course of use throughout the life span.

After identifying these use patterns, the patient might be encouraged to identify any ways in which he or she perceives that "the alcohol/cocaine/marijuana/etc. has caused negative consequences" for him or her. This interview will likely differ from interviews with patients who had a brief recent relapse after a sustained period of recovery. Elicitation of such patients' earlier history is likely to be more straightforward and to require less probing. Such patients are likely to provide an overview of their previous substance problem and of what helped them in their recovery. These interviews may be more likely to focus on the nature of the recent relapse, the particular triggers to substance use, any consequences of the relapse, and plans to help the patient return to abstinence and recovery.

As in all psychiatric interviews, the empathic stance is helpful. An empathic capacity to feel the patient's experience but at the same time to maintain objectivity is critical (Frances and Franklin 1989). Patients often feel great relief when they are asked questions about their condition, because these questions reveal that the clinician is knowledgeable about the condition, can understand what the experience of the condition might be like, and may be able to offer the patient relief through some form of treatment. It is therefore also important to reserve time at the end of the interview to summarize for the patient what the clinician has heard about the patient's history, the way in which the clinician formulates this and any diagnostic implications that the clinician is considering, and any possible treatment options and recommendations. The clinician may begin this part of the interview by saying, "I would like to save some time to give you feedback about what we have discussed and to let you know some of my thoughts. Before I do this, is there anything else that is important that we have not had a chance to discuss or that you think I haven't asked you?" After the patient has had a chance to add any further information, the clinician can then present what he or she has heard. It is often useful to first let the patient know of any particular risk factors or vulnerabilities that he or she may have. For example, the clinician might say, "It sounds to me as if you have had a number of risk factors. You have told me that both of your parents had alcohol problems, and we know that this is likely to have made you more vulnerable to the substance. Second, you have told me that you have struggled with a mood disorder, and we know that often patients with other psychiatric disorders such as mood disorders are more vulnerable to developing problems with drugs and alcohol." The clinician might then proceed to summarize the history the patient has given and to relate the key elements of the history to specific diagnostic criteria. This should then lead to a formulation of the diagnoses and the treatment implications.

To elicit key elements of the history that allow the clinician to formulate the diagnosis and to relate these elements back to the patient in a straightforward manner, it is important for the clinician to have in mind the diagnostic criteria and to use the interview to elicit history that will help establish a differential diagnosis and exclude or include the likely diagnoses for the particular patient.

Diagnosing Substance Use Disorders

Psychiatric disorders attributable to substances of abuse can generally be divided into disorders produced by the substance's pharmacological effects —such as intoxication, withdrawal, and substance-induced disorders—and disorders related to the pattern or negative consequences of such use (Woody and Cacciola 1997). In DSM-IV and DSM-IV-TR (American Psychiatric Association 1994 and 2000, respectively), both categories of these disorders are covered in the section entitled "Substance-Related Disorders," which consists of two subsections, "Substance Use Disorders" and "Substance-Induced Disorders." The substance use disorders include substance dependence and substance abuse.

Substance Use Disorders

According to DSM-IV-TR, a diagnosis of *substance dependence* is made when there has been a maladaptive pattern of substance use leading to clinically significant impairment or distress, as manifested by at least three of seven symptoms or behaviors that have occurred within the same 12-month period. The DSM-IV-TR criteria for substance dependence are listed in Table 10–1.

In DSM-IV-TR it is specified that the substance dependence diagnosis can be further characterized as being "with physiological dependence" if the substance dependence diagnosis is accompanied by evidence of tolerance or withdrawal or as being "without physiological dependence" when there is no evidence of either tolerance or withdrawal.

A diagnosis of *substance abuse* is made when the individual has never before met criteria for dependence and exhibits a maladaptive pattern of substance use leading to significant impairment or distress as manifested by any one (or more) behaviors that have occurred within a 12-month period. The DSM-IV-TR criteria for substance abuse are listed in Table 10–2.

Importantly, the criteria for substance abuse or dependence are the same regardless of the actual substance of abuse. The presence of the behaviors and symptoms listed above within the 12 months before the interview constitutes a current diagnosis, and their presence in any 12-month period earlier in the individual's life is consistent with a past diagnosis.

DSM-IV-TR also provides for a number of course specifiers. *Early full remission* is specified if for at least 1 month but for less than 12 months no criteria for dependence or abuse have been met. *Early partial remission* is specified if for at least 1 month but less than 12 months one or more criteria for dependence or abuse (but less than the full criteria for dependence) have been met intermittently or continuously. *Sustained full remission* is specified when none of the criteria have been present for 12 months or longer. *Sustained partial remission* is used when the full criteria for dependence have not been met for a period of 12 months or longer but one or more criteria for dependence or abuse have been present. The specifier *on agonist therapy* is used if the individual is taking a prescribed agonist, partial agonist, or agonist/antagonist medication and no criteria for dependence or abuse have been met for that class of medication for at least 1 month. The specifier *in a controlled environment* is similarly used when there is full remission for a month or more and the individ-

Table 10–1. DSM-IV-TR diagnostic criteria for substance dependence

A maladaptive pattern of substance use, leading to clinically significant impairment or distress, as manifested by three (or more) of the following, occurring at any time in the same 12-month period:

(1) tolerance, as defined by either of the following:
    (a) a need for markedly increased amounts of the substance to achieve intoxication or desired effect
    (b) markedly diminished effect with continued use of the same amount of the substance

(2) withdrawal, as manifested by either of the following:
    (a) the characteristic withdrawal syndrome for the substance (refer to Criteria A and B of the criteria sets for withdrawal from the specific substances)
    (b) the same (or a closely related) substance is taken to relieve or avoid withdrawal symptoms

(3) the substance is often taken in larger amounts or over a longer period than was intended

(4) there is a persistent desire or unsuccessful efforts to cut down or control substance use

(5) a great deal of time is spent in activities necessary to obtain the substance (e.g., visiting multiple doctors or driving long distances), use the substance (e.g., chain-smoking), or recover from its effects

(6) important social, occupational, or recreational activities are given up or reduced because of substance use

(7) the substance use is continued despite knowledge of having a persistent or recurrent physical or psychological problem that is likely to have been caused or exacerbated by the substance (e.g., current cocaine use despite recognition of cocaine-induced depression, or continued drinking despite recognition that an ulcer was made worse by alcohol consumption)

Specify if:

    With Physiological Dependence: evidence of tolerance or withdrawal (i.e., either Item 1 or 2 is present)
    Without Physiological Dependence: no evidence of tolerance or withdrawal (i.e., neither Item 1 nor 2 is present)

Course specifiers (see text for definitions):

    Early Full Remission
    Early Partial Remission
    Sustained Full Remission
    Sustained Partial Remission
    On Agonist Therapy
    In a Controlled Environment

ual is in an environment where there is restricted access to substances. Such an environment could be a locked hospital unit, a supervised residential setting, or a substance-free prison.

Harmful or Hazardous Substance Use

In addition to individuals who meet criteria for substance abuse or dependence, a significant number of individuals use substances in a way that is harmful or hazardous even though their use does not meet criteria for abuse or dependence or for another substance-related disorder. With respect to alcohol, the World Health Organization defines hazardous drinkers as those whose pattern of drinking poses a high risk of future damage to physical or mental health (Bohn et al. 1995; World Health Organization 1980). It defines harmful drinking as a pattern of alcohol use that is already resulting in problems (Bohn et al. 1995; World

Health Organization 1980). In addition to application of these definitions of harmful and hazardous alcohol use, in the 10th Revision of the International Statistical Classification of Diseases and Related Health Problems (ICD-10) (World Health Organization 1992), harmful substance use is defined as "clear evidence that the substance use was responsible for (or substantially contributed to) physical or psychological harm, including impaired judgment or dysfunctional behavior." This category of harmful use is the closest that ICD-10 comes to the DSM-IV-TR diagnosis of substance abuse. However, the DSM-IV-TR diagnosis of substance abuse focuses on social consequences of behavior, whereas the ICD-10 definition of harmful use focuses on psychological or physical harm. Importantly, the ICD-10 category of harmful use has greater utility cross-culturally, because the social acceptability of substance use may vary greatly from country to country (Woody and Cacciola 1997).

Table 10–2. DSM-IV-TR diagnostic criteria for substance abuse

A. A maladaptive pattern of substance use leading to clinically significant impairment or distress, as manifested by one (or more) of the following, occurring within a 12-month period:

   (1) recurrent substance use resulting in a failure to fulfill major role obligations at work, school, or home (e.g., repeated absences or poor work performance related to substance use; substance-related absences, suspensions, or expulsions from school; neglect of children or household)

   (2) recurrent substance use in situations in which it is physically hazardous (e.g., driving an automobile or operating a machine when impaired by substance use)

   (3) recurrent substance-related legal problems (e.g., arrests for substance-related disorderly conduct)

   (4) continued substance use despite having persistent or recurrent social or interpersonal problems caused or exacerbated by the effects of the substance (e.g., arguments with spouse about consequences of intoxication, physical fights)

B. The symptoms have never met the criteria for substance dependence for this class of substance.

Although the DSM-IV-TR diagnoses of substance use disorders are in wide use in the United States, the concepts of hazardous or harmful substance use defined by the World Health Organization are especially useful to consider when the patient describes the overuse or misuse of substances and the pattern of use does not meet criteria for a DSM-IV-TR definition of a substance use disorder but the patient's use of substances nevertheless increases vulnerability to developing a substance use disorder or is currently creating some difficulties. Such an ascertainment allows the clinician the opportunity to provide education and recommendations that may constitute early intervention for an individual when problem use already exists or that may constitute prevention in the case of someone whose use places them at risk. Certainly an assessment of a patient's risk factors for developing a substance use disorder (e.g., family history of substance use disorder, personal history of problems with the substance, the presence of another psychiatric disorder) may lead the clinician to advise reduction or cessation of a particular substance even if abuse or dependence is not yet present. In the case of patients with new-onset psychiatric illness such as bipolar disorder or schizophrenia, the risk of developing a substance use disorder is great and intervention that leads to cessation of any substance use is a good example of prevention (Brems et al. 2002; Greenfield and Shore 1995).

Substance-Induced Disorders

The disorders produced by the direct pharmacological effects of the substance are referred to as substance-induced disorders. These include the intoxication and withdrawal syndromes as well as syndromes such as substance-induced dementia and amnestic, psychotic, mood, anxiety, sleep, and sexual dysfunction disorders. Although all categories of substances produce an intoxication syndrome, the symptoms, signs, and durations of the syndromes vary by substance category. On the other hand, according to DSM-IV-TR, not all categories of substances produce a withdrawal syndrome or all of the other substance-induced disorders. Knowledge of the syndromes characteristic of each category of substances is important in eliciting an accurate history and clinical status.

Content of the Interview
History of the Substance Use Disorder

An understanding of the major categories of the different substances of abuse provides the interviewer with knowledge about their characteristic intoxication and withdrawal syndromes. With this knowledge, the interviewer is better able not only to assess the patient but also to make appropriate treatment recommendations. It is important to ask patients about all categories of substances and not just the patient's primary substance of abuse.

The major categories of substances of abuse are

1. Central nervous system depressants such as alcohol and sedative hypnotics such as barbiturates and benzodiazepines
2. Stimulants such as amphetamines, cocaine, and phencyclidine (PCP)
3. Cannabis (marijuana and hashish)
4. Opiates, including heroin, morphine, codeine, oxycodone, methadone, buprenorphine, and fentanyl
5. Hallucinogens such as lysergic acid diethylamide (LSD), mescaline, and psilocybin (mushrooms)

6. Nicotine in the form of cigarettes, chewing tobacco or dip, and snuff
7. Inhalants such as paint thinner, gasoline, glue, and cleaning fluids
8. "Designer drugs," including 3,4-methylenedioxymethamphetamine (MDMA; "Ecstasy"), ketamine, and γ-hydroxybutyrate (GHB)

A systematic and organized way of collecting information about the patient's history of substance use is to address the following areas:

1. Age at first substance use
2. Frequency of substance use
3. Amount of the substance taken during an episode of use
4. Route of administration for the substance
5. Consequences associated with substance use
6. Treatment history
7. Periods of abstinence
8. Relapses

The information obtained by asking about the age at first substance use serves as the framework for the history and guides the interviewer's subsequent questions. In addition, the patient's age when he or she began using substances has diagnostic and prognostic implications. Studies have shown that early onset (before age 15) of substance use is associated with the subsequent development of substance abuse and dependence (Robins and Przybeck 1985; Wills et al. 1996). The early onset of substance use disorders has also been associated with childhood psychopathology that preceded the development of the substance use disorder (Hahesy et al. 2002).

The age at first use of nicotine is also an important component of the history of the substance use disorder. Studies have shown that nicotine use often precedes experimentation with illicit drugs (Adler and Kandel 1981; Warren et al. 1997; Yamaguchi and Kandel 1984a, 1984b) and is more prevalent in individuals with other substance use disorders (Breslau et al. 1991; Budney et al. 1993; DiFranza and Guerrera 1990). Although it is incorrect to assume that all nicotine users have also used illicit drugs or have another substance use disorder, the age at first use of nicotine in a patient who uses other substances helps the interviewer have a more complete picture of the patient's history of substance use.

Once the age at first substance use is established, inquiries about the frequency of substance use as well as the amount of the substance used and the route of administration (oral, inhaled, insufflated or snorted, intravenous, subcutaneous) help the interviewer understand the progression or regression of substance use over time. For example, a patient who says she started snorting (route of administration) one bag (amount) of heroin once a week for 1 year (frequency) and then began using three bags of heroin per day by the intravenous route is reporting her progression of heroin use in all three areas. In addition, the frequency of use, the amount of the substance used, and the route of administration may be related to the development of medical disorders associated with a particular substance and will be relevant when discussing the patient's medical history.

General questions about the consequences of substance use focus on changes in academic performance, occupational functioning, and interpersonal relationships as well as medical and legal problems associated with substance abuse. The history of substance abuse treatment includes questions about hospital admissions for detoxification as well as admissions to other controlled living situations to support ongoing abstinence. Such programs include residential programs, halfway houses, sober houses, and therapeutic communities. Outpatient programs such as partial hospital programs, as well as group, individual, and pharmacological therapies (e.g., disulfiram, naltrexone, nicotine delivery systems) may also be a part of the patient's prior treatment. Understanding which earlier treatments did or did not help the patient achieve and maintain abstinence can serve as a guide for treatment recommendations. Finally, the interviewer should ask about involvement in self-help groups such as Alcoholics Anonymous, Narcotics Anonymous, Cocaine Anonymous, Self-Management and Recovery Training, Rational Recovery, and Women for Sobriety. Some patients may express positive or negative feelings about a particular type of self-help group. The interviewer should not support or discredit the patient's feelings about self-help groups but should try to understand the patient's reasons for such reactions, both to educate the patient about self-help groups and to formulate a treatment plan that will be most beneficial to the patient.

Other components of the history of substance use are the patient's periods of abstinence and the circumstances surrounding relapses. The information about abstinent periods and relapses indicates the progression or regression of substance use, the severity of the substance use disorder, and the external factors—such as relationship difficulties, psychiatric symptoms, legal or medical problems, and treatment termination—that may have influenced the return to substance use. Finally, the interviewer should review other substances of abuse with the patient to ensure that no other substances are being used currently or have been used in the past. A patient may say he only has a problem with cocaine; however, by asking about other substances of abuse, the interviewer may find that the patient has used marijuana daily for the past 10 years but did not mention the marijuana use because he does not consider it to be problematic. Although daily marijuana use may not be significant to the patient, this pattern of use could represent marijuana abuse or dependence that should be addressed with the patient.

Psychiatric History

Research studies have demonstrated an increased prevalence of substance use disorders among patients diagnosed with psychiatric disorders. For example, patients diagnosed with bipolar disorder are six times more likely than the general population to have a co-occurring substance use disorder (Regier et al. 1990). Other psychiatric disorders (Hesselbrock et al. 1985; Kessler et al. 1997; Krausz et al. 1998; Regier et al. 1990; Rounsaville et al. 1991) and personality disorders (Helzer and Pryzbeck 1988; Rounsaville et al. 1991; Weiss et al. 1993) have also been associated with substance use disorders. Conversely, patients diagnosed with substance use disorders are more likely to have a co-occurring psychiatric disorder (Brady et al. 1991; Drake and Wallach 1989; F.T. Miller et al. 1989; Mueser et al. 1992, 2000). Studies have shown that the co-occurrence of substance use disorders and psychiatric disorders can worsen the prognosis for both disorders (Greenfield et al. 1998; Sonne et al. 1994; Weiss et al. 1988). By diagnosing coexisting substance use and psychiatric disorders, however, patients can be referred to integrated treatment for both disorders. There is increasing evidence that integrated treatment improves and enhances outcomes for both disorders (Bennett et al. 2001; Mueser et al. 1992; Najavits et al. 1998; Weiss et al. 2000b). It is therefore important to assess substance use disorders in patients presenting for the treatment of their psychiatric disorder and equally important to assess psychiatric disorders among patients presenting for treatment of their substance use disorder.

If the patient reports symptoms consistent with a psychiatric disorder, the interviewer should inquire about the relationship between substance use and the emergence, exacerbation, or regression of psychiatric symptoms. Substance-induced psychiatric disorders occur when the symptoms of the disorder represent a change in affective or cognitive states that arises from the direct physiological effects of a substance. These symptoms are generally seen when the patient is intoxicated or is experiencing withdrawal symptoms. Examples of substance-induced psychiatric disorders include a patient who has exhibited symptoms of mania only when intoxicated with cocaine and a patient who has had panic attacks only when she was in benzodiazepine withdrawal. In contrast, a psychiatric disorder is independent of a substance use disorder when the patient reports a history of psychiatric symptoms that predates substance use or that does not resolve after the substance use has been stopped.

A useful way to determine whether psychiatric disorders predate or continue after abstinence from substances is to inquire about the presence or absence of psychiatric symptoms before the patient began using substances and during periods of abstinence. For example, a patient who was diagnosed with major depression 10 years ago and reports having used alcohol daily for the past 6 years in an attempt to ameliorate his untreated depressive symptoms had developed psychiatric symptoms before the initiation of substance use. Similarly, a patient who says she continues to have auditory hallucinations 6 months after her last use of marijuana demonstrates psychiatric symptoms that persist during a period of abstinence. Reviewing the patient's history of psychiatric symptoms before the onset of substance use, during episodes of intoxication with or withdrawal from substances, and after cessation of substance use can help the interviewer distinguish between substance-induced psychiatric disorders (which exist because of a substance use disorder) and co-occurring psychiatric and substance use disorders.

Medical History

Evaluating clinicians need to elicit a complete medical history—including current and past medical problems, surgical procedures, and medication allergies—from patients presenting for assessment of a substance use disorder. Regardless of their relationship to substance use, medical problems require treatment, and the interviewer would be remiss if he or she did not make inquiries about medical conditions and recommend treatment or make referrals for further evaluation for any conditions mentioned.

As the patient describes symptoms of a medical disorder, the interviewer will want to determine if the symptoms are related to or independent of substance use. Questions about a reported medical problem should include inquiries about the temporal relationship between the development of the medical condition and substance use. For example, a patient reports that her asthma, which was diagnosed at age 12, worsened about 2 years after she began smoking cigarettes at age 18. Other questions for this patient would include the continuation or resolution of symptoms after periods of abstinence. This same patient may report that when she stopped smoking for 2 weeks she had fewer asthma attacks. The role of pharmacological interventions in the treatment of medical disorders is another way to determine the effect of substance use on a medical disorder. For example, this patient may also report the failure of her previously effective steroid inhalers to treat asthma attacks in the past year. In this case, the patient's cigarette use exacerbated her asthmatic symptoms to the point where steroid inhalers were of limited therapeutic value.

It is also important to ask about current and past medical problems that are specific to use of a particular substance. A description of all the medical problems associated with each category of substances is beyond the scope of this book; the major medical problems and disorders associated with the more commonly abused substances are listed below:

- *Alcohol:* Blackouts, hangovers, withdrawal tremors, withdrawal seizures and delirium tremens, aspiration pneumonia, cardiomyopathy, cerebellar degeneration, gastritis, gastroesophageal reflux disease, hepatitis, pancreatitis, Wernicke-Korsakoff syndrome.
- *Cocaine:* Transient ischemic attacks, cerebral vascular events, ischemia of the gastrointestinal tract, chest pain, and myocardial infarctions. Ischemic necrosis of the nasal septum is associated with insufflating or snorting powder cocaine, whereas smoking crack cocaine may lead to dyspnea, pneumothorax, pneumomediastinum, and pulmonary infarction. Intravenous cocaine use may lead to use of contaminated needles, which may result in cellulitis, endocarditis, infection with the human immunodeficiency virus (HIV), and hepatitis B or C.

- *Marijuana:* The evidence for medical disorders associated with marijuana use is sparse and inconclusive. Long-term marijuana use may be associated with the earlier development of respiratory carcinomas in subjects who also use tobacco or alcohol (Taylor 1988), as well as an increased risk of prostate cancer and cervical cancer (Sidney et al. 1997).
- *Opiates:* Intravenous opiate use may result in the same medical disorders as intravenous cocaine use. Other medical problems resulting from opiate use include constipation and, in overdose, respiratory depression, coma, and death.
- *Nicotine:* Chronic obstructive pulmonary disease, emphysema, cardiovascular disease, peripheral vascular disease, and lung and oral carcinomas.
- *Sedative-hypnotics:* In overdose, respiratory depression, coma, and death; withdrawal tremors and seizures as well as a major abstinence syndrome.

Understanding the relationship between the development and exacerbation of medical disorders and substance use provides the interviewer with information that may motivate the patient to change addictive behavior. The medical history will also provide the information necessary to refer the patient to appropriate medical care regardless of the origin of the medical disorder.

Family History

The family history of substance use disorders may reveal a genetic vulnerability to the patient's own development of these disorders. In one study of 1,030 female twin pairs, it was estimated that the heritability of alcohol dependence liability ranged from 51% to 59%, with the balance being attributable to environmental factors (Kendler et al. 1992, 1994). These results are similar to the estimate reported in studies of male alcohol-dependent twins (McGue 1994; National Institute on Alcohol Abuse and Alcoholism1997). Family (Bierut et al. 1998; Kendler et al. 1997; Merikangas et al. 1998; Mirin et al. 1991), twin (Kendler and Prescott 1998a, 1998b), and adoption (Cadoret et al. 1980) studies provide compelling evidence for the relationship between genetic determinants and the development of substance use disorders. The environment created by families who have substance use disorders may also have an impact on the development of substance use disorders in their children. For example, parental modeling of drinking behavior, ethnic differences in drinking customs, parental as well as familial psychopathology, socioeconomic status, family aggression and violence, and parental cognitive impairment are risk factors that have been shown to affect the development of both alcohol dependence and other mental health problems in the children of alcoholic parents (Ellis et al. 1997). Interviewers can educate patients about genetic vulnerability to substance use disorder and risk factors in the family environment associated with the development of substance use disorder, which can provide patients with an understanding of their current problems with substances as well as compelling reasons why they should refrain from substance use.

Social and Developmental History

The social and developmental history provides information about the factors that may have influenced the development and perpetuation of substance use disorders. An important psychosocial factor to explore is the patient's relationships with others (i.e., family, friends, peers, significant others, authority figures). During adolescence, peer relationships are a powerful influence on both the initiation and continued use of substances (Hird et al. 1997). The interviewer will also want to know if the patient had any positive influences during adolescence such as emotionally supportive parents, membership in school organizations, or a focus on academic achievement; such factors are associated with a lower risk for substance use (Hird et al. 1997).

Some patients may report both initial and continued use of substances because of the effects of abusive relationships. Several studies (Brown and Anderson 1991; Greenfield et al. 2002; Rice et al. 2001; Wilsnack et al. 1997; Windle et al. 1995) have shown an association between self-reported histories of physical and sexual abuse and the development of substance use disorders. A history of abuse may also be associated with poorer drinking outcomes in alcohol-dependent subjects after treatment (Greenfield et al. 2002; Haver 1987). Conversely, the ability to have meaningful interpersonal relationships can help the patient build a social support network that might support recovery and help patients remain abstinent (Havassy et al. 1991).

Patients with substance use disorders may report the effects of substance use on their educational attainment and subsequent employment. Studies have shown that substance use may lead to school absenteeism, poor school performance, and dropout (Bray et

al. 2000; Lynskey and Hall 2000). In turn, lower educational attainment has been associated with the development of alcohol abuse and dependence in adulthood (Crum et al. 1992, 1993) and may have effects on abstinence in alcohol-dependent individuals (Curran and Booth 1999; Greenfield et al. 2003). By affecting educational attainment, alcoholism has been associated with lower income and occupational status (Crum et al. 1998; Mullahy and Sindelar 1989).

Finally, the interviewer should inquire about the patient's marital or partner status, because studies have shown that the presence or absence of a spouse or partner can be an important influence on the development and perpetuation of a substance use disorder and may also affect treatment outcomes. For example, women seeking treatment for substance use disorders are more likely than men to be single (Griffin et al. 1989; Weiss et al. 1997); to be involved with an addicted partner (Gossop et al. 1994; Griffin et al. 1989; Hser et al. 1987); and to cite interpersonal factors such as use by spouse, partner, or friend as reasons for continued substance use (Greenfield 1996; Kandel and Logan 1984). The presence of a supportive partner (Anglin et al. 1987; Eldred and Washington 1976) and the absence of an addicted partner (Nurco et al. 1982) have been shown to be the most consistent factors associated with better treatment outcomes for opiate-dependent women but not for opiate-dependent men.

The social history, therefore, helps both patient and interviewer comprehend which interpersonal relationships, negative experiences, and positive achievements shaped the development and progression of the patient's substance use disorder. These same factors may also affect the outcome of the patient's treatment for substance use disorders.

Physical and Mental Status Examinations

Physical and mental status examinations of patients presenting for an assessment of a substance use disorder are a critical part of the evaluation, because (as discussed above) both medical and psychiatric disorders are commonly found in this population. Although a mental status examination can and must be performed regardless of the treatment setting, the interviewer may be unable to perform the physical examination. Lack of appropriate space, equipment, and training can interfere with the interviewer's ability to perform the physical examination. Patient factors such as refusal to undergo an examination or inability to cooperate with the examination due to substance intoxication or withdrawal may also be reasons to defer the physical examination at the time of evaluation. Under such circumstances, the interviewer should refer the patient to the appropriate person (e.g., primary care physician) or facility (e.g., emergency room) for a complete physical examination.

The specific signs of substance use present during the physical or mental status examination will depend on the type of substance used and the presence of intoxication with or withdrawal from substances (Washburn 2002). According to DSM-IV-TR, patients who are intoxicated with amphetamines or cocaine may exhibit psychomotor agitation or retardation, diaphoresis, evidence of weight loss, and confusion. Alcohol and sedative-hypnotics can cause slurred speech, incoordination, unsteady gait, memory impairment, stupor, or coma in an intoxicated patient. Similarly, opioid intoxication is characterized by slurred speech, drowsiness, and memory impairment. One distinguishing characteristic of opioid intoxication is the appearance of pupillary constriction; severe overdose of opiates can result in pupillary dilation secondary to anoxia in the central nervous system.

Cannabis intoxication can cause motor incoordination, euphoria or anxiety, sense of slowed time, and impaired judgment. An often obvious sign of cannabis intoxication is conjunctival injection. A patient who is intoxicated with hallucinogens may be anxious, depressed, or paranoid after use. Hallucinations, illusions, perceptual distortions, incoordination, diaphoresis, and tremors can also be present. Signs of PCP intoxication include psychomotor agitation, impaired judgment, dysarthria, sensitivity to sounds, ataxia, seizures, or coma. Inhalant use may cause euphoria and impaired judgment, as well as a number of observable physical signs, including incoordination, slurred speech, lethargy, ataxia, psychomotor retardation, stupor, and coma.

Also described in DSM-IV-TR are withdrawal symptoms for the different substances of abuse. Patients withdrawing from either amphetamines or cocaine may present with dysphoria, psychomotor agitation or retardation, and signs of fatigue; they may complain of increased appetite, vivid and unpleasant dreams, insomnia, or hypersomnia. The withdrawal symptoms of alcohol and sedative-hypnotics may include diaphoresis, tremulousness, psychomotor agitation, responsiveness to internal stimuli, and seizures. Patients in withdrawal from central nervous system depressants may also report anxiety, insomnia, nausea, and vomiting. Lacrimation, rhinorrhea, pupillary dilation, piloerection, and yawning are the observable signs of opioid withdrawal; symptoms that may be reported by patients undergoing opioid withdrawal are dysphoria, fever, nausea, vomiting, muscle aches, and diarrhea. Cannabis, hallucinogens, PCP, and inhalants do not have defined withdrawal syndromes.

Although many physical signs of substance use are easily observed when the interviewer performs the mental status examination, other signs of substance use are best detected by performing a thorough physical examination. For example, small circular lesions representing the point of injection of a drug into both large and small veins, also known as tracks, may be found when examining a patient who uses drugs intravenously. If infected, these injection sites may be erythematous, purulent, and warm to the touch. Similarly, a patient with hepatic damage secondary to chronic alcohol use or with hepatitis infection as a result of intravenous drug use may present with scleral icterus or a slightly enlarged liver or, in more advanced cases of hepatic damage, jaundice, abdominal distention secondary to ascites, gynecomastia, spider angiomas, palmar erythema, and caput medusa. A complete description of all the physical findings associated with substance use is beyond of the scope of this book; these two examples are presented to illustrate the importance of a thorough physical examination to detect other signs of substance-related medical disorders that require immediate treatment.

The physical and mental status examinations of a patient presenting for an evaluation of a substance use disorder can be dramatically affected by states of intoxication or withdrawal. Alterations in mood, affect, psychiatric symptoms, thought processes, thought content, speech, memory, orientation, cognition, insight, and judgment are commonly seen when patients are intoxicated with or are withdrawing from a particular substance. Similarly, substance intoxication or withdrawal can lead to significant changes in the patient's physiological state, causing abnormalities in blood pressure, body temperature, and level of consciousness and disrupting the stability and functioning of major organ systems such as the neurological and gastrointestinal systems. In addition, the mental status examination provides important information for the diagnosis of other psychiatric disorders and for the evaluation of the current remission, recurrence, or stability of any other concurrent psychiatric disorder. A comparison of the patient's physical and mental status examinations during different stages of substance abuse treatment is one way to evaluate changes in substance use and in any concurrent medical and psychiatric disorders.

Biological Markers

Biological markers can help detect the degree and regularity of the patient's substance use (Kolodziej et al. 2002). These biological markers are most frequently tested and analyzed by sampling breath, urine, blood, hair, and saliva. The highly sensitive and specific breath alcohol testing provides immediate results at low cost and minimal discomfort to the patient. The drawbacks of breath analysis include its narrow window of assessment, which varies from minutes to hours after drinking depending on the amount of alcohol consumed and on individual differences in alcohol metabolism.

Metabolites of many substances of abuse are excreted in the urine and may be detected by urine toxicology screens. The major disadvantage of urine testing is the variations in detection time for the metabolites of different substances. For example, because cocaine metabolites remain in the urine for approximately 3 days, a urine screening test performed 5 days after the last cocaine use would not detect recent use. Conversely, cannabis metabolites may remain in the urine for a month, resulting in positive urine toxicology screens after several weeks of abstinence. In turn, the detection duration may be affected by dose, frequency of use, cutoff concentration level that results in a positive urine screen, and the patient's rate of metabolism (Cone 1997). Although quantitative urine screening may overcome some of the limitations of urine toxicology screens and reduce the numbers of false-positive and false-negative urine screens, the cost of this test may be prohibitive, and the technology involved in qualitative urine screening requires further evaluation.

Recent heavy substance use can be detected by serum testing. Alcohol exerts a direct toxic effect on hepatocytes, leading to increased levels of glycoprotein carbohydrate-deficient transferrin, γ-glutamyltransferase, serum glutamic oxaloacetic transaminase (also known as aspartate aminotransferase) and serum glutamic pyruvic transaminase (also known as alanine aminotransferase). The mean corpuscular volume of red blood cells may also be increased with heavy alcohol use, demonstrating hepatic damage as well as hematological problems such as deficiencies in vitamin B_{12} and folate. These blood markers can help clinicians monitor changes in the patient's physical health and may be used as a motivator to help the patient decrease or abstain from the use of alcohol. These markers, however, are not specific for alcohol-related medical problems and may be present with other disease states. In addition, blood markers may differ due to individual factors such as age, body mass index, gender, smoking, caffeine consumption, and the use of certain medications (Aubin et al. 1998; Daeppen et al. 1998).

A new method for evaluating biological markers of substance use is hair testing. Although it is not fully understood how drugs enter the hair, hair testing may provide a longer time to detect substance use due to the greater stability of the drug in hair samples compared with samples of bodily fluids. The disadvantages of hair testing include the possibility of false-positive results due to passive contact with a substance, the possible effect of individual hair characteristics (such as hair length) on the test results, and racial bias in hair testing. In addition, hair testing is a new technology that cannot provide information about the amount of the substance used or the temporal relationship between the presence of the substance in the hair and the use of the substance.

Saliva testing is primarily used to detect very recent substance use and is used to identify substance use in accident victims, automobile operators, and employees before their involvement in activities in which safety is paramount. The detection time for saliva testing is relatively brief, and the technology requires further evaluation to demonstrate its validity. Sweat testing may detect past substance use and may act as a cumulative measure of substance use. This test is not commonly used because of individual variations in sweat production, possible environmental contamination, and difficulties in collecting and storing sweat samples.

Testing for biological markers can serve an important function in the detection of substance use. The evaluating clinician should consider the substance used, the duration for substance detection, the invasiveness of the technique, and the expense of the test to determine which test is most appropriate for individual patients.

Screening Instruments and Standardized Interviews

Standardized instruments exist for screening, diagnostic assessment, and evaluation of severity. A number of short self-report instruments have been developed as screens for the presence of a drug or alcohol use disorder (Allen and Columbus 1995; Kolodziej et al. 2002; Rounsaville and Poling 2000). Such tests do not provide a formal diagnosis but rather provide an indication of the likely presence of substance abuse or dependence.

The four-question CAGE questionnaire (Kitchens 1994; Mayfield et al. 1974) asks "Have you ever: 1) felt you should **C**ut down on your drinking? 2) felt **A**nnoyed by criticism of your drinking? 3) felt bad or **G**uilty about your drinking? 4) taken a drink first thing in the morning (**E**ye-opener) to steady your nerves or get rid of a hangover?" The CAGE is useful because of its brevity and ease of scoring. One positively answered question has a 90% rate of detecting an alcohol-related disorder.

The Alcohol Use Disorders Identification Test (AUDIT) (Allen et al. 1997; Babor et al. 1992) was designed to screen hazardous or harmful alcohol consumption as defined by the World Health Organization in a range of clinical and nonclinical settings. This 10-item questionnaire uses a 0–5 score for each question and takes less than 2 minutes to administer and 2 minutes to score (Babor et al. 1992, 1995). A score of 8 or above has reasonably good sensitivity in detecting an alcohol use disorder (Conigrave et al. 1995).

The Michigan Alcohol Screening Test (MAST) is useful in assessing the extent of lifetime alcohol-related consequences (Allen and Columbus 1995). It is available in several versions: a 25-item self-test (Selzer 1971), a 13-item short MAST (SMAST), and a 10-item brief version (Allen and Columbus 1995).

The Drug Abuse Screening Test (DAST) (Skinner 1982; Staley and El-Guebaly 1990) is a 20-item self-test designed to detect abuse of or dependence on a wide range of substances other than alcohol.

The TWEAK test (Russell et al. 1991) (the name is derived from its five items) was originally designed to screen for high-risk drinking during pregnancy. The T-ACE (Sokol et al. 1989) is a four-item test designed to identify pregnant women at risk for drinking alcohol in quantities that might be dangerous to the fetus (Elliot and Hickam 1990). Neither the TWEAK nor the T-ACE has gender-based items, and the TWEAK has been validated in both male and female populations (Chan et al. 1993).

A number of structured interviews that are used in research settings (Kolodziej et al. 2002) may also be helpful in some clinical settings. The Timeline Follow-Back (TLFB) (Sobell and Sobell 1992) uses a calendar method that asks patients to reconstruct the type, quantity, and frequency of substance use during a specific time period. The Addiction Severity Index (ASI) (McLellan et al. 1992) was developed as a structured interview to assess problem severity in seven areas frequently affected by substance use disorders. There are several other questionnaires that measure other aspects of severity. These include the Drinker Inventory of Consequences (W. Miller et al. 1995), which assesses the adverse consequences of alcohol dependence, and the eight-item Clinical Institute Withdrawal Assessment (Sellers et al. 1991), which provides a clinical quantification of the severity of alcohol withdrawal syndrome. The Fagerstrom Test for Nicotine Dependence (Fagerstrom and Schneider 1989) was designed to provide an ordinal measure of nicotine dependence related to cigarette smoking.

Structured interviews are also reliable ways to assess diagnostic information. The Structured Clinical Interview for DSM-IV (SCID) (First et al. 1997) is a clinically based interview that aids in diagnosis of DSM-IV-TR substance-related and other psychiatric disorders. The Psychiatric Research Interview for Substance and Mental Disorders (PRISM) facilitates diagnosis of DSM-IV-TR psychiatric disorders and demonstrates good reliability for establishing psychiatric diagnoses among apatients with drug and alcohol use disorders (Hasin et al. 1996).

Involvement of Significant Others

People who seek assessment for substance use disorders often do so at the prompting of significant others such as family members, friends, coworkers, or treating clinicians who are concerned about the person's well-being. Several studies (Carroll 1995; Maisto et al. 1979; Sobell et al. 1997) have shown that significant others, serving as collateral informants, can both corroborate and provide additional information about the patient's reported substance use history. Speaking to the patient's significant others also allows for their early involvement in treatment planning. As noted above (see "Social and Developmental History"), establishing social networks may support the patient's recovery and help him or her remain abstinent (Havassy et al. 1991).

Contact with collateral informants should occur only with written permission from the patient. If the request for contact with significant others is denied, it is appropriate to explore the patient's reasons for refusal. In some cases, the patient cannot provide the name of a collateral informant because he or she is socially isolated and has no significant supports in his or her life (Weiss et al. 2000a). The patient may be ambivalent about changing his or her addictive behaviors and therefore does not want significant others involved in his or her treatment. Other reasons that a patient might refuse to authorize communication with certain individuals could include involvement of a significant other in substance use; involvement of a significant other in physical, emotional, or sexual abuse of the patient; and ability of a significant other to cause social consequences such as unemployment or loss of significant relationships.

The involvement of significant others as both collateral informants and social supports can have either a positive or a negative effect on the patient's initiation of and retention in substance abuse treatment. Because significant others may be a powerful influence in the patient's life, it is recommended that the interviewer contact only those who will support, rather than hinder, the recovery process.

Stages of Change and Motivational Interviewing

Before discussing treatment options with a patient with a substance use disorder, the interviewer will want to assess the patient's willingness to stop using substances of abuse. Prochaska and colleagues (1992) described the five stages of change that patients proceed through before giving up their addictive behavior. Patients are said to be in *precontemplation,* the first stage, if they do not want to change their addictive behavior. These patients may resist change because they do not believe they have a problem or fail to see the seriousness of their problem with substances. The second stage, *contemplation,* occurs when patients are aware of

and are thinking about changing their addictive behavior but have not yet committed to change. Patients may remain in this stage for an extended period of time as they weigh both the positive and negative aspects of continued substance use. When patients are in the *preparation* stage, they have decided to change their behavior and will do so in the near future. Patients may prepare by reducing the amount of the substance they are using or seeking a substance abuse treatment facility where they may receive help for their problem. The fourth stage, *action,* occurs when patients are modifying their addictive behavior, such as cessation of substance use. Finally, patients are in the *maintenance* stage when they sustain their changed behaviors and continuously work on relapse prevention. An example of maintenance would be a patient who achieved 6 months of sobriety and continues to attend self-help groups to receive support for his abstinence and to educate himself about relapse prevention. The standard questionnaire, the University of Rhode Island Change Assessment (URICA), is a 32-item instrument that can be used to formally assess a patient's readiness to change (McConnaughy et al. 1983).

Understanding the patient's stage of change is important for treatment recommendations. For example, a patient seeks a voluntary evaluation of marijuana use and says she is ready to stop using marijuana. Recognizing that the patient is in the preparation stage, the interviewer may refer this patient to an appropriate outpatient treatment such as psychotherapy, group therapy, or self-help groups. Giving this patient a follow-up appointment in 1 month to reevaluate her marijuana use without any other treatment recommendations would be inappropriate because she wants and is ready to change her addictive behaviors. The patient may rethink her decision to abstain from all marijuana use during that month and may not choose to seek treatment at all.

For ambivalent patients in the contemplative stage, the interviewer can use motivational interviewing techniques (W. Miller and Rollnick 2002). Motivational interviewing is a therapeutic intervention in which a therapist adopts a nonjudgmental and supportive stance to explore a patient's ambivalence about changing addictive behaviors. The desired outcome of motivational interviewing is the resolution of the patient's ambivalence and the facilitation of an increased readiness to consider change. This method of interviewing avoids confrontational questions and employs a communicative style that educes the patient's rationale for and the benefits of change. By using motivational interviewing, the interviewer circumvents a patient's defensiveness about substance use and creates an environment where the patient may speak more freely about the advantages and disadvantages of change.

Conclusion

In this chapter we have discussed the importance of assessing use and abuse of substances in all patients seen in the clinical setting. We have outlined the content areas of inquiry of the interview as well as the adjunctive use of the physical examination, mental status examination, biological markers, reports of significant others, and screening instruments. We have also provided suggestions for the style of interviewing to enhance accurate assessment as well as motivation to change. A careful and accurate assessment of the patient will provide the necessary information for intervention and treatment planning and will enhance motivation by beginning to engage the patient in the process of change.

References

Adler I, Kandel DB: Cross-cultural perspectives on developmental stages in adolescent drug use. J Stud Alcohol 42:701–715, 1981

Allen J, Columbus M: Assessing Alcohol Problems: A Guide for Clinicians and Researchers. Rockville, MD, National Institute on Alcohol Abuse and Alcoholism, 1995

Allen J, Litten R, Fertig J: A review of research on the Alcohol Use Disorders Identification Test (AUDIT). Alcohol Clin Exp Res 21:613–619, 1997

American Psychiatric Association: Diagnostic and Statistical Manual of Mental Disorders, 4th Edition. Washington, DC, American Psychiatric Association, 1994

American Psychiatric Association: Diagnostic and Statistical Manual of Mental Disorders, 4th Edition, Text Revision. Washington, DC, American Psychiatric Association, 2000

Anglin MD, Hser Y, Booth MW: Sex differences in addict careers, IV: treatment. Am J Drug Alcohol Abuse 13:253–280, 1987

Aubin H, Laureaux C, Zerah F: Joint influence of alcohol, tobacco, and coffee on biological markers of heavy drinking in alcoholics. Biol Psychiatry 44:638–643, 1998

Babor TF, Stephens RS, Marlatt GA: Verbal report methods in clinical research on alcoholism: response bias and its minimization. J Stud Alcohol 48:410–424, 1987

Babor T, Fuente JDL, Saunders J, et al: AUDIT: The Alcohol Use Disorders Identification Test: Guidelines for Use in Primary Health Care. Geneva, World Health Organization, 1992

Babor T, Bohn M, Kranzler H: The Alcohol Use Disorders Identification Test (AUDIT): validation of a screening instrument for use in medical settings. J Stud Alcohol 56:423–432, 1995

Bennett ME, Bellack AS, Gearon JS: Treating substance abuse in schizophrenia: an initial report. J Subst Abuse Treat 20:163–175, 2001

Bierut L, Dinwiddie S, Begleiter H, et al: Familial transmission of substance dependence: alcohol, marijuana, cocaine, and habitual smoking: a report from the Collaborative Study on the Genetics of Alcoholism. Arch Gen Psychiatry 59:982–988, 1998

Bohn MJ, Babor TF, Kranzler HR: The Alcohol Use Disorders Identification Test (AUDIT): validation of a screening instrument for use in medical settings. J Stud Alcohol 56:423–432, 1995

Brady K, Casto S, Lydiard RB, et al: Substance abuse in an inpatient psychiatric sample. Am J Drug Alcohol Abuse 17:389–397, 1991

Bray J, Zarkin G, Ringwalt C, et al: The relationship between marijuana initiation and dropping out of high school. Health Econ 9:9–18, 2000

Brems C, Johnson M, Namyniuk L: Clients with substance abuse and mental health concerns: a guide for conducting intake interviews. J Behav Health Serv Res 29:327–334, 2002

Breslau N, Kilbey M, Andreski P: Nicotine dependence, major depression, and anxiety in young adults. Arch Gen Psychiatry 48:1069–1074, 1991

Brown G, Anderson B: Psychiatric morbidity in adult inpatients with childhood histories of sexual and physical abuse. Am J Psychiatry 148:55–61, 1991

Budney A, Higgins S, Hughes J, et al: Nicotine and caffeine use in cocaine-dependent individuals. J Subst Abuse 5:117–130, 1993

Cadoret RJ, Cain CA, Gove WM: Development of alcoholism in adoptees raised apart from alcoholic biologic relatives. Arch Gen Psychiatry 37:561–563, 1980

Carroll K: Methodological issues and problems in the assessment of substance abuse. Psychol Assess 7:349–358, 1995

Chan AW, Pristach EA, Welte JW, et al: Use of the TWEAK test in screening for alcoholism/heavy drinking in three populations. Alcohol Clin Exp Res 17:1188–1192, 1993

Cone E: New development in biological measures of drug prevalence, in The Validity of Self-Reported Drug Use: Improving the Accuracy of Survey Estimates (NIDA Research Monograph 167). Edited by Harrison L, Hughes A. Rockville, MD, National Institute on Drug Abuse, 1997, pp 108–129

Conigrave K, Hall W, Saunders J: The AUDIT questionnaire: choosing a cut-off score. Addiction 90:1349–1356, 1995

Crum RM, Bucholz KK, Helzer JE, et al: The risk of alcohol abuse and dependence in adulthood: the association with educational level. Am J Epidemiol 135:989–999, 1992

Crum RM, Helzer JE, Anthony JC: Level of education and alcohol abuse and dependence in adulthood: a further inquiry. Am J Public Health 83:830–837, 1993

Crum R, Ensminger ME, Ro M, et al: The association of educational achievement and school dropout with risk of alcoholism: a twenty-five-year prospective study of inner-city children. J Stud Alcohol 59:318–326, 1998

Curran G, Booth B: Longitudinal changes in predictor profiles of abstinence from alcohol use among male veterans. Alcohol Clin Exp Res 23:141–143, 1999

Daeppen J, Smith T, Schuckit M: Influence of age and body mass index on gamma glutamyltransferase activity: a 15-year follow-up evaluation in a community sample. Alcohol Clin Exp Res 22:941–944, 1998

Deitz D, Rohde F, Bertolucci D, et al: Prevalence of screening for alcohol use by physicians during routine physical examinations. Alcohol Health Res World 18:162–168, 1994

DiFranza J, Guerrera M: Alcoholism and smoking. J Stud Alcohol 51:130–135, 1990

Drake R, Wallach M: Substance abuse among the chronic mentally ill. Hosp Community Psychiatry 40:1041–1046, 1989

Eldred C, Washington M: Interpersonal relationships in heroin use by men and women and their role in treatment outcome. Int J Addict 11:117–130, 1976

Elliot D, Hickam D: Use of the T-ACE questions to detect risk-drinking source. Am J Obstet Gynecol 163:684–685, 1990

Ellis DA, Zucker RA, Fitzgerald HE: The roles of family influences in development and risk. Alcohol Health Res World 21:218–226, 1997

Fagerstrom K, Schneider N: Measuring nicotine dependence: a review of the Fagerstrom Tolerance Questionnaire. J Behav Med 12:159–182, 1989

First M, Spitzer R, Gibbon M: Structured Clinical Interview for DSM-IV Axis I Disorders—Patient Version 2.0 (SCID-I/P). New York, New York State Psychiatric Institute, 1997

Frances R, Franklin J: Treatment of Alcoholism and Addictions. Washington, DC, American Psychiatric Press, 1989

Gossop M, Griffiths P, Strang J: Sex differences in patterns of drug taking behaviour: a study at a London community drug team. Br J Psychiatry 164:101–104, 1994

Greenfield SF: Women and substance use disorders, in Psychopharmacology of Women: Sex, Gender, and Hormonal Considerations. Edited by Jensvold MF, Hamilton JA. Washington, DC, American Psychiatric Press, 1996, pp 299–321

Greenfield SF, O'Leary G: Sex differences in substance use disorders, in Psychiatric Illness in Women: Emerging Treatments and Research. Edited by Lewis-Hall F, Williams TS, Panetta JA, et al. Washington, DC, American Psychiatric Publishing, 2002, pp 467–533

Greenfield SF, Shore MF: Prevention of psychiatric disorders. Harv Rev Psychiatry 3:115–129, 1995

Greenfield SF, Weiss RD, Muenz LD, et al: The effect of depression on return to drinking: a prospective study. Arch Gen Psychiatry 55:259–265, 1998

Greenfield SF, Kolodziej ME, Sugarman DE, et al: History of abuse and drinking outcomes following inpatient alcohol treatment: a prospective study. Drug Alcohol Depend 67:227–234, 2002

Greenfield SF, Sugarman DE, Muenz LR, et al: The relationship between educational attainment and relapse among alcohol-dependent men and women: a prospective study. Alcohol Clin Exp Res 27:1278–1285, 2003

Griffin ML, Weiss RD, Mirin SM, et al: A comparison of male and female cocaine abusers. Arch Gen Psychiatry 46:122–126, 1989

Hahesy A, Willens T, Biederman J, et al: Temporal association between childhood psychopathology and substance use disorders: findings from a sample of adults with opioid or alcohol dependency. Psychiatry Res 109:245–253, 2002

Hasin D, Trautman K, Miele G, et al: Psychiatric Research Interview for Substance and Mental Disorders (PRISM): reliability for substance abusers. Am J Psychiatry 153:1195–1201, 1996

Havassy B, Hall S, Wasserman D: Social support and relapse: commonalities among alcoholics, opiate users, and cigarette smokers. Addict Behav 16:235–246, 1991

Haver B: Female alcoholics, V, the relationship between family history of alcoholism and outcome 3–10 years after treatment. Acta Psychiatr Scand 76:21–27, 1987

Helzer J, Pryzbeck T: The co-occurrence of alcoholism with other psychiatric disorders in the general population and its impact on treatment. J Stud Alcohol 49:219–224, 1988

Hesselbrock MN, Meyer RE, Keene JJ: Psychopathology in hospitalized alcoholics. Arch Gen Psychiatry 42:1050–1055, 1985

Hird S, Khuri ET, Dusenbury L, et al: Adolescents, in Substance Abuse: A Comprehensive Textbook. Edited by Lowinson JH, Ruiz P, Millman RB, et al. Baltimore, MD, Williams & Wilkins, 1997, pp 683–692

Horgan C: Substance Abuse: The Number One Health Problem, Key Indicators for Policy. Princeton, NJ, Robert Wood Johnson Foundation, 1993

Horgan C: Substance Abuse: The Nation's Number One Health Problem, Key Indicators for Policy Update. Princeton, NJ, Robert Wood Johnson Foundation, 2001

Hser Y, Anglin M, McGlothin W: Sex differences in addict careers, I: initiation of use. Am J Drug Alcohol Abuse 13:33–57, 1987

Kandel DB, Logan JA: Patterns of drug use from adolescence to young adulthood, I: periods of risk for initiation, continued use, and discontinuation. Am J Public Health 74:660–666, 1984

Kendler KS, Prescott CA: Cannabis use, abuse, and dependence in a population-based sample of female twins. Am J Psychiatry 155:1016–1022, 1998a

Kendler K, Prescott CA: Cocaine use, abuse and dependence in a population-based sample of female twins. Br J Psychiatry 173:345–350, 1998b

Kendler KS, Heath AC, Neale MC: A population-based twin study of alcoholism in women. JAMA 268:1877–1882, 1992

Kendler K, Neale M, Heath A, et al: A twin family study of alcoholism in women. Am J Psychiatry 151:707–715, 1994

Kendler KS, Davis CG, Kessler RC: The familial aggregation of common psychiatric and substance use disorders in the National Comorbidity Survey: a family history study. Br J Psychiatry 170:541–548, 1997

Kessler R, Crum R, Warner L, et al: Lifetime co-occurrence of DSM-III-R alcohol abuse and dependence with other psychiatric disorders in the National Comorbidity Survey. Arch Gen Psychiatry 54:313–321, 1997

Kitchens JM: Does this patient have an alcohol problem? JAMA 272:1782–1787, 1994

Kolodziej ME, Greenfield SF, Weiss RD: Outcome measurements in substance use disorders, in Outcome Measurement in Psychiatry: A Critical Review. Edited by IsHak WW, Burt T, Sederer LI. Washington, DC, American Psychiatric Publishing, 2002, pp 207–220

Krausz M, Degkwitz P, Kuhne A, et al: Comorbidity of opiate dependence and mental disorders. Addict Behav 23:767–783, 1998

Lynskey M, Hall W: The effects of adolescent cannabis use on educational attainment: a review. Addiction 95:1621–1630, 2000

Maisto S, Sobell L, Sobell M: Comparison of alcoholics' self-reports of drinking behavior with reports of collateral informants. J Consult Clin Psychol 47:106–112, 1979

Mayfield D, McLeod G, Hall P: The CAGE questionnaire: validation of a new alcoholism screening instrument. Am J Psychiatry 131:1121–1123, 1974

McConnaughy EA, Prochaska JO, Velicer WF: Stages of change in psychotherapy: measurement and sample profiles. Psychotherapy: Theory, Research and Practice 20:368–375, 1983

McGue M: Genes, environment and the etiology of alcoholism, in The Development of Alcohol Problems: Exploring the Biopsychosocial Matrix of Risk. (NIAAA Research Monograph No 26; NIH Publ No 94-3495). Edited by Zucker RA, Boyd G, Howard J. Rockville, MD, National Institute on Alcohol Abuse and Alcoholism, 1994, pp 1–40

McLellan AT, Kushner H, Metzger D, et al: The Fifth Edition of the Addiction Severity Index. J Subst Abuse Treat 9:199–213, 1992

Merikangas KR, Stolar M, Stevens DE, et al: Familial transmission of substance use disorders. Arch Gen Psychiatry 55:973–979, 1998

Miller FT, Busch F, Tanenbaum JH: Drug abuse in schizophrenia and bipolar disorder. Am J Drug Alcohol Abuse 15:291–295, 1989

Miller W, Rollnick S: Motivational Interviewing: Preparing People for Change. New York, Guilford, 2002

Miller W, Tonigan JS, Longabaugh R: The Drinker Inventory of Consequences (DrInC): An Instrument for Assessing Adverse Consequences of Alcohol Abuse (NIAAA Project MATCH Monograph Series, NIH Publ No 95-3911). Rockville, MD, National Institute on Alcohol Abuse and Alcoholism, 1995

Mirin SM, Weiss RD, Griffin ML, et al: Psychopathology in drug abusers and their families. Compr Psychiatry 32:36–51, 1991

Mueser KT, Bellack AS, Blanchard JJ: Comorbidity of schizophrenia and substance abuse: implications for treatment. J Consult Clin Psychol 60:845–856, 1992

Mueser KT, Yarnold PR, Rosenberg SD, et al: Substance use disorder in hospitalized severely mentally ill psychiatric patients: prevalence, correlates, and subgroups. Schizophr Bull 26:179–192, 2000

Mullahy J, Sindelar J: Life cycle effects of alcoholism on education, earnings, and occupation. Inquiry 26:272–282, 1989

Najavits LM, Weiss RD, Shaw SR, et al: "Seeking safety": outcome of a new cognitive-behavioral psychotherapy for women with posttraumatic stress disorder and substance dependence. J Trauma Stress 11:437–456, 1998

National Institute on Alcohol Abuse and Alcoholism: Ninth Special Report to the U.S. Congress on Alcohol and Health. Rockville, MD, National Institute on Alcohol Abuse and Alcoholism, 1997, pp 33–63

Nurco D, Wegner N, Stephenson F: Female narcotic addicts: changing profiles. Journal on Addiction and Health 3:62–105, 1982

Prochaska J, DiClemente C, Norcross J: In search of how people change: applications to addictive behaviors. Am Psychol 47:1102–1114, 1992

Regier DA, Farmer ME, Rae DS, et al: Comorbidity of mental disorders with alcohol and other drug abuse: results from the Epidemiologic Catchment Area (ECA) study. JAMA 264:2511–2518, 1990

Rice C, Mohr C, Boca FD, et al: Self-reports of physical, sexual and emotional abuse in an alcoholism treatment sample. J Stud Alcohol 62:114–123, 2001

Robins LN, Przybeck TR: Age of onset of drug use as a factor in drug and other disorders, in Etiology of Drug Use: Implications for Prevention, Vol 56. Edited by Jones CL, Batthes RJ. Washington, DC, U.S. Government Printing Office, 1985, pp 178–192

Robins LN, Regier DA (eds): Psychiatric Disorders in America. New York, Free Press, 1991

Rounsaville B, Poling J: Substance use disorders measures, in Handbook of Psychiatric Measures. Task Force for the Handbook of Psychiatric Measures. Washington, DC, American Psychiatric Press, 2000, pp 457–484

Rounsaville BJ, Anton SF, Carroll K, et al: Psychiatric diagnoses of treatment-seeking cocaine abusers. Arch Gen Psychiatry 48:43–51, 1991

Russell M, Czarnecki D, Cowan R: Measures of maternal alcohol use as predictors of development in early childhood. Alcohol Clin Exp Res 15:991–1000, 1991

Schottenfeld R, Pantalon M: Assessment of the patient, in The American Psychiatric Press Textbook of Substance Abuse Treatment, 2nd Edition. Edited by Galanter M, Kleber H. Washington, DC, American Psychiatric Press, 1999, pp 109–120

Sellers E, Sullivan J, Somer G: Characterization of DSM-III-R criteria for uncomplicated alcohol withdrawal provides an empirical basis for DSM-IV. Arch Gen Psychiatry 48:442–447, 1991

Selzer ML: The Michigan Alcoholism Screening Test: the quest for a new diagnostic instrument. Am J Psychiatry 127:1653–1658, 1971

Senay EC: Diagnostic interview and mental status examination, in Substance Abuse: A Comprehensive Textbook. Edited by Lowinson JE, Pedro R, Millman RB, et al. Baltimore, MD, Williams & Wilkins, 1997, pp 364–369

Sidney S, Quesenberry CP, Friedman GD, et al: Marijuana use and cancer incidence (California, United States). Cancer Causes Control 8:722–728, 1997

Skinner HA: The drug abuse screening test. Addict Behav 7:363–371, 1982

Sobell LC, Sobell MB: Timeline follow-back: a technique for assessing self-reported alcohol consumption, in Measuring Alcohol Consumption. Edited by Litten R, Allen J. New York, Humana, 1992, pp 41–72

Sobell LC, Agrawal S, Sobell M: Factors affecting agreement between alcohol abusers' and their collaterals' reports. J Stud Alcohol 58:405–413, 1997

Sokol R, Martier S, Ager J: The T-ACE questions: practical prenatal detection of risk drinking. Am J Obstet Gynecol 160:863–870, 1989

Sonne S, Brady K, Morton W: Substance abuse and bipolar affective disorder. J Nerv Ment Dis 182:349–352, 1994

Staley D, El-Guebaly N: Psychometric properties of the Drug Abuse Screening Test in a psychiatric patient population. Addict Behav 15:257–264, 1990

Substance Abuse and Mental Health Services Administration: Year-End 2000 Emergency Department Data from the Drug Abuse Warning Network, DAWN Series D-18. Rockville, MD, Substance Abuse and Mental Health Services Administration, Office of Applied Studies, 2001

Taylor FM: Marijuana as a potential respiratory tract carcinogen. South Med J 81:1213–1216, 1988

Warren CW, Kann L, Small ML, et al: Age of initiating selected health-risk behaviors among high school students in the United States. J Adolesc Health 21:225–231, 1997

Washburn P: Substance use disorders: approaching the patient. Occup Med 17:67–78, 2002

Weiss RD, Mirin SM, Griffin ML, et al: A comparison of alcoholic and non-alcoholic drug abusers. J Stud Alcohol 49:510–515, 1988

Weiss RD, Mirin SM, Griffin ML, et al: Personality disorders in cocaine dependence. Compr Psychiatry 34:145–149, 1993

Weiss RD, Martinez-Raga J, Griffin ML, et al: Gender differences in cocaine dependent patients: a 6 month follow-up study. Drug Alcohol Depend 44:35–40, 1997

Weiss RD, Najavits LM, Greenfield SF, et al: Validity of substance use self-reports in dually diagnosed outpatients. Am J Psychiatry 155:127–128, 1998

Weiss RD, Greenfield SF, Griffin ML, et al: The use of collateral reports for patients with bipolar disorder and substance use disorders. Am J Drug Alcohol Abuse 26:369–378, 2000a

Weiss RD, Griffin ML, Greenfield SF, et al: Group therapy for patients with bipolar disorder and substance dependence: results of a pilot study. J Clin Psychiatry 61:361–367, 2000b

Westermeyer J: Native Americans, Asians, and new immigrants, in Substance Abuse: A Comprehensive Textbook. Edited by Lowinson JH, Ruiz P, Millman RB, et al. Baltimore, MD, Williams & Wilkins, 1997, pp 712–716

Wills TA, McNamara G, Vaccaro D, et al: Escalated substance use: a longitudinal grouping analysis from early to middle adolescence. J Abnorm Psychol 105:166–180, 1996

Wilsnack S, Vogeltanz N, Klassen A, et al: Childhood sexual abuse and women's substance abuse: national survey findings. J Stud Alcohol 58:264–271, 1997

Windle M, Windle RC, Scheidt DM, et al: Physical and sexual abuse and associated mental disorders among alcoholic inpatients. Am J Psychiatry 152:1322–1328, 1995

Woody GE, Cacciola J: Diagnosis and classification: DSM-IV and ICD-10, in Substance Abuse: A Comprehensive Textbook. Edited by Lowinson JH, Pedro R, Millman RB, et al. Baltimore, MD, Williams & Wilkins, 1997, pp 361–363

World Health Organization: Problems Related to Alcohol Consumption: Technical Report Series 650. Geneva, World Health Organization, 1980

World Health Organization: International Statistical Classification of Diseases and Related Health Problems, 10th Revision. Geneva, World Health Organization, 1992

Yamaguchi K, Kandel DB: Patterns of drug use from adolescence to young adulthood, II: sequences of progression. Am J Public Health 74:668–672, 1984a

Yamaguchi K, Kandel DB: Patterns of drug use from adolescence to young adulthood, III: predictors of progression. Am J Public Health 74:673–681, 1984b

Patient Placement Criteria

David R. Gastfriend, M.D.
Sandrine Pirard, M.D.

Patient placement criteria are decision rules that standardize treatment for optimal clinical and cost-effectiveness. Research demonstrates that substance abuse treatments reduce alcohol and drug use and relieve associated medical conditions and social, familial, and psychological problems. Nevertheless, treatment is not effective in every case, and programs vary widely in effectiveness. Beginning in the latter half of the 1980s, cost containment and managed care brought pressure on providers to justify treatment referrals for each patient. On a broader scale, effective use of resources is of interest not only in the context of the managed care process in the United States but also internationally, particularly within countries with national health care systems. In this larger context, patient placement criteria are increasingly being implemented.

Substance use disorders are heterogeneous and cause diverse biopsychosocial problems that vary by population. Standardized assessment might increase treatment effectiveness by helping to individualize treatment; however, this assumption remains to be proved.

In general, reviews of the literature on treatment outcome reveal that no single approach is superior. Principles for matching modalities of treatment to specific patients' needs have not been easily proved. At the least, this state of affairs is an annoyance, because multiple analyses indicate that the cost-effectiveness of addiction treatment is suboptimal (Institute of Medicine 1990, 1990–1992; Miller and Hester 1986b). Furthermore, when treatment components do achieve some degree of research-based support, such components often fail to gain adoption in for-profit treatment systems. These challenges have been driving studies in client-treatment matching and cost-effectiveness research.

Work for this chapter was supported by National Institute on Drug Abuse grants R01 DA08781 and K24 DA0042 (Dr. Gastfriend) and by the Belgian National Fund for Scientific Research and the Belgian American Educational Foundation (Dr. Pirard).

Rationale for Patient Placement Criteria

Level-of-care matching is the basis for cost-effective patient placement criteria. A managed care network has its best opportunity for clinical and cost optimization when level-of-care matching rules are valid and a range of settings is available. In contrast to treatment modalities, levels of care are placement options or settings that offer varying treatment intensities, structures, and degrees of restrictiveness. Levels of care have important cost implications; for example, the following settings represent decreasing levels of expense: hospital treatment, residential treatment, day treatment, and outpatient treatment.

Theoretically, certain levels of care might be expected to yield better cost savings than others; however, outcome studies have not shown conclusive benefits for inpatient versus outpatient rehabilitation or detoxification (Annis 1988; Hayashida et al. 1989; Litt et al. 1989; Miller and Hester 1986a). In fact, studies have consistently failed to prove that more-intensive treatment settings offer better outcomes than less-intensive ones. Managed care entities have used this pattern to justify eliminating higher levels of care such as hospital-based detoxification and rehabilitation. A critical point, however, is that these studies did not attempt to distinguish which patients experience the best outcomes from which level of care.

Origins and Organization of the American Society of Addiction Medicine Patient Placement Criteria

Managed care cost pressures during the 1980s prompted the development of 40–50 sets of treatment-matching protocols for addictions, many of which were proprietary and conflicting. A haphazard, confusing system arose that frustrated providers who sought admission for their patients. Among nonprofit professional provider organizations, parallel efforts arose with important differences between placement criteria. These included the Cleveland Criteria, developed for the Northern Ohio Chemical Dependency Treatment Directors Association (Hoffmann et al. 1987), and the

National Association of Addiction Treatment Providers (NAATP) Patient Placement Criteria (Weedman 1987). Despite the poor predictive validity of the Cleveland Criteria, these guidelines nonetheless became recognized as a significant contribution to the pursuit of treatment matching. Work groups of experts from internal medicine, adult and child psychiatry, pediatrics, psychology, social work, and addiction counseling subsequently critiqued the Cleveland Criteria and NAATP criteria and revised these into a single, new system.

The result of these consensus reviews was the 1991 publication of the first edition of the American Society of Addiction Medicine (ASAM) Patient Placement Criteria (PPC-1) (Hoffmann et al. 1991). This volume described four levels of care for adult and adolescent treatment. Levels of care were distinguished by the degree to which they provided medical management, structure, security, and treatment intensity. The ASAM criteria specified rules for treatment matching at three time points: admission, continued-stay review, and discharge. To place a patient, the evaluator was required to screen and diagnose the patient and then to assess patient characteristics in six dimensions encompassing all pertinent biopsychosocial aspects of addiction that determine the severity of the patient's illness and level of function. Figure 11–1 presents a schematic representation of the use of the ASAM Criteria.

Patients can be evaluated along these domains most effectively through the use of structured interviews (Gastfriend et al. 1994) such as the Addiction Severity Index (ASI) (McLellan et al. 1992), the Recovery Attitudes and Treatment Evaluator (RAATE) (Gastfriend et al. 1995; Mee-Lee et al. 1992; Najavits et al. 1997), the Clinical Institute Withdrawal Assessment (CIWA) (Sullivan et al. 1989), and the Clinical Institute Narcotics Assessment (CINA) (Fudala et al. 1991). The CIWA and CINA are standardized scales that can be used to evaluate the first assessment dimension, acute intoxication or withdrawal. The ASI and the RAATE can be used to evaluate patients on several dimensions. The ASI is a widely utilized structured interview that is designed to assess substance abuse patients on seven dimensions: medical status, employment/support status, drug use, alcohol use, legal status, family/social relationships, and psychiatric status. The RAATE was jointly developed by members of the ASAM Criteria work group to facilitate use of the criteria. Typical items from the RAATE include the following: "Does the patient demonstrate a commitment to

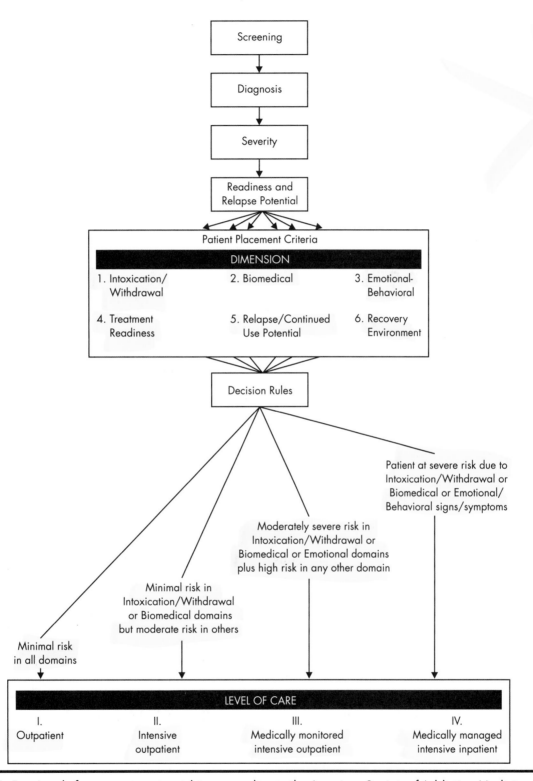

Figure 11-1. Level-of-care treatment matching according to the American Society of Addiction Medicine (ASAM) Patient Placement Criteria.

Summary of the assessment areas, dimensions, decision rules, and level-of-care settings of the ASAM Patient Placement Criteria for the Treatment of Psychoactive Substance Use Disorders. (Decision rules are an approximation only; see referenced text for detailed description.)

Source. Adapted from *Medical Clinics of North America,* Volume 81, Gastfriend DR and McClellan AT: "Treatment Matching: Theoretic Bases and Practical Implications," pp. 946–966, 1997. Used with permission from Elsevier Science.

seeking help or treatment?" "Does the patient realize that recovery is an ongoing process requiring personal responsibility?" "Does the patient have a chronic physical condition or disability which interferes with treatment or recovery efforts?" "Is the patient able to focus on addictions treatment even if he/she has psychiatric/psychological symptoms?" and "Is the work/school system accommodating or supportive of the treatment/recovery program?" The instruments listed above were the main feeders of an automated decision tree created to facilitate the use of the ASAM PPC-1 (Turner et al. 1999).

Research Findings and Automation

Publication of these nonproprietary matching criteria raised considerable interest, ranging from continuing education courses across the United States to adoption by managed care entities and 20 U.S. states. A shortcoming existed, however, because no process of field trial testing preceded the publication of the criteria. This led scientists to subject the Patient Placement Criteria to the crucial process of research testing. The literature in general strongly supports the need for patient placement criteria based on multidimensional assessment in treatment planning (Gastfriend et al. 2000; Hser et al. 1999; McLellan et al. 1997), and numerous studies have shown the predictive validity and cost-effectiveness of models such as the dimensions and levels of care of the ASAM PPC (Alterman et al. 1994; Annis 1988; Gastfriend and McLellan 1997; Hayashida et al. 1989; Mechanic et al. 1995). More specifically, a considerable body of work exists to date on the ASAM PPC itself, including at least eight evaluations involving a total of 3,440 subjects. Federal agencies—including the National Institute on Drug Abuse, the National Institute on Alcohol Abuse and Alcoholism, and the Center for Substance Abuse Treatment—have currently invested more than $7 million in this research (Gastfriend 2001).

In the earliest evaluation of the ASAM PPC, the Boston Target Cities Project used a one-page version of the ASAM Criteria in a large urban public population. Compared with direct self-referred admission to treatment programs, patients who were referred via centralized intake centers using standardized assessment with a coarse implementation of the ASAM Criteria were 38% more likely to make the transition to longitudinal treatment within 30 days and were significantly less likely to return for detoxification within 90 days (Plough et al. 1996). These findings suggested that feasibility would be within reach, because even this shortened version of the ASAM Criteria was associated with improved retention. An incomplete implementation of the original ASAM Criteria by McKay et al. (1997) was used to retrospectively test its psychosocial dimensions. This study suggested some areas of validity but highlighted a need for further revision. A prospective, naturalistic study examined the validity and impact of the PPC, comparing the placement of 287 adults within Washington State versus 240 adults within Oregon, where a statewide Patient Placement Criteria training model was fully implemented. Results showed that the use of standardized criteria such as the PPC led to better length-of-stay differentiation and improved utilization of the intensive outpatient level of care (Deck et al., in press).

To help deal with the complexity of the multidimensional branching logic of the PPC, researchers at the Massachusetts General Hospital Addiction Research Program implemented the ASAM Criteria as a comprehensive computerized interview (Turner et al. 1999). This real-time, computerized method for addiction treatment matching yielded a satisfactory degree of interrater reliability for the level-of-care assignment (intraclass correlation coefficient=0.77; $P<0.01$) (Baker and Gastfriend, in press), comparing favorably with the literature on diagnosis and severity rating (Endicott et al. 1976; Hall 1995; Regier et al. 1994).

To date, three prospective studies have tested this method. In the first one, a naturalistic study of 95 Department of Veterans Affairs patients near Boston, Massachusetts, PPC-1 matching was associated with reductions in subsequent hospital utilization (Gastfriend et al. 1998). In the second, a naturalistic study of 248 newly admitted, primarily alcohol-dependent subjects in New York City, both convergent validity and predictive validity of the PPC-1 algorithm were tested. Staines et al. (in press) examined the convergent validity by comparing level-of-care recommendations produced by the computerized algorithm with those developed by clinicians. Areas of both agreement and disagreement between the algorithm and the clinicians were found, but more importantly, the results pointed out the need for revision of the PPC to increase their clarity and to optimize their use. Magura et al. (in press) showed that outpatients who were receiving a lower level of care than that recommended by the PPC-1 had poorer alcohol use outcomes than those who were correctly matched to treatment and that overtreatment did not improve outcome. These results supported the predictive validity and cost-effectiveness of the use of Patient Placement Criteria.

The third prospective study, a multisite trial in Massachusetts, is the first randomized, controlled trial of placement criteria to be conducted to date. In this project, 700 subjects were randomized to Level II or Level III treatment, either matched or mismatched according to the recommendation of the PPC-1 algorithm. Preliminary results showed good concurrent validity (Turner et al. 1999) and evidence for predictive validity, because patients who were mismatched to a lower level of care than was recommended had higher no-show rates and less or slower improvement on several dimensions of addiction severity (Gastfriend 2001).

The ultimate goal of this ongoing research work is revision of the PPC that will emerge not simply from the current expert consensus process but also through the findings from multiple national and international research studies.

Revisions of the American Society of Addiction Medicine Patient Placement Criteria

The way that services were grouped or "bundled" in the original ASAM Criteria did not allow for great flexibility to meet individual patient needs. Between 1994 and 1995 the Coalition for National Treatment Criteria recognized that the ASAM Criteria required revision; in particular, they addressed criticism of the ASAM Criteria from managed care. These criticisms included the limitations of only four levels of care, the absence of criteria for methadone, and the required association of detoxification with inpatient care (Book et al. 1995). Most critical was the need for a method of "unbundling" the levels of care into their component services.

The second edition of the ASAM PPC (ASAM PPC-2; American Society of Addiction Medicine 1996) addressed many of these needs. This revision unbundled pharmacotherapies such as detoxification and opioid maintenance therapy (e.g., methadone) from rehabilitation services and described multilevel criteria for

both outpatient and inpatient settings. For Level II (intensive outpatient) care, new criteria were described to distinguish between evening care or day treatment programs (Level II.1) and partial hospitalization (Level II.5); for Level III (residential inpatient) care, criteria were added to distinguish between clinically managed low-intensity residential treatment (e.g., supervised domiciliary or working halfway house) (Level III.1), clinically managed medium-intensity residential treatment (e.g., modified, individualized treatment for cognitively impaired patients) (Level III.3), clinically managed high-intensity residential treatment (e.g., therapeutic community or residential treatment center) (Level III.5), and medically monitored intensive inpatient treatment (e.g., residential rehabilitation with onsite nursing supervision) (Level III.7). Criteria were added for a new level of care (Level 0.5, early intervention), which was defined as professional services for individuals who are at risk of developing substance-related problems but who may not yet qualify for a diagnosis.

The following example illustrates the growing distinctions that are being made. A patient with a history of withdrawal seizures but only mild medical conditions would be matched to Level III.7 (medically monitored inpatient detoxification). After 3–7 days without complications the patient would be "stepped down" to Level III.5 (therapeutic community) to deal with problems such as poor compliance, difficulty postponing gratification, criminal behavior, and drug-oriented relationships. This would utilize the least restrictive and least costly settings that could be expected to address the patient's needs in both phases of treatment.

The revised second edition of the ASAM PPC (ASAM PPC-2R; Mee-Lee et al. 2001) addresses the needs of patients with dual diagnoses (co-occurring mental and substance-related disorders) along a continuum of mental health and substance use service sublevels. In addition, the criteria for adolescents have been completely revised.

Significance

The changes described above were widely welcomed in the United States and resulted in adoption by payors, single-state agencies, and state Medicaid programs. In 1997, the ASAM Criteria were adopted for worldwide use by the U.S. Department of Defense and by the U.S. Department of Veterans Affairs for its 171 hospitals nationwide. International collaborations have recently been initiated to implement the use of the criteria in European, Asian, and South American countries. Yet the revised ASAM Criteria describe a desirable continuum of care that is still only in the planning stages in many regions. For example, many regions lack options such as methadone access for halfway house residents or office-based detoxification. Nevertheless, these criteria are useful guides for improving the quality and reducing the cost of patient care, particularly for capitated systems. Matching hypotheses in general should also serve as strategic guidelines for health care networks in program development and acquisition, despite the need for further methodological work and field trials of efficacy and effectiveness (Longabaugh et al. 1994).

Alternatives to Patient Placement Criteria

The ASAM Criteria orient treatment matching according to fixed levels of care. First the levels of care are described and then patients must conform to these defined settings. But level of care is a coarse distinction that lumps together heterogeneous groups of patients with a range of needs. Instead, it may be more advantageous to orient placement criteria in the opposite direction, meeting patient needs rather than fitting program requirements (Longabaugh et al. 1995; McLellan et al. 1997). This approach of "needs-to-services" matching is clinically useful whether performed formally in a research design or informally in the clinic. The key operations are a multidimensional consideration of the patient's range of needs and the provision of services to address those needs. Results from several studies have shown that matching clinical services to patient needs generally yields the best outcomes in that distinct problem area, validating needs-for-services matching (Ball and Ross 1991; Institute of Medicine 1990–1992; Joe et al. 1991; McLellan et al. 1983a, 1983b, 1993a, 1993b, 1994; Moos and Finney 1995).

Although needs-to-services treatment matching is a logical starting point for a new model of care planning, it is still necessary to consider the setting or level of care within which services can best be provided. A highly flexible, individualized approach to level-of-care assignment seems essential to clinical quality and cost efficiency. To achieve this integration with flexibil-

ity, Gastfriend (1994) proposed to the National Coalition on Placement Criteria an approach termed the Cumulative Block Increment (CBI) model. Based on a building-block concept of small service units (e.g., hour by hour of care), this approach recommended a high-resolution assessment of individual clinical needs, followed by grouping these needs together to determine the best setting for the constellation of necessary services. With the CBI model, services could be designed to taper more incrementally in an individualized fashion. This model would integrate level-of-care consideration with needs-to-services matching. Although the CBI model appears to offer face validity, as did earlier patient placement criteria models, it too awaits empirical validation.

Conclusion

Psychiatrists, physicians, and other providers can address patients' substance use problems on a rational basis with the help of published patient placement criteria. Adoption of formal rules such as the ASAM criteria is under way in numerous states, managed care entities, professional provider societies, and provider groups, and interest has been raised internationally. Initially, such criteria relied more heavily on consensus recommendations than on empirical matching data, but outcome research data drive their continuous revision. The technology for conducting psychosocial treatment matching studies has been rapidly increasing in sophistication and has been demonstrated to yield adequate reliability and concurrent validity. Although predictive validity has not yet been fully demonstrated, the national research portfolio on placement criteria is expanding. Given recent dramatic cost pressures, there is an essential public health need for further research in this area if addiction services are to continue to grow in quality and availability.

References

Alterman AI, O'Brien CP, McLellen AT, et al: Effectiveness and costs of inpatient versus day hospital cocaine rehabilitation. J Nerv Ment Dis 182:157–163, 1994

American Society of Addiction Medicine: Patient Placement Criteria for the Treatment of Substance-Related Disorders: ASAM PPC-2, 2nd Edition. Chevy Chase, MD, American Society of Addiction Medicine, 1996

Annis H: Patient-treatment matching in the management of alcoholism. NIDA Res Monogr 90:152–161, 1988

Baker SL, Gastfriend DR: Reliability of multidimensional substance abuse treatment matching: implementing the ASAM Patient Placement Criteria. J Addict Dis (in press)

Ball J, Ross A: The Effectiveness of Methadone Maintenance Treatment. New York, Springer-Verlag, 1991

Book J, Harbin H, Marques C, et al: The ASAM and Green Spring alcohol and drug detoxification and rehabilitation criteria for utilization review. Am J Addict 4:187–197, 1995

Deck D, Gabriel R, Knudson J: Impact of patient placement criteria on substance abuse treatment under the Oregon Health Plan. J Addict Dis (in press)

Endicott J, Spitzer R, Fleiss JL, et al: The Global Assessment Scale: a procedure for measuring overall severity of psychiatric diagnosis. Arch Gen Psychiatry 33:766–773, 1976

Fudala PJ, Berkow LC, Fralich JL, et al: Use of naloxone in the assessment of opiate dependence. Life Sci 49:1809–1814, 1991

Gastfriend DR: Memo to the National Consortium on Patient Placement Criteria: The Cumulative Block Increment Model. Chevy Chase, MD, American Society of Addiction Medicine, 1994

Gastfriend DR: Placement criteria come of age. Paper presented at the annual medical-scientific meeting of the American Society of Addiction Medicine, Los Angeles, A, April 20, 2001

end DR, McLellan AT: Treatment matching: theoretic s and practical implications. Med Clin North Am 045–966, 1997

end DR, Baker SL, Najavits LM, et al: Assessment in ments, in Principles of Addiction Medicine. Edited by ler N, Doot M. Chevy Chase, MD, American Society of Addiction Medicine, 1994, pp 1–8

astfriend DR, Filstead WJ, Reif S, et al: Validity of assessing treatment readiness in patients with substance use disorders. Am J Addict 4:254–260, 1995

Gastfriend DR, Sharon E, Turner W, et al: Validity of multidimensional substance abuse treatment matching using the ASAM Patient Placement Criteria. Paper presented at the annual meeting of the American Society of Addiction Medicine, April 1998

Gastfriend DR, Lu SH, Sharon E: Placement matching: challenges and technical progress. Subst Use Misuse 35(12–14):2191–2213, 2000

Hall R: Global assessment of functioning: a modified scale. Psychosomatics 36:267–275, 1995

Hayashida M, Alterman AI, McLellan AT, et al: Comparative effectiveness and costs of inpatient and outpatient detoxification of patients with mild-to-moderate alcohol withdrawal syndrome. N Engl J Med 320:358–365, 1989

Hoffmann N, Halikas J, Mee-Lee D: The Cleveland Admission, Discharge and Transfer Criteria: Model for Chemical Dependency Treatment Programs. Cleveland, OH, Northern Ohio Chemical Dependency Treatment Consortium, 1987

Hoffmann N, Halikas J, Mee-Lee D, et al: American Society of Addiction Medicine Patient Placement Criteria for the Treatment of Psychoactive Substance Use Disorders. Washington, DC, American Society of Addiction Medicine, 1991

Hser YI, Polinsky ML, Maglione M, et al: Matching clients' needs with drug treatment services. J Subst Abuse Treat 16:299–305, 1999

Institute of Medicine: Broadening the Base of Treatment for Alcohol Problems: A Report of a Study by a Committee of the Institute of Medicine, Division of Mental Health and Behavioral Medicine. Washington, DC, National Academy Press, 1990

Institute of Medicine, Committee for Substance Abuse Coverage Study: Treating Drug Problems. Edited by Gerstein DR, Harwood HJ. Washington, DC, National Academy Press, 1990–1992

Joe GW, Simpson DD, Hubbard RL, et al: Treatment predictors of tenure in methadone maintenance. J Subst Abuse 3:73–84, 1991

Litt M, Boca F, Cooney N: Matching Alcoholics to Aftercare Treatment by Empirical Clustering. Farmington, CT, University of Connecticut Health Center, 1989

Longabaugh R, Wirtz PW, DiClemente CC, et al: Issues in the development of client-treatment matching hypotheses. J Stud Alcohol Suppl 12:46–59, 1994

Longabaugh R, Wirtz PW, Beattie MC, et al: Matching treatment focus to patient social investment and support: 18-month follow-up results. J Consult Clin Psychiatry 63:296–307, 1995

Magura S, Staines GL, Kosanke N, et al: Predictive validity of the ASAM Patient Placement Criteria for naturalistically matched vs. mismatched alcohol-dependent patients. Am J Addict (in press)

McKay JR, Cacciola JS, McLellan AT, et al: An initial evaluation of the psychosocial dimensions of the American Society of Addiction Medicine criteria for inpatient vs. intensive outpatient substance abuse rehabilitation. J Stud Alcohol 58:239–252, 1997

McLellan AT, Woody GE, Luborsky L, et al: Increased effectiveness of substance abuse treatment: a prospective study of patient-treatment "matching." J Nerv Ment Dis 171:597–605, 1983a

McLellan AT, Woody GE, Luborsky L, et al: Predicting response to alcohol and drug abuse treatments. Arch Gen Psychiatry 40:620–625, 1983b

McLellan A, Kushner H, Metzger DS, et al: The fifth edition of the Addiction Severity Index. J Subst Abuse Treat 9:199–213, 1992

McLellan AT, Arndt IO, Metzger DS, et al: The effects of psychosocial services in substance abuse treatment. JAMA 269:1953–1959, 1993a

McLellan AT, Grissom GR, Brill P, et al: Private substance abuse treatments: are some programs more effective than others? J Subst Abuse Treat 10:243–254, 1993b

McLellan A, Alterman A, Metzger DS, et al: Similarity of outcome predictors across opiate, cocaine and alcohol treatments: role of treatment services. J Clin Consult Psychol 62:1141–1158, 1994

McLellan AT, Grissom GR, Zanis D, et al: Problem-service "matching" in addiction treatment: a prospective study in 4 programs. Arch Gen Psychiatry 54:730–735, 1997

Mechanic D, Schlesinger M, McAlpine DD, et al: Management of mental health and substance abuse services: state of the art and early results. Milbank Q 73:19–55, 1995

Mee-Lee D, Hoffman D, Smith M: Recovery Attitude and Treatment Evaluator (RAATE) Manual. St Paul, MN, CATOR/New Standards, 1992

Mee-Lee D, Shulman GD, Fishman M, et al: ASAM Patient Placement Criteria for the Treatment of Substance-Related Disorders, 2nd Edition, Revised (ASAM PPC-2R). Chevy Chase, MD, American Society of Addiction Medicine, 2001

Miller WR, Hester RK: The effectiveness of alcoholism treatment: what research reveals, in Treating Addictive Behaviors: Processes of Change. Edited by Miller WR, Heather N. New York, Plenum, 1986a, pp 121–174

Miller WR, Hester RK: Matching problem drinkers with optimal treatments, in Treating Addictive Behaviors: Processes of Change. Edited by Miller WR, Heather N. New York, Plenum, 1986b, pp 175–204

Moos RH, Finney JW: Substance abuse treatment programs and processes: linkages to patients' needs and outcomes. J Subst Abuse 7:1–8, 1995

Najavits LM, Gastfriend DR, Nakayama EY, et al: A measure of readiness for substance abuse treatment: psychometric properties of the RAATE research interview. Am J Addict 6:74–82, 1997

Plough AL, Shirley, Zaremba N, et al: CSAT Target Cities Demonstration Final Evaluation Report, Boston Office for Treatment Improvement. Boston, MA, Massachusetts Bureau of Substance Abuse Services, 1996

Regier DA, Kaebler CT, Roper MT, et al: The ICD-10 clinical field trial for mental and behavioral disorders: results in Canada and the United States. Am J Psychiatry 151:1340–1350, 1994

Staines GL, Kosanke N, Magura S, et al: Convergent validity of the ASAM Patient Placement Criteria using a standardized computer algorithm. J Addict Dis (in press)

Sullivan JT, Sykora K, Schneiderman J, et al: Assessment of alcohol withdrawal: the revised Clinical Institute Withdrawal Assessment for Alcohol Scale. Br J Addict 84:1353–1357, 1989

Turner WM, Turner KH, Reif S, et al: Feasibility of multidimensional substance abuse treatment matching: automating the ASAM Patient Placement Criteria. Drug Alcohol Depend 55:35–43, 1999

Weedman RD: Admission, Continued Stay and Discharge Criteria for Adult Alcoholism and Drug Dependence Treatment Services. Irvine, CA, National Association of Addiction Treatment Providers, 1987

Outcome Research

Alcoholism

Reid K. Hester, Ph.D.
Daniel D. Squires, M.S., M.P.H.

Treatments for alcohol abuse and dependence have progressed substantially during the past decade, and the scope of effective treatments offers hope with regard to these troubling problems. This chapter is a review of the current research in treatment of alcohol problems. Instead of *alcoholism,* which implies a unitary condition, we use the term *alcohol problems.* We assume that alcohol problems lie on a continuum and that effective treatments benefit many more individuals than the relatively small group at the high end of the severity spectrum.

A comprehensive and historical investigation of all alcohol treatments is beyond the scope of this chapter, so we focus primarily on current treatments that have the best empirical support. It should be remembered that there is no one treatment that is superior to all others. Rather, there are a variety of treatments that can be helpful to patients. Treatments absent from this chapter are not necessarily ineffective; rather, those treatments may not have been subjected to the careful study that the treatments considered here have undergone. Later in the chapter, we briefly discuss treatments that controlled research has shown to be ineffective.

The value of controlled trials in investigating the effectiveness of treatments for alcohol problems cannot be overstated. Historically, this field has been vulnerable to the introduction of exciting new treatments that in subsequent controlled trials are shown to have marginal or no importance for this population.

In our review, we use a rating system for treatments that was developed by W.R. Miller and colleagues (1995, 1998) for evaluating controlled studies. This rating system generates an overall score, the Cumulative Evidence Score (CES), which is the product of a methodological quality score and a rating of the strength of outcomes for a particular treatment approach. (See W.R. Miller et al. 2003 for full details of the CES for each treatment.)

Evidence of Effectiveness: What Research Reveals

Interventions With Strong Evidence of Effectiveness

For the following interventions, which are ranked according to CES, evidence of effectiveness is considered to be strong (i.e., three or more published studies exist, appropriate methodological designs were used, and outcomes were positive) (W.R. Miller et al. 2003):

- Brief interventions
- Motivational enhancement therapies
- γ-Aminobutyric acid (GABA) agonist therapy
- The community reinforcement approach
- Bibliotherapy (use of self-change manuals)
- Opioid antagonist (naltrexone) therapy
- Behavioral self-control training
- Behavior contracting
- Social skills training
- Behavioral marital therapy
- Nausea aversion therapy
- Case management

These treatments have been consistently supported by controlled research. However, some interventions have been studied more than others. For instance, there have been 34 clinical trials of brief interventions but only 5 of the GABA agonist acamprosate.

Brief interventions hold great promise for affecting the drinking behaviors of individuals with alcohol-related problems. Furthermore, such interventions can be effectively carried out in settings other than alcohol treatment programs. The Institute of Medicine (1990) concluded that brief interventions are appropriate interventions for health care providers outside the specialized treatment sector (e.g., internists, family practitioners, and psychiatrists in general practice).

Although a variety of different brief interventions have been developed, most have several features in common. The typical elements can be represented by the acronym FRAMES: **F**eedback regarding a patient's drinking is individualized and objective; **R**esponsibility is placed on the patient for deciding what to do regarding drinking; clear **A**dvice to change is given (carefully), as is a **M**enu of interventions and options for change; the counselor uses an **E**mpathic style of interacting with the patient; and there is an emphasis on **S**elf-efficacy (W.R. Miller and Sanchez 1994).

The time involved in conducting a comprehensive assessment and providing the patient with one or two brief feedback sessions is minimal, especially relative to the time involved in comprehensive inpatient and outpatient programs. A relatively new, cost-effective option is to provide the patient with a computer-based brief intervention, such as the Drinker's Check-up (R.K. Hester, D.D. Squires, and H.D. Delaney, "The Drinker's Check-up: 12-Month Outcomes of a Controlled Clinical Trial of a Stand-alone Software Program for Problem Drinkers," Sept. 2003, submitted for publication). The Drinker's Check-up is a Windows program that provides a comprehensive assessment, personalized feedback, and motivational enhancement for individuals who are ambivalent about changing their drinking. In addition to the PC-based version, the Drinker's Check-up also is available on the Internet (http://www.drinkerscheckup.com). In general, whether offered in a face-to-face or PC-based format, brief interventions have compared favorably with more extensive interventions in outcome studies, and differences between groups are usually small (e.g., Edwards et al. 1977). For more about brief interventions, see Zweben et al. (2003).

Motivational enhancement therapies are similar to brief interventions, but they usually involve several additional sessions of motivational interviewing (W.R. Miller and Rollnick 2001) beyond a brief intervention.

In the past decade, there has been an increase in the number of new medications for the treatment of alcohol problems. Two new drugs, acamprosate (a GABA analogue) and naltrexone (an opioid antagonist), appear to work by reducing the craving of abstinent patients for alcohol. Animal models indicate that the effect of these medications is mediated through the glutamatergic and opioid systems, perhaps by reducing the reinforcing value of alcohol. Clinical trials clearly show that these medications reduce relapse to heavy drinking as well as craving in patients with drinking problems.

It is clear that pharmacological interventions will be an important component of future treatments for problem drinking. Newer medications are more effective, are better tolerated by patients, and generally pose less risk in overdose because they do not potentiate the effects of alcohol. Each of these medications has been evaluated as an adjunct to ongoing treatment for problem drinking. However, their effectiveness as stand-alone agents has not been evaluated. Furthermore, each of these medications may be contraindicated for a variety of physical problems, especially liver impairment, that are common in patients with drinking problems.

The community reinforcement approach focuses on modifying contingencies in the patient's environment to reinforce abstinence. At the heart of the community reinforcement approach is functional analysis. Functional analyses help the therapist and client examine drinking behaviors to understand the triggers, thought processes, behaviors, and consequences that reinforce a particular behavior. With this perspective, the client and therapist work collaboratively using problem-solving skills to identify reinforcing alternatives to drinking. The therapist and patient also rank the patient's alcohol-related problems and choose strategies from a menu of alternatives designed to reduce or eliminate these problems. The menu includes 1) sobriety sampling (e.g., a behavior contract for periods of abstinence), 2) a behavioral compliance program to take disulfiram or naltrexone, 3) behavioral marital counseling, 4) involvement in sober leisure-time activities, 5) training in problem solving, and 6) job-finding training (if the patient is unemployed). The community reinforcement approach was originally developed and tested in the early 1970s. In these early studies, positive outcomes in patients were reported in comparison with control groups. The impact of the community reinforcement approach on the field of alcohol treatment was relatively minor until the mid-1990s. Recently, however, the community reinforcement approach has received more attention and is becoming more popular in both the United States and Europe. Meyers and Smith (1995) wrote an extensive therapist manual for clinicians interested in this approach.

Seventeen studies have been conducted on the use of self-change or self-help manuals. Most of these manuals use the protocol of behavioral self-control training (BSCT). Miller and colleagues (2003) separated the studies into two categories to distinguish the method of administration. In the BSCT category, individuals received training either through face-to-face counseling or through a computer program. However, the distinction is somewhat arbitrary, because the same skills are taught regardless of the method of administration.

BSCT involves teaching patients a set of self-management skills that can be used either to moderate consumption to nonproblematic levels or to become and remain abstinent. Most patients choose a goal of moderation, at least initially. The most common elements of self-control training are goal setting, self-monitoring, rate control and reduction, self-reinforcement of progress and goal attainment, functional analysis, and learning alternative coping skills.

If the two categories of self-change manuals and BSCT are combined, it can be said that there have been more controlled clinical trials of BSCT than of any other intervention for alcohol problems. Researchers have evaluated BSCT in a wide range of clinical populations and compared it to other effective interventions. Predictors of long-term success with BSCT include a shorter history of alcohol-related problems, lower levels of heavy drinking, and fewer signs of physical dependence (W.R. Miller et al. 1992). The picture with respect to more severely dependent patients is mixed. In some trials (e.g., Foy et al. 1984) BSCT has been found to be less effective than purely abstinence-oriented approaches for more severely dependent clients. Other trials have not found a relationship between severity of dependence and outcomes, at least with drinkers who score between 30 and 45 on the Severity of Alcohol Dependence Questionnaire (Heather et al. 2000).

Controlled comparisons have indicated that self-control training can be provided effectively in therapist-directed, computer-based, or self-help formats. Several therapist manuals are available for clinicians interested in learning how to provide this intervention (see Hester 2003 for information on these manuals).

In behavior contracting, the therapist, the patient, and often significant others set up clear contingencies for behaviors related to drinking and sobriety. A written contract specifies what kinds of reinforcers will be provided to the patient if he or she remains sober. Drinking behaviors result in a loss of those reinforcers. Although this form of contingency management seems to be more widespread in the treatment of drug abuse, controlled trials have demonstrated its potential for use with alcohol problems (P.M. Miller 1975).

Social skills training teaches patients how to form and maintain interpersonal relationships. This form of intervention often includes training in communication skills, listening skills, problem solving, and assertiveness skills. Social skills training has been considered an adjunct to treatment, not a stand-alone treatment, and has usually been conducted in groups. In studies in which its effectiveness has been evaluated, patients have typically (but not always) been selected for inclusion because they had poor social skills. Effectiveness has been evaluated in 17 studies to date. Adding this intervention has been found to improve outcomes in 11 of these studies. Some of the studies in which a difference in outcome was not found involved less severely dependent patients. An excellent manual is available for clinicians interested in learning how to provide this type of training (Monti et al. 2003).

Behavioral marital therapy emphasizes the improvement of communication skills and problem solving between partners. It also strives to increase the frequency at which each spouse gives the other positive reinforcement. Treatment has usually been provided on a conjoint basis, with one couple meeting with a therapist, but groups have also been used. Results have been positive in seven studies. A number of therapist manuals are available for interested clinicians, including a primer (O'Farrell 2003) and more advanced manuals and clinical case studies (McCrady 1982; O'Farrell 1993).

Nausea aversion therapy has been practiced in the United States since 1935. The best predictor of success with nausea aversion is the development of a classically conditioned aversive response to alcohol. In the mid-1980s there were a number of inpatient programs that treated patients with this protocol. Unfortunately with the demise of inpatient programs came a concomitant decline in facilities offering this treatment. Today the only hospital in the United States that still uses this treatment is the one that pioneered it: Shick Shadel Hospital in Seattle, Washington.

Interest in case management has increased rapidly in recent years. Case monitoring is a follow-up intervention after short-term treatment. It uses a flexible schedule of periodic brief telephone calls to support clients in maintaining abstinence and in seeking additional assistance sooner than they would have if left to their own devices.

The following treatments have demonstrated at least some modest evidence of effectiveness: cognitive therapy, covert sensitization (an aversion therapy), apneic aversion therapy, family therapy, acupuncture, and client-centered counseling.

Interventions With Indeterminate Evidence of Effectiveness

A wide variety of treatments that have been tested in controlled trials have not yielded results that are supe-

rior to those for control groups. These treatments include the following:

- Electrical aversion therapy
- Exercise therapy
- Stress management
- Antidipsotropic medication (disulfiram) therapy
- Antidepressant medication (selective serotonin reuptake inhibitor [SSRI]) therapy
- Problem-solving therapy
- Lithium therapy
- Nonbehavioral marital therapy
- Group process psychotherapy
- Functional analysis
- Relapse-prevention training
- Self-monitoring

The treatments that are considered to be of greatest interest to the reader are discussed below.

Nonbehavioral marital therapies include structural and strategic approaches. Although the terms used in this form of therapy are quite different from those used in behavioral marital therapy, in practice the two treatments seem similar. Conversely, the difficulties in operationally defining terms and strategies in nonbehavioral marital therapy may have hindered research on these approaches and contributed to equivocal outcomes.

Stress management teaches individuals how to reduce tension and manage stress. A broad-based approach usually includes relaxation strategies, systematic desensitization, and cognitive strategies. The patient learns not only how to manage his or her responses to stressful situations but also how to make changes in the external environment. Stress management training is typically considered an adjunctive treatment rather than a stand-alone treatment. To date, adding this treatment has been found to improve outcome in six studies and not to improve outcome in four studies.

The relapse-prevention protocols of Marlatt and Gordon (1985) and Annis (1986) were designed to help patients maintain gains they had made in the first few months of treatment. Both protocols are cognitive-behavioral therapies that address situations in which there is high risk for relapse. The protocol of Marlatt and Gordon (1985) also emphasizes achieving a balance in life between what one must do (responsibilities) and what one likes to do. Although the notion of directly addressing the prevention of relapse makes clinical sense, there have been more clinical trials to date in which outcomes were not improved than trials in which outcomes were improved.

Interventions With Insufficient Evidence of Effectiveness

The following treatments have consistently not been found to improve outcomes when compared with other treatments:

- Hypnosis
- Psychedelic medication therapy
- Calcium carbimide (an antidipsotropic medication) therapy
- Non-SSRI antidepressant therapy
- Standard treatment
- 12-step facilitation
- Milieu therapy
- Anxiolytic agent therapy
- Mandated attendance at Alcoholics Anonymous (AA) meetings
- Metronidazole therapy
- Relaxation training therapy
- Confrontational counseling
- Psychotherapy
- General alcoholism counseling
- Educational lectures or films

The effect of tricyclic antidepressant therapy on drinking behaviors and depression was the focus of research from the mid-1960s to the early 1970s. The evidence of the effect of these antidepressants on drinking behaviors per se is modest. On the other hand, there is more evidence of their effect on mood. However, although the incidence of affective disorders is relatively high among patients at the time of admission to alcohol treatment programs, the rate of spontaneous remission of these disorders is also high during the first few weeks of sobriety. This situation suggests that clinicians should not begin medication treatment regimens unless there is either a clear history of affective disorders predating the development of alcohol problems or a persistence of depression into sobriety.

Readers may be surprised that mandated attendance at AA meetings falls in this category. Requiring patients to attend AA meetings has been found to be effective in one study and ineffective in four studies. One conclusion of these studies is that judges should not treat mandatory attendance at AA meetings as an alternative to legal sanctions. In the original writings of AA, mandatory attendance was opposed and the importance of voluntary participation was emphasized.

Twelve-step facilitation (TSF) therapy has been evaluated in six controlled clinical trials, only one of which favored TSF over other treatments with which it was compared. However, it should be noted that most of these other treatments were well defined and have evidence of effectiveness of their own.

Interventions With the Least Evidence of Effectiveness

A number of interventions have consistently demonstrated no evidence of effectiveness, or even negative evidence. These include videotape self-confrontation; relaxation training (alone); confrontational counseling; unspecified psychotherapy; and educational lectures, tapes, or films.

Videotape self-confrontation has been shown to have negative outcomes with alcohol-abusing patients. The intervention involves taping the patient when he or she is intoxicated (usually on admission to a hospital emergency room or a treatment program) and then playing it back when the patient is sober. However, in a number of the studies, dropout rates increased among patients who underwent videotape self-confrontation. This highlights the notion that not all therapies are benign.

Educational lectures and films have occupied the bottom position in the effectiveness rankings since Drs. Hester and Miller began this series of reviews of the treatment outcome literature in 1980. Although they still appear to be common in treatment programs, their use constitutes one of the biggest wastes of resources both on the part of treatment staff and on the part of their clients.

This list of treatments might also come as a surprise to clinicians familiar with treatment services in the United States. Informal discussions with colleagues in substance abuse programs reveal that some of these interventions (e.g., educational lectures and films) are quite common and are thought to have great impact by the clinicians providing them. This discrepancy between clinicians' beliefs and the findings of controlled clinical research illustrates the pitfalls of relying solely on personal experience to draw conclusions about the effectiveness of particular treatments.

Interventions With Potential Effectiveness

There are 42 additional interventions for which only one or two controlled clinical trials have been conducted to examine their efficacy. Some are relatively new; others have been around for decades. Clearly there are a number of interventions from which to choose in helping drinkers with alcohol problems. We recommend that clinicians rely primarily on the interventions with the greatest amount of empirical support that are discussed at the beginning of this chapter.

Additional Factors Affecting Treatment Outcome

Therapist Characteristics

In retrospective analyses as well as prospective studies, therapist empathy has been shown to contribute positively to outcomes. Conversely, evidence is mounting that when therapists confront patients in an aggressive manner, outcomes suffer.

Being empathic does not mean being nondirective. An effective therapist can be directive and empathic at the same time. An approach that incorporates these elements has come to be known as *motivational interviewing* (W.R. Miller and Rollnick 2001).

Matching of Patients to Treatments

One of the most surprising developments in the area of treatment outcomes concerns the results of the Project MATCH trial (Project MATCH Research Group 1997). This experiment was designed to test the hypothesis that patients receiving alcohol treatment would respond differentially depending on how compatible certain of their own characteristics were with the kind of treatments offered. The three treatments selected for investigation were cognitive-behavioral therapy, motivational enhancement therapy, and TSF therapy. Patient-matching characteristics included severity of dependence, conceptual level, meaning-seeking by the patient, social support for drinking in the patient's life, and severity of psychiatric problems. Patients' characteristics were found not to influence response to treatment, regardless of kind of treatment received. The hypothesis that outcomes would improve if patients were matched to optimal treatments was not supported, indicating that the kind of theoret-

ical perspective used to guide treatment is less important than was previously supposed. However, it was found that patients without major psychiatric problems had fewer drinking days in the follow-up period when treated with TSF therapy than did patients who were receiving other treatments. This finding supports conventional wisdom that a 12-step approach can be successfully integrated into professional treatment. Perhaps most gratifying, the findings of Project MATCH provide evidence that all three types of treatment produced substantial improvements in patients with severe alcohol problems. Paradoxically, the excellent design and careful execution of this study, which included 8 hours of pretreatment assessment, may have favorably influenced patient outcomes and thereby obscured any differences that might otherwise have been observed between the treatments.

Conclusion

Several conclusions can be drawn from the research literature on treatments for alcohol problems. First, the data indicate that no one treatment is more effective than all others. Rather, there is good evidence of effectiveness for a number of interventions. Therefore, it would make sense for programs to offer a variety of different treatments rather than a single treatment for all patients. Second, therapist characteristics, particularly empathy, appear to have a substantial influence on outcomes. Third, Project MATCH results indicate that clinicians who adhere closely to cognitive-behavioral, motivational enhancement, or TSF therapy protocols can improve patient outcomes. In sum, it is clear that there are multiple pathways to recovery.

References

Annis HM: A relapse prevention model for treatment of alcoholics, in Treating Addictive Behaviors: Processes of Change. Edited by Miller WR, Heather NH. New York, Plenum, 1986, pp 407–433

Edwards G, Orford J, Egert S, et al: Alcoholism: a controlled trial of "treatment" and "advice." J Stud Alcohol 38:1004–1031, 1977

Foy DW, Nunn BL, Rychtarik RG: Broad-spectrum behavioral treatment for chronic alcoholics: effects of training controlled drinking skills. J Consult Clin Psychol 52:213–230, 1984

Heather N, Brodie J, Wale S, et al: A randomized controlled trial of moderation-oriented cue exposure. J Stud Alcohol 61:561–570, 2000

Hester RK: Self-control training, in Handbook of Alcoholism Treatment: Effective Alternatives, 3rd Edition. Edited by Hester RK, Miller WR. Needham Heights, MA, Allyn & Bacon, 2003, pp 152–164

Institute of Medicine: Prevention and Treatment of Alcohol Problems: Research Opportunities. Washington, DC, National Academy Press, 1990

Marlatt GA, Gordon JR: Relapse Prevention: Maintenance Strategies in the Treatment of Addictive Behaviors. New York, Guilford, 1985

McCrady BS: Conjoint behavioral treatment of an alcoholic and his spouse, in Clinical Case Studies in the Behavioral Treatment of Alcoholism. Edited by Hay WM, Nathan PE. New York, Plenum, 1982, pp 127–156

Meyers RJ, Smith JE: Clinical Guide to Alcohol Treatment: The Community Reinforcement Approach. New York, Guilford, 1995

Miller PM: A behavioral intervention program for chronic public drunkenness offenders. Arch Gen Psychiatry 32: 915–918, 1975

Miller WR, Rollnick S: Motivational Interviewing: Preparing People to Change, 2nd Edition. New York, Guilford, 2001

Miller WR, Sanchez VC: Motivating young adults for treatment and lifestyle change, in Alcohol Use and Misuse by Young Adults. Edited by Howard G, Nathan PE. Notre Dame, IN, Notre Dame Press, 1994, pp 55–81

Miller WR, Leckman AL, Delaney HD, et al: Long-term follow-up of behavioral self-control training. J Stud Alcohol 53:249–261, 1992

Miller WR, Andrews NR, Wilbourne P, et al: A wealth of alternatives: effective treatments for alcohol problems, in Treating Addictive Behaviors: Processes of Change, 2nd Edition. Edited by Miller WR, Heather N. New York, Plenum, 1998, pp 203–216

Miller WR, Wilbourne PL, Hettema JE: What works? A summary of treatment outcome research, in Handbook of Alcoholism Treatment Approaches: Effective Alternatives, 3rd Edition. Edited by Hester RK, Miller WR. Needham Heights, MA, Allyn & Bacon, 2003, pp 13–63

Monti PM, Rohsenow DJ, Colby SM, et al: Coping and social skills training, in Handbook of Alcoholism Treatment: Effective Alternatives, 3rd Edition. Edited by Hester RK, Miller WR. Needham Heights, MA, Allyn & Bacon, 2003, pp 213–236

O'Farrell TJ (ed): Treating Alcohol Problems: Marital and Family Interactions. New York, Guilford, 1993

O'Farrell TJ: Marital and family therapy, in Handbook of Alcoholism Treatment Approaches: Effective Alternatives, 3rd Edition. Edited by Hester RK, Miller WR. Needham Heights, MA, Allyn & Bacon, 2003, pp 188–212

Project MATCH Research Group: Matching alcohol treatments to client heterogeneity: Project MATCH posttreatment drinking outcomes. J Stud Alcohol 58:7–29, 1997

Zweben A, Rose SJ, Stout RL, et al: Case monitoring and motivational style brief interventions, in Handbook of Alcoholism Treatment Approaches: Effective Alternatives, 3rd Edition. Edited by Hester RK, Miller WR. Needham Heights, MA, Allyn & Bacon, 2003, pp 113–130

Outcome Research

Drug Abuse

Dean R. Gerstein, Ph.D.

Patient outcomes of treatment for drug dependence have been studied in light of the chronic, relapsing nature of the disorders—that is, not in terms of cure versus failure to cure during the course of treatment but in terms of extent of remission and degrees of improvement over time. Because the mechanisms of drug dependence are complex, because the treatment approaches in the major modalities vary systematically, and because patient populations are heterogeneous across the major modalities, an iterative presentation is needed to convey the results of outcome studies. In this chapter, current knowledge about treatment outcomes for the principal modalities of treatment is summarized in a three-part paradigm, repeated for each treatment modality: What are the concepts behind the treatment? How well does each modality work? Why and how do outcomes vary?

The major modalities of drug treatment considered here are methadone maintenance, long-term residential treatment, outpatient nonmethadone treatment, and short-term residential treatment. The observational outcome literature on these types of treatment is dominated by large multisite studies known by their acronyms: the Drug Abuse Reporting Program (DARP) in the 1970s; the Treatment Outcome Prospective Study (TOPS) in the 1980s; and the California Drug and Alcohol Treatment Assessment (CALDATA), the Drug Abuse Treatment Outcome Study (DATOS), the National Treatment Improvement Evaluation Study (NTIES), and the Services Research Outcomes Study (SROS) in the 1990s (Gerstein et al. 1994, 1997; Hubbard et al. 1989; Schildhaus et al. 2000; Sells 1974a, 1974b; Simpson and Brown 1999; Simpson and Curry 1997; Simpson et al. 1979). Some methods of treatment diverge from these general types. In particular, two well-known types of treatment are not covered here, for different reasons. Independent self-help fellowship groups such as Narcotics Anonymous (NA), Cocaine Anonymous (CA), and the Oxford Houses are not discussed because there are insufficient data to answer the critical questions about them. Although the ideas underlying the fellowships derived from Alcoholics Anonymous (AA) were incorporated into the clinical approaches of therapeutic communities and chemical dependency programs at the outset of these programs (in fact, the 12 steps of the AA creed are so fundamental to the chemical dependence modality that the latter has been referred to as the "professionalization of AA"), the fellowships have shied away from formal evaluation.

The second exclusion is detoxification, or medically supervised withdrawal. Detoxification *without subsequent treatment* has consistently been found to have no effects (in terms of reducing subsequent drug use behavior and especially relapse to dependence) that are discernibly superior to those achieved by untreated withdrawal (Cole et al. 1981; Moffet et al. 1973; Newman 1983; Resnick 1983; Sheffet et al. 1976).

Methadone Maintenance

What Is Methadone Maintenance?

Methadone maintenance is a treatment specifically designed for dependence on narcotic analgesics, particularly heroin. The controversies surrounding methadone maintenance have made it the subject of hundreds of studies, including a number of clinical trials, from which good evidence has been accumulated about the safety and efficacy of methadone.

At the base of methadone maintenance is the empirical observation, made before the biological reasons for it were well understood, that narcotic analgesics may be substituted for one another with sufficient adjustments in dosage and route of administration. Methadone, however, has several unusual pharmacological properties that make it especially suited to a maintenance approach. The drug is effective orally, and because of its particular pattern of absorption and metabolism, a single dose within a train of level doses, in the typical maintenance range of 30–100 mg/day, has a gradual onset and yields a fairly even effect across a 24-hour period or longer. Methadone is thus suitable for a regimen of single daily maintenance doses, which eliminates dramatic subjective or behavioral changes and makes it easy for the clinician and patient to fit into a routine clinic schedule. This pattern is different from the shorter action and more dramatic highs and lows of heroin, morphine, and most other opioids.

The long-term toxic side effects of methadone (like those of other opioids if taken in hygienic conditions in controlled doses) are notably benign. Since the mid-1960s, more than 2 million person-years of methadone maintenance have accumulated in the United States. The accumulated clinical experience, confirmed by thousands of carefully documented research cases, yields a well-supported conclusion that is epitomized by the following: "Physiological and biochemical alterations occur, but there are minimal side effects that are clinically detectable in patients during chronic methadone maintenance treatment. Toxicity related to methadone during chronic treatment is extraordinarily rare." (Kreek 1983, p. 474).

Although provisions for office-based practice are under development, methadone maintenance may be offered only within especially licensed and regulated programs (Rettig and Yarmolinsky 1995). These programs are largely ambulatory, involving daily visits to swallow doses under clinical observation. After several months of "clean" drug testing and compliance with other codes of proscribed behavior (e.g., no violence or threats of violence), patients may regularly take home doses between every-other-day, twice-weekly, or even weekly visits—a revocable privilege. Many patients undergoing methadone maintenance voluntarily or by program design taper their doses to abstinence and conclude treatment; others continue methadone maintenance indefinitely; and many have their doses tapered and are discharged from methadone maintenance programs because of poor response or compliance.

Methadone maintenance programs include numerous monitoring and adjustment features that emphasize the need for patients to wean themselves away from seeking street drugs. Program clinics have specific hours for dispensing, for counseling, and for medical supervision. Monitored drug tests are conducted at random intervals—at least monthly and as often as weekly—although financially strained programs test minimally. Counseling includes the assessment of patient attitudes, behavior, and service needs; these factors are evaluated in terms of their relationship to methadone dosage, employment, family matters, and criminal activities. Psychotherapy and individualized social assistance are also provided. The extent of services provided is dependent on the caseloads and the training levels of the counselors.

The longer-acting methadone congener L-α-acetylmethadol (LAAM) requires less frequent doses (i.e., every 2–3 days instead of daily). LAAM has been studied in a series of phased clinical trials, and its toxicity appears to be similar to that of methadone (Blaine et al. 1981; Ling et al. 1978; Rettig and Yarmolinsky 1995). LAAM has been approved for clinical use, but large-scale results are not yet available.

How Well Does Methadone Maintenance Work?

Early trials of methadone maintenance in New York (Dole and Nyswander 1965, 1967; Dole et al. 1966, 1968, 1969) had two striking findings: 1) most patients remained voluntarily in treatment for as long as it was available to them, in marked contrast to prior experience; and 2) methadone maintenance substantially improved the condition of patients. The most dramatic change was a sustained reduction in criminal behavior, especially in the form of drug trafficking.

The most persuasive results concerning the potential efficacy of methadone maintenance come from a handful of widely separated randomized clinical trials by Dole et al. (1969) in New York, by Newman and Whitehill (1978) in Hong Kong, and by Gunne and Gronbladh (1984) in Sweden. The latter may be taken as representative. Thirty-four heroin-dependent individuals applied for admission to the only methadone clinic in a Swedish community; 17 were randomly assigned to methadone maintenance, and 17 were assigned to outpatient nonmethadone treatment (these individuals could not apply for admission to the methadone clinic again for 24 months). After 2 years, 12 (71%) of the patients taking methadone were doing well, compared with 1 (6%) of the control patients. After 5 years, 13 (76%) of the patients taking methadone remained in treatment and were still not using heroin, and 4 (24%) had been denied treatment because of unremitting drug problems. Among the control patients, 9 had applied for admission and had entered the methadone maintenance program; of these, 8 patients were not using drugs and were socially productive. Of the 8 control patients who did not apply for methadone treatment when eligible, the authors reported that 5 had died (allegedly from overdose), 2 were in prison, and 1 was still drug free (Gunne and Gronbladh 1984, p. 211).

Similar results have been reported in California cities that abruptly closed publicly supported methadone maintenance programs for fiscal and political reasons. In cities where methadone became much less accessi-

ble, former patients at 2-year follow-up were doing appreciably less well in terms of heroin use, other criminal behavior, and (to a lesser degree) employment than were comparison groups in cities where public programs closed but private ones opened; in cities where methadone treatment remained available, those who transferred to the alternative methadone maintenance programs did much better (in terms of staying free of drugs and out of crime) than those who did not or could not continue treatment (Anglin et al. 1989; McGlothlin and Anglin 1981).

In all of the studies cited and in later multisite studies (Gerstein et al. 1994, 1997; Hubbard et al. 1989; Schildhaus et al. 2000; Simpson and Brown 1999; Simpson and Curry 1997; Simpson et al. 1979), retention in methadone maintenance as opposed to attrition was associated with reduced heroin use and crime, even after controlling for baseline conditions and covariates.

Why Do the Results of Methadone Maintenance Vary?

An appreciable proportion of patients in methadone maintenance programs do not respond well to treatment for a variety of reasons relating to the patients themselves and to the programs. This proportion averages about one in four, although there is variation from program to program (Ball et al. 1988; Gerstein et al. 1994; Hubbard et al. 1989; Simpson and Brown 1999; Simpson and Curry 1997; Simpson et al. 1979). Some patients enter methadone maintenance programs for purposes other than pursuing recovery; such patients are not compliant or responsive and are most likely to leave methadone maintenance programs after short periods. It is easier to identify these patients after the fact than at the time of entrance into a program.

The largest group of patients performs at least moderately well in response to methadone maintenance and would do poorly without it, even when other kinds of treatment are available. There is compelling evidence that program factors such as methadone dosing policies and counselor characteristics can affect patient behavior beyond any initial differences in motivation or severity of problems. Program performance (in terms of patient retention and continued use of drugs by patients) varies greatly across programs. The multisite TOPS, for example, showed a large degree of variation in clinically important patient outcomes across nine methadone maintenance programs (Hubbard et al. 1989). Twelve-month retention rates averaged 34% of admissions; five programs had rates of 7%–25%, and two programs had rates greater than 50%. Regular heroin use by patients at follow-up (approximately 3 years later) was reported by 21% of the entire follow-up sample; two programs had rates greater than 30%, and three had rates of 11%–14%. In the multisite DATOS programs, comparably large variations were observed in retention in treatment in 10 methadone maintenance programs, with 12-month retention rates ranging from 15% to 76%; these variations could not be explained by variations in patient characteristics, and there were marginal indications that greater frequency of counseling contributed to higher retention (Simpson et al. 1997).

Variation in performance has been linked most strongly to variations in methadone dosing policies. Programs that are committed to the maintenance of low average dosages (30–50 mg/day) as a virtual goal of treatment—because of therapeutic philosophy or because state regulators strongly discourage administration of higher dosages—are less tolerant of occasional patient drug use, missed counseling appointments, and other such treatment lapses and have markedly lower patient retention rates than do more tolerant, higher-dosage programs. This lower tolerance does not, however, act as a stimulant to better patient behavior or as a conveyor to move poorly responding patients out and bring in or keep better responders. There is solid, experimentally grounded evidence (Hargreaves 1983; Rettig and Yarmolinsky 1995) that higher dosage levels are fundamentally more successful than lower ones in controlling a patient's illicit drug consumption during treatment. Methadone maintenance programs in which average dosages of 60–120 mg/day are prescribed have consistently better results than do programs involving lower average dosages (Ball and Ross 1991; Ball et al. 1988; Dole 1989). Dosages in excess of 120 mg/day are seldom needed. Knowledge of and sensitivity to the clinical importance of appropriate dosage levels is probably one notable element in a constellation of clinical competencies and strategies that contribute to the greater or lesser effectiveness of methadone maintenance programs. Few research efforts have focused on the areas of competence, appropriate training, and different service arrangements in the clinical management of patients in methadone maintenance programs (McLellan et al. 1988, 1993).

Long-Term Residential Treatment

What Is Long-Term Residential Treatment?

The prototype of long-term residential treatment for drug dependence was the therapeutic community, and virtually all long-term residential treatment programs consider themselves to be therapeutic communities or modified therapeutic communities. Drug-focused therapeutic communities were initially (ca. 1960) designed to treat the same problem that methadone maintenance programs treat: the "hard-core" heroin-dependent criminal. The original drug therapeutic communities—including Synanon in California and Daytop Village and Phoenix House in New York—and their lineal descendants throughout the United States have had a broader perspective than methadone maintenance programs have had, treating individuals who are severely dependent on any illicitly obtained drug or combination of drugs and whose social adjustment to conventional family and occupational responsibilities is severely compromised as a result of drug seeking (although in most cases, social adjustment was compromised before drug seeking entered the picture). In the 1980s, cocaine dependence overtook heroin dependence in the long-term residential treatment population; patients receiving long-term residential treatment have also been younger than the predominantly heroin-dependent methadone maintenance population (Gerstein et al. 1994, 1997; Hubbard et al. 1989; Simpson and Curry 1997).

The group-centered methods of long-term residential treatment (described in greater detail in De Leon 2000 and in Chapter 38 of this volume) encompass the following elements, all grounded in an interdependent social environment, with a direct link to a specific historical foundation:

1. Firm behavioral norms across a wide range of proscriptions and specifications
2. Reality-oriented group and individual psychotherapy that extends to lengthy encounter sessions focusing on current living issues or more deep-seated emotional problems
3. A system of clearly specified rewards and punishments within a communal economy
4. A hierarchy of responsibilities, privileges, and esteem achieved by working up a "ladder" of tasks from admission to graduation
5. A degree of mobility from patient to staff status

The modifications from older therapeutic community practices now common in long-term residential treatment include accelerated (shorter) treatment plans, sharpened boundaries between patient and staff roles, and more catholic use of therapeutic imports such as psychopharmacological support and 12-step procedures. To a significant extent, long-term residential treatment simulates and enforces a model family environment that the patient lacked during developmentally critical preadolescent and adolescent years. Long-term residential treatment attempts to make up for lost years in a relatively short time; there are approximately 6–12 months of residential envelopment and an additional 6–12 months of gradual reentry to the outside community before "graduation." Continued involvement after graduation is encouraged because graduates serve as role models for new residents and gain recognition and reinforcement and because such involvement provides psychological and financial support for the program.

How Well Does Long-Term Residential Treatment Work?

Conclusions about the effectiveness of long-term residential treatment are limited by the difficulties in maintaining randomized clinical trial protocols. The most notable attempt to use a randomized design to evaluate the effectiveness of long-term residential treatment compared with no treatment or other treatments was conducted in California by Bale et al. (1980). The subjects were 585 heroin-addicted male veterans who sought and gained entry to the Veterans Administration (VA) Medical Center in Palo Alto, California, for a 5-day opioid detoxification program during an 18-month intake period in the mid-1970s. The subjects also met the study's requirements of no pending felony charges or major psychiatric complications. About one-fifth of the subjects denied any interest in transferring to a VA drug treatment program after detoxification. (Some later changed their minds.) Those who were interested were randomly assigned to one of two methadone maintenance clinics or one of three therapeutic communities.

The clinical staff invested a substantial amount of time in trying to enlist every subject in his assigned program, and the overall rate of transfers from detoxification to VA programs doubled as a result. Nevertheless, the random-assignment design was thoroughly compromised. Fewer than half of the randomly assigned subjects entered and spent as long as 1 week in any of the VA treatment programs, and only half of those subjects entered the specific programs to which they had been assigned (the other men waited out exclusion periods of at least 30 days to enter their preferred programs).

The lack of compliance affected the study so profoundly that research analysts were obliged to use multivariate statistical procedures to control for initial differences in age, ethnicity, prior treatment, drug use patterns, and criminal history among treatment and nontreatment groups. About 13% of the patients stayed less than 1 week (these individuals were considered "no-treatment" subjects), 57% dropped out within 7 weeks, and 85% left treatment before 6 months. In contrast, approximately 65% of the patients entering methadone maintenance programs were continuously in treatment for the follow-up year. The therapeutic community group was therefore divided at the median length of stay, 50 days. On average, the short-term group stayed in treatment approximately 3 weeks; the long-term group, 20 weeks; and the methadone group, 40 weeks.

At 1-year follow-up, subjects were categorized as follows: no treatment, 41%; non-VA treatment, 21%; short-term therapeutic community, 14%; long-term therapeutic community, 14%; and methadone maintenance, 11%. For purposes of analysis, the no treatment, non-VA treatment, and short-term therapeutic community groups were combined, the long-term therapeutic community and methadone maintenance groups were combined, and pretreatment characteristics were controlled for. Compared with the combined no treatment, non-VA treatment, and short-term therapeutic community groups, the combined long-term therapeutic community and methadone maintenance groups were

1. One-third less likely to have used heroin in the past month (41% versus 64%)
2. Two-fifths less likely to have been convicted during the year (22% versus 37%)
3. Two-thirds less likely to be incarcerated at year's end (7% versus 19%)
4. One and one-half times more likely to be at work or in school at year's end (59% versus 40%)

The long-term therapeutic community group ranked somewhat better than the total methadone maintenance group on each measure, but the differences were not large enough to be statistically significant in a sample of this size.

In a smaller study that is notable for its careful execution, a random sample of graduates and dropouts from a therapeutic community in Connecticut were studied in an 18- to 24-month treatment plan (Romond et al. 1975). The authors found few pretreatment differences between the graduate group and the dropout group except that women were much less likely than men to graduate. All 20 graduates in the sample were contacted, 10 of 31 dropouts in the sample were not located, and 1 dropout refused an interview; therefore, there were 20 contacts for each group. Graduates had spent on average 21 months in treatment, compared with 5.7 months for dropouts (range, 10 days to 16 months). Interview data were corroborated through formal and informal community networks.

Graduates had consistently better outcomes. Only 1 of 20 graduates relapsed to dependence for some part of the follow-up period, another 5 sometimes used nonopioid drugs, and 14 remained drug free throughout the interval. Altogether, graduates spent 0.5% of the follow-up period dependent. Of the 20 dropouts interviewed, 14 relapsed to dependence for some of the follow-up period, 2 used nonopioids occasionally, 1 was incarcerated for the entire period, and 3 had used no drugs; 35% of the dropouts' posttreatment time was spent as drug dependent. For 94% of the posttreatment time, graduates were enrolled in school or were employed; dropouts were employed or in school only 40% of the posttreatment time.

DARP, TOPS, CALDATA, DATOS, and NTIES provided further important controlled observational findings across three decades about the effectiveness of long-term residential treatment. The mean and median lengths of stay in the traditional therapeutic communities involved in DARP were close to 7 months, well below the average treatment length of 16 months, and the ultimate graduation rate was 23%. By most of the DARP outcome measures (e.g., daily opioid use, daily nonopioid use, arrests, incarceration), outcome 1 year after discharge was significantly better for patients in therapeutic communities than for patients who underwent detoxification only and patients who made no contact after program entry. As in the study by Bale et al. (1980), the multivariate-adjusted outcomes in daily opioid use, nonopioid use, and employment, as well as a composite index, for patients in long-term residential treatment programs and patients in methadone maintenance programs (matched for time since admission) were similar. The length of stay in treatment was a positive, robust, statistically significant predictor of posttreatment outcomes (e.g., drug use, employment, and crime). Among patients who stayed in treatment for more than 90 days, there was a positive and linear relationship between outcome and retention. The outcomes among patients who stayed in treatment for less than 90 days were indistinguishable from outcomes among patients who underwent detoxification only and patients who did not make any contact after program entry.

The analysis of TOPS, NTIES, and DATOS data on long-term residential treatment (Gerstein and Zhang 2001; Gerstein et al. 1997; Hubbard et al. 1989; Johnson and Gerstein 2000; Simpson and Curry 1997; Zhang et al. 2003) used multivariate regression and hierarchical linear modeling to control for pretreatment motivation and demographics, drug use, and criminality and to compare individual-level and program-level factors. These studies found strong positive relationships between typical lengths of stay and drug-use outcomes. Progressively longer durations in long-term residential treatment were significantly related to reduced use of cocaine, marijuana, and alcohol; reduced involvement in predatory crime; and reduced unemployment 12 months after treatment. In DATOS, the odds of using cocaine, for example, were about one-tenth as great for patients who stayed in treatment 12 months or longer as for patients who received treatment for less than 3 months, and the odds of having a job nearly doubled for longer-term subjects. NTIES results were similar but less dramatic. Patients with greater lengths of stay were more likely than those with shorter time in treatment to report at follow-up that they had a good relationship with a primary counselor, had attended education classes during treatment, and had participated in aftercare.

In summary, even in the absence of successful clinical trials, it is difficult to credit any explanation of the multisite and single-site research findings on long-term residential treatment other than that long-term residential treatment strongly affects the behavior of many of the drug-dependent individuals who receive it and that time in treatment is strongly related to improved outcomes as measured by drug and alcohol consumption, predatory criminal activity, and economically productive behavior.

Why Do the Results of Long-Term Residential Treatment Vary?

There are wide variations in outcome indicators across programs. In the DATOS study, 90-day retention in treatment ranged from 21% to 65% across 19 long-term residential treatment programs. Patient profile differences contributed somewhat to these differences in retention; programs with older patients and with higher proportions of alcohol-dependent patients tended to retain patients longer. However, substantial differences in outcome by program remain, after controlling for baseline patient differences, and there has been virtually no revealing research on the programmatic determinants of treatment success and failure in long-term residential treatment. It is plausible that the results of treatment depend on the quality (and quantity) of staffing and the psychosocial organization and therapeutic design of the program (De Leon 2000).

Outpatient Nonmethadone Treatment

What Is Outpatient Nonmethadone Treatment?

Outpatient nonmethadone treatment ranges from one session of assessment and referral to virtual board-out long-term residential treatment with daily psychotherapy, milieu therapy, and counseling for 1 year or longer (Kleber and Slobetz 1979). Between these extremes lie the vast majority of programs, which have treatment plans involving one to two weekly visits for 3–6 months and use a panoply of therapeutic approaches from psychiatry, counseling psychology, social work, therapeutic communities, and the 12-step paradigm. Some outpatient nonmethadone treatment programs contract extensively with probation departments, offering limited therapeutic services but monitoring compliance with probation conditions, particularly through administration of drug tests.

Some outpatient nonmethadone treatment programs prescribe ameliorants for acute withdrawal symptoms, maintenance antagonists to prevent intoxication or control drug cravings after withdrawal, or treatments for psychiatric comorbidities (e.g., depression, mood disorders, and schizophrenia). Programs with the requisite resources may deliver or link their patients to organizations offering formal education, vocational training, health care (e.g., acquired immunodeficiency syndrome [AIDS] testing or treatment), housing assistance (especially for homeless patients), support for battered spouses and children, or other social services.

The diversity of approaches to outpatient nonmethadone treatment defies easy summary and is matched by the heterogeneity of populations in outpatient nonmethadone treatment. Compared with patients in long-term residential treatment or methadone maintenance programs, these individuals are generally not abusing opioids and are less likely to be involved in the criminal justice system. Outpatient populations also include substantial proportions of drug-abusing rather than drug-dependent individuals.

How Well Does Outpatient Nonmethadone Treatment Work?

The major observation about outpatient nonmethadone treatment is familiar: the longer patients remain in treatment, the better the outcomes are at follow-up. These conclusions are based on multivariate results (statistically controlled for baseline covariates of outcome) from DARP, TOPS, and NTIES. Patients receiving outpatient nonmethadone treatment in the DARP study exhibited statistically significant follow-up improvements relative to pretreatment in terms of employment and consumption of opioids and nonopioids but not in terms of arrest rates, which were lower before treatment than they were in patients in therapeutic communities or methadone maintenance programs. The DARP comparison groups (patients in detoxification programs and patients who made no contact after program entry) reported no major pretreatment-to-posttreatment changes except in opioid consumption (Simpson et al. 1979).

In TOPS (Hubbard et al. 1989), data were collected on 1,600 patients receiving outpatient nonmethadone treatment in a total of 10 programs. Patients reported better performance during and after treatment than before admission, and multivariate analyses strongly related posttreatment outcomes to length of stay in treatment, using multivariate logistical regression to adjust for patient drug use histories and sociodemographic characteristics at admission. The analysis suggested that the critical retention threshold may be 6 months, but only 17% of patients in TOPS who underwent outpatient nonmethadone treatment were retained that long. Dropout rates for outpatient nonmethadone treatment were significantly higher than for methadone maintenance programs or therapeutic communities. Similar relationships were evident in DATOS and NTIES, although the median length of stay in outpatient nonmethadone treatment had increased to 3 months, similar to the length of stay in long-term residential treatment. Reductions in heroin use, cocaine use, criminal behavior, and AIDS risk behaviors were more substantial at lengths of stay above rather than below this median.

Why Do the Results of Outpatient Nonmethadone Treatment Vary?

There is no good answer to the question of why the results of outpatient nonmethadone treatment vary. Evidence of wide variation in program retention rates exists, with rates in DATOS ranging from 16% to 76% for stays in treatment longer than 90 days, and comparable variation occurring in NTIES. But neither study offers strong guidance about what components of outpatient nonmethadone treatment led to these variations. One can only speculate that the same factors that are beginning to emerge from methadone maintenance and therapeutic community research—in particular, staff quality and program design—may prove equally important here.

Short-Term Residential Treatment

What Is Short-Term Residential Treatment?

Short-term residential treatment is also called chemical dependency, Minnesota Model, 12-step, or Hazelden-type treatment. short-term residential treatment is the predominant therapeutic approach in inpatient and residential programs that are oriented heavily toward insured populations. Virtually all of these programs were originally oriented toward alcohol problems but have increasingly served patients who use illicit drugs. Cook (1988a, 1988b) provided a concise historical review of the development of the Minnesota Model. He noted the similarities between the underlying theories that shape short-term residential treatment and therapeutic community treatment but observed that they developed almost completely independently of each other.

Short-term residential treatment is usually an intensive, highly structured 3- to 6-week inpatient regimen. Patients begin with an in-depth psychiatric and psychosocial evaluation and are actively engaged in developing and implementing a recovery plan, which is patterned on the "step work" (working through the 12 steps of recovery) of AA. Self-help is a large part of therapy; patients work with one another and are generally required to attend AA, CA, or NA meetings. Virtually all short-term residential treatment programs incorporate daily classroom-type lectures plus two to three meetings per week in small task-oriented groups to teach patients about the disease concept of dependence, especially the harmful medical and psychosocial effects of dependence. There is usually an individual track for each patient, meetings twice a week with a focal counselor, and appointments with other professionals if medical, psychiatric, or family services are needed. Recently there has been increasing emphasis on family or codependent therapy. Aftercare is considered important, but relatively few program resources are devoted to it. Patients are urged to continue an intensive schedule of AA/CA/NA meetings through the follow-up period of 3 months to 2 years, with continued contacts thereafter at a lower rate.

Short-term residential treatment has some elements in common with the therapeutic community approach, but there are noteworthy differences. The inpatient or residential phase of the short-term residential treatment plan is much shorter, and the aftercare phase is seldom strongly integrated. Patients in short-term residential treatment programs are not required to perform housekeeping duties, so there is more time available for psychotherapy and educational tasks; in the therapeutic community process, however, performance of housekeeping and other program maintenance duties is an integral component of treatment. Short-term residential treatment program staffs, like therapeutic community staffs, are a mixture of recovering persons and licensed professionals. Many short-term residential treatment programs are attractive to patients with greater functional and social resources, particularly private health insurance, who can afford the better facilities and amenities.

How Well Does Short-Term Residential Treatment Work?

Research data on short-term residential treatment for illicit drug problems are weaker than for the other modalities. There are no relevant random-assignment trials or quasi-experimental studies. No short-term residential treatment programs were in the DARP or TOPS samples; too few of these programs were in

DATOS for more detailed analyses to be performed; short-term residential treatment–type programs in CALDATA were restricted to California's "social model" treatment of alcoholism (Gerstein et al. 1994); and the number of short-term residential treatment programs in NTIES was also small.

During the 1980s, patients in short-term residential treatment programs who presented with drug problems had poorer outcomes at posttreatment follow-up than did patients with alcohol problems (with no illicit drug consumption) in the same programs. This finding was consistent across studies by the CareUnit system (Comprehensive Care Corporation 1988), the Chemical Abuse/Addiction Treatment Outcome Registry follow-up service, and the Hazelden center in Minnesota (Gilmore 1985; Laundergan 1982).

Short-term residential treatment programs changed rapidly during the 1990s because of behavioral-health managed care protocols. Many such programs disappeared or were replaced by outpatient nonmethadone treatment programs. DATOS and NTIES results indicated that there were minimal differences between results for different substances for alcohol, cocaine, and marijuana use. Because of the short durations of treatment, length-of-stay analyses were relatively unproductive.

Why Do the Results of Short-Term Residential Treatment Vary?

No currently published studies distinguish why some patients in short-term residential treatment programs do well and others do not. As with other treatments, patient motivation and program staff quality are suspected factors. But there is no readily available information on variations in outcomes of drug-dependent patients across short-term residential treatment programs or any successful attempts to relate such differences to systematic variations among patients or in the therapeutic approach.

Conclusions About Treatment Effectiveness

Although heroin use is no longer dominant in treatment populations, methadone remains an important and well-studied treatment option. On average, heroin-dependent individuals (or those who are dependent on another opioid) have better outcomes in terms of illicit drug consumption and other criminal behavior when they are maintained on methadone than when they are not treated at all, when they are simply detoxified and released, or when methadone is tapered and treatment is terminated arbitrarily. Furthermore, longer durations are associated with better outcomes. Methadone clinics have higher rates of retention of opioid-dependent patients than other treatment modalities. Methadone doses need to be clinically monitored and individually optimized. Patients do better, generally, when they are stabilized on dosages in the range of 60–120 mg/day. Program characteristics such as inadequate methadone dose levels are significantly related to differences in patient performance during treatment.

Patients in long-term residential treatment end virtually all illicit drug taking and other criminal behavior while in residence and perform better (in terms of reduced drug taking and other criminal activity and increased social productivity) after discharge than before admission. The length of stay is the strongest predictor of outcomes at follow-up. Attrition for long-term residential treatment is typically higher than that for methadone maintenance but lower than that for outpatient nonmethadone treatment.

Despite the heterogeneity of outpatient nonmethadone treatment programs and program participants, the limited number of outcome evaluations of these programs has generated conclusions qualitatively similar to those from studies of long-term residential treatment. Patients who receive outpatient nonmethadone treatment exhibit better behavior during and after treatment than before treatment. The patients who are treated have better outcomes than patients who contact but do not enter programs or who undergo detoxification only. Outcome at follow-up is positively related to length of stay. There is increasing evidence about the outcomes of short-term residential treatment, but it remains less well understood than other modalities, and the short durations of treatment induce questions about effectiveness for more severely affected populations.

References

Anglin MD, Speckart GS, Booth MW, et al: Consequences and costs of shutting off methadone. Addict Behav 14:307–326, 1989

Bale RN, Van Stone WW, Kuldau JM, et al: Therapeutic communities vs. methadone maintenance: a prospective controlled study of narcotic addiction treatment—design and one-year follow-up. Arch Gen Psychiatry 37:179–193, 1980

Ball JC, Ross A: The Effectiveness of Methadone Maintenance. New York, Springer-Verlag, 1991

Ball JC, Lange WR, Meyers CP, et al: Reducing the risk of AIDS through methadone maintenance treatment. J Health Soc Behav 29:214–226, 1988

Blaine JD, Thomas DB, Barnett G, et al: Levo-alpha acetylmethadol (LAAM): clinical utility and pharmaceutical development, in Substance Abuse: Clinical Problems and Perspectives. Edited by Lowinson JH, Ruiz P. Baltimore, MD, Williams & Wilkins, 1981, pp 360–388

Cole SG, Lehman WE, Cole EA, et al: Inpatient vs outpatient treatment of alcohol and drug abusers. Am J Drug Alcohol Abuse 8:329–345, 1981

Comprehensive Care Corporation: Evaluation of Treatment Outcome. Irvine, CA, Comprehensive Care Corporation, 1988

Cook CCH: The Minnesota Model in the management of drug and alcohol dependency: miracle, method or myth? I: the philosophy and the programme. Br J Addict 83:625–634, 1988a

Cook CCH: The Minnesota Model in the management of drug and alcohol dependency: miracle, method or myth? II: evidence and conclusions. Br J Addict 83:735–748, 1988b

De Leon G: The Therapeutic Community: Theory, Model, and Method. New York, Springer, 2000

Dole VP: Methadone treatment and the acquired immunodeficiency syndrome epidemic. JAMA 262:1681–1682, 1989

Dole VP, Nyswander M: A medical treatment for diacetylmorphine (heroin) addiction: a clinical trial with methadone hydrochloride. JAMA 193:80–84, 1965

Dole VP, Nyswander M: Rehabilitation of the street addict. Arch Environ Health 14:477–480, 1967

Dole VP, Nyswander M, Kreek MJ: Narcotic blockade. Arch Intern Med 118:304–309, 1966

Dole VP, Nyswander M, Warner A: Successful treatment of 750 criminal addicts. JAMA 206:2708–2711, 1968

Dole VP, Robinson JW, Orraga J, et al: Methadone treatment of randomly selected criminal addicts. N Engl J Med 280:1372–1375, 1969

Gerstein DR, Zhang Z: Treatment Outcomes for Different Types of Substance Use. Washington, DC, National Opinion Research Center, 2001

Gerstein DR, Johnson RA, Harwood HJ, et al: Evaluating Recovery Services: the California Drug and Alcohol Treatment Assessment (CALDATA): General Report. Sacramento, CA, State of California Department of Alcohol and Drug Programs, 1994

Gerstein DR, Datta AR, Ingels JS, et al: The National Treatment Improvement Evaluation Study: Final Report. Washington, DC, National Opinion Research Center, 1997

Gilmore KM: Hazelden Primary Residential Treatment Program: Profile and Patient Outcome. Center City, MN, Hazelden, 1985

Gunne L, Gronbladh L: The Swedish methadone maintenance program, in The Social and Medical Aspects of Drug Abuse. Edited by Serban G. Jamaica, NY, Spectrum, 1984, pp 205–213

Hargreaves WA: Methadone dose and duration for methadone treatment, in Research on the Treatment of Narcotic Addiction: State of the Art (NIDA Treatment Research Monograph, DHHS Publ No ADM-83-1281). Edited by Cooper JR, Altman F, Brown BS, et al. Rockville, MD, National Institute on Drug Abuse, 1983, pp 19–79

Hubbard RL, Marsden ME, Rachal JV, et al: Drug Abuse Treatment: A National Study of Effectiveness. Chapel Hill, NC, University of North Carolina Press, 1989

Johnson RA, Gerstein DR: Treatment populations, services, and outcomes for cocaine and crack-cocaine dependence. Journal of Psychopathology and Behavioral Assessment 22:41–44, 2000

Kleber HD, Slobetz F: Outpatient drug-free treatment, in Handbook on Drug Abuse. Edited by Dupont RL, Goldstein A, O'Donnell J. Rockville, MD, National Institute on Drug Abuse, 1979, pp 31–38

Kreek MJ: Health consequences associated with the use of methadone, in Research on the Treatment of Narcotic Addiction: State of the Art (NIDA Treatment Research Monograph, DHHS Publ No ADM-83-1281). Edited by Cooper JR, Altman F, Brown BS, et al. Rockville, MD, National Institute on Drug Abuse, 1983, pp 456–482

Laundergan JC: Easy Does It! Alcoholism Treatment Outcomes, Hazelden and the Minnesota Model. Center City, MN, Hazelden, 1982

Ling W, Klett CJ, Gillis RD: A cooperative clinical study of methadyl acetate. Arch Gen Psychiatry 35:345–353, 1978

McGlothlin WH, Anglin MD: Shutting off methadone: costs and benefits. Arch Gen Psychiatry 38:885–892, 1981

McLellan AT, Luborsky L, Woody G, et al: Counselor differences in methadone treatment. NIDA Res Monogr 81:243–250, 1988

McLellan AT, Arndt IO, Metzger DS, et al: The effects of psychosocial services in substance abuse treatment. JAMA 269:1953–1966, 1993

Moffet AD, Soloway IH, Glick MX: Post-treatment behavior following ambulatory detoxification, in Methadone: Experience and Issues. Edited by Chambers CD, Brill L. New York, Behavioral Publications, 1973, pp 215–227

Newman RG: Critique, in Research on the Treatment of Narcotic Addiction: State of the Art (NIDA Treatment Research Monograph, DHHS Publ No ADM-83-1281). Edited by Cooper JR, Altman F, Brown BS, et al. Rockville, MD, National Institute on Drug Abuse, 1983, pp 168–171

Newman RG, Whitehill WB: Double-blind comparison of methadone and placebo maintenance treatment of narcotic addicts in Hong Kong. Lancet 2:485–488, 1978

Resnick R: Methadone detoxification from illicit opiates and methadone maintenance, in Research on the Treatment of Narcotic Addiction: State of the Art (NIDA Treatment Research Monograph, DHHS Publ No ADM-83-1281). Edited by Cooper RJ, Altman F, Brown BS, et al. Rockville, MD, National Institute on Drug Abuse, 1983, pp 160–178

Rettig RR, Yarmolinsky A (eds): Federal Regulation of Methadone. Washington, DC, National Academy Press, 1995

Romond AM, Forrest CK, Kleber HD: Follow-up of participants in a drug dependence therapeutic community. Arch Gen Psychiatry 32:369–374, 1975

Schildhaus S, Gerstein DR, Brittingham A, et al: Services Research Outcomes Study. Subst Use Misuse 35:1849–1910, 2000

Sells SB (ed): Studies of the Effectiveness of Treatments for Drug Abuse, Vol 1: Evaluation of Treatments. Cambridge, MA, Ballinger, 1974a

Sells SB (ed): Studies of the Effectiveness of Treatments for Drug Abuse, Vol 2: Research on Patients, Treatments and Outcomes. Cambridge, MA, Ballinger, 1974b

Sheffet A, Quinones M, Lavenhar MA, et al: An evaluation of detoxification as an initial step in the treatment of heroin addiction. Am J Psychiatry 133:337–340, 1976

Simpson DD, Brown BS (eds): Special Issue: Treatment Process and Outcome Studies From DATOS. Drug Alcohol Depend 57:81–176, 1999

Simpson DD, Curry SJ (eds): Drug Abuse Treatment Outcome Study (DATOS). Psychol Addict Behav 11 (special issue):211–338, 1997

Simpson DD, Savage LJ, Lloyd MR: Follow-up evaluation of treatment of drug abuse during 1969 to 1972. Arch Gen Psychiatry 36:772–780, 1979

Simpson DD, Joe GW, Broome KM, et al: Program diversity and treatment retention rates in the Drug Abuse Treatment Outcome Study (DATOS). Psychol Addict Behav 11:279–293, 1997

Zhang Z, Friedmann PD, Gerstein DR: Does retention matter? Treatment duration, pretreatment predictors, and persistent substance use outcomes. Addiction 98:673–684, 2003

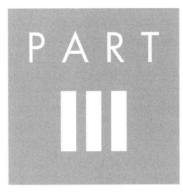

Treatment for Specific Drugs of Abuse

Alcohol

Marc A. Schuckit, M.D.
Susan Tapert, Ph.D.

At some time in their lives, 90% of American men and 75% of American women consume alcohol (Johnston et al. 2002; Schuckit 2000a). The high level of acceptance of this drug relates to a long history of use in Western societies, along with the recognition that in low doses, alcohol can have some pleasant and even healthful effects. Regular intake of modest doses (one or two drinks per day) is associated with a decreased risk for heart attacks, for one type of stroke, possibly for some old-age dementias, and for gallstones (Hendriks et al. 1998).

However, higher doses of alcohol are associated with significant problems (Dawson 2001). For example, as many as 60% of drinkers have experienced an alcohol-related adverse event such as a blackout (forgetting all or part of what occurred during heavy alcohol consumption), driving after drinking, or missing work or school to "party" or recover from drinking too much the night before. Pervasive and repetitive alcohol problems, such as those labeled *abuse* or *dependence* in DSM-IV-TR (American Psychiatric Association 2000), are seen in 15%–20% of men and 10% of women during their lives. The high rates of temporary problems and alcohol use disorders contribute to the

estimated 25,000 deaths per year from accidents and 175,000 annual deaths from heart disease, cancer, and suicide. Alcohol use disorders are seen in all races and socioeconomic strata, frequently causing or contributing to many medical and psychiatric conditions.

Not everyone has the same level of vulnerability toward alcohol abuse and dependence. Investigations over the past 50 years have suggested that genetic influences explain about 60% of the overall vulnerability (Prescott and Kendler 1999). These studies show a fourfold increased risk for alcohol abuse or dependence in alcoholic patients' close relatives, a higher risk in identical compared with fraternal twins, and a high rate of these disorders even in adopted-away sons and daughters of alcoholic patients (Prescott and Kendler 1999; Schuckit 2000b). Several genetically controlled characteristics that contribute to alcoholism risk have been identified, including alcohol metabolizing enzymes, impulsivity or disinhibition, independent psychiatric conditions such as bipolar disorder and schizophrenia, and a low level of response to alcohol (Schuckit 2000b). Environmental characteristics may interact with genetic influences to explain additional vulnerability.

These introductory comments underscore the need for clinicians to recognize that alcohol use disorders can appear in any patient and are not likely to reflect poor self-control or low moral values. It is essential to avoid stereotypes of alcoholic persons as out-of-work skid-row residents, but instead look for signs of repetitive alcohol-related problems in all men and women who come for treatment. This is especially important for alcoholic patients because, as described below, heavy problematic drinking can masquerade as almost any psychiatric symptom (American Psychiatric Association 2000; Schuckit et al. 1997). Because of the temporary nature of most psychiatric symptoms seen among alcoholic patients and the high rate of morbidity and mortality associated with alcohol use disorders, it is critical for clinicians to learn as much as possible about diagnosing and treating these syndromes. In this chapter, we review issues related to the diagnosis of alcohol use disorder, the pharmacology of alcohol, the clinical course of alcohol use disorders, assessment, and treatment, including detoxification, rehabilitation, and aftercare.

Diagnostic Issues

DSM-IV-TR Alcohol Intoxication

Intoxication from alcohol is typical of that seen with other brain depressants, including benzodiazepines and barbiturates (Schuckit 2000a). Effects of alcohol are generally observed after as little as one standard drink (i.e., 12 g of ethanol), which is likely to produce a blood alcohol concentration (BAC) of 0.015–0.020 g/dL. Most states in the United States have chosen a value of 0.080 g/dL to indicate legal intoxication, the level at which most nontolerant individuals show significant impairment in tasks such as driving. Problems with judgment and coordination increase as BAC rises, and blackouts, nystagmus, and severely disordered behavior are typically observed at BACs greater than 0.200 g/dL. Increasing the BAC above 0.300–0.400 g/dL can cause severe slowing of vital signs and death. Treating intoxication involves the passage of time because the body metabolizes approximately one drink (i.e., about 0.015 g/dL) per hour. Aggressive or difficult behavior is usually dealt with through the judicious use of cognitive and behavioral approaches, as well as calming medications, including, if BACs are low enough, benzodiazepines and antipsychotic drugs.

DSM-IV-TR Alcohol Withdrawal

Alcohol withdrawal refers to a characteristic syndrome of unpleasant effects that may occur after a heavy drinker stops or reduces the amount of alcohol intake. An alcohol withdrawal syndrome includes two or more of the following (American Psychiatric Association 2000):

1. Autonomic hyperactivity (e.g., elevated heart rate, blood pressure, respiratory rate, body temperature; sweating)
2. Anxiety
3. Insomnia
4. Psychomotor agitation
5. Nausea or vomiting
6. Tremor
7. Rarely: transient visual, tactile, or auditory hallucinations or illusions
8. Rarely: grand mal seizures

If a regular heavy drinker cuts back on alcohol intake, symptoms of withdrawal can appear within 4–8 hours, peak in intensity on day 2, and improve by day 5, although milder symptoms may take months to disappear. The symptoms are the opposite of the acute effects of the drug, and the most common are intensified autonomic nervous system activity, anxiety, and insomnia.

Only 5% of alcohol-dependent people ever develop severe withdrawal, which can include one or two grand mal convulsions or an agitated delirium (Schuckit et al. 1995b). The latter, known as *delirium tremens* or "DTs," involves severe autonomic hyperactivity, tremor, an agitated state of confusion and altered consciousness, and hallucinations (usually visual or tactile). Risk factors for experiencing these severe symptoms include advancing age, larger amounts of alcohol intake, longer periods of dependence, and concomitant medical problems.

It is important to note that acute withdrawal is just the initial, most intense form of the abstinence syndrome. Lingering symptoms of autonomic hyperactivity, anxiety, and sleep disturbance commonly continue for 1–6 months of abstinence (Drummond et al. 1998). This protracted withdrawal is not directly treated, other than educating patients that the problems will diminish with continued sobriety. Although most clinicians gauge the intensity of withdrawal clinically, standardized measures can be used. The most common is the Clinical Institute Withdrawal Assessment for Alcohol Scale—Revised (CIWA-Ar), a 10-item instrument that rates the intensity of each withdrawal symptom from zero to seven (Sullivan et al. 1989).

DSM-IV-TR Alcohol Dependence

The two major diagnostic approaches for alcohol use disorders, DSM-IV-TR and the *International Statistical Classification of Diseases and Related Health Problems,* 10th Revision (ICD-10; World Health Organization 1992), use similar methods to identify men and women with severe and persistent alcohol-related problems, focusing on repetitive difficulties related to alcohol in multiple life areas, despite which use of the drug is continued. Because past behavior is a good predictor of future behavior, this pattern of problems suggests that a return to drinking is likely to result in more difficulties.

DSM-IV-TR lists the seven problems relevant to the alcohol dependence diagnosis (see DSM-IV-TR criteria for substance dependence, Table 10–1 in Chapter 10 of this volume, "Assessment of the Patient," p. 106). Reflecting the fact that this is a syndrome, the diagnosis should be restricted to people who have shown three or more of these symptoms repetitively in the same 12-month period. This algorithm recognizes that severe problems can develop even in the absence of withdrawal or tolerance, but recent studies indicate a more severe clinical course for patients with histories of either of these physiological components, especially withdrawal (Schuckit et al. 1998). Thus, DSM-IV-TR recommends that clinicians subtype alcohol dependence as with or without a physiological component to the disorder (Schuckit et al. 1998).

Additional subtypes of alcohol dependence have been proposed. Two algorithms identify alcohol-dependent individuals with an early onset of a severe form of alcoholism often associated with criminality and multiple drug dependencies, noting them as Type II and Type B variations, respectively (Babor et al. 1992; Cloninger et al. 1996). These distinctions overlap with the DSM-IV-TR Axis II label of antisocial personality disorder. Despite these considerations, this chapter focuses on alcohol abuse or dependence in general rather than possible subtypes.

DSM-IV-TR Alcohol Abuse

Some individuals may drink without having problems, and others show severe, repetitive problems that are diagnosed as dependence. Between these extremes, *alcohol abuse* is a diagnosis applied to individuals who do not meet criteria for alcohol dependence but have repetitive interpersonal, legal, or psychosocial troubles that cluster together within a 12-month period (see DSM-IV-TR criteria for substance abuse, Table 10–2 in Chapter 10, p. 107). Prior diagnostic manuals (e.g., DSM-III-R; American Psychiatric Association 1987) assumed that this label would apply to those persons who do not yet fulfill criteria for dependence but are likely to do so, and the diagnosis was considered a "residual" (Rounsaville and Kranzler 1989). However, recent studies indicate that only 10% of the individuals with alcohol abuse go on to meet dependence criteria in the next 5 years, whereas 40% maintain their alcohol abuse diagnosis, and the remainder stop drinking or no longer show problems (Schuckit et al. 2001). Thus, the DSM-IV-TR diagnostic criteria for abuse outline a syndrome worthy of clinical recognition that is not just the prodromal phase of dependence.

The diagnostic structure of abuse and dependence allows for the possibility of a person endorsing one or two of the seven dependence criteria but not meeting criteria for abuse. These individuals, referred to as *diagnostic orphans* (Pollock and Martin 1999), were found to represent 31% of relatively high-functioning drinkers (Eng et al., submitted). A 5-year follow-up found that these men and women were significantly more likely than those with no alcohol problems at baseline to have problems at follow-up, with rates similar to those associated with abuse but significantly lower than those associated with alcohol dependence (Eng et al. 2003).

Alcohol-Induced Disorders

DSM-IV-TR warns clinicians against diagnosing major psychiatric conditions (e.g., panic disorder) when the diagnostic criteria are observed only in the context of a preexisting condition (e.g., major depression or hyperthyroidism). Such induced or secondary disorders often clear spontaneously when the first-appearing or independent condition disappears. A similar algorithm applies to psychiatric symptoms observed in the context of intoxication or withdrawal, which can temporarily mimic the same psychiatric symptomatology (see Table 14–1).

A brief background on the relations between drug types and symptoms assists in understanding substance-induced conditions. Drugs of abuse can be di-

Table 14–1. DSM-IV-TR alcohol-induced disorders

Alcohol intoxication

Alcohol withdrawal

Alcohol intoxication delirium

Alcohol withdrawal delirium

Alcohol-induced persisting dementia

Alcohol-induced persisting amnestic disorder

Alcohol-induced psychotic disorder (may be intoxication- or withdrawal-induced)

Alcohol-induced mood disorder (may be intoxication- or withdrawal-induced)

Alcohol-induced anxiety disorder (may be intoxication- or withdrawal-induced)

Alcohol-induced sexual dysfunction (may be intoxication-induced)

Alcohol-induced sleep disorder (may be intoxication- or withdrawal-induced)

Source. Adapted from American Psychiatric Association 2000.

vided into categories based on typical effects (Schuckit 2000a), including the stimulants (e.g., amphetamines, cocaine, and most weight-reducing products) and the depressants (e.g., alcohol, benzodiazepines, and barbiturates). Both of these drug types are likely to produce anxiety, depressive, and psychotic symptoms that can be mistaken for major psychiatric disorders. Repeated heavy intoxication with depressant drugs usually produces some level of mood disturbance, and in 40% of cases, the depressive symptoms are severe and pervasive enough to come close to or meet criteria for a major depressive episode (Schuckit et al. 1997). However, these substance-induced mood disorders are likely to improve markedly over the 2–4 weeks following abstinence, diminishing below the level appropriate for a major depressive episode diagnosis sooner than antidepressants are likely to work. Furthermore, no human or animal studies have clearly shown that antidepressant medications effectively treat temporary substance-induced mood disorders. Thus, clinicians should distinguish substance-induced mood disorders from major depressions that occur independent of substances because the prognoses and treatments are quite different. The same general approach applies to temporary anxiety conditions, such as panic attacks and social phobic symptoms, which are common following withdrawal from brain depressants.

One useful approach for distinguishing between substance-induced and independent psychiatric conditions is the timeline method (see Figure 14–1) (American Psychiatric Association 2000; Schuckit 2000a; Schuckit et al. 1997). First, the clinician establishes the age at onset of dependence on a substance (e.g., alcohol) capable of mimicking the major psychiatric condition (e.g., depression) by focusing on the age at which the third of the seven possible dependence criteria occurred. Determining the chronology of symptoms is facilitated by establishing the patient's age at major life events (e.g., graduation, marriage, birth of a child) and then determining whether the criterion of interest (e.g., tolerance) occurred before or after a particular life event. Second, the clinician looks for evidence of an independent psychiatric syndrome by determining whether the psychiatric disorder being considered (e.g., a major depressive episode) ever occurred before the onset of the dependence syndrome. The emphasis should be on the full DSM-IV-TR psychiatric condition, such as a major depressive episode, not just symptoms of sadness. Third, patients without a preexisting major psychiatric condition list periods since the onset of dependence when they were sober for several months or more, and the clinician probes to determine whether the psychiatric condition occurred during the extended abstinence, which would also point to a history of an independent condition. Fourth, and most critically, the clinician observes the patient over a month of abstinence to determine whether the symptoms of the depression, anxiety, or psychotic disorder improve sufficiently to drop below the diagnostic threshold. This spontaneous clearing of the disorder is highly likely if the patient never had an independent psychiatric syndrome and is less likely if he or she has a history of an independent disorder.

Patients with a major psychiatric condition predating alcohol dependence or occurring during abstinence are considered to have an independent psychiatric disorder, suggesting that the current episode reflects an independent condition. Such cases need to be carefully observed for signs of the psychiatric disorder early during abstinence, and the clinician might start medication before the recommended full month of abstinence if the psychiatric symptoms are not improving.

Pharmacology

A limited background on the pharmacology of alcohol is helpful for clinicians working with patients who have experienced intoxication and withdrawal and for identifying the manner in which alcohol affects medical disorders and medication efficacy. Alcohol is a simple

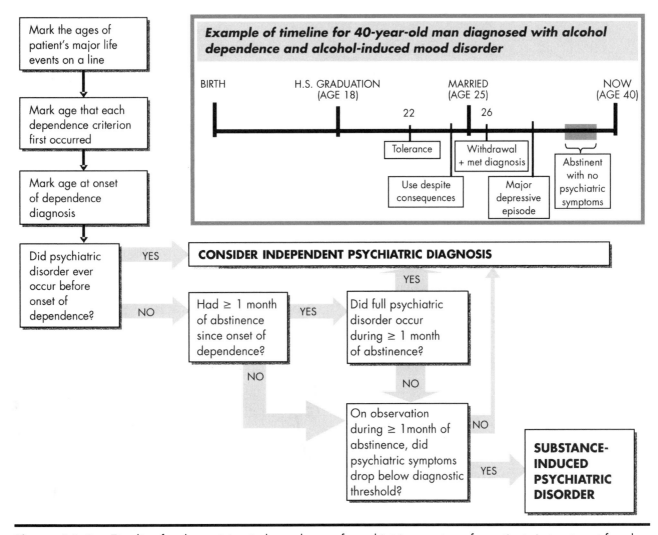

Figure 14–1. Timeline for determining independence of psychiatric symptoms for patients in treatment for alcoholism.

molecule that is partially absorbed in the lining of the mouth, esophagus, and stomach, passing quickly through the pylorus to its site of major absorption in the proximal small intestine. As with most oral fluids, anything that slows the rate of stomach emptying, including a heavy or fatty meal, delays absorption. The average drink (12 oz of beer, 4 oz of wine, or 1.5 oz of an 80-proof beverage) contains about 12 g of ethanol, as well as compounds that give the beverage its taste and smell. The latter are called congeners and include aldehydes, esters, phenols, tannins, and flavonoids. The flavonoids are found in grape products such as red wines and, in addition to the ethanol itself, may add to the decrease in heart disease associated with the intake of one to two drinks per day (Freedman et al. 2001). After absorption, the water solubility of alcohol contributes to its rapid distribution throughout the body. Ethanol is also fat soluble, which may contribute to its effects on nerve cells.

Less than 10% of absorbed alcohol is excreted directly through the lungs, kidneys, or sweat; most is broken down in the liver. Here, several pathways metabolize alcohol to its first and chemically active metabolite, acetaldehyde (see Figure 14–2), mostly through actions of various forms of the enzyme alcohol dehydrogenase (ADH). However, at higher BACs, a system residing in the microsomes (known as the microsomal ethanol oxidizing system, or MEOS) contributes. Most brain depressants cause the liver to increase production of relevant metabolizing enzymes, so that heavy repetitive drinking is associated with an increased metabolic rate of alcohol and some other drugs. This process of enzyme induction can contribute to lower blood levels of some medications.

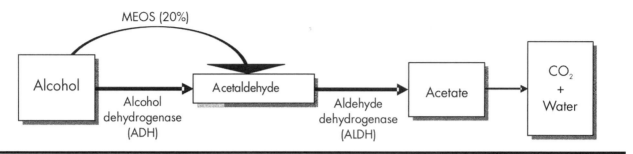

Figure 14–2. Alcohol metabolism in the liver.

MEOS=microsomal ethanol oxidizing system.

Average drinkers experience few physiological effects from acetaldehyde because it is broken down very quickly, primarily by the enzyme aldehyde dehydrogenase (ALDH) (Li 2000; Wall et al. 2001). Low levels of acetaldehyde are associated with stimulated feelings, whereas high levels contribute to nausea, vomiting, and changes in blood pressure. In fact, one medication used for treating alcoholism (disulfiram) works by inhibiting ALDH, resulting in very high levels of acetaldehyde after drinking. Among Japanese, Chinese, and Korean men and women, 10% have only an inactive form of a key ALDH and thus react very adversely to alcohol and have no risk for alcoholism (Li 2000), and another 40% have decreased activity of the relevant ALDH. The latter are likely to become drinkers, but their exaggerated response to alcohol, caused by a modest increase in acetaldehyde, reduces their risk for alcohol use disorders (Wall et al. 2001).

Tolerance

Tolerance is an important concept in understanding the pharmacology of alcohol. It is defined as either the need for significantly larger amounts of a drug to bring about the same effects previously produced by smaller amounts or the experience of diminished effects following the same dose of a drug (Schuckit 2000a). Part of tolerance can involve a very rapid adaptation to the drug, so that the effects at a given BAC are greater at rising than at declining alcohol levels (acute tolerance), and the adaptation to repeated doses over a series of drinking sessions (chronic tolerance). Components of tolerance also relate to learning (behavioral tolerance), adaptations in metabolizing systems (pharmacokinetic tolerance), and blunting of effects in the brain and other organs (pharmacodynamic tolerance). For the clinician, it is important to understand tolerance as one of the seven diagnostic criteria

for dependence and to know about this process that enables some alcoholic patients to walk and talk despite prodigiously high BACs (e.g., 0.250 g/dL).

Neurochemical Effects

Before leaving the pharmacology of alcohol, it is important to note the wide span of effects that this drug has on brain chemicals. One of the neurochemical systems most influenced by alcohol relates to the inhibitory neurotransmitter γ-aminobutyric acid (GABA), which is sensitive to the actions of all brain depressants, showing increased activity during intoxication and decreased activity during withdrawal (Ueno et al. 2001). As with all substances perceived as pleasant or reinforcing, alcohol also produces changes in dopamine functioning, especially in brain areas rich in reward recognition. Ethanol has a major effect on a third neurochemical—serotonin—and has been hypothesized to have clinically relevant relations with acetylcholine. During withdrawal, the excitatory neurotransmitter system, including glutamate and N-methyl-D-aspartate (NMDA) receptors, shows hyperactivity. Finally, alcohol has been shown to have important actions on the opioid system, which might explain the potential usefulness of opioid-blocking drugs, such as naltrexone, in treatment (Krystal et al. 2001).

Clinical Course of Alcohol Use Disorders

A major purpose of a diagnosis is to enable a clinician to use clinical experience and the scientific literature to determine whether intervention is warranted (Goodwin and Guze 1996) and which therapies have the greatest chance of doing the most good with the least harm. Understanding the usual clinical course of alcohol use disorders helps clinicians make optimal decisions.

The usual ages at first drink and first temporary problems in alcoholic persons are the early to midteens, an age range that is not much different from that in the general population of drinkers who do not become alcohol dependent (Schuckit 2000a; Schuckit et al. 1995a) (see Table 14–2). Earlier intoxication may be associated with an earlier onset of alcohol use disorders (Dawson 2000), but patterns are generally similar in those with and without alcoholism. For the average alcohol-dependent individual, the most obvious differences tend to appear in the late teens to 20s. During this time, most people moderate intake and problem patterns, but alcohol-dependent individuals have more difficulty decreasing and maintaining low levels of alcohol intake.

A clinically important aspect of the course of alcohol use disorders is their fluctuating course. Most alcoholic persons react to periods of alcohol-related problems with abstinence, which can last for days to months at a time. This abstinence is often followed by a period of temporary control, during which rules about drinking are set and followed for days to months, commonly resulting in a relaxation of rules and an escalation of problems. Thus, most alcohol-dependent people can stop drinking, often unrelated to treatment, and control intake for temporary periods, although most studies indicate that once problems are severe enough to justify a diagnosis of alcohol dependence, periods of control are highly likely to result in a resumption of problematic drinking.

In presenting an overview of the course of alcoholism, it is important to emphasize the potential for "spontaneous remission" or what might be considered a response to unspecified events (Sobell et al. 2000). Long-term studies of alcohol-dependent individuals indicate that more than 20% will permanently stop drinking even in the absence of self-help groups or formal treatment. Specific precipitants of this natural recovery remain unclear, although several studies suggest failing health, interpersonal conflicts, and legal difficulties. The high rate of spontaneous remission and the challenges in determining factors associated with good outcome highlight that recovery is possible for any patient. Even if one intervention or treatment is not effective, the alcohol-dependent person may achieve long-term and potentially permanent abstinence.

Table 14–2. Course of alcohol dependence

Event	Age (years)
First drank	13
First time intoxicated	15
First alcohol-related problem	20
First alcohol dependence symptom	22
Death	60

Source. Adapted from Schuckit et al. 1995a.

Medical Consequences

The average alcohol-dependent man or woman decreases his or her life span by 10–15 years. Remembering that the average alcoholic person has a job and a family and that, for instance, physicians have approximately the same risk for alcohol dependence as the general population, the decreased length of life is observed even in otherwise healthy and well-nourished individuals. The major cause of early mortality among alcoholic patients is heart disease, occurring at an earlier age and a higher rate than would be expected in comparable individuals. This reflects the fact that although daily consumption of one or two drinks may have some cardioprotective effects, consumption of more than two drinks has the opposite result (Hendriks et al. 1998). Repeated heavy intake of alcohol is associated with high blood pressure, increases in triglycerides and low-density lipoprotein cholesterol, and a risk for modest deterioration of heart muscle, or cardiomyopathy. These situations add to the risk for heart attack and stroke.

The second leading cause of death among alcoholic patients is cancer, related to the effects of heavy, repetitive doses of alcohol on the immune system and the irritating action of alcohol in the digestive tract and lungs. The result is a high risk for malignancies throughout the body, especially in the head, neck, esophagus, and stomach. Perhaps related to the effect on the liver overall, the cancer risk for that organ and for the colon is also high. The high rates of lung cancer occur independent of the smoking status of the patient.

The third leading cause of death is accidents. Even modest doses of alcohol influence judgment, motor coordination, and the ability to interpret relatively subtle stimuli.

The fourth leading elevated mortality factor is suicide (Preuss et al. 2002). Forty percent of alcohol-dependent men and women have periods of intense depression associated with heavy drinking, which can include all of the characteristics of major depressive disorders, such as suicidal thoughts and feelings of hopelessness, even though symptoms are likely to improve rapidly with abstinence (Schuckit et al. 1997). Coupled with the disinhibiting qualities of alcohol intoxication, it is not surprising that the risk for suicide among people with alcoholism is up to 10-fold higher than in the general population (Preuss et al. 2002).

Many additional medical conditions are prominent in alcohol-dependent individuals. The liver, taking the brunt of the effect of the alcohol absorbed from the small intestine, responds with a succession of events that includes a fatty infiltration, in which the liver cannot process fats and alcohol becomes the preferred fuel. This can contribute to a potentially reversible inflammation, alcoholic hepatitis; however, in 15% of patients with alcoholism, this condition progresses to a permanent scarring, or cirrhosis, that can severely impair liver functioning. Other problems related to the digestive system include inflammation of the pancreas, a consequence of the stimulation of digestive enzymes and the occlusion of some ducts; gastric irritation (gastritis); and an increased risk for ulcers (Schuckit 2000a).

Almost all body systems are adversely affected by high doses of alcohol. Blood-producing organs are likely to create slightly large red blood cells (responsible for high mean corpuscular volumes among alcoholic patients). Heavy doses of alcohol can impair bone production and maintenance, resulting in an increased risk for fractures, whereas nerves to the hands and feet can be compromised in a potentially irreversible condition known as *peripheral neuropathy*. The causes of all of these syndromes are complex, but most of the pathology appears to relate specifically to high doses of alcohol and its metabolite, acetaldehyde.

Neuropsychological Consequences

Approximately half of adults with alcohol dependence have at least temporary cognitive impairments, typically on tasks requiring spatial functioning, learning and memory, fast yet accurate psychomotor functioning, abstract reasoning, and planning (Parsons and Nixon 1993). Chronic heavy drinkers show increased brain ventricular and sulcal size and decreased volume of the caudate nucleus, which appear to recover partially after several months of abstinence (Pfeffer-

baum et al. 1995). Diminished brain blood flow, particularly in frontal regions (Adams et al. 1993), electrophysiological abnormalities (Holguin et al. 1999), and diminished brain response to cognitive challenges (Tapert et al. 2001) further demonstrate deleterious effects. The brain changes associated with alcohol dependence are due to both neuronal death and reversible cell shrinkage (Harper 1998). Women may have a modestly heightened vulnerability to alcohol-induced brain effects relative to men (Hommer et al. 2001).

Fetal Effects

Before leaving this brief review of morbidity and mortality, it is important to point out that alcohol easily crosses the placental barrier to a developing fetus, which cannot efficiently metabolize acetaldehyde (Eriksson 2001). The result is a range of potential difficulties, including elevated rates of spontaneous abortion, low birth weight, malformed hands and feet, small brain volume, varying levels of mental retardation, heart defects, and a facial structure that can include the absence of a philtrum and an epicanthal fold (Stratton et al. 1996). If low weight, central nervous system involvement, and facial abnormalities are observed, this is called *fetal alcohol syndrome*, whereas a less severe condition is described as *fetal alcohol effects*. No amount of alcohol intake has been established as safe for pregnant women (Stratton et al. 1996).

Identification of Patients With Alcohol Use Disorders

An essential step in identifying individuals with alcohol use disorders is to recognize the high prevalence and avoid inappropriate stereotypes. Most of the 15%–20% of the men in the United States with an alcohol use disorder have jobs and families, do not develop cirrhosis, and never have withdrawal delirium or convulsions (Schuckit 2000a). The prevalence of alcohol use disorders in the general population is amplified among patients seeking help for psychiatric symptoms or emergency medical concerns, with rates estimated to exceed 20% (Gentilello et al. 1999). Thus, any individual seeking help with life problems, insomnia, impotence, sadness, or anxiety should be screened for the pattern of repetitive problems that constitute the diagnosis of abuse or dependence. Diagnostic criteria emphasize problematic patterns, which are better predictors of future alcohol-related difficulties than the quantity or frequency of drinking because the amount of alcohol associated with psychological or physical problems differs vastly across age, gender, and the presence of medications and medical conditions.

State Markers of Heavy Drinking

Although the diagnosis of alcohol abuse or dependence rests primarily with a clinical history, the effect that alcohol has on body systems can result in temporary changes in several blood tests that can be useful markers of heavy drinking. One of the most sensitive and specific tests results from the liver induction of an enzyme important in amino acid transport, γ-glutamyltransferase (GGT). Most healthy individuals have GGT values lower than 35 U/L; thus, findings above this level should lead the clinician to search for potential causes, including drinking four or more drinks per day for 4 or more weeks. A second marker with good sensitivity and specificity (about 70%) is a value of 20 U/L for carbohydrate-deficient transferrin (CDT). These two values complement each other, as some individuals show an elevation of one but not the other. As with all state markers of heavy drinking, these usually return toward normal levels within days of alcohol cessation, often reaching cutoffs within 2 weeks (see Table 14–3).

Table 14–3. State markers of heavy drinking

| Marker | Values suggesting heavy drinking | | Accuracy |
	Men	Women	
Carbohydrate-deficient transferrin (CDT)[a]	>20 U/L	>26 U/L	Very good
γ-Glutamyltransferase (GGT)[a]	>35 U/L	>30 U/L	Very good
Mean corpuscular volume (MCV)	>91 μm^3	>91 μm^3	Good
Aspartate aminotransferase (AST)	>40 U/L	>33 U/L	Fair
Alanine aminotransferase (ALT)	>46 U/L	>35 U/L	Fair
Uric acid	>8.0 mg/dL	>6.2 mg/dL	Fair
5-Hydroxytryptophol–to–5-hydroxyindoleacetic acid ratio	>20	>20	Fair

[a]Best results when both measures are collected.

A third valuable screening test for heavy drinking involves documenting a mean red blood cell size (mean corpuscular volume) of greater than 91 μm^3. These values reside in the high-normal range and can result from heavy drinking, reflecting the effect that alcohol can have on red blood cell production. A high-normal uric acid value can also raise suspicion regarding potential heavy drinking. Liver function tests, such as aspartate aminotransferase (AST) and alanine aminotransferase (ALT), are helpful but are not very sensitive, usually increasing only after evidence of liver cell damage.

Questionnaires

Several questionnaires are available to indicate potential alcohol problems and take only a few minutes for the patient to fill out, although they do not diagnose DSM-IV-TR alcohol abuse or dependence. These include the Alcohol Use Disorders Identification Test (AUDIT), which has 10 items scored on a 0–4 scale that query about alcohol use and related problems. Scores of 8 or higher indicate a condition worthy of further evaluation in adults (Reinert and Allen 2002), whereas scores of 4 or higher are suggestive of alcohol use disorders in adolescents (Chung et al. 2000). On the 10- and 25-item Michigan Alcohol Screening Test (MAST; Conley 2001), endorsement of four or more alcohol-related problems indicates a potential alcohol use disorder. Even shorter tests, although not optimally sensitive or specific, include the four-item CAGE (**C**ut down, **A**nnoyed, **G**uilty, **E**ye openers) and five-item TWEAK (**T**olerance, **W**orried, **E**ye openers, **A**mnesia/blackouts, **K**[c]ut down).

The Process of Intervention

Perhaps the hardest step in treating alcoholism is to help the patients recognize that alcohol is causing repetitive difficulties in their lives. One of the challenges is that many people gauge their own problem and intake pattern based on the habits of those around them (Daeppen et al. 1999). Because so many alcoholic people have both alcoholic relatives and heavy-drinking friends, the process of getting them in tune with the risks of continued drinking can be daunting.

The guidelines for interventions with any condition that requires lifestyle changes are similar. Interventions for an alcoholic individual involve considerations similar to those one might use in helping an individual with diabetes recognize the need to stop smoking and modify diet or in helping a person with hypertension to exercise and take medications appropriately (O'Brien and McLellan 1996). In any of these instances, it makes sense to take advantage of the presenting concern and show how the mood, anxiety, sleep, sexual functioning, or life problem was likely to have been caused or exacerbated by alcohol use. The reasoning can be bolstered by pointing to additional difficulties and highlighting any abnormal biological markers of heavy drinking. The clinching line might be "I think you've reached a point at which alcohol may be causing problems for you. If the drinking pattern doesn't change, these difficulties are likely to get worse and worse."

These and additional considerations have been described under the label of *motivational interviewing* or *motivational enhancement* (Fleming et al. 2002). This is a brief time-limited intervention and therapeutic approach in which the clinician works with the patient to build trust by showing empathy (Fleming et al. 2002). Areas of resistance to change are noted, and the patient is encouraged to discuss why altering drinking patterns might be beneficial. The clinician explores the patient's ambivalence and offers reassurance that the patient is in charge of any decisions, while at the same time evaluating readiness for change and avoiding pushing too much too soon (see Table 14–4).

Modifications of this approach have been used in brief physician interventions (Fleming et al. 2002). One paradigm incorporates two 15-minute physician visits separated by a month. The clinician asks about drinking, reviews alcohol-related problems, and emphasizes the adverse effects of alcohol. The patient keeps a diary of his or her drinking pattern and establishes realistic goals that are then set down as a contract. In this evaluation, the interventions were followed with two 5-minute telephone conversations with a nurse to reinforce the lessons learned. With this approach, more than two-thirds of the drinking patients contacted agreed to participate, and excellent out

Table 14–4.   Features of motivational interviewing

Duration	Time-limited
Steps	1. Provide objective feedback
	2. Build motivation for patient to take responsibility to change
	3. Collaboratively develop treatment plan, giving advice and menu of options
	4. Explore ambivalence
	5. Strengthen self-efficacy and commitment to change
Clinician tasks	Develop cognitive dissonance, roll with resistance
Clinician style	Empathetic, reflective, encouraging, reassuring, nonconfrontational

comes of reduced drinking and alcohol problems were maintained over a 4-year period.

Some clinicians have advocated a more intense approach. Here, the intervention is carried out in the presence of the spouse, children, other family members, friends, and employers. As a group, they share their concern and point to instances that made them conclude that alcohol use is a problem. Usually, these family interventions are preceded by establishing a place to turn if the patient agrees to seek help. Few rigorous evaluations of this process have been published, and potential difficulties can arise.

In intervening with any medical or psychiatric difficulty, it is important to remember that the process is likely to evolve over time. Therefore, if a patient does not accept the need to consider abstinence when first approached, it is possible to return to this issue the next time a relevant opportunity appears. Usually, the summation of small cognitive events produces the actual change in behavior. Techniques for working with patients through alcohol detoxification and rehabilitation are presented next.

Detoxification

The first and most important step in detoxification, or the process of treating withdrawal, is based on studies showing that entering alcohol withdrawal while physically ill markedly increases the chances of convulsions or delirium (Schuckit et al. 1995b). Therefore, it is essential to conduct a thorough physical examination for conditions associated with alcoholism, as described previously, or any other illnesses. The second important component is to avoid doing harm. For example, few individuals in alcohol withdrawal are dehydrated, and many may be overhydrated, perhaps reflecting high levels of antidiuretic hormone during sustained intoxication and withdrawal. This, in conjunction with the possibility of alcoholic cardiomyopathy, means that intravenous fluids should be avoided unless there are solid medical indications for this approach.

The third basic element of the treatment is education and reassurance. This forms the basis of the "social model detoxification program," in which it is assumed that alcoholic persons who do not have medical problems will benefit from decent nutrition, a place to sleep comfortably, and the recognition that caregivers understand the elements of treatment. Because alcohol interferes in the absorption of B vitamins, oral multiple vitamins that include thiamine (which is not well stored in the body) can be important.

In treating depressant withdrawal, it is helpful to recognize that the symptoms have developed because the body adapted to alcohol, and levels of this drug decreased too quickly for the body to adjust. Thus, the patient is likely to benefit from any brain depressant in high enough doses on day 1 to markedly diminish symptoms. The usual 5-day course of acute withdrawal indicates that medication levels should be decreased by 20% each day to reach levels of zero by day 5. Any depressant can be useful, but the longer-acting benzodiazepines, such as diazepam or chlordiazepoxide, have many assets for patients who do not have severe brain damage or cirrhosis. For example, a typical patient showing signs of acute alcohol withdrawal might be prescribed 25 mg of chlordiazepoxide orally to be given up to five times per day, advising the patient or any caregiver to withhold the dose if the patient is sleepy or light-headed. The patient might be given an additional 25-mg dose an hour after an oral dose if significant tremor or anxiety is still present. An alternative approach is to use shorter-acting benzodiazepines, such as oxazepam. Although these drugs are as effective as longer-acting drugs and have fewer cumulative effects that might put people to sleep, they can be dangerous because the rapidly declining blood levels of these shorter-acting medications can increase the chance of a grand mal seizure. As a result, the medications must be administered every 4–6 hours without skipping a dose.

The treatment of depressant withdrawal does not usually require anticonvulsant medications unless the patient has a seizure disorder; these medications are relatively expensive, can have significant side effects, and have not been shown to be useful substitutes for benzodiazepines. Magnesium or similar elements are not usually required.

Rehabilitation

The rehabilitation approaches for all long-term relapsing disorders have many similarities (O'Brien and McLellan 1996). Education and cognitive-behavioral approaches are used to increase the motivation for behavior change, help people to rebuild their lives, and prevent relapse (Project MATCH Research Group 1998; Schuckit 2000a). For alcohol use disorders, these approaches, along with the judicious use of medications when appropriate, are associated with good outcomes (Schuckit 2000a; Smith et al. 1999). For example, among the usual alcohol-dependent individual, a person with a job and family, the chances of extended periods of abstinence (i.e., a year or longer and often permanent) are as high as 70% following completion of intensive outpatient or inpatient treatment. Even among alcohol-dependent individuals who do not have jobs or fixed incomes, continuous 1-year abstinence rates of almost 50% have been reported (Smith et al. 1999).

In evaluating treatments for alcohol dependence, the usual clinical course, described previously, is important to keep in mind. Because patients are likely to enter care at the time of the most intense symptoms, which are likely to temporarily moderate with time alone, and because spontaneous remission is possible, only controlled trials can determine whether an intervention was responsible for the outcome. Furthermore, it is important to monitor the levels of improved life functioning, and not just gauge success in terms of absolute abstinence. Several studies have attempted to determine which components of care are more or less effective for individuals with different characteristics (Project MATCH Research Group 1998). These have corroborated the generally good outcome for alcohol-dependent individuals and have highlighted some possible characteristics that might aid in matching a patient to a specific therapeutic approach. However, the overarching conclusion appears to be that once patients have reached a point at which they are willing to consider abstinence, their motivation and characteristics are likely to be better predictors of outcome than any specific aspect of the treatment program.

Basic Cognitive-Behavioral Approach to Treatment

The basic cognitive-behavioral approach forms the core of most current inpatient and outpatient treatment modalities (Schuckit 2000a). This approach is based on social learning theories, and the goal is to help the patient identify life stressors, high-risk situations for drinking, and coping skills deficits. Appropriate responses are generated and practiced by use of modeling, role-plays, and rehearsal (Morgenstern and Longabaugh 2000). Incorporated into the approach is the need to monitor ongoing relapse risk levels, anticipate risky situations, and make lifestyle adjustments to maintain positive changes. An overall goal is to promote the use of positive coping skills and mastery over managing life stresses. This is often accomplished by group therapy three to five times per week where patients describe recent stressors, cravings, and risk situations. Other patients and the group facilitator provide feedback and advice for overcoming barriers and attaining treatment goals. The trained facilitator helps maintain a supportive group environment in which patients can learn from one another and form social contacts with people who have similar goals regarding alcohol.

The family can be an important resource in this process (O'Farrell et al. 1998). Efforts should be made to optimize their understanding of the recovery process and to help them deal with their feelings about the alcoholic individual. This can be accomplished through groups for family members and friends, couples counseling, and Al-Anon (the Alcoholics Anonymous [AA] program aimed at helping families recover from living with a loved one's problem drinking).

Limited Role of Medications in Rehabilitation

As previously described, psychosocial interventions are very useful for maintaining sobriety. Three medications have demonstrated a degree of assistance toward this goal. However, for alcoholic patients without independent psychiatric disorders, double-blind, controlled trials do not support the efficacy of selective serotonin reuptake inhibitors (SSRIs), tricyclic antidepressants, lithium, benzodiazepines, or the antianxiety drug buspirone for achieving or maintaining abstinence (Fawcett et al. 2000; Kranzler et al. 1993; Schuckit 2000a).

Naltrexone.   Naltrexone, an opioid blocker hypothesized to decrease craving and the rewarding effects of alcohol, is usually prescribed in doses of 50–150 mg three times a week or more (Krystal et al. 2001). Most studies of naltrexone have involved relatively small numbers of subjects in university settings, where a great deal of additional treatment resources are available, and often these subjects were followed up for only 3 months. Although most studies support the potential efficacy of naltrexone in alcoholic patients, one large double-blind 6-month trial conducted in veterans' hospitals did not show significant effects (Krystal et al. 2001). The side-effect profile is modest, with the most frequent complaints involving gastrointestinal upset, a reversible elevation in liver function tests, and mild dysthymia. However, many clinicians believe that the bulk of the evidence supports the usefulness of this medication for patients who can afford to take it.

Acamprosate.   Acamprosate, which structurally resembles the neurotransmitter GABA and might serve as an NMDA receptor antagonist, also has been shown to have a modest effect in alcoholic patients, perhaps improving outcome by 15% (Mason 2001). Acamprosate, often prescribed at dosages approaching 2,000 mg/day, has been tested in more than 5,000 patients in Europe, with most trials continuing for 12 months. With rare exceptions, this drug generally has been reported to be modestly superior to placebo. The side effects of acamprosate appear mild, usually involving gastrointestinal upset. In small-scale studies reported to date, the combination of naltrexone and acamprosate appears to be more effective than either drug alone (Kiefer et al. 2003).

Disulfiram.   Disulfiram, an aldehyde dehydrogenase inhibitor, is usually prescribed at 250 mg/day, with instructions to patients that they cannot safely return to drinking unless disulfiram is stopped for 5 or more days. Patients are warned that the combination of alcohol and disulfiram can produce nausea, diarrhea, and blood pressure changes, with the intensity increasing at higher doses of alcohol. Perhaps because the patient's fear of a disulfiram-alcohol reaction is the effective element, double-blind, controlled trials have not convincingly confirmed its utility (Carroll et al. 2000). However, greater efficacy may result when administered by the patient's significant other, when given briefly during high-risk situations such as vacations or holiday seasons, or in the context of concomitant cocaine problems (Carroll et al. 2000). Disulfiram has a range of side effects, including some rare consequences that can be life-threatening (Schuckit 2000a).

In summary, most clinicians have reservations about the routine prescription of disulfiram.

Aftercare and Relapse Prevention

For any long-term relapsing condition, the acute phase of treatment helps return the patient to an optimal level of functioning. Yet the ongoing nature of the disorder and the many internal and external reinforcers of past alcohol use require that behavioral treatments continue at a diminishing intensity for 6–12 months after abstinence begins. AA is one of several 12-step self-help groups available around the world for assistance with alcohol use disorders. AA participation can occur as part of a formal treatment program or independent of professional assistance. In AA, participants regularly attend meetings and may try several before finding a cohort that feels comfortable, because groups vary with regard to participant demographics, smoking status, and religious belief. AA advises participants to select a sponsor, an AA member with a considerable history of abstinence, to provide guidance for achieving and maintaining sobriety through "working the steps." Twelve-step programs are named for the series of actions participants carry out, through which skills for staying sober are learned and practiced.

Relapse prevention is a conglomeration of cognitive-behavioral techniques aimed at maintaining positive treatment gains (Marlatt and Gordon 1985). As manualized (Project MATCH Research Group 1998), this integral part of treatment continues into aftercare and instructs patients to identify triggers that have been associated with a return to drinking in the past (e.g., bars, former drinking buddies) and then to develop and practice ways of avoiding such situations and managing the triggers when they arise. Patients also work through relapse situations by using homework assignments, interactions with other patients, and lecture material. The patient's responsibility for his or her own actions and behavior change is emphasized. An additional element of relapse prevention is that the occurrence of a slip should not be used as an excuse for returning to regular drinking but instead as an opportunity to learn about triggers and to correct coping skills deficits.

A Special Case: Comorbid Independent Psychiatric Disorders

As described earlier, alcohol intoxication can cause severe depressive episodes, and alcohol withdrawal can mimic most DSM-IV-TR anxiety conditions, which tend to markedly improve within days to weeks of abstinence. Medications are rarely appropriate for these alcohol-induced conditions, but long-term prescriptions are often indicated for independent psychiatric disorders (Schuckit et al. 1997). The distinction between induced and independent disorders rests with both a careful timeline of the chronology of the development of syndromes and observation of the patient over a month or so of abstinence (American Psychiatric Association 2000; Schuckit 2000a) (see Figure 14–1).

Any independent psychiatric disorder established should be treated with cognitive-behavioral, psychotherapeutic, and pharmacological approaches appropriate for the diagnosis. Thus, SSRIs and tricyclic antidepressants are appropriate treatments for depressive episodes in alcohol-dependent individuals with histories of independent major depressions whose depressive symptoms do not diminish with abstinence. In addition to cognitive-behavioral therapy, antidepressants can be effective in treating independent panic disorder or social phobia. However, benzodiazepines should be avoided in these patients because of the addictive potential.

A Special Population: Adolescents

Epidemiological studies suggest that approximately 6% of U.S. high school students meet diagnostic criteria for a current alcohol use disorder (Rohde et al. 1996). Half of the U.S. twelfth graders reported having used alcohol in the preceding month, and 33% reported having gotten drunk (Johnston et al. 2002). Unique risk factors, consequences, assessment approaches, and treatment methods are pertinent to understanding alcohol use disorders during adolescence. For youths, drinking often goes hand-in-hand with other problematic behaviors, including drug use, smoking, precocious sexual activity, and other criminal and health-threatening behaviors.

Diagnostic criteria for substance abuse and dependence are based on adult symptom patterns, and some heavy-drinking teenagers do not fit the criteria (Pollock and Martin 1999). Alcohol-involved adolescents typically use multiple intoxicants (Brown and D'Amico 2001). The diagnostic criteria of preoccupation, loss of control, and reckless behavior while using can occur in teenagers, but medical problems and severe withdrawal are unlikely (Brown and D'Amico 2001).

Optimal assessment tools for adolescents tailor wording to an appropriate reading level, accommodate the use of multiple substances, and use computer administration when possible (Winters and Henly 1989). For youths with substance use disorders, avenues to success include 1) engagement in treatment programs that incorporate family involvement and 2) participation in activities that are incompatible with substance use, such as sports, jobs, active academic involvement, and volunteer activities (Brown and D'Amico 2001). Multisystemic therapy (Henggeler et al. 1995) involves working with teenagers, parents, schools, community resources, and peers to decrease problem behaviors. Incorporating families to the extent possible helps many recovering teenagers. However, for teenagers whose parents have substance use disorders or other major problems, involvement in healthy activities outside the household that may provide role models is critical for success.

Conclusion

Alcohol use disorders affect substantial numbers of people worldwide, and the risk is even greater in persons in medical settings. Diagnostic labels of alcohol dependence and the less severe alcohol abuse indicate a need for intervention, although other indices of harmful drinking may also signal that professional attention is warranted. Symptoms of other psychiatric disorders, such as depression, anxiety, and psychosis, can be produced by heavy drinking, and establishing the presence of an independent psychiatric disorder is facilitated with a timeline approach. Alcohol detoxification, typically spanning 5 days, involves a thorough awareness of any illness in the patient, careful selection of pharmacological agents, education, and reassurance. After this period, clinicians can capitalize on the patient's recognition of problems caused by alcohol to motivate him or her toward rehabilitative efforts. Successful alcoholism treatment involves cognitive-behavioral techniques to identify risky situations for relapse and develop plans to manage these risks. This can be accomplished with professional help and self-help groups. Medications have shown modest benefits, adding almost 15% to the chance of a good outcome. Overall, most treatment trials are associated with 50% or higher success rates in the following year. Some patients will require multiple treatment attempts to achieve relevant goals.

References

Adams KM, Gilman S, Koeppe RA, et al: Neuropsychological deficits are correlated with frontal hypometabolism in positron emission tomography studies of older alcoholic patients. Alcohol Clin Exp Res 17:205–210, 1993

American Psychiatric Association: Diagnostic and Statistical Manual of Mental Disorders, 3rd Edition, Revised. Washington, DC, American Psychiatric Association, 1987

American Psychiatric Association: Diagnostic and Statistical Manual of Mental Disorders, 4th Edition, Text Revision. Washington, DC, American Psychiatric Association, 2000

Babor T, Dolinsky Z, Meyer R, et al: Types of alcoholics: concurrent and predictive validity of some common classification schemes. Br J Addict 87:1415–1431, 1992

Brown SA, D'Amico EJ: Outcomes of alcohol treatment for adolescents. Recent Dev Alcohol 15:307–327, 2001

Carroll KM, Nich C, Ball SA, et al: One-year follow-up of disulfiram and psychotherapy for cocaine-alcohol users: sustained effects of treatment. Addiction 95:1335–1349, 2000

Chung T, Colby SM, Barnett NP, et al: Screening adolescents for problem drinking: performance of brief screens against DSM-IV alcohol diagnoses. J Stud Alcohol 61:579–587, 2000

Cloninger C, Sigvardsson S, Bohman M: Type I and Type II alcoholism: an update. Alcohol Health Res World 20:18–23, 1996

Conley TB: Construct validity of the MAST and AUDIT with multiple offender drunk drivers. J Subst Abuse Treat 20:287–295, 2001

Daeppen JB, Smith TL, Schuckit MA: How would you label your own drinking pattern overall? An evaluation of answers provided by 181 high functioning middle-aged men. Alcohol Alcohol 34:767–772, 1999

Dawson DA: The link between family history and early onset alcoholism: earlier initiation of drinking or more rapid development of dependence? J Stud Alcohol 61:637–646, 2000

Dawson DA: Alcohol and mortality from external causes. J Stud Alcohol 62:790–797, 2001

Drummond SP, Gillin JC, Smith TL, et al: The sleep of abstinent pure primary alcoholic patients: natural course and relationship to relapse. Alcohol Clin Exp Res 22:1796–1802, 1998

Eng MY, Schuckit MA, Smith TL: A five-year prospective study of diagnostic orphans for alcohol use disorders. J Stud Alcohol 64:227–234, 2003

Eriksson CJ: The role of acetaldehyde in the actions of alcohol. Alcohol Clin Exp Res 25 (suppl 5):15–32, 2001

Fawcett J, Kravitz HM, McGuire M, et al: Pharmacological treatments for alcoholism: revisiting lithium and considering buspirone. Alcohol Clin Exp Res 24:666–674, 2000

Fleming MF, Mundt MP, French MT, et al: Brief physician advice for problem drinkers: long-term efficacy and benefit-cost analysis. Alcohol Clin Exp Res 26:36–43, 2002

Freedman JE, Parker C 3rd, Li L, et al: Select flavonoids and whole juice from purple grapes inhibit platelet function and enhance nitric oxide release. Circulation 103:2792–2798, 2001

Gentilello LM, Rivara FP, Donovan DM, et al: Alcohol interventions in a trauma center as a means of reducing the risk of injury recurrence. Ann Surg 230:473–483, 1999

Goodwin DW, Guze SB: Psychiatric Diagnosis, 5th Edition. New York, Oxford University Press, 1996

Harper C: The neuropathology of alcohol-specific brain damage, or does alcohol damage the brain? J Neuropathol Exp Neurol 57:101–110, 1998

Hendriks H, Veenstra J, Van Tol A, et al: Moderate doses of alcoholic beverages with dinner and postprandial high density lipoprotein composition. Alcohol Alcohol 33:403–410, 1998

Henggeler SW, Schoenwald SK, Pickrel SG: Multisystemic therapy: bridging the gap between university- and community-based treatment. J Consult Clin Psychol 63:709–717, 1995

Holguin SR, Porjesz B, Chorlian DB, et al: Visual P3a in male alcoholics and controls. Alcohol Clin Exp Res 23:582–591, 1999

Hommer D, Momenan R, Kaiser E, et al: Evidence for a gender-related effect of alcoholism on brain volumes. Am J Psychiatry 158:198–204, 2001

Johnston LD, O'Malley PM, Bachman JG: Monitoring the Future National Survey Results on Drug Use, 1975–2001, Vol 1: Secondary School Students. Rockville, MD, National Institute on Drug Abuse, 2002

Kiefer F, Jahn H, Tarnaske T, et al; Comparing and combining naltrexone and acamprosate in relapse prevention for alcoholism: a double-blind, placebo-controlled study. Arch Gen Psychiatry 60:92–99, 2003

Kranzler HR, Del Boca F, Korner P, et al: Adverse effects limit the usefulness of fluvoxamine for the treatment of alcoholism. J Subst Abuse Treat 10:283–287, 1993

Krystal JH, Cramer JA, Krol WF, et al: Naltrexone in the treatment of alcohol dependence. N Engl J Med 345:1734–1739, 2001

Li TK: Pharmacogenetics of responses to alcohol and genes that influence alcohol drinking. J Stud Alcohol 61:5–12, 2000

Marlatt GA, Gordon JR: Relapse Prevention: Maintenance Strategies in the Treatment of Addictive Behaviors. New York, Guilford, 1985

Mason BJ: Treatment of alcohol-dependent outpatients with acamprosate: a clinical review. J Clin Psychiatry 62 (suppl 20):42–48, 2001

Morgenstern J, Longabaugh R: Cognitive-behavioral treatment for alcohol dependence: a review of evidence for its hypothesized mechanisms of action. Addiction 95:1475–1490, 2000

O'Brien CP, McLellan AT: Myths about the treatment of addiction. Lancet 347:237–240, 1996

O'Farrell TJ, Choquette KA, Cutter HSG: Couples relapse prevention sessions after behavioral marital therapy for male alcoholics: outcomes during the three years after starting treatment. J Stud Alcohol 59:357–370, 1998

Parsons OA, Nixon SJ: Neurobehavioral sequelae of alcoholism. Neurol Clin 11:205–218, 1993

Pfefferbaum A, Sullivan E, Mathalon D, et al: Longitudinal changes in magnetic resonance imaging brain volumes in abstinent and relapsed alcoholics. Alcohol Clin Exp Res 19:1177–1191, 1995

Pollock N, Martin C: Diagnostic orphans: adolescents with alcohol symptoms who do not qualify for DSM-IV abuse or dependence diagnoses. Am J Psychiatry 156:897–901, 1999

Prescott C, Kendler K: Genetic and environmental contributions to alcohol abuse and dependence in a population-based sample of male twins. Am J Psychiatry 156:34–40, 1999

Preuss UW, Schuckit MA, Smith TL, et al: Comparison of 3,190 alcohol-dependent individuals with and without suicide attempts. Alcohol Clin Exp Res 26:471–477, 2002

Project MATCH Research Group: Matching alcoholism treatments to client heterogeneity: Project MATCH three-year drinking outcomes. Alcohol Clin Exp Res 22:1300–1311, 1998

Reinert DF, Allen JP: The Alcohol Use Disorders Identification Test (AUDIT): a review of recent research. Alcohol Clin Exp Res 26:272–279, 2002

Rohde P, Lewinsohn PM, Seeley JR: Psychiatric comorbidity with problematic alcohol use in high school students. J Am Acad Child Adolesc Psychiatry 35:101–109, 1996

Rounsaville B, Kranzler HR: The DSM-III-R diagnosis of alcoholism, in American Psychiatric Press Review of Psychiatry, Vol 8. Edited by Tasman A, Hales RE, Frances AJ. Washington, DC, American Psychiatric Press, 1989, pp 323–340

Schuckit MA: Drug and Alcohol Abuse: A Clinical Guide to Diagnosis and Treatment, 5th Edition. New York, Kluwer Academic/Plenum Publishers, 2000a

Schuckit MA: Vulnerability factors for alcoholism, in Neuropsychopharmacology: The Fifth Generation of Progress. Edited by Davis KL, Charney D, Coyle JT, et al. Philadelphia, PA, Lippincott Williams & Wilkins, 2000b, pp 1399–1412

Schuckit MA, Anthenelli RM, Bucholz KK, et al: The time course of development of alcohol-related problems in men and women. J Stud Alcohol 56:218–225, 1995a

Schuckit MA, Tipp JE, Reich T, et al: The histories of withdrawal convulsions and delirium tremens in 1648 alcohol dependent subjects. Addiction 90:1335–1347, 1995b

Schuckit MA, Tipp JE, Bergman M, et al: Comparison of induced and independent major depressive disorders in 2,945 alcoholics. Am J Psychiatry 154:948–957, 1997

Schuckit MA, Smith TL, Daeppen JB, et al: Clinical relevance of the distinction between alcohol dependence with and without a physiological component. Am J Psychiatry 155:733–740, 1998

Schuckit MA, Smith TL, Danko GP, et al: Five-year clinical course associated with DSM-IV alcohol abuse or dependence in a large group of men and women. Am J Psychiatry 158:1084–1090, 2001

Smith TL, Volpe FR, Hashima JN, et al: Impact of a stimulant-focused enhanced program on the outcome of alcohol- and/or stimulant-dependent men. Alcohol Clin Exp Res 23:1772–1779, 1999

Sobell LC, Ellingstad TP, Sobell MB: Natural recovery from alcohol and drug problems: methodological review of the research with suggestions for future directions. Addiction 95:749–764, 2000

Stratton K, Howe C, Battaglia F: Fetal Alcohol Syndrome: Diagnosis, Epidemiology, Prevention, and Treatment. Washington, DC, Institute of Medicine, National Academy Press, 1996

Sullivan J, Sykora K, Schneiderman J, et al: Assessment of alcohol withdrawal: the revised Clinical Institute Withdrawal Assessment for Alcohol Scale (CIWA-Ar). Br J Addict 84: 1353–1357, 1989

Tapert SF, Brown GG, Kindermann S, et al: fMRI measurement of brain dysfunction in alcohol-dependent young women. Alcohol Clin Exp Res 25:236–245, 2001

Ueno S, Harris RA, Messing RO, et al: Alcohol actions on GABA(A) receptors: from protein structure to mouse behavior. Alcohol Clin Exp Res 25 (suppl 5 ISBRA):76–81, 2001

Wall TL, Shea SH, Chan KK, et al: A genetic association with the development of alcohol and other substance use behavior in Asian Americans. J Abnorm Psychol 110:173–178, 2001

Winters KC, Henly GA: Personal Experience Inventory Test and Manual. Los Angeles, CA, Western Psychological Services, 1989

World Health Organization: International Statistical Classification of Diseases and Related Health Problems, 10th Revision. Geneva, World Health Organization, 1992

Cannabis

Mark S. Gold, M.D.
Kimberly Frost-Pineda, M.P.H.
William S. Jacobs, M.D.

Marijuana is the most frequently used illicit drug in the United States and the second most commonly smoked drug. Its use sharply increased among America's youth and young adults in the late 1960s and the 1970s, declined in the 1980s, and began increasing again in the 1990s. Among students, the increase in use appears to have leveled off in the past few years, with no significant changes in use between 2000 and 2001 and a slight decrease in 2002. However, the National Household Survey on Drug Abuse found that use of marijuana among 18- to 25-year-olds increased between 2000 and 2002. In 2001, an estimated 2.6 million Americans used marijuana for the first time (Substance Abuse and Mental Health Services Administration 2002). In 2001, an estimated 3.5 million Americans met the criteria for marijuana abuse and dependence, and approximately 974,000 persons received treatment in 2002 (Substance Abuse and Mental Health Services Administration 2002, 2003). To successfully treat these individuals, health care providers must have an understanding of why people use marijuana, the prevalence of use, the adverse consequences of marijuana use, and

how to identify, intervene, and treat marijuana abuse and dependence.

Why do people smoke marijuana? This question is complex, but it appears that no one smokes marijuana to produce a cough, bronchitis, memory problems, hoarseness, paranoia, or performance problems. The simple answer is that they smoke to obtain the euphoria that marijuana produces. However, an increasing number of people claim that they smoke marijuana for relief of a diverse range of symptoms. People generally smoke for the positive reinforcement, which makes self-administration possible and likely. Laboratory animals *will* self-administer tetrahydrocannabinol (THC), like other drugs of abuse, and receive neurochemical effects on the putative reward neuroanatomy similar to those of other drugs of abuse (Childers and Breivogel 1998; Gardner and Lowinson 1991; Tanda et al. 1997). These drugs are usually taken for the state they produce rather than the abstinence state they reverse. In this sense, the drive for marijuana intoxication is similar to that for cocaine or alcohol.

More than 50% of Americans have tried marijuana at least once (Gruber and Pope 2002). Use of marijuana is approximately equal for men and women; therefore, the historical assumption of male predominance of substance abuse does not apply to cannabis (Kendler and Prescott 1998). Women appear to develop drug dependence more rapidly than do men, and there is the additional concern for women who use drugs during pregnancy and while nursing. Both male and female use of marijuana is age related. Studies consistently report that lifetime use of marijuana increases during adolescence—from about 7% of 13-year-olds to more than 40% of 17-year-olds (Rey et al. 2002). Use increases throughout the teens, peaks in the early 20s, and declines thereafter (Bachman et al. 1997).

Forms and Types of Marijuana

Marijuana, or herbal cannabis, is the dried leaves, stalks, and flowers of *Cannabis sativa*. Cannabinoids are also found in the seeds and resin of the female plant. Marijuana is most commonly smoked via a rolled cigarette or in a pipe or bong (water pipe). Herbal cannabis contains more than 400 compounds, including in excess of 60 aryl-substituted meroterpenes unique to cannabis. Noncannabinoid constituents of the plant are similar to those found in tobacco minus the nicotine. The pharmacology of most cannabinoids is unknown, with the notable exception of delta-9-THC (Δ^9-THC), which has been isolated, synthesized, and studied (Ashton 2001). Δ^9-THC content varies depending on source and preparation of cannabis.

According to the National Institute on Drug Abuse (NIDA), most ordinary marijuana contains an average of 3% Δ^9-THC. Sinsemilla, the buds and flowering tops of female plants, has an average Δ^9-THC concentration of 7.5%, although it can be as high as 24%. Hashish, or hash, is the resin obtained from the female plant flowers and has an average of 2%–8% Δ^9-THC and can contain up to 20% Δ^9-THC. It is prepared by collecting the resin on the cannabis leaves or by boiling the plant. Hashish oil is even more potent, containing up to 30% Δ^9-THC, and involves distilling the plant in organic solvents (Gold 1989).

There is a lot of controversy over what marijuana smoke actually is and does. In comparisons between ingestion of dronabinol, the oral form of Δ^9-THC, and inhalation of cannabis, Δ^9-THC produced antinociception, catalepsy, anticonvulsive activity, hypothermia, hyperexcitability, and depression of motor activity through interaction with a specific cannabinoid receptor. However, the slower onset of dronabinol made it less reinforcing than the smoked marijuana (Beal et al. 1995; Stimmel 1995). Because many of the more than 400 compounds have not been characterized, extrapolations from Δ^9-THC to smoking are tenuous.

Cannabis potency is related to agricultural factors such as light and soil, genetic strains, and how the leaves are handled after harvesting. Cannabis growing in hotter, dryer climates produces more of the resin containing the psychoactive ingredients, whereas cannabis grown in temperate climates produces more fibrous stalk. Years of cultivation, hydroponic farming, plant breeding, and other efforts have increased the potency of cannabis. Netherweed or skinkweed may contain ≥20% Δ^9-THC (60–200 mg/joint) compared with 0.5%–3% Δ^9-THC for a typical marijuana cigarette of the 1960s (Ashton 2001).

History

Cannabis sativa is Latin for "planted hemp." Historically, cannabis use can be traced to ancient times, when it was hailed "the father of Chinese medicine" during China's Nung dynasty in 2327 B.C. It was also a staple in India in 2000 B.C. and has been throughout the Arab world since the tenth century. Cannabis may be the first non-food-bearing plant cultivated by humans (Abel 1980).

By the mid-nineteenth century, cannabis was prescribed for everything from gonorrhea to tetanus, but after it was recognized as a drug of abuse, the 1937 Marijuana Tax Act banned its use. Widespread cultivation and use preceded the discovery that Δ^9-THC, the prototypical cannabinoid, exerts many of its central effects by binding to cannabinoid-1 receptors in the peripheral and central nervous system and by binding to cannabinoid-2 receptors on immune cells (Pertwee 1998).

Epidemiology

Marijuana is the most commonly used and the most controversial illicit drug in America. Although only 2% of all Americans had ever tried an illicit drug in the early 1960s, more recent data suggest that marijuana use is an alarming fact of preteen and teenage life in America. We reported evidence of a reversal in the trend of decreasing illicit drug use each year from 1985 to 1992 (Gold et al. 1993); subsequently, marijuana smoking, cigarette smoking, and use of other illicit drugs increased in all ages of school-age children studied (Gold and Gleaton 1994).

The Monitoring the Future Study and the National Household Survey on Drug Abuse have provided estimations and trends of marijuana use, abuse, and dependence (see Figures 15–1 through 15–7).

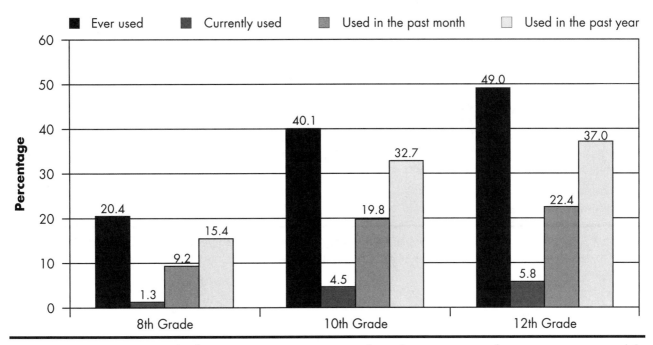

Figure 15–1. Monitoring the future: ever, current, past month, and past year use of marijuana among eighth, tenth, and twelfth graders.

Source. Data from Johnston et al. 2002.

In 1965, there were about 0.6 million new users of marijuana. The number of new users increased annually until reaching a peak in 1976 and 1977—approximately 3.2 million new users per year. Initiation rates then declined to about 1.4 million in 1990. In the early 1990s, the annual number of new marijuana users began increasing again and reached 2.5 million in 1996. In the year 2000, an estimated 2.4 million people used marijuana for the first time. Before 1970, most new users of marijuana were young adults between ages 18 and 25 years. From about 1972 to today, the number of initiates who are ages 12–17 years has been consistently greater than among young adults. The number of new marijuana users among 12- to 17-year-olds rose steadily from 0.8 million in 1990 to a level of 1.6 million annually between 1996 and 2000 (Substance Abuse and Mental Health Services Administration 2002). Average age at initiation of marijuana use in 2000 was 17.5 years.

In 2001, marijuana was used by 76% of current illicit drug users. More than half of current illicit drug users used only marijuana; another 20% used marijuana and another drug. About 12% of the past-year marijuana users smoked marijuana on 300 or more days in 2001 (Substance Abuse and Mental Health Services Administration 2002). This means that about 2.5 million persons were using marijuana on almost a daily or on a daily basis over 1 year. Of the past-month users, almost one-third (3.9 million people) used marijuana more than 20 days in the last month.

People who first use drugs at a younger age are more likely to be classified with dependence on or abuse of drugs than are adults who initiated use at a later age. The most recent National Household Survey on Drug Abuse found that of those who first tried marijuana at age 14 or younger, 11.8% were classified with dependence on or abuse of an illicit drug in the past year compared with only 2.1% of the adults who had

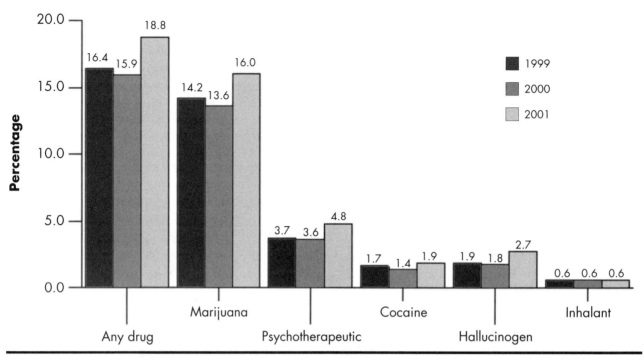

Figure 15–2.   Past month illicit drug use among young adults ages 18–25 years: 1999, 2000, and 2001.
Source.   Data from Substance Abuse and Mental Health Services Administration 2002.

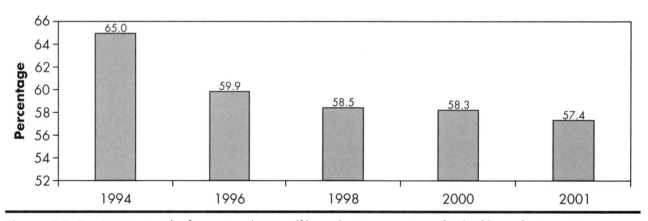

Figure 15–3.   Monitoring the future: trends in twelfth-graders' perceptions of risk of harm from marijuana use.
Source.   Data from Johnston et al. 2002.

first used marijuana at age 18 or older (Substance Abuse and Mental Health Services Administration 2002). The pattern of higher rates of dependence or abuse among persons who started using marijuana at younger ages was also found among demographic subgroups.

Of the 5.6 million Americans classified with illicit drug abuse or dependence in 2001, 3.5 million abused or were dependent on marijuana (Substance Abuse and Mental Health Services Administration 2002). This is about 1.5% of the total population and repre-

sents 62% of the persons with illicit drug abuse or dependence. Of the past-year users of marijuana, 16.5% met criteria for dependence or abuse. The National Association of State Drug and Alcohol Directors reported that 137,564 Americans received treatment for marijuana abuse in 1994 (Rueshe 1997). Among the 3.1 million persons who had received treatment for alcohol or drugs within the past year, an estimated 852,000 persons received treatment for marijuana abuse and dependence (Substance Abuse and Mental Health Services Administration 2002).

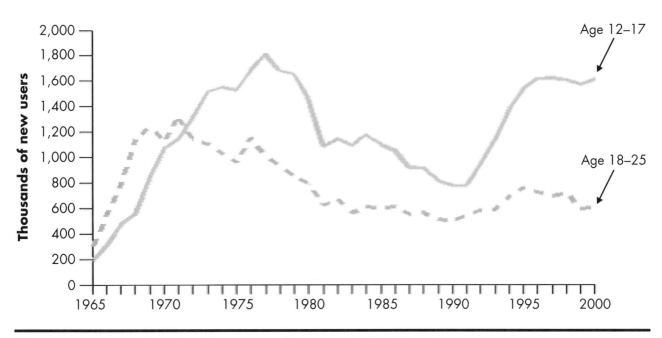

Figure 15-4. Annual number of new users of marijuana: 1965–2000.

Source. Data from Substance Abuse and Mental Health Services Administration 2002.

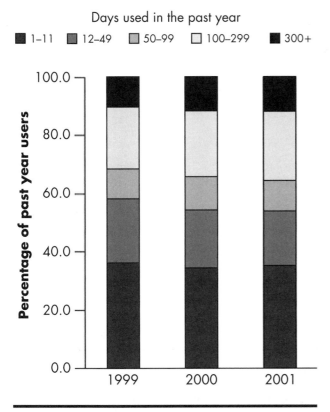

Figure 15-5. Frequency of marijuana use among past year users age 12 or older.

Source. Data from Substance Abuse and Mental Health Services Administration 2002.

Between 2000 and 2001, the percentage of the population with dependence on or abuse of marijuana increased significantly. Statistically significant increases also were noted for current use of marijuana—from 4.8% to 5.4% (Substance Abuse and Mental Health Services Administration 2002). Another measure of use is the increased number of emergency department marijuana mentions. In the 12- to 17-year-old category, Drug Abuse Warning Network (DAWN) marijuana and hashish mentions increased 622% between 1990 and 2000.

Patterns of Use and Abuse

Varying patterns of use and abuse are associated with marijuana. The continuum of use includes the experimental, occasional, daily, and chronic user. The level of abuse appears to be indigenous to the individual, but the following variables should be considered:

- Demographics: age, gender, geographic location
- Social factors: multicultural issues, socioeconomic status, parental influence, education
- Individual factors: psychological, physiological, and emotional status

The main reason that marijuana is smoked is to produce a sense of well-being, decreased anxiety, decreased alertness, and intoxication. Perceptions are

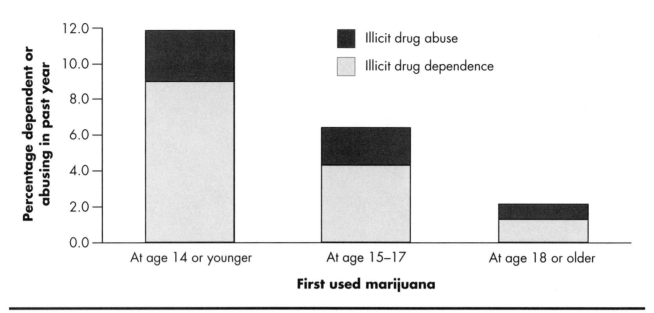

Figure 15–6. Past year marijuana dependence or abuse among adults, by age at first use: 2001.

Source. Data from Substance Abuse and Mental Health Services Administration 2002.

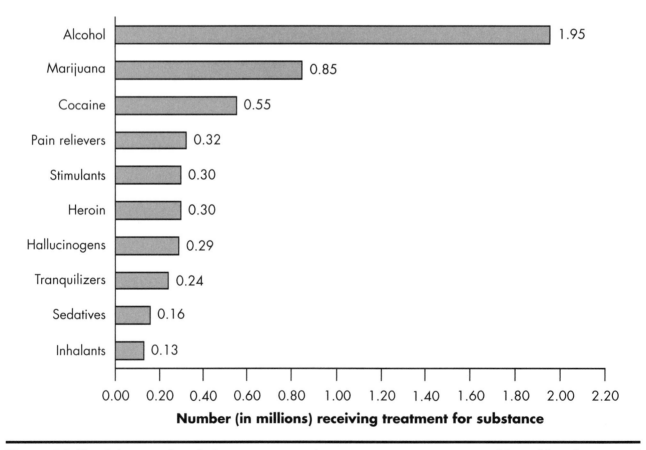

Figure 15–7. Substances for which persons received treatment among persons age 12 or older who received treatment in the past year: 2001.

Source. Data from Substance Abuse and Mental Health Services Administration 2002.

altered, with colors seeming brighter, music sounding more energetic, and emotions being more intensely felt. Perception of time and spatial awareness are distorted. The "high" is reported shortly after smoking and reaches a plateau that lasts for hours depending on dose and other factors.

Numerous variables have been studied to explain why adolescents use marijuana. Marijuana use is often related to social context and the acceptability of marijuana among peers. Exposure opportunity is an important factor in the progression from legal drugs to marijuana and then to other "harder" drugs of abuse (Wagner and Anthony 2002b). Exposure opportunity also has been described as a mechanism that links marijuana use to hallucinogen use among youths (Wilcox et al. 2002). Other researchers have suggested that sensation-seeking needs among adolescents are another risk factor (Kopstein et al. 2001). High school students who are academic achievers, are involved in athletics or school activities, are strongly religious, work few hours outside of school, and spend few evenings out during the week are less likely to use marijuana. Even when risk and protective factors are considered, alcohol and cigarette use are associated with marijuana use, and marijuana use is associated with other illicit drug use (Merrill et al. 1999).

Recent data suggest that unhealthy behaviors such as fasting and other weight-control measures are also associated with teenage marijuana and alcohol use (Neumark-Sztainer et al. 1998). Many weight-conscious young women would rather smoke marijuana than drink alcohol because of the caloric properties inherent in alcohol. Genetic and environmental factors also influence substance use (Kendler et al. 2000). In a recent study of twins, researchers found that marijuana use among females was more influenced by common environmental factors than for males (Miles et al. 2002). They also found a significant genetic correlation between conduct disorder and marijuana use, suggesting similar genetic factors for both (Miles et al. 2002). Another possible reason for teenage use may be related to Δ^9-THC's role in modifying brain function and hormones.

Some experts blame the proponents of legalization for the resurgence in marijuana use (Dupont and Voth 1995). The debate regarding medicinal use of marijuana also may play a role in increased use and decreased perception of harm. However, just as a physician would not tell a patient with ulcerative colitis to smoke tobacco cigarettes, even though nicotine has a beneficial effect on the natural history of the disease,

smoking marijuana leaves is unlikely to emerge as a "medical treatment." The outcome of controlled cannabinoid research will likely be a series of important new compounds that use cannabinoid systems to exert their effects but that are administered orally, inhaled in their pure form, or administered rectally and produce little or no euphoria. As with other potent chemicals, the U.S. Food and Drug Administration (FDA) will weigh the risks and benefits of these new compounds before approving them for medical use.

High school seniors who perceive marijuana use as dangerous and who disapprove of use among their friends are less likely to use marijuana. Marijuana has had the sharpest national decline in perceived drug danger in the last decade. In 1991, 79% of twelfth graders thought that regular marijuana users were at great risk for harming themselves. But by 2000, fewer than 60% held that opinion (Johnston et al. 2002). Peer disapproval rates also declined. For users, there appears to be a separation between acknowledging the harmfulness of marijuana and using it. Attitudes toward marijuana use affect initiation but not cessation. Simply changing users' attitudes on perceived harmfulness of a drug may not be sufficient to enable cessation of substance use. Investigators attribute increases to a decrease in cost, low rate of peer disapproval, decrease in perceived danger, and the connection with the resurgence of cigarette smoking. Changes in the Δ^9-THC content of marijuana also may play a role in the increase in teen smoking. In controlled studies, the higher the Δ^9-THC content of marijuana, the more users prefer and self-administer it (Kelly et al. 1994).

Parental influence is another factor in teen drug use. In a study published in 1996, the Center for Addiction and Substance Abuse at Columbia University found that 65% of baby boomer parents who had used marijuana regularly expected their own children to use, compared with only 29% of baby boomer parents who had never used (Luntz Research Companies 1996). Consequently, parental attitudes and expectations regarding the risks of drug use are contributing and validating factors in the growing acceptance of marijuana use among teens.

Substance use is often associated with psychological disorders. Rates of substance abuse are higher among survivors of trauma and disaster, especially those who have posttraumatic stress disorder (PTSD). One recent study reported a substantial increase in marijuana, alcohol, and tobacco use among Manhattan residents after the terrorist attacks of September

11, 2001 (Vlahov et al. 2002). In this study, persons who reported an increase in marijuana use were more likely to have PTSD and depression, and having PTSD was associated with an increased risk of marijuana use (Vlahov et al. 2002).

Learning How to Smoke and the Tobacco/Marijuana Connection

In order to smoke marijuana, one must learn to take smoke into the lungs; this is not a normal behavior for any species. To inhale and hold toxic smoke in the lungs long enough for the psychoactive constituents to be absorbed requires the user to resist the primal, biological urge to cough. Once the brain and lungs are trained, often via cigarettes, it becomes much more natural to smoke marijuana, crack, or heroin. In our recent survey of university students, virtually no one had smoked crack, heroin, or methamphetamine without smoking cigarettes or marijuana as a precursor (Tullis et al. 2003). Cigarette and marijuana smoking are strongly correlated, with cigarette smoking historically preceding onset of marijuana use.

Concurrent use with tobacco or alternating use appears to make marijuana more inviting. Cigarettes may boost and sustain the marijuana high and may also reverse some of the more negative effects of marijuana, such as decreased arousal and attention. Cigarette smoking has typically preceded marijuana smoking behavior. However, recent data from the University of Florida (Gold et al., in press) are suggesting not only a reversal in this trend but also the concurrent initiation of tobacco and marijuana smoking 2–3 years later than for those smoking only tobacco. It appears that teenagers are smoking marijuana, then rapidly initiating tobacco smoking because of the discovery that nicotine not only sustains but also enhances the marijuana high.

Factors Associated With Cessation

Much more is known about the factors associated with adolescents' initiation into drug use than about the factors associated with cessation. Aging is a potent predictor of cessation. Maturity is associated with different interests, needs, and attitudes, including decreased risk taking and increased conformity. Teen characteristics for use, such as risk taking, delinquent activities, low religiosity, depression, and low self-esteem, are less likely to appear in adults. There appears to be a relative incompatibility between using illicit drugs and par-

ticipating in conventional roles of adulthood (Chen and Kandel 1998). Chen and Kandel's study suggested that controlling for all other factors, the two most important predictors of stopping marijuana use were frequency of use and age. Infrequent users and those in their late 20s were most likely to stop using. Frequent users were more persistent in their use, and many became dependent. Using for social reasons accelerated cessation, whereas using to enhance positive feelings and reduce negative feelings was associated with persistence of use. Many of these smokers "grow out" of their marijuana use as a result of maturity, family, education, and employment. Social role participation is related to discontinuation; for example, when illicit drug users assume an expected social role, such as getting married or becoming pregnant, they are more likely to stop using a drug.

Clinical Psychopharmacology

Administration

Marijuana can be ingested orally, but the most common mode of administration is by smoking and inhalation. Smoking is a method of cannabinoid and smoke delivery that appears to be quite reinforcing in teenagers and young adults. The principal psychoactive constituents, Δ^8-THC and Δ^9-THC, were isolated in the 1960s (Gaoni and Mechoulam 1964). Marijuana smoke contains more than 400 compounds in addition to the major psychoactive component, Δ^9-THC. Many of the cannabinoids and other complex organic compounds appear to have psychoactive properties, and most have not been tested for long- or short-term safety in animals or humans. Δ^9-THC is more prevalent in marijuana and more potent than Δ^8-THC; therefore, most of the psychoactivity is attributed to Δ^9-THC. The lack of precise correlation between peak high and Δ^9-THC has suggested the importance of THC metabolism in the high. Smoking delivers THC to the brain in seconds, thereby being one of the quickest routes of administration. Intensity of central brain rewarding effects is usually correlated with the rapidity of hitting the brain. Marijuana is rapidly absorbed from the lungs, and THC and major metabolites can be traced throughout the body and brain. Up to 59% of smoked THC is absorbed, compared with only 3% when taken orally. Reports are now surfacing that marijuana users are dipping their joints and cigars ("blunts") into embalming fluid, a compound composed of formaldehyde, methanol, ethanol, and other solvents; the street name for this technique is "fry." Users believe these cigarettes burn more slowly, thereby slowing the rate of absorption. The treated cigarettes are sometimes laced with phencyclidine (PCP), and use of this combination appears to be an adolescent trend (Khun et al. 1997). (For more detailed discussion of marijuana neurobiology, see Chapter 5, "Neurobiology of Marijuana," in this volume.)

Intoxication

According to DSM-IV-TR (American Psychiatric Association 2000), acute marijuana intoxication begins with a "high" feeling followed by symptoms described in Table 15-1. In addition to euphoria, users report an increase in hunger and a state of relaxation. Individual differences in intoxication are explained on the basis of THC concentration, frequency of use, smoking abilities of the user, and genetic and psychiatric risks. Intoxication develops within minutes if smoked but usually takes at least 30 minutes if ingested orally. The effects generally last for 3–4 hours. The degree of the physiological and behavioral changes depends on the method of administration, the dose, and the individual's rate of absorption, tolerance, and sensitivity to the effects of marijuana (American Psychiatric Association 2000).

Table 15–1. DSM-IV-TR diagnostic criteria for cannabis intoxication

---

A. Recent use of cannabis.
B. Clinically significant maladaptive behavioral or psychological changes (e.g., impaired motor coordination, euphoria, anxiety, sensation of slowed time, impaired judgment, social withdrawal) that developed during, or shortly after, cannabis use.
C. Two (or more) of the following signs, developing within 2 hours of cannabis use:
   (1) conjunctival injection
   (2) increased appetite
   (3) dry mouth
   (4) tachycardia
D. The symptoms are not due to a general medical condition and are not better accounted for by another mental disorder.

Specify if:

With Perceptual Disturbances

Motor performance, concentration, alertness, and ability to drive a car or fly an airplane may be affected for hours to days. Some studies have suggested that drivers and pilots who smoke marijuana are more likely to believe that they can drive or fly than those who drink alcohol, making them more dangerous (Leirer et al. 1991). Because most cannabinoids, including Δ^9-THC, are fat soluble, the effects of cannabis or hashish may occasionally persist or recur for 12–24 hours because of a slow release of psychoactive substances from fatty tissue or to enterohepatic circulation (Naditch 1974). Visual distortions of object size and distance (Isbell et al. 1967), decrease in color discrimination, and decrease in ocular motor tracking (Adams et al. 1975) have been reported. Decreased recognition and analysis of peripheral visual field light stimuli have also been reported (Moskowitz et al. 1972). In addition, in tests of flying, using the simulated flying paradigm, the marijuana-related loss of motor and complex analysis skills and judgment decreases the pilots' ability to land safely (Janowsky et al. 1976).

Concurrent use of tobacco cigarettes or of crack appears to extend the normal course of marijuana-induced effects. Marijuana-induced vasodilation of the nasal mucosa attenuates the vasoconstrictive effects of cocaine and thus increases absorption (Lukas et al. 1994). Marijuana also impairs the emesis normally produced by acute alcohol poisoning and can be associated with youth alcohol toxicity. However, acute marijuana intoxication alone rarely results in a medical emergency. Occasionally, acute intoxication can cause psychological distress to the point that the user complains and seeks help for the unpleasant and negative affect, fearfulness, anxiety, or depression.

Adverse Psychiatric Reactions

Marijuana smoking experience, mood, dose, and route of administration determine whether the smoker becomes euphoric or dysphoric. Naive users, especially older individuals, and those exposed to high-potency marijuana tend to be the most common groups seeking treatment. Dysphoria occurs more commonly when marijuana is eaten, probably because of the facility of dose titration when marijuana is smoked rather than swallowed. Cannabis that is taken in high doses or is extremely potent has psychoactive effects that can cause emergency presentations that are difficult to differentiate from those of hallucinogens such as lysergic acid diethylamide (LSD). Paranoid ideation and persistent paranoia ranging from suspiciousness to frank delusions also may be associated with use.

Panic, anxiety, nausea, dizziness, and a general difficulty in expressing even simple thoughts in words may be associated with marijuana use. Marijuana usually does not cause psychiatric disorders, but in an individual who is predisposed to a psychiatric illness, marijuana use may trigger episodes of panic attacks, paranoia, anxiety, and even psychoses (Novak 1980). These episodes are not necessarily indicative of a psychiatric diagnosis because the symptoms typically subside after the user "comes down" from the high. However, patients with schizophrenia have relapsed to psychotic behavior after smoking marijuana. In their most extreme forms, psychiatric manifestations of marijuana intoxication may result in emergency department or student health service presentations.

Although psychiatrists, student health counselors, and college counselors suggest that cannabis use can impair motivation and learning, a clear cannabis-induced amotivational syndrome remains to be proven. Whether amotivation follows or precedes marijuana smoking is unclear. It is difficult to know a person's potential, which makes it almost impossible to determine whether, for example, a physics teacher who smokes marijuana should have been a Massachusetts Institute of Technology physicist. Still, no one has found it particularly comforting that regular marijuana smoking is compatible with a career in the sugar cane industry. Other hypotheses suggest that amotivation may be linked to coexisting psychiatric or medical conditions.

Until recently, the link between cannabis and prolonged or serious mood disorders such as depressive, dysthymic, or bipolar disorder was supported by anecdotal clinical evidence only (Swendsen and Merikangas 2000). The increased rate of cannabis use among those who attempted suicide inferred by a recent study (Beautrais et al. 1999) and the possible links between mood disorders and cannabis use suggested in other studies deserve closer attention. In a study of 302 individuals who had made serious suicide attempts, 16.2% met the criteria for cannabis dependence or abuse at the time of the attempt, compared with 1.9% of 1,028 randomly selected control subjects (Beautrais et al. 1999). Cross-sectional studies of adolescents show that depression is related to a variety of substance use behaviors, such as cigarette smoking, alcohol consumption, and illicit substance use. A recent cross-sectional

study of adolescents found that cannabis use was associated with a pattern of comorbid problems such as excessive drinking and use of other drugs, conduct problems, and depression (Rey et al. 2002). Mood problems at a young age elevate the risk for later cannabis use (McGee et al. 2000). Longitudinal studies have found that a depressed mood precedes the first use of marijuana and other illicit drugs by secondary school students (Kelder et al. 2001). A recent study suggested that marijuana use may increase the risk of psychosis (van Os et al. 2002). The researchers found that baseline marijuana use predicted the presence of any psychosis at follow-up and that more than 50% of the diagnosed psychotic disorders could be attributed to marijuana use (van Os et al. 2002).

Effects of cannabis and Δ^9-THC in humans include disruption of short-term memory, cognitive impairment, a sense of time distortion, and enhanced body awareness. Marijuana smoking causes short-term memory loss and difficulties in remembering, concentrating, and completing tasks. The effects of marijuana on cognition and psychomotor performance can be seen after a very small dose but are dose related. Many recent studies have found specific impairment of attention, memory, and executive functions in unintoxicated cannabis smokers (Rogers and Robbins 2001). In a study of marijuana-dependent patients, duration of cannabis use was correlated with memory and attention deficits during abstinence (Solowij et al. 2002). Laboratory studies have shown that cannabinoids can prevent the formation of new synapses, which may contribute to memory impairment (Kim and Thayer 2001).

Sometimes marijuana's effects may be at odds with the individual's personality and goals, leading to extremely negative reactions. For students focused on grades and time, the loss of time or time perception distortion may provoke negative affect and other reactions not generally seen in others. These idiosyncratic reactions may be caused by the particular type of marijuana smoked, the setting, or the individual's biological blueprint. In other cases, performing laboratory analysis of the substance (e.g., looking for PCP), interviewing those who smoked with the patient, and assessing for family history of substance abuse or other psychiatric disorders will help the psychiatrist to determine the causative factors. In these instances, there is almost always a "teachable moment," and even the addicted person can be receptive to medical counseling.

Cannabis and Neuroimaging

The effects of cannabis have been studied with neuroimaging techniques. Researchers from Duke University used both positron emission tomography (PET) and magnetic resonance imaging to assess the effects of Δ^9-THC infusion on brain blood flow and its behavioral correlates. Consistent with previous reports, they found a significant increase in cortical and cerebellar blood flow following THC administration, but not in all subjects. Subjects who had a decrease in cerebellar cerebral blood flow (CBF) had a significant alteration in time sense. The cerebellum has been linked to an internal timing system, which is why the relation between decreased cerebellar flow and impaired time sense is of interest (Mathew et al. 1998). Researchers examined brain morphology, including global CBF and body size, and age at first use of marijuana. Three primary findings were related to age at first use:

1. Those who started using marijuana before age 17, compared with those who initiated use later, had a smaller whole brain, a smaller percentage of cortical gray matter, and a larger percentage of white matter volume.
2. In terms of brain function, males who started using marijuana before age 17 had significantly higher CBF than did other males.
3. Males and females who started younger were physically smaller in terms of weight and height, especially in males (Wilson et al. 2000).

Two reports from the University of Iowa examined smoking marijuana and cognition via PET assessment of regional CBF (rCBF). In the first study, blood flow increased in the anterior cingulate, the cerebellum, and several paralimbic brain regions after smoking marijuana. Reductions in rCBF were observed in temporal lobe regions, which may affect auditory attention. Increased rCBF may be related to the intoxicating and mood effects of smoking marijuana, whereas reduction of rCBF in the temporal lobe may explain the impaired cognitive functions that come with acute intoxication (O'Leary et al. 2000). In the second study, smoking marijuana resulted in subjective measures of intoxication but did not significantly alter mean performance on an attention task. Both heart rate and blood pressure increased dramatically following marijuana use but did not for placebo. Mean global CBF, however, did not change significantly. The increases in rCBF in anterior brain regions were mostly in paralimbic regions. As in the previous study, reduced rCBF was observed in temporal lobe auditory regions but was also noted in the visual cortex and in regions that are thought to be part of an attentional network (parietal lobe, frontal lobe, and thalamus) (O'Leary et al. 2002). Researchers found no significant rCBF change in the reward-related brain regions, such as the nucleus accumbens, or in areas with a high density of cannabinoid receptors, such as the basal ganglia and hippocampus (O'Leary et al. 2002).

Voruganti et al. (2001) reported a case of a patient with schizophrenia who surreptitiously smoked cannabis during a single-photon emission computed tomography (SPECT) study of dopaminergic function in the brain. In this subject, a 20% decrease in striatal dopamine D_2 receptor binding occurred almost immediately, indicating increased synaptic dopamine activity (Voruganti et al. 2001).

Clinical Syndrome

Dependence

Marijuana, like other drugs of abuse, may affect the brain reward system to produce addiction in three ways: 1) through positive reinforcement, 2) by sensitization of incentive salience, and 3) by induction of new brain processes (Kelley and Berridge 2002). Almost 10% of those who ever use marijuana will eventually meet DSM-IV-TR criteria for dependence (Warner et al. 1995). An estimated 20% of the individuals who smoke several times will meet these criteria (Hall 1994). The development of dependence on marijuana is more insidious than cocaine dependence, and most users who are dependent on marijuana are between ages 15 and 25 (Wagner and Anthony 2002a). An increasing number of people in the United States are presenting for treatment of their marijuana use, complaining of loss of control of use, preoccupation, inability to stop despite adverse consequences, narrowing of interests, and an uneasy feeling that they may be addicted. Marijuana acquisition and use become primary, and school, work, other responsibilities and recreational activities become secondary. Clinicians are evaluating and treating more marijuana-dependent patients than ever before.

Chronic use sometimes results in a diminished or complete loss of the pleasurable effects of marijuana, which establishes a pattern of tolerance to the drug. Marijuana-dependent patients report that they repeatedly fail at attempts to cut down, ration, or limit their use and that they are easily angered by questions relating to their marijuana use. They often smoke their first marijuana cigarette on awakening and report feelings of guilt about their use and the consequences. Many of these patients have had losses of career, family, and friends. Some addicted persons report that they grow their own marijuana and smoke throughout the day, maintaining a personal relationship with their plants and paraphernalia. Addiction does not end when the drug is removed from the body (detoxification) or when the acute post-drug-taking illness dissipates (withdrawal). Rather, the disorder can persist and produce a tendency to relapse.

Tolerance

Chronic exposure to cannabinoids must be carefully studied for addiction and withdrawal syndrome in humans. Decreased cerebellar metabolic rates in habitual marijuana users may reflect neuroadaptive changes and also marijuana's effects on motor coordination, learning, and proprioception (Gatley and Volkow 1998). Chronic administration of cannabinoids to animals results in tolerance to many acute effects, including locomotor changes (Abood et al. 1993; Oveido et al. 1993). Tolerance to Δ^9-THC develops quickly and continues long-term after cessation of treatment (Fride 1995). Tolerance develops to anandamide (arachidonylethanolamide; ANA), a naturally occurring compound in the brain that binds with cannabinoid receptors, and cross-tolerance develops between THC and ANA. Tolerance in humans also has been reported (Hollister 1986) and usually appears with dosages of at least 3 mg/kg/day. Withdrawal can be readily produced after chronic cannabis administration (Aceto et al. 1995; Rodriquez de Fonseca et al. 1997; Tsou et al. 1995). Dependence and tolerance develop simultaneously and for some drugs are related to the severity of withdrawal symptomatology.

Withdrawal

Studies suggest that marijuana influences the brain's stress and reward systems in the same way as opiates, nicotine, and cocaine (Wickelgren 1997). The neural substrates responsible for the reinforcement of drug seeking, as well as the emotional stress of withdrawal noted in individuals addicted to cocaine and heroin, are identical. Withdrawal from cocaine, alcohol, and opiates increases intracellular corticotropin-releasing factor (CRF), producing concomitant anxiety and stress. Researchers at the Scripps Institute hastened THC withdrawal in rats with a cannabinoid antagonist, which produced increases in CRF, anxiety, and stress. These results provide a neurochemical model for marijuana withdrawal that is consistent with the current understanding of drug withdrawal and the emotional symptoms commonly observed in marijuana users who abruptly discontinue use.

The slow release of THC and active metabolites from lipid stores and other areas may explain the so-called carryover effects on driving and other reports of behavioral changes over time. THC and possibly other psychoactive ingredients accumulate in the brain and other fat-rich areas and form what has been described by N. Volkow (personal communication, June 1998) as a depot. This may explain the slow excretion and minimal acute withdrawal signs on abrupt discontinuation and also the effects on T cells and other immunological cells. Although acute withdrawal complaints are rarely reported, thoughts and dreams about marijuana smoking, mental cloudiness, irritability, and other behavioral signs are commonly reported for months after discontinuation of chronic marijuana smoking. It is logical to assume that brain cannabinoids decrease after prolonged marijuana smoking, as has been suggested in some studies (Romero et al. 1997). Dependence is easily ascertained, although cannabinoids are not avidly self-administered (Dewey 1986). Like nicotine and cocaine, cannabinoids increase dopamine levels in the mesolimbic system (Tanda et al. 1997).

Several recent studies have reported symptoms of cannabis withdrawal. In one study, most patients had 6 or more moderate to severe items on the 22-item Marijuana Withdrawal Symptom checklist, suggesting a "cluster of withdrawal symptoms" (Budney et al. 1999). In a another study that used the same checklist, consistent withdrawal symptoms included marijuana craving, sleep difficulty, decreased appetite, and weight loss; similarities to nicotine withdrawal were also noted (Budney et al. 2001). Abstinence after long-term marijuana use resulted in symptoms of irritability, anxiety, depressed mood, physical tension, and decreased appetite, which were most severe in the first 10 days but lasted for at least 28 days in one study (Kouri and Pope

2000). The results of these and other studies of cannabis withdrawal suggest that introduction of a cannabis withdrawal syndrome as a diagnostic classification may be warranted (Smith 2002).

Precipitated withdrawal with a selective antagonist in rats chronically treated with Δ^9-THC was unequivocally shown for the first time in a 1995 report (Aceto et al. 1995). A recent study also reported precipitated withdrawal with a selective cannabinoid CB_1 receptor antagonist in rats (Beardsley and Martin 2000). In another study of rats, lithium was reported to act against the cannabinoid withdrawal syndrome through oxytocinergic neuronal activation (Cui et al. 2001).

Overdose

Marijuana overdose is rare, and no deaths have been reported. The paucity of receptors in the brain stem could explain why large doses of marijuana do not lethally suppress cardiovascular and respiratory function (Herenham et al. 1990). However, the inhibition of the vomiting reflex may be associated with toxic and potentially lethal consequences caused by the combination of alcohol and marijuana. Marijuana is generally used with other drugs and alcohol and can alter the typical presentation of drug withdrawal and intoxication. Adolescents and young adults may not report drug-related problems and emergencies because they fear legal consequences, academic expulsion, and getting into trouble with parents. Often a wide range of substances is used to obtain a high, and users may be unable to describe exactly what they have ingested. Eventually, the availability of novel THC antagonists will allow us not only to treat overdoses but also to identify and treat those patients who are physiologically dependent on marijuana.

Medical Implications

Respiratory

The effects of marijuana smoking on human health have been studied since the 1970s and are similar to the effects of tobacco smoking. Marijuana smoking can also cause decreased exercise tolerance, chronic cough, bronchitis, and decreased pulmonary function (Tashkin et al. 1976; Tilles et al. 1986). Cannabis smoke is highly irritating to the nasopharynx and bronchial lining and thus increases the risk for chronic cough and other signs and symptoms of nasopharyngeal pathology. Sinusitis, pharyngitis, bronchitis, emphysema, and pulmonary dysplasia may occur with chronic, heavy use.

Much of the risk of smoked marijuana comes from the products of combustion; however, some risk may be directly attributed to the process of smoking marijuana (i.e., deep inhalation and long breath holding). Several cases of pneumothorax have been reported among marijuana smokers and attributed to this form of inhalation (Feldman et al. 1993). The risks related to products of combustion of marijuana are also comparable to those of tobacco smoke. Smoked tobacco delivers more than 3,000 chemicals, including cyanide and other toxins, directly to the lungs via carbon monoxide gas. Regular cigarettes contain 15 mg of tar each, whereas low-tar cigarettes contain 7 mg. Marijuana smoke contains 3.8 times more tar than tobacco smoke and 50% more carcinogenic hydrocarbons (Wu et al. 1988). Smoking marijuana produces a fivefold greater increase in blood carboxyhemoglobin levels compared with smoking tobacco (Tashkin et al. 1988a).

Although THC is thought to have bronchodilatory properties, work by Tashkin and colleagues (Tashkin 1977; Tashkin et al. 1988b) identified large airway bronchoconstriction following marijuana smoking similar to the effects seen in reactive airway disease. Long-term effects include lung immune system dysfunction, as evidenced by studies on pulmonary macrophages (Baldwin et al. 1997).

Immunology

Animal studies have clearly established that marijuana and synthetic and endogenous cannabinoids change the natural function of immune cells (Klein et al. 1998). Cannabinoids are immunomodulators altering immune system homeostasis. Cannabinoid receptors are found on white blood cells, but whether marijuana increases a nonimmunosuppressed or an immunosuppressed person's risk of acquiring an infection has yet to be proven. Even at low doses, marijuana suppresses natural killer cell activity and may also suppress cytotoxic T lymphocytes and macrophages. Although human studies are contradictory, several showed that marijuana use impairs the immune system; animal studies provide firmer evidence of immune system impairment. Both marijuana and THC contribute to acute phase response. THC decreases signals to helper T cells and interferes with macrophage antigen processing. Long-term impairment of the immune system may increase the risk of cancer.

Cancer

No discussion of the risks associated with marijuana smoking is complete without mention of its carcinogenic potential. Epidemiological evidence strongly implicates cigarette smoking as a causative factor in pulmonary malignancy. Barsky et al. (1998) reported that marijuana appears to cause molecular damage to the lungs similar to that of cigarettes. Smoking both marijuana and tobacco puts the smoker at greater risk for cancer than either alone. Marijuana smoke contains even larger amounts of known carcinogens than does tobacco smoke, and heavy use may increase the risk of developing malignant disease. Risk of cancer of the respiratory system from lips and mouth to pharynx, larynx, trachea, bronchi, and lung is significantly increased in smokers. Evidence correlates marijuana smoking with earlier onset of and greater dysplastic changes in several types of head and neck malignancies (Barsky et al. 1998; Denissenko et al. 1996; Fligiel et al. 1997; Matthias et al. 1997).

Cardiovascular

There is a causal relation between cardiac and pulmonary vascular diseases and smoking marijuana and tobacco (Wu et al. 1988). In fact, right heart disease and pulmonary hypertension may be more common and/or severe in marijuana smokers than in nonsmokers. Marijuana smoking almost immediately produces a significant increase in heart rate (Stillman et al. 1976), with inversion or flattening of the T wave on electrocardiogram, elevation of the ST segment, and increase in the amplitude of the P wave with occasional premature ventricular contractions. These cardiovascular effects can aggravate existing cardiac conditions or hypertension. The tachycardia associated with marijuana use appears to result from parasympathetic and sympathetic stimulation of the cardiac pacemaker; however, it is not clear whether β-adrenergic stimulation is involved (Beaconsfield et al. 1972). Fortunately, these changes in cardiac function can usually be reversed by abstinence.

A recent study reported that chronic marijuana use may increase the risk of stroke (Herning et al. 2001). Marijuana abusers had significantly increased cerebrovascular resistance and systolic velocity when compared with control subjects. The researchers suggested

that 18- to 30-year-old marijuana abusers had cerebral perfusion comparable to that of 60-year-olds who did not abuse marijuana (Herning et al. 2001).

Sexual Dysfunction and Related Issues

Initiation of marijuana smoking is occurring among younger populations. Naturally, the toxic effects of marijuana are greater on developing than on developed organisms. THC also modifies sexual hormone function and rhythm at a crucial developmental stage. THC has mainly inhibitory effects on pituitary luteinizing hormone (LH), prolactin, and growth hormone (GH) and has little or no effect on follicle-stimulating hormone (FSH) secretion. Marijuana is reported to decrease plasma testosterone, sperm count, and sperm motility (Kolodny et al. 1974). Most recently, males who smoke marijuana were found to have changes in ejaculate semen characteristics that could explain the association between infertility and marijuana smoking (Hembree et al. 2001).

Marijuana use can disrupt the female reproductive system; women who use marijuana four or more times a week have shorter menstrual cycles, elevated prolactin levels, and depressed testosterone levels, with galactorrhea occurring in as many as 20% of these patients (Cohen 1985). Animal studies also show a suppression of ovarian function, interference with gonadotropin and estrogenic activity, and amenorrhea associated with marijuana use.

Women who smoke marijuana during pregnancy often have infants with low birth weights, and those with the highest consumption of marijuana have the lowest-birth-weight infants. One study found numerous abnormal responses, including increased startle reflex, tremors, poor self-quieting, and failure to habituate to light, in newborns whose mothers used marijuana during pregnancy (Jones and Chernoff 1984). In addition, THC has been shown to cross the placental barrier, and it accumulates in mothers' milk (Fehr and Kalant 1983).

Effects on College Students and Adolescents

Neuropsychological

In college students who heavily smoke marijuana, long-lasting and demonstrable neuropsychological deficits, including problems in executive functioning, attention, new-word learning, and verbal fluency that persisted beyond intoxication, have been reported (Pope and Yurgelun-Todd 1996). Students who are or were regular smokers frequently under the influence of marijuana have poor academic performance (Jeynes 2002). In our recent survey (Gold et al. 1999), marijuana users had significantly lower grade point averages than nonusers. In addition to these studies, Lundavist (1995) studied approximately 400 cannabis users (use from 6 months to 25 years) over a 10-year period. Lundavist described a cannabis-state-dependent set of cognitive processes. Participants who used marijuana had weak analytic and synthetic skills, difficulty sorting and classifying information correctly, poor concentration, and weak psychospatial skills such as differentiating time and space. These changes were observed in individuals who used cannabis regularly or more than once every 6 weeks (the approximate elimination time of THC) for more than 2 years. These data suggest that cannabis-induced cognitive processes result from temporary prefrontal dysfunction because the symptom pattern is similar to that of prefrontal syndrome. This hypothesis is further supported by the greater density of cannabinoid receptors in the forebrain than in the hindbrain. The effects of marijuana on memory, cognition, coordination, and judgment remain long after the subjective feelings of the high have subsided.

Behavioral

Multiple brain systems are affected by marijuana use. CBF and cerebral metabolism are tightly coupled to brain function and used as indices of brain activity. In a recent study (Mathew et al. 1998), CBF response to THC showed a marked increase in bilateral frontal regions, insula, and cingulate gyrus of the right hemisphere, peaking 30–60 minutes after intravenous infusion. Marijuana users also had decreased cerebral metabolism at baseline. Marijuana intoxication impairs time perception. A PET study showed an increase in cortical blood flow and CBF following THC administration. CBF was decreased in those patients with a significantly altered time sense (Mathew et al. 1998). Additional studies may ultimately suggest that the most profound effects are on brain structures where survival drives and emotions are centered and in the prefrontal regions, which sustain attention, shift focus, and promote adaptation to environmental change and

new learning. The effects are often illusive and disguised by other addictive behaviors. For example, we noted that individuals who regularly use marijuana are vastly underemployed, working in positions that require less cognitive challenge or technological acuity. In one study, heavy users were significantly more impaired than light users when attempting attentional and executive functions. These cognitive differences remained after the researchers controlled for levels of premorbid functioning and other substance use (Pope and Yurgelun-Todd 1996). This ultimately results in a general lowering of life's goals and a decreased ability to attain or even establish goals, called the *chronic cannabis syndrome* and also known as *amotivational syndrome*.

For the millions of teenagers who use marijuana, the cumulative effects on their developing intellect and character will leave many woefully unprepared for the challenges of adulthood. Consider the educational and employment potential for a young person who has a compromised memory, limited ability to handle multiple stimuli, and lapses in motivation. The loss of human potential and the subsequent cost to society will continue to be substantial.

Treatment

Marijuana Treatment Research

Although little research has been done in the area of marijuana dependence treatment, contrary to popular belief, marijuana dependence does not always present in the context of polydrug abuse. Treatment for other drugs of abuse does not always recognize or effectively treat marijuana abuse (Budney et al. 1997). Relapse prevention appears to play a key role in the success rate of treatment. The ritualistic and behavioral components inherent in marijuana users, like tobacco smokers, raise unique concerns for the treatment provider. Issues related to environmental cues, the frequency with which the drug is dosed, and the culture surrounding marijuana use should be incorporated into any treatment protocol.

Self-efficacy, a judgment about one's ability to perform a specific behavior in a specific context, is also a consideration according to Stephens et al. (1995). Marijuana users seeking treatment appear to be motivated, and self-empowerment encourages the belief that they can live successfully without smoking marijuana. Marlatt and Gordon (1985) suggested that the availability of an alternative coping response in a high-risk situation would increase self-efficacy even more.

Presentation for Treatment

Treatment for marijuana abuse and dependence is often sought after decompensation of academic, social, and physical performance or after interaction with the legal system. Problems are usually first recognized by teachers, significant others, and friends. People often fail to make the association between their marijuana use and their social, academic, and health problems. A visit to a health care provider may be the result of poor classroom attendance and grades, confrontations with the university judicial system, or concomitant psychiatric disorders.

Drug testing may be a major reason that marijuana-smoking students seek treatment. Positive test results lead to a referral, but students also want and ask for help in quitting before an interview or a test with a major national employer. Testing fears appear to be a new major concern, and according to our recent survey (Gold et al. 1999), many students seeking internships, employment, or admittance to higher education face the prospect of failing the drug test.

Diagnosis of Marijuana Dependence

Diagnosis of marijuana dependence is not specifically addressed in DSM-IV-TR. Diagnosis of cannabis intoxication (see Table 15–1) does not immediately suggest dependence in the same way that acute alcohol intoxication does not prove dependence. However, marijuana dependence is more likely to be identified in smokers and those with recent marijuana use. DSM-IV-TR does provide general criteria for diagnosing substance dependence. The criteria in Table 15–2 have been modified for marijuana.

Table 15–2. Diagnostic criteria for marijuana dependence (adapted from DSM-IV-TR criteria for substance dependence)

A maladaptive pattern of marijuana use leading to clinically significant impairment or distress, as manifested by three (or more) of the following, occurring at any time in the same 12-month period:

- Marijuana is often taken in larger amounts or over a longer period than intended
- There is a persistent desire or unsuccessful efforts to cut down or control marijuana use
- A great deal of time is spent in activities necessary to obtain marijuana, using marijuana, or recovering from its effects
- Important social, occupational, or recreational activities are given up or reduced because of marijuana abuse
- Marijuana use is continued despite knowledge of having a persistent or recurrent psychological or physical problem that is caused or exacerbated by use of marijuana
- Tolerance, as defined by either:
    —need for greater amounts of marijuana to achieve intoxication or desired effect; or
    —markedly diminished effect with continued use of the same amount of marijuana
- Withdrawal, as manifested by either:
    —characteristic withdrawal syndrome for marijuana; or
    —the same (or closely related) substance is taken to relieve or avoid withdrawal symptoms

Source. Adapted from *Diagnostic and Statistical Manual of Mental Disorders,* 4th Edition, Text Revision. Copyright 2000, American Psychiatric Association. Used with permission.

To screen patients for marijuana dependence, we have proposed using quick office-based assessments similar to those commonly used to screen patients for alcohol dependence. The CAGE questionnaire can be administered easily in the physician's office:

- **C**—Have you felt the need to **C**ut down on your marijuana use?
- **A**—Are you easily **A**nnoyed when questioned about your drug use?

- **G**—Do you feel **G**uilty about your marijuana use?
- **E**—Do you smoke marijuana first thing in the morning (**E**ye opener)?

Pathological attachment, despite adverse consequences, and loss of control are hallmarks of marijuana dependence. However, *when* loss of control actually occurs is a question that most addicted persons cannot answer. Avoidance of activities that do not include marijuana is a good indicator, though. This avoidance is shown by changes in friends, sports, and school interests and initiation of amotivational behavior. Lack of clear thought processes, dreaming, and preoccupation with drug use provide the clinician an opportunity for intervention and treatment. These early signs are not pathognomonic and mistakes can be made, but early intervention is crucial. Urine samples can confirm evidence of recent use.

Diagnosing the use and abuse of marijuana by a clinical interview alone is often difficult. Interviews with parents and significant others combined with laboratory results will assist in the diagnosis. The user may be brought for evaluation based on marijuana use or change in motivation, behavior, and/or performance. Less often, users may come in themselves to seek a diagnosis. Finally, drug use may lead to involvement with the criminal justice system through drug courts, accidents, criminal activity, or a random drug test. Regardless, most marijuana-dependent individuals eventually come to medical attention and can then be evaluated after a positive urine sample.

Drug Testing

Self-report of marijuana use is often inaccurate. Users will often deny use or underreport frequency or amount of use. Chemical testing with radioimmunoassay screen followed by confirmation with gas chromatography/ mass spectrometry of biological samples is the objective means of detecting drug use. The presence of marijuana or one of its metabolites in a biological specimen can be used to document exposure. The most common specimen for drug testing has been a urine sample. In recent years, advanced techniques have enabled the analysis of cannabinoids in other specimens such as blood (Giroud et al. 2001), saliva (Kintz and Samyn 2002), hair (Sachs and Kintz 1998), and nails (Lemos et al. 1999).

Urine tests generally identify cannabinoid metabolites. Because these substances are fat soluble, they persist in bodily fluids for extended periods and are excreted slowly. Collection of saliva, which is relatively easy and can be done without privacy issues under close supervision, may be useful in detecting driving-under-the-influence situations. Saliva is a better specimen than urine to detect recent use, and it is more likely that the person is experiencing the pharmacological effects when the sample is taken (Kintz et al. 2000). Hair and nail analyses are markers of use that do not lose sensitivity soon after exposure, and they can be useful in providing cumulative evidence of long-term exposure to marijuana.

General Overview of Treatment Process

Today, more young people are presenting for treatment and being admitted for addiction to marijuana than for alcohol addiction. Treatment of marijuana dependence, as with that for other drugs, must be individualized for the highest probability of success. Detoxification does not address the underlying disorder and thus is not adequate treatment (O'Brien and McLellan 1996). The Stages Model of the Process of Change Model is useful in determining where a patient is in the process of changing his or her behavior (Prochaska et al. 1994). The stages in this model include precontemplation, contemplation, preparation, action, maintenance, and relapse. Twelve-step programs based on the principles of Alcoholics Anonymous are at the core of most treatments.

Crisis Intervention

Many addicted persons will seek treatment in response to a crisis, be it physical, emotional, or drug-induced panic. Patients are more likely to admit to the least "offensive" drug, often describing recent alcohol, cigarette, and marijuana use and failing to mention the heroin they have been sniffing or methylenedioxymethamphetamine (MDMA) they have been taking. After an initial assessment, admission to an inpatient treatment facility or detoxification unit may be needed if other drugs or significant medical or psychiatric problems are involved.

Inpatient Treatment

The least restrictive environment is generally recommended when patients are first attempting to stop using drugs. However, the patient's mental state, impulsivity, history, and safety influence this decision. Outpatient treatment has the advantage of enabling addicted patients or drug abusers to incorporate and confront the everyday problems they will encounter without the use of drugs. Inpatient treatment may be necessary when the patient has

- Continuing drug use after outpatient treatment
- Medical and/or psychiatric complications
- A limited support system at home
- An intent to harm self or others
- A dual diagnosis requiring expertise in dealing with multiple issues

Group Therapy

Group therapy is commonly used and is extremely effective in helping those patients who are isolated from nonusers, who are in denial, and who have limited experience with detoxification and long-term abstinence. Peers can provide a template for recovery through their own lives and experiences. Cathartic sharing, coupled with confrontation, allows users to recognize their typical defense mechanisms.

Individual and Family Psychotherapy

Individual and family psychotherapy may be particularly effective in helping patients accept the loss of time and goals, reconcile their ambitions, and plan for the future. Individual work can help with the anger the addicted person directs at self and the developmental and cognitive issues that will need to be addressed. Family psychotherapy can be a useful adjunct to individual and group counseling, especially if the patient has issues specific to the family. Individual sessions often address the following areas:

- Issues too painful to share in group therapy
- Goal-setting
- Behavioral contracts, if needed
- Identification of problems specific to patient
- Issues related to dual diagnosis, if relevant
- Discussion of feelings about group process

Pharmacotherapy

People who stop smoking marijuana often have abstinence symptoms, which they may not even associate with marijuana cessation. Multiple studies began to document these abstinence symptoms in the 1970s (Smith 2002). Symptoms such as craving, anxiety, irritability, nervousness, aggression, depression, insomnia, restlessness, sweating, nausea, and muscle aches may develop in the weeks following cessation (Gruber and Pope 2002; Smith 2002). Users who experience more severe withdrawal may benefit from pharmacotherapy to manage these symptoms. Currently, no medications are approved by the FDA for marijuana withdrawal. A recent study found that injections of lithium or oxytocin produced a strong suppressing effect on cannabinoid withdrawal in rats (Cui et al. 2001). Recently, small clinical trials have been conducted with bupropion and nefazodone. Researchers found that bupropion appeared to worsen marijuana withdrawal symptoms of insomnia, depression, irritability, and restlessness (Haney et al. 2001a). Nefazodone had no effect on marijuana withdrawal–related insomnia or irritability but was able to decrease restlessness, anxiety, and muscle aches (Haney et al. 2001b). The withdrawal pattern for marijuana is not as clear as it is for other drugs of abuse, and further research on pharmacotherapy for withdrawal is needed (Smith 2002).

Prevention and Intervention

Some researchers have focused on causes and effects to explain the current escalation in marijuana smoking, whereas others have tried to summarize what is known about risk and protective factors associated with marijuana use (Bachman et al. 1998) (Table 15–3). Studies support the conclusion that youths do pay attention to credible information about the dangers of drug use and that the reduction in demand that occurred during the 1980s was a result of this approach (Bachman et al. 1997).

Table 15–3.   Protective and risk factors associated with marijuana abstinence and use

Protective factors associated with abstinence/decreased use	Risk factors associated with increased use
Increased parental presence in the home	Easy access to illicit drugs
Student focus on school and grades	Cigarette smoking
Teenagers who are very "connected" to their parents	Peers who smoke cigarettes or marijuana
Personal importance placed on religion and prayer	Working 20 or more hours/week (ninth to twelfth graders)
Few nights out with peers	Appearing older than chronological age
High self-esteem	Low grade point average
High levels of school "connectedness"	Sexually deviant behavior
Disapproval and avoidance of peers who smoke cigarettes or marijuana	Perceived risk of untimely death

All physicians, especially pediatricians, should be cognizant of the possibility of drug use in their patients and of the importance of providing sound medical information to their patients, patients' family, and community. All annual physical examinations and hospital or office visits should also establish smoking (tobacco, marijuana) status. Simply including smoking status among the vital signs gathered at a routine physical examination may elicit important information and establish smoking prevention as an integral part of the examination.

Prevention of smoking is the first priority. If that fails, postponing onset of marijuana use, reducing the extensiveness of use, increasing the commitment to conventional social roles, and reducing delinquent participation are important interventions that appear likely to shorten any marijuana use, which, as long as use remains illegal, is most likely to stop by the person's 30s.

Conclusion

Marijuana is an important drug of abuse associated with numerous physical and psychological consequences. Marijuana use is associated with an increased likelihood of other drug use and thus serves as a potential "gateway" to other illicit drugs. Regardless of whether progression to other drug use occurs, however, the subtlety of symptoms and user denial can create substantial problems. Predicting or measuring the loss of drive, memory, and motivation and altered quality of human relationships is difficult. Pathological attachment to marijuana forms the basis of the marijuana dependence diagnosis. To the casual observer, marijuana, like alcohol, is perceived as another choice on the smorgasbord of recreational drug use. For family members and concerned others, marijuana is the focus of considerable anxiety, and they experience it as a robber of family life, relationships, motivation, potential, time, and quality of life. Health care providers can help reduce these adverse consequences by educating their patients, offering screening to identify use, and helping their patients receive appropriate treatment.

References

Abel EL: Marijuana: The First Twelve Thousand Years. New York, Plenum, 1980

Abood ME, Sauss C, Fan F, et al: Development of behavioral tolerance to delta-9-THC without alteration of cannabinoid receptor binding or mRNA levels in whole brain. Pharmacol Biochem Behav 46:575–579, 1993

Aceto MD, Scates SM, Lowe JA, et al: Cannabinoid precipitated withdrawal by the selective cannabinoid receptor antagonist SR 141716A. Eur J Pharmacol 282:R1–R2, 1995

Adams AJ, Brown B, Flom ME, et al: Alcohol and marijuana effects on static visual acuity. Am J Optom Physiol Opt 52:729–735, 1975

American Psychiatric Association: Diagnostic and Statistical Manual of Mental Disorders, 4th Edition, Text Revision. Washington, DC, American Psychiatric Association, 2000

Ashton CH: Pharmacology and effects of cannabis: a brief review. Br J Psychiatry 178:101–106, 2001

Bachman JG, Wadsworth KN, O'Malley PM, et al: Smoking, Drinking, and Drug Use in Young Adulthood: The Impacts of New Freedoms and New Responsibilities. Mahwah, NJ, Erlbaum, 1997

Bachman JG, Johnston LD, O'Malley PM: Explaining recent increases in students' marijuana use: impacts of perceived risks and disapproval, 1976 through 1996. Am J Public Health 88:887–892, 1998

Baldwin GC, Taskin DP, Buckley DP, et al: Marijuana and cocaine impair alveolar macrophage function and cytokine production. Am J Respir Crit Care Med 156:1606–1613, 1997

Barsky SH, Roth MD, Kleerup EC, et al: Histopathologic and molecular alterations in bronchial epithelium in habitual smokers of marijuana, cocaine, and/or tobacco. J Natl Cancer Inst 90:1198–1205, 1998

Beaconsfield P, Ginsburg J, Rainsbury R: Marijuana smoking: cardiovascular effects in man and possible mechanisms. N Engl J Med 287:209–212, 1972

Beal JE, Olson R, Laubenstein KL, et al: Dronabinol as a treatment for anorexia associated with weight loss in patients with AIDS. J Pain Symptom Manage 10:89–97, 1995

Beardsley PM, Martin BR: Effects of the cannabinoid CB(1) receptor antagonist, SR141716A, after delta(9)-tetrahydrocannabinol withdrawal. Eur J Pharmacol 387:47–53, 2000

Beautrais AL, Joyce PR, Mulder RT: Cannabis abuse and serious suicide attempts. Addiction 94:1155–1164, 1999

Budney AJ, Kande DB, Cherek DR, et al: Marijuana use and dependence. Drug Alcohol Depend 45:1–11, 1997

Budney AJ, Novy PL, Hughes JR: Marijuana withdrawal among adults seeking treatment for marijuana dependence. Addiction 94:1311–1322, 1999

Budney AJ, Hughes JR, Moore BA, et al: Marijuana abstinence effects in marijuana smokers maintained in their home environment. Arch Gen Psychiatry 58:917–924, 2001

Chen K, Kandel DB: Predictors of cessation of marijuana use: an event history analysis. Drug Alcohol Depend 50:109–121, 1998

Childers SR, Breivogel CS: Cannabis and endogenous cannabinoid systems. Drug Alcohol Depend 51:173–187, 1998

Cohen S: Marijuana and reproductive functions. Drug Abuse and Alcoholism News 13:1, 1985

Cui SS, Bowen RC, Gu GB, et al: Prevention of cannabinoid withdrawal syndrome by lithium: involvement of oxytocinergic neuronal activation. J Neurosci 21:9867–9876, 2001

Denissenko MF, Pao A, Tang M, et al: Preferential formation of benzo(a)pyrene adducts at lung cancer mutational hotspots in P53. Science 274:430–432, 1996

Dewey WL: Cannabinoid pharmacology. Pharmacol Rev 38:151–178, 1986

Dupont RL, Voth EA: Legalization, harm reduction and drug policy. Ann Intern Med 123:461–465, 1995

Fehr KO, Kalant H (eds): Addiction Research Foundations. World Health Organization Meeting on Adverse Health and Behavioral Consequences of Cannabis Use. Toronto, ON, Canada, Addiction Research Foundation, May 1983

Feldman AL, Sullivan JT, Passero MA, et al: Pneumothorax in poly substance abusing marijuana and tobacco smokers: three cases. J Subst Abuse 5:183–186, 1993

Fligiel SE, Roth MD, Kleerup EC, et al: Tracheobronchial histopathology in habitual smokers of cocaine, marijuana, and/or tobacco. Chest 112:319–326, 1997

Fride E: Anandamides: tolerance and cross-tolerance to delta-9-THC. Brain Res 697:83–90, 1995

Gaoni Y, Mechoulam R: Isolation, structure, and partial synthesis of an active constituent of hashish. J Am Chem Soc 86:1646–1647, 1964

Gardner EL, Lowinson JH: Marijuana's interaction with the brain reward systems: update 1991. Pharmacol Biochem Behav 40:571–580, 1991

Gatley SJ, Volkow ND: Addiction and imaging of the human living brain. Drug Alcohol Depend 51:97–108, 1998

Giroud C, Menetrey A, Augsburger M, et al: Delta(9)-THC, 11-OH-delta(9)-THC and delta(9)-THCCOOH plasma or serum to whole blood concentrations distribution ratios in blood samples taken from living and dead people. Forensic Sci Int 123:159–164, 2001

Gold MS: Drugs of Abuse: A Comprehensive Series for Clinicians: Marijuana. New York, Plenum, 1989

Gold MS, Gleaton TJ: Marked increases in USA marijuana and LSD: results of annual junior and senior high school survey (abstract). Biol Psychiatry 35:694, 1994

Gold MS, Schuchard K, Gleaton T: LSD in the USA: déjà vu again? (abstract) Biol Psychiatry 33:431, 1993

Gold MS, Tullis LM, Miller MD: Tobacco and marijuana smoking: a connection? (abstract) Biol Psychiatry 45:447, 1999

Gruber AJ, Pope HG Jr: Marijuana use among adolescents. Pediatr Clin North Am 49:389–413, 2002

Hall W: Health and Psychological Consequences of Cannabis Use (Monograph Series 25). Canberra, Australian Government Publishing Service, 1994

Haney M, Ward AS, Comer SD, et al: Bupropion SR worsens mood during marijuana withdrawal in humans. Psychopharmacology 155:171–179, 2001a

Haney M, Ward AS, Hart CL, et al: Effects of nefazodone on marijuana withdrawal in humans (abstract 241). Drug Alcohol Depend 63S:62, 2001b

Hembree WC, Nahas GG, Zeidenberg P, et al: Changes in human spermatozoa associated with high-dose marijuana smoking, in Marijuana and Medicine. Edited by Nahas GG. Totowa, NJ, Humana Press, 2001, pp 367–378

Herenham M, Lynn AB, Little MD, et al: Cannabinoid receptor localization in the brain. Proc Natl Acad Sci U S A 87:1932–1936, 1990

Herning RI, Better WE, Tate K, et al: Marijuana abusers are at increased risk for stroke: preliminary evidence from cerebrovascular perfusion data. Ann N Y Acad Sci 939:413–415, 2001

Hollister LE: Health aspects of cannabis. Pharmacol Rev 38:1–20, 1986

Isbell H, Gorodetzsky CW, Jasinski DR, et al: Effect of (–)trans-tetrahydrocannabinol in man. Psychopharmacologia 11:184–188, 1967

Janowsky DS, Meacham MP, Blaine JD, et al: Marijuana effects on simulated flying ability. Am J Psychiatry 133:384–388, 1976

Jeynes WH: The relationship between the consumption of various drugs by adolescents and their academic achievement. Am J Drug Alcohol Abuse 28:15–35, 2002

Johnston LD, O'Malley PM, Bachman JG: Monitoring the Future National Survey Results on Drug Use, 1975–2001, Vol I: Secondary School Students (NIH Publ No 02-5106). Rockville, MD, National Institute on Drug Abuse, 2002

Jones KL, Chernoff GF: Effects of chemical and environmental agents, in Maternal Fetal Medicine. Edited by Creasy RK, Resnik R. Philadelphia, PA, WB Saunders, 1984, pp 189–200

Kelder SH, Murray NG, Orpinas P, et al: Depression and substance use in minority middle-school students. Am J Public Health 91:761–766, 2001

Kelley AE, Berridge KC: The neuroscience of natural rewards: relevance to addictive drugs. J Neurosci 22:3306–3311, 2002

Kelly TH, Foltin RW, Emurian CS, et al: Effects of delta-9-THC on marijuana smoking, drug choice and verbal reports of drug liking. J Exp Anal Behav 61:203–211, 1994

Kendler KS, Prescott CA: Cannabis use, abuse, and dependence in a population-based sample of female twins. Am J Psychiatry 155:1016–1022, 1998

Kendler KS, Karkowski LM, Neale MC, et al: Illicit psychoactive substance use, heavy use, abuse and dependence in a US population-based sample of male twins. Arch Gen Psychiatry 57:261–269, 2000

Khun C, Scott S, Wilson W: Buzzed: The Straight Facts About the Most Used and Abused Drugs From Alcohol to Ecstasy. New York, WW Norton, 1997

Kim D, Thayer SA: Cannabinoids inhibit the formation of new synapses between hippocampal neurons in culture. J Neurosci 21:RC146, 2001

Kintz P, Samyn N: Use of alternative specimens: drugs of abuse in saliva and doping agents in hair. Ther Drug Monit 24:239–246, 2002

Kintz P, Cirimele V, Ludes B: Detection of cannabis in oral fluid (saliva) and forehead wipes (sweat) from impaired drivers. J Anal Toxicol 24:557–561, 2000

Klein TW, Friedman H, Specter S: Marijuana, immunity and infection. J Neuroimmunol 83:102–115, 1998

Kolodny RC, Masters WH, Kolodner RM, et al: Depression of plasma testosterone levels after chronic intensive marijuana use. N Engl J Med 290:872–874, 1974

Kopstein AN, Crum RM, Celentano DD, et al: Sensation seeking needs among 8th and 11th graders: characteristics associated with cigarette and marijuana use. Drug Alcohol Depend 62:195–203, 2001

Kouri EM, Pope HG Jr: Abstinence symptoms during withdrawal from chronic marijuana use. Exp Clin Psychopharmacol 8:483–492, 2000

Leirer VO, Yesavage JA, Morrow DG: Marijuana carry-over effects on aircraft pilot performance. Aviat Space Environ Med 62:221–227, 1991

Lemos NP, Anderson RA, Robertson JR: Nail analysis for drugs of abuse: extraction and determination of cannabis in fingernails by RIA and GC-MS. J Anal Toxicol 23:147–152, 1999

Lukas SE, Sholar M, Kouri E, et al: Marijuana smoking increases plasma cocaine levels and subjective reports of euphoria in male volunteers. Pharmacol Biochem Behav 48:715–721, 1994

Lundavist T: Specific thought patterns in chronic cannabis smokers observed during treatment. Life Sci 56:2141–2144, 1995

Luntz Research Companies: The 1996 CASA National Survey of American Attitudes on Substance Abuse II: Teens and Their Parents. Available at: http://www.casacolumbia.org

Marlatt GA, Gordon JR: Relapse Prevention. New York, Guilford, 1985

Mathew RJ, Wilson WH, Turkington TG, et al: Cerebellar activity and disturbed time sense after THC. Brain Res 797:183–189, 1998

Matthias P, Tashkin DP, Marques-Magallanes JA, et al: Effects of varying marijuana potency on deposition of tar and delta-9-THC in the lung during smoking. Pharmacol Biochem Behav 58:1145–1150, 1997

McGee R, Williams S, Poulton R, et al: A longitudinal study of cannabis use and mental health from adolescence to early adulthood. Addiction 95:491–503, 2000

Merrill JC, Kleber HD, Shwartz M, et al: Cigarettes, alcohol, marijuana, other risk behaviors, and American youth. Drug Alcohol Depend 56:205–212, 1999

Miles DR, van den Bree MB, Pickens RW: Sex differences in shared genetic and environmental influences between conduct disorder symptoms and marijuana use in adolescents. Am J Med Genet 114:159–168, 2002

Moskowitz H, Sharma SM, McGlothin W: Effects of marihuana upon peripheral vision and function of the information processing demands in central vision. Percept Mot Skills 35:875–882, 1972

Naditch MP: Acute adverse reactions to psychoactive drugs, drug usage and psychopathology. J Abnorm Psychol 83:394–403, 1974

Neumark-Sztainer D, Story M, Dixon LB, et al: Adolescents engaging in unhealthy weight control behaviors: are they at risk for other health-compromising behaviors? Am J Public Health 88:952–955, 1998

Novak W: High Culture: Marijuana in the Lives of Americans. New York, Knopf, 1980

O'Brien CP, McLellan AT: Myths about the treatment of addiction. Lancet 347:237–240, 1996

O'Leary DS, Block RI, Flaum M, et al: Acute marijuana effects on rCBF and cognition: a PET study. Neuroreport 11:3835–3841, 2000

O'Leary DS, Block RI, Koeppel JA, et al: Effects of smoking marijuana on brain perfusion and cognition. Neuropsychopharmacology 26:802–816, 2002

Oveido A, Glowa J, Herkenham M: Chronic cannabinoid administration alters cannabinoid receptor binding in rat brain: a quantitative autoradiographic study. Brain Res 616:293–302, 1993

Pertwee RG: Pharmacological, physiological and clinical implications of the discovery of cannabinoid receptors. Biochem Soc Trans 26:267–272, 1998

Pope HG, Yurgelun-Todd D: The residual cognitive effects of heavy marijuana use in college students. JAMA 275:521–527, 1996

Prochaska JO, Norcross JC, DiClemente CC: Changing for Good. New York, William Morrow, 1994

Rey JM, Sawyer MG, Raphael B, et al: Mental health of teenagers who use cannabis: results of an Australian survey. Br J Psychiatry 180:216–221, 2002

Rodriquez de Fonseca F, Carrera MRA, Navarro M, et al: Activation of corticotropin-releasing factor in the limbic system during cannabinoid withdrawal. Science 276:2050–2054, 1997

Rogers RD, Robbins TW: Investigating the neurocognitive deficits associated with chronic drug misuse. Curr Opin Neurobiol 11:250–257, 2001

Romero J, Garcia-Palormero E, Castro JG, et al: Effects of chronic exposure to delta-9-THC on cannabinoid receptor binding and mRNA levels in several rat brain regions. Mol Brain Res 46:100–108, 1997

Rueshe S: National Families in Action. 1997. Available at: http://www.nationalfamilies.org

Sachs H, Kintz P: Testing for drugs in hair: critical review of chromatographic procedures since 1992. J Chromatogr B Biomed Sci Appl 713:147–161, 1998

Smith NT: A review of the published literature into cannabis withdrawal symptoms in human users. Addiction 97:621–632, 2002

Solowij N, Stephens RS, Roffman RA, et al: Cognitive functioning of long-term heavy cannabis users seeking treatment. JAMA 287:1123–1131, 2002

Stephens RS, Wertz JS, Roffman RA: Self-efficacy and marijuana cessation: a construct validity analysis. J Consult Clin Psychol 63:1022–1031, 1995

Stillman R, Galanter M, Lemberger L, et al: Tetrahydrocannabinol (THC): metabolism and subjective effects. Life Sci 19:569–576, 1976

Stimmel B: Medical marijuana: to prescribe or not to prescribe: that is the question. J Addict Dis 14:1–4, 1995

Substance Abuse and Mental Health Services Administration: Results From the 2001 National Household Survey on Drug Abuse, Vol I: Summary of National Findings (Office of Applied Studies, NHSDA Series H-17, DHHS Publ No SMA 02-3758). Rockville, MD, Substance Abuse and Mental Health Services Administration, 2002

Substance Abuse and Mental Health Services Administration: Results From the 2002 National Survey on Drug Use and Health: National Findings, 1.1: Summary of NSDUH (Office of Applied Studies, NHSDA Series H-22, DHHS Publ No SMA 03-3836). Rockville, MD, Substance Abuse and Mental Health Services Administration, 2003. Available at: http://www.samhsa.gov/oas/nhsda.htm

Swendsen JD, Merikangas KR: The comorbidity of depression and substance use disorders. Clin Psychol Rev 20:173–189, 2000

Tanda G, Pontieri FE, DiChiara G: Cannabinoid and heroin activation of mesolimbic dopamine transmission by a common mu1 opioid receptor mechanism. Science 276:2048–2050, 1997

Tashkin DP: Bronchial effects of aerosolized delta 9 THC in healthy and asthmatic subjects. Am Rev Respir Dis 115:57–65, 1977

Tashkin DP, Shapiro BJ, Lee EY, et al: Subacute effects of heavy marijuana smoking on pulmonary function in healthy young males. N Engl J Med 294:125–129, 1976

Tashkin DP, Wu TC, Djahed B, et al: Acute and chronic effects of marijuana smoking compared with tobacco smoking on blood carboxyhemoglobin levels. J Psychoactive Drugs 20:27–31, 1988a

Tashkin DP, Simmins M, Clark V, et al: Effects of habitual smoking of marijuana alone and with tobacco on nonspecific airway hyperactivity. J Psychoactive Drugs 20:221–225, 1988b

Tilles DS, Goldenheim PD, Johnson DC, et al: Marijuana smoking as cause of reduction in single-breath carbon monoxide diffusing capacity. Am J Med 80:601–606, 1986

Tsou K, Patrick SL, Walker JM: Physical withdrawal in rats tolerant to delta-9-THC precipitated by a cannabinoid receptor antagonist. Eur J Pharmacol 280:R13–R15, 1995

Tullis LM, Dupont R, Frost-Pineda K, et al: Marijuana and tobacco: a major connection? J Addict Dis 22(3):51–62, 2003

van Os J, Bak M, Hanssen M, et al: Cannabis use and psychosis: a longitudinal population-based study. Am J Epidemiol 156:319–327, 2002

Vlahov D, Galea S, Resnick H, et al: Increased use of cigarettes, alcohol, and marijuana among Manhattan, New York, residents after the September 11th terrorist attacks. Am J Epidemiol 155:988–996, 2002

Voruganti LN, Slomka P, Zabel P, et al: Cannabis induced dopamine release: an in-vivo SPECT study. Psychiatry Res 107:173–177, 2001

Wagner FA, Anthony JC: From first drug use to drug dependence; developmental periods of risk for dependence upon marijuana, cocaine, and alcohol. Neuropsychopharmacology 26:479–488, 2002a

Wagner FA, Anthony JC: Into the world of illegal drug use: exposure opportunity and other mechanisms linking the use of alcohol, tobacco, marijuana, and cocaine. Am J Epidemiol 155:918–925, 2002b

Warner LA, Kessler RC, Hughes M, et al: Prevalence and correlates of drug use and dependence in the United States: results from the National Comorbidity Survey. Arch Gen Psychiatry 52:219–229, 1995

Wickelgren I: Marijuana: harder than we thought? Science 276 (5321):1967–1968, 1997

Wilcox HC, Wagner FA, Anthony JC: Exposure opportunity as a mechanism linking youth marijuana use to hallucinogen use. Drug Alcohol Depend 66:127–135, 2002

Wilson W, Mathew R, Turkington T, et al: Brain morphological changes and early marijuana use: a magnetic resonance and positron emission tomography study. J Addict Dis 19:1–22, 2000

Wu TC, Tashkin DP, Djahed B, et al: Pulmonary hazards of smoking marijuana as compared with tobacco. N Engl J Med 318:347–351, 1988

Stimulants

Thomas R. Kosten, M.D.
Mehmet Sofuoglu, M.D., Ph.D.

Cocaine and amphetamine are psychoactive agents that increase central nervous system (CNS) activity and produce powerful reinforcing effects (e.g., euphoria) that contribute to their high abuse liability. Since the peak of the cocaine epidemic in the mid-1980s, addiction to this stimulant has been a major public health concern. There have been localized epidemics of amphetamine abuse, particularly in the western United States. The dangers associated with stimulant use are enormous and include increased risk of human immunodeficiency virus (HIV) infection, detrimental effects on the unborn and newborn, increased crime and violence, as well as medical, financial, and psychological problems. Because of these consequences, the task of identifying, characterizing, and developing treatments is more important than ever.

Progress has been made in identifying and developing pharmacological and behavioral treatments for stimulant addiction. In this chapter, we review our current understanding of the biological basis for stimulant reinforcement and describe the clinical characteristics resulting from its use, as a foundation for a discussion of the pharmacological and behavioral treatment approaches for stimulant abuse. We conclude by providing specific treatment guidelines for managing stimulant-abusing individuals.

Neurochemical Actions Mediating Stimulant Reward

A vast behavioral and pharmacological literature indicates that the rewarding effects of stimulants are mediated through the mesocorticolimbic dopamine (DA) system, which consists of DA neurons of the ventral tegmental area and their target projections, including the nucleus accumbens and prefrontal cortex (PFC) (Johanson and Fischman 1989; Kosten 2002). The reinforcing properties of cocaine and amphetamine are associated with their ability to increase synaptic DA levels. Cocaine increases DA by binding to

Supported by National Institute on Drug Abuse grants K05 DA0454 and P50 DA12762.

the dopamine transporter (DAT) and inhibiting its activity, whereas amphetamine increases synaptic DA concentrations by actions on the vesicular monoamine transporter, which causes DA release from the vesicles into synapses (White and Kalivas 1998). Cocaine and amphetamine also have actions on norepinephrine (NE) and serotonin (5-HT) neurons, and all of these neurotransmitters are important targets for medication development (Rothman et al. 2000). However, behavioral and neurochemical studies indicate that DA is the critical neurotransmitter mediating the reinforcing effects of these stimulants and that this action is dependent on rapid entry of cocaine into the brain to raise synaptic DA levels (Volkow et al. 1996a, 1997).

Neurobiological Effects of Chronic Stimulant Abuse

In addition to the acute reinforcing effects, stimulants can produce a constellation of neurochemical, physiological, and neuropsychological impairments following chronic use. Studies examining DA receptor function show decreased postsynaptic DA receptors and reduced DA function (Sevarino et al. 2000; Volkow et al. 1992, 1996b). Single-photon emission computed tomography (SPECT) and positron emission tomography (PET) studies show increases in DAT in acutely abstinent cocaine abusers relative to control subjects (Malison et al. 1998), decreases in DA D_2 receptor binding in detoxified cocaine abusers relative to control subjects (Volkow et al. 1996b), and reduced cerebral blood flow (CBF) and cortical perfusion among chronic cocaine users (Holman et al. 1991; Kosten et al. 1998; Volkow et al. 1988). Treatment with buprenorphine or with aspirin has improved the reduced CBF in cocaine-dependent individuals, suggesting that drug-induced alterations may be reversed to some extent (Holman et al. 1993; Kosten 1998). Alterations in glucose metabolism also have been observed following stimulant administration. When tested during early withdrawal, glucose metabolism is increased among cocaine users relative to control subjects, but during late withdrawal, metabolic activity is decreased among cocaine-addicted persons (Volkow et al. 1991, 1992). Such reductions in glucose metabolism also have been observed following acute administration of cocaine (London et al. 1990).

Given the evidence of disturbances in brain structure and function following stimulant use, it is not surprising that individuals with histories of cocaine abuse also show cognitive deficits. In fact, impairments in verbal learning, memory, and attention have been well documented in cocaine-abusing individuals (Beatty et al. 1995; Bolla et al. 1998; Di Sclafani et al. 2002; Gottschalk et al. 2001), and these neuropsychological deficits have been shown to correlate with reductions in blood flow among cocaine users (Woods et al. 1991). DAT reduction is also associated with psychomotor impairment in methamphetamine abusers (Volkow et al. 2001a, 2001b). Thus, chronic stimulant use produces not only neurochemical and physiological alterations but also cognitive impairments.

Clinical Aspects of Stimulant Use

The rewarding effects of cocaine and amphetamine are influenced by the route of administration because some routes (e.g., intravenous administration) produce more immediate onset of euphoria. The preferred method of self-administering cocaine has been snorting and, more recently, smoking. Amphetamines come in a variety of forms (e.g., pill, liquid, or powder form) but are usually taken orally or intravenously. The effects of snorted cocaine generally occur within 15–20 minutes, whereas the effects from intravenously injected cocaine can be felt within 30 seconds. A smokable form of cocaine (crack cocaine), which changes cocaine hydrochloride into a free base by using baking soda and water, produces euphoria within seconds. A smokable version of amphetamine (ice amphetamine) is also available, and because of its long duration of action, it can produce euphoria lasting 12–24 hours.

Stimulant use may range from low-dose to high-dose and from infrequent to chronic or binge patterns. Depending on the dosage, pattern, and duration of use, stimulants can produce several drug-induced states that differ in clinical characteristics. Moderate to high doses of stimulants can produce stimulant intoxication that may or may not be pleasant. The intoxicated person may show signs of hyperawareness, hypersexuality, hypervigilance, and psychomotor agitation. Often, the symptoms of stimulant-induced intoxication resemble mania. The medical staff needs to monitor intoxicated persons until the symptoms of agitation and paranoia diminish. If these symptoms do not resolve within 24 hours, pharmacotherapy for the psychotic symptoms is indicated (Kosten 2002).

With increased dosage and duration of administration, stimulants can also produce a state of mental confusion and excitement known as *stimulant delirium*. Delirium is associated with becoming disoriented and confused, as well as anxious and fearful. Extreme medical caution is needed when treating delirium because such symptoms may indicate stimulant overdose. For instance, patients addicted to crack cocaine who overdose need careful monitoring for seizures, cardiac arrhythmias, stroke, and pulmonary complications. Overdose management in the past used chlorpromazine, but this agent can worsen a cocaine withdrawal syndrome of hyperthermia and agitation that resembles neuroleptic malignant syndrome (Kosten and Kleber 1988). High doses of benzodiazepines may be safer alternatives for controlling the delirium and agitation because neuroleptics will worsen the hyperthermia in some cases of overdose and lead to fatality. Acutely, benzodiazepines can also help minimize the need for physical restraints.

During high-dose stimulant use, often seen during binge episodes, individuals can experience stimulant-induced psychosis characterized by delusions, paranoid thinking, and stereotyped compulsive behavior. Delusional patients require close clinical monitoring, and use of short-term neuroleptic treatment may be necessary to ameliorate the psychosis. Psychosis is induced more commonly by amphetamine than by cocaine, perhaps because it is difficult to maintain high chronic levels of cocaine in the body (King and Ellinwood 1997). Also, stimulant-induced psychosis in humans is related to the dose and duration of administration of amphetamine and cocaine rather than psychiatric predisposition (Satel et al. 1991).

Stimulant withdrawal, which occurs following cessation of cocaine or amphetamine use, can produce a wide range of dysphoric symptoms. Following binge use, individuals may initially experience a "crash" period, which is characterized by symptoms of depression, anxiety, agitation, and intense drug craving (Gawin and Ellinwood 1988). The crash period is followed by an intermediate withdrawal phase, in which the individuals may experience fatigue, a loss of physical and mental energy, and decreased interest in the surrounding environment (Gawin and Ellinwood 1988). During the late withdrawal phase, individuals may experience brief periods of intense drug craving, such that objects and people in the addicted person's life can become a conditioned trigger for craving and relapse. These withdrawal symptoms may be a target for pharmacological agents (see "Dopaminergic Agents" below).

Treatment of Stimulant Abuse

Although a great deal has been learned about the reward mechanisms underlying stimulant abuse, the development of effective pharmacotherapy has lagged behind. The pharmacological and behavioral treatment approaches used for cocaine abuse also appear to be applicable to the treatment of amphetamine abuse, but no treatment agents have been approved by the Food and Drug Administration (FDA) for this use.

Pharmacotherapy

More than 40 medications have been investigated to treat stimulant abuse, but none has shown consistent efficacy. These medications include dopaminergic agonists; antidepressants; and, more recently, disulfiram, selegiline, and a cocaine vaccine. Studies have been relatively brief and have focused on abstinence initiation rather than on relapse prevention, but even these modest treatment targets have not been attained. Table 16–1 categorizes most of the examined agents according to their putative mechanisms.

Dopaminergic Agents

On the theoretical basis that chronic cocaine use reduces the efficiency of central DA neurotransmission, several dopaminergic compounds, including amantadine, bromocriptine, mazindol, and methylphenidate, have been examined as treatments for cocaine abuse. Investigators thought that these dopaminergic agents, which have a fast onset of action, would correct the DA dysregulation and alleviate the withdrawal symptoms that often follow cessation of stimulant use.

A recent review found little efficacy for direct DA agonists such as pergolide but some suggestion of efficacy for indirect agents such as sustained-release amphetamine, selegiline, and disulfiram (Kosten et al. 2002a; Malcolm et al. 2000). Although a controlled study found no difference between methylphenidate and placebo treatment groups in cocaine use, sustained-release amphetamine showed more promise (Grabowski et al. 1997, 2001). A recent placebo-

Table 16–1. Pharmacological agents for cocaine dependence

Type (target)	Agent
Cocaine agonists (mimic cocaine effects)	
Other stimulants	Amphetamine, methylphenidate, pemoline
Slow-onset agonist	Oral cocaine (coca tea used in South America)
Cocaine antagonists (block cocaine effects)	
Block cocaine binding at the dopamine transporter site	Bupropion, mazindol, GBR-12909
Block dopamine receptor	D_1 antagonist (ecopipam), D_2 antagonists (antipsychotics), D_1/D_3 antagonists (atypical antipsychotics)
Medications that decrease cocaine reinforcement	
Dopaminergic medications	
Dopamine agonists	D_1 agonists (ABT-431), D_2 agonists (bromocriptine, cabergoline, pergolide), D_3 agonists (amantadine, pramipexole)
Monoamine oxidase inhibitors	Phenelzine, selegiline
Inhibitor of dopamine β-hydroxylase	Disulfiram
Precursors of synthesis	Tyrosine, L-dopa
Indirect modulators of dopamine activity	
Serotonergic medications	
Reuptake blockers (selective serotonin reuptake inhibitors)	Fluoxetine, paroxetine, sertraline
Receptor agonists	Buspirone ($5-HT_{1A}$), gepirone
Receptor antagonists	Ondansetron ($5-HT_3$), mirtazapine ($5-HT_2$, $5-HT_3$, and others), ritanserin ($5-HT_2$)
Precursors of synthesis (amino acids)	L-Tryptophan
Medications that affect dopamine, serotonin, and norepinephrine	
Reuptake blockers	Desipramine, imipramine, venlafaxine
Medications that deplete dopamine, norepinephrine, and serotonin	Reserpine
Putative antikindling agents	Carbamazepine, phenytoin, valproate
Medications that decrease glutamate activity	Lamotrigine
Medications that affect the GABA (γ-aminobutyric acid) system	Baclofen, gabapentin, progesterone, tiagabine, vigabatrin
Pharmacokinetic mechanisms	
Block cocaine access to brain	Cocaine antibodies
Stress response modulators	Dehydroepiandrosterone, dexamethasone, propranolol, electroencephalogram biofeedback
Cerebral blood flow enhancers	Amiloride, hydergine, isradipine, pentoxifylline, piracetam
Cholinergic medications	
Cholinesterase inhibitor	Donepezil
Miscellaneous	
Cyclooxygenase-2 (COX-2) inhibitor	Celecoxib
Nutritional supplements and herbal products	Amino acid mixtures, ginkgo biloba, *Hypericum* (St. John's wort), ibogaine, L-carnitine/coenzyme Q10

controlled study of selegiline, a monoamine oxidase inhibitor that blocks the breakdown of DA, has not found it effective for cocaine dependence (F. Vocci, personal communication, 2003). Disulfiram has an indirect action on DA through inhibition of the enzyme DA β-hydroxylase, which converts DA to NE. Early studies with disulfiram are promising in reducing cocaine abuse (Carroll et al. 1998; George et al. 2000).

Antidepressants

The second class of medications used to treat cocaine dependence—antidepressants—are thought to down-regulate synaptic catecholamine receptors, an action opposite to the presynaptic upregulation caused by chronic stimulant use (Gawin and Ellinwood 1988). Although antidepressants have a relatively benign side-effect profile, good patient compliance rates, and lack of abuse liability, only desipramine has shown some efficacy in selected populations, and the more common serotonin reuptake inhibitors have been ineffective.

Desipramine is the tricyclic antidepressant that has been studied the most extensively as a treatment for cocaine dependence. A meta-analysis of placebo-controlled studies by Levin and Lehman (1991) showed that desipramine produced greater cocaine abstinence than placebo, but a more recent review did not concur (Lima et al. 2001). However, secondary analyses of studies with imipramine, desipramine, and bupropion have suggested that depressed cocaine abusers are more likely to show significant reductions in cocaine abuse than are nondepressed cocaine abusers (Margolin et al. 1995; Nunes et al. 1991; Ziedonis and Kosten 1991). Furthermore, recent work with desipramine has suggested its efficacy in opioid-dependent patients, particularly in combination with contingency management therapies (Kosten 2003; Oliveto et al. 1999). Early studies suggested some efficacy for fluoxetine, but this has not been confirmed in controlled trials (Grabowski et al. 1995).

Other Treatment Agents and Approaches

In addition to the dopaminergic agents and antidepressants, miscellaneous agents, including carbamazepine, buprenorphine, and γ-aminobutyric acid (GABA) agonists, have been examined for cocaine pharmacotherapy. Carbamazepine failed to show therapeutic effects in three controlled studies after initial enthusiasm (Cornish et al. 1995; Kranzler et al. 1995; Montoya et al. 1995). Buprenorphine also has had more negative than positive findings supporting its efficacy in treating cocaine-abusing, opiate-addicted persons (Kosten et al. 1989, 1993; Schottenfeld et al. 1997). The GABA agonists are showing promise following an initial study of baclofen (Ling et al. 1998).

Recent advances in understanding DA neuronal systems and in considering ways to prevent stimulants from getting into the brain have led to innovative approaches for medications. For example, although DA seems critical for reinforcement, several groups have shown that mice with the DAT deleted will still self-administer cocaine, suggesting a role for the serotonergic system (Rocha et al. 1998; Sora et al. 1998, 2001). Furthermore, the effects of κ agonists in reducing DA activity are opposite to that observed with cocaine or amphetamine, suggesting their role as potential medications (Maisonneuve et al. 1994). A cocaine vaccine also has been developed for humans and is supported by animal studies in which several different types of vaccines suppressed cocaine administration (Kosten and Biegel 2002; Kosten et al. 2002b).

Behavior Therapy

The most important component of stimulant treatment involves behavior therapies. Although a large multisite study showed little difference between drug counseling and two types of more intensive behavior therapies—cognitive and supportive expressive therapies—these therapies retain patients in treatment and can lead to abstinence (Crits-Christoph et al. 1999). These therapies form the platform for any pharmacotherapy in order to engage the patient and facilitate more long-term changes, including prevention of relapse (Carroll 1996, 1997).

A specific behavioral approach that uses positive contingencies to initiate abstinence and prevent relapse has been quite successful for managing cocaine and amphetamine abuse (Higgins et al. 1994a, 2000a, 2000b; Silverman et al. 1996). The goal of this approach has been to decrease behavior maintained by drug reinforcers and increase behavior maintained by nondrug reinforcers by presenting rewards contingent on documented drug abstinence (positive contingencies) and withdrawing privileges contingent on documented drug use (negative contingencies).

Two studies illustrate how positive contingency management procedures facilitate initial abstinence in cocaine-dependent persons. In a 24-week study (Higgins et al. 1994b), cocaine-dependent individuals were randomly assigned to receive either behavioral treatment without incentives or behavioral treatment with incentives (i.e., vouchers exchangeable for goods and services) during weeks 1–12. During weeks 13–24, clients in both groups received, in addition to behavioral treatment, a $1.00 lottery ticket for every drug-free urine sample. The group that received the incentives showed significantly greater treatment retention and longer duration of continuous abstinence than did the group not receiving the incentives. In a 12-week clinical trial among methadone-maintained cocaine abusers (Silverman et al. 1996), the contingency group also achieved significantly longer duration of sustained cocaine abstinence than did control subjects. Overall, these findings suggest that incentives contingent on drug abstinence can be a powerful intervention tool for facilitating cocaine abstinence in cocaine abusers and methadone-maintained cocaine abusers.

Treatment and Psychiatric Comorbidity

The rates of comorbid psychiatric disorders in stimulant abusers are significantly higher than community rates of depression, attention-deficit/hyperactivity disorder (ADHD), and antisocial personality disorders (Rounsaville et al. 1991; Weiss et al. 1986). Because psychiatric disorders may increase the risk for drug use (e.g., individuals may self-medicate to ease psychiatric symptomatology), treatment must address both the stimulant addiction and the comorbid disorder. Certain pharmacotherapies may be particularly useful for stimulant abusers with comorbid psychopathology. For instance, treatment with antidepressants has reduced depressive symptoms, cocaine use, and craving in depressed cocaine-addicted patients (Nunes et al. 1991; Ziedonis and Kosten 1991). Also, methylphenidate has been reported to be effective in treating cocaine-addicted patients with ADHD (Khantzian et al. 1984). Unfortunately, psychiatric comorbidity has not yet shown a specific prognostic significance for behavior therapies.

Treatment Guidelines for Stimulant Abuse

Treatment of stimulant abuse requires a comprehensive assessment of the patient's psychological, medical, forensic, and drug use history. Moreover, because information obtained from chemically dependent persons may be incomplete or unreliable, it is important that patients receive a thorough physical examination, including blood and supervised urine samples for analysis. The clinician needs to be aware that polydrug abuse is common. Patients may ingest large amounts of one or more drugs at potentially lethal doses; therefore, the physician must be aware of the dangers of possible drug combinations, such as cocaine and alcohol or heroin (Goldsmith 1996).

Pharmacological intervention may be necessary during stimulant-induced drug states. For instance, neuroleptics may be useful in controlling stimulant-induced psychosis or delirium, and anticraving agents with a fast onset of action may be helpful during the early withdrawal period. During the late withdrawal phase, when depression may set in, antidepressants may be an appropriate choice for treatment medication. Treatment medications can be given on an inpatient or outpatient basis. However, if medications are used for outpatient treatment, it is critical to warn the patient of the potential adverse interactions between cocaine and the prescribed treatment medication. For instance, high blood pressure could result from the release of epinephrine by cocaine combined with the reuptake blockade by the tricyclic, although later in the course of treatment, tricyclics decrease the sensitivity of the postsynaptic adrenergic receptors (Fischman et al. 1976; Kosten et al. 1992).

Conclusion

Dopamine neural systems appear to mediate the reinforcing effects of cocaine and amphetamine. The powerful rewarding effects make stimulants addictive and dangerous, creating a range of psychological, social, economic, and medical problems. To date, no effective treatment is available for stimulant dependence, although progress has been made in the development of pharmacological and behavioral techniques for cocaine and amphetamine addiction. Dopaminergic agents and antidepressants have shown some promise for reducing drug craving and preventing relapse. Behavioral techniques aimed at maintaining drug abstinence and preventing relapse have also shown favorable results. Although both pharmacological and behavioral interventions may be useful in treating addiction, individuals with significant medical risks, psychiatric comorbidity, and neuroadaptation from heavy stimulant use are particularly likely to benefit from pharmacological treatment (Kosten 2002). Further research is needed to address this issue and identify other effective ways to treat, manage, and prevent stimulant use.

References

Beatty WW, Katzung VM, Moreland VJ, et al: Neuropsychological performance of recently abstinent alcoholics and cocaine abusers. Drug Alcohol Depend 37:247–253, 1995

Bolla KI, Cadet JL, London ED: The neuropsychiatry of chronic cocaine abuse. J Neuropsychiatry Clin Neurosci 10:280–289, 1998

Carroll KM: Relapse prevention as a psychosocial treatment approach: a review of controlled clinical trials. Exp Clin Psychopharmacol 4:46–54, 1996

Carroll KM: Manual-guided psychosocial treatment: a new virtual requirement for pharmacotherapy trials? Arch Gen Psychiatry 54:923–928, 1997

Carroll KM, Nich C, Ball SA, et al: Treatment of cocaine and alcohol dependence with psychotherapy and disulfiram. Addiction 93:713–727, 1998

Cornish JW, Maany I, Fudala PJ, et al: Carbamazepine treatment for cocaine dependence. Drug Alcohol Depend 38:221–227, 1995

Crits-Christoph P, Siqueland L, Blaine J, et al: Psychosocial treatments for cocaine dependence: National Institute on Drug Abuse Collaborative Cocaine Treatment Study. Arch Gen Psychiatry 56:493–502, 1999

Di Sclafani V, Tolou-Shams M, Price LJ, et al: Neuropsychological performance of individuals dependent on crack-cocaine, or crack-cocaine and alcohol, at 6 weeks and 6 months of abstinence. Drug Alcohol Depend 66:161–171, 2002

Fischman MW, Schuster CR, Resnekov L, et al: Cardiovascular and subjective effects of intravenous cocaine administration in humans. Arch Gen Psychiatry 33:983–989, 1976

Gawin FH, Ellinwood EH: Cocaine and other stimulants: actions, abuse and treatment. N Engl J Med 318:1173–1182, 1988

George TP, Chawarski MC, Pakes J, et al: Disulfiram versus placebo for cocaine dependence in buprenorphine-maintained subjects: a preliminary trial. Biol Psychiatry 47:1080–1086, 2000

Goldsmith RJ: The elements of contemporary treatment, in The Principles and Practice of Addictions in Psychiatry. Edited by Miller NS. Philadelphia, PA, WB Saunders, 1996, pp 392–399

Gottschalk C, Beauvais J, Hart R, et al: Cognitive function and cerebral perfusion during cocaine abstinence. Am J Psychiatry 158:540–545, 2001

Grabowski J, Rhoades H, Elk R, et al: Fluoxetine is ineffective for treatment of cocaine dependence or concurrent opiate and cocaine dependence: two placebo-controlled double-blind trials. J Clin Psychopharmacol 15:163–174, 1995

Grabowski J, Roache JD, Schmitz JM, et al: Replacement medication for cocaine dependence: methylphenidate. J Clin Psychopharmacol 17:485–488, 1997

Grabowski J, Rhoades H, Schmitz J, et al: Dextroamphetamine for cocaine-dependence treatment: a double-blind randomized clinical trial. J Clin Psychopharmacol 21:522–526, 2001

Higgins ST, Budney AJ, Bickel WK: Applying behavioral concepts and principles to the treatment of cocaine dependence. Drug Alcohol Depend 34:87–97, 1994a

Higgins ST, Budney AJ, Bickel WK, et al: Incentives improve outcome in outpatient behavioral treatment of cocaine dependence. Arch Gen Psychiatry 51:568–576, 1994b

Higgins ST, Badger GJ, Budney AJ: Initial abstinence and success in achieving longer term cocaine abstinence. Exp Clin Psychopharmacol 8:377–386, 2000a

Higgins ST, Wong CJ, Badger GJ, et al: Contingent reinforcement increases cocaine abstinence during outpatient treatment and 1 year of follow-up. J Consult Clin Psychol 68:64–72, 2000b

Holman BL, Carvalho PA, Mendelson J, et al: Brain perfusion is abnormal in cocaine-dependent polydrug users: a study using technetium-99m-HMPAO and ASPECT. J Nucl Med 32:1206–1210, 1991

Holman BL, Mendelson J, Garada B, et al: Regional cerebral blood flow improves with treatment in chronic cocaine polydrug users. J Nucl Med 34:723–727, 1993

Johanson CE, Fischman MW: The pharmacology of cocaine related to its abuse. Pharmacol Rev 41:3–52, 1989

Khantzian EJ, Gawin F, Kleber HD, et al: Methylphenidate (Ritalin) treatment of cocaine dependence: a preliminary report. J Subst Abuse Treat 1:107–112, 1984

King GR, Ellinwood EH: Amphetamines and other stimulants, in Substance Abuse: A Comprehensive Textbook, 3rd Edition. Edited by Lowinson JH, Ruiz P, Millman RB, et al. Baltimore, MD, Williams & Wilkins, 1997, pp 207–233

Kosten TR: Pharmacotherapy of cerebral ischemia in cocaine dependence. Drug Alcohol Depend 49:133–144, 1998

Kosten TR: Pathophysiology and treatment of cocaine dependence, in Neuropsychopharmacology: The Fifth Generation of Progress. Edited by Davis KL, Charney D, Coyle JT, et al. Baltimore, MD, Lippincott Williams & Wilkins, 2002, pp 1461–1473

Kosten TR, Biegel D: Therapeutic vaccines for substance dependence. Expert Rev Vaccines 1:363–371, 2002

Kosten TR, Kleber HD: Rapid death during cocaine abuse: a variant of the neuroleptic malignant syndrome? Am J Drug Alcohol Abuse 14:335–346, 1988

Kosten TR, Kleber HD, Morgan C: Treatment of cocaine abuse with buprenorphine. Biol Psychiatry 26:637–639, 1989

Kosten TR, Gawin FH, Silverman DG, et al: Intravenous cocaine challenges during desipramine maintenance. Neuropsychopharmacology 7:169–176, 1992

Kosten TR, Schottenfeld RS, Ziedonis D, et al: Buprenorphine versus methadone maintenance for opioid dependence. J Nerv Ment Dis 181:358–364, 1993

Kosten TR, Cheeves C, Palumbo J, et al: Regional cerebral blood flow during acute and chronic abstinence from combined cocaine-alcohol abuse. Drug Alcohol Depend 50:187–195, 1998

Kosten TR, George TP, Kosten TA: The potential of dopamine agonists in drug addiction. Expert Opin Investig Drugs 11:491–499, 2002a

Kosten TR, Rosen M, Bond J, et al: Human therapeutic cocaine vaccine: safety and immunogenicity. Vaccine 20:1196–1204, 2002b

Kosten T, Oliveto A, Feingold A, et al: Desipramine and contingency management for cocaine and opiate dependence in buprenorphine maintained patients. Drug Alcohol Depend 70:315–325, 2003

Kranzler HR, Bauer LO, Hersh D, et al: Carbamazepine treatment of cocaine dependence: a placebo-controlled trial. Drug Alcohol Depend 38:203–211, 1995

Levin FR, Lehman AF: Meta-analysis of desipramine: an adjunct in the treatment of cocaine addiction. J Clin Pharmacol 11:374–378, 1991

Lima MS, Reisser AA, Soares BG, et al: Antidepressants for cocaine dependence. Cochrane Database Syst Rev 4:CD002950, 2001

Ling W, Shoptaw S, Majewska D: Baclofen as a cocaine anticraving medication: a preliminary clinical study (letter). Neuropsychopharmacology 18:403–404, 1998

London ED, Cascella NG, Wong DF, et al: Cocaine-induced reduction of glucose utilization in human brain: a study using positron emission tomography and [fluorine 18]-fluorodeoxyglucose. Arch Gen Psychiatry 47:567–574, 1990

Maisonneuve IM, Archer S, Glick SD: U50, 488, a kappa opioid receptor agonist, attenuates cocaine-induced increases in extracellular dopamine in the nucleus accumbens of rats. Neurosci Lett 181:57–60, 1994

Malcolm R, Kajdasz DK, Herron J, et al: A double-blind, placebo-controlled outpatient trial of pergolide for cocaine dependence. Drug Alcohol Depend 60:161–168, 2000

Malison RT, Best SE, van Dyck CH, et al: Elevated striatal dopamine transporters during acute cocaine abstinence as measured by [123I] beta-CIT SPECT. Am J Psychiatry 155:832–834, 1998

Margolin A, Kosten TR, Avants SK, et al: A multicenter trial of bupropion for cocaine dependence in methadone-maintained patients. Drug Alcohol Depend 40:125–131, 1995

Montoya ID, Levin FR, Fudala PJ, et al: Double-blind comparison of carbamazepine and placebo for treatment of cocaine dependence. Drug Alcohol Depend 38:213–219, 1995

Nunes EV, Quitkin FM, Brady R, et al: Imipramine treatment of methadone maintenance patients with affective disorder and illicit drug use. Am J Psychiatry 148:667–669, 1991

Oliveto AH, Feingold A, Schottenfeld R, et al: Desipramine in opioid-dependent cocaine abusers maintained on buprenorphine vs methadone. Arch Gen Psychiatry 56:812–820, 1999

Rocha BA, Fumagalli F, Gainetdinov RR, et al: Cocaine self-administration in dopamine-transporter knockout mice. Nat Neurosci 1:132–137, 1998

Rothman RB, Partilla JS, Baumann MH, et al: Neurochemical neutralization of methamphetamine with high-affinity nonselective inhibitors of biogenic amine transporters: a pharmacological strategy for treating stimulant abuse. Synapse 35:222–227, 2000

Rounsaville BJ, Anton SF, Carroll KM, et al: Psychiatric diagnosis of treatment seeking cocaine abusers. Arch Gen Psychiatry 18:43–51, 1991

Satel SL, Southwick SM, Gawin FH: Clinical features of cocaine-induced paranoia. Am J Psychiatry 148:495–498, 1991

Schottenfeld RS, Pakes JR, Oliveto A, et al: Buprenorphine vs methadone maintenance treatment for concurrent opioid dependence and cocaine abuse. Arch Gen Psychiatry 54:713–720, 1997

Sevarino KA, Oliveto A, Kosten TR: Neurobiological adaptations to psychostimulants and opiates as a basis of treatment development. Ann NY Acad Sci 909:51–87, 2000

Silverman K, Higgins ST, Brooner RK, et al: Sustained cocaine abstinence in methadone maintenance patients through voucher-based reinforcement therapy. Arch Gen Psychiatry 53:409–415, 1996

Sora I, Wichems C, Takahashi N, et al: Cocaine reward models: conditioned place preference can be established in dopamine- and in serotonin-transporter knockout mice. Proc Natl Acad Sci U S A 95:7699–7704, 1998

Sora I, Hall FS, Andrews AM, et al: Molecular mechanisms of cocaine reward: combined dopamine and serotonin transporter knockouts eliminate cocaine place preference. Proc Natl Acad Sci U S A 98:5300–5305, 2001

Volkow ND, Mullani N, Gould KL, et al: Cerebral blood flow in chronic cocaine users: a study with positron emission tomography. Br J Psychiatry 152:641–648, 1988

Volkow ND, Fowler JS, Wolf AP, et al: Changes in brain glucose metabolism in cocaine dependence and withdrawal [see comments]. Am J Psychiatry 148:621–626, 1991

Volkow ND, Hitzemann R, Wang GJ, et al: Long-term frontal brain metabolic changes in cocaine abusers [published erratum appears in Synapse 12(1):86, 1992]. Synapse 11:184–190, 1992

Volkow ND, Ding YS, Fowler JS, et al: Cocaine addiction: hypothesis derived from imaging studies with PET. J Addict Dis 15:55–71, 1996a

Volkow ND, Fowler JS, Gatley SJ, et al: PET evaluation of the dopamine system of the human brain. J Nucl Med 37:1242–1256, 1996b

Volkow ND, Wang GJ, Fischman MW, et al: Relationship between subjective effects of cocaine and dopamine transporter occupancy. Nature 386:827–830, 1997

Volkow ND, Chang L, Wang GJ, et al: Low level of brain dopamine D$_2$ receptors in methamphetamine abusers: association with metabolism in the orbitofrontal cortex. Am J Psychiatry 158:2015–2021, 2001a

Volkow ND, Chang L, Wang GJ, et al: Association of dopamine transporter reduction with psychomotor impairment in methamphetamine abusers. Am J Psychiatry 158:377–382, 2001b

Weiss RD, Mirin SM, Michael JL, et al: Psychopathology in chronic cocaine abusers. Am J Drug Alcohol Abuse 12:17–29, 1986

White FJ, Kalivas PW: Neuroadaptations involved in amphetamine and cocaine addiction. Drug Alcohol Depend 51:141–153, 1998

Woods SW, O'Malley SS, Martini BL, et al: SPECT regional cerebral blood flow and neuropsychological testing in non-demented HIV-positive drug abusers: preliminary results. Prog Neuropsychopharmacol Biol Psychiatry 15:649–662, 1991

Ziedonis DM, Kosten TR: Depression as a prognostic factor for pharmacological treatment of cocaine dependence. Psychopharmacol Bull 27:337–343, 1991

Hallucinogens

Robert N. Pechnick, Ph.D.
J. Thomas Ungerleider, M.D.

Hallucinogens that are likely to be abused include the ergot hallucinogen lysergic acid diethylamide (LSD), which is the prototype of these drugs of abuse; other indolealkylamines such as psilocybin ("magic mushrooms") and dimethyltryptamine (DMT; also contained in the South American beverage ayahuasca); and the phenalkylamines, including mescaline and dimethoxymethylamphetamine (DOM; "STP"). Other drugs with hallucinogenic activity—marijuana, phencyclidine (PCP), ketamine, and the so-called *stimulant-hallucinogens,* methylenedioxyamphetamine (MDA), and methylenedioxymethamphetamine (MDMA; "Ecstasy" or "X")—are covered elsewhere in this volume. The hallucinogens, called *psychotomimetics* or *psychedelics* (mind-manifesting), are a group of drugs that produce thought, mood, and perceptual disorders. Depending on dosage, expectation (set), and environment (setting), they also can induce euphoria and a state similar to a transcendental experience.

The term *hallucinogen* means "producer of hallucinations." Many drugs can cause auditory and/or visual hallucinations. These hallucinations may be present as part of a delirium, accompanied by disturbances in judgment, orientation, intellect, memory, and emotion (e.g., an organic brain syndrome). Such delirium also may result from drug withdrawal (e.g., sedative-hypnotic withdrawal or delirium tremens in alcohol withdrawal). When referring to substance abuse, however, the term *hallucinogens* generally refers to a group of compounds that alter consciousness without delirium, sedation, excessive stimulation, or impairment of intellect or memory. The label *hallucinogen* actually is inaccurate because true LSD-induced hallucinations are rare. What are commonly seen are illusory phenomena. An *illusion* is a perceptual distortion of an actual stimulus in the environment. To "see" someone's face melting is an illusion; to "see" a melting face when no one is present is a hallucination. Consequently, some have called these drugs *illusionogenic.* Those who use the terms *psychedelic* (coined in 1957 by Osmond) or *mind-manifesting* for hallucinogens have been criticized as being "pro-drug" much as those who use the term *hallucinogen* have been accused of being "anti-drug" (Osmond 1957). The term *psychotomimetic,* meaning "producer of psychosis," also has been widely used.

Peyote, containing mescaline, is the only hallucinogen that can be legally used in the United States, and even this practice has been challenged. Members of Native American religious communities have used it during certain ceremonies in several states and in Canada for many years.

The data on the availability of hallucinogens and the prevalence of their use must be evaluated with caution because some of the earlier studies included MDMA and PCP in the hallucinogen category. Thus, the data were confounded by changes in the patterns of use of these two drugs. From 1966 to 1970 the number of first-time hallucinogen users increased almost sixfold (Substance Abuse and Mental Health Services Administration 2003). Then the focus of illicit drug use shifted away from drugs that were once used in an attempt to enhance self-awareness and turned to drugs that were thought to elevate mood and increase work output, such as cocaine. The annual prevalence of hallucinogen use declined from the mid-1970s through the 1980s. College students, followed up 1–4 years beyond high school, showed an annual prevalence rate for LSD that steadily dropped from 6% in 1980 to 3.4% in 1989 (Johnston 1990). The estimated availability of LSD also decreased fairly steadily from 1975 to 1989 (Johnston 1990). A second period of apparent increased first-time use began in 1992. This was at least partially driven by the inclusion of MDMA in the hallucinogen category (Substance Abuse and Mental Health Services Administration 2003); however, there were clear indications that LSD was making a comeback (Johnston et al. 1996; R.H. Schwartz 1995). For example, the Washington, D.C., Board of the Drug Enforcement Administration confiscated 14 doses of LSD in 1990 and 5,600 doses in 1991. The annual survey of high school seniors found that in 1990 and 1991, for the first time since 1976, more seniors had used LSD than cocaine in the previous 12 months (Nagy 1992; Seligmann et al. 1992). In 1992, the prevalence of the use of LSD increased in school-age children and young adults. In 1994, the annual prevalence rates for LSD use were 7% in high school students and 5% in college students, and the lifetime prevalence rates for LSD and hallucinogen use were 3.7% and 2.2%, respectively, for students in the eighth grade and 13.8% and 7.4%, respectively, for young adults (Johnston et al. 1996). Other studies showed even higher rates of hallucinogen use. For example, a random survey of Tulane University undergraduates in 1990 indicated that the number of students reporting having tried LSD was more than 17% (Cuomo et al. 1994). More recently, the use of LSD has decreased in high school stu-

dents. Between 2001 and 2002, lifetime, past year, and past month use of LSD decreased in eighth, tenth, and twelfth graders (Johnston et al. 2003). In 2002 the annual prevalence rate for LSD use in twelfth graders was 3.5%. With respect to older individuals, between 2000 and 2001, the percentage reporting lifetime use of LSD increased from 14% to 15.3% in the 18–25 age group, whereas the lifetime use of other hallucinogens (peyote, mescaline, and psilocybin) remained constant (Substance Abuse and Mental Health Services Administration 2003). The percentage reporting lifetime use of hallucinogens in the 26 or older group also showed no change. There are ethnic differences in the use of hallucinogens: whites have higher use of LSD and hallucinogens compared with blacks, Asians, and Hispanics (Johnston et al. 1996; Substance Abuse and Mental Health Services Administration 2003). In recent years, the Internet has become a widely used source of information on hallucinogens (Halpern and Hope 2001) and a vehicle for obtaining the drugs (Al-Assmar 1999).

Another new development is that although from the mid-1980s to the mid-1990s little research was conducted on hallucinogen administration to humans, since that time there has been a resurgence of clinical studies carried out under highly controlled conditions (Gouzoulis-Mayfrank et al. 1999; Hermle et al. 1992; Riba et al. 2001; Strassman 1995; Strassman and Qualls 1994; Strassman et al. 1994; Vollenweider et al. 1998, 1999). The results obtained from controlled clinical studies should provide important and unbiased information, in contrast to some of the clinical data that have come from anecdotal information obtained from limited first-person accounts (Shulgin and Shulgin 1991), "street pharmacologists," or hospital emergency department records. There also has been a resumption of interest in the use of hallucinogens for the treatment of disorders (Grob 2002), such as alcoholism (Mangini 1998). The resurgence in clinical research has taken place at the same time as the major advances in the possible mechanisms of action of the hallucinogens. We may be reaching a point at which we can begin to develop a unified conceptual framework regarding the fundamental mechanisms underlying pharmacological effects of hallucinogens in humans, which might lead to advances in the pharmacological treatment of some adverse effects of these drugs and the development of new approaches to treat various mental disorders, such as obsessive-compulsive disorder (Delgado and Moreno 1998; Perrine 1999).

LSD initially was used in the 1960s primarily by those interested in its ability to alter perceptual experiences (i.e., sight, sound, and taste). Much attention was paid to "set," the expectation of what the drug experience would be like, and "setting," the environment in which the drug was used. Thus, the early drug missionaries promulgated the erroneous notion that only good LSD "trips" would result if the prospective user ensured some preconditions for his or her drug experience, including a guide. In more recent times, users have attended concerts, films (particularly psychedelic or brightly colored ones), or "rave" parties during the drug experience. Users rarely indulge more than once weekly because tolerance to LSD occurs so rapidly.

No abstinence syndrome occurs after repeated use of hallucinogens. Thus, no detoxification for the chronic effects of the hallucinogens and little direct pharmacotherapy for toxic effects are required. We therefore focus on the acute and chronic effects of these drugs and the psychosocial interventions necessary to treat the adverse reactions. LSD is discussed as the prototypical hallucinogen.

Physiological Effects

Hallucinogens such as LSD produce significant autonomic activity. They can dilate the pupils, increase the heart rate, and produce slight hypertension and hyperthermia. While under the influence, the face may flush and the deep tendon reflexes quicken. On occasion, piloerection, salivation, nausea, a fine tremor, and lacrimation may be noted. In addition, a minor degree of incoordination, restlessness, and visual blurring can occur. A stress response with elevation of 17-hydroxycorticoids may be present.

DMT and ayahuasca (which contains DMT) also increase heart rate, pupil diameter, and body temperature, and DMT elevates plasma levels of corticotropin, cortisol, and prolactin (Riba et al. 2001; Strassman and Qualls 1994). Some of these autonomic effects of the hallucinogens are variable and may be due, in part, to the anxiety state of the user. LSD also can cause nausea; nausea and sometimes vomiting are especially noteworthy after the ingestion of mescaline.

In terms of adverse physiological effects, LSD has a very high therapeutic index. The lethal dose in humans has not been determined, and fatalities that have been reported usually are secondary to perceptual distortions with resultant accidental death. Overdose with the psychotomimetic drugs is rare. Instances are known of people surviving 10,000 mg of LSD, 100 times the average dose. Hemiplegia has been reported after taking LSD, possibly a result of the production of vasospasm (Sobel et al. 1971). More recently, a fibrotic inflammatory mass located in the mesentery was reported in a chronic LSD user (Berk et al. 1999), and multifocal cerebral demyelination was reported after the use of magic mushrooms (Spengos et al. 2000). Although mescaline is often viewed as posing a minimal health risk, a case of fatal peyote ingestion associated with Mallory-Weiss lacerations, probably as a result of peyote-induced vomiting, has been reported (Nolte and Zumwalt 1999). There is no generally accepted evidence of brain cell damage, chromosomal abnormalities, or teratogenic effects after the use of the indole-type hallucinogens and mescaline (Li and Lin 1998; Strassman 1984).

Drug interactions involving the hallucinogens do not appear to be an important source of adverse reactions. In some reports, the effects of LSD were reduced after the chronic administration of monoamine oxidase inhibitors or selective serotonin reuptake inhibitor antidepressants such as fluoxetine, whereas the effects of LSD were increased after the chronic administration of lithium or tricyclic antidepressants (Bonson and Murphy 1996; Bonson et al. 1996; Resnick et al. 1964; Strassman 1992).

Psychological Effects

When the hallucinogens are taken orally, the psychic phenomena noted vary considerably, depending on the amount consumed and the set and the setting of both the subject and the observer. The overall psychological effects of the hallucinogens are quite similar; however, the rate of onset, duration of action, and absolute intensity of the effects can differ. Both Hofmann (1961) and Hollister (1978) described the effects of LSD in great detail. The absorption of LSD from the gastrointestinal tract and other mucous membranes occurs rapidly, with drug diffusion to all tissues, including the brain and across the placenta to the fetus. The onset of psychological and behavioral effects occurs approximately 30–60 minutes after oral administration and peaks at 2–4 hours after administration, with a gradual return to the predrug state in 8–12 hours. DMT produces similar effects but is inactive after oral administration and thus must be injected, sniffed, or smoked. It has a very rapid onset and short duration of action (60–120 minutes) (Strassman and Qualls 1994; Strassman et al. 1994). Thus, DMT previously was known as the "businessman's LSD" (i.e., one could have a psychedelic experience over the lunch hour and be back at work in the afternoon). The effects of psilocybin last about 2 hours (Vollenweider et al. 1998), and those of ayahuasca last approximately 4 hours (Riba et al. 2001). In contrast, the effects of DOM have been reported to last for longer than 24 hours.

The various hallucinogens also differ widely in potency and slope of the dose-response curve. Thus, some of the apparent qualitative differences between hallucinogens may be due, in part, to the amount of drug ingested relative to its specific dose-response characteristics. LSD is one of the most potent hallucinogens known, with behavioral effects occurring in some individuals after doses as low as 20 μg. Typical street doses range from 70 to 300 μg. Because of its high potency, LSD can be applied to paper blotters or to the backs of postage stamps. Some anecdotal evidence indicates that today's street LSD is less potent than that available in the 1960s: 20–80 μg versus 150–250 μg. It should be pointed out that reports of street dose are often highly inaccurate.

Perceptual alterations are notable with the hallucinogens; the initial subjective effect may be a colorful display of geometric patterns appearing before one's closed eyes. Distorted human, animal, or other forms may be projected onto the visual fields. With the eyes open, the color of perceived objects intensifies. Afterimages are remarkably prolonged; fixed objects may undulate and flow. Such illusions are common and may be given personal or idiosyncratic meaning. Auditory hallucinations are seldom described, but hyperacusis is commonly reported. Greater sensitivity to touch is regularly noticed, and sometimes taste and smell are altered. Synesthesia is frequently described, with an overflow from one sense modality into another; colors are "heard," and sounds are "seen." Subjective time is frequently affected; users often feel that time is standing still. Hypersuggestibility and distractibility are notable, perhaps because the critical functions of the ego become diminished or are absent.

The emotional responses to the hallucinogens can vary markedly. Initial apprehension or mild anxiety is common, but the most frequent response is one of euphoria. Elation and a "blissful calm" also have been de-

scribed. Less frequently, tension and anxiety culminating in panic have occurred. The mood is labile, shifting easily from happiness to depression and back. Prolonged laughter or tears may seem inappropriate emotional responses to any situation. Complete withdrawal (catatonic states) (Perera et al. 1995) and severe paranoid reactions have been encountered. An alternating intensification and fading out of the experience is present, with the subject going deeply into and out of the intoxicated state.

Performance on tests involving attention, concentration, and motivation is impaired. Thought processes are significantly altered under the influence of hallucinogenic drugs. A loosening of associations is regularly noted. Thoughts are nonlogical and fantasy laden. Thoughts flood consciousness; on the other hand, a complete absence of thought occurs on occasion. Intelligence test scores drop, but this may be due to a lack of motivation to perform or a preoccupation with the unusual experiences. Orientation is ordinarily not impaired, but judgments are not reliable. Paranoid grandiosity and, less frequently, persecutory ideation are common.

Changes in ego functioning may be imperceptible at the lower dosage ranges; however, the ego can be completely disrupted when large amounts of hallucinogens have been ingested. At first, one observes the ego's usual defense mechanisms operating to cope with these perceptions. Eventually, the ego may become overwhelmed to the point that depersonalization occurs. Current external events may not be differentiated from remote memories. The body image is frequently distorted, and the parts of the body may seem to become larger, to become smaller, or to disappear completely.

Few, if any, long-term neuropsychological deficits are attributable to hallucinogen use (Halpern and Pope 1999). Chronic personality changes with a shift in attitudes and evidence of magical thinking also can occur after the use of hallucinogens. An atypical schizophrenic-like state may persist, but whether the use of hallucinogens causes or only unmasks a predisposition to this condition is unclear. There is always the associated risk that self-destructive behavior may occur during both the acute and the chronic reaction (e.g., thinking one can fly and jumping out of a window). In addition, the hallucinogenic drugs interact in various nonspecific ways with the personality, which may particularly impair the developing adolescent (D. Miller 1973). Today, many chronic LSD users eventually come to use a variety of drugs (polydrug or multiple drug use), particularly marijuana, the sedative-hypnotics, and stimulants. This is a marked departure from the LSD users seen in the 1960s, whose entire lifestyle was organized around the use of hallucinogens and involvement in the psychedelic subculture, adopting the motto "turn on, tune in, drop out."

Diagnosis

The diagnosis of hallucinogen exposure is normally made from the patient's or an accompanying individual's report. The diagnosis can be made clinically when an individual is actively hallucinating, is having delusions, and is describing illusions, changes in body size or shape, slowing of time, and a waxing and waning of these and related symptoms. Ordinarily, the individual is able to report having taken a substance prior to the acute onset of the symptoms. The presence of dilated pupils, tachycardia, and quickened deep tendon reflexes increases the possibility that a hallucinogen has been consumed.

The routine clinical drug screen does not include testing for the hallucinogens in body fluids. However, they can be detected in the research laboratory in blood, and for longer periods in urine, by thin-layer chromatography, gas chromatography, fluorometry, or gas chromatography–mass spectrometry (Basalt 1982). A radioimmunoassay for LSD is also available. Shifts in body metabolism from hallucinogen ingestion are insufficient to induce specific abnormalities in blood chemistries, blood counts, or urine analyses.

The differential diagnosis of the psychotomimetic state includes consumption of delirium-inducing drugs such as the atropine-like agents or the atypical hallucinogens PCP and tetrahydrocannabinol (THC) in marijuana. Many drugs can produce a toxic psychosis, but this state can readily be differentiated from the psychotomimetic picture. In a toxic psychosis, confusion and loss of some aspects of orientation are present, whereas with hallucinogens, the perceptual changes occur with a clear sensorium, intact orientation, and retention of recent and remote memory. In addition, the hallucinogens produce electroencephalographic arousal, whereas drugs that cause delirium result in slowing of the electroencephalogram (Fink and Itil 1968). Atropine poisoning can be differentiated by the presence of prominent anticholinergic ef-

fects such as dry mouth and blurred vision. The THC psychosis frequently occurs with drowsiness rather than with the hyperalertness characteristic of the LSD state. PCP psychosis is accompanied by marked neurological signs (e.g., vertical nystagmus, ataxia) and more pronounced autonomic effects than are seen with the psychotomimetics. Patients with amphetamine psychoses often fail to differentiate their perceptual distortions from reality, whereas LSD users are usually aware of the difference.

The differential diagnosis also must distinguish between an acute schizophrenic reaction and a hallucinogen-induced (or other drug-induced) psychosis. The differentiation is not always easily made. It should be recalled that initial research interest in LSD arose because of the possibility that it might provide an artificially induced model of schizophrenia. The hypothesis that LSD induces a *model psychosis* similar to schizophrenia has several serious shortcomings, and investigators who used single-photon emission computed tomography (SPECT) found that the administration of mescaline to control subjects produced a "hyperfrontal" pattern, whereas "hypofrontality" has been observed in schizophrenic patients (Hermle et al. 1992). However, Gouzoulis-Mayfrank et al. (1999) used positron emission tomography and found that psilocybin produced changes in glucose metabolism similar to those in acute schizophrenia. Nevertheless, the use of the potent hallucinogens can have a variety of effects on the individual who is predisposed to schizophrenia: 1) they may cause the psychosis to become manifest at an earlier age, 2) they may produce a psychosis that would have remained dormant if drugs had not been used, or 3) they may cause relapse in an individual who has had a psychotic disorder (Bowers 1987).

It also has become more difficult to distinguish between LSD psychosis and paranoid schizophrenia, particularly because patients who are in fact paranoid often now complain of being poisoned with LSD, much as they once felt that they were being talked about on radio or on television programs. Hallucinations in schizophrenic psychosis are usually auditory, in contrast to the predominantly visual hallucinations from psychotomimetics. A history of mental illness; a psychiatric examination that indicates the absence of an intact, observing ego; auditory (rather than visual) hallucinations; and the lack of development of drug tolerance all suggest schizophrenia. An organic brain syndrome in general speaks against LSD, especially if obtunded consciousness is also present. The brief re-active schizophrenic psychosis is of sudden onset but usually follows psychosocial stressors and is associated with emotional turmoil.

Intervention

Intervention With the Acute Adverse Reactions

Once commonly reported by medical facilities (Ungerleider et al. 1968b), acute adverse LSD reactions are rarely seen today. The paucity of users seeking emergency medical treatment may reflect increased knowledge of how to deal with such situations on the part of the drug-using community, as well as a decrease in the doses of LSD currently used compared with those used in the past. An individual's experience of the effects of the drug may be either pleasant or un-pleasant; a perceptual distortion or illusion may provide intense anxiety in one individual and be a pleasant interlude for another. Social factors, media presentations, and public fear have all shaped perceptions of the drug's effects. Individuals who place a premium on self-control, planning, and impulse restriction may do particularly poorly on LSD. Prediction of who will have an adverse reaction is unreliable (Ungerleider et al. 1968a). The occurrence of multiple previous good LSD experiences renders no immunity from an adverse reaction. Traumatic and stressful external events can precipitate an adverse reaction (e.g., being arrested and read one's rights in the middle of a pleasant experience may precipitate an anxiety reaction). Thus, acute adverse behavioral reactions generally are not dose related but are a function of personal predisposition, set, and setting. Adverse reactions have occurred after doses of LSD as low as 40 μg, and no effects have been reported from using 2,000 μg, although in general the hallucinogenic effects are proportional to dosage levels.

Acute dysphoric reactions are commonly known as "bummers" or "bad trips." These reactions are caused by loss of control, the inability to cope with ego dissolution, and/or marked environmental dissonance. The result is anxiety and, in some instances, panic. The acute anxiety/panic reactions usually wear off before medical intervention is sought. Symptoms of these acute reactions are best managed by using the hypersuggestibility of the hallucinogenic state to calm and reassure the individual that he or she will be protected and that the condition will soon subside. Thus, the use years ago of a "guide," "sitter," or "baby-sitter" prevented marked anxiety from developing. Most LSD is metabolized and excreted within 24 hours, and most panic reactions are usually over within this time frame.

Acute paranoid states are adverse responses resulting from the hypervigilant state, overreading of external cues, and the unusual thoughts that occur in the course of the hallucinogenic experience. Although likely to be grandiose or megalomaniacal, they sometimes are manifested by suspiciousness and persecutory thoughts. Occasionally a confusional state (organic brain syndrome) can occur (Ungerleider 1972), and depression with suicidal ideation can develop several days after drug use (Madden 1994). Some of the adverse reactions that occur after the ingestion of hallucinogens can be caused by other contaminants in the product, such as strychnine, PCP, and amphetamine.

Treatment of the acute adverse reactions to hallucinogens first must be directed toward preventing the patient from physically harming himself or herself or others. Because the anxiety and paranoid reactions from hallucinogens may last for an hour or for a few days, the patient may require unobtrusive protection for an extended time. Reassurance and support, or the *talkdown,* is done in a quiet, pleasant environment, usually in a homelike setting. Because closing the eyes intensifies the state, the patient should sit up or walk about. Reminding the patient that a drug has produced the extraordinary ideas and feelings and that they will soon disappear may be helpful. The time sense distortion that makes minutes seem like hours also should be explained.

If drugs are needed for continuing panicky feelings, a benzodiazepine such as lorazepam can be given. Such medication can be administered orally in mildly agitated patients; however, it can be difficult to convince severely agitated and/or paranoid patients to swallow a pill, in which case parenteral administration might be necessary. Severely agitated patients who do not respond to a benzodiazepine may be given a neuroleptic agent. Caution must be used in administering neuroleptics because they can lower the seizure threshold and elicit seizures, especially if the hallucinogen has been cut with an agent that has convulsant activity, such as strychnine. Phenothiazines, such as chlorpromazine, given orally or intramuscularly can end an LSD trip and have been effective in treating LSD-induced psychosis (Cohen 1978; Dewhurst and Hatrick 1972; D. Miller 1973; Neff 1973). Because anticholinergic crises can develop with chlorpromazine in combination with other drugs with anticholinergic activity (PCP and DOM), haloperidol is a safer drug to use when the true nature of the drug ingested is unknown. Moreover, paradoxical reactions have been reported, with an increase in anxiety after the administration of phenothiazines (C.J. Schwartz 1968). It has been suggested that a combination of intramuscular haloperidol and lorazepam is particularly effective in treating acute adverse reactions (P.L. Miller et al. 1992). Theoretically, selective serotonin type 2A receptor (5-HT_{2A}) antagonists should block the acute effects of hallucinogens; however, other drugs with significant 5-HT_{2A} antagonist activity (clozapine, olanzapine, and risperidone) also might be effective (Aghajanian 1994). Vollenweider et al. (1998) found that the psychotomimetic effects of psilocybin are blocked by the 5-HT_{2A} antagonists ketanserin and risperidone; however, haloperidol *increased* the psychotomimetic effects. It should be noted that there is some indication that risperidone might exacerbate flashbacks (Abraham and Mamen 1996; Morehead 1997).

Intervention With the Chronic Adverse Reactions

Chronic adverse reactions include psychoses, depressive reactions, acting out, paranoid states, and flashbacks (Fisher 1972). The effects of the chronic use of LSD must be differentiated from the clinical picture seen with personality disorders, particularly in those who use a variety of drugs in polydrug abuse–type patterns. Personality changes that result from LSD use may occur after a single experience, unlike that with other classes of drugs—PCP, perhaps, excepted (Fisher 1972). In some individuals with well-integrated personalities and no psychiatric history, chronic personality changes also have resulted from repeated LSD use. In addition, the hallucinogenic drugs interact in various nonspecific ways with the personality, which may particularly impair the developing adolescent (D. Miller 1973). The suggestibility that may come from many experiences with LSD may be reinforced by the social values of a particular subculture in which the drug is used. For instance, if some of these subcultures embrace withdrawal from society and a noncompeti-

tive approach toward life, the person who withdraws after the LSD experience(s) may be enduring a side effect that represents more of a change in social values than a physiological drug effect. Use of hallucinogens can lead to a diminution in a variety of acceptable social behaviors.

Schizophreniform reactions lasting from weeks to years have followed the psychotomimetic experience. Closely following a dysphoric experience or developing shortly after a positive one, the manifestations of psychosis may emerge and persist. Although these reactions are most likely to be precipitated in characterologically predisposed individuals who have decompensated after the upsurge of repressed material overwhelms their ego defenses, it is unclear whether hallucinogen use can "cause" long-term psychosis or if it has a role in precipitating the onset of illness (Hekimian and Gershon 1968). Although some evidence indicates that prolonged psychotic reactions tend to occur in individuals with poor premorbid adjustment, a history of psychiatric illness, and/or repeated use of hallucinogens, severe and prolonged illness has been reported in individuals without such a history (Strassman 1984). The management of these prolonged psychotic reactions does not differ from that of schizophrenia. Neuroleptics are used, sometimes in a residential setting when behavioral dysfunction makes it necessary. These patients often attempt self-medication, and serious polydrug abuse patterns have been seen (Wesson and Smith 1978). The prognosis of these psychotic states is usually favorable; however, a few remain recalcitrant to treatment.

Chronic Anxiety and Depressive States

It is evident that to some individuals (perhaps to everyone under adverse circumstances) the LSD experience can be an unsettling one. In general, the psyche is capable of reconstituting itself surprisingly well within a reasonable period. Anxiety and depression continue for unusually long periods in a few individuals, however, and they may attribute these feelings to whatever psychotomimetic they took. The use of LSD has been found to coincide with the onset of depression, suggesting its possible role in the etiology of some depression in the young (Abraham and Fava 1999). It is difficult to know how much of the state that sometimes occurs is caused by a disruption of psychological homeostasis and how much is caused by a fragile personality that was exposed to it. At any rate, the anxiety and depression may persist despite psychiatric therapy and antianxiety and/or antidepressant medication.

Nondrug antianxiety techniques such as relaxation exercises and behavior therapy may be helpful. The clinician should not accede to the magical thinking of the patient that maybe another psychedelic session (or doubling the dose) might reshuffle the psychological fragments back into their premorbid pattern.

Flashbacks

A well-publicized adverse reaction unique to the hallucinogens is the *flashback*. Flashbacks have been renamed *hallucinogen persisting perception disorder* and have specific diagnostic criteria (American Psychiatric Association 2000). In the past, the use of variable definitions of what constitutes a flashback was a major problem (Frankel 1994), and it is hoped that the establishment of specific diagnostic criteria will facilitate studying and understanding this problem. Flashbacks are the apparently spontaneous recrudescence of the same effects that were experienced during the psychotomimetic state. These effects are usually brief visual, temporal, or emotional recurrences, complete with perceptive (time) and reality distortion, that may first appear days or months after the last drug exposure. They do not appear to be dose related and can develop after a single exposure to the drug (Levi and Miller 1990), and they can continue to recur spontaneously several weeks or months after the original drug experience. Because flashbacks appear suddenly, unexpectedly, and inappropriately, the emotional response to them may be one of dread. Even a previously pleasant drug experience may be accompanied by anxiety when the person realizes there is no way to control its recurrence. Fear of insanity may arise because no external cause for the strange, often recurrent, phenomena is apparent. However, some seem to enjoy the experience. Only a small proportion of LSD and other hallucinogen users experience flashbacks (Shick and Smith 1970). Flashbacks may or may not be precipitated by stressors, fatigue, or subsequent use of another psychedelic such as psilocybin or marijuana. Administration of selective serotonin reuptake inhibitor antidepressants (Markel et al. 1994) and risperidone (Alcantara 1998; Lerner et al. 2002b) has been reported to initiate or exacerbate flashbacks in individuals with a history of LSD use.

The exact mechanism underlying flashbacks remains obscure. These recurrences may represent a response learned during a state of hyperarousal (Cohen 1981). LSD users have been shown to have long-term changes in visual function (Abraham 1982; Abraham and Aldridge 1993; Abraham and Duffy 2001; Abraham and Wolf 1988). For example, a visual disturbance consisting of prolonged afterimages (palinopsia) has been found in individuals several years after the last reported use of LSD (Kawasaki and Purvin 1996). Such changes in visual function might underlie flashbacks. Individuals with flashbacks appear to have a high lifetime incidence of mood disorder compared with non-LSD-abusing substance abusers (Abraham and Aldridge 1994). Various pharmacological agents, such as clonidine or clonazepam (Lerner et al. 2002a), or drug combinations (e.g., fluoxetine and olanzapine; Aldurra and Crayton 2001) have been found to be useful in the treatment of flashbacks. Flashbacks also can usually be handled with psychotherapy. In time, flashbacks usually decrease in intensity, frequency, and duration (although initially they often last only a few seconds), whether treated (with pharmacotherapy and/or reassurance) or not.

Treatment of chronic hallucinogen abuse usually involves long-term psychotherapy to determine—*after* cessation of use—what needs are being fulfilled by the long-term use of the drug for this particular person. Support in the form of 12-step program meetings and family involvement also is crucial to reinforce the decision to remain abstinent. The most important aspect of treatment consists of reassurance that the condition will pass, that the brain is not damaged, and that the hallucinogen is not retained in the brain. If the patient is agitated because of repeated flashbacks, an anxiolytic drug is indicated. The patient's physical and mental status should improve with the appropriate hygienic measures, and all substances with hallucinogenic activity, including marijuana, must be avoided. If no flashbacks have occurred during the 1–2 years since the last ingestion of the hallucinogen, it is unlikely that any more will occur.

Summary

We have discussed the psychotropic drugs called hallucinogens from several perspectives, including the acute and chronic adverse effects of these drugs, their patterns of abuse, and their relation to mental illness. Diagnostic and treatment issues have been considered. We have emphasized the prototype hallucinogen LSD.

References

Abraham HD: A chronic impairment of colour vision in users of LSD. Br J Psychiatry 140:518–520, 1982

Abraham HD, Aldridge AM: Adverse consequences of lysergic acid diethylamide. Addiction 88:1327–1334, 1993

Abraham HD, Aldridge AM: LSD: a point well taken. Addiction 89:762–763, 1994

Abraham HD, Duffy FH: EEG coherence in post-LSD visual hallucinations. Psychiatry Res 107:151–163, 2001

Abraham HD, Fava M: Order of onset of substance abuse and depression in a sample of depressed outpatients. Compr Psychiatry 40:44–50, 1999

Abraham HD, Mamen A: LSD-like panic from risperidone in post-LSD visual disorder. J Clin Psychopharmacol 16:238–241, 1996

Abraham HD, Wolf E: Visual function in past users of LSD: psychophysical findings. J Abnorm Psychol 97:443–447, 1988

Aghajanian GK: Serotonin and the action of LSD in the brain. Psychiatr Ann 24:137–141, 1994

Al-Assmar SE: The seeds of the Hawaiian baby woodrose are a powerful hallucinogen (letter). Arch Intern Med 59:2090, 1999

Alcantara AG: Is there a role for the alpha2 antagonism in the exacerbation of hallucinogen-persisting perception disorder with risperidone? (comment). J Clin Psychopharmacol 18:487–488, 1998

Aldurra G, Crayton JW: Improvement of hallucinogen persisting perception disorder by treatment with a combination of fluoxetine and olanzapine: case report. J Clin Psychopharmacol 21:343–344, 2001

American Psychiatric Association: Diagnostic and Statistical Manual of Mental Disorders, 4th Edition, Text Revision. Washington, DC, American Psychiatric Association, 2000

Basalt RC: Disposition of Toxic Drugs and Chemicals in Man. Davis, CA, Biomedical Publications, 1982

Berk SI, LeBlond RF, Hodges KB, et al: A mesenteric mass in a chronic LSD user. Am J Med 107:188–198, 1999

Bonson KR, Murphy DL: Alterations in responses to LSD in humans associated with chronic administration of tricyclic antidepressants, monoamine oxidase inhibitors or lithium. Behav Brain Res 73:229–233, 1996

Bonson KR, Buckholtz JW, Murphy DL: Chronic administration of serotonergic antidepressants attenuates the subjective effects of LSD in humans. Neuropsychopharmacology 14:425–437, 1996

Bowers MB Jr: The role of drugs in the production of schizophreniform psychoses and related disorders, in Psychopharmacology: The Third Generation of Progress. Edited by Meltzer HY. New York, Raven, 1987, pp 819–828

Cohen S: Psychotomimetics (hallucinogens) and cannabis, in Principles of Psychopharmacology. Edited by Clark WG, del Gudice J. New York, Academic Press, 1978, pp 357–371

Cohen S: The Substance Abuse Problems. New York, Haworth, 1981

Cuomo MJ, Dyment PG, Gamino VM: Increasing use of "ecstasy" (MDMA) and other hallucinogens on a college campus. J Am Coll Health 42:271–274, 1994

Delgado PL, Moreno FA: Hallucinogens, serotonin and obsessive-compulsive disorder. J Psychedelic Drugs 30:359–366, 1998

Dewhurst K, Hatrick JA: Differential diagnosis and treatment of lysergic acid diethylamide-induced psychosis. Practitioner 209:327–332, 1972

Fink M, Itil TM: Neurophysiology of phantastica: EEG and behavioral relations in man, in Psychopharmacology: A Review of Progress, 1957–1967. Edited by Efrom DH. Washington, DC, U.S. Department of Health, Education, and Welfare, 1968, pp 1231–1239

Fisher DD: The chronic side effects from LSD, in The Problems and Prospects of LSD. Edited by Ungerleider JT. Springfield, IL, Charles C Thomas, 1972, pp 69–80

Frankel FH: The concept of flashbacks in historical perspective. Int J Clin Exp Hypn 42:321–335, 1994

Gouzoulis-Mayfrank E, Schreckenberger M, Sabri O, et al: Neurometabolic effects of psilocybin, 3,4-methylenedioxyethylamphetamine (MDE) and d-methamphetamine in healthy volunteers. Neuropsychopharmacology 20:565–581, 1999

Grob CS: Psychiatric research with hallucinogens: what have we learned, in Hallucinogens, A Reader. Edited by Grob CS. New York, Jeremy P Tarcher/Putnam, 2002, pp 263–291

Halpern JH, Pope HG Jr: Do hallucinogens cause residual neuropsychological toxicity? Drug Alcohol Depend 53:247–256, 1999

Halpern JH, Pope HG Jr: Hallucinogens on the internet: a vast new source of underground drug information. Am J Psychiatry 158:481–483, 2001

Hekimian LJ, Gershon S: Characteristics of drug abusers admitted to a psychiatric hospital. JAMA 205:75–80, 1968

Hermle L, Fünfgeld M, Oepen G, et al: Mescaline-induced psychopathological, neuropsychological, and neurometabolic effects in normal subjects: experimental psychosis as a tool for psychiatric research. Biol Psychiatry 32:976–991, 1992

Hofmann A: Chemical, pharmacological, and medical aspects of psychotomimetics. J Exp Med Sci 5:31–51, 1961

Hollister LE: Psychotomimetic drugs in man, in Handbook of Psychopharmacology, Vol II. Edited by Iversen LL, Iversen SD, Snyder SH. New York, Plenum, 1978, pp 389–424

Johnston L: Monitoring the Future: The National High School Senior Survey. Rockville, MD, National Institute on Drug Abuse, 1990

Johnston LD, O'Malley PM, Bachman JG: National Survey Results on Drug Use From the Monitoring the Future Study, 1975–1994, Vol II: College Students and Young Adults (NIH Publ No 96-4027). Rockville, MD, National Institute on Drug Abuse, 1996

Johnston LD, O'Malley PM, Bachman JG: Monitoring the Future National Survey Results on Drug Use, 1975–2002. Vol I: Secondary School Students (NIH Publ No 03-5385). Rockville, MD, National Institute on Drug Abuse, 2003

Kawasaki A, Purvin V: Persistent palinopsia following ingestion of lysergic acid diethylamide (LSD). Arch Ophthalmol 114:47–50, 1996

Lerner AG, Gelkopf M, Skladman I, et al: Flashback and hallucinogen persisting perception disorder: clinical aspects and pharmacological treatment approach. Isr J Psychiatry Relat Sci 39:92–99, 2002a

Lerner AG, Shufman E, Kodesh A, et al: Risperidone-associated, benign transient visual disturbances in schizophrenic patients with a past history of LSD abuse. Isr J Psychiatry Relat Sci 39:57–60, 2002b

Levi L, Miller NR: Visual illusions associated with previous drug abuse. J Neuroophthalmol 10:103–110, 1990

Li J-H, Lin L-F: Genetic toxicology of abused drugs: a brief review. Mutagenesis 13:557–565, 1998

Madden JS: LSD and post-hallucinogenic perceptual disorder. Addiction 86:762–763, 1994

Mangini M: Treatment of alcoholism using psychedelic drugs: a review of the program of research. J Psychedelic Drugs 30:381–418, 1998

Markel H, Lee A, Holmes RD, et al: LSD flashback syndrome exacerbated by selective serotonin reuptake inhibitor antidepressants in adolescents. J Pediatr 125:817–819, 1994

Miller D: The drug dependent adolescent, in Adolescent Psychiatry, Vol 2. Edited by Feinstein SC, Giovachini P. New York, Basic Books, 1973, pp 70–97

Miller PL, Gay GR, Ferris KC, et al: Treatment of acute, adverse reactions: "I've tripped and I can't get down." J Psychoactive Drugs 24:277–279, 1992

Morehead DB: Exacerbation of hallucinogen-persisting perception disorder with risperidone. J Clin Psychopharmacol 17:327–328, 1997

Nagy J: A Comparison of Drug Use Among 8th, 10th, and 12th Graders From NIDA's High School Senior Survey. Rockville, MD, National Institute on Drug Abuse, 1992

Neff L: Chemicals and their effects on the adolescent ego, in Adolescent Psychiatry, Vol 1. Edited by Feinstein S, Giovacchini P, Miller A. New York, Basic Books, 1973, pp 108–120

Nolte KB, Zumwalt RE: Fatal peyote ingestion associated with Mallory-Weiss lacerations (letter). West J Med 170:328, 1999

Osmond H: A review of the clinical effects of psychotomimetic agents. Ann N Y Acad Sci 66:418–434, 1957

Perera KMH, Ferraro A, Pinto MRM: Catatonia LSD induced? Aust N Z J Psychiatry 29:324–327, 1995

Perrine DM: Hallucinogens and obsessive-compulsive disorder (comment). Am J Psychiatry 156:7, 1999

Resnick O, Krus DM, Raskin M: LSD-25 action in normal subjects treated with a monoamine oxidase inhibitor. Life Sci 3:1207–1214, 1964

Riba J, Rodriguez-Fornells A, Urbano G, et al: Subjective effects and tolerability of the South American psychoactive beverage ayahuasca in healthy volunteers. Psychopharmacology 154:85–95, 2001

Schwartz CJ: The complications of LSD: a review of the literature. J Nerv Ment Dis 146:174–186, 1968

Schwartz RH: LSD: its rise, fall, and renewed popularity among high school students. Pediatr Clin North Am 42:403–413, 1995

Seligmann J, Mason M, Annin P, et al: The New Age of Aquarius. Newsweek, February 3, 1992, pp 66–67

Shick JFE, Smith DE: An analysis of the LSD flashback. J Psychedelic Drugs 3:13–19, 1970

Shulgin A, Shulgin A: PIKHAL: A Chemical Love Story. Berkeley, CA, Transform Press, 1991

Sobel J, Espinas O, Friedman S: Carotid artery obstruction following LSD capsule ingestion. Arch Intern Med 127:290–291, 1971

Spengos K, Schwartz A, Hennerici M: Multifocal cerebral demyelination after magic mushroom abuse. J Neurol 247:224–225, 2000

Strassman RJ: Adverse reactions to psychedelic drugs: a review of the literature. J Nerv Ment Dis 172:577–595, 1984

Strassman RJ: Human hallucinogen interactions with drugs affecting serotonergic neurotransmission. Neuropsychopharmacology 7:241–243, 1992

Strassman RJ: Hallucinogenic drugs in psychiatric research and treatment: perspectives and prospects. J Nerv Ment Dis 183:127–138, 1995

Strassman RJ, Qualls CR: Dose-response study of N,N-dimethyltryptamine in humans, I: neuroendocrine, autonomic and cardiovascular effects. Arch Gen Psychiatry 51:85–87, 1994

Strassman RJ, Qualls CR, Uhlenhuth EH, et al: Dose-response study of N,N-dimethyltryptamine in humans, II: subjective effects and preliminary results of a new rating scale. Arch Gen Psychiatry 51:98–108, 1994

Substance Abuse and Mental Health Services Administration: National Survey on Drug Use and Health. Rockville, MD, Substance Abuse and Mental Health Services Administration, Office of Applied Studies, 2003

Ungerleider JT: The acute side effects from LSD, in The Problems and Prospects of LSD. Edited by Ungerleider JT. Springfield, IL, Charles C Thomas, 1972, pp 61–68

Ungerleider JT, Fisher DD, Fuller MC, et al: The bad trip: the etiology of the adverse LSD reaction. Am J Psychiatry 125:1483–1490, 1968a

Ungerleider JT, Fisher DD, Goldsmith SR, et al: A statistical survey of adverse reactions to LSD in Los Angeles County. Am J Psychiatry 125:352–357, 1968b

Vollenweider FX, Vollenweider-Scherpenhuyzen MFI, Babler A, et al: Psilocybin induces schizophrenia-like psychosis in humans via a serotonin-2 agonist action. Neuroreport 9:3897–3902, 1998

Vollenweider FX, Vontobel P, Hell D, et al: 5-HT modulation of dopamine release in basal ganglia in psilocybin-induced psychosis in man—a PET study with [¹¹C]raclo-pride. Neuropsychopharmacology 20:424–433, 1999

Wesson DR, Smith DE: Psychedelics in Treatment Aspects of Drug Dependence. West Palm Beach, FL, CRC Press, 1978

Phencyclidine and Ketamine

Sidney H. Schnoll, M.D., Ph.D.
Michael F. Weaver, M.D.

Phencyclidine and ketamine are related substances belonging to the class of arylcyclohexylamines, often categorized as hallucinogens. Phencyclidine was synthesized in the late 1950s and was a popular drug of abuse in large United States cities in the mid-1960s, but its use has declined through the 1980s and 1990s. On the street, phencyclidine has been known by many names, including PCP, "angel dust," "animal tranquilizer," "embalming fluid," and "PeaCePill."

Ketamine is a derivative of phencyclidine that was first developed in 1965. It is less potent and shorter acting and is still used as a dissociative anesthetic in humans (Chen et al. 1959). It was classified as a Schedule III controlled substance by the Drug Enforcement Administration in 1999. It is available on the street primarily through diversion from legitimate sources, such as hospitals or veterinary clinics. Recreational use has been concentrated among adolescents, often males, and it is primarily a "party drug" at the underground social events known as "raves." Long-term use patterns are not known because questions about ketamine were just added to a national youth drug survey in 2000. Ketamine is known by several street names, including "special K," "vitamin K," "ket," "Kit Kat," and "cat Valium."

Pharmacology

Central Nervous System Actions

Phencyclidine and ketamine cause anesthesia and a range of behavioral effects. They selectively reduce the excitatory actions of glutamate on central nervous system neurons mediated by the N-methyl-D-aspartate (NMDA) receptor complex (Anis et al. 1983). NMDA receptors mediate ion flux through channels permeable to sodium, potassium, and calcium and are involved in synaptic transmission, long-term potentiation, seizure induction, ischemic brain damage, and neuronal plasticity. Phencyclidine also affects both σ and μ opioid receptors (Giannini et al. 1984), blocks uptake of dopamine equipotent to amphetamine (Bowyer et al. 1984), and inhibits serotonin uptake (R.C. Smith et al. 1977). The exact mechanism of the varied effects of phencyclidine and ketamine has not been determined.

Routes and Dosages

Phencyclidine and ketamine can be taken through various routes of administration: orally, intranasally as a spray or by insufflation ("snorting"), smoking, or intramuscular or intravenous injection. The most common method of use in social settings is ingestion as oral tablets or snorting powder. The initial onset of effects ("rush") begins in 1–10 minutes, is almost immediate after smoking, and begins instantaneously if injected intravenously (Baldridge and Besson 1990). Once the drug is taken, the subjective psychedelic experience ("trip") lasts up to an hour (Pal et al. 2002).

Metabolism takes place primarily in the liver by oxidation, hydroxylation, and conjugation with glucuronic acid (Wong and Biemann 1976). The half-life is 21–24 hours, depending on route of administration (Hurlbut 1991). Phencyclidine accumulates in adipose tissue and the brain (Misra et al. 1979), so it is one of the longest-acting drugs of abuse, and a clinical episode may take up to 6 weeks to clear (Schuckit 1984). Ketamine is shorter acting, with a half-life of approximately 75 minutes when given intravenously. Little is known of its kinetics when taken orally, taken by insufflation, or smoked.

Tolerance and Dependence

These drugs are used for relaxation, self-exploration, and pleasure (Delgarno and Shewan 1996), which are often reasons cited for experimentation with hallucinogens. Tolerance develops rapidly to desired effects, resulting in decreased length of the subjective experience, necessitating an increase in dose to maintain maximal effect (Hurt and Ritchie 1994). Users escalate the amount used to achieve the full psychedelic experience. Despite the development of tolerance, ketamine withdrawal symptoms do not appear to occur in humans (Delgarno and Shewan 1996; Pal et al. 2002), even after daily use. Physical dependence on phencyclidine appears to develop but probably requires long-term regular exposure to relatively high levels (D.A. Gorelick et al. 1986). Withdrawal has been observed in animals within 4–8 hours after discontinuation, but a withdrawal syndrome in humans has not been clearly characterized, possibly because of the long half-life. Ketamine has the potential for compulsive, repeated intravenous use (Jansen 1990), and cases of dependence have been documented (Delgarno and Shewan 1996; Hurt and Ritchie 1994; Moore and Bostwick 1999; Pal et al. 2002), but most involve recreational users who do not develop dependence.

Drug Interactions

Phencyclidine and ketamine users are polydrug abusers; nearly all report use of other substances, mainly marijuana and alcohol. The interaction with alcohol and depressants can cause respiratory and cardiac depression (Delgarno and Shewan 1996). Hypertension is significantly enhanced when other adrenergic agents are ingested, especially stimulants such as amphetamines or cocaine. The combination of phencyclidine and ketamine may enhance all psychological and physiological effects, with high potential for serious toxicity. Because these drugs are available illicitly, users may unknowingly ingest contaminants or adulterants more toxic than the original drug, or the dose may be much higher than expected.

Psychological Effects

Ketamine is a dissociative anesthetic that provides safe, effective sedation, analgesia, and amnesia (Harari and Netzer 1994). On awakening from anesthesia, patients may experience unpleasant hallucinations, termed an *emergence reaction* (Cartwright and Pingel 1984). This occurs in up to half of adults but is rare in children younger than 10 years (Bowdle et al. 1998).

Short-term effects of ketamine include profound changes in consciousness, dramatic feelings of dissociation (spiritual separation from the body), and altered perception that sometimes involves visual hallucinations (Hansen et al. 1988). Commonly reported effects include a sensation of lightness, body distortion, absence of time sense, novel experience of cosmic oneness, and out-of-body experiences. The experience is described as being very intense, especially for first-time users. The rapid onset may result in disorientation, especially in first-time users. Ketamine trips may be accompanied by a panic attack or extreme dissociation. The aftereffects of a trip include a general feeling of well-being and relaxation, mild depression, feeling mildly drained or "hung over," and nausea. Some users have reported very lucid dreams between episodes of ketamine use (Delgarno and Shewan 1996).

Long-term adverse effects include psychological problems (Hurt and Ritchie 1994) such as dysphoria, apathy, or agitation; impairment of short-term memory function (Jansen 1990); and flashbacks (Soyka et al. 1993). Regular users experience memory problems in performing daily activities (Curran and Monaghan

2001). Paranoia and egocentrism are common psychological difficulties for regular users of ketamine (Stewart 2001).

Phencyclidine produces brief dissociative psychotic reactions similar to schizophrenic psychoses. These reactions are characterized by changes in body image, thought disorder, and depersonalization. At higher doses, subjects have great difficulty differentiating between themselves and their surroundings. Other users will experience hostility, paranoia, violence, and preoccupation with death. Users may also have religious experiences while intoxicated, such as feelings of meeting God or impending death (D.A. Gorelick et al. 1986). Attention and cognitive deficits are often present. The phencyclidine experience is regarded as pleasant only half of the time and negative or aversive the rest of the time, but many chronic users report that the unpredictability of the drug's effect is one of its attractive features (Carroll 1985).

Acute phencyclidine delirium is the most common psychiatric syndrome that brings users to medical attention. The acute episode usually lasts 3–8 hours, but duration and severity are dose related. It is characterized by clouded consciousness that is frequently waxing and waning. The clinical picture is dominated by insomnia, restlessness, and behavior that is purposeless, hyperactive, bizarre, or aggressive. The mental state may include paranoia, mania, and emotional lability. Luisada and Brown (1976) observed that one-fourth of patients originally treated for phencyclidine psychosis return 1 year later with schizophrenia in the absence of drug use.

Phencyclidine organic mental disorder is a mental impairment resulting from chronic phencyclidine use, characterized by memory deficits and a state of confusion or decreased intellectual functioning with assaultiveness. This may last 4–6 weeks and improves with time if phencyclidine exposure does not recur. D.E. Smith and Wesson (1978) reported that a significant number of individuals experience profound depression from chronic use of phencyclidine.

Physiological Effects

Ketamine has been used in ambulatory medical settings for distressing procedures such as dental work or bone marrow biopsies; for burn ward procedures; and for genital examinations of children in cases of suspected sexual abuse. During ketamine anesthesia, respiration is maintained, along with protective airway reflexes (gag and cough), so that endotracheal intubation is unnecessary (Green and Johnson 1990).

Effects of recreational use result in an acute rise in blood pressure, heart rate, and respiratory rate. Serotonergic effects of phencyclidine cause dizziness, incoordination, slurred speech, and nystagmus. Ketamine causes temporary increases in intracerebral pressure and transient diplopia (Harari and Netzer 1994), and nausea is common. Ketamine can induce a state of virtual helplessness and pronounced lack of coordination (known as being in a "K-hole"), which can be problematic if the user is in a public setting (Jansen 1993).

Acute toxic effects of large doses of ketamine include emesis, seizures, respiratory depression, hypotension, and coma. The association of seizures with phencyclidine has been well documented (Alldredge et al. 1989). Ischemic and hemorrhagic stroke also have been reported (P.B. Gorelick 1990; Sloan et al. 1991). Infants exposed to phencyclidine in utero may have intrauterine growth retardation and prolonged hospitalizations but are less likely than cocaine-exposed infants to be born prematurely (Tabor et al. 1990).

Treatment

Acute Intoxication

Diagnosis of phencyclidine intoxication is based on behavioral changes, including impulsiveness, unpredictability, psychomotor agitation, impaired judgment, and assaultiveness. Low-dose intoxication induces agitation, catalepsy, and mutism (Burns and Lerner 1976). Physical findings may include hypertension, tachycardia, diminished pain sensation, ataxia, dysarthria, hyperacusis, muscle rigidity, and seizures. Severe phencyclidine intoxication is associated with patients who are unresponsive and comatose, yet their eyes remain open (Pearlson 1981). Phencyclidine is the only drug of abuse that causes a characteristic vertical nystagmus, although it can cause horizontal or rotary nystagmus, as can ketamine. The presence of hyperreflexia and hypertension differentiates phencyclidine or ketamine intoxication from sedative-hypnotic intoxication (National Institute·on Drug Abuse 1979).

Confirmation of intoxication is by toxicological analysis of blood or urine samples. However, toxicological assays for ketamine are not yet routinely available.

Other causes of behavior changes should be ruled out, such as intoxication with another drug, an acute psychotic break due to schizophrenia, or traumatic brain injury. These problems are associated with the population that abuses drugs. When possible, a careful history should be taken, including drugs taken, duration of use, time of last dose, adverse reactions to drugs, and psychiatric history. Obtaining history from companions or family members may be useful. Belongings should be carefully searched for the presence of drugs or paraphernalia.

Patients with mild to moderate intoxication should improve rapidly with minimal supportive care; most do not even come into contact with the health care system. Intoxicated patients should be observed until their mental status has remained normal for several hours (Baldridge and Besson 1990). Because of poor judgment, the patient usually will require supervision in a nonstimulating environment that should include protection from self-injury. If symptoms continue to diminish and there is no cognitive impairment after 12 hours, the patient may be discharged from the emergency department (Woolf et al. 1980).

Moderate to severe intoxication requires supportive care with special attention to respiratory and cardiac function (K.M. Smith 1999). Vital signs need to be monitored for laryngeal stridor or respiratory depression. Restraints should be avoided; the use of restraints may cause rhabdomyolysis with resultant acute renal failure (Lahmeyer and Stock 1983). The preferred method of physical restraint for combative patients is total body immobilization by rolling the patient in a sheet (Aronow et al. 1980).

If phencyclidine was taken orally, a gastric lavage should be performed to recover pill fragments. An alternative to gastric lavage is the administration of activated charcoal to adsorb the phencyclidine that is secreted back into the acid environment of the stomach. Dialysis is ineffective in removing phencyclidine from the body (Rappolt et al. 1980). Acidification of urine increases the excretion rate because phencyclidine and ketamine are weak bases. Urine acidification is controversial, so risks and benefits to the individual must be weighed. If acidification is done before toxicological screens of urine or blood, excretion of and analysis for other drugs (e.g., barbiturates or salicylates) may be adversely affected. Urine acidification is contraindicated in the presence of myoglobinuria, renal insufficiency, severe liver disease, or concomitant abuse of barbiturates or salicylates (Woolf et al. 1980).

Sedation with a benzodiazepine may be required for anxiety, agitation, or harmful behavior. Haloperidol may be given for psychotic features of intoxication. Some studies indicate that barbiturates may be more efficacious in treating the psychotomimetic effects of phencyclidine-like drugs (Olney et al. 1991). Electroconvulsive therapy may be tried in psychotic patients who have used phencyclidine if they fail to respond to antipsychotic medications after 1 week of inpatient treatment (Grover et al. 1986; Rosen et al. 1984). Other complications of intoxication are treated with additional supportive care. Hypertension may require antihypertensive medications. Death from ketamine ingestion is rare (Reich and Silvay 1989).

Chronic Use

Treatment of abuse and dependence is often difficult because of the young age of most users and their polysubstance abuse. Ketamine dependence is uncommon, so very little literature is available about appropriate long-term treatment strategies. Successful treatment involves a supportive environment in a structured program. Mixing phencyclidine and ketamine abusers with other substance abusers appears to make clinical sense because most also abuse other drugs (D.A. Gorelick and Wilkins 1989). Difficulties of treating abusers include impaired attention span and concentration, emotional lability, impulsiveness, poor group interaction, and low tolerance for confrontation (Bolter 1980). Phencyclidine and ketamine abuse, like all other chemical dependence problems, require long-term treatment.

References

Alldredge BK, Lowenstein DH, Simon RP: Seizures associated with recreational drug abuse. Neurology 39:1037–1039, 1989

Anis NA, Berry SC, Burton N, et al: The dissociative anesthetics ketamine and phencyclidine selectively reduce excitation of central mammalian neurons by N-methyl-aspartate. Br J Pharmacol 79:565–575, 1983

Aronow R, Miceli JN, Done AK: A therapeutic approach to the acutely overdosed PCP patient. J Psychedelic Drugs 12:259–267, 1980

Baldridge EB, Besson HA: Phencyclidine. Emerg Med Clin North Am 8:541–550, 1990

Bolter A: Issues for inpatient treatment of chronic PCP abuse. J Psychedelic Drugs 12:287–288, 1980

Bowdle TA, Radant AD, Cowley DS, et al: Psychedelic effects of ketamine in healthy volunteers: relationship to steady-state plasma concentrations. Anaesthesiology 88:82–88, 1998

Bowyer JF, Spuhler KP, Weiner N: Effects of phencyclidine, amphetamine and related compounds on dopamine release from and uptake into striatal synaptosomes. J Pharmacol Exp Ther 229:671–680, 1984

Burns RS, Lerner SE: Perspectives: acute phencyclidine intoxication. Clin Toxicol 9:477–501, 1976

Carroll ME: PCP, The Dangerous Angel (Encyclopedia of Psychoactive Drugs, Series 1. Edited by Snyder SH). New York, Chelsea House, 1985

Cartwright PD, Pingel SM: Midazolam and diazepam in ketamine anesthesia. Anaesthesia 59:439–442, 1984

Chen G, Ensor CR, Russell D, et al: The pharmacology of 1-(1-phenylcyclohexyl) piperidine HCl. J Pharmacol Exp Ther 127:241–250, 1959

Curran HV, Monaghan L: In and out of the K-hole: a comparison of the acute and residual effects of ketamine in frequent and infrequent ketamine users. Addiction 96:749–760, 2001

Delgarno PJ, Shewan D: Illicit use of ketamine in Scotland. J Psychoactive Drugs 28:191–199, 1996

Giannini AJ, Loiselle RH, Giannini MC, et al: Phencyclidine and the dissociatives. Psychiatr Med 3:197–217, 1984

Gorelick DA, Wilkins JN: Inpatient treatment of PCP abusers and users. Am J Drug Alcohol Abuse 15:1–12, 1989

Gorelick DA, Wilkins JN, Wong C: Diagnosis and treatment of chronic phencyclidine (PCP) abuse. NIDA Res Monogr 64:218–228, 1986

Gorelick PB: Stroke from alcohol and drug abuse: a current social peril. Postgrad Med 88:171–178, 1990

Green SM, Johnson SE: Ketamine sedation for pediatric procedures, part 2: review and implications. Ann Emerg Med 19:1033–1046, 1990

Grover D, Yeragani VK, Keshanan MS: Improvement of phencyclidine: associated psychosis with ECT. J Clin Psychiatry 47:477–478, 1986

Hansen G, Jensen SB, Chandresh L, et al: The psychotropic effect of ketamine. J Psychoactive Drugs 20:419–425, 1988

Harari MD, Netzer D: Genital examination under ketamine sedation in cases of suspected sexual abuse. Arch Dis Child 70:197–199, 1994

Hurlbut KM: Drug-induced psychoses. Emerg Med Clin North Am 9:31–52, 1991

Hurt PH, Ritchie EC: A case of ketamine dependence (letter). Am J Psychiatry 151:779, 1994

Jansen KLR: Ketamine: can chronic use impair memory? Int J Addict 25:133–139, 1990

Jansen KLR: Non-medical use of ketamine (letter). Br Med J 306:601–602, 1993

Lahmeyer HW, Stock PG: Phencyclidine intoxication, physical restraints, and acute renal failure: case report. J Clin Psychiatry 44:184–185, 1983

Luisada P, Brown B: Clinical management of phencyclidine psychosis. Clin Toxicol 9:539–545, 1976

Misra AL, Pontani RB, Bartolomeo J: Persistence of phencyclidine (PCP) and metabolites in brain and adipose tissue and implications for long-lasting behavioral effects. Res Commun Chem Pathol Pharmacol 24:431–445, 1979

Moore NN, Bostwick JM: Ketamine dependence in anesthesia providers. Psychosomatics 40:356–359, 1999

National Institute on Drug Abuse: Diagnosis and Treatment of Phencyclidine (PCP) Toxicity. Rockville, MD, National Institute on Drug Abuse, 1979

Olney JW, Labruyere J, Wang G, et al: NMDA antagonist neurotoxicity: mechanism and prevention. Science 254:1515–1518, 1991

Pal HR, Berry N, Kumar R, et al: Ketamine dependence. Anaesth Intensive Care 30:382–384, 2002

Pearlson GD: Psychiatric and medical syndromes associated with phencyclidine (PCP) abuse. Johns Hopkins Med J 148:25–33, 1981

Rappolt RT Sr, Gay GR, Farris RD: Phencyclidine (PCP) intoxication: diagnosis in stages and algorithms of treatment. Clin Toxicol 16:509–529, 1980

Reich DL, Silvay G: Ketamine: an update on the first twenty-five years of clinical experience. Can J Anaesth 36:186–197, 1989

Rosen AM, Mukherjee S, Shinbach K: The efficacy of ECT in phencyclidine-induced psychosis. J Clin Psychiatry 45:220–222, 1984

Schuckit MA: Drug and Alcohol Abuse: A Clinical Guide to Diagnosis and Treatment, 2nd Edition. New York, Plenum, 1984, pp 152–160

Sloan MA, Kittner SJ, Rigamonti D, et al: Occurrence of stroke associated with use/abuse of drugs. Neurology 41:1358–1364, 1991

Smith DE, Wesson DR: Barbiturate and other sedative hypnotics, in Treatment Aspects of Drug Dependence. Edited by Schecter A. New York, CRC Press, 1978, pp 117–130

Smith KM: Drugs used in acquaintance rape. J Am Pharm Assoc 39:519–525, 1999

Smith RC, Meltzer HY, Arora RC, et al: Effect of phencyclidine on ^{3}H-catecholamine and ^{3}H-serotonin uptake in synaptosomal preparations from rat brain. Biochem Pharmacol 26:1435–1439, 1977

Soyka M, Krupinski G, Volki G: Phenomenology of ketamine-induced psychosis. Sucht [German Journal of Addiction Research and Practice] 5:327–331, 1993

Stewart CE: Ketamine as a street drug. Emerg Med Serv 30:30–45, 2001

Tabor BL, Smith-Wallace T, Yonekura ML: Perinatal outcome associated with PCP versus cocaine use. Am J Drug Alcohol Abuse 16:337–348, 1990

Wong LK, Biemann K: Metabolites of phencyclidine. Clin Toxicol 9:583–591, 1976

Woolf DS, Vourakis C, Bennett G: Guidelines for management of acute phencyclidine intoxication. Crit Care Update 7:16–24, 1980

Tobacco

Lori Pbert, Ph.D.
Judith K. Ockene, Ph.D., M.Ed.
Sarah Reiff-Hekking, Ph.D.

Cigarette smoking is the leading preventable cause of illness and death in the United States, causing more than 430,000 deaths in the United States each year (Centers for Disease Control and Prevention 1999b). Forty-eight million adult Americans smoke cigarettes (Centers for Disease Control and Prevention 1999b). Individuals with current or past history of significant psychiatric problems, including depression, schizophrenia, and alcoholism, are much more likely to be smokers, and less likely to stop smoking, than are people in the general population (Glassman 1993; Hughes 1995a; Ziedonis et al. 1994). Despite the enormous health consequences associated with smoking, health care professionals, including mental health professionals, often do not assess or treat nicotine dependence as part of routine care, even though significant evidence indicates that brief smoking cessation treatments can be effective (Fiore et al. 1996). Mental health professionals in particular have many opportunities to address both the physiological and the psychological aspects of nicotine dependence during the course of consultations on medical services, within inpatient psychiatric settings, and during psychotherapy.

Although nicotine, the psychoactive substance in tobacco, is not dangerous as an intoxicant, it is a highly addictive substance that may control significant aspects of a person's behavior. Nicotine shares several common factors with the other recognized euphoriants (i.e., cocaine, opiates, alcohol). It produces centrally mediated effects on mood and feeling states; is a reinforcer for animals; leads to drug-seeking behavior with deprivation; and shows similar patterns of persistent use in the face of evidence that it is highly damaging to health (Benowitz 1985; Fagerstrom 1991; Hen-

This chapter was adapted from Pbert L, Reiff S, Ockene J: "Nicotine Withdrawal and Dependence," in *Treatments of Psychiatric Disorders*, Third Edition, Volume 1. Edited by Gabbard GO. Washington, DC, American Psychiatric Publishing, 2001, pp. 759–779. Used with permission.

ningfield 1984). As with other addictive substances, individual variability in the intensity of the dependence is wide, and although many smokers successfully quit on their own, many others can benefit from a variety of interventions now available.

In this chapter, current treatment strategies available to the mental health professional are examined and evidence-based treatment guidelines are presented. The guidelines offered are based on the Agency for Healthcare Research and Quality (AHRQ) *Treating Tobacco Use and Dependence* guideline (Fiore et al. 2000) and the American Psychiatric Association practice guideline for the treatment of patients with nicotine dependence (Hughes et al. 1996). Also discussed is the nicotine-dependent patient who presents with special clinical problems, such as the patient with alcoholism or other serious psychiatric problems, particularly depression.

Nicotine Dependence: Diagnostic Criteria

Nicotine dependence is classified as a substance use disorder in DSM-IV-TR (American Psychiatric Association 2000). As such, it is defined (p. 197) as "a maladaptive pattern of substance use, leading to clinically significant impairment or distress, as manifested by three (or more) of the following, occurring at any time in the same 12-month period":

1. Tolerance
2. Withdrawal
3. Taking in larger amounts of the substance or over a longer period than intended
4. Experiencing a persistent desire or unsuccessful efforts to cut down or control use
5. Spending a great deal of time obtaining, using, or recovering from nicotine's effects
6. Giving up or reducing important social, occupational, or recreational activities because of use
7. Continuing to use the substance despite knowledge of having a physical or psychological problem caused or worsened by the substance

The DSM-IV-TR diagnostic criteria for nicotine withdrawal (American Psychiatric Association 2000, p. 266) include four (or more) of the following signs or symptoms experienced within 24 hours after abrupt cessation of nicotine use or a reduction in the amount of nicotine used:

1. Dysphoric or depressed mood
2. Insomnia
3. Irritability, frustration, or anger
4. Anxiety
5. Difficulty concentrating
6. Restlessness
7. Decreased heart rate
8. Increased appetite or weight gain

Symptoms begin within a few hours of abstinence or significant reduction in tobacco use, increase over 3–4 days, and then gradually decrease over 1–3 weeks (Gritz et al. 1992; Hatsukami et al. 1990). Change in appetite and problems with concentration appear to persist longer than do feelings of restlessness and irritability. Persons who take in more nicotine typically have stronger withdrawal symptoms and a more difficult time stopping smoking, but considerable variability occurs (Hughes et al. 1990; West et al. 1989).

Several important factors affect the initiation and maintenance of nicotine dependence and smoking behavior. Understanding these factors allows the clinician to tailor the intervention strategies used to the unique needs of the individual smoker. These factors fall into three categories: physiological, psychological, and social.

Factors in Initializing and Maintaining Dependence

Physiological Factors

Nicotine exerts neurochemical effects on the brain that are believed to contribute to the maintenance of cigarette smoking. Noradrenergic effects in the locus coeruleus are thought to involve the neurotransmitter norepinephrine and to mediate symptoms of withdrawal such as craving and irritability. Dopaminergic effects in the nucleus accumbens involve the release of dopamine, which results in pleasurable feelings (Leshner 1996; Nisell et al. 1995). The smoker therefore takes in nicotine to avoid withdrawal and to obtain the pleasurable, immediate peripheral and central effects of nicotine (O. Pomerleau and Pomerleau 1984). Investigators have long noted that a smoker's primary use of cigarettes is to regulate emotional states (Tomkins 1966). Early laboratory studies concluded that smoking significantly reduces fluctuations in mood or affect during stress (C. Pomerleau and Pomerleau 1987; Schachter 1978). However, recent evidence suggests that smokers report higher stress levels than nonsmokers and recent quitters and that the perceived reduction in tension and stress may be a function of the physiological dependence on nicotine (Parrott 1999). Although desire to end the symptoms of withdrawal largely interferes with initial efforts to quit smoking, seeking out the active benefits of nicotine, such as the anorexic effect, stimulation, improved concentration, and perceived anxiolytic effects, clearly maintains the desirability of smoking and contributes to relapse for many persons.

Psychological Factors

The pleasurable physiological effects of nicotine become paired with the many activities and emotions associated with smoking (e.g., talking on the telephone, driving, being in the work setting, feeling stressed or bored). These situations and emotions become "triggers" for the urge to smoke, and for many people, smoking becomes a habitual behavior with little conscious forethought. Evaluating the functional uses of smoking for the person, such as a way to take a break from work or family chores or to handle daily stressors, can help identify areas in which the person will need to develop strategies other than smoking to help him or her function without cigarettes. In addition to identifying triggers, it is important to help the patient increase his or her self-efficacy or confidence in handling such situations and emotions without cigarettes. Considerable evidence shows that high self-efficacy predicts success in stopping smoking, whether the person is dealing with specific problem situations or with withdrawal symptoms (Ward et al. 1997).

Social Factors

The social and cultural environments of smokers affect their ability to stop smoking. Persons who experience more social support for cessation and have fewer smokers in their environment are more successful at stopping smoking (Gulliver et al. 1995; Ockene et al. 1982). In more highly educated groups, where the percentage of smokers is lowest, the "hard core" smoker may continue to smoke despite social pressures against doing so (Kristeller 1994) or may be a member of a social group in which there are social pressures to con-

tinue to smoke. The person who experiences social pressure to smoke and is one of the first in his or her group to stop smoking may have stronger personal reasons to quit than the other group members. Helping such persons address the social pressures to continue to smoke, or including spouses or significant others in treatment, may be particularly useful.

Assessment and Treatment: An Overview

Assessment of and intervention with the smoker are closely integrated because gathering information about the person's smoking history and current smoking patterns increases self-awareness in a way that facilitates behavior change. To guide the clinician, the AHRQ has developed the *Treating Tobacco Use and Dependence* clinical practice guideline (Fiore et al. 2000). This guideline provides an assessment and intervention model for the treatment of nicotine dependence, as well as evidence-based treatment strategies that incorporate the National Cancer Institute's five A's strategies: **A**sk, **A**dvise, **A**ssess, **A**ssist, and **A**rrange follow-up. In the model proposed by AHRQ (Figure 19–1), it is recommended that smoking status be routinely assessed and documented at every clinical contact (Ask). All current smokers should be given clear, strong, and personalized advice to stop smoking (Advise) and assessed for their willingness to quit at each contact (Assess). For those smokers who are willing to quit, further assessment should occur, taking into account the physiological, psychological, and social factors maintaining their smoking behavior, and brief intervention with follow-up should be provided (Assist and Arrange). When appropriate, the clinician may refer the patient for more intensive treatment. Smokers who are not willing to quit should receive a brief motivational intervention to facilitate motivation and future quitting efforts. Additionally, individuals who have recently quit should be provided intervention to prevent relapse.

Assessing Motivation and Readiness to Quit

Once a smoker has been identified through the screening process and provided personalized advice to quit, the clinician should assess the person's motivation and readiness to quit. Nicotine dependence is a

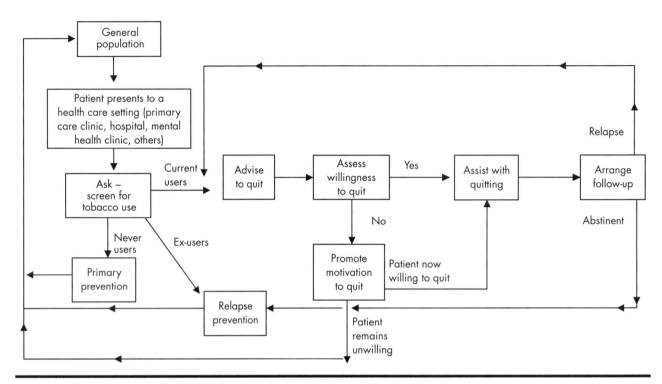

Figure 19–1. Model for nicotine dependence assessment and treatment.

Source. Adapted from Fiore et al. 2000.

chronic, relapsing disorder, and five to seven attempts are often required before maintained abstinence is achieved (U.S. Department of Health and Human Services 1990). Stopping smoking is therefore a long-term process of change that takes place in stages over time. Individuals typically proceed through the following stages of change (DiClemente et al. 1991):

1. Precontemplation
2. Contemplation
3. Preparation
4. Action
5. Maintenance

Different stages of change require different interventions on the part of the clinician.

Approximately 40% of smokers are not thinking about stopping smoking and are said to be in the *precontemplation* stage of change (Velicer et al. 1995). These smokers may be unaware of the risks of smoking, unwilling to consider making a change, or discouraged regarding their ability to quit. Many psychiatric patients fall into this stage of change (R. Hall et al. 1995; Ziedonis et al. 1994). For the precontemplator, the clinician's goal is to raise doubt in his or her

desire to continue smoking by stimulating ambivalence, such as by increasing the patient's perception of the risks and problems associated with his or her current behavior and the potential benefits of quitting. Exploring what the person perceives as the positive aspects of smoking can help overcome the natural defensiveness and resistance that can accompany this stage of change. An effective approach with the precontemplator is to develop discrepancy or a disconnect between the reasons for smoking and the reasons for quitting, encouraging the patient to consider his or her contradictory beliefs and feelings in a sensitive, nonjudgmental manner.

Another 40% of smokers express ambivalence about stopping smoking. These smokers are in the *contemplation* stage of change (Velicer et al. 1995). They report thinking about quitting and seek information about smoking and stopping but are not ready to commit to quit and express uncertainty about their desire or ability to stop. The clinician's goal with the contemplator is to help him or her resolve ambivalence by tipping the balance in favor of quitting.

With both the precontemplators and the contemplators who are unwilling to quit, the AHRQ clinical practice guideline recommends the use of the five R's:

1. **R**elevance—encouraging the patient to consider why quitting is personally important
2. **R**isk—asking the patient to identify the potential negative consequences of tobacco use, such as personal and family health risks, financial cost, and being a poor role model for children
3. **R**ewards—asking the patient to identify the potential benefits of stopping tobacco use, highlighting the most relevant for the patient
4. **R**oadblocks—asking the patient to identify barriers to quitting and noting elements of treatment that could address barriers, including reviewing past quit attempts to identify problems that led to relapse and successful coping skills used in the past that can be applied to a future quit attempt
5. **R**epetition—repeating the motivational intervention at each visit

Often, after exploring these issues, the individual may be ready to make a serious quit attempt or at least commit to an intermediate goal, such as reducing the number of cigarettes smoked or thinking about quitting.

The final 20% of current smokers are ready to stop smoking in the next month and are in the *preparation* stage of change (Velicer et al. 1995). Many of these individuals have made a serious quit attempt in the past year or have taken steps toward stopping, such as telling others of their intent to quit, cutting down on the number of cigarettes smoked, or imagining themselves as nonsmokers. The clinician's goal with the smoker in the preparation stage is to help the individual determine the best course of action to take and develop the strategies and skills needed to make a successful quit attempt.

Individuals in the *action* and *maintenance* stages of change are no longer smoking. Particularly in the action stage, previous smokers are at risk for relapse, and the best approach is to focus on relapse prevention (see section "Preventing Relapse and Maintaining Change" later in this chapter).

Assisting the Smoker Who Is Ready to Quit

For the smoker who is ready to make a quit attempt, the clinician's role is to provide assistance in developing a quit plan and arranging follow-up to support the individual through the quitting process. In developing an individual treatment plan, the physiological, psychological, and social aspects of the patient's dependence must be taken into consideration. The treatment plan should include the evidence-based strategies identified by the AHRQ clinical practice guideline (Fiore et al. 2000) and summarized in Table 19–1.

Addressing Physiological Dependence

The AHRQ and American Psychiatric Association clinical practice guidelines provide strong evidence that nicotine replacement therapy and bupropion are effective treatments for nicotine dependence and should be offered to all smokers who are interested in quitting, unless contraindicated (Fiore et al. 2000; Hughes et al. 1996). A formal evaluation of physiological dependence is not necessary in order to recommend pharmacotherapy, but it can provide information on the individual's level of physiological dependence. The Fagerstrom Test for Nicotine Dependence (FTND) (Figure 19–2) is an excellent tool for assessing level of dependence, with good reliability and validity (Heatherton et al. 1991). If the smoker reports having had significant withdrawal symptoms during prior quit attempts, has a pattern of relapsing within a few hours or days, and scores high on the FTND, nicotine dependence probably plays an important role in maintaining his or her smoking behavior. For all smokers, and especially highly dependent persons, nicotine fading, nicotine replacement therapy, or non-nicotine medication (bupropion) should be recommended. The clinician's role is to outline the benefits and drawbacks of nicotine fading and the medications available, screen for contraindications, and instruct the smoker in the appropriate use of the method or product selected.

Nicotine Fading: Brand Switching and Gradual Reduction

Nicotine fading (Foxx and Brown 1979) has two components: brand switching to a lower-nicotine-level cigarette and gradual reduction of number of cigarettes smoked. Switching to brands with lower nicotine levels one or more times over several weeks, in combination with reducing the number of cigarettes smoked by about one-half per week, can reduce withdrawal symp-

Table 19–1. Strategies for assisting smokers who are ready to quit

Action	Strategies for implementation
Help the patient develop a quit plan	*Set a quit date,* preferably within the next week.
	Tell family, friends, and co-workers of intent to quit and request understanding and support.
	Anticipate challenges to planned quit attempt, particularly during the critical first few weeks, including nicotine withdrawal symptoms, and prepare to address them.
	Remove cigarettes from environment.
Provide practical counseling (problem-solving skills training)	*Abstinence*—Total abstinence is essential. "Not even a single puff after the quit date."
	Past quit experience—Review to identify high-risk situations and what helped and hurt.
	Anticipate triggers or challenges—Discuss challenges and triggers and how patient will successfully address them.
	Alcohol—Consider limiting or abstaining from alcohol during the quitting process because alcohol is highly associated with relapse.
	Other smokers in the household—Encourage patient to quit with housemates or ask that they not smoke in his or her presence.
Provide intratreatment social support	Provide a *supportive clinical environment* while encouraging the patient in his or her quit attempt, clearly stating the clinic staff's availability to assist the patient.
Help the patient obtain extratreatment social support	Encourage the patient to *ask his or her spouse or partner, friends, and co-workers to support* his or her quit attempt.
Recommend the use of pharmacotherapy, unless contraindicated	Recommend the use of *nicotine replacement therapy or non-nicotine pill, bupropion* (see subsection "Pharmacotherapy").
Provide supplementary materials	Provide patient with *self-help materials* appropriate to his or her age, culture, race, and educational level.
Schedule follow-up contact, either in person or via telephone	*Follow-up* should occur within the first week after the quit date.
	If abstinent at follow-up, congratulate on success, address problems encountered and challenges anticipated, and monitor pharmacological aids used.
	If smoking occurred, review circumstances leading to smoking, elicit recommitment to total abstinence, address problems encountered and challenges anticipated, review pharmacological aid use and problems, and consider referral to more intensive, specialized treatment.

Source. Adapted from Fiore et al 2000. Public domain.

toms in the person who smokes heavily. However, the evidence does not support the efficacy of brand switching alone (Fiore et al. 1996; Law and Tang 1995). In fact, a recent study (Massachusetts Department of Public Health 1998) found that if smokers use compensation techniques such as vent blocking, puffing more frequently, or inhaling more deeply when smoking lower-nicotine cigarettes, their nicotine yield will be considerably higher than that suggested by the Federal Trade Commission ratings. Smokers should be cautioned about this possibility and advised to keep such compensation behaviors to a minimum during the nicotine fading process. On the other hand, despite the myth that a smoker needs to quit "cold turkey," there does not appear to be a significant difference in cessation rates between quitting "cold turkey" compared with gradually reducing the number of cigarettes smoked (Fiore et al. 1996; Hughes 1995b); therefore, patient preference should determine the approach selected. If nicotine fading is used, it should be combined with behavioral management strategies such that "lower-need" cigarettes are eliminated first and awareness of the function of each cigarette is increased; this approach also increases the individual's self-efficacy in his or her ability to eventually stop smoking.

Pharmacotherapy

Five pharmacological aids have been approved by the U.S. Food and Drug Administration for use in the

	0 Points	1 Point	2 Points	3 Points	Score
1. How soon after you wake up do you smoke your first cigarette?	After 60 minutes	31–60 minutes	6–30 minutes	Within 5 minutes	
2. Do you find it difficult to refrain from smoking in places where it is forbidden, e.g., in church, at the library, cinema, etc.?	No	Yes			
3. Which cigarette would you hate most to give up?	All others	The first one in the morning			
4. How many cigarettes/day do you smoke?	10 or less	11–20	21–30	31 or more	
5. Do you smoke more frequently during the first hours of waking than during the rest of the day?	No	Yes			
6. Do you smoke if you are so ill that you are in bed most of the day?	No	Yes			
				TOTAL	

Classification of dependence

0–2	Very low
3–4	Low
5	Moderate
6–7	High
8–10	Very high

Figure 19–2. Fagerstrom Test for Nicotine Dependence

Source. Reprinted from Heatherton T, Kozlowski L, Frecker R, et al.: "The Fagerstrom Test for Nicotine Dependence: A Revision of the Fagerstrom Tolerance Questionnaire." *British Journal of Addiction* 86:1119–1127, 1991. Used with permission.

treatment of nicotine dependence (Table 19–2). These pharmacotherapies fall into two general categories: nicotine replacement therapies and a non-nicotine pill (bupropion). (Refer to Hughes and colleagues [1999] and the 1996 American Psychiatric Association practice guideline [Hughes et al. 1996] for detailed descriptions of each of the products available and to the clinician and patient information sheets for product contraindications.) It is important to emphasize to smokers that pharmacotherapies are not "magic bullets." Rather, they are used to help minimize or dampen withdrawal symptoms while smokers work to break the conditioned connections between smoking and the activities and emotions of their daily lives and to develop coping skills to replace the many functions of smoking.

The purpose of the four nicotine replacement therapies is to prevent or minimize the symptoms of withdrawal or cravings by replacing some of the nicotine that would otherwise be obtained from smoking. This allows the individual to focus on the behavioral and emotional aspects of stopping smoking. Nicotine replacement is then gradually reduced so as to minimize withdrawal symptoms experienced. All four forms of nicotine replacement therapy have been found to be equally efficacious, approximately doubling quit rates compared with placebo. In most studies, concomitant supportive or behavior therapy has produced substantially higher quit rates than either behavior therapy or nicotine replacement alone (Hughes 1991, 1995b) and should be encouraged but not required (Hughes et al. 1999).

Nicotine gum, approved in 1984, became available over the counter in the United States in 1995. Nicotine in the gum is absorbed in the buccal mucosa. The 2-mg gum is recommended for individuals who smoke fewer than 25 cigarettes per day, and the 4-mg gum is recommended for individuals who smoke at least 25 cigarettes per day. Scheduled dosing of one or two pieces per hour has been found to be more efficacious than ad lib use (Killen et al. 1990). Proper chewing technique ("chew and park") is important to maximize the nicotine replacement obtained and to reduce potential side effects. The gum is chewed slowly for about

Table 19–2.   First-line medications for treating nicotine dependence

Characteristic	Nicotine patches[a]	Nicotine gum[a]	Nicotine inhaler	Nicotine spray	Bupropion SR
Brand name	Nicotrol, Nicoderm CQ, generic (various store brands)	Nicorette, generic (various store brands)	Nicotrol inhaler	Nicotrol NS	Zyban, Wellbutrin[b]
Product strength	7, 14, 21 mg/patch (for typical systems that deliver 17, 32, 52 mg/day of nicotine)	2 mg (for average smokers: ≤24 cigarettes/day) 4 mg (for heavy smokers: >24 cigarettes/day)	10 mg/cartridge	10 mg/mL	150 mg
Amount of nicotine delivered[c]	16-hr patch: 15 mg/day 24-hr patch: 7, 14, 21 mg/day	Up to 0.8 mg per 2-mg piece Up to 1.5 mg per 4-mg piece	Up to 2 mg/cartridge	0.5 mg=2 sprays	NA
Special directions for use	Apply to nonhairy part of body	Alternately chew and park for 20 min; nicotine absorbed through oral mucosa when gum is parked; avoid acidic beverages	Take frequent puffs over 20 min; nicotine absorbed through oral mucosa; avoid acidic beverages	1–2 sprays in each nostril	None
Dosing interval and maximum dose	16-hr patch: 16 hr on; 8 hr off 24-hr patch: replace every 24 hr (option to remove at bedtime)	1 piece every 1–2 hr and as needed for craving Maximum: 24 pieces/day	Multiple puffs on a cartridge every 1–2 hr or as needed 6–16 cartridges/day Maximum: 16 cartridges/day	1–2 doses/hr (1 dose=2 sprays or 1 per nostril)	150 mg/day (days 1–3) 150 mg twice/day (after day 3)
Time to peak plasma level	5–10 hr	20–30 min	15 min	5–7 min	3 hr
Manufacturer's recommended treatment duration[d]	16-mg patch: 6 weeks 24-hr patch: initial, 21 mg for 4 weeks; taper, 14 and 7 mg for 2 weeks each	Initial, 6 weeks Taper, 6 weeks	Initial, up to 12 weeks Taper, 12 weeks	Initial, up to 8 weeks Taper, 4–6 weeks	7–12 weeks Maintenance, up to 6 months
Adverse reactions (treatment of reaction)	50% experience mild irritant skin reactions (rotate and use steroid cream), rare allergic skin reaction, vivid dreams, sleep disturbances while using the patch 24 hr (remove at bedtime)	Mouth soreness, hiccups, dyspepsia, jaw ache (usually mild and transient; correct technique)	40% experience mouth and throat irritation (may resolve with regular use), dyspepsia	Local transient irritation in the nose and throat, watery eyes, sneezing, cough	Dry mouth, insomnia (avoid bedtime dose), shakiness

Table 19–2. First-line medications for treating nicotine dependence *(continued)*

Characteristic	Nicotine patches[a]	Nicotine gum[a]	Nicotine inhaler	Nicotine spray	Bupropion SR
Absolute contraindications	*All products:* Previous hypersensitivity reaction to any of the products (i.e., serious allergic reaction); heart attack within 6 weeks;				History of seizure; current or prior diagnosis of bulimia or anorexia nervosa; concurrent or recent use of monoamine oxidase inhibitors
	All nicotine replacement therapies: Serious heart arrhythmia; uncontrolled hypertension; active peptic ulcer disease				
	Severe eczema or other skin diseases that may be exacerbated by the patch	Severe TMJ disease or other jaw problems; dentures	Allergy to menthol	Active rhinitis; active sinusitis	
Relative contraindications/ precautions	*All products:* Moderate or severe hepatic or renal impairment				
	All nicotine replacement therapies: Active hyperthyroidism; peripheral vascular disease				
	Hot work environment (reduced patch adhesion); mild to moderate skin disease	Any jaw problem that affects gum chewing; dental appliances affected by gum	Oral or pharyngeal inflammation	Asthma, nasal polyps	Agitation, anxiety, insomnia, history of head trauma or other risk factor for seizure
Pregnancy category[e]	D	C	D	D	B

Note.   NA=not applicable; SR=sustained release; TMJ=temporomandibular joint.

[a]Available without prescription.

[b]Zyban is brand name for bupropion SR marketed for smoking cessation with support materials; Wellbutrin is brand name for bupropion SR marketed for depression.

[c]Typical cigarette delivers 1–3 mg of nicotine.

[d]Manufacturer recommendations based on duration of treatment in initial clinical trials. Many independent trials of nicotine replacement therapy suggest that treatment for 8 weeks is as effective as longer treatments for most, but shorter and longer intervals are reasonable depending on individual smoker.

[e]Pregnancy category:

B: NO EVIDENCE OF RISK IN HUMANS. Adequate, well-controlled studies in pregnant women have not shown increased risk of fetal abnormalities despite adverse findings in animals, or, in the absence of adequate human studies, animal studies show no fetal risk. The chance of fetal harm is remote but remains a possibility.

C: RISK CANNOT BE RULED OUT. Adequate, well-controlled human studies are lacking, and animal studies have shown a risk to the fetus or are lacking as well. There is a chance of fetal harm if the drug is administered during pregnancy, but the potential benefits may outweigh the potential risks.

D: POSITIVE EVIDENCE OF RISK. Studies in humans, or investigational or postmarketing data, have demonstrated fetal risk. Nevertheless, potential benefits from the use of the drug may outweigh the potential risk. For example, the drug may be acceptable if needed in a life-threatening situation or serious disease for which safer drugs cannot be used or are ineffective.

1 minute, then parked between the cheek and gum for a minute or two, then slowly chewed and parked for 30 minutes. Recommended length of treatment varies from 1 to 6 months.

The nicotine transdermal patch provides more continuous delivery of nicotine. Patches are applied daily to the upper torso in the morning and, depending on the formulation of the patch used, removed either at bedtime (16-hour patch) or on waking (24-hour patch). Starting doses are 21 mg for the 24-hour patch and 15 mg for the 16-hour patch, with dose gradually reduced over time. Six to eight weeks of treatment is reasonable for most smokers, and tapering has not been found to be necessary (Fiore et al. 1994, 2000).

The nicotine inhaler delivers nicotine bucally only to the mouth and throat, not lungs, through nicotine vapor inhaled from a plastic cartridge containing a nicotine plug. The inhaler addresses not only physical dependence but also the behavioral and sensory aspects of smoking. The recommended dose is 6–16 cartridges per day for the first 6–12 weeks, followed by gradual reduction of dose over the next 6–12 weeks. One dose is equivalent to frequent, continuous puffing for 20 minutes.

Nicotine nasal spray delivers nicotine to the bloodstream more rapidly than any other nicotine replacement therapy (although less rapidly than cigarettes), with peak blood levels occurring within 10 minutes of use (Gourlay and Benowitz 1997). Concern was raised that the nasal spray may have a significant dependency potential because of the rapid delivery of nicotine (Sutherland et al. 1992), but more recent studies have not found significant abuse liability (Hughes 1998; Schuh et al. 1997). Starting dose is one to two doses per hour (one dose=two sprays), with treatment for up to 8 weeks and then stopping or tapering the dose for 4–6 weeks.

Bupropion hydrochloride sustained-release is an atypical antidepressant believed to work on the neurochemistry of addiction by enhancing dopamine levels and affecting the action of norepinephrine in the brain; both neurotransmitters are believed to be involved in nicotine dependence (Ascher et al. 1995). As with the nicotine replacement therapies, bupropion has been found to consistently double quit rates compared with placebo. Dosing begins 1 week prior to cessation to achieve steady-state blood levels, with 150 mg/day for the first 3 days, followed by a dose increase to the recommended dose of 300 mg/day. An interval of at least 8 hours between doses is recommended to reduce the possibility of seizures. Recommended duration of treatment is 7–12 weeks. If the smoker has not made significant progress toward abstinence by the seventh week of therapy, he or she is unlikely to quit during this attempt, and treatment should be discontinued.

Addressing Psychological Dependence: Cognitive and Behavioral Interventions

Cognitive and behavioral interventions for smoking have been developed from cognitive and behavioral treatment techniques used for a wide range of behavioral and addictive disorders (Bandura 1969; Goldfried and Davison 1976) and have been found to typically double quit rates compared with control groups (Fiore et al. 1996; Law and Tang 1995; Schwartz 1992). The cognitive-behavioral approach intertwines assessment and intervention. First, past quit attempts are reviewed to identify the reasons that the quit attempts were made, what methods the smokers used (e.g., cold turkey, tapering, pharmacological aids), problems experienced (including withdrawal symptoms), strategies that helped, and what led to relapse. The key is to assist the patient in reframing past efforts to stop smoking as learning experiences and to apply what was learned to the current quit attempt. Second, current smoking patterns are assessed. In what situations and in response to what feelings or emotions does the patient most feel like smoking? These are "high-need" cigarettes. Asking the smoker to rate the level of need for each cigarette on a scale of 1 (low need) to 5 (high need) is often helpful. Behavioral self-monitoring, which involves the patient recording the time, place, situation, mood, thoughts, and need level associated with each cigarette smoked, can be very informative for both the patient and the clinician at this stage to identify specific areas needing further attention.

Once anticipated problems and triggers are identified through a review of past quit attempts and an assessment of current smoking patterns, the patient can be helped to develop specific cognitive-behavioral coping strategies to address these problems and triggers, such as the following:

1. Anticipate and avoid high-risk situations and cues that bring on an urge to smoke whenever possible.

2. Remove oneself from the trigger situation.
3. Substitute other behaviors incompatible with smoking cigarettes when urges arise (e.g., taking a walk, going to a smoke-free environment, deep breathing or other relaxation exercise).
4. Use assertiveness, refusal skills, and other skills to manage the triggers.
5. Use cognitive restructuring to reshape positive beliefs about smoking or to counteract irrational thinking, replacing maladaptive thoughts with more constructive thoughts.

Such general problem-solving and skill-building strategies (i.e., practical counseling) are one of three types of counseling and behavior therapies that have been found to result in higher abstinence rates and that are recommended by the clinical practice guideline (Fiore et al. 2000). Common elements of practical counseling are presented in Table 19–3. Two additional types of counseling and behavior therapies found to result in higher abstinence rates and recommended by the guideline are 1) providing social support as part of treatment (i.e., intratreatment social support) and 2) helping the smoker obtain social support outside of treatment from his or her spouse or significant other, co-workers, and friends (i.e., extratreatment social support). These two approaches are addressed in the next section.

Table 19–3. Common elements of practical counseling (problem-solving skills training)

Treatment component	Examples
Recognize danger situations: identify events, internal states, or activities that increase the risk of smoking or relapse.	Negative affect Being around other smokers Drinking alcohol Experiencing urges Being under time pressure
Develop coping skills: identify and practice coping or problem-solving skills; typically, these skills are intended to cope with danger situations.	Learning to anticipate and avoid temptation Learning cognitive strategies that will reduce negative moods Accomplishing lifestyle changes that reduce stress, improve quality of life, or produce pleasure Learning cognitive and behavioral activities to cope with smoking urges (e.g., distracting attention)
Provide basic information: provide basic facts about smoking and successful quitting.	That any smoking (even a single puff) increases the likelihood of a full relapse That withdrawal typically peaks within 1–3 weeks after quitting The addictive nature of smoking

Source. Reprinted from Fiore et al. 2000. Public domain.

Addressing Social Influences

Three aspects of social influence are especially important: 1) the number of smokers among the patient's friends, family, and co-workers; 2) the quality of support for cessation that can be expected by the smoker; and 3) the extent to which the smoker is able to be assertive in resisting social pressures to smoke. Exploring the concerns the smoker has about being tempted or even directly sabotaged by other smokers is important. Actively engaging the social support of friends, family, and co-workers may be easiest for the hospitalized smoker because that person is often recognized to have a heightened need to stop smoking. This is a time when a spouse also may try to quit or at least avoid smoking in the person's presence. A smoker may also have little confidence in his or her ability to refuse cigarettes if offered them or to be the first to quit in his or her social group.

Addressing Smoking Cessation and Weight Gain

Although the average weight gain of 5–6 kg for sustained quitters (Froom et al. 1998) does not present a medical risk equal to smoking a pack of cigarettes a day, weight gain is an issue that is important to many people and provides a common reason for starting, continuing, and returning to smoking. Several factors have been implicated in weight gain, including an increase in metabolism from nicotine intake (Hofstetter et al. 1986; Perkins 1992), which may cause an increase in weight while quitting even without increased caloric intake (Fiore et al. 1996), and a change in preference for sweets while smoking (Grunberg 1982). These biological factors, in combination with the use of food as a behavioral substitute, make it important to address weight gain explicitly in most treatment programs (Klesges et al. 1989; Wack and Rodin 1982). However, to date no empirically tested treatment that successfully addresses weight gain while quitting has been published. Dieting while quitting increases the rate of relapse (Ockene et al. 2000). The AHRQ guideline (Fiore et al. 2000) suggests confronting issues of weight gain with patients before they quit and preparing them for the high probability of gaining weight. Additionally, it is important to remind the patient that quitting smoking is the current priority and that support is available if the patient would like to work on weight loss after successful smoking cessation. A focus on weight loss should be delayed until the patient is no longer experiencing withdrawal symptoms and feels secure in the ability to remain smoke free. Encouraging patients to engage in sensible lifestyle changes such as increasing physical activity, eating plenty of fruits and vegetables, and avoiding alcohol is also suggested by the AHRQ guideline. Evidence indicates that increasing physical activity can help reduce weight gain and support maintenance (Bock et al. 1999; Froom et al. 1998).

Preventing Relapse and Maintaining Change

A major difficulty in smoking cessation, as with other substance abuse behaviors, is maintenance of the changed behavior. As many as 70% of those who stop smoking relapse within a year, with the strongest predictor of relapse being a slip within a relatively brief period (average between 18 and 60 days of cessation) (Ockene et al. 2000). Up to 65% of the persons who quit smoking on their own relapse within the first week after cessation (Hughes and Hatsukami 1992). Re-

lapse prevention as a treatment technique was originally developed by Marlatt and Gordon (1980) to help prevent the relapse of alcohol abuse and has been extrapolated to use in the treatment of nicotine abuse (Lichtenstein and Brown 1985). However, the success of using this approach with smokers is questionable; a recent review by Ockene and colleagues (2000) found studies showing both positive and negative results. Additionally, a recent meta-analysis (Irvin et al. 1999) concluded that relapse prevention treatment had strong and reliable effects for alcohol and polysubstance abuse but much weaker effects for smoking. The AHRQ guideline recommends that the individual be congratulated on any success, be provided strong encouragement to remain abstinent, and be encouraged to discuss 1) benefits the patient may derive from stopping smoking; 2) any success experienced such as reduced withdrawal symptoms and duration of abstinence; and 3) any problems encountered or anticipated in maintaining abstinence, such as weight gain, depression, alcohol, or other smokers in the household (Fiore et al. 2000). More intensive prescriptive relapse prevention interventions, tailored to the specific problems encountered, should be delivered when an individual experiences problems in maintaining abstinence. These interventions are presented in Table 19–4.

Summary of Treatment Recommendations

To stop smoking, a smoker must perceive this change as being beneficial and be confident that he or she can stop smoking. From a behavioral perspective, the smoker must learn new skills or enhance old skills that can be used in place of cigarettes to deal with problems as they arise. The person also needs to be able to attribute changes in smoking behavior to personal abilities and skills rather than to willpower or to the external aspects of treatment (Bandura 1977). From a pharmacological perspective, all smokers, and particularly those who show a high physiological dependency on nicotine, would benefit from nicotine replacement therapy or bupropion to allow them to work on the behavioral aspects of quitting while receiving some relief from the physiological withdrawal. Finally, the patient may benefit from intervention following a lapse to prevent relapse. For a more complete review of cognitive-

Table 19–4. Potential responses to patient-reported problems that threaten abstinence during prescriptive relapse prevention

Problem	Response
Lack of support for cessation	Schedule follow-up visits or telephone calls with the patient.
	Help the patient identify sources of support within his or her environment.
	Refer the patient to an appropriate organization that offers cessation counseling or support.
Negative mood or depression	If significant, provide counseling, prescribe appropriate medications, or refer the patient to a specialist.
Strong or prolonged withdrawal symptoms	If the patient reports prolonged craving or other withdrawal symptoms, consider extending the use of an approved pharmacotherapy or adding/combining pharmacological medications to reduce strong withdrawal symptoms.
Weight gain	Recommend starting or increasing physical activity; discourage strict dieting.
	Reassure the patient that some weight gain after quitting is common and appears to be self-limiting.
	Emphasize the importance of a healthy diet.
	Maintain the patient on pharmacotherapy known to delay weight gain (e.g., bupropion sustained-release; nicotine replacement therapies, particularly nicotine gum).
	Refer the patient to a specialist or program.
Flagging motivation/feeling deprived	Reassure the patient that these feelings are common.
	Recommend rewarding activities.
	Probe to ensure that the patient is not engaged in periodic tobacco use.
	Emphasize that beginning to smoke (even a puff) will increase urges and make quitting more difficult.

Source. Reprinted from Fiore et al. 2000. Public domain.

behavioral interventions for smoking, see the American Psychiatric Association practice guideline (Hughes et al. 1996) and the AHRQ clinical practice guideline (Fiore et al. 2000).

Smoking Cessation Treatment in Special Populations

Smoking Cessation and Alcohol

Tobacco use and alcohol abuse are moderately to strongly related (Istvan and Matarazzo 1984; Kozlowski et al. 1993). Among identified alcoholic persons, the incidence of smoking has been 80%–90% in all studies; alcoholic persons also are more likely to smoke heavily (Bien and Burge 1990; Bobo 1989). Consequently, most patients seen in an alcohol treatment program will be smokers, many of them at a level that is acutely health endangering, thereby underscoring the need to treat nicotine dependence in this patient population.

Although some individuals in alcohol abuse treatment may be interested in a smoking cessation component to their treatment (Bobo 1989), many believe that obtaining sobriety would be more difficult if trying to simultaneously stop smoking and become abstinent from alcohol (Bobo and Gilchrist 1983). Data obtained from individuals in substance abuse treatment suggest that it is difficult to quit smoking while undergoing substance abuse treatment but that working on smoking cessation does not increase relapse to alcohol use (Hughes et al. 1996; Kalman 1998). In fact, in some instances, smoking cessation was associated with a decreased relapse to alcohol use (Kalman 1998; Sobell et al. 1992). Although smoking does not appear to increase the relapse rate to alcohol use, evidence shows that alcohol may interact with nicotine, increasing some acute tolerance of alcohol effects and enhancing the reinforcing value of alcohol, and thus setting the stage for high-risk drinking (Kalman 1998).

There is support for the notion that smoking may be used as a coping strategy to avoid alcohol use in response to urges to use alcohol during early sobriety (Kalman 1998). Kalman (1998) reviewed this literature and concluded that many alcoholic smokers in alcohol abuse treatment expect that they will smoke to help remain abstinent from alcohol. Additionally, he noted that 1) those with greater nicotine dependence report more often that they cope with drinking urges by smoking; 2) those alcoholic persons with greater nicotine and alcohol dependence are more likely to have stronger urges to smoke when abstaining from alcohol; and 3) those alcoholic persons who have greater nicotine dependence are more likely to be concerned about maintaining sobriety while quitting smoking. Kalman summarized this limited literature by stating that smoking cessation will be difficult for alcoholic persons during the early phases of sobriety. In the American Psychiatric Association practice guideline for the treatment of patients with nicotine dependence (Hughes et al. 1996), the recommendation is that the timing of smoking cessation in relation to alcohol abuse treatment should be determined by the patient.

Smoking Cessation and Psychiatric Disorders

Increasing attention is being paid to the role of smoking in psychiatric disorders in regard both to the role of the central nervous system effects of nicotine and to the apparent special value of smoking to psychiatric patients (Glassman 1993). Several studies show a much higher prevalence of smoking in psychiatric populations (i.e., 50%–90%) (Breslau 1995; Hughes and Hatsukami 1986; Mathew et al. 1981; O'Farrell et al. 1983; Pohl et al. 1992), particularly in those with depression (Covey et al. 1998) and schizophrenia (Glassman 1993), than in nonpsychiatric populations. The evidence is less clear regarding the increased prevalence in those with anxiety disorders (Glassman 1993; Parrott 1999). Some psychiatric patients may be actively self-medicating through their use of cigarettes (G. Hall 1980). Evidence also indicates that smoking may interact with psychoactive medication, including antidepressants (Hughes 1993; Jusko 1981), antipsychotics (Hughes 1993; Newhouse and Hughes 1991; Pantuck et al. 1982; Perry et al. 1993; Wright et al. 1983), and minor tranquilizers (Ochs and Otter 1981). In patients with schizophrenia, smoking also may affect drug-

related movement disorders and may increase the dosage needed of antipsychotics (Goff et al. 1992; Hughes et al. 1996; Menza et al. 1991; Newhouse and Hughes 1991).

Patients who are depressed or have a history of depression are more likely to smoke, are less likely to quit (Anda et al. 1990; Covey et al. 1990; Glassman 1993), are at increased risk for experiencing dysphoric mood states and relapse of major depressive disorder after cessation (Covey et al. 1998), and may experience more extreme symptoms of withdrawal (Glassman 1993). The detrimental effect of depression on smoking cessation has been found in both men and women but may be particularly important in the treatment of women because of the increased incidence of depression and dysphoric mood states in women (Borrelli et al. 1996). The amount of time during which major depressive symptoms return after stopping smoking varies with each individual and may occur as soon as a few weeks or as long as a few months after quitting. Therefore, as noted by the American Psychiatric Association (Hughes et al. 1996), individuals with a history of depression or who have reported depression associated with past quit attempts should be advised to consider psychotherapy or pharmacological treatment of depression if they begin to experience dysphoria. Additionally, because of the interaction between nicotine and antidepressant medication, those being treated pharmacologically for depression should undergo a reevaluation of psychotropic medication because decreasing nicotine intake may increase the level of antidepressant (Hughes 1993).

A high rate of smoking and difficulty with cessation are also observed in patients with schizophrenia (Ziedonis et al. 1994). Nicotine may reduce drug-induced side effects experienced by individuals with schizophrenia, and nicotine withdrawal symptoms can mimic drug-induced side effects as well (i.e., increased restlessness). Because many patients with schizophrenia are not interested in quitting smoking, motivational treatment approaches aimed at identifying personalized reasons for quitting and at moving the individual from precontemplation through more advanced stages of change are warranted (Hughes et al. 1996).

Evidence is less strong for an association between smoking and anxiety disorders than for depression or schizophrenia (Breslau 1995; Glassman 1993). Although smoking is often reported to be relaxing and calming, smokers report higher levels of stress than nonsmokers and former smokers. Smoking likely adds to anxiety and stress by inducing mild withdrawal symptoms between cigarettes, which increases feelings of tension, stress, and anxiety. The individual then smokes in response to the anxiety and stress created by a physiological need for nicotine. Once smoking cessation has occurred for several weeks, stress and anxiety often stabilize at reduced levels when compared with precessation. The reduction in stress does not happen for the individual who simply reduces his or her cigarette consumption; therefore, smokers should be made aware that smoking likely leads to increased feelings of stress and anxiety (Parrott 1999).

Although research is beginning to document the effects of smoking in psychiatric populations, little empirical evidence is available regarding the treatment of nicotine dependence in such patients (see Hughes et al. 1996 for a discussion of intervention issues). In the psychiatric patient for whom smoking cessation is critical for medical reasons, a comprehensive intervention plan including the treatment components outlined earlier in this chapter is indicated. In particular, behavior therapy focused on the development of coping and social skills is important, and adjustment of medication may be needed, either in an attempt to decrease continued dependence on self-medicating with nicotine or in response to possible interaction effects. As more inpatient services limit access to smoking or become smoke free, use of the nicotine patch, particularly for persons who smoke heavily, is recommended. Additionally, a clear staff policy for smoking that does not undermine the smoke-free policy of the treatment unit is imperative. Providing assistance with smoking cessation within the context of a broader therapeutic alliance, monitoring for changes in psychiatric symptoms, and using motivational strategies with individuals in the precontemplation stage are also particularly important.

Modes of Intervention Delivery

Smoking interventions can be delivered through a variety of modalities, as reflected in the "Best Practices for Comprehensive Tobacco Control Programs" document produced by the Centers for Disease Control and Prevention (1999a). The Centers for Disease Control and Prevention recommends identification of smokers, advice and provision of brief counseling to smokers within the course of routine care, as well as making

available to the smoker a full range of cessation aids and services, including pharmacological aids, behavioral counseling (group and individual), and follow-up visits.

Although one role for the mental health professional may be to refer smokers to more intensive treatment programs, it is important to keep in mind that only a small minority of even motivated smokers will attend such programs. In addition, some investigations and reviews (Fiore et al. 2000; Ockene et al. 1991, 1992) have confirmed the value of brief counseling, particularly when accompanied by the use of pharmacological aids such as nicotine replacement therapy and bupropion and when some type of follow-up occurs, either in person or by telephone. Clinicians conducting brief counseling can supplement their intervention with a wide range of self-help materials and audiotapes now available.

Of additional value to the clinician is the use of behavioral contracts, which can serve as an aid in establishing realistic goals and steps by which to accomplish them. For example, the contract can specify a tapering schedule, a quit date, reasons for stopping, steps to follow in response to situational factors that could interfere with efforts to stop smoking, and a plan for follow-up.

A stepped-care approach can be used in which, for example, less dependent smokers or smokers who are ready for action may benefit from brief counseling, whereas a more dependent smoker or one who needs more intensive help can be referred to a smoking treatment specialist or a treatment group. For more intensive individual or group treatment, weekly contact for approximately 4 weeks and then biweekly contact for another 4 weeks is a reasonable frequency and one that provides the tapering of contact necessary for the patient to internalize control. For the more dependent smoker or one who has other psychiatric problems, a longer and more intensive intervention may be necessary.

References

American Psychiatric Association: Diagnostic and Statistical Manual of Mental Disorders, 4th Edition, Text Revision. Washington, DC, American Psychiatric Association, 2000

Anda R, Williamson D, Escobedo L, et al: Depression and the dynamics of smoking: a national perspective. JAMA 264:1541–1545, 1990

Ascher J, Cole J, Colin J-N, et al: Bupropion: a review of its mechanism of antidepressant activity. J Clin Psychiatry 56:395–401, 1995

Bandura A: Principles of Behavior Modification. New York, Holt, Rinehart, & Winston, 1969

Bandura A: Self-efficacy: toward a unifying theory of behavioral change. Psychol Rev 84:191–215, 1977

Benowitz N: Biochemical measurements of tobacco consumption, in Measurement in the Analysis and Treatment of Smoking (NIDA Research Monograph 48). Edited by Grabowski J, Bell C. Rockville, MD, National Institute on Drug Abuse, 1985, pp 6–26

Bien T, Burge R: Smoking and drinking: a review of the literature. Int J Addict 25:1429–1454, 1990

Bobo J: Nicotine dependence and alcoholism epidemiology and treatment. J Psychoactive Drugs 21:323–329, 1989

Bobo J, Gilchrist L: Urging the alcoholic client to quit smoking cigarettes. Addict Behav 8:297–305, 1983

Bock B, Marcus B, King T, et al: Exercise effects on withdrawal and mood among women attempting smoking cessation. Addict Behav 24:399–410, 1999

Borrelli B, Bock B, King T, et al: The impact of depression on smoking cessation in women. Am J Prev Med 12:378–387, 1996

Breslau N: Psychiatric comorbidity of smoking and nicotine dependence. Behav Genet 25:95–101, 1995

Centers for Disease Control and Prevention: Best Practices for Comprehensive Tobacco Control Programs. Atlanta, GA, U.S. Department of Health and Human Services, Centers for Disease Control and Prevention, National Center for Chronic Disease Prevention and Health Promotion, Office on Smoking and Health, March 1999a

Centers for Disease Control and Prevention: Cigarette smoking among adults—United States, 1997. MMWR Morb Mortal Wkly Rep 48:993–996, 1999b

Covey L, Glassman A, Stetner F: Depression and depressive symptoms in smoking cessation. Compr Psychiatry 31:350–354, 1990

Covey L, Glassman A, Stetner F: Cigarette smoking and major depression, in Smoking and Illicit Drug Use. Edited by Gold M, Stimmel B. Binghamton, NY, Haworth Medical Press, 1998, pp 35–46

DiClemente C, Prochaska J, Fairhurst S, et al: The process of smoking cessation: an analysis of precontemplation, contemplation, and preparation stages of change. J Consult Clin Psychol 59:295–304, 1991

Fagerstrom K: Towards better diagnoses and more individual treatment of tobacco dependence (Special Issue: Future Directions in Tobacco Research). Br J Addict 86:543–547, 1991

Fiore M, Smith S, Jorenby D, et al: The effectiveness of the nicotine patch for smoking cessation: a meta-analysis. JAMA 271:1940–1947, 1994

Fiore M, Bailey W, Cohen S, et al: Smoking Cessation: Clinical Practice Guideline No. 18. Rockville, MD, U.S. Department of Health and Human Services, Public Health Service, Agency for Health Care Policy and Research, 1996

Fiore MC, Bailey WC, Cohen SJ, et al: Treating Tobacco Use and Dependence: Clinical Practice Guideline. Rockville, MD, U.S. Department of Health and Human Services, Public Health Service, Agency for Healthcare Research and Quality, 2000

Foxx R, Brown R: Nicotine fading and self-monitoring for cigarette abstinence or controlled smoking. J Appl Behav Anal 12:111–125, 1979

Froom P, Melamed S, Benbasal J: Smoking cessation and weight gain. J Fam Pract 46:460–464, 1998

Glassman A: Cigarette smoking: implications for psychiatric illness. Am J Psychiatry 150:546–553, 1993

Goff D, Henderson D, Amico E: Cigarette smoking in schizophrenia: relationship to psychopathology and medication side effects. Am J Psychiatry 149:1189–1194, 1992

Goldfried M, Davison G: Clinical Behavior Therapy. New York, Holt, Rinehart, & Winston, 1976

Gourlay S, Benowitz N: Arteriovenous differences in plasma concentration of nicotine and catecholamines and related cardiovascular effects after smoking, nicotine nasal spray, and intravenous nicotine. Clin Pharmacol Ther 62:453–463, 1997

Gritz E, Berman B, Bastani R, et al: A randomized trial of a self-help smoking cessation intervention in a nonvolunteer female population: testing the limits of the public health model. Health Psychol 11:280–289, 1992

Grunberg N: The effects of nicotine and cigarette smoking on food consumption and taste preferences. Addict Behav 7:317–331, 1982

Gulliver S, Hughes J, Solomon L, et al: An investigation of self-efficacy, partner support and daily stresses as predictors of relapse to smoking in self-quitters. Addiction 90:767–772, 1995

Hall G: Pharmacology of tobacco smoking in relation to schizophrenia, in Biochemistry of Schizophrenia and Addiction: In Search of a Common Factor. Edited by Hemmings G. Baltimore, MD, University Park Press, 1980, pp 199–207

Hall R, Duhamel M, McClanahan R, et al: Level of functioning, severity of illness, and smoking status among chronic psychiatric patients. J Nerv Ment Dis 183:468–471, 1995

Hatsukami D, Morgan S, Pickens R, et al: Situational factors in cigarette smoking. Addict Behav 15:1–12, 1990

Heatherton T, Kozlowski L, Frecker R, et al: The Fagerstrom Test for Nicotine Dependence: a revision of the Fagerstrom Tolerance Questionnaire. Br J Addict 86:1119–1127, 1991

Henningfield J: Pharmacologic basis and treatment of cigarette smoking. J Clin Psychiatry 45:24–34, 1984

Hofstetter A, Schutz Y, Jequier E, et al: Increased 24-hours energy expenditure in cigarette smokers. N Engl J Med 314:79–82, 1986

Hughes J: Combined psychological and nicotine gum treatment for smoking: a critical review. J Subst Abuse 3:337–350, 1991

Hughes J: Possible effects of smoke-free inpatient units on psychiatric diagnosis and treatment. J Clin Psychiatry 54:109–114, 1993

Hughes J: Clinical implications of the association between smoking and alcoholism, in Alcohol and Tobacco: From Basic Science to Policy (NIAAA Research Monograph 30). Edited by Fertig J, Fuller R. Washington, DC, U.S. Government Printing Office, 1995a, pp 171–181

Hughes J: Treatment of nicotine dependence: is more better? JAMA 274:171–181, 1995b

Hughes J: Dependence on and abuse of nicotine replacement: an update, in Nicotine Safety and Toxicity. Edited by Benowitz N. New York, Oxford University Press, 1998, pp 147–160

Hughes J, Hatsukami D: Signs and symptoms of tobacco withdrawal. Arch Gen Psychiatry 43:289–294, 1986

Hughes J, Hatsukami D: The nicotine withdrawal syndrome: a brief review and update. International Journal of Smoking Cessation 1:21–26, 1992

Hughes J, Higgins S, Hatsukami D: Effects of abstinence from tobacco: a critical review, in Research Advances in Alcohol and Drug Problems. Edited by Kozlowski L, Annis H, Cappell H, et al. New York, Plenum, 1990, pp 317–398

Hughes J, Fiester S, Goldstein M, et al: American Psychiatric Association Practice Guideline for the treatment of patients with nicotine dependence. Am J Psychiatry 153:S1–S31, 1996

Hughes J, Goldstein M, Hurt R, et al: Recent advances in the pharmacotherapy of smoking. JAMA 281:72–76, 1999

Irvin J, Bowers C, Dunn M, et al: Efficacy of relapse prevention: a meta-analytic review. J Consult Clin Psychol 67:563–570, 1999

Istvan J, Matarazzo J: Tobacco, alcohol and caffeine use: a review of their interrelationships. Psychol Bull 95:301–326, 1984

Jusko W: Smoking and drug response. Pharmacology International 2:10–13, 1981

Kalman D: Smoking cessation treatment for substance misusers in early recovery: a review of the literature and recommendations for practice. Subst Use Misuse 33:2021–2047, 1998

Killen J, Fortmann S, Newman B, et al: Evaluation of a treatment approach combining nicotine gum with self-guided behavioral treatments for smoking relapse prevention. J Consult Clin Psychol 58:85–92, 1990

Klesges R, Meyers A, Klesges L, et al: Smoking, body weight and their effects on smoking behavior: a comprehensive review of the literature. Psychol Bull 106:204–230, 1989

Kozlowski L, Henningfield J, Keenan R, et al: Patterns of alcohol, cigarette, and caffeine and other drug use in two drug abusing populations. J Subst Abuse Treat 10:171–179, 1993

Kristeller J: The hard-core smoker: finding a definition to guide intervention. Health Values 18:25–32, 1994

Law M, Tang J: An analysis of the effectiveness of interventions intended to help people stop smoking. Arch Intern Med 155:1933–1941, 1995

Leshner A: Understanding drug addiction: implications for treatment. Hosp Pract (Off Ed) 31:47–54, 57–59, 1996

Lichtenstein E, Brown A: Current trends in the modification of cigarette dependence, in International Handbook of Behavior Modification and Therapy. Edited by Bellack A, Hersen M, Kazdin A. New York, Plenum, 1985, pp 575–612

Marlatt G, Gordon J: Determinants of relapse: implications for the maintenance of behavior change, in Behavioral Medicine: Changing Health Lifestyles. Edited by Davidson P, Davidson S. New York, Brunner/Mazel, 1980, pp 410–452

Massachusetts Department of Public Health: 1997 Cigarette Nicotine Disclosure Report as Required by Massachusetts General Laws. Chapter 307B, Report No CMR660.000, January 16, 1998

Mathew R, Weinman M, Mirabi M: Physical symptoms of depression. Br J Psychiatry 139:293–296, 1981

Menza M, Grossman N, Van Horn M, et al: Smoking and movement disorders in psychiatric patients. Biol Psychiatry 30:109–115, 1991

Newhouse P, Hughes J: The role of nicotine and nicotinic mechanisms in neuropsychiatric disease (Special Issue: Future Directions in Tobacco Research). Br J Addict 86:521–525, 1991

Nisell M, Nomikos G, Svensson T: Nicotine dependence, midbrain dopamine systems and psychiatric disorders. Pharmacol Toxicol 76:157–162, 1995

Ochs H, Otter H: Effects of age, sex, and smoking habits on oxazepam kinetics. Verh Dtsch Ges Inn Med 87:1205–1208, 1981

Ockene J, Benfari R, Hurwitz I, et al: Relationship of psychosocial factors to smoking behavior change in an intervention program. Prev Med 11:13–28, 1982

Ockene J, Kristeller J, Goldberg R, et al: Increasing the efficacy of physician-delivered smoking intervention: a randomized clinical trial. J Gen Intern Med 6:1–8, 1991

Ockene J, Kristeller J, Goldberg R, et al: Smoking cessation and severity of disease: the Coronary Artery Smoking Intervention Study. Health Psychol 11:119–126, 1992

Ockene J, Emmons K, Mermelstein R, et al: Relapse and maintenance issues for smoking cessation. Health Psychol 19:17–31, 2000

O'Farrell T, Connors G, Upper D: Addictive behaviors among hospitalized psychiatric patients. Addict Behav 8:329–333, 1983

Pantuck E, Pantuck C, Anderson K, et al: Cigarette smoking and chlorpromazine disposition and actions. Pharmacol Ther 31:533–538, 1982

Parrott A: Does cigarette smoking cause stress? Am Psychol 54:817–820, 1999

Perkins K: Metabolic effects of cigarette smoking. J Appl Physiol 72:401–409, 1992

Perry P, Miller D, Arndt S, et al: Haloperidol dosing requirements: the contribution of smoking and non-linear pharmacokinetics. J Clin Psychopharmacol 13:46–51, 1993

Pohl R, Yeragani V, Balon R, et al: Smoking in patients with panic disorder. Psychiatry Res 43:253–262, 1992

Pomerleau C, Pomerleau O: The effects of a psychosocial stressor on cigarette smoking and subsequent behavioral and physiological responses. Psychophysiology 24:278–285, 1987

Pomerleau O, Pomerleau C: Neuroregulators and the reinforcement of smoking: towards a biobehavioral explanation. Neurosci Biobehav Rev 8:503–513, 1984

Schachter S: Pharmacological and psychological determinants of smoking. Ann Intern Med 88:104–114, 1978

Schuh K, Schuh L, Henningfield J, et al: Nicotine nasal spray and vapor inhaler: abuse liability assessment. Psychopharmacology 130:352–361, 1997

Schwartz J: Methods of smoking cessation. Med Clin North Am 76:451–476, 1992

Sobell L, Sobell M, Toneatto T: Recovery from alcohol problems without treatment, in Self-Control and Addictive Behaviors. Edited by Heather N, Miller W, Greeley J. New York, Pergamon, 1992, pp 198–242

Sutherland G, Stapleton J, Russell M, et al: Randomised controlled trial of nasal nicotine spray in smoking cessation. Lancet 340:324–329, 1992

Tomkins S: Psychological model for smoking behavior. Am J Public Health 56:17–20, 1966

U.S. Department of Health and Human Services: The Health Benefits of Smoking Cessation: A Report of the Surgeon General (DHHS Publ No CDC 90-8416). Atlanta, GA, Center for Chronic Disease Prevention and Health Promotion, Office on Smoking and Health, 1990, pp 580–616

Velicer W, Fava J, Prochaska J, et al: Distribution of smokers by stage in three representative samples. Prev Med 48:401–411, 1995

Wack J, Rodin L: Smoking and its effects on body weight and the systems of caloric regulation. Am J Clin Nutr 35:366–380, 1982

Ward K, Klesges R, Halpern M: Predictors of smoking cessation and state-of-the-art smoking interventions. Journal of Social Issues 53:129–145, 1997

West R, Hajek P, Belcher M: Severity of withdrawal symptoms as a predictor of outcome of an attempt to quit smoking. Psychol Med 19:981–985, 1989

Wright T, Whitaker S, Welch C, et al: Hepatic enzyme induction patterns and phenothiazine side effects. Clin Pharmacol Ther 34:533–538, 1983

Ziedonis D, Kosten T, Glazer W, et al: Nicotine dependence and schizophrenia. Hosp Community Psychiatry 45:204–206, 1994

Benzodiazepines and Other Sedative-Hypnotics

David E. Smith, M.D.
Donald R. Wesson, M.D.

In this chapter, we focus on treatment of physical dependence on benzodiazepines and discuss other prescription sedative-hypnotics in terms of their similarities to or differences from benzodiazepines. Sedative-hypnotics are a chemically diverse group of compounds commonly prescribed to ameliorate symptoms of anxiety and insomnia. Although most benzodiazepines could also be classified as sedative-hypnotics, they are often grouped, as we have done here, by their chemical class name. All benzodiazepines currently marketed in the United States, except for the benzodiazepine antagonist flumazenil, share many pharmacological effects. Although clinically significant pharmacological differences exist among benzodiazepines (e.g., therapeutic indications, metabolic profile, receptor affinity, side effects, abuse potential), all benzodiazepine agonists produce little respiratory depression even in dosages much higher than those used to treat anxiety or insomnia. Even when a benzodiazepine is taken in an overdose of 20–30 times the usual therapeutic dose, fatality from respiratory depression is rare. The "safety" of benzodiazepines in the overdose situation is an important advantage of the benzodiazepines over the older sedative-hypnotics.

Despite the safety record of benzodiazepines, some combinations of medications with benzodiazepines have an increased potential for lethality. Buprenorphine is a partial opiate agonist that the U.S. Food and Drug Administration (FDA) approved in 2002 for the treatment of opiate dependence. Consistent with its pharmacological profile as a partial opiate agonist, buprenorphine has a ceiling for opiate effects and, like the benzodiazepine class of medications, is rarely lethal in overdose when taken alone. The combination of buprenorphine with a benzodiazepine (most frequently, flunitrazepam) has been implicated in deaths in France, where buprenorphine has been available since 1996 for the treatment of opiate dependence (Kintz 2001, 2002). A study in rats suggested that the combination of a benzodiazepine and buprenorphine has synergistic action in depressing respiration (Gueye et al. 2002). Benzodiazepines are commonly misused and abused among those receiving methadone maintenance and appear to be a factor in some lethal methadone-related overdoses (Ernst et al. 2002).

Benzodiazepines exert their physiological effects by attaching to a subunit of the γ-aminobutyric acid (GABA) receptor. GABA, the major inhibitory neurotransmitter in the brain and spinal cord, modulates the polarization of neurons. The GABA receptor is made up of an ion channel (an ionophore) and several subunits that bind to different drugs: one subunit binds GABA, another benzodiazepines, and another barbiturates. Benzodiazepines that enhance the effect of GABA are designated *agonists*.

Attachment of an agonist at the benzodiazepine receptor facilitates the effect of GABA (i.e., opens the chloride channel). Opening the chloride channel allows more chloride ions to enter neurons. The influx of negatively charged chloride ions increases the electrical gradient across the cell membrane and makes the neuron less excitable. The clinical effects are anxiety reduction, sedation, and increased seizure threshold. Closing the channel decreases electrical polarization and makes the cell more excitable. Substances that attach to the benzodiazepine receptor and close the channel produce an opposite effect: they are anxiogenic and lower the seizure threshold. Compounds that produce the opposite effects from benzodiazepine agonists, such as β-carboline, are designated *inverse agonists*.

Some compounds attach to the benzodiazepine receptor but neither increase nor decrease the effect of GABA. In the absence of benzodiazepine agonists or inverse agonists, they are neutral ligands (i.e., they attach to the receptor and block the effects of both the agonist and the inverse agonist). Neutral agonists are designated *antagonists*. If the receptor is already occupied by an agonist or inverse agonist, the antagonist may displace the agonist or inverse agonist. Displacement of a benzodiazepine agonist has clinical utility. For example, the benzodiazepine antagonist flumazenil is used to reverse the sedation produced by a benzodiazepine.

The long-term interaction of benzodiazepine receptors with their ligands is extremely complex. Attachment of the ligands can alter the pharmacodynamics of the receptors (e.g., altering the number of receptors or changing the affinity of the ligands for the receptors).

Benzodiazepine Abuse and Dependence

Benzodiazepines are not common primary drugs of abuse. Most people do not find the effects of benzodiazepines reinforcing or pleasurable (Chutuape and de Wit 1994). Sedative-hypnotic abusers prefer pentobarbital to diazepam, even at high dosages (Griffiths et al. 1980).

Abuse of flunitrazepam, a benzodiazepine not marketed in the United States, generated considerable media attention during the mid-1990s, particularly concerning its use as a "date rape drug" and as a drug of abuse by youths (Calhoun et al. 1996). In Europe, in experimental studies of animals and non-drug-abusing human subjects, one study found flunitrazepam to be similar to most other benzodiazepines in ability to produce drug-seeking behavior and capacity to produce physiological dependence (Woods and Winger 1997). A European study comparing flunitrazepam (0.5 and 2.0 mg) with triazolam (0.25 and 0.50 mg) in healthy male volunteers found that flunitrazepam (2.0 mg) induced significant increases in "liking" and "good effects" scales, which they suggested may indicate greater abuse potential (Farre et al. 1996).

The imidazopyridines—another chemical class of sedative-hypnotics, which includes alpidem, zolpidem, and zopiclone—attach to an ω_1 subunit of the benzodiazepine receptor and are efficacious hypnotics. Zolpidem is prescribed extensively for treatment of insomnia. It is absorbed rapidly and has a short half-life (2.2 hours). Its sedative effects are additive with alcohol. Few cases of zolpidem abuse or dependence have been reported. Some patients increase the dosage to many times that prescribed, and it appears that at very high dosage levels zolpidem produces tolerance and a withdrawal syndrome similar to that of other sedative-hypnotics (Cavallaro et al. 1993).

Studies with baboons suggested that zolpidem is reinforcing and that it produces tolerance and physical dependence (Griffiths et al. 1992). A review of the behavioral pharmacology of zolpidem can be found in Rush (1998).

Zaleplon is a pyrazolopyrimidine approved by the FDA for marketing in the United States in 1999. Like zolpidem, it is chemically unrelated to the benzodiazepines and binds to a subunit of the same complex (GABA-benzodiazepine) as the benzodiazepines. Studies in baboons (Ator et al. 2000) and healthy volunteers with a history of drug abuse (Rush et al. 1999) suggest an abuse potential similar to that of triazolam.

Patients who become physically dependent on benzodiazepines can generally be classified into one of three groups:

1. Street drug abusers who self-administer benzodiazepines as one of many substances in a pattern of polydrug abuse
2. Alcoholic individuals and prescription drug abusers who are prescribed benzodiazepines for treatment of chronic anxiety or insomnia
3. Non-drug-abusing patients with depression or panic disorders who are prescribed high dosages of benzodiazepines for long periods

Street drug abusers may take benzodiazepines to ameliorate the adverse effects of cocaine or methamphetamine, to self-medicate heroin or alcohol withdrawal, to enhance the effects of methadone, or to produce intoxication when other drugs are not available. Benzodiazepines are rarely their primary drug of abuse. Even if their use of benzodiazepines does not meet DSM-IV-TR criteria for abuse (American Psychiatric Association 2000), most people would call the use of benzodiazepines by street drug abusers *abuse* because it falls outside the context of medical treatment and is part of a polydrug abuse pattern. Furthermore, such patients often obtain the benzodiazepines by street purchase, theft, or forged prescriptions. Benzodiazepine dependency occurring among such patients must be treated in a comprehensive drug treatment program.

Alcohol and prescription drug abusers who are receiving treatment for chronic anxiety or insomnia are at significant risk for developing benzodiazepine dependency. They may receive benzodiazepines for a long time, and they may be biologically predisposed to develop benzodiazepine dependency. A study of alprazolam (1 mg) in alcoholic and nonalcoholic men found that alprazolam produced positive mood effects in alcoholic men that were not reported by the nonalcoholic men (Ciraulo et al. 1988). The difference in subjective response may be genetic. The mood-elevating effects of alprazolam were found to be greater in daughters of alcoholic parents than in those without a history of parental alcohol dependence (Ciraulo et al. 1996). Similar results have been found in sons of alcoholic parents (Cowley et al. 1992, 1994).

Patients who have depression or panic disorders may be prescribed high dosages of benzodiazepines for long periods of time. Some of these patients will develop physiological dependence on the benzodiazepines. Physiological dependency arising in the context of medical treatment does not necessarily equate with a substance abuse disorder or contraindicate benzodiazepine treatment. A history of sedative-hypnotic abuse, alcoholism, or severe symptoms following benzodiazepine discontinuation is a relative contraindication.

Other Sedative-Hypnotics

Short-acting sedative-hypnotics (e.g., secobarbital, pentobarbital) are primary drugs of abuse. Addicted persons take them alone by mouth or by injection to produce intoxication. Intoxication with sedative-hypnotics is similar to intoxication with alcohol, producing a state of disinhibition, in which mood is elevated, self-criticism, anxiety, and guilt are reduced, and energy and self-confidence are increased. During intoxication, the user's mood is often labile and may shift rapidly between euphoria and dysphoria. Users may also be irritable, hypochondriacal, anxious, or agitated, and they may have difficulty with memory. They may have poor judgment, ataxia, slurred speech, and sustained vertical and horizontal nystagmus.

Buspirone appears to have minimal abuse potential and does not produce physical dependence. Buspirone is a serotonin type 1A (5-HT_{1A}) partial agonist (Taylor and Moon 1991). Its anxiolytic effects take from days to weeks to develop. Buspirone will not prevent sedative-hypnotic withdrawal (i.e., it is not cross-tolerant with benzodiazepines), and it will not effectively treat benzodiazepine withdrawal syndromes (Schweizer and Rickels 1986). Clinical observations suggest that patients with a history of benzodiazepine abuse are resistant to the anxiolytic effects of buspirone (Schweizer et al. 1986).

Benzodiazepine and Other Sedative-Hypnotic Withdrawal Syndromes

The long-term use of benzodiazepines or sedative-hypnotics at dosages above the therapeutic dose range produces physical dependence, and both drug types have similar withdrawal syndromes that may be severe and life-threatening. Therapeutic doses of benzodiazepines taken daily for months to years also may produce physiological dependence.

High-Dose Sedative-Hypnotic Withdrawal Syndrome

Human studies have established that large doses of chlordiazepoxide (Hollister et al. 1961) and diazepam (Hollister et al. 1963), taken for 1 month or more, produce a sedative-hypnotic withdrawal syndrome. Other benzodiazepines have not been studied under such precise conditions, but case reports leave no doubt that they produce a similar withdrawal syndrome.

Signs and symptoms of sedative-hypnotic withdrawal include anxiety, tremors, nightmares, insomnia, anorexia, nausea, vomiting, postural hypotension, seizures, delirium, and hyperpyrexia. Abrupt discontinuation of sedative-hypnotics in patients who are severely physically dependent on them can result in serious medical complications and even death. The syndrome is qualitatively similar for all sedative-hypnotics; however, the time course and intensity of signs and symptoms may vary depending on the drug. With short-acting sedative-hypnotics (e.g., pentobarbital, secobarbital, meprobamate, methaqualone) and short-acting benzodiazepines (e.g., oxazepam, alprazolam, triazolam), withdrawal symptoms typically begin 12–24 hours after the last dose and peak in intensity between 24 and 72 hours. (Symptoms may develop more slowly in patients who have liver disease and in the elderly because of decreased drug metabolism.) With long-acting drugs (e.g., phenobarbital, diazepam, and chlordiazepoxide), withdrawal symptoms peak on the fifth to eighth day.

During untreated sedative-hypnotic withdrawal, the electroencephalogram may show paroxysmal bursts of high-voltage, slow-frequency activity that precedes the development of seizures. Withdrawal delirium may include confusion and visual and auditory hallucinations. Delirium generally follows a period of insomnia. Some patients may have only delirium, others have only seizures, and some may have both.

Low-Dose Benzodiazepine Withdrawal Syndrome

In the medical literature, the low-dose benzodiazepine withdrawal syndrome is variously referred to as *thera-*

peutic-dose withdrawal, normal-dose withdrawal, or *benzodiazepine discontinuation syndrome.*

Through the 1960s and early 1970s, it was generally believed that benzodiazepines taken within the usual recommended therapeutic dose range did not produce physical dependence. The knowledge that some patients had a withdrawal syndrome emerged from clinical observations. In 1978, investigators at the Addiction Research Center in Lexington, Kentucky, published a detailed case study of an incarcerated 37-year-old man who had been prescribed 30–45 mg/day of diazepam for 20 months (Pevnick et al. 1978). Five days after the subject was crossed over to placebo, he reported muscle twitches, muscle cramps, facial numbness, and abdominal cramping. The patient lost weight and had an increased pulse rate. Symptoms occurred primarily between days 5 and 9 and had abated by day 16.

Winokur et al. (1980) reported a similar placebo crossover study of a 32-year-old man who had been taking 15–25 mg/day of diazepam for 6 years. Two days after crossover to placebo, the patient began complaining of anxiety, dizziness, blurred vision, constipation, and palpitations. During the next 2 days, he became increasingly anxious and irritable, diaphoretic, and grossly tremulous, and he had difficulty expressing his thoughts coherently. His auditory and olfactory senses were "at times so hypersensitive that normally unobtrusive sounds (a watch ticking) or odors (an orange peel) were acutely uncomfortable to him" (p. 103). He was also hypersensitive to tactile stimuli, to the point that he could not stand to have clothes on his body. His symptoms subsided over the next 30 days.

Standard medical texts prior to 1980 generally concurred that therapeutic doses of benzodiazepines produced minimal withdrawal. During the 1980s, additional clinical studies and case reports established that therapeutic doses of benzodiazepines could produce physical dependency (Ladner 1991). Many patients experienced a transient increase in symptoms for 1–2 weeks after withdrawal. A few patients experienced a severe, protracted withdrawal syndrome that included symptoms, such as paresthesia and psychosis, that were not present before. The American Psychiatric Association formed a task force that reviewed the issues and published its report in book form (American Psychiatric Association Task Force on Benzodiazepine Dependency 1990). The conclusions of the task force were unambiguous about therapeutic dose dependency:

Physiological dependence on benzodiazepines, as indicated by the appearance of discontinuance symptoms, can develop with therapeutic doses. Duration of treatment determines the onset of dependence when typical therapeutic anxiolytic doses are used: clinically significant dependence indicated by the appearance of discontinuance symptoms usually does not appear before four months of such daily dosing. Dependence may develop sooner when higher antipanic doses are taken daily. (p. 56)

The chronology of therapeutic dose dependency is important for medical-legal reasons. During the 1980s, some patients who developed therapeutic dose dependency sued their physicians for malpractice, claiming that their physicians were negligent in not warning them about the possibility of therapeutic dose dependency and in treating them with benzodiazepines for extended periods, often many years. Some of these patients were treated, however, during the 1960s and 1970s. During those decades, therapeutic dose dependency was not part of mainstream medical knowledge.

Some patients who have taken a benzodiazepine in therapeutic doses for months to years can abruptly discontinue it without developing withdrawal symptoms. Others, taking similar amounts of a benzodiazepine, develop symptoms ranging from mild to severe when the benzodiazepine is stopped or the dosage is reduced substantially. Characteristically, patients tolerate a gradual tapering of the benzodiazepine until they are at 10%–20% of the peak dosage. Further reduction in benzodiazepine dose causes patients to become increasingly symptomatic.

At least three reasons explain symptoms that emerge after benzodiazepine cessation. Two of these, *symptom rebound* and the *protracted withdrawal syndrome*, are the result of dependence; the other, *symptom reemergence*, is not.

Symptom Rebound

Symptom rebound is an intensified return of the symptoms for which the benzodiazepine was prescribed (e.g., insomnia or anxiety). The term comes from sleep research in which rebound insomnia may occur after discontinuation of a hypnotic. Symptom rebound, the most common consequence of prolonged benzodiazepine use, may last a few days to weeks after discontinuation (American Psychiatric Association Task Force on Benzodiazepine Dependency 1990, p. 16).

Protracted Withdrawal From Benzodiazepines

Protracted withdrawal from benzodiazepines should be distinguished from the protracted withdrawal syndrome that has been described for most drugs, including alcohol. The symptoms generally attributed to protracted withdrawal syndromes consist of relatively mild symptoms such as irritability, anxiety, insomnia, and mood instability. The protracted withdrawal syndrome from benzodiazepines can be severe and disabling and may last many months.

Many symptoms are nonspecific, and they may mimic an obsessive-compulsive disorder with psychotic features. Symptoms such as increased sensitivity to sound, light, and touch and paresthesia are particularly suggestive of low-dose withdrawal.

The waxing and waning symptom intensity illustrated in the waviness of the line in the phase IV section of Figure 20–1 is characteristic of the low-dose protracted benzodiazepine withdrawal syndrome. Patients are sometimes asymptomatic for several days, then, without apparent reason, they become acutely anxious. Often, concomitant physiological signs (e.g., dilated pupils, increased resting heart rate and blood pressure) are present.

Protracted benzodiazepine withdrawal has no pathognomonic signs or symptoms, and the broad range of nonspecific symptoms produced by the protracted benzodiazepine withdrawal syndrome also mimic agitated depression, generalized anxiety disorder, panic disorder, complex partial seizures, and schizophrenia. The time course of symptom resolution is the primary differentiating feature between the symptoms generated by withdrawal and symptom reemergence. The symptoms from withdrawal subside gradually with continued abstinence, whereas symptom reemergence and symptom sensitization do not.

Symptom Reemergence (Recrudescence)

Patients' symptoms of anxiety, insomnia, or muscle tension abate during benzodiazepine treatment. When the benzodiazepine is stopped, symptoms return to the same level as before benzodiazepine therapy. A distinction is made between symptom rebound and symptom reemergence because symptom reemergence suggests underlying psychopathology, whereas symptom rebound suggests a withdrawal syndrome (American Psychiatric Association Task Force on Benzodiazepine Dependency 1990, p. 17).

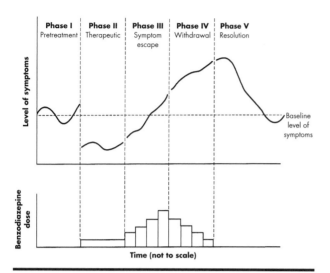

Figure 20–1. The treatment–dependence cycle.

Schematic illustration of a hypothetical patient's symptoms over time with continued benzodiazepine treatment. For some patients, the therapeutic phase may last for many years, and symptom escape is not an inevitable consequence of long-term treatment.

Risk Factors for Low-Dose Withdrawal

Some drugs or medications may facilitate neuroadaptation by increasing the affinity of benzodiazepines for their receptors. Patients at increased risk for development of the low-dose withdrawal syndrome are those with a family or personal history of alcoholism, those who use alcohol daily, or those who concomitantly use other sedatives. Case-control studies suggest that patients with a history of addiction, particularly to other sedative-hypnotics, are at high risk for benzodiazepine dependence. The short-acting, high-potency benzodiazepines appear to produce a more intense withdrawal syndrome (Rickels et al. 1990b).

The Dependence/Withdrawal Cycle

When dependence arises during therapeutic treatment, a sequence of phases often occurs (see Figure 20–1). The clinical course described here most often occurs during long-term treatment of a generalized anxiety disorder, panic disorder, or severe insomnia.

Pretreatment Phase

The first panel on Figure 20–1 represents the time before the patient was treated with benzodiazepines. Patients' symptoms generally vary in intensity from day to day depending on life stresses and the waxing and

waning of their underlying disorder. For purposes of the illustration, the average symptom level, shown by the horizontal dotted line, illustrates the patient's baseline level of symptoms.

Therapeutic Phase

When treatment with a benzodiazepine is started, patients often have initial side effects, such as drowsiness, psychomotor impairment, or memory impairment. Tolerance to such side effects usually develops within a few days, and afterward the patient's overall level of symptoms decreases. The therapeutic phase, illustrated in phase II of Figure 20–1, may last for months to years.

Symptom Escape and Dosage Escalation Phase

During long-term treatment, benzodiazepines may suddenly lose their effectiveness in controlling symptoms. For some patients, the *symptom escape* coincides with a period of increased life stress; for others, no unusual psychological stressor is apparent. Patients are often aware that the medication "no longer works" or that its effect is qualitatively different. The increasing symptoms are represented by the ascending wavy line in phase III of Figure 20–1.

As the usual dosages of benzodiazepines lose effectiveness, patients may increase their benzodiazepine consumption in the hope of regaining symptom amelioration. As the daily dosage of benzodiazepine increases, patients may develop subtle neuropsychological impairment that is difficult to diagnose without psychometric assessment.

Benzodiazepine-induced memory impairment may be a common clinical problem that generally goes unrecognized. It has not received sufficient research attention. Although many studies have reported that acute doses of benzodiazepines impair cognitive function, there has been little study of the effects of benzodiazepines with prolonged use. One psychometric study, which compared long-term benzodiazepine users with subjects who were benzodiazepine abstinent, found that the long-term benzodiazepine users performed poorly on tasks involving visual-spatial ability and sustained attention (Golombok et al. 1988). Patients may not be aware that their impairment is benzodiazepine induced. Coping skills that were previously bolstered by the benzodiazepine may become compromised. In a study of long-term benzodiazepine users taking 5–20 mg/day of diazepam, the neurocognitive effects of a 10-

mg oral dose of diazepam had no measurable effect on psychomotor performance; however, it did produce measurable effects on memory. The authors concluded that tolerance to the memory effects of benzodiazepines does not fully develop (Gorenstein et al. 1994).

The symptom escape phase is not an invariable consequence of long-term benzodiazepine treatment. Patients who have experienced symptom escape and dosage escalation may also be the most likely to have a protracted withdrawal syndrome.

Withdrawal Phase

When patients stop taking the benzodiazepine or the daily dosage falls below 25% of the peak maintenance dosage, patients become increasingly symptomatic. The symptoms, represented by the ascending wavy line in phase IV of Figure 20–1, may be the result of symptom rebound, symptom reemergence, or the beginning of a protracted withdrawal syndrome. The symptoms that occur during this phase may be a mixture of symptoms that were present during the pretreatment phase and new symptoms. During the first few weeks, it is not possible to determine the exact cause of the symptoms or to accurately predict their duration. Symptoms of the same type that occurred during the pretreatment phase suggest symptom rebound or symptom reemergence. New symptoms, particularly alterations in sensory perception, suggest the beginning of a protracted withdrawal syndrome. Increasing the benzodiazepine dosage will reduce symptoms because benzodiazepines have not completely lost effectiveness and because the withdrawal syndrome is reversed; however, symptom reduction will not be as complete as during the initial therapeutic phase.

Resolution Phase

The duration of the resolution phase is highly variable. Most patients will have only symptom rebound lasting a few weeks; others will have a severe, protracted abstinence syndrome lasting months to more than 1 year. During early abstinence, the patient's symptoms will generally vary in intensity from day to day. If abstinence from benzodiazepines is maintained, symptoms will gradually return to their baseline level. An encouraging finding of one discontinuation study was that "patients who were able to remain free of benzodiazepines for at least 5 weeks obtained lower levels of anxiety than before benzodiazepine discontinuation" (Rickels et al. 1990b, p. 899).

Pharmacological Treatment of Benzodiazepine Withdrawal

The physician's response during the withdrawal phase is critical to achieving a satisfactory resolution of the physical dependency. One common response is to declare the patient "addicted to benzodiazepines" and refer him or her for chemical dependency treatment; however, referral to a chemical dependency program is not appropriate unless the patient has a substance abuse disorder. Some physicians interpret the patient's escalating symptoms as evidence of the patient's "need" for benzodiazepine treatment and reinstitute higher dosages of benzodiazepines or switch the patient to another benzodiazepine. Reinstitution of any benzodiazepine agonist usually does not achieve satisfactory symptom control and may prolong the recovery process. Benzodiazepine withdrawal, using one of the strategies described in this section, generally achieves the best long-term outcome.

The salient features of the various benzodiazepine withdrawal syndromes are summarized in Table 20–1. Benzodiazepine withdrawal strategies must be tailored to suit three possible dependency situations:

1. A high-dose withdrawal (i.e., doses greater than the recommended therapeutic doses for more than 1 month)
2. A low-dose withdrawal (i.e., doses below those in the upper range of Table 20–2)
3. A combined high-dose and low-dose withdrawal (i.e., following daily high dosages for more than 6 months, both a high-dose sedative-hypnotic withdrawal syndrome and a low-dose benzodiazepine withdrawal syndrome may occur)

High-Dose Sedative-Hypnotic Withdrawal

Four general strategies may be used for withdrawing patients from sedative-hypnotics, including benzodiazepines. The first is to use decreasing dosages of the agent of dependence. The second is to substitute phenobarbital or some other long-acting barbiturate for the addicting agent and gradually withdraw the substitute medication (Smith and Wesson 1970, 1971, 1983). The third, used for patients with a dependence on both alcohol and a benzodiazepine, is to substitute a long-acting benzodiazepine, such as chlordiazepoxide, and taper it over 1–2 weeks. Finally, valproate

Table 20–1. Characteristics of syndromes related to benzodiazepine withdrawal

Syndrome	Signs and symptoms	Time course	Response to reinstitution of benzodiazepine
High-dose withdrawal	Anxiety, insomnia, nightmares, major motor seizures, psychosis, hyperpyrexia, death	Begins 1–2 days after a short-acting benzodiazepine is stopped; 3–8 days after a long-acting benzodiazepine is stopped	Signs and symptoms reverse 2–6 hours after a hypnotic dose of a benzodiazepine
Symptom rebound	Same symptoms that were present before treatment	Begins 1–2 days after a short-acting benzodiazepine is stopped; 3–8 days after a long-acting benzodiazepine is stopped; lasts 7–14 days	Signs and symptoms reverse 2–6 hours after a hypnotic dose of a benzodiazepine
Protracted, low-dose withdrawal	Anxiety, agitation, tachycardia, palpitations, anorexia, blurred vision, muscle cramps, insomnia, nightmares, confusion, muscle spasms, psychosis, increased sensitivity to sounds and light, paresthesia	Signs and symptoms emerge 1–7 days after a benzodiazepine is stopped or after a benzodiazepine is reduced to below the usual therapeutic dose	Signs and symptoms reverse 2–6 hours after a sedative dose of high-potency benzodiazepine
Symptom reemergence	Recurrence of the same symptoms that were present before taking a benzodiazepine (e.g., anxiety, insomnia)	Symptoms emerge when a benzodiazepine is stopped and continue unabated with time	Signs and symptoms reverse 2–6 hours after usual therapeutic dose of a benzodiazepine

or carbamazepine may be prescribed. The method selected will depend on the particular benzodiazepine, the involvement of other drugs of dependence, and the clinical setting in which the detoxification program takes place.

Phenobarbital Substitution

Phenobarbital substitution has the broadest use for all sedative-hypnotic drug dependencies. Substitution of phenobarbital can also be used to withdraw patients who have lost control of their benzodiazepine use or who are dependent on multiple sedative-hypnotics, including alcohol.

The pharmacological rationale for phenobarbital substitution is that phenobarbital is long acting, and little change in blood levels of phenobarbital occurs between doses. This allows the safe use of a progressively smaller daily dose. Phenobarbital is safer than the shorter-acting barbiturates; lethal doses of phenobarbital are many times higher than toxic doses, and the signs of toxicity (i.e., sustained nystagmus, slurred speech, and ataxia) are easy to observe. Phenobarbital has low abuse potential (Griffiths and Roache 1985), and intoxication usually does not produce behavioral

disinhibition. Most patients view phenobarbital as a medication, not as a drug of abuse. Phenobarbital is excreted primarily by the kidneys, is not toxic to the liver, and can used in the presence of significant liver disease.

Stabilization phase. The patient's history of drug use during the month before treatment is used to compute the initial stabilization dosage of phenobarbital. Although many addicted patients exaggerate the number of pills they are taking, patient history is the best guide to initiating pharmacotherapy. Patients who have overstated the amount of drug they are taking will become intoxicated during the first day or two of treatment. Intoxication is easily managed by omitting one or more doses of phenobarbital and downwardly adjusting the daily dosage. The key is close monitoring of the patient for signs and symptoms of intoxication or toxicity.

The patient's average daily sedative-hypnotic dosage is converted to phenobarbital withdrawal equivalents, and the daily amount is divided into three doses. (The conversion equivalents for various benzodiazepines are listed in Table 20–2 and for other sedative-hypnotics in Table 20–3.)

The computed daily phenobarbital dosage is given in divided doses three times daily. If the patient is us-

Table 20–2. Benzodiazepines and their phenobarbital withdrawal equivalents

Generic name	Trade name	Common therapeutic indication(s)	Therapeutic dose range (mg/day)	Dose equal to 30 mg phenobarbital for withdrawal (mg)[a]
Alprazolam	Xanax	Sedative, antipanic	0.75–6	1
Chlordiazepoxide	Librium	Sedative	15–100	25
Clonazepam	Klonopin	Anticonvulsant	0.5–4	2
Clorazepate	Tranxene	Sedative	15–60	7.5
Diazepam	Valium	Sedative	4–40	10
Estazolam	ProSom	Hypnotic	1–2	1
Flumazenil	Romazicon	Benzodiazepine antagonist	N/A	N/A
Flunitrazepam[b]	Rohypnol[b]	Hypnotic	0.5–1	0.5
Flurazepam	Dalmane	Hypnotic	15–30[c]	15
Halazepam	Paxipam	Sedative	60–160	40
Lorazepam	Ativan	Sedative	1–6	2
Midazolam	Versed	Intravenous sedation	2.5–7	2.5
Nitrazepam[b]	Mogadon[b]	Hypnotic	5–10	5
Oxazepam	Serax	Sedative	10–120	10
Prazepam	Centrax	Sedative	15–30	15
Quazepam	Doral	Hypnotic	15	15
Temazepam	Restoril	Hypnotic	15–30	15
Triazolam	Halcion	Hypnotic	0.125–0.50	0.25

Note. N/A=not applicable.
[a]Phenobarbital withdrawal conversion equivalence is not the same as therapeutic dose equivalency. Withdrawal equivalence is the amount of the drug that 30 mg of phenobarbital will substitute for and prevent serious high-dose withdrawal signs and symptoms.
[b]Although not marketed in the United States, these benzodiazepines are commonly used in many countries.
[c]Usual hypnotic dose.

ing significant amounts of other sedative-hypnotics (including alcohol), the amounts of all the drugs are converted to phenobarbital equivalents and added together (30 cc of 100-proof alcohol is equated to 30 mg of phenobarbital for withdrawal purposes). The maximum starting phenobarbital dosage, however, is 500 mg/day.

Before receiving each dose of phenobarbital, the patient is checked for signs of phenobarbital toxicity: sustained nystagmus, slurred speech, or ataxia. Sustained nystagmus is the most reliable sign of phenobarbital toxicity. If nystagmus is present, the scheduled dose of phenobarbital is withheld. If all three signs are present, the next two doses of phenobarbital are withheld, and the daily dosage of phenobarbital for the following day is halved.

If the patient is in acute withdrawal and has had or is in danger of having withdrawal seizures, the initial dose of phenobarbital is administered by intramuscular injection. If nystagmus and other signs of intoxication develop 1–2 hours after the intramuscular dosage, the patient is in no immediate danger from barbitu-

rate withdrawal. Patients are maintained on the initial dosing schedule of phenobarbital for 2 days. If the patient has signs of neither withdrawal nor phenobarbital toxicity, then the patient enters the withdrawal phase of treatment.

Withdrawal phase. Unless the patient develops signs and symptoms of phenobarbital toxicity or sedative-hypnotic withdrawal, phenobarbital is decreased by 30 mg/day. Should signs of phenobarbital toxicity develop during withdrawal, the daily phenobarbital dose is decreased by 50% and the 30 mg/day withdrawal is continued from the reduced phenobarbital dosage. Should the patient have objective signs of sedative-hypnotic withdrawal, the daily dosage is increased by 50% and the patient is restabilized before continuing the withdrawal.

Low-Dose Benzodiazepine Withdrawal

In low-dose benzodiazepine withdrawal, most patients experience only mild to moderate symptom rebound

Table 20–3. Sedative-hypnotics and their phenobarbital withdrawal equivalents

Generic name	Trade name	Common therapeutic indication(s)	Therapeutic dose range (mg/day)	Dose equal to 30 mg phenobarbital for withdrawal (mg)[a]
Barbiturates				
Amobarbital	Amytal	Sedative	50–150	100
Butabarbital	Butisol	Sedative	45–120	100
Butalbital	Fiorinal, Sedapap	Sedative/analgesic[b]	100–300	100
Pentobarbital	Nembutal	Hypnotic	50–100[b]	100
Secobarbital	Seconal	Hypnotic	50–100[b]	100
Other sedative-hypnotics				
Buspirone	BuSpar	Sedative	15–60	NC
Chloral hydrate	Noctec	Hypnotic	250–1,000	500
Ethchlorvynol	Placidyl	Hypnotic	500–1,000	500
Glutethimide	Doriden	Hypnotic	250–500	250
Meprobamate	Miltown, Equanil, Equagesic, Deprol	Sedative	1,200–1,600	400
Methyprylon	Noludar	Hypnotic	200–400	200
Zaleplon	Sonata	Hypnotic	5–20	5
Zolpidem	Ambien	Hypnotic	5–10	5

Note. NC=not cross-tolerant with barbiturates.
[a]Phenobarbital withdrawal conversion equivalence is not the same as therapeutic dose equivalency. Withdrawal equivalence is the amount of the drug that 30 mg of phenobarbital will substitute for and prevent serious high-dose withdrawal signs and symptoms.
[b]Butalbital is usually available in combination with opiate or nonopiate analgesics.

that disappears after a few days to weeks. No special treatment is needed. During early abstinence, patients need support and reassurance that rebound symptoms are common and that with continued abstinence the symptoms will subside.

Some patients experience severe symptoms that may be quite unlike preexisting symptoms. The phenobarbital regimen described earlier will not suppress symptoms to tolerable levels, but increasing the phenobarbital dose to 200 mg/day and then tapering the phenobarbital over several months can be an effective protocol for treating low-dose withdrawal. There are other protocols for discontinuation.

Gradual Reduction of the Benzodiazepine

The gradual reduction of the benzodiazepine of dependence is used primarily for treatment of physiological dependence on long-acting benzodiazepines arising from treatment of an underlying condition. The patient must be cooperative and able to adhere to dosing regimens and must not be abusing alcohol or other drugs.

Carbamazepine and Valproate

Medications used for treatment of seizure disorders have found clinical utility in treatment of mood and anxiety disorders (Keck et al. 1992) and in patients with comorbid anxiety and alcohol dependence (Brady et al. 1994). The medications most studied have been carbamazepine and valproate, although gabapentin and lamotrigine are receiving scrutiny. Carbamazepine and valproate enhance GABA function, seemingly by a different mechanism than the benzodiazepines. Neither carbamazepine nor valproate produces subjective effects that sedative-hypnotic abusers find desirable.

Valproate has received some clinical attention for treatment of alcohol withdrawal (Hammer and Brady 1996; Hillbom et al. 1989) and has been proposed for benzodiazepine withdrawal (Roy-Byrne et al. 1989). Clinical case reports of its use in benzodiazepine withdrawal have appeared (Apelt and Emrich 1990; McElroy et al. 1991). For low-dose benzodiazepine withdrawal, a valproate dosage of 500–1,500 mg/day can be used. The most common side effect of valproate is gastrointestinal upset.

Carbamazepine is used widely in Europe for treatment of alcohol withdrawal. Case reports and controlled studies suggest its utility in treating benzodiazepine withdrawal (Klein et al. 1986; Lawlor 1987; Neppe and Sindorf 1991; Rickels et al. 1990a; Ries et al. 1989; Schweizer et al. 1991). Withdrawal protocols use carbamazepine in a dosage of 200–800 mg/day.

In clinical experience with treating benzodiazepine withdrawal and in the controlled clinical trials in the treatment of epilepsy, valproate appears to be better tolerated than carbamazepine (Richens et al. 1994).

Outpatient Treatment of Withdrawal

Although withdrawal from high dosages of barbiturates and other sedative-hypnotics should generally be done in a hospital, the realities of managed care often mean that many patients must be treated in part, if not exclusively, as outpatients. With patients who are withdrawing from therapeutic doses of benzodiazepines, a slow outpatient taper is a reasonable strategy and should be continued as long as the patient can tolerate withdrawal symptoms.

Conclusion

Benzodiazepines have many therapeutic uses, and in the treatment of some conditions, such as panic disorder, benzodiazepine treatment for months or years is appropriate. Dependency is not always an avoidable complication. Physicians should discuss with patients before initiating a course of prolonged therapy the possibility of their developing new or intensified symptoms when the benzodiazepines are discontinued.

References

American Psychiatric Association: Diagnostic and Statistical Manual of Mental Disorders, 4th Edition, Text Revision. Washington, DC, American Psychiatric Association, 2000

American Psychiatric Association Task Force on Benzodiazepine Dependency: Benzodiazepine Dependency, Toxicity, and Abuse. Washington, DC, American Psychiatric Association, 1990

Apelt S, Emrich HM: Sodium valproate in benzodiazepine withdrawal (letter). Am J Psychiatry 147:950–951, 1990

Ator NA, Weerts EM, Kaminski BJ, et al: Zaleplon and triazolam physical dependence assessed across increasing doses under a once-daily dosing regimen in baboons. Drug Alcohol Depend 61:69–84, 2000

Brady KT, Sonne S, Lydiard RB: Valproate treatment of co-morbid panic disorder and affective disorders in two alcoholic patients (letter). J Clin Psychopharmacol 14:81–82, 1994

Calhoun SR, Wesson DR, Galloway GP, et al: Abuse of flunitrazepam (Rohypnol) and other benzodiazepines in Austin and south Texas. J Psychoactive Drugs 28:183–189, 1996

Cavallaro R, Regazzetti MG, Covelli G, et al: Tolerance and withdrawal with zolpidem (letter). Lancet 342(8867): 374–375, 1993

Chutuape MA, de Wit H: Relationship between subjective effects and drug preferences: ethanol and diazepam. Drug Alcohol Depend 34:243–251, 1994

Ciraulo DA, Barnhill JG, Greenblatt DJ, et al: Abuse liability and clinical pharmacokinetics of alprazolam in alcoholic men. J Clin Psychiatry 49:333–337, 1988

Ciraulo DA, Sarid-Segal O, Knapp C, et al: Liability to alprazolam abuse in daughters of alcoholics. Am J Psychiatry 153:956–958, 1996

Cowley DS, Roy-Byrne PP, Godon C, et al: Response to diazepam in sons of alcoholics. Alcohol Clin Exp Res 16: 1057–1063, 1992

Cowley DS, Roy-Byrne PP, Radant A, et al: Eye movement effects of diazepam in sons of alcoholic fathers and male control subjects. Alcohol Clin Exp Res 18:324–332, 1994

Ernst E, Bartu A, Popescu A, et al: Methadone-related deaths in Western Australia 1993–99. Aust N Z J Public Health 26:364–370, 2002

Farre M, Teran MT, Cami J: A comparison of the acute behavioral effects of flunitrazepam and triazolam in healthy volunteers. Psychopharmacology (Berl) 125:1–12, 1996

Golombok S, Moodley P, Lader M: Cognitive impairment in long-term benzodiazepine users. Psychol Med 18:365–374, 1988

Gorenstein C, Bernik MA, Pompeia S: Differential acute psychomotor and cognitive effects of diazepam on long-term benzodiazepine users. Int Clin Psychopharmacol 9:145–153, 1994

Griffiths R, Roache J: Abuse liability of benzodiazepines: a review of human studies evaluating subjective and/or reinforcing effects, in The Benzodiazepines: Current Standards for Medical Practice. Edited by Smith D, Wesson D. Hingham, MA, MTP Press, 1985, pp 209–225

Griffiths RR, Bigelow GE, Liebson I, et al: Drug preference in humans: double-blind choice comparison of pentobarbital, diazepam and placebo. J Pharmacol Exp Ther 215:649–661, 1980

Griffiths RR, Sannerud CA, Ator NA, et al: Zolpidem behavioral pharmacology in baboons: self-injection, discrimination, tolerance and withdrawal. J Pharmacol Exp Ther 260:1199–1208, 1992

Gueye PN, Borron SW, Risede P, et al: Buprenorphine and midazolam act in combination to depress respiration in rats. Toxicol Sci 65:107–114, 2002

Hammer BA, Brady KT: Valproate treatment of alcohol withdrawal and mania (letter). Am J Psychiatry 153:1232, 1996

Hillbom M, Tokola R, Kuusela V, et al: Prevention of alcohol withdrawal seizures with carbamazepine and valproic acid. Alcohol 6:223–226, 1989

Hollister L, Motzenbecker E, Degan R: Withdrawal reactions from chlordiazepoxide (Librium). Psychopharmacologia 2:63–68, 1961

Hollister LE, Bennett LL, Kimbell I, et al: Diazepam in newly admitted schizophrenics. Dis Nerv Syst 24:746–750, 1963

Keck PE Jr, McElroy SL, Friedman LM: Valproate and carbamazepine in the treatment of panic and posttraumatic stress disorders, withdrawal states, and behavioral dyscontrol syndromes. J Clin Psychopharmacol 12 (suppl):36S–41S, 1992

Kintz P: Deaths involving buprenorphine: a compendium of French cases. Forensic Sci Int 121:65–69, 2001

Kintz P: A new series of 13 buprenorphine-related deaths. Clin Biochem 35:513–516, 2002

Klein E, Uhde TW, Post RM: Preliminary evidence for the utility of carbamazepine in alprazolam withdrawal. Am J Psychiatry 143:235–236, 1986

Ladner M: History of benzodiazepine dependence. J Subst Abuse Treat 8:53–59, 1991

Lawlor BA: Carbamazepine, alprazolam withdrawal, and panic disorder (letter). Am J Psychiatry 144:265–266, 1987

McElroy SL, Keck PE Jr, Lawrence JM: Treatment of panic disorder and benzodiazepine withdrawal with valproate (letter). J Neuropsychiatry Clin Neurosci 3:232–233, 1991

Neppe VM, Sindorf J: Carbamazepine for high-dose diazepam withdrawal in opiate users. J Nerv Ment Dis 179:234–235, 1991

Pevnick JS, Jasinski DR, Haertzen CA: Abrupt withdrawal from therapeutically administered diazepam. Arch Gen Psychiatry 35:995–998, 1978

Richens A, Davidson DL, Cartlidge NE, et al: A multicentre comparative trial of sodium valproate and carbamazepine in adult onset epilepsy. J Neurol Neurosurg Psychiatry 57:682–687, 1994

Rickels K, Case WG, Schweizer E, et al: Benzodiazepine dependence: management of discontinuation. Psychopharmacol Bull 26:63–68, 1990a

Rickels K, Schweizer E, Case WG, et al: Long-term therapeutic use of benzodiazepines, I: effects of abrupt discontinuation [published erratum appears in Arch Gen Psychiatry 48(1):51, 1991]. Arch Gen Psychiatry 47:899–907, 1990b

Ries RK, Roy-Byrne PP, Ward NG, et al: Carbamazepine treatment for benzodiazepine withdrawal. Am J Psychiatry 146:536–537, 1989

Roy-Byrne PP, Ward NG, Donnelly PJ: Valproate in anxiety and withdrawal syndromes. J Clin Psychiatry 50 (suppl):44–48, 1989

Rush CR: Behavioral pharmacology of zolpidem relative to benzodiazepines: a review. Pharmacol Biochem Behav 61:253–269, 1998

Rush CR, Frey JM, Griffiths RR: Zaleplon and triazolam in humans: acute behavioral effects and abuse potential. Psychopharmacology (Berl) 145:39–51, 1999

Schweizer E, Rickels K: Failure of buspirone to manage benzodiazepine withdrawal. Am J Psychiatry 143:1590–1592, 1986

Schweizer E, Rickels K, Lucki I: Resistance to the anti-anxiety effect of buspirone in patients with a history of benzodiazepine use (letter). N Engl J Med 314:719–720, 1986

Schweizer E, Rickels K, Case WG, et al: Carbamazepine treatment in patients discontinuing long-term benzodiazepine therapy: effects on withdrawal severity and outcome. Arch Gen Psychiatry 48:448–452, 1991

Smith DE, Wesson DR: A new method for treatment of barbiturate dependence. JAMA 213:294–295, 1970

Smith DE, Wesson DR: Phenobarbital technique for treatment of barbiturate dependence. Arch Gen Psychiatry 24:56–60, 1971

Smith DE, Wesson DR: Benzodiazepine dependency syndromes. J Psychoactive Drugs 15:85–95, 1983

Taylor DP, Moon SL: Buspirone and related compounds as alternative anxiolytics. Neuropeptides 19 (suppl):15–19, 1991

Winokur A, Rickels K, Greenblatt DJ, et al: Withdrawal reaction from long-term, low-dosage administration of diazepam: a double-blind, placebo-controlled case study. Arch Gen Psychiatry 37:101–105, 1980

Woods JH, Winger G: Abuse liability of flunitrazepam. J Clin Psychopharmacol 17 (3, suppl 2):1S–57S, 1997

Inhalants

Thomas J. Crowley, M.D.
Joseph T. Sakai, M.D.

Inhalants, also called *volatile substances, volatile solvents, volatile compounds,* and *organic solvents,* are substances that are volatile at room temperature and are deliberately inhaled to cause intoxication. Common household products, such as rubber cement, nail polish remover, spray paints, and cleaning agents, can contain volatile solvents (Table 21–1), meaning that these products are widely available to children and adolescents. Once obtained, inhalants can be 1) sprayed (spraying directly into the mouth), 2) huffed (holding a cloth soaked in the substance to the mouth and taking several breaths), or 3) bagged (concentrating vapors in a bag and inhaling them).

Epidemiology

Prevalence of Inhalant Use

Inhalant use is common among adolescents. In 2001, 17.1% of eighth graders reported using inhalants at least once in their lifetime (Johnston et al. 2001), and in 1999, there were 1 million new inhalant users in the United States (Substance Abuse and Mental Health Services Administration 2002). However, past-year inhalant use declines from about 4% during adolescence to 0%–0.5% among those in their mid-20s and older (National Household Survey on Drug Abuse 2002), and of 12- to 17-year-olds who reported ever using inhalants, about 70% had used fewer than six times (Neumark et al. 1998). Although about one in six adolescents tries inhalants, it appears that most use only once or a few times.

Prevalence of Inhalant Abuse and Dependence

Inhalant dependence is relatively uncommon, and only a small proportion of those who try inhalants progress to inhalant dependence. The prevalence of DSM-III-R–defined (American Psychiatric Association 1987) lifetime inhalant dependence was estimated from the National Comorbidity Survey at 0.3%, compared with 24.1% for nicotine dependence and 14.1% for alcohol dependence (Anthony et al. 1994). On average, about 1 in 27 lifetime inhalant users met criteria for inhalant dependence, whereas about 1 in 4 people who had tried heroin were dependent (Anthony et al.

Table 21–1. Some household products and possible contents

Product	Possible contents
Air freshener	Amyl, butyl, cyclohexyl nitrite
Air freshener (spray)	Butane; propane
Carburetor cleaning fluid	Propane; toluene; 1,1,1-trichloroethane
Cigarette lighter fluid	Butane
Cleaning agents	n-Hexane; tetrachloroethylene; 1,1,1-trichloroethane; trichloroethylene
Computer/electronics cleaner (spray)	Butane; n-hexane; propane
Gasoline	Benzene; n-hexane; toluene; xylene; sometimes lead
Gum/adhesive remover	1,1,1-Trichloroethane; xylene
Hair spray	Butane; propane
Mothballs	Naphthalene; paradichlorobenzene
Nail polish remover	Acetone; toluene
Paint thinner/stripper	Toluene; trichloroethylene; xylene
Permanent markers	Xylene
Pipe cement	Methyl ethyl ketone; trichloroethylene
Refrigerant	Freon
Rubber cement	Acetone; benzene; n-Hexane; toluene
Rust preventer	Xylene
Solvent-based paints	Toluene; xylene
Spray paint	Butane; propane; toluene
Varnishes/lacquers	Toluene; xylene
Video head cleaner	Amyl, butyl, cyclohexyl nitrite
Whipped cream canisters	Nitrous oxide

Note. Ingredients vary by brand. Some labels do not list ingredients, but an Internet search for MSDS (material safety data sheets) and the product may help to identify hazardous ingredients.

1994). More recently, past-year prevalence of DSM-IV-TR-defined inhalant abuse or dependence (American Psychiatric Association 2000) has been estimated at 0.1% (0.4% of 12- to 17-year-olds) (Substance Abuse and Mental Health Services Administration 2003).

Prevalence of Treatment Seeking

A small proportion of adolescents in substance treatment programs nationally have problematic use of inhalants. In 1999, of 131,000 adolescents admitted to federally monitored substance abuse treatment facilities, only 2,091 (1.6%) had an identified problem with inhalants, and more than 90% of these adolescents also had problematic use of substances other than inhalants (Drug and Alcohol Services Information System 2002). We and our colleagues treat adolescents ages 13–19 years with conduct and substance use problems in a program with outpatient, day treatment, and residential services. Since 1995, the program has had almost 800 patient admissions who completed a standardized diagnostic interview—the CIDI-SAM (Composite International Diagnostic Interview, Substance Abuse Module; Cottler et al. 1989). In this sample, 16 patients (2%) met criteria for inhalant abuse, and 8 (1%) met criteria for inhalant dependence. Of those with inhalant dependence, 7 of 8 (88%) also had cannabis dependence, 7 of 8 (88%) had nicotine dependence, 6 of 8 (75%) had alcohol dependence, and 4 of 8 (50%) were dependent on any other substance (such as hallucinogens, cocaine, or opiates), suggesting that inhalant abuse and dependence are relatively uncommon and often co-occur with alcohol, cannabis, and nicotine dependence.

Comorbidity

Despite the relatively low prevalence of inhalant dependence, a strong association exists between inhalant use and antisocial personality disorder (Dinwiddie et al. 1990), polysubstance use (Dinwiddie and Reich 1991), and later injection drug use (Johnson et al. 1995; Schultz et al. 1994). This suggests that for a subgroup of inhalant users, especially those with comorbid conduct disorder, inhalant use presages or co-occurs with serious polysubstance involvement.

Pharmacology

Pharmacokinetics

Because inhalants encompass many different substances, in-depth discussion of the pharmacology of each of these substances is beyond the scope of this chapter. Generally, inhalants consist of hydrocarbon chains that are highly lipophilic. When inhaled, they are quickly absorbed into the bloodstream through the extensive pulmonary vasculature, readily cross the blood-brain barrier, and accumulate in lipid-rich organs, such as the brain. Some inhalants (such as toluene) undergo extensive hepatic metabolism; these metabolites are then more slowly excreted in the urine. Other inhalants (such as 1,1,1,-trichloroethane) are mostly exhaled unchanged.

Pharmacodynamics

Although individuals may briefly experience euphoria, disinhibition, and hallucinations, inhalants are central nervous system (CNS) depressants and result in subsequent drowsiness that lasts a few hours. It is not well understood how inhalants exert their psychoactive effect. Cross-tolerance to other CNS depressants and limited animal research suggest that inhalants' effects, like those of other CNS depressants, may be mediated through γ-aminobutyric acid (GABA) and *N*-methyl-D-aspartate (NMDA) receptors (Balster 1998). Animal studies show that toluene alters activity in the ventral tegmental dopamine system and increases extracellular dopamine in the prefrontal cortex, and the reinforcing effects of inhalants may be mediated through these changes (Gerasimov et al. 2002; Riegel and French 1999).

Toxicology

Chronic use of inhalants is associated with medical, neurological, and psychiatric problems. Inhalants readily cross the placenta, and inhalant use is also associated with several congenital problems.

Medical Problems

Inhalants can affect various systems: cardiac (arrhythmia, cardiomyopathy, heart block), dermatological (burns, perioral infection, rash), gastrointestinal (hepatitis, hepatorenal failure, nausea, vomiting, anorexia), genitourinary (glomerulonephritis, Goodpasture's syndrome, hypokalemia, type I renal tubular acidosis), hematopoietic (aplastic anemia, bone marrow suppression, leukemia), musculoskeletal (rhabdomyolysis), and pulmonary (chemical pneumonitis, emphysema, hypoxia, aspiration pneumonia).

Associations between particular solvents and certain medical sequelae have been described through animal research and occupational exposures. For example, toluene can cause renal tubular acidosis, hypokalemia, hypophosphatemia, and Goodpasture's syndrome. Benzene, a gasoline additive, has been linked to bone marrow suppression, aplastic anemia, and leukemia. Chlorinated hydrocarbons can cause hepatotoxicity (Brouette and Anton 2001; Sharp and Rosenberg 1997).

Neurological Problems

Inhalant use also has been associated with neurological problems, including a multiple sclerosis–like syndrome, parkinsonism, peripheral neuropathy (*n*-hexane and methyl butyl ketone), trigeminal neuropathy (trichloroethylene), optic neuropathy (toluene), and delirium and dementia (toluene). Because of cerebellar atrophy, chronic users may present with tremors, ataxia, and gait abnormalities. Neuroimaging has shown an association between chronic toluene use and white matter changes, as well as general cerebral, cerebellar, and brain stem atrophy (Rosenberg et al. 2002). Degree of white matter change is correlated with severity of neuropsychological impairment (Filley et al. 1990), and the presence of white matter changes among inhalant users is associated with lower performance IQ scores on the Wechsler Adult Intelligence Scale—Revised (WAIS-R) (Yamanouchi et al. 1997). Neuropsychological testing has shown poorer performance on working memory tasks and tests of executive function among inhalant users compared with users of noninhalant drugs (Rosenberg et al. 2002).

Psychiatric Problems

According to DSM-IV-TR (American Psychiatric Association 2000), inhalants can induce several psychiatric disorders, including inhalant intoxication, inhalant-induced persisting dementia, inhalant-induced psychotic disorder, inhalant-induced mood disorder, and inhalant-induced anxiety disorder.

Congenital Effects

Inhalants cross the placenta and can present dangers to the fetus. But linking associated birth abnormalities with inhalant use is more difficult because most persons with inhalant dependence are also dependent on other substances. Alcohol dependence, for example, commonly co-occurs and makes elucidation of a distinct syndrome more difficult. However, occupational exposures to solvents usually are uncomplicated by other substances, and occupational exposures have been associated with higher rates of spontaneous abortions, esophageal stenosis, omphalocele, gastroschisis, CNS defects, oral cleft malformations, and ventricular septal defects (Jones and Balster 1998). Inhalant-abusing women are exposed to much higher concentrations of solvents than occurs in most occupational exposures, and some offspring of such women show growth retardation, as well as craniofacial and limb abnormalities (Dinwiddie 1994). These children may have developmental delays and language deficits (Jones and Balster 1998). Animal studies of toluene also report fetotoxicity, such as abnormal neuronal migration and proliferation (Gospe and Zhou 2000). Clinically dangerous renal tubular acidosis occurs among pregnant inhalant users and in their heavily exposed neonates.

Recognition and Initial Assessment

Recognition of recent or regular use is imperative because inhalant-induced symptoms can resemble various psychiatric syndromes. Misdiagnosis can lead to fruitless efforts at treatment of the induced syndrome (Miller et al. 2002).

Inhalant intoxication resembles ethanol intoxication, and individuals intoxicated with inhalants can show irritability, slurred speech, tremulousness, psychomotor retardation, weakness, and euphoria and, with increasing doses, can progress to stupor or coma. Signs of recent use also may include perioral or nasal rash, burns, conjunctival injection, poor hygiene, an odor of inhalants, as well as solvent stains and paint or correction fluid on the clothing or the face. Patients may complain of loss of appetite, nausea, respiratory problems, and chronic sore throat. Parents may note worsening school performance and loss of interest in activities and may find products such as spray paints or glues in the child's room.

Once inhalant use is suspected, a careful history will attend to the products used and extent of use. A psychiatrist also should examine adolescent patients for comorbid diagnoses, such as conduct disorder, attention deficit disorder, major depression, posttraumatic stress disorder, inhalant-induced psychotic disorder, and inhalant-induced persisting dementia. Clinicians should assess the general history of drug and alcohol use because other substance problems often coexist with inhalant dependence. Clinicians should also carefully evaluate dangerousness because intoxication with inhalants is associated with both impaired self-care and suicidality. A history of childhood abuse or neglect should be assessed because such histories commonly antedate inhalant problems.

Appropriate staff should take a medical history and perform a physical examination. Inhalant use can result in several medical problems, and careful consideration should be given to laboratory workup of concerning signs or symptoms, especially in chronic users. Tests indicated by history and examination might include urine drug screen (general), complete blood count, chemistries (especially potassium, phosphorus, creatine kinase, and liver function tests), urinalysis, electrocardiogram or cardiac monitoring, chest X ray, magnetic resonance imaging of the brain for white matter abnormalities and old traumatic injuries, neuropsychological testing, and urine and blood testing for inhalants or inhalant metabolites. In countries where leaded gasoline is available, a lead level also may be indicated.

Treatment

Inhalant users may present intoxicated, in withdrawal, with induced psychiatric symptomatology, or for treatment of inhalant abuse and dependence.

Inhalant Intoxication

Care for patients during intoxication is generally supportive. Some evidence suggests that inhalants sensitize the heart to catecholamines, and startling an intoxicated patient may therefore induce arrhythmias and sudden sniffer's death (Bass 1970). Caregivers should attempt to keep intoxicated individuals calm and in an environment with low stimulation; bronchodilators should be used with caution, and epinephrine should be avoided (Seymour and Henry 2001). Breath, blood, or urine tests for inhalants or their metabolites may be helpful in confirming a diagnosis of inhalant intoxication. In an inhalant-free atmosphere, intoxication from inhalation is generally short-lived (although with ingestion of toxic amounts of petroleum products, serious symptoms may persist for days) (Seymour and Henry 2001). Clothes smelling of solvents should be removed, and solvents on skin or hair should be washed away with a mild soap and water. Gastric emptying is not recommended for solvent ingestion because the risk of aspiration is believed to outweigh the potential benefits (Seymour and Henry 2001). Level of alertness, mental status, and vital signs (and pulse oximetry for blood oxygen saturation) should be monitored. Rehydration, supplemental oxygen, and electrolyte repletion may be required. Marked agitation may be controlled, when necessary, with low-dose antipsychotics. Benzodiazepines may potentiate the effects of inhalants and thus should be avoided.

Inhalant Withdrawal

Inhalant withdrawal has been described by some clinicians; symptoms include a few to several days of irritability, anxiety, inattention, diaphoresis, diarrhea, restlessness, insomnia, and tremor (Keriotis and Himanshu 2000), but DSM-IV-TR concludes that withdrawal is infrequent, not well documented, and probably clinically insignificant. No pharmacological treatment is universally recommended, although some clinicians believe that benzodiazepines may be helpful (Brouette and Anton 2001; Westermeyer 1987). However, chronic inhalant users will often have polysubstance involvement, and careful monitoring and treatment of withdrawal from other substances (such as alcohol) should be undertaken.

Inhalant-Induced Persisting Dementia

Much of the research on cerebral damage from inhalants has focused on toluene and its associated white matter changes. Patients with chronic toluene use have characteristically showed attentional problems, impaired learning, slowed processing of information, apathy, and poor memory, but usually they do not have cortical gray matter signs (prominent aphasia) or the movement disorders (resting tremors, chorea, athetosis, dystonia) seen in many subcortical dementias (Filley et al. 1989). No treatments have been studied for inhalant-induced persisting dementia. Discontinuing inhalant use likely stops the progression of cerebral damage, but most cognitive deficits that persist for days to weeks are probably irreversible. Careful assessment of the patient's ability for self-care is important, and appropriate steps should be taken to support the patient's limitations, including consideration of sheltered living or nursing home placement.

Inhalant-Induced Psychotic Disorder, Mood Disorder, and Anxiety Disorder

Inhalant users sometimes present with inhalant-induced symptoms. When these psychotic, mood, or anxiety symptoms are the result of the direct physiological effects of an inhalant, are out of proportion to what would normally be expected during intoxication or withdrawal, and are not better accounted for by a primary disorder or a delirium, the appropriate diagnosis is inhalant-induced psychotic disorder, inhalant-induced mood disorder, or inhalant-induced anxiety disorder. Generally, the symptoms may last a few days to at most 1 month. In some countries, tetraethyl lead in gasoline may be an important factor in producing psychotic symptoms; switching to unleaded gasoline in an indigenous community in Australia reportedly eliminated previously frequent inhalant-induced psychotic emergencies among users (Cairney et al. 2002).

There is no research on the effectiveness of psychosocial treatments for inhalant-induced psychotic disorders. Psychotic symptoms abate equally well during treatment with either carbamazepine or haloperidol, but carbamazepine produced fewer extrapyramidal side effects in a study by Hernandez-Avila et al. (1998). However, no placebo-controlled trials for this condition have been done, leaving open the possibility that the psychotic symptoms would resolve on a time course independent of medication.

Inhalant-induced mood and anxiety symptoms are also sometimes seen. No scientific research on psychosocial or pharmacological treatments of inhalant-induced mood and anxiety disorders has been published. We believe that antidepressants are rarely useful in treating these time-limited mood disorders. Benzodiazepine drugs usually are not indicated because they exacerbate inhalant intoxication.

Inhalant Abuse and Dependence

Although some clinicians say that those with inhalant abuse and dependence require specialized inhalant treatment programs, we suggest a more general approach to treatment of these disorders. We suggest this because 1) no evidence indicates that specialized treatments are more effective; 2) establishing specialized programs is impractical because nationally, only a small percentage of those entering treatment have problematic use of inhalants; and 3) most of those who are dependent on inhalants are also dependent on several other substances such as alcohol and cannabis.

Adolescents

We and our colleagues treat adolescents who have inhalant abuse or dependence together with adolescents who have abuse or dependence on other substances. Adolescents undergo extensive assessments with structured diagnostic interviews and clinical interviews. These interviews assess for substance abuse and dependence diagnoses, comorbid psychiatric diagnoses (such as conduct disorder, attention deficit disorder, major depression, and posttraumatic stress disorder), histories of abuse and neglect, safety, cognitive deficits, and medical or neurological issues. Careful consideration is given to what level of care is most appropriate (outpatient, day treatment, or residential). The treatment programs have on-site schools, where further assessments are completed. Academic testing and teacher observations are used in setting realistic educational and vocational goals. Treatment includes individual counseling and behaviorally oriented groups. Family therapists meet with the family at times that are convenient for the parents, usually in the home, and are available by pager 24 hours a day, 7 days a week. The family therapists are trained in multisystemic therapy (Henggeler et al. 2002). They assess the family's strengths and weaknesses and attempt to shape the home environment in ways that reward sobriety and add quick but fair punitive consequences to delinquent behavior and substance use. Counselors work closely with probation officers and social services to get patients into treatment and to keep them engaged in treatment. They also help patients to develop prosocial activities and drug-free peer groups. Random urine drug screens and breath tests for alcohol are collected.

Adults

We also treat inhalant-dependent adults. Treatment includes individual counseling, group therapy, and random urine drug screens. Therapists use motivational interviewing, cognitive-behavioral therapy, and/or contingency management and work closely with state agencies (such as probation and social services) to keep clients in treatment. They sometimes assess the patient's family members and peers and, when appropriate, engage these people in the patient's treatment. Medical and psychiatric evaluations can be quickly obtained within the program, and neuropsychological testing also can be done if indicated. Nursing home placement is considered for patients with severe cognitive deficits.

Laboratory Monitoring

Objective monitoring for substance use, via testing, is an integral part of drug treatment. Unfortunately, testing for inhalant use presents some complications (some adolescent patients have remarked to us that they had started using inhalants after their urine had begun to be monitored because they were aware that inhalant testing was difficult). First, the drug category "inhalants" encompasses several different substances. Second, inhalants are rapidly exhaled and excreted, meaning that they cannot be detected very long after the end of the period of intoxication. Third, inhalants can bind to or cross plastic walls of urine cups, reducing the quantity available for detection.

Expired air, blood, and urine can all be used to monitor for recent inhalant use. Expired air can be collected in glass traps or tubes, and the samples are examined through gas chromatography and mass spectroscopy. Unfortunately, this can cost two to three times more than a standard urine drug screen, and in some laboratories, samples are only run weekly. Additionally, inhalants are rapidly exhaled, and one manufacturer recommends that breath samples be captured within 2 hours of exposure. Inhalants also can be identified through collection of blood samples. Generally, collection tubes should be made of glass, a minimal amount of headspace should be left in the tube after collection, and the sample should be refrigerated until testing. However, blood draws two to three times per week are impractical. Urine samples also can be used to test for inhalants (again, using glass containers, leaving minimal headspace, and refrigerating the sample), but for some inhalants, a minimal amount is excreted in the urine unchanged. Many inhalants undergo hepatic metabolism, and many of these metabolites remain in the body much longer than their volatile parent compounds (Table 21–2). Urine samples can be tested for specific metabolites, but inhalant users may sometimes switch products, leading to different urinary metabolites. There is also a risk of false-positive re-sults (any food product with benzoic acid may cause false-positive results for hippuric acid), and tests for me-tabolites are expensive, sometimes costing 6–17 times a standard urine drug screen. Finally, in some cases the parent compound is mostly exhaled unchanged.

Table 21–2.   Metabolites of common inhalants

Inhalant	Urinary metabolites
Automotive gasoline	Urinary thioether can be tested, but results are confounded by smoking.
Benzene	Urinary phenol can be tested.
	Urinary muconic acid can be tested, but sorbic acid ingestion can cause false-positive results.
n-Hexane	Urinary 2,5-hexanedione can be detected about 2–3 days following exposure.
Toluene	Urinary hippuric acid can be tested.
	Urinary orthocresol also can be tested.
1,1,1-Trichloroethane	Urinary trichloroethane
	Urinary trichloroacetic acid
Trichloroethylene	Urinary trichloroethanol
	Urinary trichloroacetic acid can be detected up to 1 week from exposure.
Xylene	Urinary methylhippuric acid can be detected 1–2 days after exposure (methylhippuric acid is also known as toluric acid).

Note.   Rates of metabolism have been reported for occupational exposure and not within inhalant abusers. Rates of metabolism will vary with body fat percentage and with concurrent use of other substances, such as alcohol. The Agency for Toxic Substances and Disease Registry (an agency of the U.S. Department of Health and Human Services) publishes thorough toxicological profiles for a number of volatile substances. These profiles include biomarkers for exposure.

Laboratory testing for inhalants may be helpful as a one-time confirmation of the diagnosis of inhalant intoxication. For assessing patients' possible relapse to inhalant use, we recommend educating staff, reliable family members, and significant others about the signs of recent inhalant use and using immediate testing to confirm suspicions of very recent use.

Nitrous Oxide and Amyl or Butyl Nitrite

Nitrous oxide (N_2O) and amyl or butyl nitrite are not classified in DSM-IV-TR under inhalant use disorders; instead, they are termed *other or unknown substance-related disorders* because characteristic users, modes of action, and associated problems are distinctly different from those of inhalant abusers.

Nitrous Oxide

N_2O, known as "laughing gas," was discovered in the eighteenth century and was used along with ether and chloroform at parties to reduce inhibitions and pro-vide intoxicating entertainment. In the nineteenth century, it was introduced as an anesthetic. N_2O is still used for this purpose and also is used as a propellant in whipped cream dispensers. N_2O reinforces self-administration in some individuals (Walker and Zacny 2001), and abuse of N_2O appears to occur more commonly among those with greater access, such as health care and food service workers. Sequelae of repeated N_2O use include depression, psychosis, memory loss, peripheral neuropathy, and bone marrow suppression (Brouette and Anton 2001). N_2O can also mimic symptoms of pernicious anemia; administration of vitamin B_{12} and folate, in conjunction with abstinence, may mitigate these symptoms. No data are available on the treatment of N_2O abuse and dependence; therefore, we recommend general approaches like those used with persons dependent on other substances.

Amyl and Butyl Nitrite

Amyl nitrite, butyl nitrite, and isobutyl nitrite are in-haled to cause vasodilation, smooth muscle relaxation, and intoxication. Amyl nitrite was once widely used to treat angina and was sold in bulbs that could be broken to release the vapors, thus the street name "poppers" or "snappers." In 1960, the U.S. Food and Drug Administration (FDA) dropped prescription requirements for amyl nitrite, and during that decade it became more widely used as a sexual enhancer, especially by homosexual men. Therefore, in the late 1960s, the FDA reinstituted the requirement of a prescription for amyl nitrite, but soon butyl nitrite began to be marketed under the names "Rush," "Jolt," "Locker Room," and "Jack Hammer" and was sometimes marketed as an air freshener or liquid incense. Its utility in such applications is suspect, and this likely constitutes a method of avoiding legal entanglements. In fact, some patients remark that butyl nitrite smells something like soiled gym socks. Although it is now illegal, sale of amyl and butyl nitrite continues. They are often sold in sex shops as room deodorizers and video head cleaners.

In the 1980s, an association between nitrite use and Kaposi's sarcoma was noted, and with this information, widespread use of the nitrites declined. Subsequently, human immunodeficiency virus (HIV) was identified and was linked to acquired immunodeficiency syndrome (AIDS); the association between nitrite use and Kaposi's sarcoma may be related to high-risk behavior in nitrite users. Amyl and butyl nitrite have been linked to bradycardia, hemolytic anemia, methemoglobinemia, impaired immune system functioning (Sharp and Rosenberg 1997), and headaches and are highly flammable and have caused flash burns. Again, in the absence of any research on the treatment of amyl and butyl nitrite–related disorders, we recommend a general approach like that used with persons dependent on other substances.

References

American Psychiatric Association: Diagnostic and Statistical Manual of Mental Disorders, 3rd Edition, Revised. Washington, DC, American Psychiatric Association, 1987

American Psychiatric Association: Diagnostic and Statistical Manual of Mental Disorders, 4th Edition, Text Revision. Washington, DC, American Psychiatric Association, 2000

Anthony JC, Warner LA, Kessler RC: Comparative epidemiology of dependence on tobacco, alcohol, controlled substances, and inhalants: basic findings from the National Comorbidity Survey. Exp Clin Psychopharmacol 2:244–268, 1994

Balster RL: Neural basis of inhalant abuse. Drug Alcohol Depend 51:207–214, 1998

Bass M: Sudden sniffing death. JAMA 212:2075–2079, 1970

Brouette T, Anton R: Clinical review of inhalants. Am J Addict 10:79–94, 2001

Cairney S, Maruff P, Burns C, et al: The neurobehavioral consequences of petrol (gasoline) sniffing. Neurosci Biobehav Rev 26:81–89, 2002

Cottler L, Robins L, Helzer J: The reliability of the CIDI-SAM. Addiction 84:801–814, 1989

Dinwiddie S: Abuse of inhalants: a review. Addiction 89:925–939, 1994

Dinwiddie SH, Reich T: The relationship of solvent use to other substance use. Am J Drug Alcohol Abuse 17:173–186, 1991

Dinwiddie SH, Reich T, Cloninger CR: Solvent use and psychiatric comorbidity. Addiction 85:1647–1656, 1990

Drug and Alcohol Services Information System: Adolescent admissions involving inhalants. March 14, 2002. Available at: http://www.samhsa.gov/oas/facts.cfm. Accessed August 27, 2002

Filley CM, Franklin GM, Heaton RK, et al: White matter dementia. Neuropsychiatry Neuropsychol Behav Neurol 1:239–254, 1989

Filley CM, Heaton RK, Rosenberg NL: White matter dementia in chronic toluene abuse. Neurology 40:532–534, 1990

Gerasimov MR, Schiffer WK, Marstellar D, et al: Toluene inhalation produces regionally specific changes in extracellular dopamine. Drug Alcohol Depend 65:243–251, 2002

Gospe SM, Zhou SS: Prenatal exposure to toluene results in abnormal neurogenesis and migration in rat somatosensory cortex. Pediatr Res 47:362–368, 2000

Henggeler SW, Clingempeel WG, Brondino MJ, et al: Four-year follow-up of multisystemic therapy with substance-abusing and substance-dependent juvenile offenders. J Am Acad Child Adolesc Psychiatry 41:868–874, 2002

Hernandez-Avila CA, Ortega-Soto HA, Jasso A, et al: Treatment of inhalant-induced psychotic disorder with carbamazepine versus haloperidol. Psychiatr Serv 49:812–815, 1998

Johnson EO, Schutz CG, Anthony JC, et al: Inhalants to heroin: a prospective analysis from adolescence to adulthood. Drug Alcohol Depend 40:159–164, 1995

Johnston LD, O'Malley PM, Bachman JG: Monitoring the Future National Results on Adolescent Drug Use: Overview of Key Findings, 2001. Rockville, MD, National Institute on Drug Abuse, 2002

Jones HE, Balster RL: Inhalant abuse in pregnancy. Obstet Gynecol Clin North Am 25:153–167, 1998

Keriotis AA, Himanshu U: Inhalant dependence and withdrawal symptoms. J Am Acad Child Adolesc Psychiatry 29:679–680, 2000

Miller PW, Mycyk MB, Leikin JB, et al: An unusual presentation of inhalant abuse with dissociative amnesia. Vet Hum Toxicol 44:17–19, 2002

Neumark YD, Delva J, Anthony JC: The epidemiology of adolescent inhalant drug involvement. Arch Pediatr Adolesc Med 152:781–786, 1998

Riegel AC, French ED: An electrophysiological analysis of rat ventral tegmental dopamine neuronal activity during acute toluene exposure. Pharmacol Toxicol 85:37–43, 1999

Rosenberg NL, Grigsby J, Dreisbach J, et al: Neuropsychiatric impairment and MRI abnormalities associated with chronic solvent abuse. Clin Toxicol 40:21–34, 2002

Schutz CG, Chilcoat HD, Anthony JC: The association between sniffing inhalants and injecting drugs. Compr Psychiatry 35:99–105, 1994

Seymour FK, Henry JA: Assessment and management of acute poisoning by petroleum products. Hum Exp Toxicol 20:551–562, 2001

Sharp CW, Rosenberg NL: Inhalants, in Substance Abuse: A Comprehensive Textbook, 3rd Edition. Edited by Lowinson JH, Ruiz P, Millman RB, et al. Baltimore, MD, Williams & Wilkins, 1997, pp 246–264

Substance Abuse and Mental Health Services Administration: The NHSDA Report: inhalant use among youths. March 22, 2002. Available at: http://www.samhsa.gov/oas/facts.cfm. Accessed August 27, 2002

Substance Abuse and Mental Health Services Administration: Results From the 2002 National Survey on Drug Use and Health: Detailed Tables (Office of Applied Studies, NHSDA Series H-22, DHHS Publ No SMA 03-3836). Rockville, MD, Substance Abuse and Mental Health Services Administration, 2003

Walker DJ, Zacny JP: Within- and between-subject variability in the reinforcing and subjective effects of nitrous oxide in healthy volunteers. Drug Alcohol Depend 64:85–96, 2001

Westermeyer J: The psychiatrist and solvent-inhalant abuse: recognition, assessment, and treatment. Am J Psychiatry 144:903–907, 1987

Yamanouchi N, Okada S, Kodama K, et al: Effects of MRI abnormalities on WAIS-R performance in solvent abusers. Acta Neurol Scand 96:34–39, 1997

Anabolic-Androgenic Steroids

Harrison G. Pope Jr., M.D.
Kirk J. Brower, M.D.

The anabolic-androgenic steroids (AAS) are a family of drugs that includes testosterone, the natural male hormone, and dozens of synthetic derivatives of testosterone developed over the last 50 years (Pope and Brower 2003). In the United States, data from the National Household Survey suggest that about 1 million men have used these drugs at some time (Substance Abuse and Mental Health Services Administration Office of Applied Studies 1997); many began using AAS as teenagers (Johnston et al. 2002). Although AAS use was formerly confined largely to elite athletes, increasing numbers of boys and young men have now begun to use these drugs to gain muscle and lose fat, often simply for the sake of personal appearance (Kanayama et al. 2001). The number of women using AAS is much smaller because women are less likely to desire muscle gain and women are vulnerable to the masculinizing effects of AAS. For example, in the 1994 National Household Survey (the most recent to collect AAS data), the number of American men estimated to have used AAS in the past 3 years was 413,458, as compared with only 31,316 women—a ratio of 13 to 1 (U.S. Department of Health and Human Services 1997). For these reasons, we focus primarily on treatment of male AAS use—although the general principles expressed would presumably apply to the relatively rare cases of female use as well (Gruber and Pope 2000).

Although AAS pose a range of medical and psychiatric risks as described in this chapter, AAS users rarely seek treatment. First, they often perceive their use of AAS to be a positive and healthy activity when it is combined with intensive exercise and optimal diet as part of the "bodybuilding lifestyle." Societal forces are partly to blame for this misperception of AAS (Kanayama et al. 2001); muscular male bodies are portrayed as an ideal in advertising, magazines, television, and movies. Even children's action toys, such as G.I. Joe, have grown from ordinary-looking men in the 1960s and 1970s to muscle-bound specimens in the 1990s (Pope et al. 1999). We think nothing of seeing an advertisement promoting a powerful car or truck as being "on steroids," whereas no one would advertise the same vehicle as being "on cocaine" or "on marijuana." Given this societal milieu, it is not surprising that AAS users have difficulty regarding their drug use as a disorder requiring psychiatric treatment.

Second, AAS are very different from conventional drugs of abuse. Most drugs of abuse described in this volume deliver an immediate reward, in the form of intoxication, within minutes or hours of ingestion. However, with "body image" drugs such as AAS, the immediate reward is negligible (except perhaps in "stage 2" AAS dependence; see "Anabolic-Androgenic Steroid Dependence" section later in this chapter); instead, the user is seeking a long-term reward in the form of a more muscular body, athletic success, or admiration from peers or potential sexual partners. Thus, conventional methods of treating substance abuse are usually inadequate unless modified specifically for AAS users (Kanayama et al. 2001).

Third, AAS users often have little respect for doctors. Underground guides and Internet sites for illicit AAS users are replete with derogatory remarks about health professionals—and with some justification. For decades, the medical profession asserted that AAS were ineffective for gaining muscle mass. This claim, based on two decades of seriously flawed studies, undermined the credibility of doctors among many athletes (Pope and Brower, in press). Now, most professionals finally concede that AAS are effective for gaining muscle mass, but they remain largely uninformed about the extent and nature of the AAS-using subculture.

Given the above considerations, it is understandable that AAS users almost never voluntarily request treatment to stop using these drugs. Nevertheless, several specific situations bring AAS users to the attention of clinicians, and some attempt at treatment may then be initiated. These situations include 1) AAS dependence syndromes, 2) hypomanic and manic syndromes during AAS exposure, 3) syndromes of depression and anxiety associated with AAS withdrawal, 4) progression from AAS use to opioid abuse and dependence, 5) body image disorders associated with AAS use, and 6) forensic situations, such as cases of AAS-induced violence or criminality. In the following sections, we begin with a general discussion of the initial identification and assessment of AAS users and continue with each of the six clinical issues enumerated.

Identification and Assessment

Identification

AAS use is one of the few types of substance use in which a diagnosis is often suggested simply by looking at the patient as he walks through the door. As we have

described elsewhere (Kouri et al. 1995), there is a fairly sharp upper limit of muscularity that can be achieved by a lean individual without the help of drugs. We have published a formula to calculate muscularity, expressed as the "fat-free mass index," which clinicians can apply if they know the height, weight, and approximate percentage of body fat of the patient (Kouri et al. 1995). Men who have low body fat, have a fat-free mass index of greater than approximately 26 kg/m^2, and claim that they have not used drugs are almost certainly lying. We have published photographs comparing bodybuilders who have used AAS with those who have not to aid the clinician in making this distinction (Pope and Brower, in press). Clinicians who suspect AAS use in any patient should follow several guidelines to take a specific history.

History

The clinician may lead into the topic of AAS by asking about athletic or fitness-related activities. Young men who lift weights regularly are at the greatest risk for use of AAS. Other lead-in questions include the use of over-the-counter and mail-order dietary supplements ranging from vitamins, minerals, and creatine to ephedrine, ginseng, androstenedione, and dehydroepiandrosterone. The use of such legal substances is commonly associated with using AAS. Does the patient know other people who use AAS? Potential users learn about AAS from other users. Finally, has the patient ever tried AAS or thought about using them? Patients thinking about AAS use are good candidates for prevention. Why is the patient interested in using, and what has prevented the patient from using to date? In addressing these questions, it is particularly critical for the clinician to be nonjudgmental, while still discouraging use.

For patients who admit having tried AAS, both the perceived benefits and any adverse consequences from using are important to determine. The dates of first and last use, names and doses of AAS used, sources of drugs, and routes of administration should be ascertained. Patients who inject AAS should be asked about needle sharing. Sources of drugs include prescriptions (including transdermal testosterone patches), diversion from the legal market (including the veterinary market), and the illicit market. Patients and clinicians should remember that drugs obtained from the illicit market are frequently adulterated, falsely labeled, and sometimes nonsterile. In short, the user does not necessarily know what and how much he is taking.

Inquiry into the patterns of use is also important. Illicit AAS users typically combine ("stack") multiple AAS drugs, including both oral and injected intramuscular forms, to achieve doses that are 10–100 times the amounts ordinarily prescribed for therapeutic indications. AAS are usually taken in "cycles" (courses) of 4–16 weeks or more, often characterized by taking small doses at the beginning, building to large doses and combinations in the middle, and tapering doses at the end—a pattern referred to as a *pyramid.* The clinician gains useful information when exploring the role of cycling with an individual AAS user. Does the patient cycle off AAS to avoid testing positive on drug screening? Does the patient cycle off AAS to give his body a rest, allowing his endogenous hormonal system a chance to regain its normal functioning? Does the patient experience depression or other withdrawal symptoms during "off periods"? Dependent users may eliminate cycling altogether in favor of prolonged, continuous use to avoid withdrawal symptoms.

Finally, a history of other drug abuse should be obtained. Users often combine other drugs with AAS to augment their effects (e.g., human growth hormone, human chorionic gonadotropin, clenbuterol), to reduce unpleasant side effects (e.g., clomiphene, tamoxifen), and to mask urine testing (e.g., probenecid, diuretics). Traditional drugs of abuse may be used either to enhance performance (such as stimulants) or to get high (such as ethanol). Concomitant opioid use is discussed later in this chapter (see "Syndromes Associated With Anabolic-Androgenic Steroid Use").

Physical Examination

The physical examination is essential to detect the somatic consequences of using AAS. Generalized muscle hypertrophy with a disproportionately large upper torso (neck, shoulders, arms, and chest) is readily apparent. The skin is examined for acne (on the face, shoulders, and back) and needle marks in large muscles (especially the gluteals, but sometimes the thigh and deltoids). Gynecomastia, caused by metabolic conversion of excess testosterone to estrogen, may be detectable by palpation or even simple observation in some men. By contrast, the testicles become atrophic as they shut down testosterone production when exogenous AAS are administered in high doses. Male pattern baldness, hirsutism, hypertension, hepatomegaly, right upper quadrant tenderness, jaundice, and prostatic hypertrophy are also possible but are not reliably

associated with AAS use. In women, hirsutism, deepening of the voice, and clitoral hypertrophy may be detected.

Mental Status Examination

The clinician should assess the patient's appearance for excessive muscularity (as described above under "Identification") sometimes disguised by oversized clothes, especially in patients with muscle dysmorphia who become preoccupied that they do not look big enough (Pope et al. 1997). The patient's cooperation may vary depending on his defensiveness or denial of AAS use. Speech and sensorium are generally normal. However, if the patient is experiencing hypomanic symptoms from current AAS use may show irritability, agitation, and possibly grandiose beliefs. Patients experiencing depression from AAS withdrawal may have depressed mood, dysphoria, anxiety, psychomotor retardation, and possible suicidal ideation.

Laboratory Examination

Laboratory abnormalities reported in AAS users are summarized in Table 22–1. Standard urine screens for drugs of abuse do not include AAS, so urine testing for AAS must be performed at a reference laboratory. Such testing can detect only recent AAS use: orally active AAS disappear from the urine within weeks, and most intramuscular preparations disappear within a few months. However, given the association between AAS use and other illicit drug use, standard urine screens for illicit drugs also should be ordered.

Important blood chemistries include skeletal muscle enzymes, but these can be elevated even in non-AAS users after intensive weight training. AAS users may occasionally have extreme elevations of creatine kinase from rhabdomyolysis (Braseth et al. 2001; Pertusi et al. 2001). Standard liver function tests, such as transaminases and lactic dehydrogenase, are nonspecific because these enzymes are also present in muscle and may be elevated from weight training. Elevation of chemistries specific to the liver, such as bilirubin and γ-glutamyltransferase, may suggest true hepatic abnormalities, whereas elevated creatine kinase (an enzyme largely specific to muscle) may suggest muscle damage (Braseth et al. 2001).

Blood testosterone concentrations may be grossly elevated in patients who are administering exogenous testosterone or grossly depressed in patients who are

Table 22–1. Laboratory abnormalities in anabolic-androgenic steroid users

Measure	Abnormality
Blood work	
Muscle enzymes	↑ALT, AST, LDH, and CK
Liver function tests	↑ALT, AST, LDH, GGT, and total bilirubin
Cholesterol levels	↑HDL-C, ↓LDL-C, ↑or no change in total cholesterol and triglycerides
Hormonal levels	↑Testosterone and estradiol (with use of testosterone esters)
	↓Testosterone (without use of testosterone esters or during withdrawal)
	↓LH and FSH
Complete blood count	↑RBC count, hemoglobin, and hematocrit
Urine testing	
AAS	Positive
Other drugs of abuse	May be positive
Cardiac testing	
Electrocardiogram	Left ventricular hypertrophy (seen in intensive weight trainers also)
Echocardiogram	Impaired diastolic function
Semen analysis	↓Sperm count and motility, abnormal morphology

Note. ALT=alanine aminotransferase; AST=aspartate aminotransferase; CK=creatine kinase; FSH=follicle-stimulating hormone; GGT=γ-glutamyltransferase; HDL-C=high-density lipoprotein cholesterol; LDH=lactate dehydrogenase; LDL-C=low-density lipoprotein cholesterol; LH=luteinizing hormone; RBC=red blood cell.
Source. Reprinted from Brower KJ: "Anabolic Steroid Abuse and Dependence." *Current Psychiatry Reports* 4:377–387, 2002. Used with permission.

administering other types of AAS and hence inhibiting their own endogenous testosterone production. Testosterone levels may remain depressed for weeks and sometimes months during AAS withdrawal.

General Considerations

Although many health consequences of using AAS are readily detectable by performing a comprehensive history, physical examination, and laboratory tests, the long-term health consequences are poorly studied (Parssinen and Seppala 2002). Therefore, the clinician should be alert to heretofore-undocumented sequelae of AAS use as the first generation of users advances in age. In the meantime, the following syndromes resulting from long-term use are most likely to bring AAS users to the attention of psychiatrists.

Anabolic-Androgenic Steroid Dependence

Although the "anabolic steroid addiction hypothesis" (Kashkin and Kleber 1989) remains subject to debate (Bahrke and Yesalis 1994; Midgley et al. 1999), AAS are included and discussed in DSM-IV and its text revision, DSM-IV-TR (American Psychiatric Association 1994, 2000), under the category of "Other (or Unknown) Substance-Related Disorders." A recent review of the medical literature has documented at least 165 AAS users who met DSM-III-R (American Psychiatric Association 1987) or DSM-IV criteria for AAS dependence (Brower 2002).

We have hypothesized a two-stage model of dependence on AAS (Brower 2002; Pope and Brower, in press). During stage 1, users are primarily interested in developing muscle size and power to improve their body image or athletic performance. Training and diet at this stage have a compulsive quality to them that extends to using AAS. The AAS user may appear to meet DSM-IV-TR criteria for substance dependence at this stage because of the compulsive nature of drug taking. This stage of dependence, however, can be explained without invoking any psychoactive properties of AAS because AAS *are* strongly "myoactive" and they *do* help users to achieve their muscle-related goals when combined with proper training and diet. Addiction-specialized treatment is not likely to be needed at this stage, although treatment for a body image disorder such as muscle dysmorphia may be (Pope et al. 1997).

According to the model, some AAS users will eventually develop stage 2 dependence, due in part perhaps to genetic vulnerability and in part to cumulative, high-dose exposure to AAS. Chronically consumed high doses of AAS are postulated to stimulate brain reward systems and to result in neuroadaptations in other brain systems that manifest as withdrawal symptoms on discontinuation. Thus, users take AAS for both their psychoactive and their myoactive effects at this stage. Clinically, stage 2 dependence resembles dependence on traditional drugs of abuse, and it meets formal DSM-IV-TR criteria for substance dependence. In addition, stage 2 dependent users may have co-occurring dependence on other drugs of abuse such as opioids, alcohol, and stimulants.

Stage 2 users have difficulty with stopping drug use on their own and are likely to require addiction-specialized treatment. The first step in such treatment is to initiate, and motivate the patient for, abstinence. As with other drugs of abuse, motivational techniques include providing empathic feedback and encouraging self-efficacy as well as involving family and friends (Brower and Rootenberg 1999). Feedback, given in a nonjudgmental manner, about findings from the physical examination and laboratory abnormalities allows for engagement around bodily concerns. Encouraging self-efficacy takes advantage of the patient's need to see himself as big, powerful, and strong. Initiating abstinence also involves the treatment of withdrawal symptoms, which is discussed in detail later in this chapter (see "Anabolic-Androgenic Steroid Withdrawal Depression").

After initiating abstinence, the principles of relapse prevention may be applied as with other addicted individuals, but unique therapeutic issues also must be addressed in AAS users. One is the overreliance on physical attributes for self-esteem—a feature that resembles the dynamics of patients with eating disorders and body dysmorphic disorder (Pope et al. 1997). Some evidence indicates that patients with body dysmorphic disorder respond well to selective serotonin reuptake inhibitors (Phillips 2000). Therefore, the diagnosis of comorbid mental disorders not ordinarily observed in patients with substance dependence is important. Another therapeutic issue concerns the psychological response to giving up AAS, which have likely served the patient in achieving some measure of competitive success. The patient will likely feel smaller and weaker, both literally and figuratively, without AAS. In helping the patient mourn the loss of AAS, the clinician appreciates that 1) the patient's goals were culturally congruent (the bigger, better, stronger winner), and 2) AAS are potently myoactive and really can facilitate those goals.

Anabolic-Androgenic Steroid Hypomania and Mania

A substantial literature over the last 15 years has established that AAS produce hypomanic or manic syndromes in some individuals, sometimes accompanied by aggressive or violent behavior and, very rarely, psychotic symptoms (Pope and Katz 1988, 1994, 2003). These effects are rare in individuals taking the equivalent of 300 mg of testosterone per week or less, but they appear to become progressively more common with higher doses, especially doses greater than 1,000 mg/week. These syndromes were initially noted in field studies of illicit AAS users, and some investigators questioned whether the effects were actually due to AAS themselves, as opposed to expectational factors, personality variables, or subcultural influences (Bahrke and Yesalis 1994; Riem and Hursey 1995). Recently, however, several studies have reported that such syndromes can develop even in volunteers taking supraphysiological doses of AAS under placebo-controlled, double-blind laboratory conditions (Pope et al. 2000; Su et al. 1993; Yates et al. 1999). Therefore, the mood-altering effects of AAS almost certainly have a biological basis, even though they can undoubtedly be modified by contextual factors (Rubinow and Schmidt 1996).

Little has been written about the treatment of such episodes beyond anecdotal reports (Pope and Katz 1988; Stanley 1994). Thus, the best treatment recommendations would seem to include removal of the offending agent and temporary treatment, if necessary, with neuroleptics or other antimanic drugs. In general, it appears that manic or hypomanic episodes will remit quickly when AAS are stopped and that clinicians should be alert for the onset of depressive symptoms associated with abrupt AAS withdrawal. If a patient reports a history of mood disorder prior to AAS use, or continues to have manic or psychotic symptoms for more than a week or two after AAS are stopped, it would seem important to consider the possibility of an underlying major mood disorder independent of AAS.

Anabolic-Androgenic Steroid Withdrawal Depression

The withdrawal syndrome from AAS is primarily depressive in nature and includes symptoms of fatigue, restlessness, anorexia, insomnia, decreased libido, and a desire to take more AAS (craving) in addition to depressed mood (Brower 2000). The syndrome typically lasts for several weeks and usually does not require specific pharmacological treatment. However, some individuals may develop severe or persistent depressive symptoms, sometimes accompanied by suicidal ide-ation (Malone et al. 1995). Such cases appear to re-spond well to selective serotonin reuptake inhibitors such as fluoxetine (Malone and Dimeff 1992). These drugs are also the agents of choice for treating muscle dysmorphia and other forms of body dysmorphic dis-order that may accompany AAS use (Phillips 2000).

The hypothalamic-pituitary-gonadal axis can be depressed during the withdrawal period for many months, resulting in sterility in some cases and contrib-uting to depressive symptoms in others. In men who continue to have impaired sexual function or persis-tent depressive symptoms despite pharmacotherapy, consultation with an endocrinologist should be con-sidered. Endocrine pharmacotherapy—including in-jected testosterone esters, human chorionic gonado-tropin, and antiestrogens—may be indicated to restore functioning of the hypothalamic-pituitary-gonadal axis in such cases (Brower 2000).

Syndromes Associated With Anabolic-Androgenic Steroid Use

Recent years have seen the appearance of two impor-tant syndromes that appear associated with AAS use. The first, termed *muscle dysmorphia,* is a form of body dysmorphic disorder in which the individual perceives himself to be small and frail, even though he is actually large and muscular (Olivardia et al. 2000; Pope et al. 1997). Men with muscle dysmorphia will often engage in compulsive weight lifting and bodybuilding, even to the exclusion of other activities that they enjoy; they frequently will avoid situations in which their body will be seen by others, such as going to the beach or chang-ing in a locker room, for fear that they look too small. Not surprisingly, such individuals may use AAS to "treat" their preoccupation, but paradoxically, many describe even more severe symptoms of muscle dys-morphia following initiation of AAS use. In rare cases, women may also develop muscle dysmorphia and use AAS. No systematic studies of treatment of muscle dys-morphia per se have been done, but it seems reason-able to follow general principles of treatment for other forms of body dysmorphic disorder, relying on cogni-tive-behavioral and pharmacological interventions (Neziroglu et al. 1996; Phillips 2000; Phillips et al. 1997).

Another ominous syndrome associated with AAS use has been progression from AAS to opioid abuse and dependence. Specifically, AAS users learn about opioids from fellow bodybuilders in the gym and often first purchase opioids from the same individual who had sold them AAS (Arvary and Pope 2000; Kanayama et al. 2003; McBride et al. 1996; Wines et al. 1999). AAS users often start by experimenting with the opioid agonist-antagonist nalbuphine, followed by progres-sion to pure opioid agonists, including heroin. We are personally aware of several deaths among AAS users who developed opioid abuse or dependence and then inadvertently overdosed on intravenous opioids. Opi-oid abuse or dependence in current or former AAS us-ers should be aggressively treated. (See the chapters on opioids in this volume, Chapters 23–25, regarding principles of treatment.)

Anabolic-Androgenic Steroids in Forensic Situations

AAS users may occasionally come to clinical attention through the courts as the result of violent or criminal behavior. Specifically, some articles have described in-dividuals, often with no history of psychiatric disorder, violence, or criminal behavior, who became unchar-acteristically violent, and sometimes committed murder, while intoxicated with AAS (see Pope and Katz 2003). In some such cases, the diagnosis of AAS use may be missed because the possibility is never considered. However, AAS use should be suspected in any unusu-ally muscular man apprehended for violent behavior, especially if it appears that this violence is not charac-teristic of his usual personality. The clinician's index of suspicion should be particularly raised when such a man rapidly develops vegetative symptoms of depres-sion after being incarcerated but then improves a few weeks or months later. This pattern may indicate AAS withdrawal, precipitated by the abrupt discontinuation of AAS following incarceration, with a gradual re-mission of depressive symptoms as suppressed hypo-thalamic-pituitary-gonadal function gradually returns to normal. Of course, this pattern of biological depres-sion must be distinguished from the situational de-pression associated with incarceration itself.

In cases in which AAS use is openly acknowledged by the defendant, and appears to have been a clear precipitant of criminal behavior, forensic clinicians may be asked to offer an opinion that the defendant had "involuntary intoxication" or "diminished capacity" from AAS. The legal aspects of this defense have been discussed in detail elsewhere (Bidwell and Katz 1989). If an individual is released and placed on probation after a crime believed to be associated with AAS, it may be wise to require random, unannounced, observed urine tests for AAS to ensure that he does not resume use of these drugs.

Conclusion

Of the various forms of substance abuse and dependence described in this volume, AAS abuse and dependence may be the least likely to come to the attention of the average clinician. However, the frequency of surreptitious AAS abuse and dependence, together with the various psychiatric syndromes associated with it, is very likely underestimated, and many cases doubtless go unrecognized. Greater awareness of this problem among clinicians may lead to the detection of many more cases and a better understanding of how best to treat them.

References

American Psychiatric Association: Diagnostic and Statistical Manual of Mental Disorders, 3rd Edition, Revised. Washington, DC, American Psychiatric Association, 1987

American Psychiatric Association: Diagnostic and Statistical Manual of Mental Disorders, 4th Edition. Washington, DC, American Psychiatric Association, 1994

American Psychiatric Association: Diagnostic and Statistical Manual of Mental Disorders, 4th Edition, Text Revision. Washington, DC, American Psychiatric Association, 2000

Arvary D, Pope HG Jr: Anabolic steroids: a possible gateway to opioid dependence (letter). N Engl J Med 342:1532, 2000

Bahrke MS, Yesalis CE: Weight training: a potential confounding factor in examining the psychological and behavioral effects of anabolic-androgenic steroids. Sports Med 18:309–318, 1994

Bidwell M, Katz DL: Injecting new life into an old defense: anabolic steroid-induced psychosis as a paradigm of involuntary intoxication. University of Miami Entertainment and Sports Law Review 7:1–63, 1989

Braseth NR, Allison EJ Jr, Gough JE: Exertional rhabdomyolysis in a body builder abusing anabolic androgenic steroids. Eur J Emerg Med 8:155–157, 2001

Brower KJ: Assessment and treatment of anabolic steroid abuse, dependence, and withdrawal, in Anabolic Steroids in Sport and Exercise, 2nd Edition. Edited by Yesalis CE. Champaign, IL, Human Kinetics, 2000, pp 305–332

Brower KJ: Anabolic steroid abuse and dependence. Curr Psychiatry Rep 4:377–387, 2002

Brower KJ, Rootenberg JH: Counseling for substance abuse problems, in Counseling in Sports Medicine. Edited by Ray R, Wiese-Bjornstal D. Champaign, IL, Human Kinetics, 1999, pp 179–204

Gruber AJ, Pope HG Jr: Psychiatric and medical effects of anabolic-androgenic steroid use in women. Psychother Psychosom 69:19–26, 2000

Johnston LD, O'Malley PM, Bachman JG: Monitoring the Future: National Survey Results on Drug Use, 1975–2001, Vol 1: Secondary School Students (NIH Publ No 02-5106). Rockville, MD, National Institute on Drug Abuse, 2002

Kanayama G, Pope HG Jr, Hudson JI: "Body image" drugs: a growing psychosomatic problem. Psychother Psychosom 70:61–65, 2001

Kanayama G, Cohane GH, Weiss RD, et al: Past anabolic-androgenic steroid use among men admitted for substance abuse treatment: an underrecognized problem? J Clin Psychiatry 64:156–160, 2003

Kashkin KB, Kleber HD: Hooked on hormones? An anabolic steroid addiction hypothesis. JAMA 262:3166–3170, 1989

Kouri E, Pope HG, Katz DL, et al: Fat-free mass index in users and non-users of anabolic-androgenic steroids. Clin J Sport Med 5:223–228, 1995

Malone DA Jr, Dimeff RJ: The use of fluoxetine in depression associated with anabolic steroid withdrawal: a case series. J Clin Psychiatry 53:130–132, 1992

Malone DA Jr, Dimeff R, Lombardo JA, et al: Psychiatric effects and psychoactive substance use in anabolic-androgenic steroid users. Clin J Sport Med 5:25–31, 1995

McBride AJ, Williamson K, Petersen T: Three cases of nalbuphine hydrochloride dependence associated with anabolic steroid abuse. Br J Sports Med 30:69–70, 1996

Midgley SJ, Heather N, Davies JB: Dependence producing potential of anabolic-androgenic steroids. Addiction Research 7:539–550, 1999

Neziroglu F, McKay D, Todaro J, et al: Effect of cognitive-behavior therapy on persons with BDD and comorbid Axis II diagnoses. Behav Ther 27:67–77, 1996

Olivardia R, Pope HG Jr, Hudson JI: "Muscle dysmorphia" in male weightlifters: a case-control study. Am J Psychiatry 157:1291–1296, 2000

Parssinen M, Seppala T: Steroid use and long-term health risks in former athletes. Sports Med 32:83–94, 2002

Pertusi R, Dickerman RD, McConathy WJ: Evaluation of aminotransferase elevations in a bodybuilder using anabolic steroids: hepatitis or rhabdomyolysis? J Am Osteopath Assoc 101:391–394, 2001

Phillips KA: Pharmacologic treatment of body dysmorphic disorder: a review of empirical data and a proposed treatment algorithm, in The Psychiatric Clinics of North America Annual of Drug Therapy, Vol 7. Edited by Dunner DL, Rosenbaum JF. Philadelphia, PA, WB Saunders, 2000, pp 59–82

Phillips KA, O'Sullivan RL, Pope HG Jr: Muscle dysmorphia (letter). J Clin Psychiatry 58:361, 1997

Pope HG Jr, Brower KJ: Anabolic-androgenic steroid abuse, in Comprehensive Textbook of Psychiatry/VIII. Edited by Sadock BJ, Sadock VA. Philadelphia, PA, Lippincott Williams & Wilkins (in press)

Pope HG Jr, Katz DL: Affective and psychotic symptoms associated with anabolic steroid use. Am J Psychiatry 145:487–490, 1988

Pope HG Jr, Katz DL: Psychiatric and medical effects of anabolic-androgenic steroid use. Arch Gen Psychiatry 51:375–382, 1994

Pope HG Jr, Katz DL: Psychiatric effects of exogenous anabolic-androgenic steroids, in Psychoneuroendocrinology: The Scientific Basis of Clinical Practice. Edited by Wolkowitz OM, Rothschild AJ. Washington, DC, American Psychiatric Publishing, 2003, pp 331–358

Pope HG Jr, Gruber AJ, Choi PY, et al: Muscle dysmorphia: an underrecognized form of body dysmorphic disorder. Psychosomatics 38:548–557, 1997

Pope HG Jr, Olivardia R, Gruber A, et al: Evolving ideals of male body image as seen through action toys. Int J Eat Disord 26:65–72, 1999

Pope HG Jr, Kouri EM, Hudson JI: Effects of supraphysiologic doses of testosterone on mood and aggression in normal men: a randomized controlled trial. Arch Gen Psychiatry 57:133–140, 2000

Riem KE, Hursey KG: Using anabolic-androgenic steroids to enhance physique and performance: effects on moods and behavior. Clin Psychol Rev 15:235–256, 1995

Rubinow DR, Schmidt PJ: Androgens, brain, and behavior. Am J Psychiatry 153:974–984, 1996

Stanley A: Anabolic steroids—the drugs that give and take away manhood: a case with an unusual physical sign. Med Sci Law 34:82–83, 1994

Su T-P, Pagliaro M, Schmidt PJ, et al: Neuropsychiatric effects of anabolic steroid in male normal volunteers. JAMA 269:2760–2764, 1993

Substance Abuse and Mental Health Services Administration Office of Applied Studies: National Household Survey on Drug Abuse, 1994 (computer file). ICPSR version. Research Triangle Park, NC, Research Triangle Institute/Chicago, IL, National Opinion Research Center [producers], 1997. Ann Arbor, MI, Inter-university Consortium for Political and Social Research [distributor], 1997. Available at: http://www.icpsr.umich.edu:8080/ICPSR-STUDY/06949.xml.

Wines JD Jr, Gruber AJ, Pope HG Jr, et al: Nalbuphine hydrochloride dependence in anabolic steroid users. Am J Addict 8:161–164, 1999

Yates WR, Perry P, MacIndoe J, et al: Psychosexual effects of three doses of testosterone in cycling and normal men. Biol Psychiatry 45:254–260, 1999

Opioids

Detoxification

Eric D. Collins, M.D.
Herbert D. Kleber, M.D.

The history of the treatment of narcotic withdrawal is a long and mainly dishonorable one. The trail is strewn with cures enthusiastically received and then quietly dropped when they turned out to be relatively ineffective or, even worse, productive of greater morbidity and mortality. Because of this history, one must be especially careful in proposing new techniques that they meet the twin demands of safety and efficacy. Any claims for a new method should be put forward with modesty and viewed with skepticism until amply documented by careful experimental procedures (Kleber and Riordan 1982).

Opioid detoxification continues to be used for most heroin abusers as a pretreatment procedure before residential therapeutic community treatment, outpatient drug-free treatments, and opioid antagonist maintenance treatment. It is also used by some who do not seek long-term treatment either because they expect that they can remain abstinent from opioids without additional help or because they do not se-

riously intend to remain abstinent. Although therapeutic community and antagonist maintenance treatments are effective for many patients, the prerequisite detoxification and associated withdrawal discomfort can be a barrier to entering such treatment for many patients.

Despite improvements over the last 30 years, most current approaches to detoxification continue to be plagued by patient discomfort, high dropout rates, and high relapse rates. Many patients fear the physical discomfort of opioid withdrawal and delay or avoid detoxification altogether. Others attempt detoxification, either with medical assistance or on their own, but they frequently do not complete the process, usually because withdrawal symptoms become too uncomfortable. Finally, even those who successfully complete detoxification have a high relapse rate. These problems have given rise to the "ultrarapid" or anesthesia-assisted detoxification and antagonist induction procedures, which are offered at high cost without evidence of improved patient outcomes, despite increased risk. Thus, detoxification is a necessary part of treatment for many patients, but it has not achieved its full potential for the transition from opioid dependence to drug-free and/or antagonist maintenance treatments. The advent of buprenorphine for opioid detoxification may improve this transition and enable more patients both to enter treatment and to achieve sustained abstinence from opioids.

Dependence, Tolerance, and Detoxification

Physical dependence refers to the physiological state that follows chronic, regular use of a substance. It is clinically evidenced by the emergence of a characteristic withdrawal syndrome (for that drug or class of drugs) following a significant reduction in the amount of the drug regularly ingested. The withdrawal syndrome can be understood to be the physiological manifestation of nervous system changes that are unmasked when the drug is no longer present. Tolerance almost always accompanies physical dependence.

Tolerance describes the phenomenon by which a drug's effectiveness diminishes over time with regular use of the drug. This is seen either when the effects of a fixed amount of drug lessen or when an individual needs greater amounts of the drug to produce the same effects initially produced by smaller amounts of the drug. Tolerance typically occurs by reduced end organ response to the drug (pharmacodynamic tolerance) or by increased metabolism of the drug (pharmacokinetic tolerance), although other physiological mechanisms may uncommonly play a role.

Addiction is a less precise term, sometimes used synonymously with the DSM-IV-TR (American Psychiatric Association 2000) diagnosis of substance dependence, to describe compulsive use of a drug and overwhelming involvement with its procurement and use. Tolerance, physical dependence, and withdrawal may be present in the absence of addiction or a DSM-IV-TR diagnosis of dependence (as will occur commonly in individuals receiving chronic treatment with opioids for analgesia).

Detoxification refers to the process of taking an individual off a drug on which he or she has become physically dependent. The detoxification may be done abruptly or gradually (Kleber 1981). A variety of medication options are available for use in opioid detoxification: 1) the drug on which the individual is dependent, 2) other drugs that produce cross-tolerance, 3) medications to provide symptomatic relief, and 4) drugs that affect the mechanisms by which withdrawal is expressed. Settings for detoxification can include inpatient, residential, day, or outpatient programs.

Given the current armamentarium of medications, opioid detoxification can be accomplished safely, relatively quickly, and with a minimum of discomfort. Unfortunately, the method chosen often depends more on what is available than on what is ideal. This is a consequence of many factors: physician or patient preference or bias, the availability of physicians trained in detoxification methods, federal and state regulations, insurance or other funding mechanisms, and the methods available in a given setting in a particular geographic area.

Goals of Detoxification

The goals of the detoxification process are as follows:

1. To rid the body of the acute physiological dependence associated with chronic daily opioid use
2. To diminish, or ideally to eliminate, the pain and discomfort of opioid withdrawal
3. To provide a safe and humane treatment to enable the individual to remain abstinent during the acute phase of withdrawal
4. To provide an environment that increases the likelihood that a patient continues treatment after detoxification and to make referrals to such treatment centers
5. To identify any medical problems and to treat them or make referrals for additional care following detoxification
6. To begin educating the patient about issues related to health and relapse prevention, and to begin exploring issues related to family, vocational, and legal problems that may need referral

When Is Detoxification Successful?

Because relatively few opioid-dependent individuals can sustain abstinence from opioids without additional help immediately after detoxification, detoxification should be viewed as the first stage of treatment. It is unrealistic to expect detoxification alone to produce the more ambitious goals, beyond abstinence, of long-term treatment, including improvements in employment, criminal behavior, interpersonal relationships, and general physical and psychological well-being. Success is a function not only of safety and comfort but also of treatment retention and participation in longer-term treatment. This does not mean that detoxification is necessarily a failure if the person does not agree to long-term treatment. Younger patients often believe that detoxification is all they need to eradicate their habit and remain off drugs. They may see no need for longer-term treatment. When they return for a second or third detoxification, they are frequently more realistic about what is involved in staying drug free and more willing to consider longer-term treatment. Because of the relapsing nature of opioid dependence, formal detoxification may be required many times over the course of the disorder.

Setting Choice

Detoxification can take place in an outpatient, an inpatient, or a partial hospitalization setting. Outpatient detoxification is the least expensive setting and may enable the patient to continue working or otherwise carry on his or her life. It has the potential advantage of forcing a person to confront his or her home environment, with all of its usual cues to drug use, and immediately find alternatives to drug use in response to these cues; going from the protected inpatient setting to everyday reality is often accompanied by rapid relapse because a patient has not found adequate alternatives. The disadvantages of outpatient detoxification include immediate access to drugs at a time when drug craving may be extremely high, more difficulty assessing and dealing with other medical conditions, and the possible need for detoxification to proceed more slowly in the unprotected environment.

During inpatient detoxification, access to drugs or to craving-inducing stimuli can be minimized, the patient can be observed more closely for medical problems or complications of withdrawal, and the withdrawal can be more rapid. If the program is a comprehensive one, more attention can be focused on other aspects of the patient's life—in the family, vocational, medical, and psychiatric arenas. The disadvantages are primarily the cost and the disruption of the patient's life in the need to be away from work and home.

Partial hospitalization programs are considerably less expensive than inpatient programs, while retaining some of the inpatient advantages; nevertheless, they are not widely available. The clinician is usually forced to choose between inpatient and outpatient settings, and the choices are often limited by factors such as insurance coverage and the availability of programs in the community. As a result of managed care restrictions, inpatient detoxification has become primarily for those patients who have serious medical or psychiatric problems or who have repeatedly failed outpatient detoxification. Although inpatient detoxification has a much higher completion rate (up to 80%) compared with outpatient programs (as low as 17%) (Gossop et al. 1986), its long-term advantages related to relapse are less definite. Some patients need inpatient detoxification to achieve initial abstinence. Work is still needed in accurately identifying which patients require inpatient treatment and which would do well with an outpatient approach.

Historical Overview

In the past century, many treatments have been introduced for relieving the symptoms of opioid withdrawal. Many of these treatments have proven either more addicting than the drug being withdrawn or more dangerous than untreated withdrawal. In a masterful review, Kolb and Himmelsbach (1938) looked back on 40 years of mostly futile attempts to treat narcotic withdrawal, including the use of autohemotherapy (injection of blood previously withdrawn from the patient), water balance therapy, and numerous toxic chemicals, alone or in combination. Kleber and Riordan (1982) reviewed the earlier work by these writers and updated it with the techniques that had been used in the 40 years since their article. Since that review, the most common approach—methadone substitution and gradual withdrawal—has declined slightly in popularity and the newer approaches described in this chapter have gained favor. Some of these newer approaches may yet be discarded if they are found wanting.

Clinical Characteristics of the Opioid (μ Agonist) Withdrawal Syndrome

Naturally occurring opiates such as opium, morphine, and codeine; derivatives such as heroin, hydromorphone, and dihydrocodeine; and synthetics such as methadone, meperidine, and fentanyl are capable of creating physical dependence and may require detoxification if they have been taken in sufficient quantities over time. In general, clinically significant withdrawal syndromes do not develop after less than 2 weeks of daily opiate use (Jaffe and Martin 1975), but individuals previously dependent on opioids may redevelop physical dependence much more quickly.

Factors Influencing Symptom Severity

The nature and severity of withdrawal symptoms when opioid-type drugs are halted relate to a variety of factors:

- *Specific drug used.* Rapidly metabolized drugs such as heroin are generally associated with more severe but shorter-lived withdrawal phenomena, whereas drugs that dissociate slowly from the opioid receptor, such as buprenorphine, or that are slowly excreted from the body, such as methadone, have a slower onset with a less intense but more protracted withdrawal syndrome. In general, the longer the duration of drug action, the less intense but longer lasting the withdrawal symptoms.
- *Total daily amount used.* In general, the more opioids ingested daily, the more severe the withdrawal syndrome. However, some researchers have suggested that dosage does not correlate well with severity of withdrawal symptoms (Gossop et al. 1987).
- *Duration and regularity of use.* Although some withdrawal can be seen when a single dose of morphine is followed a few hours later by a narcotic antagonist (Heishman et al. 1989), clinically significant withdrawal usually requires daily use of an adequate amount of the opioid for at least 2–3 weeks (Jaffe and Martin 1975). In contrast, duration of use much beyond 2–3 months does not appear to be associated with any greater severity. A good rule of thumb regarding the regularity of use and its as-

sociation with symptom severity is that the more intermittent the drug use, the less severe the withdrawal.
- *Psychological and individual factors.* In general, the greater the patient's expectation that his or her suffering would be relieved by an available medication, the more severe the reported withdrawal symptoms. Thus, if an individual expects little symptom relief, there seems to be a diminution in the withdrawal intensity reported. Anticipatory anxiety appears to increase withdrawal severity (Phillips et al. 1986). The patient's personality and state of mind can also influence withdrawal severity, as can his or her general physical health and ability to handle stress. Finally, some individuals appear to be far more sensitive to opioid withdrawal symptoms than others.

Signs and Symptoms of Opioid Withdrawal

The μ agonist withdrawal syndrome can be conceptualized as rebound hyperactivity in the biological systems suppressed by the agonists. (For a more detailed description of the neurochemical mechanisms involved, see Chapter 2, "Neurobiology of Opiates/Opioids," in this volume.) Withdrawal phenomena are generally the opposite of the acute agonistic effects of the opioid (e.g., acute opioids cause constipation and pupillary constriction, whereas withdrawal is associated with diarrhea and pupillary dilatation). The clinical characteristics of opioid withdrawal may be described in several ways. Some authors separate objective signs from subjective symptoms, whereas others separate signs and symptoms into grades on the basis of severity. No single classification is totally satisfactory.

Subjective symptoms, even under controlled conditions, are often more distressing than objective signs. It also has been shown that opioid-dependent patients may experience major withdrawal symptoms with minimal or no objective signs to confirm this discomfort. Table 23–1 lists the most common signs and symptoms, which are divided into two categories based on their approximate order of appearance.

When a short-acting opioid such as heroin has been taken chronically, the onset of withdrawal begins with anxiety and craving about 8–12 hours after the last dose (see Table 23–2). If an opioid is not ingested, this progresses to dysphoria, yawning, lacrimation, rhinorrhea, perspiration, restlessness, and broken

Table 23–1. Signs and symptoms of opioid withdrawal

Early to moderate	Moderate to advanced
Anorexia	Abdominal cramps
Anxiety	Broken sleep
Craving	Hot or cold flashes
Dysphoria	Increased blood pressure
Fatigue	Increased pulse
Headache	Low-grade fever
Increased respiratory rate	Muscle and bone pain
Irritability	Muscle spasm (hence the term *kicking the habit*)
Lacrimation	
Mydriasis (mild)	Mydriasis (with dilated fixed pupils at the peak)
Perspiration	
Piloerection (gooseflesh)	Nausea and vomiting
Restlessness	
Rhinorrhea	
Yawning	

sleep. Later, there are waves of gooseflesh, hot and cold flashes, aching of bones and muscles, nausea, vomiting, diarrhea, abdominal cramps, weight loss, and low-grade fever. An untreated individual in opioid withdrawal may lie in a fetal position (to ease abdominal cramping) and request blankets, even on warm days (because of the hot and cold flashes). The individual's skin may be exquisitely sensitive to the touch. The heroin withdrawal syndrome typically reaches its peak between 36 and 72 hours after the last dose, and the acute symptoms subside substantially within 5 days. With methadone withdrawal, in contrast, the peak occurs between days 4 and 6, and symptoms do not substantially subside until 14–21 days (Kleber 1996). With a somewhat more short-acting opioid, such as meperidine, craving may be intense, but the autonomic signs, such as pupillary dilatation, are not particularly prominent. Usually, little nausea, vomiting, or diarrhea occurs, but, at peak intensity, the muscle twitching, restlessness, and nervousness may be worse than during morphine withdrawal (Jaffe and Martin 1975). Regardless of which opioid is used, even after the acute symptoms have subsided, evidence indicates a more protracted abstinence syndrome with subtle disturbances of mood and sleep that can persist for 6–8 months (Martin and Jasinski 1969). Therefore, an addicted individual may not feel that he or she has returned to normal for months after the last ingestion of the drug. Fatigue, dysphoria, irritability, and insomnia may all increase the likelihood of relapse. Protracted abstinence may involve both conditioning and physiological factors (Satel et al. 1993).

Evaluation and Diagnosis

When a patient is first seen by the clinician, he or she should be evaluated to determine whether detoxification is needed. Once this is determined and the patient is accepted for treatment, a more complete assessment is necessary to devise an individual treatment plan. Thus, information needs to be gathered on a wider range of areas, including psychological, psychosocial, and physical status.

Table 23–2. Duration of effects and first appearance of withdrawal

Drug	Effects wear off (hours)[a]	Appearance of nonpurposive withdrawal symptoms	Peak withdrawal effects	Majority of symptoms over
Meperidine	2–3	4–6 hours	8–12 hours	4–5 days
Hydromorphone	4–5	4–5 hours	36–72 hours	Approximately the same as morphine
Heroin	4[b]	8–12 hours	36–72 hours	7–10 days
Morphine	4–5	8–12 hours	36–72 hours	7–10 days
Codeine	4	8–12 hours	36–72 hours	Approximately the same as morphine
Methadone	8–12	36–72 hours	96–144 hours	14–21 days

[a]Duration may vary with chronic dosing.
[b]Usually taken two to four times per day.

The Interview

While gathering the information detailed below, especially the drug history, a nonjudgmental attitude is more likely to elicit accurate data. Disdainful behavior is likely to create ongoing difficulties and to produce false information, and it may even drive the patient away.

Drug History

A review of current and past drug and alcohol use and abuse is necessary for adequate patient assessment. The following information should be obtained for each current substance or group of substances, with special emphasis on substance use during the past week:

- Name of drug used, length of time used, frequency of use
- Date or time of last use
- Route of administration
- Amount
- Cost
- Purpose (e.g., to get high, to relieve depression or boredom, to sleep, for energy, to relieve side effects of other drugs, to avoid withdrawal)
- For drugs previously used: name, age at which drug use started, length of time used, adverse effects
- Previous treatment experiences: where, what kind, outcome
- Prescription drugs currently used: name; reason for use; amount, frequency, and duration of use; last dose

Other Medical History

The medical history includes serious illnesses, accidents, and hospitalizations. In addition to the usual medical history, special attention should be given to the possible medical complications of drug abuse. The medical history also includes the existence of current symptoms in the various body systems. It is important to look for illnesses that may complicate withdrawal and those that previously may have been ignored or missed because of the patient's chaotic lifestyle.

Social Functioning

Information should be gathered on the following topics: 1) living arrangements (e.g., alone, with family); 2) marital status; 3) sexual orientation and function-

ing; 4) employment and/or educational status; 5) family members' (e.g., parents, siblings, spouse, other key members) occupations, education, psychological state, history of drug or alcohol problems; 6) friends (in particular, are there non-drug-using ones?); 7) recreational and leisure-time activities; and 8) current and past legal status. The Addiction Severity Index is a useful instrument for gathering this information (McLellan et al. 1985).

The interviewer should try to get a feel for the emotional and factual aspects of the interview topics. For example: What is the patient's attitude toward his or her job, and what type of job is it? What is the quality of the patient's marital or family relationships? How does the patient cope with spare time at nights and on weekends, when relapse is most likely to occur? Such questions can identify the nature and degree of the patient's social supports and aid in planning for post-detoxification treatment. Prior attempts at withdrawal and factors associated with relapse should be especially explored.

Psychological Status

When carried out by a nonpsychiatrist physician, psychological evaluation may single out patients who need early psychiatric referral for possible psychosis, delirium, psychiatric syndromes secondary to medical conditions, serious depression, suicide, or being violence prone. The psychiatrist, in addition to exploring factors that could complicate withdrawal, should evaluate for the presence of less obvious comorbid psychiatric syndromes. When possible, the evaluator should ascertain whether psychiatric conditions preceded or followed the drug abuse. Some patients take drugs to self-medicate dysphoric states of loneliness, depression, or anxiety or to control unacceptable, usually aggressive, impulses. Conversely, continued use of certain drugs may lead to or exacerbate psychiatric states not previously evident. Opioids seem to have antipsychotic effects in some patients, and withdrawal can lead to an exacerbation or sudden appearance of psychotic symptoms.

As part of the psychological state evaluation, a mental status examination should be carried out and include orientation for place, person, and date; presence or absence of hallucinations, delusions, or suicidal ideation; memory; intelligence, mood, and affect; thought processes; preoccupations and behavior during interview; judgment; and insight.

Physical Examination

Although there is no special physical examination for opioid-dependent individuals, the clinician should remember that certain conditions can be either direct or indirect sequelae of drug abuse. Although some of these findings appear in nondependent individuals, and some dependent individuals may have few or none of them, their presence aids proper diagnosis.

Cutaneous Signs

The following cutaneous signs may be directly or indirectly associated with drug abuse:

- *Needle puncture marks.* Needle marks are usually found over veins, especially in the antecubital area, back of the hands, and forearms, but can be found anywhere on the body where a vein is reachable, including the neck, tongue, and dorsal vein of the penis.
- *"Tracks."* Tracks, or track marks, are one of the most common and readily recognizable signs of chronic injection drug abuse. They are usually hyperpigmented linear scars located along veins. They result both from frequent unsterile injections and from the deposit of carbon following needle sterilization performed with a match or other sooty heating procedure. Tracks tend to lighten over time but may never totally disappear.
- *Tattoos.* Because tracks are such a well-known indication of drug abuse, addicted individuals may try to hide them with tattoos over the area.
- *Hand edema.* When addicted individuals run out of antecubital and forearm veins, they often turn to veins in the fingers and back of the hands, which can lead to hand edema. Such edema can persist for months.
- *Thrombophlebitis.* Thrombophlebitis (blockage or inflammation of veins) may be found on the limbs of injection drug users because their injections are often unsterile and because irritation is produced by adulterants.
- *Abscesses and ulcers.* Abscesses and ulcers are particularly common among individuals who inject barbiturates because of the irritating quality of these chemicals. When secondary to heroin injection, they are more likely to be septic and in the vicinity of veins.
- *Ulceration or perforation of the nasal septum.* Frequent snorting of heroin can lead to ulceration of the septum, whereas similar chronic use of cocaine can cause septal perforation secondary to vasoconstriction and loss of blood supply.
- *Cigarette burns or scars from old burns.* Cigarette burns or scars can result from drug-induced drowsiness. It has been estimated that more than 90% of drug- and alcohol-dependent individuals smoke tobacco.
- *Piloerection.* Piloerection, a sign of opioid withdrawal, is usually found on the arms and trunk. Truncal piloerection is unusual in the absence of opioid withdrawal.
- *Cheilosis.* Cheilosis (cracking of skin at the corners of the mouth) is especially seen in chronic amphetamine-using individuals and in opioid-addicted individuals prior to or during detoxification.
- *Contact dermatitis.* In solvent-abusing individuals, contact dermatitis is seen around the nose, mouth, and hands and is sometimes called *glue-sniffer's rash.* In other abusers, it may occur around areas of injection secondary to use of chemicals to cleanse the skin.
- *Jaundice.* Jaundice, due to hepatitis, is usually secondary to use of unsterilized shared needles and syringes. Rates of hepatitis C infection among injection drug users in New York City have been reported to be between 80% and 90%.
- *Monilial infection.* Monilial infection, typically oral thrush, is a common finding in acquired immunodeficiency syndrome (AIDS).

Laboratory Tests

The following laboratory tests should usually be performed:

- Urine screen for drugs, including opioids, barbiturates, amphetamines, cocaine, benzodiazepines, phencyclidine, and marijuana. Most routine urine tests, however, do not detect the prescription opioids oxycodone, hydrocodone, fentanyl, and buprenorphine.
- Complete blood count and differential; leukocytosis is common, and white blood cell counts greater than $14,000/mm^3$ are not unusual.
- Urinalysis
- Blood chemistry profile (e.g., sequential multiple analysis 20 with serum amylase and magnesium)
- Syphilis serology
- Human immunodeficiency virus (HIV) test (permission from the patient is necessary in many states)

- Hepatitis antigen and antibody test
- Chest X ray
- Electrocardiogram in patients older than 40 years
- Pregnancy test in women (hold chest X ray until test is complete)
- Tuberculin skin test (purified protein derivative)
- Any other necessary test suggested by the history or physical examination

Opioid Agonist Substitution and Taper

Because of cross-tolerance and cross-dependence among all opioids, one could, in theory, use almost any opioid to prevent withdrawal and gradually detoxify opioid-dependent individuals. Two opioids, however, deserve special attention for this purpose: methadone and buprenorphine.

Methadone

Until the recent approval of buprenorphine for opioid detoxification, the most common detoxification method was methadone substitution and taper, although the method declined in popularity even before buprenorphine became widely available. Methadone has several advantages over most other agents for detoxification:

- It is orally effective, which eliminates the need for continued injection drug use, thus avoiding continuation of a needle habit.
- It is long acting, which allows for once-daily dosing and a milder, albeit longer-lasting, withdrawal syndrome (longer-acting opioids produce withdrawal syndromes that are milder but longer lasting, and they need to be given less often, thus producing smoother withdrawal).
- It is safe, provided that appropriate care is taken with initial dosing.

In general, a more addictive drug should not be used to detoxify a patient from a less addictive one. In practice, this means that although methadone can be used to withdraw patients from narcotics such as heroin, morphine, hydromorphone, oxycodone, or meperidine, it should be avoided for drugs such as propoxyphene or pentazocine, for which the withdrawal should be handled by gradually decreasing the dosage

of the agent itself or by an agent such as clonidine. Buprenorphine, given sublingually, will probably become the opioid of choice for withdrawal from most opioids.

U.S. Food and Drug Administration (FDA) guidelines for narcotic detoxification describe two types of detoxification: short term and long term. Short-term detoxification is for a period not more than 30 days; long-term detoxification is for a period not more than 180 days. Short-term detoxification is most likely to occur with individuals currently dependent on opioids other than methadone. Long-term detoxification is used for individuals already taking methadone and wishing to stop it, although in some programs, individuals are taken directly from heroin to long-term detoxification with methadone over a 6-month period. Prolonged detoxification avoids some of the withdrawal symptoms that occur in more rapid detoxification and provides a setting in which psychosocial rehabilitation can take place. However, the long-term effectiveness of this option, as opposed to shorter-term detoxification or methadone maintenance, has not been shown.

Initiation of Detoxification

If the patient has been taking opioids for medical purposes, and the physician is reasonably sure about the amount being ingested, Table 23–3 can be used to convert the narcotic dosage into a methadone dosage. With illicit drug use, the picture is very different. Knowledge of the exact dosage is usually not available. The amount of narcotics in illegal "bags" can vary from dealer to dealer, week to week, city to city, and even day to day. Under these circumstances, the physician must guess at the initial methadone dosage. Given that the purity of heroin on the street has ranged from 60% to 80% or more in recent years, the choice of an initial dosage is very important. It needs to be high enough to suppress withdrawal symptoms so that the patient does not leave the program but low enough so that if the patient's habit is lower than presumed, the dosage would not be health or life threatening. Because 40 mg of methadone can be a fatal dose in some nontolerant individuals, the initial dose should be less than 40 mg. One common approach to ensuring safety is to start with a dose of 10–20 mg, large enough to control many heroin habits yet small enough to be safe for virtually everyone. The patient should be kept under observation to assess the effect of the initial methadone dose. If withdrawal symptoms are initially present, the dose should suppress them within 30–60 minutes; if withdrawal symptoms persist an hour after dosing, an addi-

Table 23–3.	Drug relationships for withdrawal

Methadone 1 mg is equivalent to:
- Codeine 30 mg
- Dromoran 1 mg
- Heroin 1–2 mg
- Hydrocodone 0.5 mg
- Hydromorphone 0.5 mg
- Laudanum (opium tincture) 3 mL
- Levorphanol 0.5 mg
- Meperidine 20 mg
- Morphine 3–4 mg
- Oxycodone 1.5 mg
- Paregoric 7–8 mL

tional 5–10 mg of methadone can be given. When withdrawal symptoms are not initially present, the patient should be observed for drowsiness or depressed respiration an hour after dosing. When 10–20 mg is given as the initial dose, a similar amount may be given 12 hours later if necessary. This split-dosing approach is usually not practical in outpatient detoxification but is used at times in inpatient settings. Unless evidence of narcotic use in excess of 40 mg of methadone equivalent per day is documented, the initial dose should not exceed 30 mg, and the total 24-hour dose should not exceed 40 mg the first few days. A safe initial dose in a nontolerant individual can become dangerous if continued beyond 1 or 2 days because of rising blood levels of methadone. A dangerous dose manifests itself in drowsiness and/or signs of motor impairment, as well as miosis, nausea, and possible mild hypothermia.

Some clinicians disagree as to whether to start the withdrawal regimen in the absence of withdrawal signs and symptoms. It is sometimes difficult to know with certainty that an individual is currently physically dependent. The information gathered through the interview, physical examination, and laboratory tests does not always establish the presence of physical dependence sufficient to require medical detoxification, unless the clinician has observed the signs and symptoms of opioid withdrawal. The history of drug taking may be unreliable, as a result of overreporting drug use to increase the dose of prescribed opioid or underreporting to conceal a habit (the latter appears more common among addicted health care professionals). The drug history may be misleading even when the patient is trying to be honest because of the variable nature of illicitly obtained drugs. Physical signs such as tracks tell of past drug use, not necessarily current use. Fresh needle marks may provide little information about the frequency, nature, and amount of what was injected. Urinalyses positive for drugs suggest recent use but do not establish the need for detoxification. Heroin, detected as morphine in the urine, can be found up to approximately 48 hours after the last use among infrequent users.

Definitive evidence of physical dependence can be collected in two ways: 1) by waiting until the patient develops withdrawal signs and symptoms or 2) by producing withdrawal through administration of naloxone. Parenteral naloxone can distinguish opioid-dependent from nondependent individuals through the severity of withdrawal related to the naloxone dose. A common method is to inject 0.2 mg of naloxone subcutaneously, followed by 0.4 mg 30 minutes later if the results from the smaller dose are inconclusive. Some physicians recommend an initial dose of 0.6–0.8 mg to speed up the process and rule out false-negative results. Because of the possibility of fetal injury or induced miscarriage, the naloxone test should not be done if the patient is pregnant.

Whether the program is inpatient or outpatient, the availability of trained medical personnel will often determine how the program will establish the need for medical detoxification. If, as is commonly the case, the program uses the combined evidence of the medical history, physical examination, and urine toxicology screen, it should still be prepared to wait for withdrawal signs or administer a naloxone challenge test in borderline or doubtful situations. Once the need for medical detoxification has been established, decisions still have to be made regarding the setting, the specific method of detoxification, and the need for concurrent treatment of comorbid physical or emotional problems. When serious physical or emotional problems are present, it is not uncommon to delay the opioid taper by temporarily maintaining the individual on methadone, attending to the acute problem, and then beginning the methadone taper once some stability has been achieved in the other areas.

Length of Withdrawal

The total methadone dosage necessary to stabilize a patient for the first 24 hours should be repeated on day 2, either in one dose for outpatients or in divided doses for inpatients. Dosage adjustments can then be made if the patient is sedated or remains in some withdrawal. Revision to a higher dosage should preferably be made on the basis of objective signs of opioid withdrawal rather than on subjective complaints alone. This is not always easy because certain signs, including pupillary dilatation, may be modified by the methadone, even when the patient is undermedicated. After the patient is stabilized, the dosage can then be gradually reduced. Two common approaches are either to decrease the methadone by 5 mg/day until zero dosage is reached (*linear withdrawal method*) or to decrease it by 10 mg/day until a dosage of 10 mg/day is reached and then decrease it more slowly (e.g., by 2 mg/day) (*inverse exponential withdrawal method*). For individuals who have large initial habits, the linear method may be better, whereas in those with a starting dosage of less than 50 mg/day of methadone, the inverse exponential method leads to more rapid passing of the withdrawal syndrome without any significant increase in withdrawal severity or dropout rate (Strang and Gossop 1990).

Inpatient methadone substitution and taper is usually accomplished in 5–7 days, whereas outpatient detoxification is often extended to minimize withdrawal symptoms and to decrease the likelihood of dropout and relapse. Some inpatient programs complete the process in as few as 4 days, whereas some outpatient programs last for months. Symptoms of insomnia, fatigue, and irritability or anxiety may linger for weeks or months. The acute phase of opioid withdrawal may be considered complete and the patient discharged from the detoxification program when no objective signs of opioid withdrawal occur for 48 hours in the absence of any opioid.

Withdrawal From Methadone Maintenance

For a patient withdrawing from methadone maintenance, the detoxification approach used tends to be a function of the reasons for terminating methadone maintenance treatment. Patients in good standing who desire to become drug free should be tapered off methadone slowly over a 3- to 6-month period. The most difficult period usually occurs at methadone dosages less than 25 mg/day because at these lower dosages, withdrawal symptoms may emerge sooner than 24 hours following a dose. Split doses, typically given twice daily, may help counter this problem, but they are not always possible or practical. The methadone dosage is usually reduced by 5–10 mg/week until the dosage reaches 25 mg/day. At that point, a reduction of no more than 5 mg/week is often recommended. If the patient needs to be withdrawn more rapidly because he or she is being discharged in bad standing,

must leave the geographic area, or may be going to prison, then withdrawal usually takes place during a 10- to 30-day period. For example, the patient dosage may be decreased by 10 mg/day until a total dosage of 40 mg/day is reached, then it is decreased by 5 mg/day until the dosage of 5 mg/day is reached, at which point that dosage is given for 2–3 days. If the patient is on an inpatient or residential unit, divided doses are helpful, especially when the total dosage is less than 25 mg/day.

Other Drugs and Supportive Measures

Even with gradual withdrawal, some withdrawal symptoms usually emerge, and certain mild symptoms may persist for many days after treatment has been completed. There is no consensus on the use of other drugs during these periods. Tranquilizers or bedtime sedation can help allay the patient's anxiety and minimize the craving for opioids, but nonopioid medications are, at best, only partially effective in relieving the specific symptoms of opioid abstinence, with the exception of α_2-adrenergic agonists (e.g., clonidine or lofexidine; see section "Other Detoxification Agents and Methods" later in this chapter). If insomnia and other withdrawal symptoms are unusually severe, especially in older patients, an incremental increase in the next dose of methadone and, therefore, a slower withdrawal schedule can provide relief.

Insomnia is often one of the more debilitating withdrawal symptoms. It is difficult to tolerate in and of itself, and it also diminishes a patient's ability to cope with other withdrawal symptoms. Barbiturates should generally not be used to treat insomnia because of their abuse liability and low therapeutic index. Sedating medications, including flurazepam, clonazepam, oxazepam, diphenhydramine, hydroxyzine, and antidepressants such as trazodone, have all been proposed for withdrawal-related insomnia. Because many opioid-dependent individuals may also abuse benzodiazepines, the choice of such agents needs to be made carefully. Generally, few or no problems result when benzodiazepines are used for up to a week in inpatient detoxification settings. Outpatient detoxification presents more problems because there is no control over benzodiazepine use, misuse, or diversion.

Comfort medications used to treat ancillary withdrawal symptoms include nonsteroidal anti-inflammatory drugs (e.g., ibuprofen 600–800 mg every 6–8 hours or ketorolac tromethamine 30 mg intramuscularly every 6 hours for no more than 5 days) for muscle cramps or pain; dicyclomine 10 mg every 6 hours for abdominal cramps; bismuth subsalicylate 30 cc after each loose stool; and prochlorperazine 10 mg intramuscularly three times a day or ondansetron 8 mg orally every 8 hours for nausea and vomiting.

Psychosocial support can also play an important role. A warm, kind, and reassuring attitude from the treatment staff is most helpful. Involvement of patients in their own detoxification schedule helps with inpatient, but not outpatient, detoxification (Dawe et al. 1991). The fewer the struggles over medication dosing, the better the alliance can be with the patient. Visitors, however, can be a problem, and a firm stand is often necessary. Visitors should be limited to immediate family members (i.e., parents or spouse) who are known not to abuse drugs. Even parents have been known to smuggle in drugs under the pressure of a patient's entreaties that the staff does not understand his or her distress. A watchful presence is therefore necessary around all visitors. Such attempts at deception may be less likely to occur if family meetings are held and parents and significant others are well informed about the approach to detoxification.

Other potentially helpful measures include warm baths, exercise (when the patient feels up to it), and various diets. Except when specific nutritional deficiencies are present, there is no evidence for benefits from any particular dietary regimen. However, because opioid-dependent patients are often malnourished, general vitamin and mineral supplements should be given.

Buprenorphine

Buprenorphine is a partial μ-receptor agonist and μ-receptor antagonist. Although initially marketed in the United States as a parenteral analgesic (Buprenex), buprenorphine was approved by the FDA in late 2002 in sublingual tablet formulations for both detoxification and maintenance treatment of opioid dependence. Buprenorphine sublingual tablets are available with buprenorphine only (Subutex) and in combination with naloxone (Suboxone). The addition of naloxone to the tablet is intended to reduce the risk of buprenorphine abuse by injection. Naloxone is not readily bioavailable with sublingual administration because the potency ratio of parenteral-to-sublingual naloxone is 15:1. Therefore, the small quantities of naloxone absorbed by the sublingual route will not

precipitate withdrawal. If, however, the sublingual tablet is crushed and snorted or dissolved and injected, it may precipitate withdrawal, especially among heroin users, and thus significantly reduce the risk of buprenorphine diversion. It is not entirely clear whether even injected naloxone will precipitate withdrawal in individuals receiving buprenorphine maintenance (Kosten et al. 1990) because buprenorphine has a long receptor half-life and greater affinity for opioid receptors than does naloxone.

Many of the advantages noted above for methadone in detoxification apply equally to buprenorphine, which is also long-acting, safe, and effective by a nonparenteral route of administration. Initiation of buprenorphine for detoxification differs from methadone initiation, in that buprenorphine may precipitate withdrawal symptoms if it is given too soon following use of a pure opioid agonist. Thus, the better approach in using buprenorphine for detoxification is to wait until the patient shows some withdrawal symptoms, at which point buprenorphine usually serves to relieve these symptoms. When some of the older literature on buprenorphine is considered, one must keep in mind that until the mid-1990s, buprenorphine was usually administered in an aqueous-alcohol solution, which is approximately twice as bioavailable as the tablet formulations now available.

A typical approach to managing heroin detoxification is to administer buprenorphine 4 mg sublingually after the emergence of mild to moderate withdrawal (usually at least 10–12 hours after the last use of heroin). Another dose of buprenorphine 4 mg sublingually may be administered approximately 1 hour later, depending on the patient's comfort level. On subsequent days, doses of buprenorphine between 8 and 12 mg sublingually are usually sufficient to relieve withdrawal symptoms. Data are insufficient to make definitive recommendations about the optimal subsequent duration of buprenorphine treatment in detoxification, although abrupt cessation of buprenorphine is generally mild because the slow dissociation of buprenorphine from opioid receptors provides a self-tapering effect. For some patients, it may be beneficial to continue a buprenorphine taper for several days or more. In one study comparing 5 days of buprenorphine with 8 days of clonidine, buprenorphine appeared to be better than clonidine (see section "Other Detoxification Agents and Methods" later in this chapter for more on clonidine) for detoxification of heroin dependence (Lintzeris et al. 2002).

When buprenorphine is stopped abruptly, the exact duration of withdrawal is not well known and may vary considerably from patient to patient. Various periods have been reported, ranging from no signs of abstinence after being maintained for 10 days on 8 mg (Mello and Mendelson 1980) to mild symptoms appearing after 2–3 days and peaking at approximately 2 weeks after the last dose (Jasinski et al. 1978) to mild symptoms peaking at 3–5 days and going away after another 5 days (Fudala et al. 1990). Individual differences may be quite important because a recent study suggested that about one-fifth of the patients maintained on daily buprenorphine 16 mg sublingually for 10 days experienced significant end of dose withdrawal symptoms (Lopatko et al. 2003). However, some studies have suggested that opioid withdrawal symptoms in less-than-daily buprenorphine maintenance regimens are minimal to very mild for up to 96 hours (Gross et al. 2001; Petry et al. 1999).

As the dosage of buprenorphine is increased, a ceiling effect comparable to approximately 20–30 mg of parenteral morphine is reached. Buprenorphine is thus less likely to produce the severe respiratory depression found with full μ agonists. Nevertheless, deaths have been attributed to respiratory depression in patients treated with buprenorphine, but, in most cases, the respiratory depression was attributed to concomitant use or abuse of benzodiazepines (Reynaud et al. 1998; Tracqui et al. 1998).

It may be possible to use buprenorphine to help individuals detoxify from methadone maintenance, either to achieve a drug-free state or to transition to buprenorphine maintenance, although scant information is available about how this procedure can be optimized or whether the mono and combination forms are interchangeable for this purpose. A handful of laboratory studies (Mendelson et al. 1997; Preston et al. 1988; Strain et al. 1992, 1995; Walsh et al. 1995) of the effects of buprenorphine in methadone-maintained populations have been done. The results from these studies have been mixed and conflicting, with some suggesting that higher doses of methadone and higher doses of buprenorphine produce more severe precipitated withdrawal when buprenorphine is given to methadone-maintained individuals and others suggesting that higher doses of buprenorphine produce more agonist effect and make the transition easier. The timing of buprenorphine administration relative to the last use of methadone is another important variable, but little is known about how exactly this affects the tolerability of the transition from methadone to buprenorphine. Very little clinical literature exists on making this transition. In general, however, as with detoxification from heroin, the patient should be at least in mild withdrawal, suggesting a minimum of 36 hours after the last full methadone dose. Also, most researchers suggest tapering the methadone dose down to 40 mg or less prior to buprenorphine induction. Two studies that used this procedure tapered methadone nearly to zero before buprenorphine induction (Janiri et al. 1994; Levin et al. 1997).

The possibility of using buprenorphine in rapid antagonist induction also has been studied. In one study, 23 patients maintained for 1 month at a dosage of 3–6 mg/day of buprenorphine solution (more bioavailable than the tablets) were abruptly given increasing dosages of naltrexone over 4 days, starting 24 hours after the last buprenorphine dose (Kosten et al. 1991). Minimal withdrawal occurred, and 20 of the patients took the initial 6-mg naltrexone dose. However, only 4 patients continued the naltrexone at 50 mg/day beyond the 2 weeks. More recently, patients were given buprenorphine solution 3 mg/day sublingually for 3 days followed by 25 mg of naltrexone plus clonidine on day 4 and naltrexone 50 mg on day 5 (O'Connor et al. 1997). The individuals in the buprenorphine group had milder withdrawal and were more likely to complete detoxification (81%) than were those in the clonidine group (65%). The buprenorphine group had detoxification completion rates comparable to the clonidine-naltrexone comparison group (also 81%), but no difference in naltrexone retention was found at 8 days. Finally, a small study used a 7-day buprenorphine stabilization prior to anesthesia-assisted naltrexone induction, with less postprocedure morbidity than a historical control population inducted onto naltrexone under anesthesia without buprenorphine stabilization (Bochud Tornay et al. 2003). It would appear that a rapid detoxification method involving buprenorphine as a bridge to antagonist induction and maintenance may ultimately be the least painful and the most successful.

Summary

Studies examining gradual methadone withdrawal suggest the following:

- Inpatient withdrawal has a significantly higher retention rate (about 80%) than short-term outpatient withdrawal (as low as 13%–17%).

- Although little evidence indicates that this initial higher rate is associated with better sustained abstinence 4–6 months later, more research is necessary to determine which patients need inpatient withdrawal.
- The success rate for short-term outpatient withdrawal appears about the same as reported by addicted individuals attempting self-withdrawal.
- The success rate for outpatient withdrawal appears to be improved substantially (up to 62%) if longer periods (e.g., 4–6 months) and higher dosages are used.
- Attention to psychosocial factors during outpatient withdrawal is associated with better retention and less use of heroin.
- Regardless of duration or dosage, once the methadone is stopped, a rebound in withdrawal symptoms lasting somewhat longer than 1 month occurs, and these symptoms are probably connected with the high postwithdrawal relapse rate.

Studies of buprenorphine in opioid detoxification suggest the following:

- Buprenorphine shares many of the advantages of methadone in opioid detoxification—it is safe, long-acting, and available for sublingual administration, thus diminishing the potential for misuse and abuse of the drug.
- Detoxification from buprenorphine is less severe than heroin or methadone withdrawal, even with abrupt cessation of buprenorphine, but there are conflicting reports as to the timing of peak withdrawal intensity, ranging between several days and several weeks.
- Buprenorphine may play important roles in two procedures related to detoxification: 1) the transition of patients in methadone maintenance to buprenorphine maintenance and potentially to drug-free treatments and 2) the rapid induction of naltrexone in heroin-dependent patients who desire antagonist maintenance treatment. More research is needed in both of these areas.

Other Detoxification Agents and Methods

Clonidine

The α_2-adrenergic agonist drug clonidine, marketed as an antihypertensive, has been used to facilitate opioid withdrawal in both inpatient and outpatient settings (Charney et al. 1986; Gold et al. 1978; Kleber et al. 1985). Clonidine in doses of 0.6–2.0 mg/day reduces many of the autonomic components of the opioid withdrawal syndrome, although craving, lethargy, insomnia, restlessness, and muscle aches are not well suppressed (Charney et al. 1981; Jasinski et al. 1985). Clonidine is believed to exert its ameliorative actions by binding to α_2 autoreceptors in the brain (e.g., locus coeruleus) and spinal cord. Both opioids and clonidine can suppress the activity of the locus coeruleus, which is hyperactive during opioid withdrawal.

Inpatients stabilized at 50 mg/day or less of methadone can be switched abruptly to clonidine. Dosages reaching 2.5 mg/day during precipitated withdrawal and antagonist induction have been used, with careful monitoring of heart rate and blood pressure to minimize the risk of significant hypotension and/or syncope. Sedation and hypotension have been the major side effects.

Clonidine also has been used for outpatient detoxification from either heroin or methadone maintenance. Patients maintained on 20 mg/day or less of methadone are about as successful after abrupt substitution of clonidine as after reduction of methadone by 1 mg/day (Kleber et al. 1985). With experienced personnel, street addicted persons also can be successfully withdrawn by using clonidine. O'Connor et al. (1997) found that 65% of such patients completed detoxification and entered the next phase of treatment. Clonidine has not been given official FDA approval for use in controlling withdrawal, but it has been used so widely now, both in the United States and abroad, that it has become accepted as an alternative to gradual methadone reduction.

Although many of the clonidine studies were conducted by the group that originated the techniques, a number of both open and controlled studies have been published since the mid-1980s (Cami et al. 1985; Gerra et al. 1995; Pini et al. 1991; San et al. 1990). Studies show that clonidine (and other α_2-adrenergic agonists such as lofexidine and guanfacine) is about as effective as gradual methadone withdrawal with the following differences: 1) methadone detoxification has fewer symptoms early in withdrawal and more at the end; 2) clonidine has the opposite profile: dropouts are more likely to occur early with clonidine and later with methadone; 3) clonidine has more side effects, especially hypotension and sedation; and 4) clonidine is less likely to be associated with postwithdrawal rebound. It also appears that clonidine is more effective if given in the context of abrupt opioid withdrawal rather than as an adjunct during gradual methadone tapering (Ghodse et al. 1994). In a direct comparison of clonidine with buprenorphine for short-term heroin detoxification, however, the group receiving buprenorphine fared better on measures of retention in detoxification, heroin use, and withdrawal severity scores than did the clonidine group (Lintzeris et al. 2002).

Techniques of Clonidine-Aided Detoxification

On the day before the start of clonidine detoxification, the usual dosage of opioid is given. On day 1 of the detoxification, the opioid is stopped abruptly, and clonidine is given in divided doses as shown in Table 23–4. Clonidine is to be used with caution in patients who have hypotension or who are taking antihypertensive medications. Use of tricyclic antidepressants within 3 weeks precludes use of clonidine because these agents render the α_2 receptors hyposensitive to clonidine. Other exclusions include pregnancy, history of psychosis, cardiac arrhythmias, or other medical conditions in which use of clonidine might aggravate the associated medical problems. Because clonidine can cause sedation, patients should be cautioned about driving and operating equipment.

Table 23–4. Clonidine-aided detoxification

Schedule for heroin, morphine, oxycodone, meperidine, and other short-acting opioids

Outpatient/inpatient

    Day 1: 0.1–0.2 mg orally every 4–6 hours up to 1 mg

    Days 2–4: 0.2–0.4 mg orally every 4–6 hours up to 1.2 mg

    Day 5 to completion: Reduce by 0.2 mg/day, given in two or three divided doses; the nighttime dose should be reduced last; or reduce total dosage by one-half each day, not to exceed 0.4 mg/day reduction

Schedule for methadone-maintained patients (20–30 mg/day methadone)

Day 1: 0.3 mg ⎤

Day 2: 0.4–0.6 mg ⎟

Day 3: 0.5–0.8 mg ⎬ Total daily dosage, given in divided doses every 4–6 hours

Day 4: 0.5–1.2 mg ⎦

Days 5–10: Maintain on day 4 dosage

Day 11 to completion: Reduce by 0.2 mg/day, given in two or three divided doses; the nighttime dose should be reduced last; if the patient complains of side effects, the dosage can be reduced by one-half each day, not to exceed 0.4 mg/day reduction

---

When clonidine is used on an outpatient basis, it is usually advisable not to give the patient more than a 2-day supply at one time. The patient should not drive during the first few days. The patient's blood pressure should be checked at the next visit. If dizziness occurs, the clinician should instruct the patient to cut back on the dosage, increase fluid intake, and/or lie down.

Lower clonidine dosages are used on day 1 because opioid withdrawal is less severe at that point, and the patient usually needs time to adjust to the sedative effects of clonidine. It is useful to give 0.1 mg of clonidine as the initial dose and observe the patient's reaction and blood pressure over the next hour or two. The total daily dosage should be divided into three doses given at 4- to 6-hour intervals. Unless the patient is either very thin or very obese, standard dosages are used rather than basing the dosage on body weight. The dosages from days 2 to 10 usually do not exceed 17 µg/kg/day (approximately 1.3 mg/day).

During withdrawal from long-acting opioids such as methadone, clonidine dosages can be increased gradually over several days. In treating withdrawal from short-acting opioids, however, dosages of clonidine are increased (i.e., titrated to symptoms) as rapidly as side effects permit because serious withdrawal symptoms appear earlier. However, the total duration of clonidine dosing is shorter.

Antiwithdrawal effects usually begin within 30 minutes and peak at 2–3 hours following oral administration of clonidine. For inpatients, blood pressure should be checked before each dose; if it is 85/55 mm Hg or lower, subsequent doses should be withheld until the pressure stabilizes. Dizziness between doses is best handled by monitoring blood pressure and having the patient lie down and increase fluid intake. If the pressure is too low, the dosage should be reduced. Sedation is commonly experienced, especially within the first few days, but usually remits by day 3 or 4. Dry mouth and facial pain are less common.

Insomnia is not usually a problem until day 3 or 4 of methadone withdrawal but occurs by day 2 or 3 with short-acting opioids. Paradoxically, clonidine may worsen the insomnia associated with detoxification even while causing sedation during the day. Other withdrawal symptoms not relieved by clonidine are primarily muscle aches, nervousness, and irritability. Benzodiazepines may be used for both the muscle aches and the insomnia, but they should be given with caution, particularly in outpatients, because many substance-dependent individuals abuse this class of drugs.

Clonidine is known to have mild analgesic effects. Thus, in withdrawing *medical opioid addicts,* analgesia may not be needed during the withdrawal period, even though the original painful condition persists to some extent. Pain usually returns 24–48 hours after the last clonidine dose; if naltrexone is to be used, pain needs to be treated with nonopioid analgesics.

Clonidine Patches

In some settings, clonidine is administered via transdermal patches (Spencer and Gregory 1989). The clonidine patch is a 0.2-mm square applied as a self-adhesive bandage. It comes in three sizes that deliver an amount of clonidine equal to daily dosing with 0.1, 0.2, or 0.3 mg of oral clonidine. The technique involves the following: Patients showing objective withdrawal signs are given 0.2 mg of oral clonidine every 6 hours during the first 24 hours. During the second 24 hours, the oral dose is halved. On day 1, patients are given one #2 patch if they weigh less than 100 pounds (0.2 mg in a 24-hour period), two #2 patches if they weigh 100–200 pounds, and three #2 patches if they weigh more than 200 pounds. The patch supplies clonidine for up to 7 days, is placed on a hairless area of the upper body, and is removed if systolic blood pressure falls below 80 mm Hg or diastolic blood pressure falls below 50 mm Hg. The patches are removed after the first week of treatment and replaced by half the dosage on another area of the upper body, if needed. The clonidine patches are removed after the second week of treatment or when the patient feels the patches are no longer needed.

Transdermal clonidine offers several advantages over the oral form:

- Patches can be applied by medical staff weekly; patients are not required to self-administer pills several times daily.
- Patients require fewer supplemental medications.
- The patches supply an even blood level of medication without peaks and troughs.
- The buildup of withdrawal symptoms during the night is prevented.
- Diversion and patient misuse are minimized.

Oral clonidine is given during the first 2 days because the steady-state levels of transdermal clonidine are not reached for 24–48 hours after application of the patch. The patches are used for 7–10 days for heroin withdrawal and 10–21 days for methadone withdrawal. To treat symptoms not relieved by clonidine, ibuprofen can be given for musculoskeletal pain, and other medications (described earlier in this chapter in the section "Other Drugs and Supportive Measures") can be given for insomnia.

In summary, clonidine appears to be a safe and effective alternative to the gradual reduction of methadone for opioid detoxification. Its disadvantages include more side effects and less coverage of the entire spectrum of withdrawal symptoms. Its advantages include much lower potential for diversion, because it is not an opioid, and more important, avoidance of the long residual withdrawal symptoms that persist for weeks after methadone withdrawal. Use of the transdermal patch in selected patients may lead to smoother withdrawal, but the oral form must be used for the first 24–48 hours until a steady blood level is achieved. The availability of buprenorphine for office-based prescribing may decrease interest in and use of clonidine for opioid detoxification.

Lofexidine

The optimal dosing of clonidine for opioid withdrawal may be limited by hypotensive effects because some patients cannot safely receive the recommended doses of clonidine without experiencing significant hypotension. The α_2-adrenergic agonist lofexidine, an analogue of clonidine, may be as effective as clonidine for opioid withdrawal while producing less hypotension and sedation. Three subtypes of the α_2-adrenergic receptor have been cloned: A, B, and C. Herman and O'Brien (1997) suggested that although clonidine has equal affinity for all three subtypes, lofexidine has a higher affinity for A and consequently has less hypotensive effects.

Although lofexidine was initially studied in the United States in the early 1980s for opioid withdrawal, its lack of adequate hypotensive effect (the major desired indication) led its manufacturer to discontinue efforts for FDA approval. Since that time, the drug has been approved in England for opioid withdrawal, and it is estimated that more than 70,000 patients have received it to date. The controlled studies published so far suggest that it is approximately as efficacious as clonidine with less hypotension and sedation (Carnwath and Hardman 1998; Kahn et al. 1997). Bearn et al. (1996) found that at a maximum dosage of 2 mg/day, lofexidine was approximately equivalent to methadone detoxification for overall symptom relief, although the lofexidine group had slightly greater self-rated withdrawal symptoms. Lofexidine is being studied by the National Institute on Drug Abuse's Medication Development Division for possible submission to the FDA for use in opioid withdrawal.

Utility of α_2-Adrenergic Agonists

A recent systematic review of α_2-adrenergic agonists in opioid detoxification (Gowing et al. 2002) reported the following: these drugs are associated with similar or slightly greater opioid withdrawal than a methadone taper, although withdrawal signs and symptoms resolved sooner with the α_2 agonists; completion of detoxification is also slightly higher with methadone, and there are more adverse effects with clonidine or lofexidine. This meta-analysis also confirmed that lofexidine produces less hypotension than clonidine but is otherwise similar. The utility of the α_2 agonists alone may not be as great as that of buprenorphine alone, but they will continue to be useful adjuncts in heroin detoxification.

Clonidine-Naltrexone Detoxification and Antagonist Induction

Although clonidine can be an effective alternative to methadone for opioid withdrawal, it does not shorten substantially the time required for withdrawal. Furthermore, the success rate in outpatient withdrawal leaves much to be desired. To solve these two problems, researchers first combined clonidine and naloxone and then subsequently clonidine and naltrexone

to provide a safe, effective, and more rapid withdrawal with quick induction of antagonist maintenance for patients detoxifying from either heroin or methadone. The method (Riordan and Kleber 1980) combines the rapid, precipitated displacement of opioids from endogenous opioid receptors and consequent severe withdrawal symptoms with aggressive use of clonidine prior to and following naltrexone to provide withdrawal symptom relief. For those symptoms not adequately controlled by clonidine, other medications are used, such as clonazepam or oxazepam for muscle spasms and insomnia and antiemetics for nausea and vomiting.

Vining et al. (1988) described the method in detail, and O'Connor et al. (1995) provided an update aimed at primary practitioners. Other authors (Gerra et al. 1995; Senft 1991) have also successfully used this procedure. The patient is premedicated with clonidine and oxazepam or clonazepam, and then the naltrexone is started—12.5 mg on day 1, 25 mg on day 2, and 50 mg on day 3. Clonidine is given every 4 hours as needed and oxazepam every 4–6 hours as needed. Table 23–5 describes the method in detail. In the O'Connor study ($N=68$), 94% of the patients were able to complete detoxification successfully and move on to the next phase of treatment. By 1 month later, however, there was no difference in treatment retention between the clonidine-alone and the clonidine-naltrexone groups. The biggest limitation of this method is the need to monitor patients for at least 8 hours on day 1 because of the potential severity of withdrawal that typically occurs after the first dose of naltrexone, including possible delirium, and because of the need for careful blood pressure monitoring during the detoxification procedure. Thus, trained staff and appropriate space are necessary for this procedure.

An even more rapid version of the clonidine-naltrexone method was developed for inpatient use (Brewer et al. 1988). Use of higher dosages of naltrexone and clonidine on day 1 as well as heavy doses of diazepam reduced the average detoxification time from approximately 3 days to a little more than 2 days. It has been hypothesized that because the dosage of clonidine needed decreases after the first day, even though the dosage of naltrexone is increasing, naltrexone is rapidly normalizing the number and sensitivity of opioid receptors and reversing the opioid-induced central noradrenergic hypersensitivity (Kleber et al. 1987).

Table 23–5. Clonidine-naltrexone rapid detoxification

Day	Time	Drug[a]
0		Use of heroin or methadone as usual
1	9:00 A.M.	Clonidine, 0.2–0.4 mg
		Oxazepam, 30–60 mg
	10:00–11:00 A.M.	Naltrexone, 12.5 mg
		Clonidine, 0.1–0.4 mg every 4–6 hours up to 1.2 mg
		Oxazepam, 30–60 mg every 4–6 hours as needed
	Patient in clinic until 5:00 P.M.	
2	9:00 A.M.	Clonidine, 0.1–0.2 mg (then every 4–6 hours as needed up to 1.2 mg)
		Oxazepam, 30–60 mg (then every 4–6 hours as needed)
	10:00 A.M.	Naltrexone, 25 mg
	Patient may leave 2 hours after naltrexone administration	
3	9:00 A.M.	Clonidine, 0.1–0.2 mg (then every 4–6 hours as needed, tapering total dosage by 0.2–0.4 mg/day)
		Oxazepam, 15–30 mg (then every 4–6 hours as needed)
	10:00 A.M.	Naltrexone, 50 mg
	Patient may leave 1 hour after naltrexone administration	
After day 3[b]		Clonidine, continue 0.1–0.2 mg every 4–6 hours as needed over next 2–3 days[b]
		Oxazepam, continue 15–30 mg every 4–6 hours as needed over next 2–3 days
		Naltrexone, 50 mg/day orally

[a]Clonidine, oxazepam, and naltrexone administered orally.
[b]Adjuvant medications as needed. For muscle cramps: nonsteroidal anti-inflammatory drugs (e.g., ibuprofen 600 mg orally every 6 hours or ketorolac 30 mg intramuscularly every 6 hours while on site); for nausea/vomiting: antiemetics (e.g., prochlorperazine 5 mg intramuscularly or 10 mg orally every 4–6 hours while on site or ondansetron 8 mg orally every 8 hours); for anxiety, insomnia, or muscle cramps: benzodiazepines (e.g., oxazepam 30–60 mg as needed, not to exceed 120 mg/day after day 1).

The clonidine-naltrexone detoxification and antagonist induction technique appears to be a safe, effective, and economical alternative to either gradual methadone taper or clonidine detoxification. Its advantages, in trained hands, include a dramatic reduction in the time necessary to complete detoxification, high completion rates (e.g., 55%–95%), and the ability to move rapidly to the next stage of rehabilitation with fewer lingering withdrawal symptoms. The shortened time frame also has economic advantages independent of the detoxification setting. Its disadvantages include generally poorer patient acceptance, compared with other techniques; the need for intensive monitoring by experienced staff, especially during the first day of treatment; and the need for sufficient space in outpatient settings to accommodate potentially very sick patients. More intensive variations on this approach, which may shorten the duration of symptoms, tend to require hospitalization and do not appear to offer any significant advantage. No significant evidence indicates that the technique is associated with any longer abstinence or retention on naltrexone. A recent review of 12 rapid clonidine-naltrexone studies found only 3 with outcome data after the acute detoxification (O'Connor and Kosten 1998).

Rapid Antagonist Induction Under General Anesthesia

The rate-limiting factor of the clonidine-naltrexone method is the ability to find medications that adequately relieve the symptoms of the precipitated withdrawal in the conscious patient. The approach to the clonidine-naltrexone procedure used initially by

Brewer et al. (1988) represented one of the earliest attempts to address this problem. The procedure was further shortened and advanced by carrying it out under general anesthesia (Loimer et al. 1989) (an ironic throwback to the hibernation therapy of 1941, in which the patient was kept asleep from 1 to 3 days). Since that time, the technique has been modified and improved (for review, see Brewer 1997). The current method commonly uses naltrexone, propofol anesthesia, the antiemetic ondansetron, the antidiarrheal octreotide, and clonidine and benzodiazepines for other withdrawal symptoms. Heavy sedation via midazolam has been used instead of anesthesia. Endoctracheal intubation is usually used with general anesthesia but not with heavy sedation. Occasionally, the opioid antagonist nalmefene or naloxone is used prior to or instead of naltrexone. Some clinicians do the procedure on an inpatient basis, others on an outpatient basis; some encourage naltrexone maintenance and/or therapy after detoxification, and others simply refer the patient to Narcotics Anonymous. What tends to be common is high price, usually ranging from $3,000 or more for the outpatient approach to more than $10,000 for the inpatient procedure. Claims of high rates of abstinence months after detoxification have been made, but no objective verification exists, and the samples are not representative of the heroin-dependent population as a whole.

Although some clinicians argue that these techniques are a magic bullet, others see them as exploitation of heroin-dependent individuals and the general public: use of a technique with potential serious morbidity and mortality to achieve opioid detoxification when safer (essentially no mortality) and less expensive methods may readily be used instead (Kleber 1998). Advocates of these approaches have argued that it is acceptable to expose individuals to significant risks, including mortality, given the potentially life-threatening consequences of their underlying illness. The high levels of patient interest in these approaches reflect the nearly universal desire for a pain-free detoxification procedure. Some practitioners of these approaches suggest that their patients are "detoxified in a day." Recent research with these procedures suggests that significant withdrawal symptoms persist for several days and up to a week after the procedure (Scherbaum et al. 1998). Follow-up data on withdrawal symptomatology suggest that withdrawal symptoms persist for days following the procedure (Collins et al., in press). Furthermore, intermediate- and long-term outcome data are limited. In a review of nine published anesthesia studies, only two had outcome data beyond 7 days (O'Connor and Kosten 1998). The authors deplored the lack of randomized design or control groups, the short-term outcomes studied, and the inadequate assessment of risks. In one recently published randomized trial of anesthesia-assisted antagonist induction/detoxification, the anesthesia technique offered no advantage in treatment outcomes at 3 months following detoxification (McGregor et al. 2002). Another randomized trial (Collins et al., in press) comparing anesthesia-assisted antagonist induction with buprenorphine-mediated naltrexone induction and clonidine-assisted antagonist induction found the highest level of withdrawal symptoms in the anesthesia group, with no benefit at 1 or 3 months following detoxification over the buprenorphine-mediated induction of naltrexone.

The morbidity of the procedure continues to raise the level of concern about its ultimate utility, even if one were to accept that the procedure might offer a means to attract highly resistant patients into treatment. Several studies suggest that the procedure produces profound increases in plasma catecholamines (Kienbaum et al. 1998, 2000). A series of six cases of individuals presenting to Philadelphia-area emergency departments cited complications of pulmonary edema, prolonged withdrawal, drug toxicity, rupture of varices, aspiration pneumonia, and death (Hamilton et al. 2002). In fact, at least seven deaths have occurred within 72 hours of the procedure (Gevirtz 2002). Obviously, more deaths could occur if the approach were extended to dual-dependent patients or those with cardiac or liver disease. More research on the procedure is emerging, but the early studies suggest that it will ultimately have no more than a limited place in the treatment armamentarium for opioid dependence.

Special Problems

Seizures

Opioid withdrawal or intoxication usually does not lead to seizures; however, seizures may occasionally occur with chronic use of meperidine or intoxication with propoxyphene. A seizure may signify undiagnosed sedative-hypnotic withdrawal, stimulant intoxication, another medical condition (e.g., head injury or epilepsy), or a faked or hysterical seizure. Because most addicted individuals are polydrug users, possible abuse of sedative-type drugs (including alcohol, barbiturates, and benzodiazepines) must be considered when providing treatment. If a patient is suspected of sedative-hypnotic dependence, a pentobarbital challenge will help clarify the picture (Smith and Wesson 1970; Wikler 1968). The challenge involves administration of pentobarbital 200 mg orally. An hour later, a nontolerant individual administered this dose will either be asleep or show coarse nystagmus, gross ataxia, a positive Romberg's sign, and dysarthria. If these signs are lacking, physical dependence on one or more sedative-hypnotic drugs should be presumed and treated correspondingly.

Mixed Addictions

Sedative-hypnotic (e.g., alcohol, benzodiazepines, barbiturates) dependence can lead to serious hazards, including seizures, toxic psychosis, hyperthermia, and even death. Withdrawal from stimulant-type drugs is much less of a physical hazard, although it can be associated with severe depression and even suicide. If sedative-hypnotic dependence is present, it may be preferable to maintain the patient on methadone or buprenorphine, withdraw the sedative gradually, and then withdraw the methadone.

Vomiting

Although vomiting can be a symptom of withdrawal, it can occur with no relation to the degree of physical abstinence and in spite of all kinds of support measures, including reintoxication with opioids. It usually can be handled by intramuscular injections of a drug such as trimethobenzamide or prochlorperazine. As noted earlier in this chapter, ondansetron, available in both oral and parenteral forms, also may be used and can be very effective in alleviating severe nausea and vomiting. Patients sometimes vomit so that they will receive repeat medication or intramuscular doses (especially when opioids may be given). Observation for 15–30 minutes after an opioid medication dose usually eliminates this behavior.

Intoxication

Dosing to opioid intoxication is not necessary to prevent withdrawal symptoms and can prolong and complicate the detoxification. If intoxication occurs, the next opioid dose should be decreased sufficiently to prevent it at the next medication administration. Smoking while intoxicated or otherwise impaired from the withdrawal-suppressing medications being used should not be permitted for obvious safety reasons, and when patients are ambulatory, they should be assisted so as to avoid injury.

Repetitive Withdrawal

Addicted individuals often have a characteristic withdrawal syndrome focused on a particular organ system. For one patient, withdrawal may involve the gastrointestinal system, commonly with significant abdominal cramping; for another, it may involve the musculoskeletal system, typically with aching in the bones or muscles. A supportive, reassuring, but firm approach usually helps patients with these symptoms. In the absence of psychosis, antipsychotic medications are rarely necessary.

Other Medical Conditions

Opioid withdrawal is usually not accompanied by high fevers, although low-grade temperature elevation can occur (rarely above 100.4°F or 38°C). Acute febrile illnesses may temporarily increase the severity of withdrawal symptoms, thus necessitating more methadone. When serious medical or surgical problems are present, withdrawal should be delayed or done very gradually to minimize the degree of stress. The patient should be brought to the point of tolerance, kept there for several days, and then slowly withdrawn. With certain illnesses (e.g., acute myocardial infarction, renal colic), the patient should be maintained on methadone until stable enough to permit withdrawal. The patient also should be evaluated carefully to determine whether longer-term agonist maintenance is preferable to detoxification. When withdrawal does take place, giving methadone three or four times per day instead of once or twice can minimize the patient's discomfort and stress.

Pregnancy

When pregnancy is complicated by heroin addiction, the patient and her physician are forced to choose from several relatively undesirable alternatives. The ideal outcome would be for the woman to abstain totally from drugs, licit and illicit, during the entire pregnancy. Unfortunately, this usually does not occur. On an outpatient drug-free regimen, many patients cycle in and out of heroin use, subjecting the fetus to periods of intoxication and withdrawal and a risk of spontaneous abortion, stillbirth, prematurity, and possible developmental anomalies. The drug effects are compounded by the patient's lifestyle, poor prenatal care, inadequate diet, and drug adulterants. Residential placement to ensure drug-free status is usually resisted, especially if other children are at home, or it may be difficult to find, even when desired. The optimal practical approach to the heroin-dependent pregnant woman avoids the risks of miscarriage and premature birth associated with detoxification, although some have suggested that carefully selected women may be safely withdrawn from opioids (Dashe et al. 1998).

No agonist or antagonist maintenance therapies have been approved by the FDA for use in the management of opioid dependence during pregnancy. Antagonist (naltrexone) maintenance is typically avoided because the prerequisite detoxification increases the risk of miscarriage and premature birth and because compliance problems increase the likelihood of cycling between dependence and withdrawal. Nevertheless, some authors have reported successful outcomes of naltrexone maintenance with small numbers of pregnant women (Hulse et al. 2001). Methadone maintenance has been used for many years and is generally accepted as the standard approach to the pregnant patient (Jarvis and Schnoll 1994). Dosing can be problematic because the increased metabolism of methadone during pregnancy can render the usual dosage inadequate and require an increased dosage rather than a decreased one (Jarvis et al. 1999). This can often be handled by split dosing during the day. The infant will be born physically dependent on methadone and will need to be withdrawn, but if prenatal care is adequate, no known birth defects are associated with prenatal methadone exposure. If withdrawal from methadone maintenance is necessary, it should occur during the second trimester at a rate no greater than 5 mg/week. During the first trimester, withdrawal may be especially deleterious to fetal development; during the third trimester, withdrawal may trigger premature labor.

A relatively recent alternative for the pregnant heroin-dependent patient is maintenance on buprenorphine. There is much less experience with buprenorphine than with methadone in pregnancy, but there have been various reports of treatment success with pregnant heroin users, with good fetal outcomes (Johnson et al. 2001; Schindler et al. 2003). Therefore, buprenorphine may be reasonably safe in pregnancy, with a risk profile comparable to that of methadone maintenance for pregnant heroin users. However, more research is needed to help establish the parameters of its use in pregnancy and to define its effects on newborns, particularly with respect to any potential need for treatment of opioid withdrawal in the newborn.

Experimental Medications

Some investigators have suggested the possibility of other detoxification agents, none of which has been researched thoroughly enough to be recommended at this time but for which there may be some efficacy in the future (Herman and O'Brien 1997). These agents include low-affinity, noncompetitive N-methyl-D-aspartate (NMDA) receptor antagonists such as dextromethorphan and memantine; serotonergic agents such as the serotonin type 1A (5-HT$_{1A}$) partial receptor agonist buspirone; and the neutral endopeptidase inhibitor acetorphan. One recent imperfectly controlled study suggested that massive doses of vitamin C (300 mg/kg), supplemented with vitamin E, reduced opioid withdrawal symptoms in most patients studied (Evangelou et al. 2000). We expect that advances in neuropharmacology and other areas of brain science will continue to provide promising candidate medications for use in opioid detoxification.

Alternative/Complementary Medicine

Despite considerable attention to alternative/complementary medicine approaches in other areas of medicine, opioid detoxification has received little of this attention, outside of the focus given over the last 30 years to acupuncture (discussed in the next section). A recent controlled study of the traditional Chinese medicine practice of qigong suggested that it produce better withdrawal relief than lofexidine (Li et al. 2002). In addition, some plant preparations, such as the West African hallucinogen ibogaine and the Vietnamese herbal mixture heanta, have developed enthusiastic followings, but they lack support in controlled studies of safety and efficacy. An ibogaine derivative, which may be safer than the original ibogaine plant extract, is currently under study. The Chinese herbal compound WeiniCom compared favorably with buprenorphine on measures of withdrawal severity and heroin craving (Hao and Zhao 2000). Of course, much more research is needed to assess what role, if any, complementary medicine may play in the future of opioid detoxification.

Acupuncture

Although acupuncture has been used for thousands of years in Chinese medicine to relieve pain, its use in the treatment of narcotic withdrawal is much more recent. Wen and Cheung (1973) reported more or less favorable results in 40 patients who received acupuncture with electrical stimulation. A review 5 years later (Whitehead 1978) concluded that because the studies used inadequate controls, they did not prove that the procedure worked.

Acupuncture consists of the use of thin needles inserted subcutaneously at points on the body believed to be related to the body functions that need to be stimulated. For detoxification, points on the external ear are usually used. Electroacupuncture involves applying small amounts of electricity to needles, which are inserted in those acupuncture points on the external ear believed to affect opioid withdrawal. Evidence from animal studies indicates that electroacupuncture is mediated through the endorphin system, and its effects can be blocked by the use of naloxone. A small laboratory study with heroin-dependent volunteers suggested that auricular acupuncture effects are mediated through the endogenous opioid system, and it noted that 20% of patients are resistant to acupuncture effects (Timofeev 1999).

Research studies of these approaches have several methodological problems, including high dropout rates, inconsistent placement of electrodes, inconsistent electrical parameters, and problems in blinding patients and staff. Thus, we are not as far along as we should be since Whitehead (1978) concluded that the existing evidence for acupuncture in opioid detoxification was inadequate.

Some studies or reviews have asserted that acupuncture and its closely related variants, including electroacupuncture, are effective, while others have asserted that they are not (Alling et al. 1990; Brewington et al. 1994; NCAHF 1991; Ter Riet et al. 1990; Ulett 1992). Most studies have been flawed by the lack of random assignment or the lack of a placebo control. One recent sham-controlled study of electroacupuncture suggested that both objective and subjective symptoms of opioid withdrawal were reduced with active treatment compared with the inactive control (Zhang et al. 2000). Although some studies suggest that acupuncture detoxification can be as effective as gradual methadone withdrawal in symptom alleviation, retention, and relapse rates, better controlled studies are needed to confirm this conclusion.

In general, programs that use acupuncture and its related variants tend to be enthusiastic about the results; published reviews tend to be more critical. Acupuncture may be useful for some patients, but many questions remain about its use. The optimal technique for detoxification remains to be clarified. It also remains to be determined how acupuncture compares with other detoxification methods described earlier in this chapter, especially methadone, buprenorphine, and clonidine detoxifications. For those who prefer not to use medications, clearly there is something appealing about a nonpharmaceutical technique. Additional questions include the following: What are the characteristics of individuals most likely to benefit from acupuncture during opioid withdrawal? For example, Washburn et al. (1993) suggested that heroin users with smaller habits stay in treatment longer than those with larger habits. What are the optimal circumstances and complementary approaches to be used during the procedure? As Brumbaugh (1993, p. 36) noted, "Acupuncture is not a panacea, and it loses much of its efficacy…when practiced in isolation from the more traditional Western modalities of counseling, pharmaceutical therapies, 12-Step Programs, and urine testing. It is best seen as an adjunct or a complement to these other forms." Acupuncture will become an important and standard part of opioid detoxification treatments only after well-controlled studies establish its utility and begin to answer some of these more specific questions.

Conclusion

For most opioid-dependent individuals, detoxification is only the first step in the long process of remaining abstinent from illicit drugs. Success is a function not only of how comfortable the procedure can be made but also of how well patients can be retained in both detoxification and longer-term treatment. Whatever method is chosen, appropriate psychosocial interventions and education must be available to prepare the patient for this next step. More information is needed as to the best combinations of withdrawal techniques and patient characteristics. The ideal detoxification method would be relatively rapid, inexpensive, comfortable, safe, and available on an outpatient basis; it would also increase the likelihood that patients seek longer-term help. Although none of the techniques reviewed in this chapter meets this ideal, significant progress has been made in improving the pharmacology of opioid withdrawal. The recent FDA approval of buprenorphine for opioid detoxification and maintenance therapy should make opioid dependence treatments much more widely available. The more urgent area for future research is in improving treatment retention at all phases of opioid dependence treatment. Compared with 60 years ago, the current detoxification methods are faster and more comfortable. In the future, there may be pharmacological approaches that decrease relapse by restoring the disordered neurochemistry associated with protracted withdrawal, cue-induced craving, and comorbid psychiatric illness.

References

Alling FA, Johnson BD, Elmoghazy E: Cranial electrostimulation (CES) use in the detoxification of opiate-dependent patients. J Subst Abuse Treat 7:173–180, 1990

American Psychiatric Association: Diagnostic and Statistical Manual of Mental Disorders, 4th Edition, Text Revision. Washington, DC, American Psychiatric Association, 2000

Bearn J, Gossop M, Strang J: Randomised double-blind comparison of lofexidine and methadone in the in-patient treatment of opiate withdrawal. Drug Alcohol Depend 43:87–91, 1996

Bochud Tornay C, Favrat B, Monnat M, et al: Ultra-rapid opiate detoxification using deep sedation and prior oral buprenorphine preparation: long-term results. Drug Alcohol Depend 69:283–288, 2003

Brewer C: Ultra-rapid, antagonist-precipitated opiate detoxification under general anaesthesia or sedation. Addict Biol 2:291–302, 1997

Brewer C, Rezae H, Bailey C: Opioid withdrawal and naltrexone induction in 48–72 hours with minimal drop-out, using a modification of the naltrexone-clonidine technique. Br J Psychiatry 153:340–343, 1988

Brewington V, Smith M, Lipton D: Acupuncture as a detoxification treatment: an analysis of controlled research. J Subst Abuse Treat 11:289–307, 1994

Brumbaugh AG: Acupuncture: new perspectives in chemical dependency treatment. J Subst Abuse Treat 10:35–43, 1993

Cami J, de Torres S, San L, et al: Efficacy of clonidine and of methadone in the rapid detoxification of patients dependent on heroin. Clin Pharmacol Ther 38:336–341, 1985

Carnwath T, Hardman J: Randomised double-blind comparison of lofexidine and clonidine in the out-patient treatment of opiate withdrawal. Drug Alcohol Depend 50:251–254, 1998

Charney DS, Sternberg DE, Kleber HD, et al: The clinical use of clonidine in abrupt withdrawal from methadone: effects on blood pressure and specific signs and symptoms. Arch Gen Psychiatry 38:1273–1277, 1981

Charney DS, Heninger GR, Kleber HD: The combined use of clonidine and naltrexone as a rapid, safe, and effective treatment of abrupt withdrawal from methadone. Am J Psychiatry 143:831–837, 1986

Collins ED, Whittington RA, Heitler NE, et al: Randomized trial of anesthesia-assisted heroin detoxification and naltrexone induction: an update. Drug Alcohol Depend (in press)

Dashe JS, Jackson GL, Olscher DA, et al: Opioid detoxification in pregnancy. Obstet Gynecol 92:854–858, 1998

Dawe S, Griffiths P, Gossop M, et al: Should opiate addicts be involved in controlling their own detoxification? A comparison of fixed versus negotiable schedules [published erratum appears in Br J Addict 87(8):1221, 1992]. Br J Addict 86:977–982, 1991

Evangelou A, Kalfakakou V, Georgakas P, et al: Ascorbic acid (vitamin C) effects on withdrawal syndrome of heroin abusers. In Vivo 14:363–366, 2000

Fudala PJ, Jaffe JH, Dax EM, et al: Use of buprenorphine in the treatment of opioid addiction, II: physiologic and behavioral effects of daily and alternate-day administration and abrupt withdrawal. Clin Pharmacol Ther 47:525–534, 1990

Gerra G, Marcato A, Caccavari R, et al: Clonidine and opiate receptor antagonists in the treatment of heroin addiction. J Subst Abuse Treat 12:35–41, 1995

Gevirtz C: Anesthesiological safety of ultrarapid detoxification. Paper presented at the 7th Stapleford International Conference on Addiction Management, Nijmegen, The Netherlands, 2002

Ghodse H, Myles J, Smith SE: Clonidine is not a useful adjunct to methadone gradual detoxification in opioid addiction. Br J Psychiatry 165:370–374, 1994

Gold MS, Redmond DE Jr, Kleber HD: Clonidine blocks acute opiate-withdrawal symptoms. Lancet 2(8090):599–602, 1978

Gossop M, Johns A, Green L: Opiate withdrawal: inpatient versus outpatient programmes and preferred versus random assignment to treatment. Br Med J 293(6539):103–104, 1986

Gossop M, Bradley B, Phillips GT: An investigation of withdrawal symptoms shown by opiate addicts during and subsequent to a 21-day in-patient methadone detoxification procedure. Addict Behav 12:1–6, 1987

Gowing LR, Farrell M, Ali RL, et al: Alpha2-adrenergic agonists in opioid withdrawal. Addiction 97:49–58, 2002

Gross A, Jacobs EA, Petry NM, et al: Limits to buprenorphine dosing: a comparison between quintuple and sextuple the maintenance dose every 5 days. Drug Alcohol Depend 64:111–116, 2001

Hamilton RJ, Olmedo RE, Shah S, et al: Complications of ultrarapid opioid detoxification with subcutaneous naltrexone pellets. Acad Emerg Med 9:63–68, 2002

Hao W, Zhao M: A comparative clinical study of the effect of WeiniCom, a Chinese herbal compound, on alleviation of withdrawal symptoms and craving for heroin in detoxification treatment. J Psychoactive Drugs 32:277–284, 2000

Heishman SJ, Stitzer ML, Bigelow GE, et al: Acute opioid physical dependence in postaddict humans: naloxone dose effects after brief morphine exposure. J Pharmacol Exp Ther 248:127–134, 1989

Herman BH, O'Brien CP: Clinical medications development for opiate addiction: focus on nonopioids and opioid antagonists for the amelioration of opiate withdrawal symptoms and relapse prevention. Seminars in Neuroscience 9:158–172, 1997

Hulse GK, O'Neill G, Pereira C, et al: Obstetric and neonatal outcomes associated with maternal naltrexone exposure. Aust N Z J Obstet Gynaecol 41:424–428, 2001

Jaffe JH, Martin WR: Narcotic analgesics and antagonists, in The Pharmacological Basis of Therapeutics. Edited by Goodman LS, Gilman A. New York, Macmillan, 1975, pp 245–324

Janiri L, Mannelli P, Persico AM, et al: Opiate detoxification of methadone maintenance patients using lefetamine, clonidine and buprenorphine. Drug Alcohol Depend 36:139–145, 1994

Jarvis MA, Schnoll SH: Methadone treatment during pregnancy. J Psychoactive Drugs 26:155–161, 1994

Jarvis MA, Wu-Pong S, Kniseley JS, et al: Alterations in methadone metabolism during late pregnancy. J Addict Dis 18:51–61, 1999

Jasinski DR, Pevnick JS, Griffith JD: Human pharmacology and abuse potential of the analgesic buprenorphine: a potential agent for treating narcotic addiction. Arch Gen Psychiatry 35:501–516, 1978

Jasinski DR, Johnson RE, Kocher TR: Clonidine in morphine withdrawal: differential effects on signs and symptoms. Arch Gen Psychiatry 42:1063–1066, 1985

Johnson RE, Jones HE, Jasinski DR, et al: Buprenorphine treatment of pregnant opioid-dependent women: maternal and neonatal outcomes. Drug Alcohol Depend 63:97–103, 2001

Kahn A, Mumford JP, Rogers GA, et al: Double-blind study of lofexidine and clonidine in the detoxification of opiate addicts in hospital. Drug Alcohol Depend 44:57–61, 1997

Kienbaum P, Thurauf N, Michel MC, et al: Profound increase in epinephrine concentration in plasma and cardiovascular stimulation after mu-opioid receptor blockade in opioid-addicted patients during barbiturate-induced anesthesia for acute detoxification [see comments]. Anesthesiology 88:1154–1161, 1998

Kienbaum P, Scherbaum N, Thurauf N, et al: Acute detoxification of opioid-addicted patients with naloxone during propofol or methohexital anesthesia: a comparison of withdrawal symptoms, neuroendocrine, metabolic, and cardiovascular patterns. Crit Care Med 28:969–976, 2000

Kleber HD: Detoxification from narcotics, in Substance Abuse: Clinical Issues and Perspectives. Edited by Lowinson JH, Ruiz P. Baltimore, MD, Williams & Wilkins, 1981, pp 317–339

Kleber HD: Outpatient detoxification from opiates. Primary Psychiatry 3:42–52, 1996

Kleber H: Ultrarapid opiate detoxification. Addiction 93:1629–1633, 1998

Kleber HD, Riordan CE, Rounsaville B, et al: Clonidine in outpatient detoxification from methadone maintenance. Arch Gen Psychiatry 42:391–394, 1985

Kleber HD, Topazian M, Gaspari J, et al: Clonidine and naltrexone in the outpatient treatment of heroin withdrawal. Am J Drug Alcohol Abuse 13:1–17, 1987

Kolb L, Himmelsbach CK: Clinical studies of drug addiction, III: a critical review of the withdrawal treatment with method of evaluating abstinence syndromes. Am J Psychiatry 94:759–799, 1938

Kosten TR, Krystal JH, Charney DS, et al: Opioid antagonist challenges in buprenorphine maintained patients. Drug Alcohol Depend 25:73–78, 1990

Kosten TR, Morgan C, Kleber HD: Treatment of heroin addicts using buprenorphine. Am J Drug Alcohol Abuse 17:119–128, 1991

Levin FR, Fischman MW, Connerney I, et al: A protocol to switch high-dose, methadone-maintained subjects to buprenorphine. Am J Addict 6:105–116, 1997

Li M, Chen K, Mo Z: Use of qigong therapy in the detoxification of heroin addicts. Altern Ther Health Med 8:50–54, 56–59, 2002

Lintzeris N, Bell J, Bammer G, et al: A randomized controlled trial of buprenorphine in the management of short-term ambulatory heroin withdrawal. Addiction 97:1395–1404, 2002

Loimer N, Schmid RW, Presslich O, et al: Continuous naloxone administration suppresses opiate withdrawal symptoms in human opiate addicts during detoxification treatment. J Psychiatr Res 23:81–86, 1989

Lopatko OV, White JM, Huber A, et al: Opioid effects and opioid withdrawal during a 24 h dosing interval in patients maintained on buprenorphine. Drug Alcohol Depend 69:317–322, 2003

Martin WR, Jasinski DR: Physiological parameters of morphine dependence in man: tolerance, early abstinence, protracted abstinence. J Psychiatr Res 7:9–17, 1969

McGregor C, Ali R, White JM, et al: A comparison of antagonist-precipitated withdrawal under anesthesia to standard inpatient withdrawal as a precursor to maintenance naltrexone treatment in heroin users: outcomes at 6 and 12 months. Drug Alcohol Depend 68:5–14, 2002

McLellan AT, Luborsky L, Cacciola J, et al: New data from the Addiction Severity Index: reliability and validity in three centers. J Nerv Ment Dis 173:412–423, 1985

Mello NK, Mendelson JH: Buprenorphine suppresses heroin use by heroin addicts. Science 207:657–659, 1980

Mendelson J, Jones RT, Welm S, et al: Buprenorphine and naloxone interactions in methadone maintenance patients. Biol Psychiatry 41:1095–1101, 1997

NCAHF: Acupuncture: the position paper of the National Council Against Health Fraud. Clin J Pain 7:162–166, 1991

O'Connor PG, Kosten TR: Rapid and ultrarapid opioid detoxification techniques. JAMA 279:229–234, 1998

O'Connor PG, Waugh ME, Carroll KM, et al: Primary care-based ambulatory opioid detoxification: the results of a clinical trial. J Gen Intern Med 10:255–260, 1995

O'Connor PG, Carroll KM, Shi JM, et al: Three methods of opioid detoxification in a primary care setting: a randomized trial. Ann Intern Med 127:526–530, 1997

Petry NM, Bickel WK, Badger GJ: A comparison of four buprenorphine dosing regimens in the treatment of opioid dependence. Clin Pharmacol Ther 66:306–314, 1999

Phillips GT, Gossop M, Bradley B: The influence of psychological factors on the opiate withdrawal syndrome. Br J Psychiatry 149:235–238, 1986

Pini LA, Sternieri E, Ferretti C: Dapiprazole compared with clonidine and a placebo in detoxification of opiate addicts. Int J Clin Pharmacol Res 11:99–105, 1991

Preston KL, Bigelow GE, Liebson IA: Buprenorphine and naloxone alone and in combination in opioid-dependent humans. Psychopharmacology (Berl) 94:484–490, 1988

Reynaud M, Petit G, Potard D, et al: Six deaths linked to concomitant use of buprenorphine and benzodiazepines. Addiction 93:1385–1392, 1998

Riordan CE, Kleber HD: Rapid opiate detoxification with clonidine and naloxone (letter). Lancet 1(8177):1079–1080, 1980

San L, Cami J, Peri JM, et al: Efficacy of clonidine, guanfacine and methadone in the rapid detoxification of heroin addicts: a controlled clinical trial. Br J Addict 85:141–147, 1990

Satel SL, Kosten, TR Schuckit MA, et al: Should protracted withdrawal from drugs be included in DSM-IV? Am J Psychiatry 150:695–704, 1993

Scherbaum N, Klein S, Kaube H, et al: Alternative strategies of opiate detoxification: evaluation of the so-called ultra-rapid detoxification. Pharmacopsychiatry 31:205–209, 1998

Schindler SD, Eder H, Ortner R, et al: Neonatal outcome following buprenorphine maintenance during conception and throughout pregnancy. Addiction 98:103–110, 2003

Senft RA: Experience with clonidine-naltrexone for rapid opiate detoxification. J Subst Abuse Treat 8:257–259, 1991

Smith DE, Wesson DR: A new method for treatment of barbiturate dependence. JAMA 213:294–295, 1970

Spencer L, Gregory M: Clonidine transdermal patches for use in outpatient opiate withdrawal. J Subst Abuse Treat 6:113–117, 1989

Strain EC, Preston KL, Liebson IA, et al: Acute effects of buprenorphine, hydromorphone and naloxone in methadone-maintained volunteers. J Pharmacol Exp Ther 261:985–993, 1992

Strain EC, Preston KL, Liebson IA, et al: Buprenorphine effects in methadone-maintained volunteers: effects at two hours after methadone. J Pharmacol Exp Ther 272:628–638, 1995

Strang J, Gossop M: Comparison of linear versus inverse exponential methadone reduction curves in the detoxification of opiate addicts. Addict Behav 15:541–547, 1990

Ter Riet G, Kleijnen J, Knipschild P: A meta-analysis of studies into the effect of acupuncture on addiction. Br J Gen Pract 40:379–382, 1990

Timofeev MF: Effects of acupuncture and an agonist of opiate receptors on heroin dependent patients. Am J Chin Med 27:143–148, 1999

Tracqui A, Kintz P, Ludes B: Buprenorphine-related deaths among drug addicts in France: a report on 20 fatalities. J Anal Toxicol 22:430–434, 1998

Ulett GA: Beyond Yin and Yang: How Acupuncture Really Works. St Louis, MO, Warren H Green, 1992

Vining E, Kosten TR, Kleber HD: Clinical utility of rapid clonidine-naltrexone detoxification for opioid abusers. Br J Addict 83:567–575, 1988

Walsh SL, June HL, Schuh KJ, et al: Effects of buprenorphine and methadone in methadone-maintained subjects. Psychopharmacology (Berl) 119:268–276, 1995

Washburn AM, Fullilove RE, Fullilove MT, et al: Acupuncture heroin detoxification: a single-blind clinical trial. J Subst Abuse Treat 10:345–351, 1993

Wen HL, Cheung SYC: Treatment of drug addiction by acupuncture and electrical stimulation. Am J Acupunct 1:71–75, 1973

Whitehead PC: Acupuncture in the treatment of addiction: a review and analysis. Int J Addict 13:1–16, 1978

Wikler A: Diagnosis and treatment of drug dependence of the barbiturate type. Am J Psychiatry 125:758–765, 1968

Zhang B, Luo F, Liu C: [Treatment of 121 heroin addicts with Han's acupoint nerve stimulator]. Zhongguo Zhong Xi Yi Jie He Za Zhi 20:593–595, 2000

Opioids

Maintenance Treatment

Richard Steven Schottenfeld, M.D.

Opioid dependence (i.e., dependence on opiate or opiate-like drugs) is a chronic and severe psychiatric disorder that is associated with substantial risk of mortality; medical and other psychiatric morbidity; and adverse social, vocational, familial, and legal consequences. As with other chronic and severe medical or psychiatric disorders, the goals of treatment are to prevent or reduce the adverse medical, psychiatric, and other consequences of the disorder and to improve the patient's functioning, quality of life, and overall well-being.

Since its development in the 1960s as a treatment for opioid dependence, opioid agonist maintenance treatment, initially with methadone and more recently with L-α-acetylmethadol (LAAM) or the partial μ agonist buprenorphine, has proven to be the most effective treatment for opioid dependence. This treatment greatly reduces the risk of mortality, morbidity, and other adverse consequences of the disorder. Methadone or other opioid agonist maintenance treatment refers to a comprehensive treatment approach that in-

cludes the continuing administration of opioid medications under medical supervision in combination with drug counseling, behavioral monitoring and intervention, and provision of other psychiatric, medical, and vocational services as clinically indicated. Although other treatments (e.g., medically supervised withdrawal followed by opioid antagonist maintenance treatment or long-term residential therapeutic community) are efficacious for some patients, the widespread patient appeal of opioid agonist maintenance treatment, high treatment retention, substantial reductions of illicit drug use and criminal activity, and improvement in medical, social, family, and vocational functioning during opioid agonist maintenance treatment combine to make it the most effective approach for individuals meeting eligibility requirements for it.

Nevertheless, the rationale for methadone or other opioid agonist maintenance treatment is often misunderstood; social and political opposition to methadone maintenance treatment limits its use in many regions of the world and within the United States; access to the treatment is often limited by inadequate treatment resources (lack of programs or treatment "slots") and reimbursement; and methadone or other opioid agonist maintenance treatment is often suboptimal and provided without adhering to research-based principles that are known to improve its efficacy.

In this chapter, I review the rationale for opioid agonist maintenance treatment and the clinical pharmacology, medication interactions, and adverse effects of methadone and LAAM; the research supporting the efficacy and effectiveness of opioid agonist maintenance treatment overall and the efficacy of specific components of treatment (dose, counseling, duration of treatment); special treatment issues (comorbid other substance use, psychiatric disorders, and medical disorders; pain management; pregnancy); federal rules governing opioid agonist maintenance treatment; and opioid agonist maintenance treatment in primary care clinics and physician offices.

The clinical pharmacology of buprenorphine, the third medication approved by the U.S. Food and Drug Administration (FDA) for opioid agonist maintenance treatment, is reviewed in Chapter 23, "Opioids: Detoxification," in this volume.

Opioid Dependence: Epidemiology and Natural History

Recent studies point to an increase in illicit opioid use and dependence in the United States during the past several years and indicate that an estimated 1 million adults are dependent on heroin or other opioids (Rhodes et al. 2001). Initiation of illicit opioid use most often begins in late adolescence and early adulthood and is generally preceded by use of cigarettes, alcohol, and other drugs. The latency period for the transition from occasional use to dependence is variable and may last only a few weeks to several years or more. Regional epidemics of dependence on various prescription opioids among high school students and young adults have been reported in recent years, and the availability of high-purity heroin, which may be used by nasal insufflation or smoking, also may have lowered the threshold for initial experimentation and attracted many new users (Bach and Lantos 1999). Although heroin was used primarily by injection until

the late 1980s in the United States, most patients addicted to heroin who are entering treatment in many regions of the country now report noninjection routes of administration (National Institute on Drug Abuse 1997). Although these other routes of administration reduce the risk of infectious diseases (e.g., human immunodeficiency virus [HIV], hepatitis, endocarditis), the risk of transition from noninjection to injection use is high (estimated 15% per year in one study [Neaigus 1998]), and the incidence of infectious diseases increases dramatically following transition to injection use. Drug overdose is also a significant risk with insufflation or smoking, although many users are not aware of this risk.

The transition from opioid use to dependence carries a dire prognosis, with a risk of dying of approximately 2% per year, and sustained remission is difficult to achieve. A little more than 30 years after admission to compulsory drug abuse treatment in California, nearly half of the 581 heroin-addicted men followed up in one cohort study had died (Hser et al. 2001). At the time of admission, most of these heroin-addicted men were in their 20s and 30s, and the results of this and other studies indicate that, in comparison to their peers, matched for age, gender, and socioeconomic status, the annual risk of dying for a heroin-addicted person is increased 6- to 20-fold. Most of the excess mortality is due to drug overdose, suicide, violence, accidents, infection, or chronic liver disease. Only 23% of the original cohort of California addicted men were not currently using illicit opiates 33 years after admission; the rest were currently using (9%), refused to provide a urine specimen for toxicology testing (4%), were in prison (6%), were not interviewed (10%), or were dead (49%). Notably, only about one out of six of those who were continuing to use 20 years after admission and about the same proportion of those who had been abstinent for less than 5 years at that time point were abstinent 10 years later. One-quarter of those who had been abstinent for more than 15 years at the 20-year follow-up also relapsed over the next 10 years. These findings point to the persistence of the disorder and the high risk of relapse even following long periods of remission. Less than 10% of the cohort participated in methadone maintenance treatment in any given year, but heroin use was reduced in those who participated in this treatment. As so vividly demonstrated in the results of this and other long-term follow-up studies (Vaillant 1973), following its onset, the course of heroin or other opioid dependence is chronic and persistent, marked by periods of abstinence that are often followed by relapse, and associated with a severe risk of death or disability.

Clinical Pharmacology of Methadone and LAAM

Methadone is a synthetic, long-acting, orally available opioid that acts primarily as a high-affinity agonist at μ and δ opiate receptors; methadone also acts as an N-methyl-D-aspartate (NMDA) antagonist (Gutstein and Akil 2001). Following oral administration, methadone is rapidly and nearly completely (85%–90%) absorbed in the intestine. Absorption can be delayed by reductions in gastric emptying, caused by food, by hypertonic sucrose solutions often used to dissolve methadone (in order to deter its injection), or by methadone itself. Peak plasma levels of methadone occur 2–6 hours after oral administration. Methadone is highly lipophilic, has a large volume of distribution, and accumulates in high concentrations in solid organs (liver, kidney, lungs, and brain) (Wolff et al. 1997).

Generally administered as a racemic mixture, R-methadone has substantially higher affinity and efficacy at μ and δ opioid receptors and lower protein binding in plasma compared with the S-enantiomer. Methadone undergoes N-demethylation to a highly unstable compound, which undergoes rapid and spontaneous cyclization and dehydration to the major inactive methadone metabolites. Methadone is metabolized primarily by cytochrome P450 (CYP) enzymes, predominantly through the CYP3A4 pathway but also involving CYP2C19, CYP2C9, and possibly also CYP2D6; methadone also inhibits CYP2D6 (Eap et al. 2001). Following oral administration, methadone and its metabolites are excreted in approximately equal amounts in urine, and urinary excretion accounts for about 50% of the dose.

The long plasma half-life of methadone (averaging 24 hours, with a range of 13–50 hours) following repeated daily dosing results in part from accumulation of methadone in organ systems, and achievement of steady-state plasma levels may take 5–10 days. Its long half-life permits once-a-day methadone dosing during maintenance treatment. During maintenance treatment, peak-to-trough plasma ratios generally range from 2:1 to 4:1 (Foster et al. 2001). Trough concentrations exceeding 200 ng/mL are usually sufficient to prevent withdrawal, although some studies suggest that an increased rate of decline, even with adequate trough levels, also may be associated with withdrawal symptoms (Dyer et al. 1999). Although clinically significant diurnal alterations in mood state are not generally observed or reported during methadone maintenance treatment, mood changes associated with changes in methadone plasma concentration have been observed following administration of a sensitive assessment measure, the Profile of Mood States, and these changes are more pronounced in patients who report experiencing withdrawal symptoms even while taking a stable methadone dose compared with patients who do not report withdrawal (Dyer et al. 2001).

LAAM, a methadone derivative also approved by the FDA for opioid agonist maintenance treatment, has a longer half-life than methadone (2 days) and is metabolized by cytochrome P450 enzymes (primarily CYP3A4) to two active metabolites, with half-lives of 2 days (nor-LAAM) and 4 days (dinor-LAAM) (Neff and Moody 2001). Like methadone, LAAM acts as a full agonist at opiate receptors and is absorbed from the gastrointestinal tract following oral administration, with initial effects appearing after 1–2 hours. Because LAAM is slowly metabolized to two active metabolites, which are somewhat more potent than LAAM, steady-state levels of LAAM and its active metabolites and its full effects are achieved after 1–3 weeks. Daily dosing can lead to excessive accumulation of active medication and metabolites, and Monday-Wednesday-Friday dosing is recommended. The longer period required to achieve a full maintenance dose is thought to be responsible for the greater early attrition from treatment found during induction onto LAAM compared with methadone. The abuse liability of LAAM is comparable to that of methadone, and, consequently, use of LAAM is restricted to approved narcotic treatment programs, which has diminished its appeal to patients.

Medication Interactions

Knowledge of possible interactions between opioid agonist medications used for maintenance treatment and other prescribed medications is essential to ensure the safety and efficacy of methadone dosing and dosing with other medications. Medication interactions with methadone have been more thoroughly evaluated than with buprenorphine or LAAM, and interaction effects with LAAM are complicated because its major metabolites are active.

Methadone metabolism may be increased substantially by concomitant administration of medications that induce cytochrome P450 hepatic enzymes (e.g., carbamazepine, phenytoin, rifampin, efavirenz, nevirapine, phenobarbital, and possibly risperidone), and initiation of treatment with any of these medications may lead to withdrawal symptoms in a methadone-maintained patient (Rainey 2002). Initiation of risperidone treatment during methadone maintenance also has been associated with precipitation of opioid withdrawal, possibly through induction of methadone metabolism, interference with methadone absorption, or a direct effect of risperidone on opioid receptors (Wines and Weiss 1999). Medications that inhibit cytochrome P450 enzymes also may cause inhibition of

methadone metabolism and symptoms associated with increased methadone plasma levels, including sedation, confusion, or possibly respiratory depression, as illustrated by a recent case report of a methadone-maintained woman treated with ciprofloxacin, a potent inhibitor of CYP1A2 and CYP3A4 (Herrlin et al. 2000). Fluoxetine and fluvoxamine, inhibitors of CYP2D6 and CYP1A2, respectively, and fluconazole cause delayed metabolism and increases in plasma methadone half-life (Begre et al. 2002). Methadone treatment also affects the metabolism of other medications and causes increased plasma levels of desipramine, amitriptyline, and zidovudine. Table 24–1 shows some of the reported and possible medication interactions with methadone.

Table 24–1. Medication interactions

May reduce plasma methadone	May increase plasma methadone	Methadone may increase plasma levels of	Methadone may decrease plasma levels of
Carbamazepine	Amiodarone	Amitriptyline	Didanosine
Efavirenz	Cimetidine	Desipramine	Stavudine
Nelfinavir	Ciprofloxacin	Zidovudine	
Phenytoin	Erythromycin		
Rifampin	Fluconazole		
Risperidone	Fluoxetine		
Ritonavir	Fluvoxamine		
St. John's wort	Saquinavir		

Methadone interactions with antiretroviral medications are of particular interest because of the high prevalence of HIV infection among injection drug users (Rainey 2002). Although protease inhibitors are potent inhibitors of CYP3A4, nelfinavir causes substantial decreases (40%) in plasma methadone, which can be associated with withdrawal symptoms, possibly as a result of inducing cytochrome P450 enzymes or increasing the free (unbound) fraction of methadone in plasma. Methadone inhibition of the glucuronidization of zidovudine increases the plasma concentrations of this medication and the potential for dose-related toxicity. Methadone-induced decreased gastrointestinal motility, however, leads to increased gastrointestinal degradation of stavudine and didanosine and significant decreases in plasma concentrations of these medications.

The effects of medication interactions are further complicated by the need to take into consideration the effects of medication discontinuation. For example, discontinuation of a medication that inhibits metha-

done metabolism, such as fluoxetine, can lead to increased methadone metabolism and the occurrence of withdrawal symptoms in an otherwise stable methadone-maintained patient.

Rationale for Opioid Agonist Substitution Treatment With Methadone, LAAM, or Buprenorphine

The main, planned, and desired pharmacological effects of methadone, LAAM, or buprenorphine when used for opioid agonist maintenance treatment are to prevent withdrawal and craving and to block or attenuate the euphoric or other rewarding effects of heroin or other illicit opioid use. Daily oral methadone dosages of 20–40 mg are generally sufficient to prevent or at least greatly attenuate opiate withdrawal symptoms. Because craving for opiates is one of the earliest and most powerful hallmarks of withdrawal, preventing withdrawal greatly reduces craving or the urge to use illicit opioids. Preventing withdrawal also eliminates the repeated negative reinforcement that occurs when heroin or other illicit opioids are self-administered to relieve withdrawal. Chronic administration of higher doses of methadone, LAAM, or buprenorphine may directly reduce craving (possibly by preventing more subtle manifestations of withdrawal) and induce tolerance to the effects of street doses of heroin and other illicit opioids, so that individuals maintained at sufficiently high doses experience little or no direct reinforcement from illicit opioid use.

Additional advantages of the medications used for opioid agonist maintenance treatment are that all of them substitute a less dangerous and less reinforcing method of administration (oral or sublingual) for more dangerous and reinforcing routes (injection, smoking, nasal insufflation) and that, unlike the fluctuations in mood and consciousness associated with repeated illicit administration of heroin and other short-acting opioids, administration of maintenance medications during maintenance treatment does not substantially alter mood or alertness throughout the day. Oral or sublingual routes of administration lead to a relatively slow rate of increase in plasma (and brain) levels and are thus less euphorigenic and inherently less reinforcing than routes associated with faster rates of increase. By preventing withdrawal, attenuating euphoric effects of illicit opioid use, reducing illicit opioid use, and stabilizing mood, opioid agonist substitution treatment also provides a stable medication platform facilitating provision of drug abuse counseling and other effective rehabilitation services.

Safety and Toxicity

Nearly 40 years of clinical experience with methadone maintenance treatment, involving hundreds of thousands of patients worldwide, has established the overall safety of methadone when used for opioid agonist maintenance treatment. When used for maintenance treatment, methadone has not been found to produce any long-term damage to heart, lung, kidney, liver, brain, or other organ systems (Kreek 2000). Heroin and other opioid dependence is associated with alter-

ations of hypothalamic-pituitary-adrenal axis and immune system functioning, whereas methadone maintenance treatment generally leads to normalization of most measures of hypothalamic-pituitary-adrenal axis and immune system functioning and overall improvement in health status. The most commonly reported adverse effects of methadone when used for maintenance treatment include constipation, which may be quite severe; sweating; and urinary retention.

Although generally quite safe, methadone can cause severe respiratory depression in individuals who are not tolerant to the methadone dose (Wolff 2002). This is particularly a problem with regard to accidental ingestion by children and use by nondependent opioid users who experiment with methadone or self-administer it. There are reports of apnea and coma in children following ingestion of 5 mg of methadone and of death following ingestion of 10 mg of methadone, although prompt treatment of overdose has led to complete recovery in children following ingestion of much higher doses. Because of its long elimination half-life and the possibility of delayed absorption, methadone overdose requires prolonged treatment. Death has been reported to occur more than 24 hours after ingestion (and several hours after discontinuation of naloxone treatment). Overdose deaths can also occur at the onset of methadone maintenance treatment if induction onto methadone occurs too rapidly. Methadone dosages in excess of 40–50 mg/day at the onset of methadone maintenance treatment may lead to overdose death even in individuals reporting large heroin habits but who are not fully tolerant to the full effects at both μ and Δ receptors of methadone. Fatalities may occur after several days of dosing if the methadone dose is started too high or increased too rapidly (Buster et al. 2002). The risk of methadone overdose is increased by concomitant use of medications interfering with methadone metabolism (e.g., medications that inhibit CYP3A4) or in individuals with reduced methadone metabolism due to genetic factors or liver disease.

Recent reports indicate an association between very high doses of methadone and cardiac conduction defects (prolonged QT interval) and torsades de pointes (Krantz et al. 2002), an association previously noted for LAAM. Because of its potential for prolonging the QT interval, LAAM should not be administered to patients with prolonged QT intervals or in conjunction with medications that can prolong the QT interval or are associated with an increased risk for cardiac arrhythmias (Deamer et al. 2001).

Effectiveness of Opioid Agonist Maintenance Treatment

The effectiveness of methadone and other opioid agonist maintenance treatments for reducing illicit drug use, reducing mortality and morbidity, and improving social, vocational, and legal functioning has been established in randomized controlled clinical trials and quasi-experimental and observational studies and has been validated in several recent meta-analyses. Mortality rates are reduced substantially during methadone maintenance treatment, although they remain somewhat higher than for the general population because of the impaired health of many patients at treatment entry (e.g., HIV infection, hepatitis C). The risk of new infection with HIV is substantially reduced in methadone-maintained patients compared with untreated heroin-addicted patients in the same geographic setting (Metzger et al. 1993). Criminal activity decreases during treatment and has been found to increase substantially among individuals discharged from treatment because of the closing of public methadone programs after financial cutbacks (Anglin et al. 1989). Follow-up data from the National Treatment Outcome Study confirm the findings of previous national studies of drug abuse treatment regarding the effectiveness of methadone maintenance treatment for reducing illicit drug use and criminal activity (Hubbard et al. 1997).

Most studies of the long-term effects of treatment are based on methadone maintenance, but shorter-term studies (generally lasting up to 6 months) suggest that the effectiveness of maintenance treatment with LAAM or buprenorphine is comparable to that of maintenance treatment with methadone. Early attrition from LAAM compared with methadone has been a problem in some studies (Clark et al. 2002), but in a recent study, maintenance with LAAM was associated with the greatest reductions in illicit opioid use compared with patients randomly assigned to comparable doses of methadone or buprenorphine (Johnson et al. 2000). In many studies, methadone compared with buprenorphine maintenance was associated with somewhat greater reductions in illicit opiate use, although sufficient doses of both methadone and buprenorphine are more efficacious than low maintenance doses of either medication. Advantages of buprenorphine compared with methadone, resulting in buprenorphine being classified as a Schedule III narcotic, whereas methadone is a Schedule II narcotic,

suggest that buprenorphine maintenance will have an important role in the treatment of opioid dependence.

Despite the overwhelming scientific evidence establishing the efficacy and effectiveness of opioid agonist maintenance treatment, misunderstanding of, prejudice toward, and political opposition to methadone treatment persist and continue to interfere with efforts to increase access to and availability of this treatment modality in the United States and elsewhere in the world. At present, only about 200,000 of the estimated 1 million heroin-dependent individuals in the United States are enrolled in opioid agonist maintenance treatment. When methadone maintenance treatment has been made widely available, free or at low cost, and publicized, 90% or more of the heroin-addicted population have been attracted into treatment (Hartgers et al. 1992). These findings indicate that the low "market penetration" of methadone maintenance treatment results from the lack of its availability in many geographic areas, the long waiting lists and costs of treatment even in areas where programs are available, and the continued stigma often associated with narcotic treatment program attendance.

Considerable program-to-program variability in how treatment is provided and in the effectiveness of agonist maintenance treatment (as measured by the prevalence of continued illicit drug use during treatment and other outcome measures) has drawn attention to identifying the key components of methadone maintenance treatment (e.g., dose, duration of treatment, counseling, program structure) and improving the quality of treatment programs (Ball and Ross 1991). The most recent national survey of methadone treatment practices found that substantial progress had been made in improving treatment practices compared with earlier surveys but still pointed to continuing problems with inadequate methadone doses in many programs (D'Aunno and Pollack 2002).

Methadone Dose and Treatment Duration

The efficacy and effectiveness of maintenance treatment with methadone, LAAM, and buprenorphine are dose dependent, and effective doses generally fall within a targeted range of 60–100 mg/day for methadone, 8–16 mg/day sublingually for buprenorphine, and 80–140 mg three times per week for LAAM. The optimal dose for a given patient, however, should be based on the patient's response to treatment.

Early observational studies pointed to the dose-dependent efficacy of methadone for maintenance treatment, and more recent randomized, double-blind clinical trials and experimental studies confirmed the earlier observations with regard to methadone and established the dose-dependent efficacy of buprenorphine and LAAM. Although daily methadone doses of 20–30 mg lead to greater retention in treatment compared with placebo doses, illicit opioid use is dose-dependently reduced at moderate (60–75 mg) daily doses and reduced even more at higher (100 mg) daily doses (Strain et al. 1993, 1999). In experimental studies, daily doses of 30 and 60 mg are sufficient to suppress most withdrawal symptoms for more than 48 hours, but full attenuation of the effects of heroin (up to 20 mg/70 kg) occurs only with a higher daily methadone dose (120 mg) (Donny et al. 2002). Increased craving for opiates has been observed 24 hours after a 25% reduction in the daily methadone dose, consistent with clinical observations and patient reports of withdrawal-related discomfort and increased risk for resumption of illicit opioid use following a missed daily methadone dose (Greenwald 2002). Clinically, patients who continue illicit opioid use at a given daily methadone dose often reduce or eliminate illicit opioid use when the daily methadone dose is increased gradually over several weeks to a sufficiently high dose. Several studies suggest that some poor responders to even relatively high methadone doses (e.g., 80–100 mg/day) have increased metabolism of methadone and suboptimal trough plasma methadone levels or increased rates of clearance; increasing the methadone dose to achieve trough levels greater than 200 ng/mL, or providing methadone in split doses to prevent trough levels from declining too rapidly or below this target, can help to reduce or eliminate continued illicit opiate use (Dyer et al. 2001).

Duration of treatment is also a critical factor, and premature discontinuation of methadone treatment leads to relapse. In a recent randomized clinical trial, tapering of methadone dose to zero over 60 days (methadone detoxification) after 4 months of methadone maintenance treatment led to accelerated attrition from treatment and significant increases in illicit opioid use, compared with a group assigned to continued methadone maintenance treatment (Sees et al. 2000). The risk of relapse following discontinuation of methadone maintenance remains high even for pa-

tients who have been maintained on methadone for prolonged periods and have made substantial changes in lifestyle and achieved stable recovery while receiving treatment. Because of the high risk of relapse and the very high risk of severe adverse consequences associated with relapse, many patients may benefit optimally from lifetime maintenance, and decisions about whether or when to discontinue methadone treatment for patients who are benefiting from it should always be made collaboratively and with the patient's fully informed and voluntary consent.

Taken together, the results of observational studies, experimental human laboratory studies, and randomized clinical trials are compelling: methadone maintenance dose-dependently decreases illicit opioid use, and the effectiveness of methadone maintenance treatment diminishes substantially when methadone doses are lowered or discontinued, even when patients can continue to receive enhanced psychosocial services.

Drug Counseling and Behavioral Components of Agonist Maintenance Treatment

As with many other medical or psychiatric disorders, the effectiveness of medication treatment can be greatly enhanced by combining medication administration with counseling aimed at promoting treatment adherence and lifestyle change. The seminal study establishing the treatment effects of counseling evaluated treatment outcomes for 92 patients randomly assigned to one of three levels of services (minimal counseling, standard drug counseling, or standard drug counseling plus enhanced vocational, legal, and medical services) (McLellan et al. 1993). All patients were maintained on identical standard daily methadone doses. The prevalence of continued illicit opioid use and of cocaine use was substantially higher among patients in the minimal counseling group, who received only brief contact with a counselor once per month, compared with patients in the standard counseling group, who received weekly or more frequent counseling until achieving sustained abstinence, or the enhanced services group. By the end of 12 weeks, 69% of the patients in the minimal counseling group had triggered the criteria for protective transfer (unremitting drug use, as evidenced by 8 consecutive weeks of illicit opiate or cocaine use or three emergency situations requiring immediate health care interventions), whereas 41% of those receiving standard counseling and 19% of those receiving enhanced services met the criteria. Although enhanced services led to the best outcomes overall, standard drug counseling was found to be the most cost-effective approach. Subsequent studies have found no overall advantage for requiring an intensive day treatment program at program entry compared with weekly drug counseling, and some patients (e.g., those with social anxiety) may benefit more from weekly individual drug counseling than from day treatment (Avants et al. 1998, 1999). A variety of different types of counseling approaches, including cognitive and behavioral treatment, the community reinforcement approach, 12-step facilitation counseling, and counseling combining the different approaches, can be effective, as long as they are performed consistently and with a high degree of competence. In addition to the specific counseling provided, behavioral monitoring (e.g., urine toxicology testing) during treatment and consistent behavioral responses to patient's behavior (e.g., providing take-home methadone to patients who become abstinent or increasing the frequency and intensity of required counseling for patients with continued illicit drug use) contributes greatly to improved treatment outcomes.

Co-occurring Psychiatric Disorders

The prevalence of co-occurring substance use and other psychiatric disorders among opiate-dependent individuals entering methadone maintenance treatment greatly exceeds the prevalence found in the general population, even controlling for age, gender, socioeconomic status, and other factors, as has consistently been shown in studies conducted over the past 20 years in several different geographic areas (Brooner et al. 1997). Left untreated, many of these disorders are associated with an adverse prognosis and an overall poorer response to methadone maintenance treatment. Thus, careful psychiatric assessment of patients entering methadone or other agonist maintenance treatment and early institution of treatment interventions for co-occurring disorders are essential.

A high prevalence of co-occurring alcohol abuse or dependence was noted in early studies of methadone-

maintained patients, and several studies suggested that treatment with disulfiram (after detoxification, if necessary), with disulfiram administration supervised at the time of methadone ingestion, led to improvement of alcohol dependence, illicit drug use, and social functioning. Marijuana use is also very common among opioid agonist–maintained patients, but the clinical significance of marijuana use in this population is a matter of some controversy. Some studies suggest that marijuana use is not associated with other illicit drug use during opioid agonist maintenance treatment, but marijuana use still may interfere with full participation in treatment and rehabilitation (Nirenberg et al. 1996; Saxon et al. 1993).

Beginning in the early 1980s, cocaine abuse and dependence became epidemic among opioid-dependent individuals. Although the prevalence of cocaine abuse and dependence has declined substantially in the general population since then, these problems have remained endemic among opioid-dependent individuals. The reported prevalence of cocaine abuse or dependence among new admissions to methadone treatment ranges from 15% to 40% or more in the United States. Although the prevalence of frequent cocaine use decreases substantially during opioid agonist maintenance treatment (from 36% at treatment entry to 22% after 1 year in the Treatment Outcome Prospective Study; Fairbank et al. 1993), continued cocaine abuse is associated with continued illicit opiate use, injection drug use, increased risk of HIV and other infectious diseases, and criminal activity.

Promising treatment interventions for cocaine abuse during opioid agonist maintenance treatment include behavioral treatments, such as contingency management, in which vouchers with a monetary value are used to reward cocaine-free urine tests. Several studies suggest that supervised administration of disulfiram also reduces cocaine use during methadone or buprenorphine maintenance treatment (George et al. 2000; Petrakis et al. 2000), independent of its effects on reducing alcohol use, but this is not an FDA-approved indication for disulfiram.

Benzodiazepine abuse and dependence are also a problem for a high proportion (generally comparable to the prevalence of cocaine abuse) of opioid agonist–maintained individuals. As with concurrent cocaine abuse and dependence, benzodiazepine abuse and dependence are associated with injection drug use, continued heroin or other illicit drug use, increased risk of infection, and continued involvement in drug subcultures (Darke et al. 1993). Benzodiazepine use during agonist maintenance treatment poses a difficult challenge for psychiatrists and treatment programs because many patients experience anxiety disorders that could be treated with benzodiazepines, but benzodiazepines are frequently misused by opioid agonist–maintained patients (Spiga et al. 2001). Approximately one-third of the benzodiazepine-using patients in one study reported taking higher benzodiazepine doses than prescribed, and many took very high doses around the time of ingesting their daily methadone to boost the methadone effects (Stitzer et al. 1981). Gradual tapering and then discontinuation of benzodiazepines may be possible on an ambulatory basis, but many patients require inpatient treatment to complete detoxification successfully.

Mood disorders, anxiety disorders, and personality disorders, which are also considerably more prevalent among opioid agonist–maintained patients than in the general population, also may adversely affect response to agonist maintenance treatment. Treatment of current depression, found in approximately 15%–25% of those entering treatment, leads to improvements in mood and other depression outcome measures and also to reductions in illicit drug use (Nunes et al. 1998). Treatment of anxiety disorders in agonist-maintained patients is complicated by the high abuse liability of benzodiazepines in this population. Cognitive and behavioral treatments for anxiety disorders either alone or, when indicated, in combination with medications with little or no abuse liability (e.g., buspirone, citalopram) can be beneficial for patients. Antisocial personality disorder, found in approximately 25% of patients, has in some but not all studies been associated with a relatively poor prognosis (Alterman et al. 1996).

Co-occurring Medical Disorders and Provision of Medical Care

Patients receiving opioid agonist maintenance treatment may experience health problems associated with opioid dependence (e.g., acquired immunodeficiency syndrome [AIDS], hepatitis B or C, tuberculosis) or common in the general population (e.g., hypertension, diabetes, heart and lung disease), and the stabilizing effects of maintenance treatment on patients' overall functioning facilitate implementation of effective medical treatment for these health problems and preventive health services. A study conducted by the Centers for Disease Control and Prevention (CDC) among 1,717 injection drug users entering treatment in six cities in the United States found that 50%–81% had evidence of hepatitis B, 66%–93% had hepatitis C, and infection with HIV ranged from 3% to 5% in cities in the Midwest and West to 28%–29% in the Northeast (Murrill et al. 2002). The prevalence of infection with hepatitis B, hepatitis C, or HIV was significantly higher for older injection drug users than for younger users. With the advent of effective treatments for HIV and hepatitis C, it is essential to screen patients for these conditions at admission and at regular intervals during opioid agonist maintenance treatment and to refer patients with these disorders for treatment.

Coordination of addiction treatment and medical treatments can improve medication adherence, adherence to medical treatment recommendations, and the response to medical treatment. Interactions between opioid agonist maintenance medications and medications to treat medical conditions may necessitate dose adjustments or consideration of alternative medication treatments. Other preventive health services that benefit patients include immunizations (e.g., for hepatitis B, for antibody- and antigen-negative patients who are at risk for infection; for tetanus; and for pneumococcal pneumonia) and testing for tuberculosis and syphilis and treatment for those with evidence of infection. Adherence to medical treatment, such as prophylactic isoniazid treatment, can also be improved through directly observed treatment at the time of methadone dispensing.

Because of the extremely high prevalence of cigarette smoking among opioid-dependent individuals, health problems associated with cigarette smoking (e.g., emphysema, cancer, cardiovascular disease) are common among opioid agonist–maintained patients, and smoking cessation interventions may lead to considerable health benefits.

Pain Management During Opioid Agonist Maintenance Treatment

Considering the prevalence of medical conditions associated with chronic pain in opioid agonist–maintained patients, pain management is an important clinical issue. Because methadone is used for the treatment of chronic pain, some physicians mistakenly assume that methadone-maintained patients do not require analgesic medications in addition to their daily methadone dose to treat painful conditions. To the contrary, methadone-maintained patients develop tolerance to the analgesic effects of their daily dose and may require even higher doses or more frequent administration of opioid analgesic medications to ameliorate pain. Several recent studies documented an increased sensitivity to pain among methadone-maintained patients (Compton et al. 2001). When opioid analgesics are required, it is important to use only medications that act as full (rather than partial) agonists at opioid receptors; administration of a partial agonist (e.g., pentazocine) may precipitate withdrawal in a methadone-maintained patient.

Pregnancy and Opioid Dependence

Opioid dependence during pregnancy has adverse health effects on the pregnant woman, fetus, and neonate, resulting from a combination of direct drug effects, withdrawal, infections associated with injection drug use and addiction, and the detrimental effect of addiction on nutrition and the possible exposure to violence. Opiate withdrawal during pregnancy, especially when it occurs without medical treatment or supervision, causes significant fetal stress and is associated with spontaneous abortion and fetal demise (Archie 1998). Early studies found that methadone maintenance treatment led to substantial reductions in opiate use and improvements in nutrition, health status, and participation in prenatal care for heroin-dependent pregnant women and also to improved fetal growth and perinatal outcomes in their offspring. These findings led to the recommendation to provide comprehensive methadone treatment to heroin-dependent pregnant women, with services including prenatal and obstetrical treatment, nutritional supplementation, and counseling in addition to methadone maintenance medications.

Determination of the optimal methadone dose during pregnancy requires careful balancing between the risks of continued illicit opiate use, if the methadone dose is too low, and the risks of neonatal withdrawal associated with higher methadone doses. Opiate dependence and opioid agonist maintenance treatment during pregnancy are both associated with a risk of neonatal withdrawal, and higher dosages of methadone (greater than 40 mg/day) are associated with the greatest risk, although withdrawal has been reported in neonates whose mothers received considerably lower daily doses. Higher doses or split dosing may be needed during pregnancy because of the increased volume of distribution and increased methadone metabolism associated with pregnancy, which might otherwise increase the possible occurrence of withdrawal symptoms and the possibility of relapse to illicit opioid use.

In recent years, some experts have called for a reappraisal of the role of methadone maintenance treatment during pregnancy (Brown et al. 1998). High rates of continued illicit opioid use and concurrent other illicit or harmful substance use (including cocaine, benzodiazepines, marijuana, cigarettes, and alcohol) during methadone maintenance treatment in pregnant women have reduced some of the beneficial effects of methadone maintenance treatment during pregnancy on fetal growth and perinatal outcome. Additionally, methadone maintenance treatment is not available even for pregnant women in some areas of the United States and elsewhere. Finally, some opioid-dependent pregnant women may refuse methadone maintenance treatment or may request medical withdrawal. Some studies suggest that opiate detoxification can be performed safely during pregnancy under careful medical supervision (Dashe et al. 1998). Based on earlier studies suggesting that the risk of miscarriage or fetal demise is highest when withdrawal occurs during the first or third trimester, withdrawal during the second trimester is often advised when medical withdrawal is warranted. Of course, withdrawal during pregnancy reduces the likelihood of neonatal abstinence and other perinatal complications only if the pregnant woman remains abstinent following completion of withdrawal and adheres to other medical and nutritional recommendations.

Federal Rules Governing Opioid Agonist Maintenance Treatment

Many aspects of opioid agonist maintenance treatment, including patient eligibility criteria, medications that can be used for opioid agonist maintenance treatment, medication dispensing, and program guidelines, are tightly regulated by federal and state rules and guidelines. The regulations are designed to ensure appropriate use of this treatment modality, maintain effectiveness by encouraging optimal treatment and program structure, and limit diversion of prescribed medications to illicit use. Recent revisions in federal regulations (42 CFR part 8) regarding maintenance treatment with methadone or LAAM have introduced quality assurance monitoring and program certification requirements and also have made changes in the provisions for take-home medications. The new regulations define the required administrative and organizational structure of the program, including the need for a medical director, and require the availability of counseling and medical services and referral for other service needs. Eligibility for maintenance treatment with methadone or LAAM generally remains restricted to individuals age 18 or older who have been dependent on opioids for a minimum of 1 year before admission. The 1-year history of dependence may be waived for pregnant or previously treated patients or following prison release. Individuals younger than 18 may be admitted if they have a history of repeated treatment failure (two or more documented attempts at short-term detoxification or drug-free treatment within past 12 months); parent or guardian consent is required for individuals younger than 18. Depending on their response to treatment, patients may receive up to a 6-day supply of take-home medications by the end of the first year in treatment, up to a 2-week supply after 1 year in treatment, and a maximum of a 1-month supply after 2 years in treatment.

A recent amendment to the Controlled Substances Act (Drug Addiction Treatment Act of 2000) enables qualified physicians meeting defined training and certification criteria to prescribe office-based opioid agonist detoxification or maintenance treatment using Schedule III, IV, or V medications that have been approved for these indications by the FDA. In October 2002, buprenorphine became the first Schedule III narcotic to be approved for these indications by the FDA (Drug Enforcement Administration, 21 CFR part 1308) and is now available through office-based prescription by physicians. The current regulations governing narcotic treatment programs also permit office-based physicians to become part of the medical staff of a narcotic treatment program, obtain a license as a satellite medication dispensing unit, and thereby provide a form of office-based prescription of methadone

maintenance treatment. Individual physicians also may obtain a special narcotic treatment program license, but the requirements for obtaining the license and operating as a narcotic treatment program are considered too cumbersome for most physicians to make use of this mechanism.

Office-Based Opioid Agonist Maintenance Treatment

Currently, opioid agonist maintenance treatment in the United States is provided almost entirely to patients enrolled in licensed narcotic treatment programs, whereas physician's-office-based treatment is widely available in Canada, England, France, and other countries. Despite the laudable goals of restricting opioid agonist maintenance treatment to specially licensed narcotic treatment programs (e.g., facilitating quality improvement goals and adherence to patient eligibility criteria and decreasing the likelihood of diversion of prescribed opioid agonist medications to illicit use), the restriction contributes to the lack of availability and difficulties in gaining access to this treatment. Recent studies suggest that some opioid-dependent individuals refrain from enrolling in narcotic treatment programs because of concerns about being recognized by others in the program and identified as an addicted person and the possibility that this might jeopardize their employment, family, or social situation. Additionally, some patients who have achieved sustained recovery from illicit drug use during opioid agonist maintenance treatment indicate a strong preference for "medical maintenance" by an office-based physician in order to move away from continuing contact in clinics with many active drug users, to reduce the perceived stigma of continuing attendance in a narcotic treatment program, and to gain greater flexibility in prescribing and dispensing procedures (Fiellin et al. 2001).

The effectiveness of medical maintenance for stable methadone-maintained patients has been evaluated in several studies, and many patients who have been abstinent from illicit drugs for prolonged periods are able to make the transition to medical maintenance successfully (Fiellin et al. 2001; King et al. 2002). In one recent study that used hair toxicology testing, a surprisingly high prevalence of previously undetected, recent illicit drug use was found among patients meeting clinical criteria for medical maintenance (Fiellin et al. 2001). Patients with recent illicit drug use were substantially more likely than documented abstinent patients to use illicit drugs in the following 6 months, but the likelihood of illicit drug use did not differ between patients randomly assigned to medical maintenance in a physician's office and patients receiving continued treatment in the narcotic treatment program.

Qualified physicians who obtain special Drug Enforcement Administration registrations can now provide office-based buprenorphine maintenance treatment for new admissions to maintenance treatment, but relatively few studies have evaluated this setting and approach in the United States. Initial, small pilot studies of buprenorphine maintenance in a primary care clinic suggest the feasibility and potential efficacy of this approach. Adherence to buprenorphine was a problem for many patients, however, and adherence is associated with reductions in illicit drug use and retention in treatment. As we enter an era of expanded access to opioid agonist maintenance treatment and approval of new medications, settings, and dispensing options for this treatment, it will be essential to evaluate the counseling requirements and the treatment protocols and treatment algorithms that lead to optimal outcomes for patients.

References

Alterman AI, Rutherford MJ, Cacciola JS, et al: Response to methadone maintenance and counseling in antisocial patients with and without major depression. J Nerv Ment Dis 184:695–702, 1996

Anglin MD, Speckart GR, Booth MW, et al: Consequences and costs of shutting off methadone. Addict Behav 14:307–326, 1989

Archie C: Methadone in the management of narcotic addiction in pregnancy. Obstet Gynecol 10:435–440, 1998

Avants SK, Margolin A, Kosten TR, et al: When is less treatment better? The role of social anxiety in matching methadone patients to psychosocial treatments. J Consult Clin Psychol 66:924–931, 1998

Avants SK, Margolin A, Sindelar JL, et al: Day treatment versus enhanced standard methadone services for opioid-dependent patients: a comparison of clinical efficacy and cost. Am J Psychiatry 156:27–33, 1999

Bach PB, Lantos J: Methadone dosing, heroin affordability, and the severity of addiction. Am J Public Health 89:662–665, 1999

Ball JC, Ross A: The Effectiveness of Methadone Maintenance Treatment. New York, Springer-Verlag, 1991

Begre S, von Bardeleben U, Ladewig D, et al: Paroxetine increases steady-state concentrations of (R)-methadone in CYP2D6 extensive but not poor metabolizers. J Clin Psychopharmacol 22:211–215, 2002

Brooner RK, King VL, Kidorf M, et al: Psychiatric and substance use comorbidity among treatment-seeking opioid abusers. Arch Gen Psychiatry 54:71–80, 1997

Brown HL, Britton KA, Mahaffey D, et al: Methadone maintenance in pregnancy: a reappraisal. Am J Obstet Gynecol 179:459–463, 1998

Buster MC, van Brussel GH, van den Brink W: An increase in overdose mortality during the first 2 weeks after entering or re-entering methadone treatment in Amsterdam. Addiction 97:993–1001, 2002

Clark N, Lintzeris N, Gijsbers A, et al: LAAM maintenance vs methadone maintenance for heroin dependence. Cochrane Database Syst Rev 2:CD002210, 2002

Compton P, Charuvastra VC, Ling W: Pain intolerance in opioid-maintained former opiate addicts: effect of long-acting maintenance agent. Drug Alcohol Depend 63:139–146, 2001

Darke S, Swift W, Hall W, et al: Drug use, HIV risk-taking and psychosocial correlates of benzodiazepine use among methadone maintenance clients. Drug Alcohol Depend 34:67–70, 1993

Dashe JS, Jackson GL, Olscher DA, et al: Opioid detoxification in pregnancy. Obstet Gynecol 92:854–858, 1998

D'Aunno T, Pollack HA: Changes in methadone treatment practices: results from a national panel study, 1988–2000. JAMA 288:850–856, 2002

Deamer RL, Wilson DR, Clark DS, et al: Torsades de pointes associated with high dose levomethadyl acetate (ORLAAM). J Addict Dis 20:7–14, 2001

Donny EC, Walsh SL, Bigelow GE, et al: High-dose methadone produces superior opioid blockade and comparable withdrawal suppression to lower doses in opioid-dependent humans. Psychopharmacology 161:202–212, 2002

Drug Addiction Treatment Act of 2000, Pub. L. No. 106-310 (October 17, 2000)

Drug Enforcement Administration, 21 CFR part 1308. Schedules of Controlled Substances: Rescheduling of Buprenorphine From Schedule V to Schedule III (2002). Federal Reporter, October 7, 2002, Vol. 67, No. 194, pp 62354–62370

Dyer KR, Foster DJ, White JM, et al: Steady-state pharmacokinetics and pharmacodynamics in methadone maintenance patients: comparison of those who do and do not experience withdrawal and concentration-effect relationships. Clin Pharmacol Ther 65:685–694, 1999

Dyer KR, White JM, Foster DJ, et al: The relationship between mood state and plasma methadone concentration in maintenance patients. J Clin Psychopharmacol 21:78–84, 2001

Eap CB, Broly F, Mino A, et al: Cytochrome P450 2D6 genotype and methadone steady-state concentrations. J Clin Psychopharmacol 21:229–234, 2001

Fairbank JA, Dunteman GH, Condelli WS: Do methadone patients substitute other drugs for heroin? Predicting substance use at 1-year follow-up. Am J Drug Alcohol Abuse 19:465–474, 1993

Fiellin DA, O'Connor PG, Chawarski M, et al: Methadone maintenance in primary care: a randomized controlled trial. JAMA 286:1724–1731, 2001

Foster DJ, Somogyi AA, Dyer KR, et al: Steady-state pharmacokinetics of (R)- and (S)-methadone in methadone maintenance patients. Br J Clin Pharmacol 50:427–440, 2001

George TP, Chawarski MC, Pakes J, et al: Disulfiram versus placebo for cocaine dependence in buprenorphine-maintained subjects: a preliminary trial. Biol Psychiatry 47:1080–1086, 2000

Greenwald MK: Heroin craving and drug use in opioid-maintained volunteers: effects of methadone dose variations. Exp Clin Psychopharmacol 10:39–46, 2002

Gutstein HB, Akil H: Opioid analgesics, in Goodman and Gilman's The Pharmacological Basis of Therapeutics. Edited by Hardman JG, Limbird LL. New York, McGraw-Hill, 2001, pp 569–619

Hartgers C, van den Hoek A, Krijnen P, et al: HIV prevalence and risk behavior among injecting drug users who participate in "low-threshold" methadone programs in Amsterdam. Am J Public Health 82:547–551, 1992

Herrlin K, Segerdahl M, Gustafsson LL, et al: Methadone, ciprofloxacin, and adverse drug reactions. Lancet 356 (9247):2069–2070, 2000

Hser YI, Hoffman V, Grella CE, et al: A 33-year follow-up of narcotics addicts. Arch Gen Psychiatry 58:503–508, 2001

Hubbard RL, Craddock SG, Flynn PM, et al: Overview of 1-year follow-up outcomes in Drug Abuse Treatment Outcome Study (DATOS). Psychol Addict Behav 11:261–278, 1997

Johnson RE, Chutuape MA, Strain EC, et al: A comparison of levomethadyl acetate, buprenorphine, and methadone for opioid dependence. N Engl J Med 343:1290–1297, 2000

King VL, Stoller KB, Hayes M, et al: A multicenter randomized evaluation of methadone medical maintenance. Drug Alcohol Depend 65:137–148, 2002

Krantz MJ, Lewkowiez L, Hays H, et al: Torsade de pointes associated with very-high-dose methadone. Ann Intern Med 137:501–504, 2002

Kreek MJ: Methadone-related opioid agonist pharmacotherapy for heroin addiction: history, recent molecular and neurochemical research and future in mainstream medicine. Ann N Y Acad Sci 909:186–216, 2000

McLellan AT, Arndt IO, Metzger DS, et al: The effects of psychosocial services in substance abuse treatment. JAMA 269:1953–1959, 1993

Metzger DS, Woody GE, McLellan AT, et al: Human immunodeficiency virus seroconversion among intravenous drug users in- and out-of-treatment: an 18-month prospective follow-up. J Acquir Immune Defic Syndr 6:1049–1056, 1993

Murrill CS, Weeks H, Castrucci BC, et al: Age-specific seroprevalence of HIV, hepatitis B virus, and hepatitis C virus infection among injection drug users admitted to drug treatment in 6 US cities. Am J Public Health 92:385–387, 2002

National Institute on Drug Abuse: Research Report: Heroin Abuse and Addiction. Rockville, MD, National Institute on Drug Abuse, 1997

Neaigus A: Trends in the noninjected use of heroin and factors associated with the transition to injecting, in Heroin in the Age of Crack Cocaine. Edited by Inciardi JA, Harrison LD. Thousand Oaks, CA, Sage Publications, 1998, pp 131–159

Neff JA, Moody DE: Differential N-demethylation of l-alpha-acetylmethadol (LAAM) and norLAAM by cytochrome P450s 2B6, 2C18, and 3A4. Biochem Biophys Res Commun 284:751–756, 2001

Nirenberg TD, Cellucci T, Liepman MR, et al: Cannabis versus other illicit drug use among methadone maintenance patients. Psychol Addict Behav 10:222–227, 1996

Nunes EV, Quitkin FM, Donovan SJ, et al: Imipramine treatment of opiate-dependent patients with depressive disorders: a placebo-controlled trial. Arch Gen Psychiatry 55:153–160, 1998

Petrakis IL, Carroll KM, Nich C, et al: Disulfiram treatment for cocaine dependence in methadone-maintained opioid addicts. Addiction 95:219–228, 2000

Rainey PM: HIV drug interactions: the good, the bad, and the other. Ther Drug Monit 24:26–31, 2002

Rhodes W, Layne M, Bruen AM, et al: What America's Users Spend on Illegal Drugs 1988–2000. Washington, DC, Office of National Drug Control Policy, December 2001

Saxon AJ, Calsyn DA, Greenberg D, et al: Urine screening for marijuana among methadone-maintained patients. Am J Addict 2:207–211, 1993

Sees KL, Delucchi KL, Masson C, et al: Methadone maintenance vs 180-day psychosocially enriched detoxification for treatment of opioid dependence: a randomized controlled trial. JAMA 283:1303–1310, 2000

Spiga R, Huang DB, Meisch RA, et al: Human methadone self-administration: effects of diazepam pretreatment. Exp Clin Psychopharmacol 9:40–46, 2001

Stitzer ML, Griffiths RR, McLellan AT, et al: Diazepam use among methadone maintenance patients: patterns and dosages. Drug Alcohol Depend 8:189–199, 1981

Strain EC, Stitzer ML, Liebson IA, et al: Dose-response effects of methadone in the treatment of opioid dependence. Ann Intern Med 119:23–27, 1993

Strain EC, Bigelow GE, Liebson IA, et al: Moderate- vs high-dose methadone in the treatment of opioid dependence: a randomized trial [see comments]. JAMA 281:1000–1005, 1999

Vaillant GE: A 20-year follow-up of New York narcotic addicts. Arch Gen Psychiatry 29:237–241, 1973

Wines JD Jr, Weiss RD: Opioid withdrawal during risperidone treatment. J Clin Psychopharmacol 19:265–267, 1999

Wolff K: Characterization of methadone overdose: clinical considerations and the scientific evidence. Ther Drug Monit 24:457–470, 2002

Wolff K, Rostami-Hodjegan A, Shires S, et al: The pharmacokinetics of methadone in healthy subjects and opiate users. Br J Clin Pharmacol 44:325–334, 1997

Opioids

Antagonists and Partial Agonists

Charles P. O'Brien, M.D., Ph.D.
Kyle M. Kampman, M.D.

Researchers have studied opioid drugs since the earliest days of pharmacology because of their importance in the treatment of pain. Over the past 25 years, this intense research produced discoveries in the endogenous opioid system that have increased knowledge about the way these drugs act. Our understanding of the biology of opioid effects, including opioid dependence, is well developed and probably more complete than our understanding of any other class of drugs of abuse (see O'Brien 1992). Although much remains to be learned about the chronic changes produced in opioid receptors and second messenger systems during dependence, considerable knowledge exists about the interaction between these receptors and both opiates (derivatives of the opium plant) and opioids (synthetic substances or peptides acting at opiate receptors). This knowledge has led to the classification of drugs according to their interactions with these receptors. The three basic categories are the following:

1. *Agonists* (e.g., heroin, methadone), which activate specific opiate receptors
2. *Antagonists* (e.g., naloxone, naltrexone), which occupy opiate receptors but do not activate them; antagonists with high affinity may displace agonists in a dependent subject, causing an immediate withdrawal syndrome
3. *Partial agonists* (e.g., buprenorphine), which occupy opiate receptors but activate them only in a limited way so that there is a ceiling to their agonist effects. Partial agonists may also block the occupation of receptors by full agonists with lesser affinity, thus producing antagonist effects in certain circumstances.

Of all the medications used in the treatment of opioid dependence, methadone, a long-acting agonist at the μ subtype of the opioid receptor, has had the greatest effect (see Chapter 24, "Opioids: Maintenance Treatment," in this volume). Naltrexone, which became available for general use in 1985, is an antagonist and therefore offers a treatment distinctly different from that of methadone. Naltrexone specifically blocks opiate receptors. While this medication is present, readdiction to heroin and any other drug that acts via opiate receptors is prevented. Because it is so different from other available treatments, naltrexone is commonly misunderstood. Clinicians tend to confuse it with disulfiram in the treatment of alcoholism or methadone for agonist maintenance of opioid-addicted patients. As an antagonist, naltrexone has a specific mechanism of action, and to use this tool effectively, clinicians should understand this mechanism completely.

Although pharmacologically distinctive, naltrexone does not change the fundamental requirements for good treatment of addiction. Rehabilitation requires a comprehensive treatment program with attention to the nonpharmacological variables that play a critical role in the complex problem of addiction. Thus, the prescription of naltrexone alone will not work. It should be part of an overall treatment program that includes individual or group psychotherapy, family therapy, contingency contracting, and possibly behavioral extinction of drug-conditioned responses.

In considering this new treatment, it should be recognized that naltrexone will not appeal to most opioid-dependent individuals. Of all street heroin-addicted subjects presenting for treatment, not more than 10%–15% show any interest in a drug that "keeps you from getting high" (Greenstein et al. 1984). The vast majority prefer methadone treatment, but for certain patients, naltrexone is an excellent alternative. Patients such as health care professionals, middle-class addicted individuals, and formerly addicted persons given an early parole from prison may find naltrexone to be the treatment of choice. It also may be a form of "insurance" for patients who are graduating from a therapeutic community (see Chapter 38, "Therapeutic Communities," in this volume) and preparing to live in the "outside world," where heroin is readily available.

It also should be emphasized that naltrexone acts specifically only at opiate receptors. It does not block the effects of nonopioid drugs, although evidence indicates that it reduces the high from alcohol (discussed later in this chapter under "Naltrexone in the Treatment of Alcoholism"). Cocaine abuse in association with heroin became a common problem during the 1980s. Patients dependent on both opioids and co-

caine may be treated with naltrexone, but they will need additional therapy to deal with their cocaine dependence.

Receptor Interactions With Drugs

Opiates such as heroin and morphine and the synthetic opioids such as methadone and meperidine act through specific opiate receptors; these drugs are referred to as *agonists*. Antagonists such as naloxone or naltrexone also bind to these receptors, but they do not activate the receptor to initiate the chain of cellular events that produce so-called *opiate effects*. Naloxone and naltrexone are relatively pure antagonists in that they produce little or no agonist activity at usual doses. This is in contrast to mixed partial agonists, such as nalorphine or buprenorphine, which produce significant agonist effects. Not only do pure antagonists fail to produce opiate effects, but their presence at the receptor also prevents opiate agonists from binding to the receptor and producing opiate effects. Because the antagonist competes for a binding site with the agonist, the degree of blockade depends on the relative concentrations of each and their relative affinity for the receptor site. Naltrexone has high receptor affinity, and thus it can block virtually all the effects of the usual doses of opioids and opiates such as heroin. In the presence of naltrexone, there can be no opiate-induced euphoria, respiratory depression, pupillary construction, or any other opiate effect (O'Brien et al. 1975).

There are four categories of medical uses for opiate antagonists:

1. To reverse the effects of an opiate or opioid, particularly in the treatment of an opioid overdose. Naloxone is commonly used to reverse the effects of high-dose morphine anesthesia and to reverse opioid-induced respiratory depression in newborns whose mothers have received opioids during labor. Naloxone is preferable for this purpose because its short duration of action allows dose titration, but it may need to be given continuously.

2. To diagnose physical dependence on opioid drugs. An antagonist such as naloxone will displace the opioid from the receptors in a dependent individual and produce an immediate withdrawal syn-

drome. Naloxone rather than naltrexone is typically used for this purpose because its brief duration of action will produce discomfort for only a short time. The absence of a withdrawal syndrome implies that the subject is not dependent on opioids, and thus it is safe to begin treatment with a long-acting antagonist such as naltrexone. Persons currently dependent on opioids are exquisitely sensitive to opioid antagonists. The degree of sensitivity depends on the time since the last dose of opioid and the size of the dose. Even a very small amount of naloxone or naltrexone can rapidly displace enough opioid from opiate receptors to precipitate a withdrawal syndrome. Therefore, in starting a patient on naltrexone, it is important to make certain that the opioid-dependent patient is fully detoxified prior to the initiation of antagonist treatment.

3. To prevent readdiction in an individual who has been detoxified from opioid drugs. This is the principal reason for the development of naltrexone and is discussed later in this chapter under "Benefits of Naltrexone."

4. To block the effects of endogenous opioids when there is a disease state consisting of high levels of these substances (Myer et al. 1990). Blocking endogenous opioids is also the presumed mechanism of naltrexone in reducing the effects of alcohol.

Effects of Antagonists

If a person not currently dependent on an opioid agonist receives an opioid antagonist, usually no obvious effects occur. Theoretically, something should happen because the antagonist blocks certain endogenous opioids (e.g., endorphins) that may regulate mood, pain perception, and various neuroendocrine and cardiovascular functions. Dysphoric reactions and endocrine changes have been reported in experimental subjects given naltrexone (Ellingboe et al. 1980). Spiegel et al. (1987) reported small decreases in appetite produced by naltrexone in human volunteers. Hollister et al. (1982) found adverse mood effects in nonaddicted volunteers given naltrexone. Crowley et al. (1985) noted similar effects in recently detoxified opioid-addicted subjects. These dysphoric effects of naltrexone were reported after brief treatment (1 day to 3 weeks), and the number of subjects was small. In contrast, another study of nonaddicted subjects reported no differences in mood effects between naltrexone and placebo (O'Brien et al. 1978). Moreover, most large-scale studies of recovering opioid-addicted patients have not found dysphoria or other mood changes to be a significant problem in the clinical use of naltrexone (Brahen et al. 1984). Since 1995, larger numbers of alcoholic patients have received naltrexone, and up to 10% report dysphoric effects including nausea. A possible explanation is that the basal state of some patients includes relatively high levels of endogenous opioids whose access to receptors is blocked abruptly when naltrexone is taken. Such patients would likely constitute a significant portion of the early dropouts. Those who continue taking naltrexone for months or even years generally report no mood effects, although careful long-term studies of mood have not been conducted.

Among opiate-addicted patients, reduced drug craving has been reported in naltrexone-maintained patients, but it is not clear that this is a pharmacological effect. It may simply be a reduction in craving caused by the security that patients feel knowing that they are protected from the temptation to experience opioid effects. Reduced craving for alcohol also has been reported among alcoholic patients receiving naltrexone under double-blind conditions (O'Malley et al. 1992, 2002; Volpicelli et al. 1992).

Clinical Use of Naltrexone

Naloxone Versus Naltrexone

Naloxone and naltrexone differ in several important ways. Naloxone is poorly absorbed from the gut; when given parenterally, it is metabolized rapidly. Naloxone, therefore, is useful only for the acute reversal of opioid effects as in the emergency treatment of opioid overdoses and in the diagnosis of physical dependence. If the presence of physical dependence is in question, a small (0.2–0.8 mg) injection of naloxone can be given. In a dependent individual, a withdrawal syndrome would occur immediately, but it would be short lived (i.e., 20–40 minutes).

In contrast to naloxone, naltrexone is well absorbed when given by mouth, and it has a long duration of action. Pharmacokinetic studies of naltrexone show a plasma half-life of the parent compound of 4 hours. An important active metabolite, 6-β-naltrexol, has a plasma half-life of 12 hours. With repeated dosing over time, both peak and trough levels of 6-β-nal-trexol increase. The pharmacological duration of naltrexone is longer than might be predicted by the plasma kinetics. Double-blind studies showed antagonism of injected opioids up to 72 hours after a 150-mg dose, but the degree of antagonism was less than that seen at 24 and 48 hours (O'Brien et al. 1975). This observation is consistent with a positron emission tomography study of naltrexone's occupation of brain μ receptors showing 80% blockade at 72 hours following a single dose (Lee et al. 1988).

A long-acting drug such as naltrexone is ideal for use in preventing relapse to opioid use. In the presence of naltrexone, heroin self-administration is no longer rewarding, and under experimental conditions, addicted individuals stop taking heroin even when it is available. Although daily ingestion of naltrexone would provide the most secure protection against opioid effects, naltrexone can be given as infrequently as two or three times per week, with adequate protection against readdiction to street heroin. The reduced frequency makes monitoring of the medication more practical over the long term. Tolerance does not appear to develop to the antagonism of opioid effects even after more than 1 year of regular naltrexone ingestion (Kleber et al. 1985).

Benefits of Naltrexone

Naltrexone was approved by the U.S. Food and Drug Administration (FDA) on the basis of its clear pharmacological activity as an opioid antagonist. It has never been shown in large-scale double-blind trials to be more effective than placebo in the rehabilitation of opioid-addicted patients. In large-scale studies, the dropout rate is very high, just as it is in drug-free outpatient treatment of heroin addiction. Naltrexone is not effective when simply prescribed as a medication for street-heroin-addicted patients in the absence of a structured rehabilitation program. Within a structured program, naltrexone appears to be effective, particularly with specific motivated populations. A randomized controlled study conducted with federal probationers suggested that the impressions of efficacy can be confirmed by data collected in individuals who are at risk to return to prison (Cornish et al. 1997). Naltrexone can permit recently detoxified addicted patients to return to their usual environments secure in the knowledge that they cannot succumb to an impulsive wish to get high. For many patients, this may be

the first time in years that they have been able to exist outside of a hospital or prison in an opioid-free state.

The subtle manifestations of the opioid withdrawal syndrome are known to persist for months (Martin and Jasinski 1969). During this protracted withdrawal syndrome, the patient's autonomic nervous system is unstable, and symptoms such as anxiety and sleep disturbances are common. Conditioned responses to environmental cues produced by previous drug use (O'Brien et al. 1986; Wikler 1965) also may contribute to relapse. Maintenance on naltrexone provides an ideal situation to extinguish these conditioned responses (O'Brien et al. 1980, 1992) and to permit the protracted withdrawal syndrome to subside.

For someone recovering from addiction who works in a field such as nursing, pharmacy, or medicine, naltrexone maintenance has an added benefit: it reduces the concerns about relapse felt by colleagues who are aware of the person's history. Because these medical occupations often require individuals to work with opioid drugs, they face a daily temptation to resume drug use. Of course, return to work is very important to rehabilitation, but it presents problems in a medical setting. Colleagues tend to regard any hint of unusual behavior as a sign that relapse to addiction has occurred. However, with a program of verified naltrexone ingestion as part of a comprehensive treatment program, the professional can return to work. Physicians who are recovering from addiction often cite this reduction of suspicion from colleagues as an important reason to continue naltrexone, some for 5 years or more. Of course, the opioid-free period also permits the use of psychotherapy to deal with underlying or superimposed psychosocial problems.

Comparison With Other Treatment Approaches

As with other treatments for addiction, naltrexone works best within a comprehensive program that deals with all aspects of the patient's problems. Naltrexone is similar to methadone in this sense: both medications can reduce relapse to illicit drug use. There are significant differences, however. Methadone is an excellent treatment for most street heroin users because it satisfies their drug craving. Methadone also enables them to stop committing crimes because they no longer have an expensive drug habit to support. Former heroin users can thus stabilize their lives, take care of their families, and find legal employment. Methadone does not "block" heroin's effects, however. There is cross-tolerance between heroin and methadone, and an adequate dosage of methadone will produce sufficient tolerance so that there will be little reward from the usual dose of heroin. In addition to satisfying opioid craving, methadone may produce beneficial psychoactive effects.

In contrast to methadone, naltrexone cannot be given until all opioids have been metabolized and cleared from the body. Naltrexone does not produce opioid effects or any psychoactive benefits; patients are therefore without any of the feeling of opioids in their bodies. During the 24–72 hours of naltrexone's effects, it will effectively block or diminish the actions of any opioid drug; thus, if the patient decides to resume heroin use, he or she cannot experience euphoria or calming from the use of heroin as in the past.

Another important distinction between methadone and naltrexone is the absence of dependence on naltrexone. Naltrexone can be stopped abruptly at any time without concern for withdrawal symptoms. In a sense, this lack of physical dependence is a drawback to naltrexone in clinical practice because the patient perceives no direct drug effect, as is the case with methadone. Thus, there is no built-in reward, and there is no immediate penalty for stopping. One way to overcome this problem is to provide an external reward for medication adherence, such as a small payment contingent on the patient ingesting naltrexone. Such a contingency management system has been used successfully in the treatment of other addictive disorders. Coupling naltrexone with small payments (Grabowski et al. 1979) or contingency management programs significantly improved treatment retention and abstinence rates among opiate-dependent patients (Carroll et al. 2001; Preston et al. 1999).

Another treatment strategy that is often confused with naltrexone is disulfiram. The medications are similar only in that both are taken to prevent relapse and both are nonaddicting. Disulfiram blocks the metabolism of alcohol, not its effects. If a person receiving disulfiram ingests alcohol, the normal degradation of alcohol is inhibited and acetaldehyde accumulates. Acetaldehyde produces flushing, nausea, and other noxious symptoms. Avoiding alcohol while taking disulfiram, of course, can prevent these effects. In contrast, no such noxious effects result from the use of opioids in association with naltrexone treatment. The opioid effects are simply blocked or neutralized in an individual receiving naltrexone treatment.

Target Populations

Health Care Professionals

Health care professionals generally have done well in naltrexone treatment programs. For example, Ling and Wesson (1984) reported the use of naltrexone in the management of 60 health care professionals for an average of 8 months. Forty-seven (78%) were rated as "much improved" or "moderately improved" at follow-up. Washton et al. (1984) found that 74% of opioid-dependent physicians completed at least 6 months of treatment with naltrexone and were opioid free and practicing medicine at 1-year follow-up. More recently, Roth et al. (1997) reported on the use of naltrexone in a specialized treatment program for opiate-addicted health care professionals. This program combined supervised naltrexone administration and group therapy. In a sample of 18 subjects, 94% achieved long-term abstinence. These studies involved comprehensive treatment programs, with naltrexone providing a kind of structure around which psychotherapy was built.

The comprehensive treatment program should involve a full medical evaluation, detoxification, psychiatric evaluation, family evaluation, and provision for ongoing therapy along with confirmed regular ingestion of naltrexone. Ongoing therapy usually involves marital and individual therapy. By use of this approach, the physician, whose drug use may have been discovered during a crisis, can be detoxified, started on naltrexone, and back at work practicing medicine in as little as 2 weeks. Of course, therapy including naltrexone may continue for several years, but avoiding a prolonged inpatient stay minimizes the disruption of family life and medical practice.

Employed Individuals

Studies of psychotherapy outcome consistently show that patients coming into treatment with the greatest psychosocial assets tend to respond best to treatment. Thus, it is not surprising that patients with a history of recent employment and good educational backgrounds do well on naltrexone. Some patients avoid methadone because of the required daily clinic visits, especially at the beginning of treatment. Because naltrexone is not a controlled substance, greater flexibility is permitted. Although these patients may be strongly motivated to be drug free, they remain susceptible to impulsive drug use. Using naltrexone as a kind of "insurance" is often a very appealing idea.

Another practical reason that naltrexone has been successful in this population is that it can be prescribed by any licensed physician. Naltrexone use is not restricted to a special program for the treatment of addiction. Middle-class patients may object to coming to such a clinic. It is recommended, however, that naltrexone be prescribed only by physicians who are familiar with the psychodynamics and behavior patterns of the addicted individual. Patients may appreciate the opportunity for treatment by an experienced practitioner from a private office rather than being restricted to a drug treatment clinic.

Tennant et al. (1984) described a group of suburban practitioners treating opioid dependence in a wide range of socioeconomic groups in southern California. They reported on 160 addicted patients with an average history of opioid use of 10.5 years. The majority (63.8%) were employed, and all expressed a desire for abstinence-oriented treatment. Treatment was on an outpatient basis, and a naloxone challenge was given after completion of detoxification. After a graduated dosage increase, naltrexone was given three times per week. Patients paid a fee or had the treatment covered by insurance. Each week the patients were subjected to a urine screen for all drug classes and an alcohol breath test. Counseling sessions were held weekly. The 160 patients remained in treatment a mean of 51 days, with a range up to 635 days, but most were in short-term treatment. Only 27 (17%) remained longer than 90 days. Tests for illicit drug or alcohol use were only 1%–3% positive during treatment. Although this program was considered successful, it must be remembered that despite long remissions on naltrexone, relapse to opioid use can still occur after naltrexone is stopped. Based on follow-up results of naltrexone patients, Greenstein et al. (1983) found that although treatment with naltrexone tends to be short term, even as little as 30 days of treatment is associated with a significant improvement in overall rehabilitative status at 6-month follow-up.

A study of patients in a higher socioeconomic group predictably found even better results. Washton et al. (1984) reported on the treatment with naltrexone in 114 businessmen dependent for at least 2 years on heroin, methadone, or prescription opioids. They were mainly white men of about age 30 years, with a mean income of $42,000 per year in 1983 dollars. A critical feature of this group was that there was considerable external pressure for them to receive treat-

ment, and almost half were in jeopardy of losing their jobs or facing legal consequences.

The Washton et al. (1984) treatment program was oriented toward complete abstinence. It began with 4–10 weeks of inpatient treatment, during which detoxification and induction onto naltrexone was accomplished. Intensive individual psychotherapy and involvement in self-help groups were part of the program. The importance of the posthospital phase was stressed, and all patients signed a contract for aftercare treatment.

Of the 114 patients who began the program, all completed naltrexone induction; 61% continued taking the medication for at least 6 months with no missed visits or positive urine tests. An additional 20% took naltrexone for less than 6 months but remained in the program with drug-free urine tests. Of the entire group, at 12- to 18-month follow-up, 64% were still opioid free. Those patients who had stipulated pressure from their employers to get treatment did significantly better than the group without a clear-cut risk of job loss.

Probationers in a Work-Release Program

It is a well-known fact that a large proportion of prison inmates throughout the United States have been convicted of drug-related crimes. Of course, relapse to drug use and consequent crime is common among these prisoners after they are released. One way to approach this recidivism and perhaps also alleviate some of the overcrowding of our prison system is to use a work-release or halfway house program that enables prisoners to obtain an early release with the stipulation that they work in the community and live in a prison-supervised house. Naltrexone can be prescribed for those prisoners who are addicted to heroin. A pioneering model of such a program was started in Nassau County, New York, in 1972, first with cyclazocine and later with naltrexone.

Dr. Leonard Brahen, the founder and director of this program, has reported on the results of 691 former inmates whom he treated with naltrexone (Brahen et al. 1984). The treatment is set within a work-release program during which the members live in a transitional house outside the prison and obtain employment in the community. Prior to the introduction of naltrexone, the success of former opioid-addicted patients in the program was limited because of their high relapse rate when placed in an environment where drugs were freely available.

An inmate with a history of opioid addiction who wishes to volunteer for the program must first be stabilized on naltrexone. Random urine tests are also used to monitor the participants. Uncashed paychecks must be turned in as proof that attendance at work has been regular; a portion of the salary is applied to the cost of room and board. The participants are given supervision and counseling for problems that develop during this reentry period. Some try to use street heroin to get high despite the naltrexone, but because the heroin effects are blocked, they eventually abandon this behavior. Participants are also offered continued treatment after their sentences have been served.

Since the introduction of naltrexone, the rehabilitation success rate of the formerly addicted inmates is equal to that of inmates without a drug history. Although a controlled study with random assignment to naltrexone was not conducted, the staff of the work-release program were enthusiastic about the benefits of the medication. Follow-up data suggested that even after completing their terms and leaving the program, the individuals who received naltrexone had fewer drug arrests than did inmates with a history of opioid abuse who did not receive naltrexone treatment.

More recently, Cornish and colleagues (1997) conducted a random assignment study among federal probationers convicted of drug-related crimes in Philadelphia, Pennsylvania. The probationers all received the same amount of parole counseling, but half were randomly selected to receive naltrexone. At follow-up 6 months after leaving prison, the group randomly selected for naltrexone had approximately half the reincarceration rate of the control group.

Heroin-Addicted Patients

Among street heroin users involved in crime to support their drug habit, it is difficult to predict who will respond well to treatment with naltrexone. Certainly, the proportion of former heroin-using individuals currently being treated with naltrexone is low. One possible reason for this is that publicly funded treatment programs may be discouraged by the cost of naltrexone (currently $4–$5 per tablet). Of course, the main cost of the treatment is the counseling required to support patients after detoxification. Most programs that use naltrexone have focused on patients who are employed or who have good employment prospects, have a stable relationship with spouse or family, and express willingness to enter long-term psychotherapy or family therapy. As stated earlier in this chapter, even short-

term (30 days or more) treatment with naltrexone has been associated with improved outcome at 6-month follow-up. Patients willing to continue taking the antagonist for 6 to 12 months generally do well, but it is difficult to know to what degree the success is influenced by the patient's strong motivation as evidenced by his or her remaining in treatment. A good outcome probably involves interaction of several factors, and any single factor might not have been adequate by itself.

How to Use Naltrexone in a Comprehensive Treatment Program

Detoxification

An abstinence-oriented program begins with detoxification. This process facilitates the performance of a complete medical evaluation and the recognition of any additional health problems that may be present. Detoxification, which should be accomplished on an inpatient basis if possible, also allows for family and individual psychological evaluations.

Several pharmacological options are available for detoxification. Gradually reducing doses of methadone for 5–10 days constitutes one approach. At the other end of the spectrum, a rapid clonidine-aided detoxification can ready the patient for naltrexone in as little as 48 hours after being opioid dependent (Kleber and Kosten 1984). The choice depends on the type of opioid agonist the patient was using (short acting vs. long acting), the patient's motivation, and the need for speed in returning the patient to work.

Because many patients fail to be inducted onto naltrexone because they leave during detoxification or relapse almost immediately after detoxification, rapid clonidine-aided detoxification or ultrarapid detoxification with heavy sedation or general anesthesia has been proposed as an improved means of starting naltrexone. Some studies have found that rapid and ultrarapid detoxification can be done safely and lead to high rates of long-term abstinence. For instance, Gerra et al. (2000) showed that compared with a traditional methadone detoxification, significantly more patients who used a clonidine-aided rapid detoxification were inducted onto naltrexone (75% vs. 26%). Two recent studies of ultrarapid detoxification in which general anesthesia was used found good patient acceptance in all of the 192 subjects completing the procedure (Albanese et al. 2000; Hensel and Kox 2000). Long-term abstinence rates were also impressive, with one study reporting 6-month abstinence rates of 55% (Albanese et al. 2000) and the other reporting a 12-month abstinence rate of 68% (Hensel and Kox 2000).

However, other studies have not found relapse rates to be reduced after ultrarapid detoxification compared with traditional detoxification techniques, and controversy exists as to whether any long-term advantage is gained by ultrarapid detoxification (Lawental 2000). (See Chapter 23, "Opioids: Detoxification," in this volume for a discussion of the different types of detoxification techniques.)

Naloxone Testing for Residual Dependence

Various methods are available for beginning treatment with naltrexone. In all cases, there should be no residual physical dependence on opioid agonists. If the patient has been using a long-acting opioid such as methadone, it may be necessary to wait 7–10 days after the last dose before initiating treatment with naltrexone. With dependence on short-acting drugs such as heroin or hydromorphone, the time between detoxification and starting naltrexone can be much shorter. If naltrexone is started too soon, precipitated withdrawal will occur. Even mild withdrawal, consisting of only abdominal cramps or periods of nausea, may be enough to discourage the patient from further treatment. In contrast, the eagerness of some patients to be protected by naltrexone and to return to work results in their willingness to tolerate mild withdrawal symptoms.

Most clinicians who work with naltrexone have found it helpful to administer a naloxone test to determine whether the patient has any residual physical dependence before he or she is given the first dose of naltrexone. A positive test indicating physical dependence consists of symptoms of opioid withdrawal, such as perspiration, nausea, or cramps, that last for 20–40 minutes. A positive test indicates that the patient should wait at least another day before starting naltrexone. Naloxone can be given parenterally, 0.2–0.8 mg subcutaneously or intramuscularly. It can also be used intravenously if very rapid results are desired.

Some clinicians prefer to test for residual opioid dependence by using a very small oral dose of naltrexone rather than a naloxone injection. They recommend a half or a quarter of a tablet (12.5–25 mg) as a safe dose. Certainly this approach is safe, but if even a mild withdrawal syndrome is precipitated, it will be of long duration (at least several hours and perhaps more than a day) and will possibly discourage the patient from further naltrexone treatment.

Generally, it is better to wait a longer time between the end of detoxification and the beginning of naltrexone rather than risk evoking a precipitated withdrawal reaction. This period is critical, however, because the patient is vulnerable to relapse, as yet unprotected by naltrexone. Therefore, the clinician must exercise judgment in balancing the benefits of a rapid transition to naltrexone against the risks of discouraging the patient with a recurrence of physical withdrawal symptoms. Rapid and ultrarapid detoxification techniques using clonidine, sedation, or general anesthesia to treat withdrawal symptoms and effect a more rapid induction of naltrexone were developed because of this problem and may be helpful for some patients.

Naltrexone to Prevent Relapse

When the naloxone challenge is negative, naltrexone can be started with an initial dose of 25 mg (one-half tablet). If no side effects occur within an hour, another 25 mg may be administered. The recommended dosage subsequently is 50 mg/day. After the first 1 to 2 weeks, it is usually possible to graduate the patient to three doses per week (e.g., 100, 100, and 150 mg given on Monday, Wednesday, and Friday, respectively). It is critical that psychotherapy sessions be initiated early in treatment and that these sessions involve family members and other significant figures in the patient's life.

Naltrexone ingestion should be monitored. Confirmed dosing can occur in the clinic, but it is usually disruptive to the patient's rehabilitation to be required to come to the clinic for every dose. For this reason, it is important to involve significant figures in the patient's life to observe the ingestion of naltrexone and to report periodically to the therapist. In the case of physicians, for example, a colleague may have already confronted the patient with his or her drug problem and helped steer the patient into therapy. This has sometimes been the chief of staff of the hospital where the patient works or the chairperson of the patient's department. A family member or co-worker also can be enlisted after determining the existence of a constructive relationship.

Progress in treatment is determined by engagement in psychotherapy, performance on the job, and absence of drug abuse as confirmed by urine tests. The patient should be asked to agree to random urine tests arranged by telephoning the patient and asking him or her to come in that day without prior notification. Patients who are doing well can eventually graduate to a schedule of only two doses of naltrexone per week, even though this would not provide full antagonist coverage over the entire interval between doses. However, the reduced frequency of visits decreases the patient's dependence on the therapist and reduces the treatment's interference with the patient's life. Although the degree of pharmacological blockade is diminished by the third or fourth day after receiving the drug, at this stage of therapy the patient is less likely to be testing limits by taking opioids. Moreover, the random urine testing should detect opioid use between naltrexone doses, which would necessitate a return to more frequent dosing. A slip should not be treated as a treatment failure but rather as a symptom to be examined in therapy (i.e., grist for the therapeutic mill).

In private practice, patients are often given a prescription for naltrexone that can be filled at a pharmacy. Patients can eventually be trusted to take doses of naltrexone at home, but it is best that some doses be taken in the physician's office under direct observation. If a patient is pretending to take naltrexone and is using opioids, a dose in the office would precipitate a withdrawal reaction. Also, the treating physician should keep a supply of naltrexone tablets in his or her office to administer to patients. Physician and pharmacist patients have been known to attempt to deactivate their supply of naltrexone tablets by treating them in a microwave oven. They could then appear to consume naltrexone in the presence of the treating physician or nurse, but they would be taking a relatively inert tablet.

Side Effects

Considering that naltrexone is a very specific and potent drug that acts on opioid receptors throughout the body, it is surprising that it has so few side effects. Most patients report no symptoms at all; however, when the drug was first introduced in clinical trials, various effects were reported. These effects included abdominal pain, headache, and mild increases in blood pressure. Many of these symptoms were probably related to precipitation of opioid withdrawal symptoms in recently detoxified heroin-addicted individuals. Because of the

recognition of naltrexone's potency in producing withdrawal, these complaints have now become much less common.

Because naltrexone blocks endogenous opioid peptides in addition to injected opioid drugs, one would expect to find multiple symptoms related to blockage of the wide-ranging functions of the endorphin systems. Endocrine changes have been reported following naltrexone ingestion, although these changes are less dramatic than those produced by opioids themselves. For example, Ellingboe et al. (1980) reported a prompt rise in luteinizing hormone and a delayed rise in testosterone after naltrexone ingestion. The subjective effects probably depend on the baseline level of endogenous opioids. In infants with apparent excess endogenous opioids, naltrexone can be lifesaving (Myer et al. 1990).

Most former opioid-dependent patients do not report subjective effects that can be related to naltrexone. Of course, these patients have just discontinued heroin or a similar opioid that has altered for the past several years the normal patterns of endocrine function, libido, mood, and pain thresholds. They could be expected to experience some rebound phenomena simply because of the absence of heroin, to which they had been adapted. Some patients and their spouses report that the use of naltrexone increased the patient's sex drive, a finding that also has been observed in rodents. Some patients report decreased appetite, whereas others gain weight. Thus, the effects of naltrexone are probably confounded with those of protracted opioid withdrawal, and they are further influenced by the contrast with the patient's prior life on varying doses of opioids. Consistent subjective effects have been lacking even in patients who have been maintained on naltrexone for several years. Certainly, the fear that long-term blocking of opioid receptors will inevitably lead to problems such as depression has not been realized.

Effects on Opioid Receptors

Rodent studies have shown that repeated doses of naloxone or naltrexone produce upregulation of μ opioid receptors and a transient increased sensitivity to morphine. If this phenomenon were present in humans treated with naltrexone, former opioid-addicted individuals would be at risk for overdose should they stop naltrexone, wait for the drug to be metabolized, and inject their usual dose of heroin. This question was addressed in an experiment by Cornish et al. (1993) that used healthy volunteers with no history of opioid use. A standard dose of morphine depressed the brain stem and reduced the respiratory response to a CO_2 stimulus. The degree of depression was measured, and after 2 weeks of naltrexone at 50 mg/day, the subjects were retested. No change in morphine's effects was found at varying times after the last dose of naltrexone, indicating lack of detectable change in receptor sensitivity. Thus, the theoretical risk of overdose based on upregulation of opioid receptors does not seem to present a clinical problem for the use of naltrexone in preventing relapse to opioid dependence. Of course, patients taking naltrexone will lose their tolerance to opioids just as will drug-free patients. This means, by definition, that they will be more sensitive and thus vulnerable to overdose if they resume heroin use at previous levels.

Effects on Blood Chemistry

Changes in laboratory tests also have been examined in more than 2,000 patients involved in clinical trials with naltrexone (Pfohl et al. 1986). Although addicted individuals are generally unhealthy to begin with, studies in addiction treatment programs have not identified significant laboratory abnormalities resulting from naltrexone treatment. Liver function tests are a matter of great concern because of the high frequency of hepatitis among addicted individuals. As many as 70%–80% of patients in methadone programs have some liver abnormalities, usually ascribed to past or present hepatitis.

Studies of patients given high-dose naltrexone for experimental treatment of conditions such as obesity have noted dose-related increments in transaminase levels that were all reversible when the drug was stopped. These subjects generally received 300 mg/day of naltrexone, or about six times the therapeutic dosage for prevention of addiction relapse (Pfohl et al. 1986). This finding raises cautions in the treatment of addiction, although in practice, naltrexone-related transaminase elevations have not been observed at the lower dosage levels used in recovering addicted patients (Arndt et al. 1986). Three recent naltrexone studies in different clinical patients were conducted to investigate the hepatic effects of the medication. Naltrexone, 50–300 mg/day, was used for periods between 10 and 36 months to treat dyskinesia in 10 patients with Huntington's disease and had no hepatic effects

(Sax et al. 1994). Marrazzi et al. (1997) reported no adverse clinical or laboratory hepatic changes for subjects in a double-blind study of high-dose naltrexone, 200–400 mg/day, for the treatment of eating disorders. Naltrexone was also studied in 865 alcoholic patients; 570 patients received naltrexone, and 295 were in a reference group (Croop et al. 1997). The results from this large trial failed to show any hepatic toxicity related to naltrexone.

Opioid-addicted individuals in liver failure should not be given naltrexone, although those with minor abnormalities in liver function tests may receive naltrexone. Baseline laboratory tests must include a full battery of liver function studies, and monthly retesting should occur for the first 3 months. Assays for serum transaminases (e.g., aspartate aminotransferase, alanine aminotransferase) and serum γ-glutamyltransferase, total bilirubin, and uric acid are routinely used to assess damage to the liver from disease and heavy drinking. Caution should be exercised in administering naltrexone to patients whose serum chemistry results are five times or more above normal. Because total bilirubin appears to be the most sensitive of these measures of naltrexone-induced hepatic toxicity, it can be used to evaluate and monitor the development of liver problems. This is particularly important in the use of naltrexone for alcoholic patients in whom alcohol-induced liver damage is frequent and treatment with naltrexone can spare the liver if it helps to reduce or eliminate drinking. In most cases, if no evidence of rising enzymes exists, the tests can be repeated at intervals of 2–6 months.

Safety in Pregnant Women and in Children

Another set of issues regarding the safety of any new drug concerns its use in pregnant women and in children. No clinical trials have been done in these groups; thus, no definitive statements can be made. Studies of naltrexone in animals generally have not shown signs of potential risks for pregnant subjects at clinical doses, but a teratogenic effect specific to humans is always possible.

Drug Interactions

There have been no systematic studies of nonopioid drug interactions with naltrexone, but with more than 20 years of clinical trials and 15 years of postmarketing experience, much anecdotal information is available. Naltrexone has been used safely in combination with disulfiram, lithium, and antidepressants, both tricyclics and selective serotonin reuptake inhibitors; if these agents are indicated, they apparently can be used in their normal way at their usual dosages. In an unpublished report, naltrexone plasma levels were increased by the coprescription of ibuprofen, but toxicity was not noted.

An adverse interaction has been reported between thioridazine and naltrexone. Maany et al. (1987) reported that sedation occurred when naltrexone was added to the regimens of two patients stabilized on thioridazine. No thioridazine plasma levels were available, but a likely explanation is that naltrexone impaired the degradation of thioridazine, resulting in increased plasma levels and increased sedation. If a neuroleptic were required in combination with naltrexone, a nonsedating neuroleptic would be preferable.

Treatment of Pain During Naltrexone Maintenance

Patients are expected to continue taking naltrexone for months or years to prevent relapse to opioid abuse. During this time, they may require surgery or treatment of trauma caused by an accident. The presence of naltrexone would not interfere with inhalation anesthesia, but the use of morphine during anesthesia would be affected. Also, opioids for immediate postoperative pain would be precluded in usual doses. If the surgery is elective, the naltrexone could be stopped several days before the date of the operation. For emergency surgery, nonopioid anesthesia and postoperative pain medication can be used. If opioid medication is necessary, high doses of a short-acting opioid could be used to override the competitive antagonism produced by naltrexone. As naltrexone and its active metabolites are metabolized, the problem would be resolved. In practice, this issue is rarely a problem because nonopioid alternatives can be used for these patients.

New Therapeutic Prospects

Depot Naltrexone

A major impediment to the more widespread use of naltrexone is the early dropout rate. Often patients express an apparently genuine desire for opioid-free treatment, but during the extremely vulnerable period within the first month after detoxification, they miss an appointment, act on an impulse, and take a dose of heroin. Stopping naltrexone does not produce withdrawal symptoms. Other patients simply become overconfident and feel that they do not need the protection of naltrexone. Even though the patient may later regret the sudden decision to stop naltrexone, the treatment process must start all over again with detoxification.

A delivery system for naltrexone that provides adequate antagonist protection for 30–60 days would take the patient through the period when relapse is most likely. Several sustained-release injectable naltrexone compounds are currently under development. In these products, naltrexone is embedded in a polymer that gradually dissolves, releasing the medication over time. Preliminary clinical testing suggests that these products are well tolerated and provide a gradual release of naltrexone for up to 30 days. Other studies have confirmed the ability of these injectable compounds to block the effects of injected opioids for up to 4 weeks (Comer et al. 2002). Much more testing is necessary, but this delivery system holds promise for increasing the efficacy of naltrexone in the rehabilitation of opioid-addicted patients.

Buprenorphine: Qualities of Methadone and Naltrexone

Buprenorphine is a partial μ opioid agonist that is currently approved by the FDA in an injectable form to treat pain. As an agonist, it is 25–50 times more potent than morphine, but because it is a partial agonist, its opioid effects are limited. Unlike agonists such as morphine and methadone, higher dosages of buprenorphine do not produce progressively greater opioid effects; thus, buprenorphine is less likely to produce an overdose. In fact, in France, where buprenorphine is available as an alternative to methadone for opioid agonist treatment, the death rate attributable to buprenorphine is three times less than the death rate associated with methadone (Auriacombe et al. 2001).

In clinical trials, buprenorphine shows some of the features of methadone and naltrexone. The agonist properties of buprenorphine cause it to be attractive as a maintenance treatment for a large proportion of opioid-addicted patients. It blocks opioid withdrawal and satisfies craving for opioids. If buprenorphine is discontinued abruptly, the withdrawal syndrome is very mild. Heroin, in contrast, has an intense but short-lived withdrawal syndrome depending on the dose. The methadone withdrawal syndrome is milder than that of heroin but significantly longer in duration. In addition to these opioid agonist effects, buprenorphine antagonizes the effects of other opioids in a manner comparable to naltrexone.

Based on clinical trials to date, buprenorphine appears to be useful in the treatment of heroin addiction. Because of its good safety profile and less severe abuse liability, buprenorphine will have significantly fewer restrictions placed on its use compared with methadone and should improve access to effective treatment for opiate-dependent patients. Once approved, buprenorphine will be available to qualified physicians to dispense from their offices. Because of the benefits of making it available for prescription outside of methadone treatment programs, it is important to reduce the risk of abuse of this medication. Therefore, the product proposed for use by office-based physicians is a combination of buprenorphine and naloxone. The addition of naloxone would block the μ effects of buprenorphine if injected, but because of the poor oral bioavailability of naloxone, it would not impair the sublingual administration of buprenorphine. A large multicenter clinical trial of the combination of buprenorphine and naloxone showed that this medication was significantly better than placebo at reducing heroin craving and heroin use in opiate-dependent patients. Buprenorphine-naloxone has been approved for use as both an agonist treatment and an aid for opiate detoxification.

Naltrexone in the Treatment of Alcoholism

We discuss here an additional approved indication for naltrexone in the treatment of alcoholism because the mechanism is believed to involve the endogenous opioid system. Numerous animal studies have shown that alcohol drinking produces activation of the endogenous opioid system and increases in dopamine in the reward pathways of the ventral striatum. Opioids have been reported to increase alcohol consumption in rodents, and opioid antagonists block or antagonize preference for alcohol. The mechanism of these effects is not clear, but blocking opioid receptors consistently tends to decrease the ingestion of alcohol by an-

imals previously choosing to drink this substance. The effect of alcohol on increasing dopamine in reward pathways is blocked by naltrexone.

Although the effects of alcohol consumption on endogenous opioids appear to be quite complex and incompletely understood, experiments with naltrexone in alcoholic humans suggest a practical clinical application from this line of animal research. Volpicelli and colleagues (1990, 1992) found significant reductions in relapse to alcohol dependence in alcoholic outpatients receiving naltrexone after detoxification. The study was conducted under double-blind, placebo-controlled conditions, and all patients received intensive outpatient rehabilitation counseling in addition to the study medication. Naltrexone-treated patients had about as many small slips to alcohol use as did the patients randomly assigned to placebo. However, significantly fewer of the naltrexone patients continued to drink and to relapse to alcohol dependence during the 3-month trial. Those who did drink alcohol while receiving naltrexone reported less pleasure than expected, an effect predicted by the animal research. One interpretation of these results is that alcohol activates endogenous opioids, which form part of the reinforcement of continued alcohol drinking. Because naltrexone blocks opioid receptors, the reinforcement via the opioid system would be attenuated, and the probability of continued alcohol drinking would be reduced. O'Malley and colleagues (1992) essentially replicated these results.

Subsequent controlled trials also have been mainly positive. (However, two trials failed to show a significant advantage for naltrexone over placebo.) These seemingly conflicting results may be attributable to the fact that although effective for alcohol dependence, naltrexone is far from a "magic bullet," and in clinical trials, its effectiveness may be affected by numerous factors, including patient selection, concurrent psychosocial treatment, and medication adherence. Naltrexone effectiveness is especially sensitive to medication adherence. In order for naltrexone to be most effective, patients must take it regularly. In several trials, the superiority of naltrexone over placebo was evident only in a subgroup of patients who took their medication regularly (Chick et al. 2000; Monti et al. 2001; Volpicelli et al. 1997).

Patients with a positive family history of alcoholism are more likely to have an endogenous opioid response to alcohol in the laboratory (Gianoulakis et al. 1996). Because naltrexone has no significant effects other than blocking opiate receptors, it would not be surprising if it were useful only in those patients whose endogenous opioids were increased by alcohol. Some clinical trials suggest that alcoholic patients with a positive family history are more likely to benefit from naltrexone.

Mason et al. (1994) reported good results with alcoholic patients who were given another opiate receptor antagonist, nalmefene. Our understanding of the mechanism of opiate antagonists such as naltrexone and nalmefene is increasing because of laboratory research such as that of King et al. (1997) showing that naltrexone reduces the alcohol high in heavy drinkers who have a family history of alcoholism. As in the treatment of opioid dependence, medication alone is not sufficient; rather, naltrexone requires a comprehensive treatment program including psychotherapy and attention to all facets of the alcohol dependence syndrome. Unfortunately, a good deal of resistance remains to using a medication in the treatment of alcoholism; thus, naltrexone use is increasing slowly as word of its efficacy spreads among practitioners.

Conclusion

Naltrexone is a specific opioid antagonist that has a relatively long duration of action such that it can be used in the prevention of relapse to opioid dependence. Naltrexone is safe and relatively nontoxic. The antagonist treatment option is important to make available to well-motivated opiate-addicted individuals who desire to become drug free. As with all medications in the treatment of addiction, naltrexone must be used within a comprehensive treatment program, including individual or family psychotherapy and urine testing for illicit drugs. Treatment should continue for at least 3 months after detoxification—and in many cases longer, because a significant risk of relapse continues for several years.

The National Institute on Drug Abuse is conducting an active program in medications development that will continue to add options for the treatment of opioid dependence. The partial agonist buprenorphine combines features of methadone and naltrexone and is now FDA approved. A depot form of naltrexone that gives protection against relapse for at least 30 days is already in clinical trials for both alcoholism and heroin addiction.

References

Albanese AP, Gevritz C, Oppenheim B, et al: Outcome and six month follow up of patients after ultra rapid opiate detoxification (UROD). J Addict Dis 19:11–27, 2000

Arndt IO, Cacciola JS, McLellan AT, et al: A re-evaluation of naltrexone toxicity in recovering opiate addicts, in Problems of Drug Dependence 1985 (NIDA Research Monograph 67; Publ No ADM-86-1448). Edited by Harris LS. Rockville, MD, National Institute on Drug Abuse, 1986, p 525

Auriacombe M, Franques P, Tignol J: Deaths attributable to methadone vs. buprenorphine in France (letter). JAMA 285:45, 2001

Brahen LS, Henderson RK, Copone T, et al: Naltrexone treatment in a jail work-release program. J Clin Psychiatry 45:49–52, 1984

Carroll KM, Ball SA, Nich C, et al: Targeting behavioral therapies to enhance naltrexone treatment of opioid dependence: efficacy of contingency management and significant other involvement. Arch Gen Psychiatry 58:755–761, 2001

Chick J, Anton R, Checinski K, et al: A multicentre, randomized, double-blind, placebo-controlled trial of naltrexone in the treatment of alcohol dependence or abuse. Alcohol Alcohol 35:587–593, 2000

Comer SD, Collins ED, Kleber HD, et al: Depot naltrexone: long-lasting antagonism of the effects of heroin in humans. Psychopharmacology 159:351–360, 2002

Cornish JW, Henson D, Levine S, et al: Naltrexone maintenance: effect on morphine sensitivity in normal volunteers. Am J Addict 2:34–38, 1993

Cornish JW, Metzger D, Woody GE, et al: Naltrexone pharmacotherapy for opioid dependent federal probationers. J Subst Abuse Treat 14:529–534, 1997

Croop RS, Faulkner EB, Labriola DF: The safety profile of naltrexone in the treatment of alcoholism: results from a multicenter usage study. The Naltrexone Usage Study Group. Arch Gen Psychiatry 54:1130–1135, 1997

Crowley T, Wagner J, Zerbe G, et al: Naltrexone-induced dysphoria in former opioid addicts. Am J Psychiatry 142:1081–1084, 1985

Ellingboe J, Mendelson JH, Kuehnle JC: Effects of heroin and naltrexone on plasma prolactin levels in man. Pharmacol Biochem Behav 12:163–165, 1980

Gerra G, Zaimovic A, Rustichelli P, et al: Rapid opiate detoxification in outpatient treatment relationship with naltrexone compliance. J Subst Abuse Treat 18:185–191, 2000

Gianoulakis C, Krishnan B, Thavundayil J: Enhanced sensitivity of pituitary β-endorphin to ethanol in subjects at high risk of alcoholism. Arch Gen Psychiatry 53:250–257, 1996

Grabowski J, O'Brien CP, Mintz J: Increasing the likelihood that consent is informed. J Exp Anal Behav 24:283–284, 1979

Greenstein RA, Evans BD, McLellan AT, et al: Predictors of favorable outcome following naltrexone treatment. Drug Alcohol Depend 12:173–180, 1983

Greenstein RA, Arndt IC, McLellan AT, et al: Naltrexone: a clinical perspective. J Clin Psychiatry 45:25–28, 1984

Hensel M, Kox WJ: Safety, efficacy, and long-term results of a modified version of rapid opiate detoxification under general anesthesia: a prospective study in methadone heroin, codeine and morphine addicts. Acta Anaesthesiol Scand 44:326–333, 2000

Hollister L, Johnson K, Boukhabza D, et al: Aversive effects of naltrexone in subjects not dependent on opiates. Drug Alcohol Depend 8:37–42, 1982

King AC, Volpicelli JR, Frazer A, et al: Effect of naltrexone on subjective alcohol response in subjects at high and low risk for future alcohol dependence. Psychopharmacology (Berl) 129:15–22, 1997

Kleber HD, Kosten TR: Naltrexone induction: psychologic and pharmacologic strategies. J Clin Psychiatry 45:29–38, 1984

Kleber HD, Kosten TR, Gaspari J, et al: Nontolerance to the opioid antagonism of naltrexone. Biol Psychiatry 2:66–72, 1985

Lawental E: Ultra rapid opiate detoxification as compared to 30-day inpatient detoxification program: a retrospective follow-up study. J Subst Abuse 11:173–181, 2000

Lee MC, Wagner HN, Tanada S, et al: Duration of occupancy of opiate receptors by naltrexone. J Nucl Med 29:1207–1211, 1988

Ling W, Wesson DR: Naltrexone treatment for addicted health-care professionals: a collaborative private practice experience. J Clin Psychiatry 45:46–48, 1984

Maany I, O'Brien CP, Woody G: Interaction between thioridazine and naltrexone (letter). Am J Psychiatry 144:966, 1987

Marrazzi MA, Wroblewski JM, Kinzie J, et al: High-dose naltrexone and liver function safety. Am J Addict 6:21–29, 1997

Martin WR, Jasinski DR: Physiological parameters of morphine in man: tolerance, early abstinence, protracted abstinence. J Psychiatry Res 7:9–16, 1969

Mason BJ, Ritvo EC, Morgan RO, et al: A double-blind, placebo-controlled pilot study to evaluate the efficacy and safety of oral nalmefene HCl for alcohol dependence. Alcohol Clin Exp Res 18:1162–1167, 1994

Monti PM, Rohsenow DJ, Swift RM, et al: Naltrexone and cue exposure with coping and communication skills training for alcoholics: treatment process and 1-year outcomes. Alcohol Clin Exp Res 25:1635–1647, 2001

Myer EC, Morris DL, Brase DA, et al: Naltrexone therapy of apnea in children with elevated cerebrospinal fluid beta-endorphin. Ann Neurol 27:75–80, 1990

O'Brien CP: Opioid addiction, in Handbook of Experimental Pharmacology. Edited by Herz A, Akil H, Simon EJ. Berlin, Springer-Verlag, 1992, pp 803–823

O'Brien CP, Greenstein R, Mintz J, et al: Clinical experience with naltrexone. Am J Drug Alcohol Abuse 2:365–377, 1975

O'Brien CP, Greenstein R, Ternes J, et al: Clinical pharmacology of narcotic antagonists. Ann N Y Acad Sci 311:232–240, 1978

O'Brien CP, Greenstein R, Ternes J, et al: Unreinforced self-injections: effects on rituals and outcome in heroin addicts, in Proceedings of the 41st Annual Scientific Meeting, The Committee on Problems of Drug Dependence (NIDA Research Monograph 27; Publ No ADM-80-901). Edited by Harris LS. Rockville, MD, National Institute on Drug Abuse, 1980, pp 275–281

O'Brien CP, Ehrman R, Ternes J: Classical conditioning in human opioid dependence, in Behavioral Analysis of Drug Dependence. Edited by Goldberg S, Stolerman I. San Diego, CA, Academic Press, 1986, pp 329–356

O'Brien CP, Childress AR, McLellan AT, et al: A learning model of addiction, in Addictive States, Vol 70. Edited by O'Brien CP, Jaffe J. New York, Raven, 1992, pp 157–177

O'Malley SS, Jaffe A, Chang G, et al: Naltrexone and coping skills therapy for alcohol dependence: a controlled study. Arch Gen Psychiatry 49:881–887, 1992

O'Malley SS, Krishnan-Sarin S, Farren C, et al: Naltrexone decreases craving and alcohol self-administration in alcohol-dependent subjects and activates the hypothalamo-pituitary-adrenocortical axis. Psychopharmacology (Berl) 160:19–29, 2002

Pfohl D, Allen J, Atkinson R, et al: Trexan (naltrexone hydrochloride): a review of hepatic toxicity at high dosage, in Problems of Drug Dependence 1985 (NIDA Research Monograph 67; Publ No ADM-86-1448). Edited by Harris LS. Rockville, MD, National Institute on Drug Abuse, 1986, pp 66–72

Preston KL, Silverman K, Umbricht A, et al: Improvement in naltrexone treatment compliance with contingency management. Drug Alcohol Depend 54:127–135, 1999

Roth A, Hogan I, Farren C: Naltrexone plus group therapy for the treatment of opiate-abusing health care professionals. J Subst Abuse Treat 14:19–22, 1997

Sax DS, Kornetsky C, Kim A: Lack of hepatotoxicity with naltrexone treatment. J Clin Pharmacol 34:898–901, 1994

Spiegel F, Stunkard AJ, Shrager E, et al: Effect of naltrexone on food intake, hunger, and satiety in obese men. Physiol Behav 40:135–141, 1987

Tennant F, Rawson R, Cohen A, et al: A clinical experience with naltrexone in suburban opioid addicts. J Clin Psychiatry 45:42–45, 1984

Volpicelli JR, O'Brien CP, Alterman AI, et al: Naltrexone and the treatment of alcohol dependence: initial observations, in Opioids, Bulimia, and Alcohol Abuse and Alcoholism. Edited by Reid LB. New York, Springer-Verlag, 1990, pp 195–214

Volpicelli JR, Alterman AI, Hayashida M, et al: Naltrexone in the treatment of alcohol dependence. Arch Gen Psychiatry 49:876–880, 1992

Volpicelli JR, Rhines KC, Rhines JS, et al: Naltexone and alcohol dependence: role of subject compliance. Arch Gen Psychiatry 54:737–742, 1997

Washton AM, Pottash AC, Gold MS: Naltrexone in addicted business executives and physicians. J Clin Psychiatry 45:39–41, 1984

Wikler A: Conditioning factors in opiate addiction and relapse, in Narcotics. Edited by Wilner DI, Kassebaum GG. New York, McGraw-Hill, 1965, pp 85–100

CHAPTER 26

MDMA, Ketamine, GHB, and the "Club Drug" Scene

David M. McDowell, M.D.

Methylenedioxymethamphetamine (MDMA), ketamine, and γ-hydroxybutyrate (GHB) are unique compounds, differing in terms of their pharmacological properties and their phenomenological effects. The common thread linking these disparate drugs is the people who use them. These substances are taken throughout the world, most frequently by a sophisticated adolescent or 20-something constituency, as well as within a subculture of the gay community. The drugs are used and abused widely at urban social gatherings in both commercial and informal settings. They are most commonly used at nightclubs and all-night dance parties known as *raves* and at gay *circuit parties*. Attended primarily by affluent gay men, circuit parties are large social gatherings held in many different countries, usually on weekends and holidays. Both raves and circuit parties became very popular during the 1990s and have remained so. Hence, these drugs, which we discuss extensively in this chapter, and several other drugs that we describe more briefly are sometimes known as *party drugs* but are widely known as *club drugs* and are here referred to as such.

In recent years, the popularity of the club drugs has been linked inextricably with the rise of the rave phenomenon. Anecdotal reports suggest that raves were "created" in Ibiza, an island off the coast of Spain (Bellis et al. 2000). They first became noticeably popular in England during the late 1980s and then spread to the United States and the rest of the world. Raves have periodically been considered "the next big thing," and their popularity has remained relatively constant. Raves have remained a locus where young people are introduced to and use drugs.

At raves, groups of young people, who are typically in their teens, dance to rapid electronically synthesized music called *techno* that has no lyrics. These events traditionally take place in unregulated and unlicensed locations such as stadiums, abandoned warehouses, and other surreptitious places. In recent years, the venues have become increasingly mainstream. Teenagers and young adults consider the club drugs the perfect match for this scene. At some of these events, a substantial majority of rave participants are using MDMA, ketamine, GHB, or other drugs, such as marijuana and lysergic acid diethylamide (LSD)

321

(McDowell and Kleber 1994; Winstock et al. 2001). Polysubstance use is the norm at such events, with more than 80% of the participants using more than one substance (Boys et al. 1997; Winstock et al. 2001). Such rampant drug use has inspired efforts at "harm reduction" and more responsible use of the drugs, with some organizations offering on-site verification of the authenticity of these drugs. Perhaps the most prominent and well funded of these organizations, Dancesafe (http://www.dancesafe.org), offers a wide variety of services and advice (Koesters et al. 2002). In addition, law enforcement agencies have begun to focus on the trafficking and marketing of these substances, with organized attempts at cracking down on the events themselves.

MDMA

Do not get married within three weeks of doing Ecstasy.

—*Bumper sticker popular in California during the 1980s*

MDMA, better known as Ecstasy, also has been called Adam, XTC, and X. A synthetic amphetamine analogue with stimulant properties, the drug is easily distinguishable from chemically related substances in terms of its subjective effects (Hermle et al. 1993; Shulgin 1986). Recreational use of MDMA has been illegal since it was made a Schedule I drug on July 1, 1985. Despite its illegal status, the use of MDMA has skyrocketed in recent years (Cohen 1998; Morgan 2000). This rise in use has been particularly marked among adolescents, and MDMA has been strongly linked to raves.

MDMA's appeal rests primarily on its psychological effect, a dramatic and consistent ability to induce a profound feeling of attachment and connection in the user. The compound's street name is perhaps a misnomer; the Los Angeles drug dealer who coined the term *Ecstasy* wanted to call the drug Empathy but asked, "Who would know what that means?" (Eisner 1986).

MDMA has long been known to damage brain serotonin (5-HT) neurons in laboratory animals (McCann and Ricaurte 1993; Montoya et al. 2002). Although a minority disputes this, it has become increasingly apparent that MDMA is neurotoxic to humans. Furthermore, the neurotoxicity has real and functional implications (McCann et al. 2000; Montoya et al. 2002; Morgan 2000; Sprague et al. 1998). Ecstasy use is associated with sleep, mood, and anxiety distur-

bances; elevated impulsiveness; memory deficits; and attention problems. Many of these disturbances appear to be permanent; they seem likely to depend on the overall amount of MDMA consumed over time but may be caused by as little as a single dose (Rodgers 2000; Turner and Parrott 2000).

History

MDMA was patented in 1914 by Merck in Darmstadt, Germany (Shulgin 1990). MDMA was not, as is sometimes thought, intended as an appetite suppressant but was probably developed as an experimental compound. Except for a minor chemical modification in a patent in 1919, there is no other known historical record of MDMA until the 1950s. At that time, the United States Army experimented with MDMA. The resulting information was declassified and became available to the general public in the early 1970s. These findings consisted primarily of a number of LD_{50} (median lethal dose) determinations for a variety of laboratory animals.

Humans probably first used MDMA in the late 1960s. It was discovered as a recreational drug by free-thinking pop aficionados (New Age seekers), people who liked its properties of inducing feelings of well-being and connection (Watson and Beck 1986). Given MDMA's capacity to induce feelings of warmth and openness, some practitioners and researchers interested in insight-oriented psychotherapy believed it would be an ideal agent to enhance the therapeutic process. The drug was introduced into clinical psychotherapy practice on the West Coast of the United States early in 1976 and on the East Coast about 6 months later (Shulgin 1990). Before the compound became illegal in 1985, it was used extensively for this purpose (Beck 1990).

MDMA became increasingly popular in the early 1980s. In 1984, the year before it became illegal, production reached at least 30,000 tablets per month. The drug's capacity to induce feelings of connection, and a psychomotor agitation that can be pleasurably relieved by dancing, made it the ideal "party drug." Despite widespread use during the early 1980s, the drug did not attract much attention from the media or from law enforcement officials (Beck and Rosenbaum 1994; Cohen 1998).

This lack of widespread notoriety was changed by events that occurred in Texas. Until 1985, MDMA was not scheduled or regulated and was completely legal. A distribution network in Texas began an aggressive marketing campaign, and the drug was available for a time over the counter at bars, at convenience stores, and even through a toll-free number. This widespread distribution attracted the attention of then–Texas Senator Lloyd Bentsen. He petitioned the U.S. Food and Drug Administration (FDA), and the compound was placed on Schedule I on an emergency basis as of July 1, 1985.

A series of three hearings was scheduled to determine MDMA's permanent status. FDA officials were reportedly surprised that a substantial number of people, including therapists and clergymen, supported a less restrictive categorization. The administrative judge recommended that the compound be placed on Schedule III. This recommendation was overruled. The growing evidence of neurotoxicity, combined with concern about illicit drug use in general, resulted in MDMA's permanent placement on Schedule I. Its clinical use is prohibited, and because of the intense regulation of Schedule I compounds, research with MDMA is very difficult to execute. It remains on Schedule I today, and although some individuals believe that the drug should be more widely available for research, especially given the increasingly clear evidence of the neurotoxic effects of MDMA, its status will not likely change in the foreseeable future (Cohen 1998).

Synthesis of MDMA is relatively simple, and it can be made in illicit laboratories or even in domestic locations such as garages. Most supplies in the United States are imported and then distributed by organized crime networks. In addition, it is often cut with other substances so that the purity varies substantially. In England, this impure MDMA is known as *Snide-E*. Its price, usually $25–$40 for a 125-mg tablet, the amount producing the sought-after effect in most intermittent users (Green et al. 1995), has remained remarkably stable since the 1980s.

Physiological Effects

MDMA is usually ingested orally. Other methods of administration are much less popular. The usual single dose is 100–150 mg. The onset of effect begins about 20–40 minutes after ingestion and is experienced as a sudden, amphetamine-like "rush." Nausea, which is usually mild, but sometimes severe enough to cause vomiting, may accompany this initial feeling, as may the urgent need to defecate ("disco dump").

The plateau stage of drug effects lasts 3–4 hours. The principal desired effect, according to most users, is a profound feeling of relatedness to the rest of the world. Most users experience this feeling as a powerful connection to those around them, but this may include the larger world. In general, people taking the drug appear to be less aggressive and less impulsive. Users also experience a drastically altered perception of time and a decreased inclination to perform mental and physical tasks (Leister et al. 1992). Although the desire for sex can increase, the ability to achieve arousal and orgasm is greatly diminished in both men and women (Buffum and Moser 1986). MDMA has thus been described as a sensual, not a sexual, drug. The prescription drug sildenafil may be taken to counteract diminished arousal and may be sold along with MDMA (Weir 2000). In addition, people taking MDMA experience mild psychomotor restlessness, bruxism, trismus, anorexia, diaphoresis, hot flashes, tremor, and piloerection (Peroutka et al. 1988). The array of physical effects and behaviors produced by MDMA is remarkably similar across mammalian species (Green et al. 1995).

Common aftereffects can be pronounced, sometimes lasting 24 hours or more. The most dramatic hangover effect is a sometimes severe anhedonia. The hangover effects of MDMA share many similarities with amphetamine withdrawal. MDMA users can experience lethargy, anorexia, decreased motivation, sleepiness, depressed mood, and fatigue, occasionally lasting for days.

Severe, immediate effects appear to be rare but definitely occur. These include altered mental status, convulsions, hypo- or hyperthermia, severe changes in blood pressure, tachycardia, coagulopathy, acute renal failure, hepatotoxicity, rhabdomyolysis, and death (Demirkiran et al. 1996; Kalant 2001). The combination of paramethoxyamphetamine and MDMA has been associated with several serious adverse events and deaths (Ling et al. 2001). Another acute adverse event, hyponatremia, followed by seizure and coma, appears to be an unintended consequence of the harm reduction strategy of ingesting copious amounts of water prior to and while taking MDMA (Holmes et al. 1999). This phenomenon may be linked to the syndrome of inappropriate antidiuretic hormone secretion (Ajaelo et al. 1998). There are numerous case reports of a single dose of MDMA precipitating severe psychiatric illness. MDMA probably induces a range of depressive symptoms and anxiety in some individuals, and for that reason people with affective illness should be specifically cautioned about the dangers of using MDMA (McCann et al. 1994; McDowell 1998; Ricaurte).

Mechanism of Action

MDMA's primary mechanism of action is as an indirect serotonergic agonist (Ames and Wirshing 1993). However, MDMA is considered a "messy drug" because it affects serotonin- and dopamine-containing neurons and a host of other neurotransmitter systems (Rattray 1991; Sprague et al. 1998). After ingestion, MDMA is taken up by the serotonin cell through an active channel where it induces the release of serotonin stores. The drug also blocks reuptake of serotonin, contributing to its length of action. Although it inhibits the synthesis of new serotonin, this is an aftereffect and does not contribute to the intoxication phase. It may, however, contribute to sustained feelings of depression reported by some users and to a diminished magnitude of subjective effects when the next dose is taken within a few days of the first dose. The drug's effects, and side effects (an arbitrary distinction), including anorexia, psychomotor agitation, difficulty in achieving orgasm, and profound feelings of empathy, can be explained as a result of the flooding of the serotonin system (Beck and Rosenbaum 1994).

People who use MDMA on a regular basis tend not to increase their use as time goes on (Cohen 1998; Peroutka 1990). Because the drug depletes serotonin stores and inhibits synthesis of new serotonin, subsequent doses produce a diminished high and a worsening of the drug's undesirable effects such as psychomotor restlessness and teeth gnashing. MDMA users quickly become aware of this consequence and adjust their usage patterns. Many users who are at first enamored with the drug subsequently lose interest, usually citing the substantial side effects. An adage about Ecstasy reported on college campuses captures this phenomenon: "Freshmen love it, sophomores like it, juniors are ambivalent, and seniors are afraid of it" (Eisner 1993). Those who continue to use the drug over longer periods usually tend to take the drug only periodically.

MDMA's effects can be characterized as short term (lasting less than 24 hours) and long term (lasting more than 24 hours) (McKenna and Peroutka 1990). The short-term effects presumably result from the acute release of serotonin and are associated with a decrease in serotonin and 5-hydroxyindoleacetic acid (5-HIAA), a decrease in tryptamine hydroxylase (TPH) activity, and recovery of 5-HIAA levels, usually within 24 hours. The long-term effects are manifested by a persistent, slow decrease in serotonin and 5-HIAA after initial recovery, persistently depressed TPH activity, and a decrease in serotonin terminal density (Demirkiran et al. 1996; Ricaurte et al. 2000).

MDMA and Neurotoxicity

The ingestion of MDMA in laboratory animals causes a decrease in the serum and spinal fluid levels of 5-HIAA in a dose-dependent fashion (McCann et al. 2000; Shulgin 1990) and damages brain serotonin neurons (Burgess et al. 2000; McCann and Ricaurte 1993; Montoya et al. 2002). The dosage necessary to cause permanent damage to most rodent species is many times greater than that normally ingested by humans (Shulgin 1990). In nonhuman primates, the neurotoxic dosage approximates the recreational dosage taken by humans (McCann and Ricaurte 1993). Like its close structural relative methylenedioxyamphetamine (MDA or "Eve"), MDMA has been found to damage serotonin neurons in all animal species tested to date (McCann et al. 1996). The closer a given mammal is phylogenetically to humans, the less MDMA is required to induce this permanent damage.

In addition, MDMA produces a 30%–35% decline in serotonin metabolism in humans (McCann et al. 1994). Even one dose of MDMA may cause lasting damage to the serotonin system. There have been reports of individuals with lasting neuropsychiatric disturbances after MDMA use (Creighton et al. 1991; McCann and Ricaurte 1991; Schifano 1991). Furthermore, such damage might become apparent only with time or under conditions of stress. Users with no initial complications may manifest problems over time (McCann et al. 1996).

Some disagreement among researchers remains as to the permanence and functional implications of MDMA's neurotoxicity. The impressive and growing literature on this subject makes the neurotoxicity of MDMA very apparent and the experimental evidence overwhelming and irrefutable. (Because this is a general chapter dealing with all aspects of club drugs and MDMA, the reader is directed to several excellent and extensive reviews of this particular subject: McCann et al. 2000; Montoya et al. 2002 and Verkes et al. 2001.)

Human studies are, for obvious reasons, more difficult to execute and offer more fodder for critique. The bulk of evidence that MDMA is neurotoxic in humans is indirect, but it is convincing and alarming

(Burgess et al. 2000; Green et al. 1995). This evidence includes metabolite studies, which quantify the levels of serotonin and metabolites in populations of Ecstasy users. An increasing number of investigations show that metabolite levels of serotonin are much lower in chronic users, even when abstinent for a long time. The difficulties of the studies notwithstanding, the available clinical evidence suggests that repeated ingestion of high doses of MDMA might produce long-term reductions in serotonergic activity and degeneration of serotonergic terminals in humans (Montoya et al. 2002). Extensive cognitive studies in individuals who use MDMA, although rife with methodological problems, show a consistent and compelling pattern of cognitive dysfunction in the frontal cortex and the hippocampus. This phenomenon is consistent with that found in animals exposed to MDMA (Fox et al. 2001; Montoya et al. 2002). Psychiatric problems, such as depression, anxiety, panic, increased impulsiveness, and sleep disturbances, are significantly higher in MDMA users, even when abstinent and when the last use is remote. Although causality is very difficult to prove, the level of cognitive and psychiatric disturbance seen in the populations of heavy Ecstasy users is about what would be expected from the degree of serotonergic dysfunction shown to be the result of MDMA use in both humans and nonhuman primates (Kalant 2001; McGuire 2000).

Functional brain imaging studies (Buchert et al. 2001) and results from animal studies (Ricaurte et al. 2000) are consistent with significant and lasting damage to serotonergic structures. These studies cumulatively imply the possibility that the use of Ecstasy in humans may have lasting effects on central nervous system (CNS) functioning (Ricaurte and McCann 2001). In a symposium titled "Is MDMA a Human Neurotoxin?" Turner and Parrott (2000) concluded the following:

> Novel studies…confirmed and extended the range of cognitive, behavioral, EEG, and neurological deficits, displayed by drug-free Ecstasy users. Moreover, these deficits often remained when other illicit drug use was statistically controlled. In conclusion: If MDMA neurotoxicity in humans is a myth, then it is a myth with a heavy serotonergic component. (p. 233)

A recent study by Ricaurte et al. (2002) implicated MDMA as causal of dopaminergic neurotoxicity as well. The involvement of the dopamine system has im-portant implications in terms of increased vulnerability of a variety of motor and cognitive functions.

Treatment

The treatment of MDMA abuse may be divided into the treatment of acute reactions to the drug and the treatment of chronic abuse.

Urgent Treatments

Fatalities from Ecstasy use and overdose, although rare, do occur. Because polydrug use is the norm at many of the venues where Ecstasy is popular, it is sometimes difficult to ascertain the contribution of MDMA compared with that of other substances ingested. Fatalities can be caused by hyperpyrexia, rhabdomyolysis, intravascular coagulopathy, hepatic necrosis, cardiac arrhythmias, cerebrovascular accidents, and a variety of behaviors associated with confusion and impaired judgment (Kalant 2001).

Ecstasy has many chemical similarities to amphetamine, and many commercially available products will indicate a positive presence of amphetamine. MDMA intoxication or overdose may be suspected in any individual with alterations of sensorium, hyperthermia, muscle rigidity, and fever. Because the drug is used in specific settings and by specific subgroups, the level of suspicion should be commensurate with the identity of the individual patient. If an individual patient has been to a rave, or some clublike event, this should raise the clinician's suspicion that MDMA was ingested. In addition, the clinician should have a high degree of suspicion that the patient may have taken multiple drugs. Drugs that might have been substituted for Ecstasy tablets, such as ephedrine, ma-huang (herbal Ecstasy), and caffeine, should be considered.

MDMA overdose is very similar to classic stimulant intoxication. Signs of overdose are tachycardia, agitation, tremor, mydriasis, and diaphoresis. Ecstasy ingestion may mimic LSD or other classic hallucinogen ingestion. In addition, MDMA overdose may mimic the ingestion of an anticholinergic agent (Padkin 1994). The notable exception to this is the presence of diaphoresis after Ecstasy ingestion (except in the case of dehydration). Anticholinergic agents induce dry, hot skin.

MDMA overdose or toxic reaction is a diagnosis by exclusion. Ecstasy overdose would most likely involve the ingestion of multiple doses and also would most likely occur in an environment that induced dehydration. A differential diagnosis would include infections such as meningitis, trauma, and other drug intoxications. Supportive measures such as providing effective hydration with intravenous fluids and lowering the temperature of the patient with cooling blankets or an ice bath are often necessary. Standard gastric lavage should be used (Ajaelo et al. 1998; Schwartz and Miller 1997).

In patients with significant MDMA intoxication, vascular access should be established to provide hydration and anticipation of more serious effects. Cardiac arrhythmias can be treated according to standard protocols; the patient should be paralyzed to reduce the chance of further thermogenesis (Larner 1992; Schwartz and Miller 1997). An anesthesiologist should be present, as well as a comprehensive team of professionals, and transfer should be made to an intensive care unit setting.

Physical restraint may be necessary for agitated patients but should be used sparingly and replaced with chemical restraint as soon as is possible. Benzodiazepines are the preferred choice for sedation (Holland 2001). Hypertension often resolves with sedation. If it persists, nitroprusside or a calcium channel blocker is preferred over a β-blocker, which may worsen vasospasm and hypertension (Holland 2001).

Nonurgent Treatments

MDMA intoxication is associated with several psychiatric symptoms, particularly anxiety, panic, and depression. These symptoms are usually short-term sequelae and subside in a matter of days. Support and reassurance are often all that is needed to help the individual through what may be a distressing experience. If the symptoms are severe, brief pharmacotherapy to alleviate symptoms is recommended.

Although classic physiological dependence on MDMA does not occur, some individuals use the drug compulsively. For these people, the standard panoply of treatments, based on external resources and the patient's characteristics, is recommended.

Patients with problems involving MDMA may present some unique challenges. They are often adolescents, and the many complications involved with this population must be considered (McDowell and Spitz 1999). Furthermore, they are more likely to be involved with the subculture that is enmeshed with MDMA and that views the drug as harmless at worst and life transforming at best (Beck and Rosenbaum 1994; Winstock 2001).

Ketamine

I remember dancing on the pier and looking way up at an apartment and thinking I could be there in five minutes and it wouldn't surprise me. It's like you're on a different plane. Anything seems possible.

—Ketamine user

Ketamine, also known as Special K, Super K, Vitamin K, or just plain K, was first manufactured in 1965. It is still legally manufactured, primarily for use by veterinarians and pediatric surgeons as a nonanalgesic anesthetic. It is often via these manufacturers and suppliers that illegal supplies are diverted to recreational users. Law enforcement officials have traditionally used fewer resources for regulating and monitoring medications intended for veterinary use, although there are indications that this trend is changing. The recreational use of ketamine probably began in the 1960s and was first described in detail by Lilly (1978). Since that time, its popularity has continued to rise (Cooper 1996; Dotson et al. 1995; Graeme 2000).

Ketamine is classified as a dissociative anesthetic. As its name implies, the drug causes a dose-dependent dissociative episode with feelings of fragmentation, detachment, and what one user described as "psychic/physical/spiritual scatter." It induces a lack of responsive awareness not only to pain but also to the general environment, without a corresponding depression of autonomic reflexes and vital centers in the diencephalon.

History

Ketamine was first manufactured in 1965 at the University of Michigan and was first marketed by Parke, Davis under the brand name Ketalar. Since that time, it has been commercially available under various brand names. It is most commonly available in 10-mL (100 mg/mL) liquid-containing vials (Fort Dodge Laboratories 1997). It is a close chemical cousin of phencyclidine, also known as PCP or angel dust. PCP was the first of a new class of general anesthetics known as cataleptoid anesthetics or dissociative anesthetics. PCP had physiological properties that made it advantageous as an anesthetic, the most significant being that it was quite effective without the great risk of cardiac or respiratory depression typical of classic general anesthetic agents.

PCP also had some severe limitations as an anesthetic, most significantly that it caused a high degree of psychotic and violent reactions (National Institute on Drug Abuse 1979). At least half of the patients subjected to PCP anesthesia developed several perioperative reactions, including agitation and hallucinations. Some of these patients developed severe psychotic reactions that persisted for as long as 10 days (Crider 1986; Meyer et al. 1959). Ketamine produces minimal cardiac and respiratory effects, and its anesthetic and behavioral effects remit soon after administration (Moretti et al. 1984; Pandit et al. 1980). The medication has found a place in the pharmacopoeia, principally with children and animals.

Since the 1970s, ketamine has been popular with two types of users. The first type uses ketamine in a solitary fashion and seeks a paranormal experience or uses it to enhance a spiritual journey. The second type uses the drug socially. These are the young club-goers and "ravers" (Weir 2000). Ketamine is especially popular at circuit parties. Epidemiological evidence about the use of ketamine is difficult to obtain. Reports in the media, anecdotal evidence, and my clinical observations indicate that ketamine is quite popular in urban clubs and at raves.

Ketamine is commercially available as a liquid. About 90% of ketamine comes from diverted veterinary sources. The liquid form is easily converted to a powder, the form in which it is most often sold. Ketamine can be administered in a variety of ways. In its most potent form, it is mixed with water and injected. At clubs, most people snort lines of the powder. Ketamine also may be dabbed on the tongue or mixed with a liquid and imbibed.

Physiological Effects

Ketamine has been studied extensively in humans. It is a noncompetitive N-methyl-D-aspartate (NMDA) antagonist (Verheyden et al. 2002). Recreational users of ketamine report feeling anesthetized and sedated. This is clearly a dose-dependent phenomenon (Krystal et al. 1994). For example, ketamine can induce tangential thinking and ideas of reference. At higher dosages, it distorts perception of the body, the environment, and time. Ketamine can influence all modes of sensory function (Garfield et al. 1994; Óye et al. 1992). At typical dosages, ketamine distorts sensory stimuli, producing illusions (Garfield et al. 1994). In higher-than-typical dosages, hallucinations and paranoid delusions can occur (Malhotra et al. 1996).

Ketamine substantially disrupts both attention and learning. Research volunteers using the drug fail to modify behavior in response to feedback, take longer to learn initial tasks, and have a decreased ability to apply strategy. Retrieval, long-term recall, and the consolidation of memory are all altered, as are recognition, memory, and attention (Krystal et al. 1994; Verheyden et al. 2002).

The recreational dose is approximately 0.4 mg/kg, and the anesthetic dose is almost double that. The LD_{50} is nearly 30 times the anesthetic dose. The minimal risk of overdosing is one of the drug's attractive properties.

Individuals injecting the drug recreationally begin to feel the effects in about 5 minutes. Intranasal users experience the effects of the drug in about 10 minutes. Chronic users develop tolerance. Although tingling sensations are present initially, and mild effects occur almost immediately, the principal dissociative effect occurs about 10 minutes later. In the first half-hour after ingestion, the peak effects of the drug occur and then subside gradually. The bulk of the "trip" lasts about 1 hour (Delgarno and Shewan 1996). This is known as the *emergence state,* and it is here that the perception of time is significantly altered. Users describe a sense of "eternity" and a heightened capacity to discern causal connections in all things. The effects diminish gradually over another hour. Larger doses last longer and have a more intense effect (Malhotra et al. 1996). Flashbacks have been reported, and their incidence may be higher than with many other hallucinogens (Siegel 1984).

Someone who has recently used ketamine may have catatonia, a flat face, an open mouth, fixed staring with dilated pupils, "sightless staring," and rigid posturing. At higher doses, the user enters a catatonic state colloquially known as a *K-hole* and characterized by social withdrawal, autistic behavior, an inability to maintain a cognitive set, impoverished and idiosyncratic thought patterns, and bizarre responses. Motor impairment is a marked feature of this state, and people in a K-hole are found on the edge of the dance floor, staring blankly into space, appearing nondistressed but seemingly incapable of communication (GMHC 1997).

Mechanism of Action

The mechanism of action of ketamine has been extensively studied. Ketamine is a congener of PCP and has some similar properties (Jansen 2000). It interferes with the actions of the excitatory amino acid neurotransmitters, especially glutamate and aspartate, the most prevalent excitatory neurotransmitters in the brain. These neurotransmitters regulate numerous functions of the CNS and are particularly important in cortical-cortical and cortical-subcortical interactions (Cotman and Monaghan 1987). The excitatory amino acid receptor subtype to which ketamine binds with the most affinity is the NMDA receptor complex, which regulates calcium flow through its ion channel. Ketamine binds to the NMDA receptor complex on the same site as PCP, located inside the calcium channel. Therefore, the direct action of ketamine is the blockade of calcium movement through this channel (Hampton et al. 1982).

Noncompetitive antagonism of NMDA receptors by the channel blockers induces changes of perception, memory, and cognition throughout the brain. In addition, the channel blockers affect dopaminergic transmission, inhibiting cocaine-induced increases in extracellular dopamine in the nucleus accumbens (Pap and Bradberry 1995). NMDA blockade causes an increase in dopamine release in the midbrain and prefrontal cortex (Bubser et al. 1992). NMDA blockade also causes activation of serotonin systems specifically targeting the 5-HT$_{1A}$ receptor (Loscher and Honack 1993). Agents such as ketamine work globally, directly or indirectly affecting numerous neurotransmitter systems, but ketamine's action as an NMDA antagonist is likely the cause of its schizotypal and dissociative symptoms.

Ketamine is well documented to produce acute impairments of working, episodic, and semantic memory along with schizotypal and dissociative symptoms. These are produced with as little as a single dose. Furthermore, persisting memory deficits have been shown to be present 3 days after one initial dose (Curran and Monaghan 2000). Whether these changes persist after that is an unanswered and worrisome question.

Treatment

Because of its high therapeutic index, only ingestion of massive amounts of ketamine would be considered dangerous. Such occurrences are quite rare. Perhaps the most dangerous effects of ketamine are behavioral. Individuals may become withdrawn, paranoid, and very uncoordinated. In such cases, the physician must treat the individual symptomatically. Calm reassurance and a low-stimulation environment are usually most helpful. The patient should be placed in a part of the clinic or emergency department with the least amount of light and stimulation. Neuroleptics should be used in only the rarest of cases because their side-effect profile may cause discomfort and therefore provoke the patient. If necessary, the patient may be given benzodiazepines to control the associated anxiety (Graeme 2000).

Ketamine is reinforcing in the classical sense. Numerous reports exist of individuals who became dependent on the drug and use it daily (Galloway et al. 1997; Jansen 2000). Such dependence should be treated in the manner of any other chemical dependency. The clinician should be alert to other psychological conditions and treat them appropriately. If such a condition is not found, then individual treatment should focus on the drug use issues.

GHB

> I only meant to take a little, but when I woke up, I didn't remember what had happened.
>
> *—GHB user*

GHB is sold as "liquid Ecstasy" and in Great Britain as GBH, or "grievous bodily harm." It is found naturally in many mammalian cells. In the brain, the highest amounts are found in the hypothalamus and basal ganglia (Gallimberti et al. 1989). It may function as a neurotransmitter (Galloway et al. 1997). GHB is closely linked to γ-aminobutyric acid (GABA) and is both a precursor and a metabolite of GABA. GHB, however, does not act directly on GABA receptor sites (Chin et al. 1992).

In the 1970s, GHB was used with little fanfare as a sleep aid. It has some demonstrated therapeutic efficacy, particularly in the treatment of narcolepsy (Lammers et al. 1993; Mamelak et al. 1986; Scrima et al. 1990). In addition, bodybuilders sometimes use it, hoping it will promote muscle growth because it increases episodic secretion of growth hormone. In 1990, after reports indicated that GHB might have contributed to the hospitalization of several California youths, the FDA banned it.

The legal status of GHB is complicated. Recently, GHB, under the brand name Xyrem, was classified as a Schedule III controlled substance. In addition, its distribution is governed by the FDA's Subpart H regulations. To comply with these regulations, the company that makes and markets the medication—Orphan Medical—has developed a rigorous system that makes Xyrem available to patients from a single, specialty pharmacy. Both physicians and patients must receive an education program from the company before obtaining Xyrem. Orphan Medical has worked closely with the FDA, Drug Enforcement Agency, and law enforcement agencies to develop strict distribution and risk management controls designed to restrict access to Xyrem to the intended patient population (Tunnicliff and Raess 2002).

Xyrem has been designated as a Schedule III controlled substance for medical use, meaning that it cannot be sold, distributed, or provided to anyone other than for its prescribed use. Illicit use of Xyrem is subject to penalties reserved for Schedule I drugs.

Most of the GHB sold in the United States is of the bootleg variety, manufactured by nonprofessional kitchen chemists. In fact, it is relatively easy to manufacture, and Internet sites devoted to explaining the process can be found readily, although they are sometimes cleverly concealed.

GHB has an extremely small therapeutic index, and as little as double the euphorigenic dose may cause serious CNS depression. In recent years, it has been associated with several incidents of respiratory depression and coma. Increasing numbers of deaths have been linked to GHB (Li et al. 1998).

History

GHB was first synthesized about 30 years ago by Dr. H. Laborit, a French researcher interested in exploring the effects of GABA in the brain. Laborit was attempting to manufacture a GABA-like agent that would cross the blood-brain barrier (Vickers 1969). During the 1980s, GHB was widely available in health food stores. It came to the attention of authorities in the late 1980s as a drug of abuse, and the FDA banned it in 1990 after reports of several poisonings with the drug (Chin et al. 1992). In the past decade, it has become more widely known as a drug of abuse associated with nightclubs and raves.

Physiological Effects

GHB is ingested orally, is absorbed rapidly, and reaches peak plasma concentrations in 20–60 minutes (Vickers 1969). The typical recreational dose is 0.75–

1.5 g; higher doses result in increased effects. The high lasts for no more than 3 hours and reportedly has few lasting effects. Repeated use of the drug can prolong its effects.

Users of the drug report that GHB induces a pleasant state of relaxation and tranquility. Frequently reported effects are placidity, mild euphoria, and an enhanced tendency to verbalize. GHB, like MDMA, also has been described as a sensual drug. Its effects have been likened to those of alcohol, another GABA-like drug (McCabe et al. 1971). Users report a feeling of mild numbing and pleasant disinhibition. This effect may account for the reports that GHB enhances the experience of sex. The dose-response curve for GHB is exceedingly steep. The LD_{50} is estimated at perhaps only five times the intoxicating dose (Vickers 1969). Furthermore, the drug has synergistic effects with alcohol and probably other drugs as well. Therefore, small increases in the amount ingested may lead to significant intensification of the effects and to the onset of CNS depression. Overdose is a real danger. Users drinking alcohol, which impairs judgment and with which synergy is likely, are at greater risk.

The most commonly experienced side effects of GHB are drowsiness, dizziness, nausea, and vomiting. Less common side effects include weakness, loss of peripheral vision, confusion, agitation, hallucinations, and bradycardia. The drug is a sedative and can produce ataxia and loss of coordination. As doses increase, patients may experience loss of bladder control, temporary amnesia, and sleepwalking. Clonus, seizures, and cardiopulmonary depression can occur. Coma and persistent vegetative states may occur, and death may result from overdose (Chin et al. 1992; Gallimberti et al. 1989; Takahara et al. 1977; Vickers 1969).

Mechanism of Action

Several lines of evidence support the hypothesis that GHB is a neurotransmitter (Galloway et al. 1997). Specific high-affinity binding sites for GHB have been found in the rat brain (Hechler et al. 1992). GHB temporarily suppresses the release of dopamine in the mammalian brain. This is followed by a marked increase in dopamine release, especially in the nigrostriatal pathway, and is accompanied by the increased release of endogenous opioids (Hechler et al. 1992).

GHB also stimulates pituitary growth hormone release. One study (Takahara et al. 1977) reported 9-fold and 16-fold increases in growth hormone 30 and 60 minutes, respectively, after intravenous administration of 2.5 g of GHB in six healthy adult men. Growth hormone levels were still 7-fold higher than baseline after 120 minutes. The mechanism by which GHB stimulates growth hormone release is not known. Dopamine activity in the hypothalamus stimulates pituitary release of growth hormone, but GHB inhibits dopamine release while it stimulates growth hormone release. While growth hormone is being released, serum prolactin levels also rise, in a similar time-dependent fashion. GHB has several different actions in the CNS, and some reports indicate that it antagonizes the effects of marijuana (Galloway et al. 1997). The consequences of these physiological changes are unclear, as are the overall health consequences for individuals who use GHB.

Treatment

Clinicians should remember to ask about GHB use, especially in younger people, for whom it has become a drug of choice. Because GHB is not detectable by routine drug screening, this history is that much more important. In cases of acute GHB intoxication, physicians should provide physiological support and maintain a high index of suspicion for intoxication with other drugs. A review (Li et al. 1998) suggested the following guidelines for the management of GHB ingestion with a spontaneously breathing patient:

- Maintain oxygen supplementation and intravenous access.
- Maintain comprehensive physiological and cardiac monitoring.
- Attempt to keep the patient stimulated.
- Use atropine for persistent symptomatic bradycardia.
- Admit the patient to the hospital if he or she is still intoxicated after 6 hours.
- Discharge the patient if he or she is clinically well in 6 hours (with plans for follow-up).

Patients whose breathing is labored should be managed in the intensive care unit. Most patients who overdose on GHB recover completely if they receive proper medical attention. The most dangerous effects of GHB use often occur with the use of other drugs. For example, concurrent use of sedatives or alcohol may increase the risk of vomiting, aspiration, or cardiopulmonary depression. For this reason, clinicians treating individuals who abuse or are dependent on GHB should be aware of its interactions with other drugs. The use of GHB and methamphetamine or cocaine may increase the risk of seizure.

Some individuals have developed physiological dependence on GHB. The symptoms of withdrawal include anxiety, tremor, insomnia, and "feelings of doom," which may persist for several weeks after stopping the drug (Galloway et al. 1997). Anecdotal evidence, such as the proliferation of support groups and help lines for GHB-dependent individuals, indicates that the number of GHB-dependent individuals is rising. The treatment of GHB withdrawal has received scant attention. Its complex symptomatology suggests that benzodiazepines may be useful in treating GHB withdrawal. Because data are lacking, clinicians must exercise their most prudent judgment regarding what will be most helpful in a given situation. Health care professionals should be alert for this potentially dangerous drug.

Conclusion

MDMA, ketamine, and GHB are by no means the only drugs found at clubs, raves, or circuit parties. They are, however, the most emblematic. Attendees also use more traditional drugs such as LSD and other hallucinogens. Marijuana is perennially popular, and alcohol use is also common. Some drug users have begun to experiment with flunitrazepam, a short-acting benzodiazepine better known by its street names, "Rohypnol," "Roofies," or "Ro." Because of the ability of this drug to interfere with short-term memory, it has become known in the media as the "date rape drug." Slipped into the drink of someone unsuspecting, it may indeed make the person feel very disinhibited and unable to remember much of what happened after ingestion. Furthermore, each week seems to bring a report of some "new" drug of abuse. Often this is just an older, well-known drug, packaged differently or with a new name.

When the evidence of MDMA's neurotoxicity was lacking, and what existed was not as compelling, individuals concerned with the public's safety could afford to be less alarmed. The mounting body of evidence, however, and the possible public health implications call for effective prevention and education interventions.

These drugs are used at clubs, often in combination, and often by very young people. This is cause for concern for several reasons. The younger a person is when he or she begins to use drugs, and the more often use occurs, the more likely it becomes that he or she will develop serious problems with these or other substances. In the future, we are likely to see increasing use of such drugs and the problems that come with their use.

References

Ajaelo I, Koenig K, Snoey E: Severe hyponatremia and inappropriate antidiuretic hormone secretion following ecstasy use. Acad Emerg Med 5:939–940, 1998

Ames D, Wirshing W: Ecstasy, the serotonin syndrome, and neuroleptic malignant syndrome: a possible link? JAMA 269:869–870, 1993

Beck J: The public health implications of MDMA use, in Ecstasy: The Clinical, Pharmacological and Neurotoxicological Effects of the Drug MDMA. Edited by Peroutka S. Boston, MA, Kluwer Academic, 1990, pp 77–103

Beck J, Rosenbaum M: Pursuit of Ecstasy: The MDMA Experience. SUNY Series in New Social Studies on Alcohol and Drugs. New York, State University of New York Press, 1994

Bellis MA, Hale G, Bennett A, et al: Ibiza uncovered: changes in substance use and sexual behavior amongst young people visiting an international nightlife resort. Int J Drug Policy 11:235–244, 2000

Boys A, Lenton S, Norcross K: Polydrug use at raves by a Western Australian sample. Drug Alcohol Rev 16:227–234, 1997

Bubser M, Keseberg U, Notz PK, et al: Differential behavioral and neurochemical effects of competitive and noncompetitive NMDA receptor antagonists in rats. Eur J Pharmacol 229:75–82, 1992

Buchert R, Obrocki J, Thomasius R, et al: Long term effects of "ecstasy" MDMA abuse on the human brain studied by FDG PET. Nucl Med Commun 22:425–489, 2001

Buffum J, Moser C: MDMA and human sexual function. J Psychoactive Drugs 18:355–359, 1986

Burgess C, O'Donoghoe A, Gill M: Agony and Ecstasy: a review of MDMA effects and toxicity. Eur Psychiatry 15:287–294, 2000

Chin MY, Kreutzer RA, Dyer JE: Acute poisoning from gamma-hydroxybutyrate in California. West J Med 156:380–384, 1992

Cohen R: The Love Drug: Marching to the Beat of Ecstasy. Binghamton, NY, Hayworth Press, 1998

Cooper M: "Special K:" rough catnip for clubgoers. The New York Times, January 28, 1996, p 6

Cotman CW, Monaghan DT: Chemistry and anatomy of excitatory amino acid systems, in Psychopharmacology: The Third Generation of Progress. Edited by Meltzer HY. New York, Raven, 1987, pp 194–210

Creighton F, Black D, Hyde C: Ecstasy psychosis and flashbacks. Br J Psychiatry 159:713–715, 1991

Crider R: Phencyclidine: Changing Abuse Patterns (NIDA Res Monogr 64). Rockville, MD, National Institute on Drug Abuse, 1986, pp 163–173

Curran HV, Monaghan L: In and out of the K-hole: a comparison of the acute and residual effects of ketamine in frequent and infrequent ketamine users. Addiction 96:749–760, 2000

Delgarno PJ, Shewan D: Illicit use of ketamine in Scotland. J Psychoactive Drugs 28:191–199, 1996

Demirkiran M, Jankovic J, Dean J: Ecstasy intoxication: an overlap between serotonin syndrome and neuroleptic malignant syndrome. Clin Neuropharmacol 19:157–164, 1996

Dotson J, Ackerman D, West L: Ketamine abuse. J Drug Issues 25:751–757, 1995

Eisner B: Ecstasy: The MDMA Story. Boston, MA, Little, Brown, 1986

Eisner B: Ecstasy: The MDMA Story, 2nd Expanded Edition. Berkeley, CA, Ronin Publishing, 1993

Fort Dodge Laboratories: Ketaset package insert. Fort Dodge, IA, Ketamine HCL INJ USP, 1997

Fox HC, Parrott AC, Turner JJ: Ecstasy use: cognitive deficits related to dosage rather than self reported problematic use of the drug. J Psychopharmacol 15:273–281, 2001

Gallimberti L, Gentile N, Cibin M, et al: Gamma-hydroxybutyric acid for treatment of alcohol withdrawal syndrome. Lancet 30:787–789, 1989

Galloway GP, Frederick SL, Staggers FE, et al: Gamma-hydroxybutyrate: an emerging drug of abuse that causes physical dependence. Addiction 92:89–96, 1997

Garfield JM, Garfield FB, Stone JG, et al: A comparison of psychologic responses to ketamine and thiopental-nitrous oxide-halothane anesthesia. Anesthesiology 36:329–338, 1994

GMHC (McDowell D, consultant): Drugs in Partyland (educational brochure). New York, GMHC Press, 1997

Graeme KA: New drugs of abuse. Emerg Med Clin North Am 18:625–636, 2000

Green A, Cross A, Goodwin G: Review of pharmacology and clinical pharmacology of 3,4-methylenedioxymethamphetamine (MDMA or "Ecstasy"). Psychopharmacology (Berl) 119:247–260, 1995

Hampton RY, Medzihradsky F, Woods JH, et al: Stereospecific binding of ^3H phencyclidine in brain membranes. Life Sci 30:2147–2154, 1982

Hechler V, Goebaille S, Maitre M: Selective distribution pattern of gamma-hydroxybutyrate receptors in the rat forebrain and mid-brain as revealed by quantitative autoradiograph. Brain Res 572:345–348, 1992

Hermle L, Spitzer M, Borchardt K, et al: Psychological effects of MDE in normal subjects. Neuropsychopharmacology 8:171–176, 1993

Holland J: Ecstasy: The Complete Guide. Rochester, VT, Park Street Press, 2001

Holmes SB, Banerjee AK, Alexander WD: Hyponatremia and seizures after ecstasy use. Postgrad Med J 75:32–43, 1999

Jansen K: A review of the nonmedical uses of ketamine: use, uses, and consequences. J Psychoactive Drugs 32:419–433

Kalant H: The pharmacology and toxicology of "ecstasy" (MDMA) and related drugs. Can Med Assoc J 165:917–928, 2001

Koesters SC, Rogers PD, Rajasingham CR: MDMA ("ecstasy") and other "club drugs": the new epidemic. Pediatr Clin North Am 49:415–433, 2002

Krystal JH, Karper LP, Seityl JP, et al: Subanesthetic effects of the noncompetitive NMDA antagonist ketamine in humans. Arch Gen Psychiatry 51:199–214, 1994

Lammers GJ, Arends J, Deckerck AC, et al: Gammahydroxybutyrate and narcolepsy: a double blind placebo controlled study. Sleep 16:216–220, 1993

Larner AJ: Complications of "Ecstasy" misuse (letter). Lancet 340:726, 1992

Leister M, Grob C, Bravo G, et al: Phenomenology and sequelae of 3,4-methylenedioxymethamphetamine use. J Nerv Ment Dis 180:345–354, 1992

Li J, Stokes S, Woeckener A: A tale of novel intoxication: a review of the effects of γ-hydroxybutyric acid with recommendations for management. Ann Emerg Med 31:729–736, 1998

Lilly JC: The Scientist: A Novel Autobiography. New York, JB Lippincott, 1978

Ling LH, Marchant C, Buckley NA, et al: Poisoning with the recreational drug paramethoxyamphetamine ("death"). Med J Aust 174:453–455, 2001

Loscher W, Honack D: Effects of the novel 5-HT$_{1A}$ receptor antagonist, (+)-WAY 100135, on the stereotyped behavior induced by NMDA receptor antagonist dizocilpine in rats. Eur J Pharmacol 242:99–104, 1993

Malhotra AK, Pinals DA, Weingartner H, et al: NMDA receptor function and human cognition: the effects of ketamine in healthy volunteers. Neuropsychopharmacology 14:301–307, 1996

Mamelak M, Scharf MB, Woods M: Treatment of narcolepsy with gamma-hydroxybutyrate: a review of clinical and sleep laboratory findings. Sleep 9(1 pt 2):285–289, 1986

McCabe E, Layne E, Sayler D, et al: Synergy of ethanol and a natural soporific: gamma hydroxybutyrate. Science 171:404–406, 1971

McCann U, Ricaurte G: Lasting neuropsychiatric sequelae of methylenedioxymethamphetamine ("Ecstasy") in recreational users. J Clin Psychopharmacol 11:302–305, 1991

McCann U, Ricaurte G: Reinforcing subjective effects of 3,4-methylenedioxymethamphetamine ("Ecstasy") may be separable from its neurotoxic actions: clinical evidence. J Clin Psychopharmacol 13:214–217, 1993

McCann UD, Ridenour A, Shaham Y, et al: Serotonin neurotoxicity after (±)3,4-methylenedioxymethamphetamine (MDMA; "Ecstasy"): a controlled study in humans. Neuropsychopharmacology 10:129–138, 1994

McCann U, Slate S, Ricaurte G: Adverse reactions with 3,4-methylenedioxymethamphetamine (MDMA: "Ecstasy"). Drug Saf 15:107–115, 1996

McCann UD, Eligulashvili W, Ricaurte GA: (±) 3,4-Methylenedioxy-methamphetamine ("Ecstasy") induced serotonin neurotoxicity: clinical studies. Neuropsychology 42:11–16, 2000

McDowell DM: Testimony to House Judiciary Committee, 1998. Available at: http://www.house.gov/judiciary/mcdo0615.htm.

McDowell D, Kleber H: MDMA, its history and pharmacology. Psychiatr Ann 24:127–130, 1994

McDowell D, Spitz H: Substance Abuse: From Principles to Practice. New York, Brunner/Mazel, 1999

McGuire P: Long term psychiatric and cognitive effects of MDMA use. Toxicol Lett 112–113:153–156, 2000

McKenna D, Peroutka S: The neurochemistry and neurotoxicity of 3,4-methylenedioxymethamphetamine, "Ecstasy." J Neurochem 54:14–22, 1990

Meyer JS, Greifenstein F, DeVault M: A new drug causing symptoms of sensory depravation. J Nerv Ment Dis 129:54–61, 1959

Montoya A, Sorrentino R, Lucas S, et al: Long-term neuropsychiatric consequences of "Ecstasy" (MDMA): a review. Harv Rev Psychiatry 10:212–220, 2002

Moretti RJ, Hassan SZ, Goodman LI, et al: Comparison of ketamine and thiopental in healthy volunteers: effects on mental status, mood, and personality. Anesth Analg 63:1087–1096, 1984

Morgan MJ: Ecstasy (MDMA): a review of its possible persistent psychological effects. Psychopharmacology (Berl) 152:230–248, 2000

National Institute on Drug Abuse: Diagnosis and Treatment of Phencyclidine (PCP) Toxicity. Rockville, MD, National Institute on Drug Abuse, 1979

Óye N, Paulsen O, Maurset A: Effects of ketamine on sensory perception: evidence for a role of N-methyl-D-aspartate receptors. J Pharmacol Exp Ther 260:1209–1213, 1992

Padkin A: Treating MDMA ("ecstasy") toxicity (letter). Anaesthesia 49:259

Pandit SK, Kothary SP, Kumar SM: Low dose intravenous infusion technique with ketamine. Anesthesia 35:669–675, 1980

Pap A, Bradberry CW: Excitatory amino acid antagonists attenuate the effects of cocaine on extracellular dopamine in the nucleus accumbens. J Pharmacol Exp Ther 274:127–133, 1995

Peroutka S (ed): Ecstasy: The Clinical, Pharmacological and Neurotoxicological Effects of the Drug MDMA. Boston, MA, Kluwer Academic, 1990

Peroutka S, Newman H, Harris H: Subjective effects of 3,4-MDMA in recreational abusers. Neuropsychopharmacology 11:273–277, 1988

Rattray M: Ecstasy: towards an understanding of the biochemical basis of the actions of MDMA. Essays Biochem 26:77–87, 1991

Ricaurte GA, McCann UD: Assessing long-term effects of MDMA (Ecstasy). Lancet 358:1831–1832, 2001

Ricaurte GA, McCann UD, Szabo Z, et al: Toxicodynamics and long-term toxicity of the recreational drug 3,4-methylenedioxymethamphetamine (MDMA, "Ecstasy"). Toxicol Lett 112–113:143–146, 2000

Ricaurte GA, Yuan J, Hatzidiitrious G, et al: Severe dopaminergic neurotoxicity in primates after a common recreational dose regimen of MDMA ("Ecstasy"). Science 297(5590):2260–2263, 2002

Rodgers J: Cognitive performance amongst recreational users of "ecstasy." Psychopharmacology (Berl) 151:19–24, 2000

Schifano F: Chronic atypical psychosis associated with MDMA ("Ecstasy") abuse. Lancet 338:1335, 1991

Schwartz RH, Miller NS: MDMA (Ecstasy) and the rave: a review. Pediatrics 100:705–708, 1997

Scrima L, Hartman P, Johnson F, et al: The effects of gamma-hydroxybutyrate on the sleep of narcolepsy patients: a double-blind study. Sleep 13:479–490, 1990

Shulgin A: The background and chemistry of MDMA. J Psychoactive Drugs 18:291–304, 1986

Shulgin A: History of MDMA, in Ecstasy: The Clinical, Pharmacological and Neurotoxicological Effects of the Drug MDMA. Edited by Peroutka S. Boston, MA, Kluwer Academic, 1990, pp 1–20

Siegel RK: The natural history of hallucinogens, in Hallucinogens: Neurochemistry, Behavioral, and Clinical Perspectives. New York, Raven, 1984, pp 1–18

Sprague JE, Everman SL, Nichols DE: An integrated hypothesis for the serotonergic axonal loss induced by 3,4-methylenedioxymethamphetamine. Neurotoxicology 19:427–441, 1998

Takahara J, Yunoki S, Yakushiji WL: Stimulatory effects of gamma-hydroxybutyric acid on growth hormone and prolactin release in humans (letter). J Clin Endocrinol Metab 44:1014, 1977

Tunnicliff G, Raess BU: Gamma-hydroxybutyrate (orphan medical). Curr Opin Investig Drugs 3:278–283, 2002

Turner JJ, Parrott AC: "Is MDMA a human neurotoxin?" Diverse views from the discussants. Neuropsychobiology 42(1):42–48, 2000

Verheyden SL, Hadfield J, Calin T, et al: Sub-acute effects of MDMA (+/-3,4-methylenedioxymethamphetamine, "ecstasy") on mood: evidence of gender differences. Psychopharmacology (Berl) 161:23–31, 2002

Verkes RJ, Gijsman HJ, Pieters MS, et al: Cognitive performance and serotonergic function in users of ecstasy. Psychopharmacology (Berl) 153:196–202, 2001

Watson L, Beck J: New Age seekers: MDMA use as an adjunct to spiritual pursuit. J Psychoactive Drugs 23:261–270, 1986

Weir E: Raves: a review of the culture, the drugs and the prevention of harm. Can Med Assoc J 162:1843–1848, 2000

Winstock A, Griffiths P, Stewart D: Drugs and the dance music scene: a survey of current drug use patterns among a sample of dance music enthusiasts in the UK. Drug Alcohol Depend 64:9–17, 2001

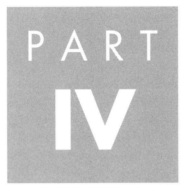

Treatment Approaches

Psychodynamics

Richard J. Frances, M.D.

Avram H. Mack, M.D.

Lisa Borg, M.D.

John E. Franklin, M.D.

Psychoanalysis and psychodynamic theory have had a wide effect on psychiatric treatment, including addiction treatment. Although some investigators have argued that psychodynamic treatment has only a minor role in the treatment of substance abuse (Vaillant 1995), psychodynamic understanding can indeed add depth to work with individuals and groups, further the rehabilitation process (Dodes and Khantzian 1998; Frances et al. 1989; Khantzian 1997), and increase the usefulness of 12-step programs (Dodes 1988). In this chapter, we develop a rationale for the application of dynamic concepts in addiction treatment, examine its indications and contraindications, and explore how psychodynamic theory can be used to enhance standard treatment techniques and deepen understanding of addiction treatment. Finally, we provide a psychodynamic approach to addiction that includes neurobiological findings.

Psychodynamic Theories of Addiction

Classical and Early Psychoanalysis

Psychoanalytic understanding of addiction derives from general psychoanalytic theory. Psychodynamic treatment is based on Freud's work in discovering the importance of unconscious phenomena; the development of a theory of the relationship between id, ego, and superego, with an emphasis on resistance, defenses, and conflict; and the use of techniques such as free association, clarification, and interpretation. Freud (1905/1949), Abraham (Abraham 1908/1960), and Rado (1984) each posited trauma-related developmental issues—including orality, regression toward infantile fixations, defenses against homosexuality, sexual and social inferiority, emotional immaturity, depressive tendencies, and insecurity—as psychopathological pathways leading to substance abuse (Lorand 1948). On the other hand, Freud (1930/1964) also connected the elation of intoxication, which he believed relaxed superego repression, to manic states. Glover (1932/1956) noted the important role of aggressive drives in substance abuse.

The questions of primary versus secondary effects of alcoholism were originally raised by Hippocrates and were raised again in 1911, when Bleuler (1911/1921) hypothesized that drinking was often the cause of neurotic disturbances and that clinicians should not be taken in by the "stupid excuses" of heavy drinkers. Ferenczi (1912/1916) and Freud and Ferenczi (1908–1914/1993), on the other hand, viewed alcoholism as an "escape into narcosis" from underlying psychodynamic causes, the theory from which the self-medication hypothesis originated.

Modern Psychoanalysis and Psychodynamics

As the focus of psychoanalytic theory has moved from drives to developmental and structural deficits and affective experience, psychoanalytic approaches to addictions have been redrawn as well. A number of theorists have contributed important ideas on the role of ego defenses, defense deficit, and affective experience in drug abuse and alcoholism.

Affective control has been a major area of interest among those studying the psychodynamics of addiction. Krystal (1982–1983) emphasized a defective stimulus barrier resulting from psychic trauma and the attempt to use substances to fortify against the onslaught of overwhelming affects. He described the inability of patients to label affects, which he called alexithymia, and the inability of addicted individuals to verbalize affective states. McDougall (1984) focused on drug use as a dispersion of affects into action. Lewis (1987) highlighted pathological shame, affecting one's core sense of self, as an affect associated with substance abuse. Dodes and Khantzian (1998) emphasized the addicted individual's sense of helplessness and powerlessness, often in the face of intolerable affects, and the need to restore through drug use a sense of power and control to which the individual feels entitled. Pharmacological control or change of one's affect state is the goal, despite often unpredictable psychological, behavioral, or physiological drug or alcohol effects.

Addictions have also been explained in terms of fixation or delay of psychosexual development. Krystal (1982–1983) described an inability in addicted individuals to take over the internal maternal functions associated with care of the self. Bean-Bayog (1988) described the addiction itself and the resultant loss of control as a sort of severe psychic trauma that leads to characteristic defensive patterns. Wurmser (1984) and Meissner (1986) emphasized narcissistic collapse as a cause of substance use; in other words, individuals use substances to compensate for a punctured grandiose or idealized self. According to Wurmser (1984), feelings of emptiness, boredom, rage, shame, depression, and guilt are symptoms of narcissistic wounds and superego regression, which prompt substance use. Furthermore, Wurmser characterized addiction as self-medication for claustrophobia, a feeling of being trapped; that is, substance use is a means of escape. These authors stressed the severity of psychopathology underlying drug dependence. Silber (1974) emphasized the alcoholic individual's pathological identification with destructive or psychotic parents. Some authors have attempted to analyze the substance itself, framing alcohol as a fetish object (Keller 1992), or have described alcohol abuse in terms of falling in love with the reward state of intoxication (DuPont 1998).

Both object relations and self psychology perspectives have been applied to addictions. According to Kohut and Wolf (1978), drugs serve as substitute idealized selfobjects for selfobjects missing developmentally in addicted individuals, and drug problems are considered *narcissistic behavior disorders*. Kernberg (1991) described addictive behavior as a reunion with a forgiving parent, an activation of "all good" selfobject images, and a gratification of instinctual needs. Kernberg (1991) identified subsets of addicted individuals with *malignant narcissism*, associated with strong antisocial features.

The self-medication hypothesis has evolved over several decades and is based on observations of patients with dual diagnoses. Theorists such as Wieder and Kaplan (1969), Milkman and Frosch (1973), and Khantzian (1997) have discussed the importance of the specific effects of particular drugs on affect and the choice of a particular substance on the basis of specific sought-after effects. Khantzian (1997) highlighted this self-medication hypothesis in describing the use of opioids to assuage end-point feelings of rage and aggression and the use of cocaine to counter feelings of depressive anergic restlessness or to augment grandiosity. Alcohol has been related to deep-seated fears of closeness, dependence, and intimacy, with the alcohol effect promoting toleration of loving or aggressive feelings.

Moving the self-medication hypothesis beyond strict psychiatric diagnoses and toward underlying psychological states, Khantzian (1997) emphasized affect regulation, tolerance, self-regulation of affect, self-esteem, need satisfaction, relationships, and self-care. He also related psychodynamic concepts to the total care of addicted patients, providing a better understanding of how 12-step programs are helpful. He described substance-abusing individuals as lacking an internal, comforting sense of self-validation. These individuals also have difficulty obtaining nurturance and validation from others in a consistent, mature way. Self-care relates to the individual's developmental inability to anticipate danger or to worry about, anticipate, or consider the consequences of his or her actions, resulting in self-defeating and self-destructive behavior.

Some other psychodynamic views of addiction have been promulgated. Dodes (1996) suggested that addictions are in the same category as compulsions, and because compulsions have been seen as treatable with traditional psychodynamic psychotherapy, addictions should also be treatable by similar approaches. Luborsky (1984) and Klerman et al. (1984) stressed the importance of clarifying the impact of drugs on the addicted individual's interpersonal relationships. Empirical research (using structured instruments) has failed to demonstrate high levels of dissociation among previously traumatized adults with substance use disorders, and the theory has been promoted that alcohol subsumes the expected dissociation (Langeland et al. 2002). Galanter (2002) emphasized the value of self-help groups and religious and social networks in providing a calming, soothing release of anxiety and a support for failing functioning of the individual's ego and superego.

Application of Psychodynamics to Treatment

Applied psychodynamic principles must be distinguished from psychoanalysis. Psychodynamic principles can be used to understand individual and group treatment, rehabilitation, and other aspects of treatment, whereas psychoanalysis is a more specific technique that is suited for a small number of recovering addicted patients. Most patients cannot tolerate certain aspects of psychoanalysis, such as seeing an analyst four or five times per week with the analyst providing relatively little feedback, being quite neutral, and providing little reassurance in order to allow the patient to experience frustration and have regressive fantasies. In contrast, psychodynamic psychotherapy usually occurs one to two times per week, possibly in addition to other modalities, and the patient sits up, facing the therapist. (Use of a couch is generally avoided because it facilitates regression.) Abstinence is essential for successful treatment. Vigilant efforts at relapse prevention and helping patients get back on track after relapse are very much a part of psychodynamic psychotherapy with addicted patients. Psychodynamic psychotherapy and 12-step mutual self-help programs are compatible approaches for the maintenance of long-term abstinence.

Today, the focus of psychodynamic approaches tends to be on current conflicts as they relate to the past rather than on childhood experience. The therapist, aware of the patient's characteristic defenses and particular ego weaknesses and strengths, more often provides empathic interpretations and takes an active and supportive role. The therapist-patient relationship is discussed openly in order to work through resistance, and no effort is made to foster further regression. Psychodynamic techniques aimed at increased self-awareness, growth, and working through of conflicts can be combined with cognitive approaches, case finding, relapse prevention, motivational techniques, suggestions, education, and provision of support and reassurance as indicated.

Indications and Rationale for Psychodynamic Psychotherapy

Psychodynamic principles are applicable throughout psychiatry and are relevant to addiction treatment. Insight-oriented therapy may be especially sought out by individuals for whom this kind of approach represents a particularly good fit. Individual psychodynamic psychotherapy may be the sole treatment or may be combined with group, family, psychopharmacological, self-help, cognitive-behavioral, and other treatment approaches. It may be reserved for treatment-resistant cases, or it may be the treatment of choice because of patient factors. Some patients refuse to participate in group or self-help programs and seek out individual psychodynamic therapy because of a wish for privacy, confidentiality, and insight. Patients with certain characteristics may especially seek out psychodynamic psychotherapy. Positive characteristics may include high intelligence, interest, and insight; psychological mindedness; a wish to understand or find meaning in behavior; a capacity for intimacy; identification with a therapist; ample time; ample funds; and a wish to change aspects of self that are not acceptable.

As with most forms of psychotherapy, positive prognostic indicators are higher socioeconomic status, marital stability, less severe psychopathology, and minimal sociopathy (Woody et al. 1986). Some relatively negative characteristics associated with other treatments are social phobia, avoidance, and fears, which make attendance at Alcoholics Anonymous (AA) and Narcotics Anonymous (NA) meetings difficult. Factors that may lead some individuals to consider psychodynamic psychotherapy instead of other treatments include initial reactions of distaste toward spirituality, as may occur in some atheists; strong negative reactions to groups in general; unwillingness to take medication when indicated; and a lack of a rational approach to the world (patients with such a lack might benefit from cognitive-behavioral treatment).

Adolescents and young adults sorting out identity issues, problems regarding individuation, and a need for independence may especially benefit from an insight-oriented approach. For patients in whom denial, projection, splitting, and projective identifications are prominent defenses, consistent interpretation of defenses may be needed to form a working alliance that can be used to achieve sobriety and growth.

Patients who continue to be anxious, depressed, and troubled after detoxification are more likely to seek out additional psychotherapy. In many ways, patients who benefit from psychodynamic psychotherapy and have abused substances are similar to those who benefit from such therapy and have not abused substances. At the same time, many patients who failed to respond to psychodynamic psychotherapy when they were drinking find that they do benefit from this form of treatment when they are sober. Insight-oriented psychotherapy may be used to achieve or maintain the benefits of abstinence and to prevent relapse.

Those affected by disasters, such as the Oklahoma City bombing or the September 11, 2001, terrorist attacks, often turn to substances for relief of painful affects. Alcohol and substance use can increase vulnerability to posttraumatic stress disorder, and the disorder itself can increase alcohol and drug problems. In one study of alcohol use among victims of the Oklahoma City bombing, alcohol did not alleviate symptoms but in fact increased functional impairment in these individuals (Pfefferbaum and Doughty (2001). Psychotherapy might prevent addiction or relapse in vulnerable individuals in these contexts.

Recovering addicted patients are often members of families with heavy addiction, and the danger of relapse is greater among patients who have conflicts about enjoying and enhancing their success. These patients may fear being more successful than an addicted parent or sibling, and insight into the sources of self-defeating behavior can be essential to preventing relapse.

In the case of patients for whom self-care, self-destructiveness, suicidality, and masochism are major issues, an awareness of unconscious forces of self-destructive behavior can be useful to both patient and therapist. Many patients are not aware that their alcoholism may be what Menninger (1938) called "a slow form of suicide." Awareness of risk-taking aspects of behavior may lead the patient to take greater caution. Addiction and suicide are long-term solutions to what are often short-term problems, and the therapist's job is to help the patient realize this.

The rationale for using psychodynamic principles is frequently based on an in-depth clinical understanding of a particular patient's life situation. There is good evidence that alcoholism is influenced by genetic and environmental factors. Biological factors, such as the dopamine reward pathways and the mesolimbic reward system, have also enhanced understanding of the brain basis of addiction (Koob and Le Moal 1997; Kreek and Koob 1998; Leshner 1997; O'Brien 1997a, 1997b; Volkow et al. 1997). Studies indicate that medications such as lithium and valproate may be neurotrophic for patients with bipolar disorder, and it will be interesting to see which forms of psychotherapy may also have neurotrophic effects (Manji et al. 2000). The study of temperament is leading to intriguing implications for psychiatric treatment, including treatment of addictions (Cloninger 1987). Psychodynamic understanding takes into account the patient's childhood history; temperament; existing conflicts at the oral, anal, phallic, or genital levels; development of defenses; and ego and superego development, including object relations and relationships with parents, siblings, and friends (Khantzian 1997).

Psychodynamics are used to deepen the patient's understanding of the rehabilitation process and group psychotherapy and to help him or her understand how self-help groups work (Frances et al. 1989). Awareness of the importance of an unconscious wish to return to drinking, especially during periods of stress, is used in treatment. When unconscious factors have repeatedly led to relapse, exploratory psychotherapy may be particularly useful (Dodes and Khantzian 1998). For example, a patient's discussion of a "lost weekend," a drunk dream, or a planned vacation to a location where relapses frequently occurred in the past may be a warning sign of a possible relapse and can be used to help the patient to recognize that craving still exists and should be addressed.

An awareness of reasons not to drink and the strengthening of that side of the conflict may help, along with increased insight into the sources of the internal struggle. The greatest focus of attention has been on how substances may be used to self-medicate for other psychiatric disorders or to self-regulate affect and on how their use may be a symptom of an underlying problem (Khantzian 1997). Abused substances may be used to push painful thoughts from one's consciousness and to numb feelings associated with painful knowledge, or they may be used to gain access to unconscious material and to facilitate experience or expression of anger and other feelings that may be avoided during sobriety. For patients for whom affect regulation is an issue, psychodynamic psychotherapy may be especially valuable. A patient with an underlying dysthymia, depression, or affective disorder may need to understand how he or she has used substances to cope with unmanageable feelings. Given that alcohol and drugs invariably cause additional life difficulties, psychodynamic approaches may help the patient deal with the psychosocial effects associated with the toxic metabolic complications of substance use.

The application of psychodynamic theory to the treatment of comorbid psychiatric problems such as Axis II personality disorders (including borderline, narcissistic, and avoidant personality disorders) is important, especially because alcoholism and drug abuse are overrepresented in these patients. The literature on comorbidity of Axis I and Axis II disorders is extensive, and a presentation of findings is beyond the scope of this chapter (for further discussion, see Kessler et al. 1997). It may be especially hard to identify the boundaries of temperament, acute substance-induced personality change, other Axis I disorders, secondary personality features, and independent personality disorders. Exploratory psychotherapy with borderline personality disorder patients who have a history of addiction must be informed by a good knowledge of addiction psychiatry and an emphasis on structure and limit-setting in treatment, including the vital parameter of abstinence.

Kernberg (1991) discussed the deception and projection often seen in the initial therapeutic alliance with borderline and narcissistic personality disorder patients, as well as the need to confront distorted views of reality in the therapeutic relationship. The use of insight in interpreting negative transference and acting out may deepen a positive transference and ultimately foster open expression. As a patient develops a clearer picture of his or her life through exploratory psychotherapy, the value of openness and honesty becomes apparent, and the tie to the therapist is cemented. Frequently, addicted patients have lied to themselves and others and are tired of feeling false and phony. The therapist's healthy ability to tolerate being conned by highly skilled, manipulative patients may minimize damaging countertransference reactions. If the therapist finds himself or herself doing something with a patient (either positive or negative) that is out of the ordinary, some examination of countertransference is warranted.

Early in treatment, it may be hard to tell whether personality change is resulting from a gradual return to better function because of physical, social, and psychological recovery from addiction effects; whether the initial diagnosis of personality disorder was correct; or whether psychodynamic and/or 12-step programs have effected personality change. Some patients experience a rebound high that is analogous to the practicing subphase of development in the second year of life, when there is a burst of autonomous development (Mahler et al. 1975).

Many addicted patients who have narcissistic traits or personality disorder, and in whom the toxic effects of addiction heighten narcissism, feel a sense of specialness and entitlement, have no empathy for others, are unable to allow gratification of dependence needs, and experience loneliness. For these patients, rehabilitation often involves acceptance of vulnerability and of being ordinary and similar to others with the same problem; a reaching out for help; and encouragement to develop a new humility. Whether this rehabilitation is achieved through 12-step programs, application of Beck's cognitive therapy (A.T. Beck et al. 1993; J.S. Beck and Liese 1998), or psychodynamic exploration of the narcissistic vulnerability, these issues should be dealt with in this substantial subpopulation.

A real danger of psychodynamic theory has been a reductionism in which attempts are made to apply one theory or approach to every situation. A broad and flexible use of psychodynamic thinking takes into account the total range of structural issues, including id, ego, and superego; developmental factors; conflict theory; self psychology; affect regulation; and cognitive deficits. Perry et al. (1987) clarified how three psychodynamic theoretical models—self psychology; object relations; and classical ego, id, and superego conflict theory—can be used to find the metaphor most useful to a particular patient or psychodynamic history.

Evidence indicates that alcohol problems can either cause or result from anxiety disorders and that more often than not, agoraphobia, social phobia, and obsessive-compulsive disorder precede rather than follow an alcohol problem (Kushner et al. 1990). Although cognitive-behavioral and pharmacological approaches may be first-line treatments for panic disorder, agoraphobia, and social phobia, psychodynamic approaches are often used with patients whose conditions have been resistant to, or have only partially responded to, other psychotherapies and medications (Frances and Borg 1993).

Partial day hospitals (sometimes in conjunction with halfway houses) are increasingly being used after the patient has been stabilized and detoxified. In one series of studies, researchers found that treatment in day hospitals was as effective as inpatient treatment for addiction (Alterman et al. 1994).

Contraindications for Psychodynamic Psychotherapy

Contraindications for psychodynamic psychotherapy include active use of substances, severe organicity, psychosis, and, for the most part, antisocial personality disorder. Some patients who regress too readily in individual therapy, who develop psychotic transferences, or who develop negative therapeutic reactions benefit from the diffusion of transference that takes place in group therapy. If the principal problem is marital, family therapy is the treatment of choice.

Initiation of Treatment

Some authors recommend waiting 6 months to 1 year before beginning psychodynamic psychotherapy (Bean-Bayog 1988). We believe that psychodynamic treatment can be initiated early; however, timing should be tailored to the patient. The greatest opportunity to develop a treatment alliance is often early, while the patient is in crisis. Supportive elements, such as confrontation, clarification, support of defenses, and building on ego strengths, may be more prominent early in treatment. The therapist should also take into account state-related problems of organicity, physical illness, and affective vulnerability, all of which can lead to an inability to utilize interpretations. In their work on initiating treatment, Prochaska et al. (1992) discussed the stages in which patients develop awareness of their addiction problems. Focusing on motivational aspects of treatment and confronting denial of a need for help are essential elements in initiating treatment. Promoting identification as a recovering person can boost self-esteem and provide stability.

The psychodynamic psychotherapist needs to consider the effects of intoxication and withdrawal and the chronic organic effects of alcohol. However, during intoxication or withdrawal, there are patients for whom psychodynamic interpretations are indicated from the very outset of treatment, regardless of the stage of addiction. Interpretations may help the patient work through resistances to accepting help. They may also provide a meaningful explanation for destructive patterns, one that can inspire a wish for change.

Timing of interpretations is crucial. A patient who may need to project blame and responsibility for his or her actions onto substances early in recovery may later be able to accept responsibility for those actions. For example, one patient later admitted that having an affair, embezzling money, and being abusive were things he wanted to do anyway and that he used alcohol and cocaine abuse as an excuse. The individual may not be ready to take full responsibility for his or her actions early in abstinence, but over time, these issues can be explored and pointed out, denial can be worked through, and acceptance of responsibility can be achieved. Defenses may need to be supported at first, including denial of affect related to some of the losses. Confrontation should concentrate initially on denial surrounding addictive behaviors. Ultimately, clarifications, confrontations, and interpretations of denial, lying, splitting, and projective defenses in other areas need to be expanded. However, in selected cases, with repeated treatment failure, an initial intervention may require active, across-the-board confrontation and interpretation of inconsistencies and denial in order to help the patient accept a need for change. In patients with alexithymia or constricted affect, interpretations are aimed at increasing the patient's awareness of feeling states and helping him or her connect thoughts and feelings without the use of substances.

Session Frequency, Setting, and Goals

Psychodynamic psychotherapy with alcoholic patients is usually conducted one to two times per week, is often combined with group psychotherapy, and includes a parameter of abstinence and a long-term goal of sobriety. It can be done during an inpatient stay or in an organized outpatient or office practice, and it can be time-limited and focused or long-term.

It is foolhardy for psychotherapists to promise that once underlying causes of a "symptom of drinking" are dealt with, the patient will be able to return to controlled drinking. Similarly, it is unwise to promise that once a patient is fully treated with psychoanalytically oriented psychotherapy, he or she will never need additional help through 12-step programs or additional psychotherapy.

For most alcoholic individuals, shifting from dependence on a chemical such as alcohol to dependence on a therapist, group, or spiritual belief or involvement with anything human is a major step in the direction of growth. Although issues of dependence may be worked through partially, an ongoing positive identification with a therapist, a sponsor, and/or recovering friends may be a major positive outcome of treatment. Active dialogue with the patient and an attitude of empathic concern and sharing on the part of the therapist are optimal. Issues of termination of individual therapy or graduation from phases of treatment may bring earlier conflicts back to the surface and trigger relapse. The goal of psychodynamic treatment for addicted patients is to help them maintain abstinence, provide them with a richer understanding of and control of their inner lives, and reduce psychological triggers for relapse. Achieving this goal helps improve pa-

tient self-esteem, self-care, and affect regulation (Khantzian 1997).

General Technical Aspects of Treatment

Advances in object relations theory, ego psychology, and modern psychodynamic understanding of conflicts and affect regulation can be applied to addiction treatment. Psychodynamic principles are applied in conjunction with an understanding of the clinical exigencies of addiction treatment. Techniques need to be modified, especially those related to attaining and sustaining abstinence, and the effects of regression should be monitored carefully. However, well-established techniques and principles of brief and long-term psychodynamic treatment are generally maintained. The therapist listens for themes relating to the patient's intrapsychic conflicts, developmental impairments, and defenses, paying special attention to how they may relate to substance abuse and relapse potential.

The therapist has some important objectives: to obtain a careful developmental history of the patient, with attention to achievement of milestones of ego development; to evaluate temperament in the patient and significant caretakers; to examine the patient's capacity to identify with and to separate from important figures of identification, including parents, siblings, and admired peers; and to explore the patient's affect regulation, especially in relation to substance use. The therapist's tools include free association, "slips," and dreams, which are examined to find meaning in the unconscious derivatives of behavior (such as an unconscious wish to drink, expressed in a drunk dream).

Treatment Parameters

Treatment parameters for patients with addictions (parameters such as structure, clear boundaries, and abstinence) are similar to those used effectively in treating borderline personality disorder. Structure and boundaries help the patient reestablish control and self-regulation and help him or her express feelings verbally rather than by acting them out. The conventional practice of psychodynamic psychotherapy with limit-setting is generally helpful, although on rare occasions a more active approach may be needed. For example,

a therapist may need to mobilize a family to bring a suicidal alcoholic patient to the emergency room or to
the physician's office after a relapse.

While the therapist works through the patient's resistance and defenses, he or she should be aware of
how alcohol provides the patient with an escape, can
numb or facilitate expression, and can itself alter defensive operations, especially in terms of heightening
denial. The therapist should watch closely the interplay of ego function, feeling states, and chemical effects in the patient.

Most therapists in the addiction field believe that
abstinence is necessary for psychotherapy to be effective. Many think it is best to first develop a solid relationship with the patient and then aim for gradual
achievement of abstinence (Dodes and Khantzian
1998). We believe that although flexibility is often
needed for patients with severe psychiatric illness, psychiatric problems for the most part must be treated in
synchrony with the addiction disorder, and abstinence
is vital with this approach. Unfortunately, sometimes
continuation of psychodynamic psychotherapy can enable the addicted patient to continue substance use.
Psychodynamic psychotherapy can also raise conflicts
that may lead to worsening of the addiction, and thus
the treatment can be contraindicated. The following
case illustrates such a situation:

> A 37-year-old successful journalist was in psychoanal-
> ysis 5 days per week for a severe alcohol addiction.
> He frequently arrived at sessions intoxicated or
> missed them altogether. During years of analysis, his
> addiction to alcohol progressed. His family tried to
> convince him to see an addiction psychiatrist. He
> protested that he had a good relationship with his an-
> alyst, thought that he was being helped, and used this
> as a rationale to avoid effective treatment.

This patient achieved poor results in treatment because his psychoanalyst was not knowledgeable about
addictions and was adhering to a technique that was
wrong for the patient. The issue of abstinence was crucial here, but it was ignored.

Other Treatment Tools

A combination of psychodynamic approaches such as
clarification, interpretation, and genetic reconstruc-
tion may be used along with directive approaches such
as assertiveness training, social skills training, self-

efficacy groups, modeling, positive reinforcement, cognitive awareness, and suggestion. A sophisticated familiarity with typical problems that occur in alcoholic or
drug-abusing individuals and their families and the use
of psychoeducation about these issues help the therapist establish a positive alliance with his or her patient.
The literature on adult children of alcoholic patients
can aid the therapist's understanding and be used in
educating patients and their families. The following
case illustrates the use of combined approaches:

> A 42-year-old recovering alcoholic woman with panic
> attacks and agoraphobia had special problems when
> flying. Psychodynamic psychotherapy was useful
> when added to desensitization, relaxation therapy,
> exposure to flying, and closely monitored medica-
> tion for panic attacks (paroxetine and benzodiaze-
> pines 2 hours before airplane trips). The anxiety per-
> sisted at a significant level, frequently interfering
> with the patient's plans. Her fears of flying were re-
> lated to childhood conflicts about having to take
> planes to visit her father after her parents divorced.
> She was the "apple of her father's eye" and had clearly
> won out over her mother, although she had consid-
> erable guilt over her especially favored position. Her
> oedipal guilt persisted, contributing to difficulty in
> reaching orgasm with her husband and feelings of
> guilt about enjoying her sexuality. At the time of
> treatment, the flights she feared most were those re-
> lated to visits with her father and those involved in
> pleasure trips with her husband. Although none of
> the treatments totally allayed her fears, she was able
> to travel without drinking and was better able to un-
> derstand and cope with her fears of flying, having
> gained enhanced insight into the roots of her fears.
> She was increasingly allowing herself to enjoy grad-
> ual steps toward success without relapsing (see Bal-
> lenger 1999 for a discussion of anxiety disorder treat-
> ments).

Initial Focus and Phases of Treatment

The phases of intervention include initial screening,
evaluation and intervention, rehabilitation, and aftercare. The initial focus is often on conflicts related to
the acceptance of addiction as a problem, the patient's
reluctance to acknowledge dependence and the need
for treatment, and conflicts resulting from the complications of alcoholism (including the loss of relationships, health, and jobs) and from missing alcohol itself. As emphasized above in "Treatment Parameters,"
the first goal is abstinence.

More often than is usually the case in insight-oriented psychotherapy, the patient may initially be forced into the consultation by an employer, probation officer, family member, or physician. Especially when coercion has occurred, the therapist must make a considerable effort to develop trust and a working alliance with the patient. This is achieved through careful review of the patient's history and the ways in which addiction has interfered with work, family relationships, and other relationships or has caused legal problems, all of which have contributed to pain and the need to escape it. The therapist's integrity, adherence to confidentiality, and ability to be helpful all contribute to the establishment of trust.

The patient is helped to accept a diagnosis and to accept the need for help, which may lead to positive transference. These steps are similar to the first two AA steps, in which patients admit their powerlessness over alcohol and accept their need for help or acknowledge their own dependence needs, which in AA is called "accepting a higher power." A psychodynamic perspective may aid in the confrontation of denial and other defenses, and through interpretations patients achieve a deeper understanding of certain destructive patterns that have led to the present problem. It is especially challenging to help the patient acknowledge dependence needs that have been channeled into the addiction.

Therapy is a process in which a need for substances is shifted back into a need for people, including the therapist. Patients who abuse drugs often refuse to take medications because of fears of using them in compulsive ways, becoming dependent on drugs for relief, and becoming dependent on the therapist to obtain the medications. From early in treatment, issues of trust, dependence, separation, loss, disappointment, and truthfulness are frequent themes.

In the later stages, the focus of exploratory psychotherapy should not be imposed from the outside—that is, it should not be based on purely theoretical considerations. Rather, the focus should be on the most pressing issue of the moment that may relate to the patient's drinking: a particular conflict; a relationship with a family member or employer; a problem with self-esteem, self-destructiveness, or self-medication for panic; or other painful affects.

Other major themes include specific conflicts over assertiveness, handling of aggression, and issues of control and inhibition. The disinhibiting role of addiction, leading to risk-taking behavior (including increased sexual activity), may be an issue. Alternatively, alcohol may play a role in distancing the individual from sexual life or drinking may substitute for sexual activity.

Relapse

Patients should be observed carefully for drinking or drug use behavior. Laboratory tests may be useful, and meeting with family and other sources of collateral information may be essential to get a true picture before confronting patients who dissimulate.

As mentioned above in the section "Indications and Rationale for Psychodynamic Psychotherapy," psychodynamic therapy can help in relapse prevention. Consider the following case:

> A 47-year-old pediatric surgical nurse frequently relapsed in her addiction to diazepam on evenings after she had had to deal with families of children with disastrous surgical results. As a child, she had been traumatized by a younger sister's postoperative death due to a brain tumor. Her parents had tried to protect her by never discussing her sister's death, and she had always found this to be strange. Her relapses were triggered by unresolved conflicts and grief regarding her dead sister, whom she envied, loved, and, at self-destructive moments, wished to join in death. Her initial treatment plan involved detoxification, support, and an aim of abstinence. However, the effectiveness of relapse prevention was enhanced by psychodynamic treatment that helped her mourn her sister and eliminate an important trigger for relapse.

Acceptance of Self in Recovery

An important part of recovery is a change in self-awareness and self-perception. An enormous shift for the patient is the acceptance of a diagnosis of alcoholism as an illness. This entails not only shifting from a moral model (in which the patient sees himself or herself as weak, shameful, and bad for being alcoholic) but also being aware that a problem exists about which a great deal is known, that the problem is treatable, and that it does not have to lead to hopelessness and despair. Sometimes this awareness leads to reaction formation, in which the patient feels grateful for being alcoholic and turns a disability into an advantage. There may have been real advantages in terms of broadening of experience, overcoming a vulnerability, and developing a pride that can occur in any group that finds a way to overcome a stigma. The patient's feeling of relief after he or she is no longer experiencing the consequences of alcoholism and addiction often leads to a rebound after initial abstinence—a rebound that can approach euphoria. This euphoria is often followed by a letdown when awareness of the multitude of problems that the addiction caused occurs as denial wanes.

An Ego Psychological Model of Rehabilitation

Assessment of ego function needs to include a search for strengths, talents, and positive qualities that can be used to help the patient. All too often, therapists miss opportunities to enhance self-esteem in patients whose self-criticism leads them to overlook real and potential opportunities for growth. One way to combine positive insight with support is to help patients recall periods in which their values were in place and to give them hope for a return to a higher level of function. Even very damaged, impaired individuals in inner cities often have dreams in their lives that they have buried. Rekindled dreams can foster renewed hope and improve self-esteem. The stigma of the illness can also be lessened by discussing positive role models, such as Betty Ford, who have struggled with the same illness and have worked hard at recovery.

An ego psychological model can be applied to the biopsychosocial effects of addiction and to rehabilitation. Chemicals and psychosocial consequences have effects and may lead to regression and impairment of defenses, object relatedness, judgment, reality testing, and superego. It may take time and practice for good ego and superego function to return. The following case demonstrates recovery of function:

> A 47-year-old narcissistic man who had drunk heavily for 25 years had disuse atrophy of ego functions and was pushed to function better as part of rehabilitation. He thought of his wife only in terms of what she could do for him, as a part object or a need-satisfying object, and only with practice and with time sober could he relate to her in a more complex way as having needs of her own. He would idealize or devalue everyone and everything, and it took him a long time to relate to others as having both good and bad qualities. To develop friendships and break isolation, he had to practice relatedness in individual therapy, couples therapy, group therapy, and self-help groups.

The superego had been dissolved in chemicals for years, and it took external structure and parameters to gradually awaken the sleeping policeman within— that is, for the superego to start working again. The program requirements and the external norms of the groups helped him regain structure. His superego was initially inconsistent and vacillated from a lack of restraint and self-indulgence to a primitive punitive masochistic rigidity. Cognitive impairment, especially in the nondominant hemisphere functions of spatial and temporal relationships, was present and improved over time with abstinence.

The defenses initially encountered are usually the most primitive and include denial, rationalization, splitting, projection, and projective identification. With time and treatment, higher-level defenses such as intellectualization, reaction formation, repression, and sublimation may be more in the forefront. For example, instead of denying alcoholism and projecting poor self-esteem, a patient may feel grateful to have alcoholism and honored to have been part of a group that initially was perceived as stigmatizing. Denial of alcohol's harmful effects on the liver, which can be addressed through psychoeducation, can be replaced with curiosity and intellectualization about how liver damage occurs. Denial of losses related to addiction may be replaced with repression over time, after grieving over the losses has occurred.

Applications of Psychodynamics to Groups and Self-Help

The addition of group psychotherapy, AA, or NA is especially needed when individual therapy alone is not helping the patient maintain abstinence. Group treatments help diffuse some of the powerful negative transference that may be impossible to overcome early in treatment. Groups can focus on self-care, self-esteem, affect regulation, sharing, and exposure to feared social situations. They can provide social support and models for identification and coping skills, and they can help patients work through family problems. They can be targeted to specific additional diagnoses such as anxiety disorders or to specific subpopulations such as persons with chronic mental illness, those with medical complications, women, and adolescents. Groups can be homogeneous (e.g., recovering physicians with anxiety disorders) or heterogeneous (e.g., all patients in a detoxification unit).

Khantzian (1997) described a model of modified psychodynamic group therapy for substance-abusing patients involving self-care, self-esteem, and affect regulation. Together the patient and the individual therapist can look at how the patient projects feelings toward other AA, NA, or group members who, for example, remind the patient of his or her alcoholic relatives. Character flaws can be actively worked on, with immediate and multiple feedback from group members. If the individual therapist is also the group therapist, the individual work may be used to encourage the patient to try a new behavior in the group; conversely, conflicts observed in the group can be worked on individually.

Aspects of 12-step programs may readily lend themselves to incorporation into psychodynamic treatment. These aspects include accepting a diagnosis, accepting dependence needs, being aware that one cannot control drinking alone, taking a personal inventory (often discussed in terms of a higher power), working at change, dealing with sobriety one day at a time, accepting the structure of a treatment program, and enhancing self-esteem by helping others with the problem, thus living up to an ego ideal.

The 12-step programs provide education, auxiliary ego and superego support, and powerful role models for positive identification. Steps in AA that involve taking a personal inventory and making amends can be used in conjunction with the psychotherapeutic process of self-exploration and insight aimed at behavioral change. The addition of AA is especially helpful during periods of relapse and during periods when the therapist is unavailable because either the patient or the therapist is away. Because alcoholism and drug abuse are often chronic relapsing illnesses, both the patient and the therapist must be prepared for the possibility of a relapse. The therapist should be both nonjudgmental and unafraid of confrontation.

The Patient-Therapist Relationship

Many problems related to working with addicted patients concern the challenge of establishing a positive therapeutic relationship between the patient and the therapist. Frequently, errors in treatment occur because of negative feelings and attitudes that therapists have toward addicted patients. Typical mistakes include providing inadequate empathy or overly identifying with patients. A major source of countertransference is the uncritical acceptance by a clinician of roles projected onto him or her in the patient's transference.

In many cases, an understanding of the patient's specific transference that may either evoke countertransference problems or prevent compliance with treatment may be essential for good management and a successful alliance with the patient. Typical transference may result from growing up in a household in which the parents were addicted, inconsistent, and either overly harsh or indulgent. Children of alcoholic parents frequently have authority problems and will often trust siblings, peers, and other alcoholic individuals more readily than they will trust teachers, nurses, doctors, or police. When a patient describes a therapist as cold, neglectful, uninvolved, or detached, this may be transference from a parent who fits this description and may lead the therapist to behave in this way.

It is helpful for the therapist to be able to interpret negative transference and to know how to manage and appropriately use therapist countertransference. Alcoholic patients frequently will try to evoke feelings of fear, anger, and despair in their therapists and will reenact relationships with alcoholic parents, siblings, and spouses through the transference. They may project critical attitudes onto the therapist and keep secrets out of fear that the therapist will respond like a parent. When the patient feels that the therapist is like a parent, sibling, or friend, this feeling may have been evoked for specific reasons. The greater the therapist's awareness of what is happening, the more this issue can be brought into the treatment in a constructive way.

A second major source of countertransference in treating addicted patients is a therapist's weak knowledge base about addiction and its treatment. The more knowledgeable the therapist is about addiction psychiatry and about the patient, the less likely the therapist is to project his or her own problems onto the patient. Attitudinal problems on the part of the therapist can be reduced by good training and the experience of having worked through issues related to stigma. The more the therapist is in command of a treatment armamentarium, the less frightened he or she is in the face of what can be a dreadful disease. Ultimately, patients are the best teachers. By listening carefully, the therapist can learn about the addictive experience, addictive practices, and the street language of addiction.

A third source of countertransference is based on a therapist's mostly unconscious transference, related to his or her past or present problems. Transference may relate to the therapist's attitudes about substances; present or past problems with addiction; or experience with a parent, spouse, or child with a substance use problem. The therapist's own envy, fear, hopes, and needs can adversely affect his or her prescribing practices and lead to overinvolvement, avoidance, hopelessness, jealousy, and burnout. Some clinicians who have chosen to work in the addiction field because of their wish to overcome personal problems related to addictions may have special difficulty dealing with patients' problems if they have not worked out their own. Frequent mistakes include excessive self-revelation of personal problems and a tendency not to see the specifics of patients' problems clearly because of a need to see everyone as similar to the self. A recovering clinician might consider a patient's problem minor compared with his or her own. Alternatively, some clinicians see every problem only in relation to addictive problems. This results in misdiagnosis and overdiagnosis. One extreme of overinvolvement is sexual or aggressive acting out with a vulnerable substance-abusing patient; this has disastrous consequences for both patient and therapist.

Seeking out second opinions from or supervision by experienced practitioners is advisable when working with difficult patients. Thorough self-exploration by the therapist in personal therapy also helps. Clinicians with maturity, a good support system, and a secure personal life are better protected against countertransference problems. Additional protection is given by working in a team: team members can point out one another's blind spots and assist in improving one another's technique. Feedback from patients and their families can be another means of supervision for the clinician who listens carefully. A wise clinician admits his or her mistakes, learns from them, and tries to avoid future mistakes (Committee on Alcoholism and Addictions 1998).

Myths and Pitfalls to Avoid in Psychodynamic Psychotherapy

Myths

- One can first develop a therapeutic relationship and then gradually wean the patient off substances.

- Substance use will disappear with understanding.
- Once conflicts have been resolved, the patient can safely return to drinking.
- If the problem is narcotic addiction, alcohol is a safer and legal alternative.
- Addiction is always a symptom, not a primary problem.

Pitfalls

- Believing the patient's explanation for drinking, without awareness of rationalization and a patient's need to justify his or her behavior
- Not checking out the patient's story
- Conducting treatment as if psychodynamic interpretations were "golden" and other interventions less valuable. Treatment and sequence should be selected on the basis of the patient's needs.
- Not having a healthy respect for the patient's dependence needs, and having too high expectations for resolving these needs. It is better for the patient to depend on therapists or on AA than on substances, and an endless relationship with AA is a desirable goal—not a compromise of a therapist's goal of self-reliance on the patient's part.
- Being overinvolved or overly distant. Therapists in recovery themselves sometimes have blind spots or may share with the patient more than the patient needs to know.
- Having a bias toward one or another form of treatment and lacking theoretical and practical flexibility. Even moderate biases of this type can be a disservice to the patient.

Treatment Outcome Research

The state of the art in addiction treatment involves being aware of the results of treatment outcome studies but also selecting a combination of treatments that takes into account current knowledge and patient characteristics. Treatment recommendations depend on a wide range of considerations, and trial results are only one factor. The American Psychiatric Association (1995) developed practice guidelines for the treatment of substance use disorders based on reviews of the literature on treatment and outcomes. These guidelines recommend individualizing treatment planning and include the treatment of comorbid conditions. Woody et al. (1990) showed meaningful differences in efficacy between supportive-expressive psychotherapy and cognitive-behavioral therapy in methadone-maintained patients. Carroll et al. (1994) pointed out that there is a delayed emergence of effects of psychotherapy after cessation of short-term treatments in cocaine-dependent patients. O'Malley et al. (1996) compared psychotherapy with and without naltrexone therapy in alcoholic patients and found that the combined treatment had favorable results.

With managed care entering the arena of health care, studies of cost-effectiveness and outcomes are becoming increasingly important. Humphreys and Moos (1996) found reduced substance-related health care costs in a study involving veterans participating in AA. O'Brien (1997a) compared specific treatment approaches for addictive disorders with other chronic disorders such as diabetes and asthma, and O'Brien (1997b) also pointed to studies that have shown a cost saving of $4–$12 for every dollar spent on substance abuse treatment.

It is too early in addiction outcome research to make hard-and-fast recommendations regarding treatments to be used. Treatment guidelines and the treatment outcome studies discussed in this volume provide useful information but are not definitive instructions to clinicians. Although clinicians agree on some points (e.g., the usefulness of abstinence as a goal, pharmacological treatment of comorbid disorders such as panic attacks, the value of adding education and cognitive and behavioral approaches), the value of 12-step programs and psychodynamic psychotherapy has not been strongly proved in controlled studies, although each treatment has a commonsense rationale. Where definite answers are still lacking, clinicians need to be aware of a growing literature of outcome study findings, of the methodological problems involved in conducting good studies, and of the problems in reliability and validity in applying these results. Uncertainties about the exact value of psychodynamic and combined treatments should not deter clinicians from using what has seemed useful, especially with patients who have specific favorable characteristics such as motivation and capacity for insight and who have destructive patterns amenable to interpretation. When definitive conclusions about the effectiveness of treatment components have been drawn, targeting of treatment will improve.

Neurobiology

Psychodynamics integrated with neurobiological models of addiction provide a deeper understanding of the patient, and researchers are clarifying the biological factors that appear to modulate both the predisposition to addiction to illicit drugs and the risk of relapse; these factors include genetic polymorphisms and neuroendocrine pathways (including the mesolimbic system and the ventral tegmental area) that modulate the effects of substances of abuse (Kreek 2000).

There is a growing body of evidence (e.g., as demonstrated by neuroimaging studies) that psychotherapy influences biological activity in the brain. Psychological factors and a psychodynamic perspective clearly must be integrated with current scientific understanding of brain mechanisms in relation to the etiology and treatment of addictions. Further knowledge about the relation of brain mechanisms to the psyche will advance psychoanalytic understanding (Leshner 1997).

Greater understanding of the process and psychology of addiction is achieved through psychodynamic psychotherapy. This understanding may add to the development of treatment methods, such as improved cognitive-behavioral techniques (A. T. Beck et al. 1993), that take into account more complex human motivating factors and that may be tailored specifically to an individual's conflicts and defenses. In a patient with a dual diagnosis (a term most commonly used to indicate addiction plus another mental illness), an integrated approach geared toward treating both the mental illness and substance abuse yields better results. A psychodynamic understanding frequently enhances the treatment of anxiety disorders, depression, and personality disorders occurring with substance abuse.

Implications for Research

New research is needed to identify the patients for whom psychodynamic treatment is appropriate. Specifically, investigators must determine which Axis I or Axis II disorders, which age group, what timing, and which patient characteristics are best suited for this approach, and they must determine which psychodynamic interventions should be used, and combined with what other treatments. It is hard to find good databases of what is often clinically subjective material. Premature closure on any of these questions because of the challenge and expense of studying the particular area may lead to overly narrow, poorer-quality treatment approaches. It will take time, the pooling of large amounts of clinical data, and the collaboration of many clinician researchers to obtain these answers. Initially, nonrandomized, noncontrolled, and descriptive studies will be needed. Ultimately, randomized studies will best exclude even moderate biases, and with large samples, it will be possible to correct for both false-positive and false-negative results.

Conclusion

Psychodynamic theory can play an important role in enriching and informing substance abuse treatment and improving the therapeutic relationship. However, rigid application of psychoanalytic technique is inappropriate in substance abuse treatment and can be counterproductive. Application of psychodynamic understanding—including attending to the unconscious, child development, ego function, affect regulation, and efforts to enhance self-esteem and to deal with shame and other narcissistic vulnerability—widens the range of patients that can be treated.

Greater academic and scientific attention is needed if progress is to be made in this area of the addictions. Currently, definitive outcome studies of psychodynamic psychotherapy in substance-abusing patients are rare. A rich descriptive clinical experience in this area will bring improved understanding of addicted patients in both theoretical and practical settings.

References

Abraham K: The psychological relation between sexuality and alcoholism (1908), in Selected Papers of Karl Abraham. New York, Basic Books, 1960, pp 80–89

Alterman AI, O'Brien CP, McLellan AT, et al: Effectiveness and costs of inpatient versus day hospital cocaine rehabilitation. J Nerv Ment Dis 182:157–163, 1994

American Psychiatric Association: Practice guideline for the treatment of patients with substance use disorders: alcohol, cocaine, opioids. Am J Psychiatry 152:5–59, 1995

Ballenger JC: Current treatments of the anxiety disorders in adults. Biol Psychiatry 46:1579–1594, 1999

Bean-Bayog M: Alcoholism as a cause of psychopathology. Hosp Community Psychiatry 39:352–354, 1988

Beck AT, Wright FD, Newman CF, et al: Cognitive Therapy of Substance Abuse. New York, Guilford, 1993

Beck JS, Liese BS: Cognitive therapy for substance abuse, in Clinical Textbook of Addictive Disorders, 2nd Edition. Edited by Frances RJ, Miller SI. New York, Guilford, 1998, pp 547–574

Bleuler E: Alcohol and the neuroses (1911), in Jahrbuch für psychoanalytische und psychopathologische Forschungen; Jahrbuch der Psychoanalyse 3:848. Abstracted by Blungart L. Psychoanal Rev 8:443–444, 1921

Carroll KM, Rounsaville BJ, Nich C, et al: One-year follow-up of psychotherapy and pharmacotherapy for cocaine dependence: delayed emergence of psychotherapy effects. Arch Gen Psychiatry 51:989–997, 1994

Cloninger CR: A systematic method for clinical description and classification of personality variants: a proposal. Arch Gen Psychiatry 44:573–588, 1987

Committee on Alcoholism and Addictions, Group for the Advancement of Psychiatry: Addiction Treatment: Avoiding Pitfalls—A Case Approach (Report/Group for the Advancement of Psychiatry, no 142). Washington, DC, American Psychiatric Press, 1998

Dodes LM: The psychology of combining dynamic psychotherapy and Alcoholics Anonymous. Bull Menninger Clin 52:283–293, 1988

Dodes LM: Compulsion and addiction. J Am Psychoanal Assoc 44:815–835, 1996

Dodes LM, Khantzian EJ: Individual psychodynamic psychotherapy, in Clinical Textbook of Addictive Disorders, 2nd Edition. Edited by Frances RJ, Miller SI. New York, Guilford, 1998, pp 479–496

DuPont RL: Addiction: a new paradigm. Bull Menninger Clin 62:231–242, 1998

Ferenczi S: On the part played by homosexuality in the pathogenesis of paranoia (1912), in First Contributions to Psycho-analysis. Boston, MA, Richard G Badger, 1916, pp 154–184

Frances RJ, Borg L: The treatment of anxiety in patients with alcoholism. J Clin Psychiatry 54 (suppl):37–43, 1993

Frances RJ, Khantzian EJ, Tamerin JS: Psychodynamic psychotherapy, in Treatments of Psychiatric Disorders: A Task Force Report of the American Psychiatric Association, Vol 2. Washington, DC, American Psychiatric Association, 1989, pp 1103–1111

Freud S: Three essays on the theory of sexuality (1905), in The Standard Edition of the Complete Psychological Works of Sigmund Freud, Vol 7. Translated and edited by Strachey J. London, Hogarth Press, 1953, pp 125–245

Freud S: Civilization and Its Discontents (1930). New York, WW Norton, 1964

Freud S, Ferenczi S: The Correspondence of Sigmund Freud and Sándor Ferenczi, Vol 1: 1908–1914. Translated by Hoffer PT. Edited by Brabant E, Falzeder E, Giampieri-Deutsch P. Cambridge, MA, Belknap Press of Harvard University Press, 1993

Galanter M: Healing through social and spiritual affiliation. Psychiatr Serv 53:1072–1074, 2002

Glover E: On the etiology of drug addiction (1932), in Selected Papers on Psycho-analysis, Vol 1: On the Early Development of Mind. New York, International Universities Press, 1956, pp 187–215

Humphreys K, Moos RH: Reduced substance-abuse-related health care costs among voluntary participants in Alcoholics Anonymous. Psychiatr Serv 47:709–713, 1996

Keller LE: Addiction as a form of perversion. Bull Menninger Clin 56:221–231, 1992

Kernberg OF: Transference regression and psychoanalytic technique with infantile personalities. Int J Psychoanal 72:189–200, 1991

Kessler RC, Crum RM, Warner LA, et al: Lifetime co-occurrence of DSM-III-R alcohol abuse and dependence with other psychiatric disorders in the National Comorbidity Survey. Arch Gen Psychiatry 54:313–321, 1997

Khantzian EJ: The self medication hypothesis of substance use disorders: a reconsideration and recent applications. Harv Rev Psychiatry 4:231–244, 1997

Klerman GL, Weissman MM, Rounsaville BH, et al: The Theory and Practice of Interpersonal Psychotherapy for Depression. New York, Basic Books, 1984

Kohut H, Wolf ES: The disorders of the self and their treatment: an outline. Int J Psychoanal 59:413–425, 1978

Koob GF, Le Moal M: Drug abuse: hedonic homeostatic dysregulation. Science 278:52–58, 1997

Kreek MJ: Opiates, opioids, SNP's and the addictions: Nathan B. Eddy Memorial Award for Lifetime Excellence in Drug Abuse Research lecture, in Problems of Drug Dependence, 1999 (National Institute on Drug Abuse Research Monograph 180; DHHS Publ No ADM-00-4737). Edited by Harris LS. Rockville, MD, National Institute on Drug Abuse, 2000, pp 3–22

Kreek MJ, Koob GF: Drug dependence: stress and dysregulation of brain reward pathways. Drug Alcohol Depend 51:23–47, 1998

Krystal H: Alexithymia and the effectiveness of psychoanalytic treatment. Int J Psychoanal Psychother 9:353–378, 1982–1983

Kushner MA, Sher KJ, Bertman BD: The relation between alcohol problems and anxiety disorders. Am J Psychiatry 147:685–695, 1990

Langeland W, Draijer N, van den Brink W: Trauma and dissociation in treatment-seeking alcoholics: towards a resolution of inconsistent findings. Compr Psychiatry 43:195–203, 2002

Leshner A: Addiction is a brain disease, and it matters. Science 278:45–47, 1997

Lewis HB: Shame and the narcissistic personality, in The Many Faces of Shame. Edited by Nathanson DL. New York, Guilford, 1987, pp 93–132

Lorand J: A summary of psychoanalytic literature on problems of alcoholism. Yearbook of Psychoanalysis 1:359–378, 1948

Luborsky L: Principles of Psychoanalytic Psychotherapy: A Manual for Supportive-Expressive Treatment. New York, Basic Books, 1984

Mahler M, Pine R, Bergman A: The Psychological Birth of the Human Infant: Symbiosis and Individuation. New York, Basic Books, 1975

Manji HK, Moore GJ, Chen G: Clinical and preclinical evidence for the neurotrophic effects of mood stabilizers: implications for the pathophysiology and treatment of manic-depressive illness. Biol Psychiatry 48:740–754, 2000

McDougall J: The "dis-affected" patient: reflections on affect pathology. Psychoanal Q 53:386–409, 1984

Meissner WW: Psychotherapy and the Paranoid Process. New York, Jason Aronson, 1986

Menninger KA: Man Against Himself. New York, Harcourt Brace, 1938

Milkman H, Frosch WA: On the preferential abuse of heroin and amphetamine. J Nerv Ment Dis 156:242–248, 1973

O'Brien CP: Progress in the science of addiction (editorial). Am J Psychiatry 154:1195–1197, 1997a

O'Brien CP: A range of research-based pharmacotherapies for addiction. Science 278:66–69, 1997b

O'Malley SS, Jaffe AJ, Chang G, et al: Six-month follow-up of naltrexone and psychotherapy for alcohol dependence. Arch Gen Psychiatry 53:217–224, 1996

Perry S, Cooper A, Michels R: The psychodynamic formulation: its purpose, structure, and clinical application. Am J Psychiatry 144:543–550, 1987

Pfefferbaum B, Doughty DE: Increased alcohol use in a treatment sample of Oklahoma City bombing victims. Psychiatry 64:296–303, 2001

Prochaska JO, DiClemente CC, Norcross JC: In search of how people change: applications to addictive behaviors. Am Psychol 47:1102–1114, 1992

Rado S: The psychoanalysis of pharmacothymia (drug addiction). J Subst Abuse Treat 1:59–68, 1984

Silber A: Rationale for the technique of psychotherapy with alcoholics. Int J Psychoanal Psychother 3:28–47, 1974

Vaillant GE: The Natural History of Alcoholism Revisited. Cambridge, MA, Harvard University Press, 1995, pp 362–373

Volkow ND, Wang GJ, Fischman MW, et al: Relationship between subjective effects of cocaine and dopamine transporter occupancy. Nature 386:827–830, 1997

Wieder H, Kaplan EH: Drug use in adolescents. Psychoanal Study Child 24:399–431, 1969

Woody GE, McLellan AT, Luborsky L, et al: Psychotherapy for substance abuse. Psychiatr Clin North Am 9:547–562, 1986

Woody G[E], Luborsky L, McLellan AT, et al: Corrections and revised analyses for psychotherapy in methadone maintenance patients (letter). Arch Gen Psychiatry 47:788–789, 1990

Wurmser L: The role of superego conflicts in substance abuse and their treatment. Int J Psychoanal Psychother 10:227–258, 1984

Network Therapy

Marc Galanter, M.D.

In this chapter, I define aspects of addiction relevant to ambulatory therapy and describe a treatment technique developed to help addicted patients achieve recovery. Network therapy (Galanter 1999) can be defined as a multimodal approach to rehabilitation in which specific family members and friends are enlisted to provide ongoing support and promote attitude change. The goal of this approach is the prompt achievement of abstinence, with relapse prevention and the development of a drug-free adaptation. Network members are part of the therapist's working team and are not recipients of treatment.

Most mental health professionals are ill prepared to help alcoholic or drug-abusing patients achieve recovery, even though addicted patients and their families regularly turn to them for help. Furthermore, few alcoholic or drug-addicted individuals are willing to go to 12-step programs such as Alcoholics Anonymous (AA) until they have endured their illness for a long time, and most drop out before becoming involved. A pointed question inevitably arises: How can health care providers engage and treat these troubled addicted individuals more effectively?

In recent years, length of stay in inpatient rehabilitation facilities for substance-abusing patients has become increasingly limited. Programs at these facilities have been useful in that they terminate patients' access to drugs and create a safe environment for detoxification and education. Nonetheless, family and social ties are often disrupted while patients are hospitalized. The programs also do not allow patients to deal with drinking cues in the home environment. The practitioner should therefore attempt to support a patient's rehabilitation by means of the social ties available in his or her own community.

An individual's network enhances the effectiveness of ambulatory therapy and includes his or her spouse, friends, and/or family of origin. Components of the network are parts of the natural support system that usually operates without professional involvement, and if these components can be brought to act in concert, the network can serve as a therapeutic device. The network can complement individual or group therapy and AA.

Addressing Relapse and Loss of Control

To develop a social therapy involving network support, one must first define the target problem clearly and then consider the effect of the network on the problem. From a clinician's perspective, the problems of *relapse* and *loss of control,* embodied in the third and fourth criteria for substance dependence in DSM-IV-TR (American Psychiatric Association 2000), are central to the difficulty in treating addiction. Because addicted patients are typically under pressure to relapse, they are unlikely to attend treatment sessions regularly, and they tend to drop out of treatment precipitously. *Loss of control* has been used to describe an addicted individual's inability to reliably limit consumption once an initial dose is taken.

A Conditioning Model

These clinical phenomena are generally described anecdotally but can also be explained mechanistically, using the model of conditioned withdrawal, which relates the psychopharmacology of dependence-producing drugs to the behaviors they produce. Wikler (1973), an early investigator of addiction pharmacology, developed this model to explain the spontaneous appearance of drug craving and relapse. He pointed out that drugs of dependence typically produce compensatory responses in the central nervous system at the same time that their direct pharmacological effects are felt, and these compensatory effects partly counter the drugs' direct actions. Thus, when an opioid antagonist is administered to addicted subjects who are maintained on morphine, latent withdrawal phenomena are unmasked. Similar compensatory effects are observed in alcoholic subjects maintained on alcohol, who, while still clinically intoxicated, manifest evoked response patterns characteristic of withdrawal (Begleiter and Porjesz 1979).

O'Brien et al. (1977) found that addicted subjects could be conditioned to experience opioid withdrawal responses to neutral stimuli such as sound and odor. This conditioning, produced in a laboratory setting, lent support to Wikler's hypothesis. Furthermore, for the alcoholic subject, the alcohol dose itself can serve as a conditioned stimulus for enhancing craving, as can the appropriate drinking context.

Clinical interviews show that withdrawal feelings, and hence craving, can be elicited by cues previously associated with the addicted subject's use of the drug. Hence, exposure to the smell of liquor in a bar can precipitate the "need" to drink, and seeing the "works" for injecting heroin, or going by a "shooting gallery," can lead a heroin-addicted individual to relapse.

The conditioned stimulus of a drug or an environmental cue, or even the affective state regularly associated with the drug, can lead directly to the behavioral response before the addicted individual consciously experiences withdrawal feelings. The individual may automatically seek out drugs on experiencing anxiety, depression, or narcissistic injury, all of which may have become conditioned stimuli.

Often, modulations of mood are the conditioned stimuli for drug seeking, and the substance-abusing individual can become vulnerable to relapse through reflexive response to a specific affective state. Khantzian (1985) described such phenomena clinically as *self-medication.* Such mood-related cues, however, are not necessarily mentioned spontaneously by the patient in conventional therapy, because the triggering feeling may not be associated with a memorable event and the drug use may avert memorable distress.

More dramatic is the phenomenon of *affect regression,* which Wurmser (1977) observed among addicted patients who were studied in a psychoanalytic context. He pointed out that when addicted subjects sustain narcissistic injury, they are prone to a precipitous collapse of ego defenses, followed by intense and unmanageable affective flooding. In the face of such vulnerability, these subjects handle stress poorly and may turn to drugs for relief. This vulnerability can be considered in light of the model of conditioned withdrawal, whereby drug seeking can become an immediate reflexive response to stress, undermining the stability and effectiveness of a patient's coping mechanisms. Drug seeking can occur quite suddenly in patients who have long associated drug use with their attempts to cope with stress, as illustrated in the following case:

> In the course of therapy, an alcoholic lawyer found that his drinking had often been precipitated by situations that threatened his self-esteem. After 6 months of sobriety, he had a relapse that was later examined in a session as follows: immediately before his relapse, he had received an erroneous report that his share of the partnership's profits would be cut back, which he took to be evidence of failure. He reported feeling humiliated and then very anxious. Without weighing the consequences, he went out and purchased a bottle of liquor, returned to his office, and began drinking. He said that he had not thought to control this behavior at the time.

This model helps to explain why relapse is such a frequent and unanticipated aspect of addiction treatment. Exposure to conditioned cues, ones that were repeatedly associated with drug use, can precipitate reflexive drug craving during the course of therapy, and such cue exposure can also initiate a sequence of conditioned behaviors that lead addicted individuals to relapse unwittingly into drug use.

Loss of control can be the product of conditioned withdrawal. The sensations associated with ingestion of an addictive drug, such as the odor of alcohol or the euphoria produced by opioids, are temporally associated with the pharmacological elicitation of a compensatory response to that drug and can later produce drug-seeking behavior. For this reason, the first drink can serve as a conditioned cue for further drinking. These phenomena lead to relapse in patients who have very limited capacities to control consumption once a single dose of drug has been taken.

Dealing With the Issue of Relapse

What minimally noxious aversive stimuli are specific for the conditioned stimuli associated with drug craving and can thus provide a maximally useful learning experience? To answer this question, one may look at Wikler's (1971) initial conception of the implications of his conditioning theory:

> The user would become entangled in an interlocking web of self-perpetuating reinforcers, which perhaps explain the persistence of drug abuse, despite disastrous consequences for the user, and his imperviousness to psychotherapy which does not take such conditioning factors into account, because neither the subject nor the therapist is aware of their existence. (p. 611)

Since Wikler's time, specific techniques have been developed to overcome this problem. The model of conditioned drug-seeking has been applied in training patients to recognize drug-related cues and avert relapse. Annis (1986), for example, used a self-report schedule to assist patients in identifying the cues, situations, and moods most likely to lead to alcohol craving. Marlatt evolved the approach he described as *relapse prevention* (Marlatt and Gordon 1985), in which patients are taught strategies for avoiding the consequences of the alcohol-related cues they have identified, and a similar approach has been used to extinguish cocaine craving through cue exposure in a clinical laboratory (Childress et al. 1988).

These approaches can be introduced as part of a single-modality behavioral regimen, but they also can be used in expressive or family-oriented psychotherapy. By means of *cognitive labeling*, drinking cues can be associated with readily identified guideposts to aid the patient in consciously averting the consequences of prior conditioning. Similarly, *guided recall* can be used to explore the sequence of antecedents of given episodes of craving or drinking "slips" that were not previously clear to a patient. These approaches can be applied concomitantly with an examination of general adaptive problems in exploratory therapy.

A problem can occur, however, when such an approach is applied. If a patient is committed to becoming abstinent from an addictive drug but is in jeopardy of making occasional slips, cognitive labeling can facilitate consolidation of an abstinent adaptation. However, such an approach is less valuable in the context of inadequate motivation for abstinence, fragile social supports, or compulsive substance abuse unmanageable by the patient in his or her usual social settings. Hospitalization or replacement therapy (e.g., methadone therapy) may be necessary in these situations because ambulatory stabilization through psychotherapeutic support is often not feasible. Under any circumstances, cognitive labeling is an adjunct to psychotherapy and not a replacement for group supports such as AA, family counseling, or community programs.

Use of Network Therapy

Having examined the need for behavioral techniques in the ongoing treatment of addiction, I now consider the model of network therapy for addiction. This model enhances the effectiveness of office-based individual therapy by drawing on the recent advances described in the preceding section.

Network therapy has been validated in general terms. In an evaluation of family treatment for alcohol problems, it was concluded that "research data support superior outcomes for family involved treatment, enough so that the modal approach should involve family members and carefully planned interventions" (Institute of Medicine 1990, p. 84). Indeed, the idea of the therapist intervening with the patient's family and friends to start treatment was introduced by Johnson (1986) as one of the early ambulatory techniques in the addiction field. More broadly, greater social support for patients contributes to positive outcome in addiction.

In a clinical trial involving 60 patients, network therapy was associated with a positive outcome (Galanter

1993). Patients attended one session of network therapy per week for the first month; subsequent sessions were less frequent, typically every other month after 1 year of ambulatory care. Individual therapy was carried out concomitantly once or twice a week. On average, networks had 2.3 members, and the most frequent participants were mates, peers, parents, or siblings.

The Couple as a Network

A cohabiting couple serves as an example of how natural affiliative ties can be used to develop a network to support the patient in rehabilitation. Couples therapy for addiction has been described in both ambulatory and inpatient settings, and a favorable marital adjustment is associated with a diminished likelihood of dropping out and with a positive overall outcome (McCrady et al. 1986).

In controlled trials, disulfiram has produced relatively little benefit overall when prescribed for patients to take on their own. This agent is effective only if ingested as instructed, typically daily. Alcoholic patients who forget to take required doses will likely resume drinking in time. Such forgetting often reflects initiation of a sequence of conditioned drug-seeking behaviors.

Although patient characteristics have not been shown to predict compliance with a disulfiram treatment regimen, changes in the format of patient management have been beneficial. For example, involvement of a spouse in observing the patient's consumption of disulfiram considerably improves outcome because such involvement introduces a system of monitoring (Azrin et al. 1982). Patients alerted to take disulfiram each morning by this external reminder are less likely to experience conditioned drug-seeking when exposed to addictive cues and are more likely to comply with the dosing regimen on subsequent days.

The technique also helps clearly define the roles in therapy of both the alcoholic patient and his or her spouse. The spouse does not need to monitor drinking behaviors he or she cannot control, nor does the spouse actively remind the alcoholic patient to take each disulfiram dose. The spouse merely notifies the therapist if he or she does not observe the pill being ingested on a given day. Decisions concerning management of compliance are then allocated to the therapist, thereby preventing entanglement of the couple in a dispute over the patient's attitude and the possibility of drinking in secret.

Other behavioral devices demonstrated to improve outcome can be incorporated into this couples therapy format. For example, setting the first appointment as soon as possible after an initial telephone contact can improve outcome by undercutting the possibility of early loss of motivation. Spouses can also be engaged in history taking at the outset of treatment, to minimize introduction of denial into the patient's presentation of his or her illness. The initiation of treatment with such a regimen is illustrated in the following case:

> A 39-year-old alcoholic man was referred for treatment. The psychiatrist initially engaged both the patient and his wife in an exchange on the telephone, so that all three could plan for the patient to remain abstinent on the day of the first session. They agreed that the wife would meet the patient at his office at the end of the workday on the way to the appointment. This would ensure that cues presented by the patient's friends going out for a drink after work would not lead him to drink. In the session, an initial history was obtained from both the patient and his wife, an approach that allowed the wife to expand on ill consequences of the patient's drinking, thereby avoiding minimization of the problem by the patient. A review of the patient's medical status revealed no evidence of relevant organ damage, and the option of initiating treatment with disulfiram at that time was discussed. The patient, with encouragement from his wife, agreed to take his first dose that day and to continue under her observation. Subsequent sessions with the couple were dedicated to dealing with implementation of this plan, and concurrent individual therapy was initiated.

The Network's Membership

Networks generally consist of a number of members. Once the patient has come for an appointment, establishment of a network is undertaken with active collaboration between the patient and the therapist. The two, aided by those parties who join the network initially, must search for the right balance of members. The therapist, however, must carefully promote the choice of appropriate network members, just as the platoon leader selects those who will go into combat. The network will be crucial in determining the balance of the therapy. This process is not without problems, and the therapist must think strategically of the interactions that may occur among network members. The following case illustrates the nature of the therapist's task:

A 25-year-old graduate student had been abusing drugs since high school, in part drawing on funds from his affluent family, who lived in a remote city. At two points in the process of establishing his support network, the reactions of his live-in girlfriend were particularly important. They both agreed to bring in his 19-year-old sister, a freshman at a nearby college. He then mentioned a "friend" of his, a woman whom he had apparently found attractive, even though there was no history of an overt romantic involvement. The expression on his girlfriend's face suggested that she was uncomfortable with this option. The therapist temporarily put aside the idea of the friend and moved on to evaluating the patient's uncle. Initially, the patient was reluctant to include him in the network because he perceived the uncle as a potentially disapproving representative of the parental generation. The therapist and the girlfriend nonetheless encouraged him to accept the uncle as a network member to round out the range of relationships within the group. The uncle was caring and supportive, particularly after he was helped to understand the nature of the addictive process.

The Network's Task

The therapist's relationship to the network is one of a task-oriented team leader rather than of a family therapist oriented toward restructuring relationships. The network is established to implement a straightforward task, that of aiding the therapist to sustain the patient's abstinence. The network must be directed with the same clarity of purpose that a task force is directed in any effective organization. Competing and alternative goals must be suppressed or at least prevented from interfering with the primary task.

Unlike family members involved in traditional family therapy, network members are not led to expect symptom relief or self-realization for themselves. This approach prevents development of competing goals for the network's meetings. It also protects members from having their own motives scrutinized and thereby supports their continuing involvement without the threat of an assault on their psychological defenses. Because network members have kindly volunteered to participate, their motives must not be impugned. Their constructive behavior should be commended. Network members should be acknowledged for the contribution they are making to the therapy. Network members have a counterproductive tendency to minimize the value of their contribution. The network must therefore be structured as an effective working group with good morale. This approach is illustrated below:

A 45-year-old single woman served as an executive in a large family-held business, except when her alcohol problem led her into protracted binges. Her father, brother, and sister were prepared to banish her from the business but decided first to seek consultation. The father was a domineering figure who intruded in all aspects of the business, evoking angry outbursts from his children. The children typically reacted with petulance, provoking him in return. The situation came to a head 2 months into treatment, when the patient's siblings angrily petitioned the therapist to exclude the father from the network. This presented a problem because the father's control over the business made his involvement important in securing the patient's compliance. Relapse by the patient was still a real possibility. The father implied that he might compromise his son's role in the family business. The father's potentially coercive role, however, was an issue that the group could not deal with easily. The therapist supported the father's membership in the group, pointing out the constructive role he had played in getting the therapy started. It was clear to the therapist that the father could not deal with a situation in which he was not accorded sufficient respect and that there was no place in this network for addressing the father's character pathology directly. The children became less provocative as the group responded to the therapist's pleas for civil behavior.

Some Specific Techniques

Yalom (1974) described anxiety-reducing tactics that he used in therapy groups with alcoholic patients to avert disruptions and promote cohesiveness. These tactics included setting an agenda for the session and using instruction. In the network format, a cognitive framework can be achieved in each session by starting out with the patient recounting events related to cue exposure or substance use since the last meeting. Network members are then expected to comment on this report; this ensures that all members are engaged in a mutual task with correct, shared information. Their reactions to the patient's report are also addressed. Here is one example of how this was done:

An alcoholic man began one of his early network sessions by reporting a minor lapse into drinking. His report was disrupted by an angry outburst from his older sister. She said that she had "had it up to here" with his frequent unfulfilled promises of sobriety. The psychiatrist addressed this source of conflict by explaining in a didactic manner how behavioral cues affect vulnerability to relapse. This didactic approach was adopted to deal with the assumption that relapse is easily controlled and to relieve consequent resentment. The psychiatrist then led members in planning concretely with the patient how he might avoid further drinking cues in the period preceding their next conjoint session.

Patients undergoing detoxification from depressant medication taken for long periods often experience considerable anxiety, even when dose reduction is gradual. The expectation of distress, coupled with conditioned withdrawal phenomena, may cause patients to balk at completing a detoxification regimen. In individual therapy alone, the psychiatrist has little leverage on this point. When individual therapy is augmented by network therapy, however, the added support can be invaluable in securing compliance under these circumstances, as indicated below:

> A patient elected to undergo detoxification from chronic use of diazepam; she had been taking approximately 60 mg/day. In network meetings with the patient, her husband, and a friend, the psychiatrist discussed the need for added support toward the end of her detoxification. As her daily dosage was brought to 2 mg three times daily, she became anxious, said that she had never intended to stop completely, and insisted on being maintained permanently on that low dose. Network members supportively but explicitly pointed out that this had not been the plan. She then relented, and the dose was reduced to zero over 6 weeks.

Contingency contracting as used in behavioral treatment stipulates that an unpalatable contingency will be applied should a patient engage in a prohibited symptomatic behavior. Crowley (1984) successfully applied this technique to rehabilitating cocaine-addicted patients by preparing a written contract with each patient that indicated a highly aversive consequence that would be initiated for any use of the drug. For example, for an addicted physician, a signed letter admitting addiction was prepared for mailing to the state licensing board. This approach can also be adapted to the network setting.

Patients are strongly inclined to deny drinking problems during relapse. The network may be the only resource the psychiatrist has for communicating with a relapsing patient and for assisting in reestablishing abstinence, as occurred in this situation:

> A patient began drinking again after 6 months of abstinence. One of the network members consulted with the psychiatrist and then stayed with the patient in his home for a day to ensure that he would not drink. The network member then brought the patient to the psychiatrist's office along with the other members of the network, to reestablish a plan for abstinence.

Use of Alcoholics Anonymous

Use of AA is desirable. For the alcoholic individual, certainly, participation in AA is strongly encouraged. Groups such as Narcotics Anonymous, Pills Anonymous, and Cocaine Anonymous are modeled after AA and play a similarly useful role among drug-abusing individuals. One approach is to tell the patient that he or she is expected to attend at least two AA meetings each week for at least 1 month to familiarize himself or herself with the program. If after 1 month the patient is quite reluctant to continue, and other aspects of the treatment are going well, his or her nonparticipation may have to be accepted.

Some patients are easily convinced to attend AA meetings. Others may be less compliant. The therapist should mobilize the support network as appropriate in order to continue pressing the patient to give participation in AA a reasonable try. It may take considerable time, but ultimately the patient may experience something of a conversion, wherein he or she adopts the group ethos and expresses a deep commitment to abstinence—a measure of commitment rarely observed in patients who only undergo psychotherapy. When this conversion occurs, the therapist may assume a more passive role in monitoring the patient's abstinence and should keep an eye on the patient's ongoing involvement in AA.

Contrasts With Family Therapy

Like family and group therapy, network therapy brings several people together to address a psychological problem. Approaches vary among practitioners of group and family therapies: the therapist may focus on the individual patient or try to shape the family or group overall. In network therapy, however, the focus is always on the individual patient and his or her addictive problem.

In network therapy, unlike in family therapy, the practitioner avoids focusing on the patient's family history in the network sessions themselves, because involvement in family conflicts can hinder the network in performing its primary task of helping the therapist maintain the patient's abstinence. Such a focus would establish an additional agenda and set of goals, potentially obliging the therapist to assume responsibility for resolving conflicts that are not necessarily tied to the addiction itself. Family and interpersonal dynamics can be addressed individually with the patient on his or her own, as illustrated below:

A patient brought his estranged wife and his brother in as network members as he embarked on treatment for prescription drug abuse. The tension between the patient and his spouse was considerable because both were competitive and controlling. She interrupted too often, offering her opinions, and he was dismissive of her and sat with his back to her. His brother tried his best to remain neutral. By listening with interest and respect to both husband and wife, letting each play a positive role in framing the treatment, the therapist could tap their initiative and their desire to shine in the session. This approach allowed the therapist to draw on the wife's knowledge of the patient's drug use and focused all three participants on the task of considering more members for this emerging network. The traits that might have served as grist for a family therapist were not discussed.

A technique of family therapy that bears considerable similarity to the network format is the *strategic family approach* (Haley 1977). The focus of this approach, like the focus of network therapy, is on the current problem rather than on the dynamics of the family system. Treatment is begun with a careful examination of the nature of the symptoms, their time course, and the events that take place as they emerge. As in other behaviorally oriented therapies, the focus is a relatively narrow one, and an understanding of behavioral sequences associated with the problematic situation is of primary importance. This identification of circumstances surrounding the problem's emergence can be likened to ferreting out conditioned cues that lead to the addicted subject's sequence of drug use. The assumption in both strategic family therapy and the behavioral approach is that these circumstances will suggest options for bringing about resolution of the problem. Indeed, as he developed this strategic model, Haley (1977) observed that certain behaviors within a family can unintentionally promote the symptoms they are designed to suppress, similar to the conception of the alcoholic subject's spouse unwittingly serving as an enabler.

Rules of Network Therapy: A Summary

Network therapy is meant to be straightforward and uncomplicated by theoretical bias. In this section, I summarize the main points to be observed in treatment.

Determine Who Needs Network Therapy

- Network therapy is appropriate for individuals who cannot reliably control their intake of alcohol or drugs once they have taken their first dose; those who have tried to stop and relapsed; and those who have not been willing or able to stop.
- Individuals whose problems are too severe for the network approach in ambulatory care include those who cannot stop their drug use even for a day or who cannot comply with outpatient detoxification.
- Individuals who can be treated with conventional therapy and without a network include those who have demonstrated the ability to moderate their consumption without problems.

Start a Network as Soon as Possible

- It is important to see the alcohol- or drug-abusing patient promptly, because the window of opportunity for openness to treatment is generally brief.
- If the patient is married, the spouse should be engaged early on, preferably at the time of the first telephone call. The clinician should point out that addiction is a family problem. In the case of most drugs, the therapist can enlist the spouse in ensuring that the patient arrives at the therapist's office with a day's sobriety.
- In the initial interview, the exchange should be framed so that a good case is built for the grave consequences of the patient's addiction, and this should be done before the patient can introduce a system of denial. That way, the therapist does not put the spouse or other network members in the awkward position of having to contradict a close relation. Then the clinician must make it clear that the patient needs to be abstinent, starting now.
- When seeing an alcoholic patient for the first time, the clinician should prescribe disulfiram as soon as possible—in the office if possible. The patient should continue taking disulfiram under observation of a network member.
- At the first session, the clinician should make arrangements for a network to be assembled, generally involving a number of the patient's family members or close friends.
- From the first meeting, the clinician should consider whatever is necessary to ensure sobriety until the next meeting, and these tactics should be

planned with the network. Initially, the plan might consist of the network's immediate company and a scheme for daily AA attendance.

- People who are close to the patient, who have a long-standing relationship with him or her, and who are trusted should be included in the network. Members with substance abuse problems should be avoided because they will let the clinician down when he or she needs their unbiased support.
- The group should be balanced. A network composed solely of the parental generation, of younger people, or of people of the opposite sex should be avoided.
- The tone should be directive. The therapist must give explicit instructions to support and ensure abstinence.

Highlight Three Priorities During Therapy

1. *Maintain abstinence.* At the outset of each session, the patient and the network members should report any events related to the patient's exposure to alcohol and drugs. The patient and network members should be instructed about the nature of relapse and should plan with the therapist how to sustain abstinence. Cues to conditioned drug-seeking should be examined.
2. *Support the network's integrity.* The patient is expected to make sure network members keep their meeting appointments and stay involved. The therapist sets meeting times explicitly and summons the network when there is an emergency, such as a relapse; he or she does whatever is necessary to secure membership stability if the patient is having trouble doing so.
3. *Secure future behavior.* The therapist should combine all modalities necessary to ensure the patient's stability, such as a stable, drug-free residence; avoidance of substance-abusing friends; attendance at 12-step-group meetings; compliance in taking medications such as disulfiram or blocking agents; observed urinalysis; and ancillary psychiatric care.

Also, the patient should meet with the therapist as frequently as necessary to ensure abstinence—perhaps once a week for 1 month, every other week for the next few months, and every month or two by the end of 1 year. Individual sessions run concomitantly. The therapist should make sure that the mood of meetings

is trusting and that meetings are free of recrimination. He or she should explain issues of conflict in terms of the problems presented by addiction rather than get into personality conflicts. Once abstinence is stabilized, the network can help the patient plan for a new drug-free adaptation.

End Network Therapy Appropriately

- Network sessions can be terminated after the patient has been stably abstinent for at least 6 months to 1 year. Before network therapy is stopped, the therapist should discuss with the patient and network the patient's readiness to handle sobriety.
- An understanding is established with the network members that they will contact the therapist at any point in the future if the patient becomes vulnerable to relapse. The network members can also be summoned by the therapist. These points should be made clear to the patient before termination, in the presence of the network, but they also apply throughout treatment.

Research on Network Therapy

In the American Psychiatric Association (1995) practice guidelines for the treatment of substance use disorders, network therapy is included as an approach for facilitating adherence to a treatment plan. Four studies have demonstrated the effectiveness of network therapy in treatment and training. Each study addressed the technique's validation from a different perspective: a trial in office management; studies of its effectiveness in the training of psychiatry residents and of counselors who work with cocaine-addicted persons; and an evaluation of acceptance of the network approach in an Internet technology transfer course.

An Office-Based Clinical Trial

A chart review was conducted involving a series of 60 substance-dependent patients, with follow-up appointments scheduled through the period of treatment and up to 1 year thereafter (Galanter 1993). For 27 patients, the primary drug of dependence was alcohol; for 23, it was cocaine; for 3, it was marijuana; and for 1, it was nicotine. Opiates were the primary drugs of dependence for 6 patients. For all but 8 of the patients, networks were fully established. Of the 60 patients, 46 experienced full improvement (i.e., abstinence for at least 6 months) or major improvement (i.e., a marked decrease in drug use to nonproblematic levels). The study demonstrated the viability of establishing networks and applying them in the practitioner's treatment setting. It also served as a basis for the ensuing developmental research supported by the National Institute on Drug Abuse.

Treatment by Psychiatry Residents

We developed and implemented a network therapy training sequence in the New York University psychiatry residency program and then evaluated the clinical outcomes of a group of cocaine-dependent patients treated by the residents. The psychiatry residency was chosen because of the growing importance of clinical training in the management of addiction in outpatient care in residency programs, in line with the standards set for specialty certification.

A training manual was prepared on the network technique, defining the specifics of the treatment in a manner allowing for uniformity in practice. The manual was developed for use as a training tool and then as a guide for the residents during the treatment phase. Network therapy tape segments drawn from a library of 130 videotaped sessions were used to illustrate typical therapy situations. A network therapy rating scale was developed to assess the technique's application, with items emphasizing key aspects of treatment (Keller et al. 1997). The scale was evaluated for reliability in distinguishing two contrasting addiction therapies (network therapy and systemic family therapy), both of which were presented to faculty and residents on videotape. The internal consistency of responses for each of the techniques was high for both the faculty and the resident samples, and both groups consistently distinguished the two modalities. The scale was then used by clinical supervisors as an aid in training and to monitor therapist adherence to the study treatment manual.

We trained third-year psychiatry residents to apply the network therapy approach, and we emphasized distinctions in technique between treatment of addiction and treatment of other major mental illnesses or personality disorder. The residents then worked with a sample of 47 cocaine-addicted patients. Once treatment was initiated, 77% of subjects established a network (i.e., brought in at least one member for a network therapy session). In fact, an average of 1.47 collaterals attended any given network therapy session, across all subjects and sessions. This is notable, given that compliance after initial screening was not necessarily assured. Of the patients who completed a 24-week regimen, almost all (15 of 17 patients) tested negative for cocaine in their last three urine toxicology screenings. On the other hand, only a minority of those who attended the first week but did not complete the sequence (4 of 18 subjects) met this outcome criterion (Galanter et al. 2002). The residents, inexperienced in drug treatment, achieved results similar to those reported for experienced professionals (Carroll et al. 1994; Higgins et al. 1993; Shoptaw et al. 1994). These comparisons supported the feasibility of successful training of psychiatry residents new to administration of addiction treatment, as well as the efficacy of the treatment in their hands (Galanter et al. 1997a).

Treatment by Addiction Counselors

Another study was conducted in a community-based addiction treatment clinic, and the network therapy training sequence was essentially the same as the one applied to the psychiatry residents (see "Treatment by Psychiatry Residents") (Keller and Galanter 1999). A cohort of 10 cocaine-dependent patients received treatment in the community program with a format that included network therapy, along with the clinic's usual package of modalities. An additional 20 cocaine-dependent patients received treatment as usual and served as control subjects. Network therapy was found to enhance the outcome of the experimental patients. Of the 107 urinalyses conducted in the network therapy group, 88% yielded negative results, but only 66% of the 82 urine samples from the control subjects were negative for cocaine, a significantly lower proportion. The mean retention in treatment was 13.9 weeks for the network therapy patients, reflecting a trend toward greater retention than the 10.7 weeks for control subjects.

The results of this study supported the feasibility of transferring the network technique into community-based settings, with the potential for enhancing outcomes. Addiction counselors working in a typical outpatient rehabilitation setting were able to learn the technique and then incorporate it into their largely 12-step-group-oriented treatment regimens without undue difficulty and with improved outcome.

Use of the Internet

We studied ways in which psychiatrists and other professionals could be offered training by a distance learning method using the Internet. An advertisement was placed in *Psychiatric News,* the newspaper of the American Psychiatric Association, offering an Internet course combining network therapy with the use of naltrexone for the treatment of alcoholism.

The material presented on the Internet was divided into three didactic "sessions," followed by a set of questions, with a hypertext link to download relevant references and a certificate of completion. The course took about 2 hours for the student to complete. Our assessment was based on 679 sequential counts, representing 240 unique respondents who went beyond the introductory Web page (Galanter et al. 1997b). Of these respondents, 154 were psychiatrists, who responded positively to the course. A majority of them responded "a good deal" or "very much" (a score of 3 or 4 on a 4-point scale) to the following statements about the course: "It helped me understand the management of alcoholism treatment" (56%), "It helped me learn to use family or friends in network treatment for alcoholism" (75%), and "It improved my ability to use naltrexone in treating alcoholism" (64%).

Conclusion

The four studies described in this section support the use of network therapy as a treatment for addictive disorders. The studies are especially encouraging given the relative ease with which different types of clinicians were engaged and trained in the network approach. Because the approach combines a number of well-established clinical techniques that can be adapted to delivery in typical clinical settings, it is apparently suitable for use by general clinicians and addiction specialists.

References

American Psychiatric Association: Practice guideline for the treatment of patients with substance use disorders: alcohol, cocaine, opioids. Am J Psychiatry 152:5–59, 1995

American Psychiatric Association: Diagnostic and Statistical Manual of Mental Disorders, 4th Edition, Text Revision. Washington, DC, American Psychiatric Association, 2000

Annis HM: A relapse prevention model for treatment of alcoholics, in Treating Addictive Behaviors: Processes of Change. Edited by Miller WR, Heather NH. New York, Plenum, 1986, pp 407–434

Azrin NH, Sisson RW, Meyers R: Alcoholism treatment by disulfiram and community reinforcement therapy. J Behav Ther Exp Psychiatry 13:105–112, 1982

Begleiter H, Porjesz B: Persistence of a "subacute withdrawal syndrome" following chronic ethanol intake. Drug Alcohol Depend 4:353–357, 1979

Carroll KM, Rounsaville BJ, Gordon LT, et al: Psychotherapy and pharmacotherapy for ambulatory cocaine abusers. Arch Gen Psychiatry 51:177–187, 1994

Childress AR, McLellan AT, Ehrman R, et al: Classically conditioned responses in opioid and cocaine dependence: a role in relapse? in Learning Factors in Substance Abuse (NIDA Research Monograph 84). Edited by Ray BA. Rockville, MD, National Institute on Drug Abuse, 1988, pp 25–43

Crowley TJ: Contingency contracting treatment of drug-abusing physicians, nurses, and dentists, in Behavioral Integration Techniques in Drug Abuse Treatment (NIDA Research Monograph 46). Edited by Grabowski J, Stitzer ML, Henningfeld JF. Rockville, MD, National Institute on Drug Abuse, 1984

Galanter M: Network therapy for substance abuse: a clinical trial. Psychotherapy 30:251–258, 1993

Galanter M: Network Therapy for Addiction: A New Approach, Expanded Edition. New York, Guilford, 1999

Galanter M, Keller DS, Dermatis H: Network therapy for addiction: assessment of the clinical outcome of training. Am J Drug Alcohol Abuse 23:355–367, 1997a

Galanter M, Keller DS, Dermatis H: Using the Internet for clinical training: a course on network therapy for substance abuse. Psychiatr Serv 48:999–1000, 1008, 1997b

Galanter M, Dermatis H, Keller D, et al: Network therapy for cocaine abuse: use of family and peer supports. Am J Addict 11:161–166, 2002

Haley J: Problem-Solving Therapy. San Francisco, CA, Jossey-Bass, 1977

Higgins ST, Budney AJ, Bickel WK, et al: Achieving cocaine abstinence with a behavioral approach. Am J Psychiatry 150:763–769, 1993

Institute of Medicine: Broadening the Base of Treatment for Alcohol Problems: Report of a Study by a Committee of the Institute of Medicine, Division of Mental Health and Behavioral Medicine. Washington, DC, National Academy Press, 1990

Johnson VE: Intervention: How to Help Someone Who Doesn't Want Help. Minneapolis, MN, Johnson Institute Books, 1986

Keller DS, Galanter M: Technology transfer of network therapy to community-based addictions counselors. J Subst Abuse Treat 16:183–189, 1999

Keller DS, Galanter M, Weinberg S: Validation of a scale for network therapy: a technique for systematic use of peer and family support in addiction treatment. Am J Drug Alcohol Abuse 23:115–127, 1997

Khantzian EJ: The self-medication hypothesis of addictive disorders: focus on heroin and cocaine dependence. Am J Psychiatry 142:1259–1264, 1985

Marlatt GA, Gordon J (eds): Relapse Prevention: Maintenance Strategies in the Treatment of Addictive Behaviors. New York, Guilford, 1985

McCrady BS, Noel NE, Abrams DB, et al: Comparative effectiveness of three types of spouse involvement in outpatient behavioral alcoholism treatment. J Stud Alcohol 47:459–467, 1986

O'Brien CP, Testa T, O'Brien TJ, et al: Conditioned narcotic withdrawal in humans. Science 195:1000–1002, 1977

Shoptaw S, Rawson RA, McCann MJ, et al: The Matrix model of outpatient stimulant abuse treatment: evidence of efficacy. J Addict Dis 13:129–141, 1994

Wikler A: Some implications of conditioning theory for problems of drug abuse. Behav Sci 16:92–97, 1971

Wikler A: Dynamics of drug dependence: implications of a conditioning theory for research and treatment. Arch Gen Psychiatry 28:611–616, 1973

Wurmser L: Mrs. Pecksniff's horse? Psychodynamics of compulsive drug use, in Psychodynamics of Drug Dependence (NIDA Research Monograph 12). Edited by Blaine JD, Julius DS. Rockville, MD, National Institute on Drug Abuse, 1977, pp 36–72

Yalom ID: Group therapy and alcoholism. Ann N Y Acad Sci 233:85–103, 1974

Cognitive, Behavioral, and Motivational Therapies

Kathleen M. Carroll, Ph.D.
Samuel A. Ball, Ph.D.
Steve Martino, Ph.D.

Behavioral, cognitive-behavioral, and motivational treatments are among the most well-defined and rigorously studied psychotherapeutic interventions for substance use disorders. These three general approaches almost entirely encompass the universe of scientifically validated behavioral therapies for a range of alcohol and drug use disorders and hence should be a component of any substance abuse clinician's repertoire. In this chapter, we review the three treatments' theoretical bases, briefly summarize their empirical support, and provide an overview of their major defining techniques and strategies for implementation.

Behavioral, cognitive-behavioral, and motivational approaches share several important features. First, they are applicable across a broad range of substance use disorders. That is, well-controlled trials have sup-

ported their efficacy in alcohol-, stimulant-, marijuana-, and opioid-dependent populations. Second, these approaches were developed from well-founded theoretical traditions with established theories and principles of human behavior: cognitive-behavioral approaches from cognitive psychology and social learning theory, behavioral approaches from principles of operant and classical conditioning, and motivational approaches from motivational psychology and stage of change models. These solid theoretical roots closely link these treatments to other behavioral, cognitive-behavioral, and motivational treatments that are used across a range of problems and disorders other than substance abuse and posit clear mediating variables critical to the recovery process. Third, these approaches are highly flexible and can be implemented in a wide range of clinical modalities and settings.

Support was provided by National Institute on Drug Abuse grants P50-DA09241, U10-DA13038, and K05-DA00457.

Moreover, they are compatible with a variety of pharmacotherapies and in many cases enhance and foster compliance with pharmacotherapies, including methadone, naltrexone, and disulfiram therapies. Finally, all three are relatively brief and highly focused approaches that emphasize rapid mobilization of motivation and targeted change in substance use behaviors. Thus, the treatments are compatible with a health care environment increasingly influenced by managed care, best clinical practice models, and professional accountability.

Behavioral Therapies

Theoretical Background

Behavioral treatments have their roots in classical behavioral theory and the pioneering work of Pavlov, Watson, Skinner, and Bandura (see reviews by Craighead et al. [1995] and Rotgers [1996]). Pavlov's work on classical conditioning demonstrated that a previously neutral stimulus could elicit a conditioned response after being paired repeatedly with an unconditioned stimulus. Furthermore, repeated exposure to the conditioned stimulus without the unconditioned stimulus eventually leads to extinction of the conditioned response. The power of classical conditioning in drug abuse was demonstrated by Wikler (1973), who confirmed that opioid-addicted individuals exhibit conditioned withdrawal symptoms when exposed to drug paraphernalia. Today, classical conditioning theory is the basis of several behavioral approaches to substance use treatment, such as cue exposure (Childress et al. 1999; Monti et al. 1993) and stimulus avoidance, which is used as a component of many addiction counseling approaches.

Skinner's work on operant conditioning demonstrated that behaviors that are positively reinforced are likely to be exhibited more frequently. The field of behavioral pharmacology, which has convincingly demonstrated the reinforcing properties of abused substances in both humans and animals (Aigner and Balster 1978; Bigelow et al. 1984; Thompson and Pickens 1971), is grounded in operant conditioning theory and principles. The assumption in behavior therapies is that drug use and related behaviors are learned through their association with the positively reinforcing properties of the drugs themselves, as well as through their secondary association with other environmental stimuli. Behavior therapies attempt to disrupt this learned association between drug-related cues or stimuli and drug craving or use. A wide range of behavioral interventions, including those that seek to provide alternative reinforcers or to reduce reinforcing aspects of abused substances, are also based on operant conditioning theory. Examples include the community reinforcement approach (Azrin 1976), contingency management voucher incentive systems (Budney and Higgins 1998; Higgins et al. 1991), and the use of incentives as in the work of Stitzer and colleagues (1993), who demonstrated that methadone-maintained, opioid-addicted individuals will reduce illicit drug use when incentives such as take-home methadone are offered for abstinence.

In both cognitive-behavioral and behavior therapies, substance abuse is conceived as a complex behavior, with a number of etiological influences playing a role. These influences may include family history and genetic factors; comorbid psychopathology; personality traits such as sensation seeking or sociopathy; and environmental factors, including substance availability and a lack of countervailing influences and rewards. In cognitive-behavioral and behavior therapies, the reinforcing properties of substances are considered central to the development and maintenance of substance abuse and dependence, but these etiological influences are seen as heightening the risk of or vulnerability to substance use problems. For example, individuals may find substances particularly rewarding because of comorbid depression, a family history of alcoholism, or a high need for sensation seeking; because of modeling by family and friends who use substances; or because of environments devoid of alternative reinforcers (Carroll 1999).

Empirical Support

As a rule, behavior therapies are effective for reducing substance use and craving or urges to use. Research tends to suggest that extinction, stimulus avoidance, and counterconditioning approaches are effective, but the effects are durable only when the techniques are part of broader behavioral approaches. For example, there are several limitations to the use of behavioral techniques based exclusively on an extinction approach. First, findings of some laboratory clinical analogue studies do not generalize to real-life situations. Second, the specific cue associations usually need to be extinguished one at a time, and some cues are difficult to extinguish because of their centrality in the person's life. Third, the later re-pairing of one cue with drug use tends to reinstate previously extinguished cues through a phenomenon called *reinstatement liability*.

Consistent with behavior therapy principles, positive reinforcement is a generally better shaper of behavior than is nonreward, negative reinforcement, or punishment. Investigators have evaluated a variety of contingency management approaches for reducing illicit substance use among methadone-maintained, opiate-addicted persons. Several features of standard methadone maintenance treatment (e.g., daily attendance, regular urine monitoring, reinforcing properties of methadone) have offered behavioral researchers the opportunity to control reinforcers available to patients and hence to evaluate the effects of both positive and negative contingencies on outcome within methadone maintenance programs (Higgins and Silverman 1999; Stitzer and Bigelow 1978; Stitzer et al. 1992).

Several studies have evaluated negative contingency contracting, in which specific improvements in behavior (typically, production of drug-free urine samples) are required for continued methadone treatment, with failure to improve or comply resulting in dose reduction, detoxification, or termination of treatment, or other negative consequences associated with informing a referral source (e.g., a probation officer). Liebson and colleagues (1978) found that this procedure increased compliance with disulfiram treatment among methadone-maintained alcoholic individuals with opiate addiction. Several other research groups demonstrated that approximately 40%–60% of subjects reduce or stop illicit substance use under threat of dose reduction or treatment termination (Dolan et al. 1985; McCarthy and Borders 1985; Nolimal and Crowley 1990). However, many patients in such studies do not reduce their substance use under these conditions and are forced to withdraw from treatment; often these patients have more frequent or severe polysubstance use (Dolan et al. 1985; Saxon et al. 1993). Thus, these studies demonstrate that although negative contingencies may reduce or stop illicit substance use in some methadone-maintained patients, these procedures may also have the undesirable effect of terminating treatment for more severely impaired patients who may need treatment most (Stitzer et al. 1986).

Thus, much of the recent emphasis on contingency management has been on providing rewards for desired behavior. Methadone take-home privileges contingent on reduced drug use is an attractive approach because it capitalizes on an inexpensive reinforcer that is potentially available in all methadone maintenance programs. Stitzer and colleagues (1993) have extensively evaluated methadone take-home privileges granted as a reward for decreased illicit drug use. In a series of well-controlled trials, this group of researchers demonstrated 1) the relative benefits of positive versus negative contingencies (Stitzer et al. 1986), 2) the attractiveness of take-home privileges compared with other incentives available in methadone maintenance clinics (Stitzer and Bigelow 1978), 3) the effectiveness of aiming for and rewarding patients for drug-free urine samples versus other less directly related behaviors such as group attendance (Iguchi et al. 1996), and 4) the benefits of using take-home privileges contingent on drug-free urine samples versus using noncontingent take-home privileges (Stitzer et al. 1992). A recent meta-analysis of 30 studies of contingency management approaches in the context of methadone maintenance suggested an overall effect size of 0.25, indicative of the robust and meaningful changes associated with this type of intervention (Griffith et al. 2000). However, this positive incentive system obviously can work only when paired with administration of a medication that patients are highly motivated to take, and the system requires modification for other drugs of abuse such as cocaine.

Some of the most innovative and exciting findings pertaining to the effectiveness of behavioral treatments have been reported by Higgins and colleagues (Higgins and Silverman 1999; Higgins et al. 1991, 1999), who evaluated contingency management approaches among cocaine-dependent patients. Patients received vouchers redeemable for goods and services contingent on demonstrated targeted outcomes such as absence of cocaine in urine specimens. In a series of well-controlled clinical trials, Higgins and co-workers 1) demonstrated high acceptance, retention, and rates of abstinence among patients assigned to this approach (e.g., 85% completed a 12-week course of treatment, 65% achieved 6 or more weeks of abstinence) relative to standard counseling approaches (Higgins et al. 1991, 1993), 2) determined that rates of abstinence do not decrease when less valuable incentives, such as lottery tickets, are substituted for the voucher system (Higgins et al. 1993), 3) found, through comparisons of the behavioral system with and without vouchers, that the voucher system itself (as opposed to other program elements) produces good outcomes (Higgins et al. 1994), and 4) demonstrated the durability of treatment effects after cessation of the contingencies (Higgins et al. 2000). The effectiveness of this approach (see summaries in Higgins et al. 2002) has also been noted in studies involving methadone-maintained, cocaine-abusing, opioid-addicted individuals (Silverman et al. 1996), homeless substance abusers (Milby et al. 1996), and freebase cocaine users (Kirby et al. 1998).

These findings are of great importance because contingency management procedures are potentially applicable to a wide range of target behaviors and problems. For example, Iguchi and colleagues (1996) showed that contingency management can be used to reinforce desired treatment goals (e.g., looking for a job) in addition to abstinence. Contingency management has also been demonstrated to improve compliance with and outcome of pharmacotherapies such as naltrexone therapy (Carroll et al. 2001a, 2002; Preston et al. 1999).

However, despite the compelling evidence of the effectiveness of these procedures in promoting retention in treatment and reducing cocaine use, these approaches are rarely implemented in clinical treatment programs. One major impediment to broader use of contingency management is the expense associated with the voucher program: average earnings by patients are equivalent to about $600 over the course of a program and can be over $1,000 (Higgins et al. 1994; Silverman et al. 1996). Recently developed low-cost contingency management procedures may help bring this effective approach into general clinical practice. Petry and colleagues (Petry and Martin 2002; Petry et al., in press) demonstrated that a variable ratio schedule of reinforcement (in which rewards are given after varying numbers of specific target behaviors are demonstrated) that provides access to large reinforcers (but at low probabilities) is effective in retaining subjects in treatment and reducing substance use at rates similar to those achieved in the earlier voucher studies. Rather than earning vouchers, subjects earn the chance to draw from a bowl and win prizes ranging from small $1 prizes (bus tokens, McDonald's coupons) to large $20 prizes (portable audio players, watches, phone cards) to jumbo $100 prizes (small televisions). This system is far less expensive than the standard voucher system (which costs roughly $200–$400 per patient) because only a proportion of behaviors are reinforced with a prize (Petry et al. 2000).

Techniques and Interventions

Several detailed manuals and books describe a range of contingency management interventions (Budney and Higgins 1998; Higgins and Silverman 1999). The "classic" strategy developed by Higgins and colleagues (1994) has four organizing features that are grounded in principles of behavioral pharmacology: 1) drug use and abstinence must be swiftly and accurately detected, 2) abstinence is positively reinforced, 3) drug use results in a loss of reinforcement, and 4) emphasis is placed on the development of reinforcers that compete with drug use. In this program, urine specimens are required three times weekly. Abstinence, assessed by urinalysis, is reinforced through a voucher system in which patients receive points redeemable for items consistent with a drug-free lifestyle, such as movie tickets or sporting goods, but patients never receive money directly. To encourage longer periods of abstinence, the value of the points earned by the patients increases with each successive drug-free urine specimen, and the value of the points returns to its original level when the patient produces a drug-positive urine sample or does not come in for treatment.

Contingency management procedures can be highly effective and applicable to a wide range of target behaviors, including abstinence from drugs, compliance with treatment plans, treatment attendance, and compliance with pharmacotherapy. Moreover, reinforcers need not be limited to cash or high-value vouchers. Less expensive and more practical alternatives such as on-site retail items, small prizes, and clinic privileges have been shown to be effective reinforcers, as have employment, housing, and public assistance (Kirby et al. 1999). Petry and colleagues (Petry 2000; Petry et al. 2001) articulated several important principles for applying contingency management effectively in clinical settings. These include establishing clear and unambiguous behavioral targets and goals, identifying behavioral targets that can be objectively quantified, being consistent in monitoring target behaviors and providing reinforcers, reinforcing successive approximations for difficult-to-achieve targets (e.g., reinforcing small steps that are components of larger goals), providing reinforcers immediately after a target behavior is demonstrated, providing reinforcers of sufficient magnitude, and increasing the value of the reinforcement over time.

Contingency management interventions can be applied alone or as part of a multimodal treatment program. For example, in a "pure" contingency management approach, the therapist and the patient might meet infrequently, or not at all, while the contingency is in place. Alternatively, behavioral contingencies can be added to a full-spectrum treatment approach (see Budney et al. 2000) encompassing standard counseling, medical services, family or couples counseling, use of medication, or other treatments such as cognitive-behavioral therapy.

Cognitive-Behavioral Therapies

Theoretical Background

Cognitive-behavioral therapies (CBTs) are grounded in behavioral theory and reflect the pioneering work of Ellis and Beck, which emphasized the importance of the person's thoughts and feelings as determinants of behavior. CBT evolved in part from dissatisfaction with the extreme positions of radical behaviorism (e.g., emphasis on overt behaviors) and classical psychoanalysis (emphasis on unconscious conflicts or representations). In cognitive therapy, the individual's perception of and interpretation of life events are emphasized as important determinants of behavior (Meichenbaum 1995). A person's conscious thoughts, feelings, and expectations mediate his or her response to the environment. A key concept in CBT is reciprocal determinism, which emphasizes the interdependence of cognitive, affective, and behavioral processes. Goals of CBT are to help patients become aware of maladaptive cognitions and to "teach them how to notice, catch, monitor, and interrupt the cognitive-affective-behavioral chains and to produce more adaptive coping responses" (Meichenbaum 1995, p. 147).

Empirical Support

CBT has been shown to be effective across a wide range of substance use disorders (Carroll 1996; Irvin et al. 1999), including alcohol dependence (Miller and Wilbourne 2002; Morgenstern and Longabaugh 2000), marijuana dependence (MTP Research Group, in press; Stephens et al. 2000), cocaine dependence (Carroll et al. 1994a, 1998; McKay et al. 1997; Rohsenow et al. 2000), and nicotine dependence (Fiore et al. 1994; Hall et al. 1998; Patten et al. 1998). CBT has also been shown to be compatible with a number of other treatment approaches, including pharmacotherapy (Anton et al. 1999; O'Malley et al. 1992) and traditional counseling approaches (Morgenstern et al. 2001), and thus can be implemented in a wide range of settings. CBT is effective for a number of other psychiatric disorders as well, including depression, anxiety disorders, and eating disorders (DeRubeis and Crits-Christoph 1998).

Among scientifically validated treatments for drug dependence, CBT has emerged as an approach with particularly durable effects. That is, a number of studies have demonstrated, in a range of populations, continuing improvement after treatment termination among patients treated with CBT (Carroll et al. 1994b, 2000; McKay et al. 1999; Monti et al. 1997). Recently, Rawson and colleagues (2002) directly contrasted CBT and contingency management in two independent clinical trials, one involving cocaine abusers treated as outpatients and another involving cocaine-dependent patients enrolled in a methadone maintenance program. Although end-of-treatment outcomes favored contingency management over CBT (both were superior to usual treatment), 1-year follow-up findings indicated significant continuing improvement among patients assigned to CBT, in contrast to weakening effects among patients assigned to contingency management.

Techniques and Strategies

Specific techniques vary widely with the type of cognitive-behavioral treatment used, and a variety of manuals and protocols describe the techniques associated with each approach (Annis and Davis 1989; Carroll 1998; Kadden et al. 1992; Marlatt and Gordon 1985; Monti et al. 1989). Simply put, the aim of most CBTs is to help patients 1) recognize the situations in which they are most likely to use substances, 2) avoid these situations when appropriate, and 3) cope more effectively with a range of problems and problematic behaviors associated with substance use.

Two defining features of most cognitive-behavioral approaches for substance use disorders are an emphasis on functional analysis of drug use (that is, on understanding drug use with respect to its antecedents and consequences) and an emphasis on skills training. Cognitive-behavioral approaches include development of a range of skills and strategies to foster or maintain abstinence. Strategies typically include the following:

- Understanding the patterns that maintain drug use and developing strategies for changing these patterns (this often involves self-monitoring of thoughts and behaviors that take place before, during, and after high-risk situations)

- Fostering the resolution to stop substance use through exploring positive and negative consequences of continued use (also known as a *decisional balance*)
- Understanding craving and craving cues, and developing skills for coping with craving when it occurs (including a variety of affect regulation strategies, such as distraction, talking through a craving, and "urge surfing")
- Recognizing and challenging the cognitions that accompany and maintain patterns of substance use
- Increasing awareness of the consequences of even small decisions (e.g., which route to take home from work) and identifying seemingly irrelevant decisions that can culminate in high-risk situations
- Developing problem-solving skills and practicing application of those skills to substance-related and more general problems
- Planning for emergencies and unexpected problems and situations that can lead to high-risk situations
- Developing skills for assertively refusing offers of drugs, as well as reducing exposure to drugs and drug-related cues

Broad-spectrum cognitive-behavioral approaches, such as those described by Monti and colleagues (1989) and adapted for use in Project MATCH (Kadden et al. 1992), include interventions directed toward other problems in the individual's life that are seen as functionally related to substance use. These interventions include teaching general problem-solving skills, giving assertiveness training, teaching strategies for coping with negative affect, creating awareness of anger and teaching anger management, teaching the patient how to cope with criticism, having the patient increase pleasant activities, enhancing social support networks, and teaching job-seeking skills (Carroll 1999).

Cognitive-behavioral treatment typically is highly structured. These treatment approaches are generally brief (12–24 weeks) and are organized closely around well-specified treatment goals. Usually there is an articulated agenda for each session, and the clinical discussion remains focused on issues directly related to substance use. Progress toward treatment goals is monitored closely and frequently, and the therapist takes

an active stance throughout treatment. Generally, sessions take place within a weekly, scheduled therapy "hour." In broad-spectrum cognitive-behavioral approaches, sessions often are organized roughly in thirds, with the first third of the session devoted to assessment of the patient's substance use and general functioning in the past week and to a report of current concerns and problems; the second third is more didactic and is devoted to skills training and practice; and in the final third, the therapist and the patient plan for the week ahead and discuss how new skills will be implemented (Carroll 1998). The therapeutic relationship is seen as principally collaborative. Thus, the role of the therapist is one of consultant, educator, and guide who can lead the patient through a functional analysis of his or her substance use, aid in identifying and prioritizing target behaviors, and help select and implement strategies to foster desired behavioral changes.

Although structured and didactic, CBT is a highly individualized and flexible treatment. Rather than treating CBT as straight psychoeducation, the therapist carefully matches the content of the material—as well as the timing and nature of presentation of that material—to the individual patient. The therapist attempts to provide skills training at the moments when the patient is most in need of them. That is, when treating a patient who is highly motivated and has been abstinent for several weeks, the therapist does not belabor topics such as breaking ties with cocaine suppliers. The therapist also does not race through material in an attempt to cover all of it in a few weeks; some patients may take several weeks to master a basic skill.

In CBT, the therapist encourages the patient to practice new skills; such practice is a central, essential component of treatment. Whether the treatment is a skills training approach rather than merely a skills exposure approach has to do with the amount of opportunity to practice and implement coping skills. It is critical that the patient have the opportunity to try out new skills within the supportive context of treatment. Through firsthand experience, the patient can learn what new approaches work or do not work for him or her, where the patient has difficulty or problems, and so on. There are many opportunities for practice in CBT, both within sessions and outside them. Within each session, there are opportunities for the patient to rehearse and review ideas, raise concerns, and obtain feedback from the therapist. Also, a key component of

CBT is developing and practicing skills outside sessions, through tasks developed collaboratively (Carroll 1998).

Motivational Approaches

Theoretical Background

Motivational approaches are brief treatment approaches designed to produce rapid, internally motivated change in addictive behavior and other problem behaviors. Motivational interviewing, developed by William Miller and his colleagues (Miller and Rollnick 1991, 2002), best represents these treatment approaches. Grounded in principles of motivational psychology and patient-centered counseling, motivational interviewing arose out of several recent theoretical and empirical advances (Miller 2000).

First, several studies of problem drinking found that very brief interventions (e.g., lasting one or two sessions) were associated with reductions in drinking that were as robust and enduring as reductions associated with much more intensive treatments (Bien et al. 1993). These studies highlighted that change in addictive behavior can occur with relatively little treatment.

Second, research on how people change problem behaviors led to greater interest in natural recovery and the transtheoretical model (Prochaska et al. 1992), also called the *stage of change* model. In this model, individuals attempting to change problem behaviors move through a sequence of stages: from precontemplation (a stage associated with individuals who are not considering changing their behavior) to contemplation (recognition of the need to change and consideration of the costs and feasibility of behavioral change) to determination (the act of making the decision to take action and change) to action and maintenance. Motivation for change was seen as a critical variable in understanding how people move from one stage to another (DiClemente et al. 1999). The model emphasized the need for developing interventions matched to different stages of change.

Third, research among substance users indicated that drinking outcomes were associated with therapist style: high levels of therapist confrontation were associated with poorer outcomes, whereas high levels of empathy were associated with better outcomes (Miller et al. 1993). Empathic listening became a central feature in the development of motivational interviewing.

Finally, and importantly, ambivalence was conceptualized as a crucial concept in understanding why people become stuck in addictive behaviors that are associated with clear risks and have negative consequences (Miller and Rollnick 1991, 2002). Helping people become unstuck by resolving ambivalence, and skillfully handling patient resistance to change along the way, became a hallmark of the motivational interviewing approach.

Empirical Support

Motivational interviewing has a high level of empirical support across a wide range of substance use disorders, with particularly strong support for alcohol-abusing and alcohol-dependent populations (Miller and Wilbourne 2002; Swanson et al. 1999; Wilk et al. 1997). Several recent studies have suggested that brief motivational approaches enhance engagement and outcome in drug-abusing populations, including methadone-maintained, opioid-addicted persons (Saunders et al. 1995), cocaine-dependent patients (Stotts et al. 2001), nicotine-dependent persons (Butler et al. 1999), marijuana-dependent individuals (MTP Research Group, in press; Stephens et al. 2000), patients with both psychiatric illness and substance abuse problems (Martino et al. 2000; Swanson et al. 1999), and drug-abusing parents referred to treatment through the child protection system (Carroll et al. 2001b).

Techniques and Interventions

Although several techniques are used in motivational interviewing, this therapeutic approach is more often seen as a specific interviewing style designed to facilitate a patient's movement toward change rather than resistance. Patient resistance is considered to be caused either by collision between the therapist's and the patient's views of reality or by the therapist's being out of step with where the patient is on the stages of change continuum. Confrontation is regarded as counterproductive because it leads to a defensive movement away from change on the part of the patient. Although the therapist may not always agree with the patient, the therapist accepts the patient's position and perspective. The therapist is not globally neutral, given that education is sometimes provided and advice is given if specifically requested, but he or she is neutral about what the patient does with this education or advice.

The core principles of motivational interviewing include expression of empathy, development of discrepancy, avoidance of argument, patience in the face of resistance, and support of self-efficacy. In motivational interviewing, the important assumption is made that ambivalence and fluctuating motivations define substance abuse recovery and need to be explored rather than harshly confronted. Ambivalence is considered a normal event, not an indication that the patient is unsuitable for treatment or needs vigorous confrontation in order to force a sudden change. The patient's point of view is respected, which in some cases means accepting that major change—or even any change—is not what the patient wants, at least at present.

Miller and Rollnick (2002) emphasized four core techniques ("microskills"), represented by the acronym *OARS:* **O**pen-ended questions (e.g., "What do you make of this?"), **A**ffirmation (e.g., "You are really putting a lot of effort into our work"), **R**eflective statements (e.g., "A lot has happened, but you still haven't made up your mind that this is really a problem"), and **S**ummary statements (e.g., "Let me see if I have this right. It sounds like you don't feel good about how much you're drinking and like you haven't been able to decide whether you need to stop, cut down, or maybe just keep going like you are and see what happens. Does that sound right?"). Another group of techniques is used specifically to manage resistance to change and involves the sophisticated use of several of these microskills (simple reflection, amplified reflection, double-sided reflection, shifting focus, agreement with a twist, reframing, and siding with the negative).

In addition, the following techniques are used in motivational interviewing to increase awareness, self-efficacy, and the intention to change: 1) personal feedback, 2) elicitation of self-motivational statements, 3) decision balance, and 4) development of alternatives and options through a change plan. Personal feedback involves increasing awareness and giving feedback but leaving conclusions to the patient. Eliciting self-motivational statements involves the sophisticated use of language (e.g., open-ended questions) and techniques (e.g., importance and confidence rulers) to steer the patient to verbalize an intention or commitment to change. Decision balance involves a process of listing the advantages and positive consequences of continuing or stopping substance use versus the disadvantages and negative consequences of

continuing or stopping substance use. A balance metaphor is used to emphasize ambivalence and heightening of discrepancy between a person's goals and values and his or her substance use. When alternatives and a change plan are developed, the therapist focuses on assessing what steps have already been taken or tried and what went wrong and why. Throughout this process of change planning, the therapist serves as a resource person, helping the patient decide what to do about a potential problem. The therapist does not force the patient to change but provides information, perspective, alternatives, and possibilities and lets the patient decide what to do.

Motivational interviewing typically occurs over the course of one to four sessions, with earlier work focusing on building the patient's motivation for change and subsequent work focusing on strengthening the patient's commitment to change. During the initial part of the interview, the therapist most often uses the four core techniques (OARS), with minimal introduction of other motivational interviewing techniques. In brief, the core techniques help the patient explore his or her substance use and ambivalence about changing it. Open-ended questions or requests (e.g., "How did you get referred to treatment?" or "Tell me about your cocaine use") invite patient discussion and reduce the amount of time that the therapist spends talking. As the patient talks, the therapist reflects back to the patient what the patient has said, so that the therapist can understand the patient's perceptions about his or her substance use and clarify reasons for change. As the conversation continues, the therapist becomes increasingly selective in reflecting the patient's statements, choosing those that highlight the change dilemmas faced by the patient and that reinforce change-related talk. Similarly, the therapist frequently links patient statements in summary reflections, to achieve these same aims. Throughout this carefully attentive and interactive process, the therapist looks for genuine opportunities to affirm the patient's strengths, personal qualities, or efforts that might promote the patient's change attempts.

In motivational interviewing, it is recognized that part of any effort to change is resistance to change. Resistance is seen not as a trait within the patient but as an interpersonal phenomenon that is affected by how the therapist responds to it. A highly confrontational therapeutic style is likely to promote further patient resistance. A variety of therapeutic techniques are used to navigate patient resistance when it occurs, particularly when the four core techniques (OARS) alone have not been successful in this regard (Miller and Rollnick 1991, 2002). These techniques include asking direct open-ended questions to increase problem awareness, concern, intention to change, or optimism about change; using increasingly sophisticated forms of reflection (double-sided reflections, agreeing with a twist) that help reduce resistant reactions; offering objective personalized feedback in an overall motivational interviewing style; exploring the costs and benefits of remaining the same or trying to change; heightening discrepancies between the patient's current behavior and his or her goals, values, or self-perceptions; and emphasizing the patient's personal choice and control over what he or she concludes or does.

Conclusion

Behavioral, cognitive-behavioral, and motivational approaches have strong theoretical and empirical support in a variety of substance-abusing populations. In recent years, clinical researchers have emphasized extending these approaches more broadly into the clinical community, and thus a range of practical resources (e.g., books, videotapes, manuals, training resources and programs) on implementing these treatments in clinical practice have become available. Moreover, these approaches can be combined and integrated effectively with each other (Barrowclough et al. 2001; Budney et al. 2000) and with a range of other approaches. Thus, cognitive-behavioral, behavior, and motivational therapies should be a component of all substance abuse clinicians' repertoires.

References

Aigner TG, Balster RL: Choice behavior in rhesus monkeys: cocaine versus food. Science 201:534–535, 1978

Annis HM, Davis CS: Relapse prevention, in Handbook of Alcoholism Treatment Approaches. Edited by Hester RK, Miller WR. New York, Pergamon, 1989, pp 170–182

Anton RF, Moak DH, Waid LR, et al: Naltrexone and cognitive-behavioral therapy for the treatment of outpatient alcoholics: results of a placebo-controlled trial. Am J Psychiatry 156:1758–1764, 1999

Azrin NH: Improvements in the community-reinforcement approach to alcoholism. Behav Res Ther 14:339–348, 1976

Barrowclough C, Haddock G, Tarrier N, et al: Randomized controlled trial of motivational interviewing, cognitive behavior therapy and family intervention for patients with comorbid schizophrenia and substance use disorders. Am J Psychiatry 158:1706–1713, 2001

Bien TH, Miller WR, Tonigan JS: Brief interventions for alcohol problems: a review. Addiction 88:315–335, 1993

Bigelow GE, Stitzer ML, Liebson IA: The role of behavioral contingency management in drug abuse treatment, in Behavioral Intervention Techniques in Drug Abuse Treatment. Edited by Grabowski J, Stitzer ML, Henningfield JE. Rockville, MD, National Institute on Drug Abuse, 1984, pp 36–52

Budney AJ, Higgins ST: A Community Reinforcement Plus Vouchers Approach: Treating Cocaine Addiction. Rockville, MD, National Institute on Drug Abuse, 1998

Budney AJ, Higgins ST, Radonovich KJ, et al: Adding voucher-based incentives to coping skills and motivational enhancement improves outcomes during treatment for marijuana dependence. J Consult Clin Psychol 68:1051–1061, 2000

Butler CC, Rollnick S, Cohen D, et al: Motivational consulting versus brief advice for smokers in general practice: a randomised trial. Br J Gen Pract 49:611–616, 1999

Carroll KM: Relapse prevention as a psychosocial treatment approach: a review of controlled clinical trials. Exp Clin Psychopharmacol 4:46–54, 1996

Carroll KM: A Cognitive-Behavioral Approach: Treating Cocaine Addiction. Rockville, MD, National Institute on Drug Abuse, 1998

Carroll KM: Behavioral and cognitive behavioral treatments, in Addictions: A Comprehensive Guidebook. Edited by McCrady BS, Epstein EE. New York, Oxford University Press, 1999, pp 250–267

Carroll KM, Rounsaville BJ, Gordon LT, et al: Psychotherapy and pharmacotherapy for ambulatory cocaine abusers. Arch Gen Psychiatry 51:177–187, 1994a

Carroll KM, Rounsaville BJ, Nich C, et al: One year follow-up of psychotherapy and pharmacotherapy for cocaine dependence: delayed emergence of psychotherapy effects. Arch Gen Psychiatry 51:989–997, 1994b

Carroll KM, Nich C, Ball SA, et al: Treatment of cocaine and alcohol dependence with psychotherapy and disulfiram. Addiction 93:713–727, 1998

Carroll KM, Nich C, Ball SA, et al: One year follow-up of disulfiram and psychotherapy for cocaine-alcohol abusers: sustained effects of treatment. Addiction 95:1335–1349, 2000

Carroll KM, Ball SA, Nich C, et al: Targeting behavioral therapies to enhance naltrexone treatment of opioid dependence: efficacy of contingency management and significant other involvement. Arch Gen Psychiatry 58:755–761, 2001a

Carroll KM, Libby B, Sheehan J, et al: Motivational interviewing to enhance treatment initiation in substance abusers: an effectiveness study. Am J Addict 10:335–339, 2001b

Carroll KM, Sinha R, Nich C, et al: Contingency management to enhance naltrexone treatment of opioid dependence: a randomized clinical trial of reinforcement magnitude. Exp Clin Psychopharmacol 10:54–63, 2002

Childress AR, Mozley PD, McElgin W, et al: Limbic activation during cue-induced cocaine craving. Am J Psychiatry 156:11–18, 1999

Craighead WE, Craighead LW, Ilardi S: Behavioral therapies in historical perspective, in Comprehensive Textbook of Psychotherapy: Theory and Practice. Edited by Bongar BM, Beutler LE. New York, Oxford University Press, 1995, pp 64–83

DeRubeis RJ, Crits-Christoph P: Empirically supported individual and group psychological treatments for adult mental disorders. J Consult Clin Psychol 66:37–52, 1998

DiClemente CC, Bellino LE, Neavins TM: Motivation for change and alcoholism treatment. Alcohol Res Health 23:86–92, 1999

Dolan MP, Black JL, Penk WE, et al: Contracting for treatment termination to reduce illicit drug use among methadone maintenance treatment failures. J Consult Clin Psychol 53:549–551, 1985

Fiore MC, Smith SS, Jorenberg DE, et al: The effectiveness of the nicotine patch for smoking cessation: a meta-analysis. JAMA 271:1940–1947, 1994

Griffith JD, Rowan-Szal GA, Roark RR, et al: Contingency management in outpatient methadone treatment: a meta-analysis. Drug Alcohol Depend 58:55–66, 2000

Hall SM, Reus VI, Munoz RF, et al: Nortriptyline and cognitive-behavioral therapy in the treatment of cigarette smoking. Arch Gen Psychiatry 55:683–690, 1998

Higgins ST, Silverman K: Motivating Behavior Change Among Illicit Drug Abusers: Research on Contingency Management Interventions. Washington, DC, American Psychological Association, 1999

Higgins ST, Delany DD, Budney AJ, et al: A behavioral approach to achieving initial cocaine abstinence. Am J Psychiatry 148:1218–1224, 1991

Higgins ST, Budney AJ, Bickel WK, et al: Achieving cocaine abstinence with a behavioral approach. Am J Psychiatry 150:763–769, 1993

Higgins ST, Budney AJ, Bickel WK, et al: Incentives improve outcome in outpatient behavioral treatment of cocaine dependence. Arch Gen Psychiatry 51:568–576, 1994

Higgins ST, Wong CJ, Badger GJ, et al: Contingent reinforcement increases cocaine abstinence during outpatient treatment and 1 year of follow-up. J Consult Clin Psychol 68:64–72, 2000

Higgins ST, Alessi SM, Dantona RL: Voucher-based incentives: a substance abuse treatment innovation. Addict Behav 27:887–910, 2002

Iguchi MY, Lamb RJ, Belding MA, et al: Contingent reinforcement of group participation versus abstinence in a methadone maintenance program. Exp Clin Psychopharmacol 4:1–7, 1996

Irvin JE, Bowers CA, Dunn ME, et al: Efficacy of relapse prevention: a meta-analytic review. J Consult Clin Psychol 67:563–570, 1999

Kadden R, Carroll KM, Donovan D, et al: Cognitive-Behavioral Coping Skills Therapy Manual: A Clinical Research Guide for Therapists Treating Individuals With Alcohol Abuse and Dependence. Rockville, MD, National Institute on Alcohol Abuse and Alcoholism, 1992

Kirby KC, Marlowe DB, Festinger DS, et al: Schedule of voucher delivery influences initiation of cocaine abstinence. J Consult Clin Psychol 66:761–767, 1998

Kirby KC, Amass L, McLellan AT: Disseminating contingency management research to drug abuse treatment practitioners, in Motivating Behavior Change Among Illicit Drug Abusers: Research on Contingency Management Interventions. Washington, DC, American Psychological Association, 1999, pp 327–344

Liebson IA, Tommasello A, Bigelow GE: A behavioral treatment of alcoholic methadone patients. Ann Intern Med 89:342–344, 1978

Marlatt GA, Gordon JR (eds): Relapse Prevention: Maintenance Strategies in the Treatment of Addictive Behaviors. New York, Guilford, 1985

Martino S, Carroll KM, O'Malley SS, et al: Motivational interviewing with psychiatrically ill substance abusing patients. Am J Addict 9:88–91, 2000

McCarthy JJ, Borders OT: Limit setting on drug abuse in methadone maintenance patients. Am J Psychiatry 142:1419–1423, 1985

McKay JR, Alterman AI, Cacciola JS, et al: Group counseling versus individualized relapse prevention aftercare following intensive outpatient treatment for cocaine dependence. J Consult Clin Psychol 65:778–788, 1997

McKay JR, Alterman AI, Cacciola JS, et al: Continuing care for cocaine dependence: comprehensive 2-year outcomes. J Consult Clin Psychol 63:70–78, 1999

Meichenbaum DH: Cognitive-behavioral therapy in historical perspective, in Comprehensive Textbook of Psychotherapy: Theory and Practice. Edited by Bongar BM, Beutler LE. New York, Oxford University Press, 1995, pp 140–158

Milby JB, Schumacher JE, Raczynski JM, et al: Sufficient conditions for effective treatment of substance abusing homeless persons. Drug Alcohol Dependence 43:39–47, 1996

Miller WR: Rediscovering fire: small interventions, large effects. Psychol Addict Behav 14:6–18, 2000

Miller WR, Rollnick S: Motivational Interviewing: Preparing People to Change Addictive Behavior. New York, Guilford, 1991

Miller WR, Rollnick S: Motivational Interviewing: Preparing People for Change, 2nd Edition. New York, Guilford, 2002

Miller WR, Wilbourne PL: Mesa Grande: a methodological analysis of clinical trials of treatments for alcohol use disorders. Addiction 97:265–277, 2002

Miller WR, Benefield RG, Tonigan JS: Enhancing motivation for change in problem drinking: a controlled comparison of two therapist styles. J Consult Clin Psychol 61:455–461, 1993

Monti PM, Rohsenow DJ, Abrams DB, et al: Treating Alcohol Dependence: A Coping Skills Training Guide in the Treatment of Alcoholism. New York, Guilford, 1989

Monti PM, Rohsenow DJ, Rubnis AV, et al: Cue exposure with coping skills treatment for male alcoholics: a preliminary investigation. J Consult Clin Psychol 61:1011–1019, 1993

Monti PM, Rohsenow DJ, Michalec E, et al: Brief coping skills treatment for cocaine abuse: substance abuse outcomes at three months. Addiction 92:1717–1728, 1997

Morgenstern J, Longabaugh R: Cognitive-behavioral treatment for alcohol dependence: a review of the evidence for its hypothesized mechanisms of action. Addiction 95:1475–1490, 2000

Morgenstern J, Morgan TJ, McCrady BS, et al: Manual-guided cognitive-behavioral therapy training: a promising method for disseminating empirically supported substance abuse treatments to the practice community. Psychol Addict Behav 15:83–88, 2001

MTP Research Group: Treating cannabis dependence: findings from a multisite study. J Consult Clin Psychol (in press)

Nolimal D, Crowley TJ: Difficulties in a clinical application of methadone-dose contingency contracting. J Subst Abuse Treat 7:219–224, 1990

O'Malley SS, Jaffe AJ, Chang G: Naltrexone and coping skills therapy for alcohol dependence: a controlled study. Arch Gen Psychiatry 49:881–887, 1992

Patten CA, Martin JE, Myers MG, et al: Effectiveness of cognitive-behavioral therapy for smokers with histories of alcohol dependence and depression. J Stud Alcohol 59:327–335, 1998

Petry NM: A comprehensive guide to the application of contingency management procedures in clinical settings. Drug Alcohol Depend 58:9–25, 2000

Petry NM, Martin B: Low-cost contingency management for treating cocaine- and opioid-abusing methadone patients. J Consult Clin Psychol 70:398–405, 2002

Petry NM, Martin B, Cooney JL, et al: Give them prizes and they will come: contingency management treatment of alcohol dependence. J Consult Clin Psychol 68:250–257, 2000

Petry NM, Petrakis I, Trevisan L, et al: Contingency management interventions: from research to practice. Am J Psychiatry 20:33–44, 2001

Petry NM, Tedford J, Austin M, et al: Prize reinforcement contingency management for treating cocaine abusers: you get what you pay for. Addiction (in press)

Preston KL, Silverman K, Umbricht A, et al: Improvement in naltrexone treatment compliance with contingency management. Drug Alcohol Depend 54:127–135, 1999

Prochaska JO, DiClemente CC, Norcross JC: In search of how people change: applications to addictive behaviors. Am Psychol 47:1102–1114, 1992

Rawson RA, Huber A, McCann M, et al: A comparison of contingency management and cognitive-behavioral approaches during methadone maintenance treatment for cocaine dependence. Arch Gen Psychiatry 59:817–824, 2002

Rohsenow DJ, Monti PM, Martin RA, et al: Brief coping skills treatment for cocaine abuse: 12-month substance use outcomes. J Consult Clin Psychol 68:515–520, 2000

Rotgers F: Behavioral theory of substance abuse treatment: bringing science to bear on practice, in Treating Substance Abusers: Theory and Technique. Edited by Rotgers F, Keller DS, Morgenstern J. New York, Guilford, 1996, pp 174–201

Saunders B, Wilkinson C, Phillips M: The impact of a brief motivational intervention with opiate users attending a methadone programme. Addiction 90:415–424, 1995

Saxon AJ, Calsyn DA, Kivlahan DR, et al: Outcome of contingency contracting for illicit drug use in a methadone maintenance program. Drug Alcohol Depend 31:205–214, 1993

Silverman K, Higgins ST, Brooner RK, et al: Sustained cocaine abstinence in methadone maintenance patients through voucher-based reinforcement therapy. Arch Gen Psychiatry 53:409–415, 1996

Stephens R, Roffman RA, Curtin L: Comparison of extended versus brief treatments for marijuana use. J Consult Clin Psychol 68:898–908, 2000

Stitzer M[L], Bigelow G: Contingency management in a methadone maintenance program: availability of reinforcers. Int J Addict 13:737–746, 1978

Stitzer ML, Bickel WK, Bigelow GE, et al: Effect of methadone dose contingencies on urinalysis test results of polydrug abusing methadone maintenance patients. Drug Alcohol Depend 18:341–348, 1986

Stitzer ML, Iguchi MY, Felch LJ: Contingent take-home incentive: effects on drug use of methadone maintenance patients. J Consult Clin Psychol 60:927–934, 1992

Stitzer ML, Iguchi MY, Kidorf M, et al: Contingency management in methadone treatment: the case for positive incentives, in Behavioral Treatments for Drug Abuse and Dependence. Edited by Onken LS, Blaine JD, Boren JJ. Rockville, MD, National Institute on Drug Abuse, 1993, pp 19–36

Stotts AL, Schmitz JM, Rhoades HM, et al: Motivational interviewing with cocaine-dependent patients: a pilot study. J Consult Clin Psychol 69:858–862, 2001

Swanson AJ, Pantalon MV, Cohen KR: Motivational interviewing and treatment adherence among psychiatric and dually diagnosed patients. J Nerv Ment Dis 187:630–635, 1999

Thompson T, Pickens RW: Stimulus Properties of Drugs. New York, Appleton-Century-Crofts, 1971

Wikler A: Dynamics of drug dependence: implications of a conditioning theory for research and treatment. Arch Gen Psychiatry 28:611–616, 1973

Wilk AI, Jensen NM, Havighurst TC: Meta-analysis of randomized control trials addressing brief interventions in heavy alcohol drinkers. J Gen Intern Med 12:274–283, 1997

Individual Psychotherapy

Delinda Mercer, Ph.D.
George E. Woody, M.D.
Lester Luborsky, Ph.D.

Counseling and psychotherapy are critical components of effective treatments for addiction and are among the most widely used interventions. They often constitute the entire program (Onken and Blaine 1990), although methadone, L-α-acetylmethadol (LAAM), and buprenorphine are used in combination with them in patients with opioid dependence. Several types of psychotherapy and counseling are used. Given the heterogeneity of patients with addictions, no single treatment could be universally acceptable and effective. For example, addicted patients often use more than one substance, resulting in behavioral patterns that may produce mixtures of pharmacological and psychological effects. Furthermore, the social, economic, and familial aspects that contribute to the development and maintenance of addiction and recovery also vary, as does the presence or absence of co-occurring psychiatric and medical problems.

The field of addiction treatment has evolved rapidly over the last decade. This has been due in part to increased recognition of addiction as a public health problem, particularly in terms of the spread of HIV. Interest in determining what treatments are most effective has led to increased research, including studies of psychotherapy and counseling used alone or, in the case of opioid dependence, with methadone maintenance.

In this chapter, we provide an overview of the rationale for and efficacy of individual psychotherapy and counseling in addicted individuals. We begin with a discussion of the differences between psychotherapy and counseling. We then review the rationale for using psychotherapy to treat addictive disorders and discuss the pharmacological effects of abused drugs; 12-step and other self-help programs; treatment settings, frequency, and intensity; family involvement; the therapeutic alliance; HIV risk reduction; major models of psychotherapy; and research on treatment for specific addictions. Finally, we outline some practical treatment implications.

Definitions of Psychotherapy and Counseling

Throughout this chapter, we use the term *psychotherapy* to describe a psychological treatment that aims to change problematic thoughts, feelings, and behaviors by creating a new understanding that relates them to the patient's addiction. Psychotherapy focuses on behaviors, thoughts, and feelings that appear to promote, maintain, or occur in association with the addiction. In psychotherapy, the emphasis is on identifying and addressing problematic aspects, both past and present, of the patient's life that contribute to the drug use; thus, the focus is internal and interpersonal processes rather than external events.

Drug counseling is the most widely used intervention in addiction treatment. In contrast to psychotherapy, counseling is much less focused on identifying and changing internal psychological processes and is much more focused on managing current problems related to drug use and its immediate complications. Counseling involves the regular management of addiction, primarily through giving support, providing structure, monitoring behavior, encouraging abstinence, and providing concrete services such as referrals for job counseling, housing, medical services, or legal aid. Counseling directly addresses addictive behavior, often using the language and concepts of the 12-step program developed by Alcoholics Anonymous.

Increasingly, addiction counseling and psychotherapy have become somewhat merged in the actual practice of treatment. Regardless of therapeutic orientation, effective therapists and counselors often use similar basic interpersonal skills, including active listening, empathy, and support. Beyond these interpersonal skills, however, there are particular strategies and tools associated with specific types of psychotherapy. Addiction counseling usually is more pragmatic and less theoretically based than psychotherapy.

Rationale for Using Psychotherapy to Treat Substance Disorders

The idea of using psychotherapy in addiction treatment emerged from clinical observations that addicted patients have psychological and psychiatric problems that appear to contribute to the initiation and continuation of dependence. These observations were discussed at professional meetings and were published, mainly by psychiatrists working in methadone maintenance programs (Khantzian 1985; Khantzian and Khantzian 1984). In retrospect, it is not surprising that psychiatrists treating methadone-maintained patients were impressed with the self-medication aspects of addiction; methadone and other opioids are known to have potent antianxiety, sedative, and analgesic effects.

These observations were confirmed in later studies that found high levels of comorbidity between substance use and psychiatric disorders (Kessler et al. 1996; Khantzian and Treece 1985; Rounsaville et al. 1982, 1991; Weiss et al. 1986; Woody et al. 1983, 1990a, 1990b). The conditions most often found were major depression, dysthymia, anxiety disorders, and antisocial personality. Because chronic use of most abused drugs can magnify or even produce psychiatric symptoms, it is often difficult to determine which symptoms are substance induced and which are caused by disorders not related to substance use. Researchers also found that patients with high levels of psychiatric symptoms were more difficult to treat and, in general, had worse drug use and overall adjustment when assessed at a later time compared with patients with lower levels of psychiatric symptoms (Carroll et al. 1995; Woody et al. 1985, 1990a, 1990b). This finding is especially relevant to psychotherapeutic approaches, because most psychotherapies that have been studied in addiction treatment were initially developed to treat non-addiction-related psychiatric disorders. When viewed in this way, the presence of psychiatric symptoms in the context of a substance use disorder, especially if they are not substance induced, identifies a subgroup of patients that may benefit from an approach (such as psychotherapy) that focuses on reducing psychiatric symptoms.

Pharmacological Effects of Abused Drugs

Therapists treating addiction, regardless of their approach or orientation, need a basic knowledge of drugs of abuse and their pharmacological and psychosocial effects. An excellent overview of these effects is found in the substance-related disorders section of DSM-IV (American Psychiatric Association 1994) and

DSM-IV-TR (American Psychiatric Association 2000). Common adverse effects are depression, antisocial behavior, and hepatitis C, among persons addicted to opioids; paranoia and depression, among persons addicted to cocaine and/or alcohol; and HIV infection, among persons who have injected drugs (mainly opioids) or have engaged in frequent unprotected sexual activity to obtain drugs (mainly cocaine). It is also important to be familiar with the pharmacological effects of the most common drug combinations. Examples include opioids and cocaine (speedballs); opioids and benzodiazepines (especially among methadone-maintained patients); and cocaine used with alcohol. New combinations can emerge at any time because persons with addictions often experiment.

Twelve-Step and Other Self-Help Programs

Twelve-step programs such as Alcoholics Anonymous and Narcotics Anonymous are widely available, free of charge, and part of most successful addiction treatment programs (Fiorentine and Anglin 1996). Research has shown that frequency of attendance at and participation in 12-step meetings are positively associated with outcome (Etheridge et al. 1999; Hoffmann et al. 1983; Weiss et al. 1996). These programs can be combined with psychotherapy or counseling, which seems to have an additive effect on enhancing outcomes (Fiorentine and Hillhouse 2000). Crits-Christoph et al. (in press) found that belief in the philosophy of 12-step programs appeared to mediate drug use outcomes among patients receiving addiction counseling: patients endorsing these beliefs had more positive outcomes. In addition to their immediate positive effects, 12-step programs help prevent relapse after a structured program of psychotherapy or counseling (Fiorentine 1999). These programs are abstinence oriented, foster a network of healthy social support, and impart ideas that many recovering persons find useful in dealing with everyday life and in establishing and maintaining a sober lifestyle.

Key aspects of the 12-step philosophy are the belief that addiction is a disease rather than simply bad or immoral behavior; the idea that addiction damages the whole person—physically, mentally, and spiritually—and that recovery must address all those domains; the idea that healing or recovery comes from connecting to something larger than oneself; the paradox that one must surrender power in order to be empowered to attain sobriety; the idea that interpersonal support is critical for recovery; and the belief that recovery is a lifelong process and that there should be continued personal growth.

Treatment Settings

Treatment of substance use disorders can occur in almost any type of setting. The settings most commonly used are 1) inpatient settings, in psychiatric or general hospitals; 2) outpatient settings, in clinics or private practice; 3) intensive day treatment settings; 4) halfway houses; 5) therapeutic communities; and 6) penal institutions. Drug treatment programs vary greatly in basic aspects, such as treatment philosophy, availability of psychiatric and medical services, control of behavioral problems, level of illicit drug use treated, type of physical facilities, use of psychotropic drugs, level of staff morale, educational level of staff, and types of patients (Ball et al. 1986). These qualities can greatly affect the feasibility, efficacy, or relative importance of psychotherapy in different settings. Individual psychotherapy is unlikely to be accepted or to be effective in settings in which it is strongly believed that all psychiatric symptoms are substance induced; settings in which there are strong behavioral contingencies, such as immediate suspension of patients for continuing drug use; settings in which staff have strong negative feelings toward psychotherapy; and settings in which all therapy is conducted in groups.

Psychotherapy probably has the best chance to work when it is integrated into an ongoing program that focuses directly on reducing or eliminating drug use but that is also open to addressing psychiatric symptoms that may accompany the dependence. Both psychotherapy and counseling are probably most effective when combined with random urine testing done at intervals specific to the stage in treatment (that is, more frequent testing until abstinence is established). Urine testing encourages honesty and helps hold the patient accountable for his or her behavior. (Urine testing may also encourage attempts to evade detection and thus should involve observation or temperature testing, to assure validity of the specimen.) Newer technologies such as saliva testing may be very useful in the future because they avoid the embarrassment and other problems that can be associated with urine testing. Prompt feedback on test results is an excellent way to monitor therapy outcome and can also help patients feel that the therapist is concerned with his or her progress. It can also facilitate appropriate confrontation and analysis of what led to drug use, and it can help establish positive rewards, such as take-home privileges in a methadone maintenance program.

Frequency and Intensity of Psychotherapy and Counseling

The "dose" of psychotherapy or counseling necessary to produce improvement is unclear. According to research involving methadone-maintained patients, psychotherapy has typically been offered once a week, but patients have attended, on average, only once every 1.5–2 weeks (Woody et al. 1983). However, patients in these studies received daily doses of methadone, so the intensity of the combined pharmacotherapy and psychotherapy was high, involving daily or near daily visits. Research looking at intensity and content of drug counseling and psychiatric services for methadone-maintained patients found that when maintenance was combined with weekly drug counseling or enhanced treatment (i.e., treatment including individual psychotherapy or family therapy), patients achieved a greater reduction in drug use and greater overall improvement compared with those who received brief, monthly counseling (McLellan et al. 1993).

In a study involving cocaine-dependent outpatients, Kleinman et al. (1990) compared weekly family therapy, supportive-expressive psychotherapy, and group drug counseling. In the sample of mainly urban users of crack cocaine, attrition was high and there was no evidence of a treatment effect for any of the modalities. It was concluded that weekly therapy was of insufficient intensity to create a significant effect in these crack cocaine users. In another study, Hoffman et al. (1991) combined individual, family, and group drug counseling at different frequencies for treatment of cocaine dependence. Results indicated that intensive day treatment involving group or individual counseling produced better outcomes than did weekly therapy, a finding consistent with implications drawn from the study by Kleinman et al. (1990). In a study of more intensive treatments, Alterman (1990) found an absti-

nence rate of 50%–60% at 6-month follow-up among cocaine-dependent patients who had been randomly assigned to 1 month of 12-step-program-oriented drug counseling in inpatient treatment or in intensive day treatment (5 days per week) followed by twice-weekly therapy. This study showed a likely treatment effect and also demonstrated that intensive day treatment is a viable alternative to inpatient treatment. These three studies suggest that for cocaine-dependent patients, drug counseling should be relatively intense initially, with a decrease in intensity over time if the patient progresses.

Two controlled studies of psychotherapy—one of group therapy (Stephens et al. 1994) and one of individual therapy (Grenyer et al. 1996)—found a substantial reduction in marijuana use and related problems in marijuana-dependent patients treated with once-weekly therapy. With regard to alcohol dependence, the least intensive, effective treatment was seen in Project MATCH, in which motivational enhancement therapy had a positive effect when offered only once a month (Project MATCH Research Group 1997).

These data suggest that the intensity of psychotherapy and counseling needed to produce a treatment effect varies with the drug, with the patient's associated psychiatric problems, and according to whether the psychotherapy or counseling is used with an effective pharmacotherapy. In most cases, opioid or cocaine dependence appears to require more intense treatment than does marijuana or alcohol dependence. In the methadone studies, psychotherapy was most useful in patients with moderate to high levels of psychiatric symptoms.

Family Involvement

Most addiction treatment programs try to involve significant family members. A variation on this theme is involvement of significant others, an approach that is being used increasingly in addiction programs as an adjunct to individual therapy. One purpose of involvement of family members or significant others is to explain the treatment process and obtain support for it. Family meetings, a multifamily session, or a family workshop usually accomplishes these goals. Family involvement also allows the therapist to explore factors that might undermine treatment. These include addiction in other family members, enabling behaviors, and development of family crises in response to the patient's improvement. Family involvement is encouraged by staff, in treatment manuals, and by the Joint Commission on Accreditation of Healthcare Organizations. One of the earliest controlled studies of family therapy showed positive effects when it was added to drug counseling among methadone-maintained patients (Stanton and Todd 1982).

Therapeutic Alliance

Therapist qualities clearly have an effect on therapy outcome (Luborsky et al. 1985, 1986). Kleinman et al. (1990) found that therapist assignment was the strongest predictor of treatment retention, a variable that has been associated with treatment success. Among the qualities that have been associated with better outcome are therapist adjustment, therapist skill, and therapist interest in helping patients (Luborsky et al. 1985). Research has not identified the types of therapists who are more (or less) effective in treating addiction (Crits-Christoph et al. 1990). This lack of a clear description could mean that there are no specific types of effective therapists or that there is something in the therapist-patient relationship that is predictive of outcome.

This relationship has been referred to as the therapeutic alliance or the "helping alliance." Studies have shown that a therapist who is able to establish a positive connection with the patient at the beginning of treatment, and who is perceived by the patient as helpful, is more likely to achieve a successful outcome, as evidenced by better retention in treatment and greater reductions in drug use (Luborsky et al. 1985). The relationship between a positive alliance and outcome holds across different modalities (Horvath and Symonds 1991) and for a variety of psychiatric problems, including substance abuse (Conners et al. 1997). Generally, patients' ratings of the therapeutic alliance are stronger predictors of outcome than are therapists' ratings (Horvath and Symonds 1991), but patient and therapist ratings are usually somewhat consistent.

According to data gathered from several sites as part of Project MATCH, the alliance (rated by the therapist or the patient) consistently predicted treatment participation, days abstinent, and drinks per drinking day in a large outpatient sample ($N=952$) of patients seeking treatment for alcohol dependence (Conners et al. 1997). These changes were all in the expected direc-

tion; that is, a positive alliance predicted greater participation in treatment and greater reduction in alcohol use. Project MATCH also assessed patients after discharge from inpatient rehabilitation programs and found that their ratings of the aftercare therapist were not significant predictors of treatment participation or drinking-related outcomes; therapist ratings predicted only the percentage of days abstinent. The lack of an association between alliance and outcome in the inpatient group could be due to the fact that patients who entered outpatient treatment after inpatient treatment had already achieved abstinence and were compliant and/or motivated enough to continue. It is also possible that the inpatient group in Project MATCH established a positive alliance with inpatient staff, and that the strength of the alliance (which was not studied) promoted continued treatment participation and recovery.

It has been theorized that therapists' emotional reactions to patients are important determinants of the helping alliance. This may be true to some extent in all psychotherapy, but it is considered particularly true in the treatment of patients with substance use disorders, because therapists' emotional responses can be more intense or negative and thus have the potential for a greater effect (Imhof 1991). For example, in one study of alcoholism treatment, the more anger and anxiety there was in the clinician's voice in the initial session, the less likely the patient was to remain in treatment (Milmoe et al. 1967). Negative reactions can be minimized or avoided if the therapist is honestly interested in and comfortable with addiction-related problems, which can have manipulative, impulsive, demanding, or self-abusing aspects. Simply stated, it is probably helpful to be interested in working with substance abusers and to respect the severity of their problems (Woody et al. 1990a). Washton and Stone-Washton (1990) offered more specific suggestions, recommending that therapists convey a high degree of empathy, confidence, and hope, along with a low wish to control the patient.

In clinical practice, to promote a positive therapeutic alliance, therapists should refrain from being judgmental and may occasionally need to extend themselves more with addicted patients than with persons who have other types of psychiatric disorders. The dependence needs of addicted patients often express themselves in the therapist-patient relationship, and occasional appropriate, concrete, supportive responses can be useful, especially in the early phases of treatment. This therapeutic posture may consist of greeting the patient warmly on entering the office, actively seeking to reestablish contact when an appointment is missed, being generous with reinforcement for improvement, or seeing the patient occasionally at unscheduled times if necessary.

HIV Risk Reduction

Drug users are at increased risk for HIV infection and other infections transmitted by blood and body fluids, such as hepatitis B and hepatitis C. Treatment of opioid dependence using methadone maintenance, and treatment of cocaine dependence using outpatient counseling or psychotherapy, are associated with reductions in HIV risk behavior, and treatment of opioid dependence using methadone maintenance has been shown to decrease the actual incidence of HIV infection (Metzger et al. 1998; Shoptaw et al. 1997). In the National Institute on Drug Abuse (NIDA) Collaborative Cocaine Treatment Study—in which treatment consisted of an initial session of HIV risk reduction counseling followed by 6 months of outpatient psychotherapy and counseling—treatment participation was associated with a 49% decrease in HIV risk across all treatment, gender, and ethnic groups, mainly due to participants' having fewer sexual partners and less unprotected sex (Woody et al. 2003). Shoptaw and Frosch (2000) reviewed studies of substance abuse treatment and its relationship to HIV risk among men who have sex with men. The authors concluded that treatment combined with risk reduction counseling has significant value as an intervention for reducing HIV risk because this approach is associated with less unprotected sexual activity. An outreach study of motivational interviewing among female sex workers who were using drugs found reductions in drug use and in HIV risk behaviors and increases in time spent in lawful employment (Yahne et al. 2002). These studies expand on the known effects of methadone maintenance on HIV risk and indicate that counseling and psychotherapy can have similar effects in persons addicted to cocaine or, possibly, other substances.

Major Models of Psychotherapy

A number of individual psychotherapy and counseling approaches have been tested for efficacy in NIDA-supported investigations. Key concepts of the most commonly studied approaches are as discussed here.

Cognitive-Behavioral Therapy and Relapse Prevention Therapy

Cognitive-behavioral therapy (CBT) (Beck et al. 1993; Carroll et al. 1991) and relapse prevention therapy (Marlatt and Gordon 1985) are closely related and are based on the theory that learning processes play a critical role in the development of addiction. These approaches involve strategies and techniques to enhance self-control and foster abstinence. The techniques and strategies include self-monitoring to recognize false beliefs and drug cravings, identification of situations in which one is at high risk for substance use, and development of strategies for avoiding or coping with affects or situations that stimulate drug craving. A central element of CBT and relapse prevention therapy is learning to anticipate the problems one may meet in recovery and developing effective coping strategies before reoccurrence of these problems.

Individual Drug Counseling

Individual drug counseling (Mercer and Woody 1999) helps the patient to set present-oriented, behavioral goals and to focus directly on reducing or stopping drug use. This approach also addresses related areas of impaired functioning (such as employment problems, illegal activity, and impaired social and family relations) and the structure and content of the patient's personal recovery program. Like relapse prevention therapy, counseling helps the patient develop behavioral tools and basic coping strategies to abstain from drug use and maintain abstinence. Counseling typically employs the philosophy of the 12-step program, and participation in 12-step groups is encouraged.

Supportive-Expressive Psychotherapy

Supportive-expressive psychotherapy (Luborsky 1984) derives from psychoanalytic theory and has been modified to address substance use disorders—specifically, opioid and cocaine dependence (Luborsky 1984; Luborsky et al. 1995). It has two main components: supportive techniques to help the patient feel comfortable, and expressive or interpretive techniques to help the patient identify and work through problematic interpersonal issues. Special attention is given to the role of drugs in relation to feelings and behaviors and to how problems may be solved without resorting to drug use.

Interpersonal Psychotherapy

As the phrase implies, interpersonal psychotherapy focuses on resolving interpersonal problems. It has elements of supportive-expressive psychotherapy, but attempts are not made to relate current problems to past experiences; rather, the focus is on the patient's current situation. Interpersonal psychotherapy has been adapted for use in treating opioid and cocaine use disorders (Rounsaville et al. 1983, 1985).

Motivational Enhancement Therapy and Motivational Interviewing

Motivational enhancement therapy and motivational interviewing (Miller 1996; Miller et al. 1992) are the only psychotherapies that were developed specifically for substance use disorders. Each is a client-centered therapy rooted in the concept of stages of change, and each attempts to facilitate abstinence by helping the patient resolve the ambivalence he or she typically feels about stopping substance use. Specific techniques are used to help the patient explore the pros and cons of using drugs and to help him or her move from precontemplation or contemplation to action and maintenance. In contrast to traditional drug counseling, in which the focus often is on exhortation or setting external limits, motivational enhancement therapy and motivational interviewing attempt to create internally motivated change. Motivational enhancement therapy is usually brief, often lasting only one to four sessions, and it was as effective as cognitive therapy and 12-step-program-oriented approaches in the alcohol-dependent patients studied in Project MATCH (Miller 1996; Miller et al. 1992).

Treatment of Opioid Dependence

Clinical experience with psychotherapy before the development of methadone maintenance indicated that psychotherapy was not effective for opioid dependence. Dropout rates were extremely high, and few patients showed meaningful benefits (Nyswander et al. 1958).

This conclusion changed significantly after the introduction of methadone, which substantially reduces opioid use in most patients and keeps them in treatment. In one of the first controlled psychotherapy studies, involving methadone-maintained patients in a Veterans Administration treatment program, drug counseling alone was compared with drug counseling plus supportive-expressive psychotherapy and CBT (Woody et al. 1983, 1985). Patients who received additional psychotherapy improved more than those who received counseling alone, but these benefits were mainly due to improvements among psychotherapy patients who had high levels of psychiatric symptoms; patients with low symptom levels improved as much with counseling alone as with the extra psychotherapy. As in psychotherapy studies involving nonaddicted patients, neither of the two psychotherapies was superior to the other.

A parallel study done in New Haven, Connecticut, did not find a psychotherapy effect (Rounsaville et al. 1983). Reasons for the differences in outcome were unclear, but the differences may have been the result of low enrollment at the New Haven site, of programmatic differences related to the degree to which therapists were integrated into the program in New Haven, or of the use of suspension from methadone maintenance for patients who did not stop drug use at the New Haven site (Woody et al. 1998, 2003).

A follow-up study in Philadelphia, Pennsylvania, which studied participants in three non–Veterans Affairs methadone maintenance programs, also showed that patients with high levels of psychiatric symptoms did better with counseling plus psychotherapy than with counseling alone (Woody et al. 1995). The results were similar to those obtained earlier by Resnick et al. (1981), who found that psychotherapy was effective when used with methadone maintenance or with naltrexone therapy for opioid dependence. Another study of naltrexone treatment of opioid dependence showed that a manual-based psychosocial intervention designed to enhance the clinical value of naltrexone therapy was associated with greater treatment retention, greater intake of naltrexone, use of more psychosocial services, and greater reduction of opiate use (Rawson et al. 2001).

Collectively, these controlled studies involving heroin-addicted patients found that psychotherapy can be helpful when used in conjunction with pharmacotherapy, particularly for patients with high levels of psychiatric symptoms. The specific advantage of psychotherapy appears to be evident when psychotherapy is used in combination with drug counseling in patients with high levels of psychiatric symptoms.

Treatment of Cocaine Use Disorders

One of the earliest studies of psychotherapy and counseling for cocaine dependence compared a 12-week course of relapse prevention therapy (conducted weekly on an outpatient basis) and a course of interpersonal psychotherapy (Carroll et al. 1991). Fifty-seven percent of patients who received relapse prevention therapy achieved more than 3 weeks of abstinence, compared with 33% of interpersonal psychotherapy patients. These differences were not significant but suggest that relapse prevention might be more effective than interpersonal psychotherapy for patients with cocaine dependence.

The largest study of psychotherapy and counseling for cocaine dependence was the NIDA Collaborative Cocaine Treatment Study. It investigated the efficacy of four psychosocial treatments that were delivered in outpatient settings: 1) cognitive therapy plus group drug counseling, 2) supportive-expressive psychotherapy plus group drug counseling, 3) individual drug counseling plus group drug counseling, and 4) group drug counseling alone (Crits-Christoph et al. 1997). Four hundred eighty-seven patients were randomly assigned to one of these four manually guided treatments. Treatment was intensive, with 36 possible individual and 24 possible group sessions over 6 months. At the time of admission to the study, patients were using cocaine (mainly crack) 10 days per month on average. Most had low levels of psychiatric symptoms, although there was a subgroup with higher symptom levels. Patients were assessed monthly during treatment and 9 and 12 months after randomization. Although all groups showed substantial reductions in cocaine use (i.e., frequency of use changed from an average of 10 days per month at baseline to 1 day per month at the 6-month assessment), patients receiving individual and group drug counseling reduced cocaine use to a greater degree than did those in the other three treatment groups. Patients with higher levels of psychiatric symptoms had poorer outcomes across all treatments, but psychotherapy did not provide additional benefits to this more psychiatrically im-

paired group (a finding unlike those obtained in the methadone studies and similar to Project MATCH findings).

In other studies, behavioral interventions such as community reinforcement (Higgins et al. 1993), voucher-based reinforcement (Silverman et al. 1996), and reinforcement for completing treatment-plan-related tasks (Iguchi et al. 1997) had positive effects in patients with cocaine dependence. Behavioral interventions were compared with psychotherapy and counseling in a study by Rawson et al. (2002), who randomly assigned 120 methadone-maintained, cocaine-dependent patients to contingency management, CBT, contingency management plus CBT, or standard treatment (methadone maintenance and drug counseling). Patients who received either contingency management or CBT improved more than did those who received standard methadone maintenance, a finding that indicates the efficacy of each of these interventions in methadone-maintained patients.

Although no pharmacotherapies have been consistently effective in treating cocaine dependence, an early study done by Gawin et al. (1989) suggested that desipramine therapy might be a useful adjunct to counseling or psychotherapy. As a follow-up to this early finding, a study of methadone-maintained, cocaine-abusing patients showed that desipramine had an effect on depression but not on cocaine use (Arndt et al. 1992). Similar results were obtained in another follow-up study, which compared relapse prevention therapy plus desipramine therapy, clinical management plus desipramine therapy, relapse prevention therapy plus placebo, and clinical management plus placebo, all in ambulatory patients with cocaine dependence: all groups improved, but there were no main effects connected with pharmacotherapy or psychotherapy (Carroll et al. 1994). However, relapse prevention therapy was associated with better outcomes than was clinical management in patients with heavier cocaine use, and further analyses suggested that desipramine therapy was effective in reducing depressive symptoms but not in reducing cocaine use (Carroll et al. 1995). Also of interest, relapse prevention therapy was more effective in reducing cocaine use in the depressed group than was clinical management.

Overall, these findings indicate that the combination of individual and group drug counseling is as effective or more effective than professional psychotherapy in patients with cocaine dependence (Crits-Christoph et al. 1999). The finding by Carroll et al.

(1995) of an additional benefit from relapse prevention therapy for patients with more severe cocaine dependence or depression suggests that relapse prevention therapy may be additionally useful for these subtypes of cocaine-dependent patients. However, neither supportive-expressive psychotherapy nor cognitive therapy was more effective than drug counseling in patients in the NIDA study who had high levels of psychiatric symptoms (Crits-Christoph et al. 1999).

Treatment of Alcohol Use Disorders

Project MATCH compared CBT, 12-step facilitation therapy (Nowinski et al. 1992), and motivational enhancement therapy (Miller et al. 1992) for the treatment of alcohol dependence. With all treatments, patients decreased alcohol use significantly and maintained improvement 1 year posttreatment, and there was no significant difference in outcome between treatments. Although higher levels of psychiatric symptoms were associated with worse outcome, the psychiatrically focused treatments did not alter this relationship. As in the NIDA Collaborative Cocaine Treatment Study, standard, 12-step-program-oriented drug counseling compared favorably with the psychotherapies, at least when drug counseling was used alone without psychotherapy or effective pharmacotherapy.

Treatment of Marijuana Use Disorders

A few studies have examined psychotherapy for marijuana use disorders. Grenyer et al. (1996) compared a one-session intervention and a modification of supportive-expressive psychotherapy (Grenyer et al. 1995) delivered over 12 weeks. At 16 weeks, the supportive-expressive psychotherapy group showed significantly greater decreases in marijuana use, depression, and anxiety and significantly greater increases in psychological health than did the brief intervention group.

In a study by Stephens et al. (1994), patients were randomly assigned to either a relapse prevention (Marlatt and Gordon 1985) group or a social support group. Both groups met weekly for the first 8 weeks and then every other week for the next 4 weeks, for a total of ten 2-hour sessions. Patients in both groups achieved and maintained reductions in marijuana use and related problems; however, outcomes did not differ between the two treatments.

Budney et al. (2000) compared motivational enhancement therapy, motivational enhancement therapy plus behavioral coping skills therapy, and motivational enhancement plus behavioral coping skills therapy plus voucher-based incentives. The incentives included vouchers that could be exchanged for retail goods or services such as movie passes, sporting equipment, or vocational classes. During the 14-week study, 40% of patients in the incentives group achieved at least 7 weeks of continuous abstinence from marijuana, compared with 5% of patients in each of the other groups. At the end of the 14-week treatment, 35% of the incentives group had stopped using marijuana, compared with 10% of patients who had received motivational enhancement therapy plus behavioral coping skills therapy and 5% of patients who had received motivational enhancement therapy alone.

Given the small number of studies of psychotherapy for marijuana use disorders, and the different outcome measures (reduction in use vs. abstinence) used in these studies, it is difficult to generalize about treatment effects other than to say psychotherapy and counseling seem to help.

Implications for Treatment

Although the relative benefits of psychotherapy and counseling varied in the studies reviewed in this chapter, many studies agree that both can be effective in the treatment of substance use disorders (Carroll et al. 1991; Crits-Christoph et al. 1997; Resnick et al. 1981; Woody et al. 1983) and, moreover, that some type of psychosocial intervention is a necessary component of substance abuse treatment. However, it appears that other conditions must be met for positive outcomes to occur.

The chemically dependent patient usually requires more structure and a greater frequency of visits than traditional psychotherapy provides or involves. The intensity of therapy necessary to produce positive effects seems to vary according to the type of addiction, with cocaine and opioid dependence requiring the most intensive treatment, especially at the beginning of treatment. For these disorders, it seems necessary to have sessions twice a week to daily at the beginning, followed by a reduction in frequency as progress is achieved.

In addition, psychotherapy appears to be most effective when combined with drug-focused treatment that is administered either within the context of a structured addiction program or in sessions organized by an individual psychotherapist. Additional services, including vocational counseling, are also helpful for patients who are not working, and family involvement tends to support treatment retention and compliance. In the case of outpatient treatment for opioid dependence, methadone maintenance or some other type of substitution therapy is nearly essential for psychotherapy or counseling to be helpful. This combined approach—that is, offering psychotherapy and/or counseling with an effective medication—is likely to keep the greatest number of patients in treatment and to have the most pervasive benefits. Studies indicate that the more traditional psychotherapies, such as CBT, supportive-expressive psychotherapy, and interpersonal psychotherapy, are primarily useful in methadone-maintained patients with clinically significant psychiatric symptoms (Woody et al. 1985, 1995).

Research has not clearly indicated that one kind of psychotherapy is superior to any other for the treatment of addiction or any other psychiatric disorder. The most commonly used psychotherapies in addiction treatment are cognitive therapy, CBT, interpersonal psychotherapy, motivational enhancement therapy, motivational interviewing, and supportive-expressive psychotherapy. New approaches are being developed and tested. Currently, there is much interest in combining psychological and pharmacological treatments, and it appears that this may be a valuable approach for many addictions. It is important to recognize the value of participation in 12-step and other self-help groups. Consistent with the idea of continuing self-help, it is probably best to view treatment of and recovery from substance use disorders as a process that extends well beyond the end of formal treatment and that involves personal commitment and continued growth by the patient.

The following guidelines may be helpful to the clinician interested in treating substance use disorders:

- Be familiar with the pharmacology of abused drugs, the subculture of addiction, and self-help programs.
- Formulate clear goals early in treatment, and keep abreast of the patient's success with abstinence and with compliance in other aspects of the treatment.
- Establish a positive, supportive therapeutic alliance with the patient.
- Ensure that drug-focused interventions are part of the treatment program.
- Consider using an effective pharmacotherapy, when available, in combination with psychotherapy or counseling.
- Recognize that because the recovering patient usually requires structure and treatment resources in addition to psychotherapy, therapy is most effective when administered within the context of a structured program that can provide additional services or refer the patient to such services.
- Acknowledge the importance of urine drug testing and alcohol breath testing with prompt feedback to the patient.
- Understand that for many patients, addiction is a chronic condition, and be pleased if the patient shows significant improvement, even if he or she is not "cured."
- Remember that the special role for psychotherapy in preference to drug counseling is probably limited to patients with high levels of psychiatric symptoms who are on methadone maintenance.

References

Alterman AI: Day hospital versus inpatient cocaine dependence rehabilitation: an interim report, in Problems of Drug Dependence 1990 (NIDA Research Monograph 105). Edited by Harris L. Rockville, MD, National Institute on Drug Abuse, 1990, pp 363–364

American Psychiatric Association: Diagnostic and Statistical Manual of Mental Disorders, 4th Edition. Washington, DC, American Psychiatric Association, 1994

American Psychiatric Association: Diagnostic and Statistical Manual of Mental Disorders, 4th Edition, Text Revision. Washington, DC, American Psychiatric Association, 2000

Arndt IO, Dorozynsky L, Woody GE, et al: Desipramine treatment of cocaine dependence in methadone-maintained patients. Arch Gen Psychiatry 49:888–893, 1992

Ball JC, Corty E, Petroski SP, et al: Medical services provided to 2394 patients at methadone programs in three states. J Subst Abuse Treat 3:203–209, 1986

Beck AT, Wright FD, Newman CF, et al: Cognitive Therapy of Substance Abuse. New York, Guilford, 1993

Budney AJ, Higgins ST, Radonovich KJ, et al: Adding voucher-based incentives to coping skills and motivational enhancement improves outcomes during treatment for marijuana dependence. J Consult Clin Psychol 68:1051–1061, 2000

Carroll KM, Rounsaville BJ, Treece FH: A comparative trial of psychotherapies for ambulatory cocaine abusers: relapse prevention and interpersonal psychotherapy. Am J Drug Alcohol Abuse 17:229–247, 1991

Carroll KM, Rounsaville BJ, Gordon LT, et al: Psychotherapy and pharmacotherapy for ambulatory cocaine abusers. Arch Gen Psychiatry 51:177–187, 1994

Carroll KM, Nich C, Rounsaville BJ: Differential symptom reduction in depressed cocaine abusers treated with psychotherapy and pharmacotherapy. J Nerv Ment Dis 183:251–259, 1995

Conners GJ, Carroll KM, DiClemente CC: The therapeutic alliance and its relationship to alcoholism treatment participation and outcome. J Consult Clin Psychol 65:588–598, 1997

Crits-Christoph P, Beebe KL, Connolly MB: Therapist effects in the treatment of drug dependence: implications for conducting comparative treatment studies, in Psychotherapy and Counseling in the Treatment of Drug Abuse (NIDA Research Monograph 104). Edited by Onken LS, Blaine JD. Rockville, MD, National Institute on Drug Abuse, 1990, pp 39–48

Crits-Christoph P, Siqueland L, Blaine J, et al: The National Institute on Drug Abuse Collaborative Cocaine Treatment Study: rationale and methods. Arch Gen Psychiatry 54:721–726, 1997

Crits-Christoph P, Siqueland L, Blaine J, et al: Psychosocial treatments for cocaine dependence: National Institute on Drug Abuse Collaborative Cocaine Treatment Study. Arch Gen Psychiatry 56:493–502, 1999

Crits-Christoph P, Connolly MB, Barber J, et al: Mediators of outcome for psychosocial treatment for cocaine dependence. J Consult Clin Psychol (in press)

Etheridge RM, Craddock SG, Hubbard RL, et al: The relationship of counseling and self-help participation to patient outcomes in DATOS. Drug Alcohol Depend 57:99–112, 1999

Fiorentine R: After drug treatment: are 12-step programs effective in maintaining abstinence? Am J Drug Alcohol Abuse 25:93–116, 1999

Fiorentine R, Anglin MD: More is better: counseling participation and the effectiveness of outpatient drug treatment. J Subst Abuse Treat 13:341–348, 1996

Fiorentine R, Hillhouse MP: Drug treatment and 12-step program participation: the additive effects of integrated recovery activities. J Subst Abuse Treat 18:65–74, 2000

Gawin FH, Kleber HD, Byck R, et al: Desipramine facilitation of initial cocaine abstinence. Arch Gen Psychiatry 46:117–121, 1989

Grenyer BFS, Luborsky L, Solowij N: Treatment Manual for Supportive-Expressive Dynamic Therapy: Special Adaptation for Treatment of Cannabis (Marijuana) Dependence (Technical Report 26). Sydney, Australia, National Drug and Alcohol Research Centre, 1995

Grenyer BFS, Solowij N, Peters R: Psychotherapy for marijuana addiction: a randomized controlled trial of brief versus intensive treatment. Paper presented at the international meeting of the Society for Psychotherapy Research, Amelia Island, FL, June 19–23, 1996

Higgins ST, Budney AJ, Bickel WK, et al: Achieving cocaine abstinence with a behavioral approach. Am J Psychiatry 150:763–769, 1993

Hoffman JA, Caudill BD, Moolchan ET, et al: Effective treatments for cocaine abuse and HIV risk: the cocaine abuse treatment strategies (CATS) project. Plenary lecture given at the 5th International Congress on Drug Abuse, Jerusalem, Israel, September 1–6, 1991

Hoffmann NG, Harrison PA, Belille CA: Alcoholics Anonymous after treatment: attendance and abstinence. Int J Addict 18:311–318, 1983

Horvath AO, Symonds BD: Relation between working alliance and outcome in psychotherapy: a meta-analysis. Journal of Counseling Psychology 38:139–149, 1991

Iguchi MY, Belding MA, Morral AR, et al: Reinforcing operants other than abstinence in drug abuse treatment: an effective alternative for reducing drug use. J Consult Clin Psychol 65:421–428, 1997

Imhof J: Countertransference issues in alcohol and drug addiction. Psychiatric Annals 21:292–306, 1991

Kessler RC, Nelson CB, McGonagle KA, et al: The epidemiology of co-occurring addictive and mental disorders: implications for prevention and service utilization. Am J Orthopsychiatry 66:17–31, 1996

Khantzian EJ: The self-medication hypothesis of addictive disorders: focus on heroin and cocaine dependence. Am J Psychiatry 142:1259–1264, 1985

Khantzian EJ, Khantzian NJ: Cocaine addiction: is there a psychological predisposition? Psychiatric Annals 14:753–759, 1984

Khantzian EJ, Treece C: DSM-III psychiatric diagnosis of narcotic addicts: recent findings. Arch Gen Psychiatry 42:1067–1071, 1985

Kleinman PH, Woody GE, Todd TC, et al: Crack and cocaine abusers in outpatient psychotherapy, in Psychotherapy and Counseling in the Treatment of Drug Abuse (NIDA Research Monograph 104). Edited by Onken LS, Blaine JD. Rockville, MD, National Institute on Drug Abuse, 1990, pp 24–34

Luborsky L: Principles of Psychoanalytic Psychotherapy: A Manual for Supportive-Expressive Treatment. New York, Basic Books, 1984

Luborsky L, McLellan AT, Woody GE, et al: Therapist success and its determinants. Arch Gen Psychiatry 42:602–611, 1985

Luborsky L, Crits-Christoph P, McLellan AT: Do therapists vary in their effectiveness? Findings from four outcome studies. Am J Orthopsychiatry 66:501–512, 1986

Luborsky L, Woody GE, Hole A, et al: Supportive-expressive dynamic psychotherapy for treatment of opiate drug dependence, in Dynamic Therapies for Psychiatric Disorders (Axis I). Edited by Barber JP, Crits-Christoph P. New York, Basic Books, 1995, pp 131–160

Marlatt GA, Gordon J (eds): Relapse Prevention: Maintenance Strategies in the Treatment of Addictive Behaviors. New York, Guilford, 1985

McLellan AT, Arndt IO, Metzger DS, et al: Are psychosocial services necessary in substance abuse treatment? JAMA 269:1953–1959, 1993

Mercer DE, Woody GE: An Individual Counseling Approach to Treat Cocaine Addiction: The Collaborative Cocaine Treatment Study Model (NIDA Therapy Manuals for Drug Addiction, Manual 3). Rockville, MD, National Institute on Drug Abuse, 1999

Metzger DS, Navaline H, Woody GE: Drug abuse treatment as AIDS prevention. Public Health Rep 113 (suppl 1):97–106, 1998

Miller WR: Motivational interviewing: research, practice and puzzles. Addict Behav 61:835–842, 1996

Miller WR, Zweben A, DiClemente CC, et al: Motivational Enhancement Therapy Manual: A Clinical Research Guide for Therapists Treating Individuals With Alcohol Abuse and Dependence (DHHS Publ No ADM-92-1894) (Project MATCH Monograph Series, Vol 2). Rockville, MD, National Institute on Alcohol Abuse and Alcoholism, 1992

Milmoe S, Rosenthal R, Blane HT, et al: The doctor's voice: postdictor of successful referral of alcoholic patients. J Abnorm Psychol 72:78–84, 1967

Nowinski J, Baker S, Carroll K: Twelve-Step Facilitation Therapy Manual: A Clinical Research Guide for Therapists Treating Individuals With Alcohol Abuse and Dependence (DHHS Publ No ADM-92-1893) (Project MATCH Monograph Series, Vol 1). Rockville, MD, National Institute on Alcohol Abuse and Alcoholism, 1992

Nyswander M, Winick C, Bernstein A, et al: The treatment of drug addicts as voluntary outpatients: a progress report. Am J Orthopsychiatry 28:714–729, 1958

Onken LS, Blaine JD: Psychotherapy and counseling research in drug abuse treatment: questions, problems, and solutions, in Psychotherapy and Counseling in the Treatment of Drug Abuse (NIDA Research Monograph 104). Edited by Onken LS, Blaine JD. Rockville, MD, National Institute on Drug Abuse, 1990, pp 1–5

Project MATCH Research Group: Matching alcoholism treatments to client heterogeneity: Project MATCH posttreatment drinking outcomes. J Stud Alcohol 58:7–29, 1997

Rawson RA, McCann MJ, Shoptaw SJ, et al: Naltrexone for opioid dependence: evaluation of a manualized psychosocial protocol to enhance treatment response. Drug and Alcohol Review 20:67–78, 2001

Rawson RA, Huber A, McCann M, et al: A comparison of contingency management and cognitive-behavioral approaches during methadone maintenance treatment for cocaine dependence. Arch Gen Psychiatry 59:817–824, 2002

Resnick RB, Washton AM, Stone-Washton N, et al: Psychotherapy and naltrexone in opioid dependence, in Problems of Drug Dependence (NIDA Research Monograph 34). Edited by Harris LS. Rockville, MD, National Institute on Drug Abuse, 1981, pp 109–115

Rounsaville BJ, Weissman MM, Kleber HD, et al: Heterogeneity of psychiatric diagnoses in treated opiate addicts. Arch Gen Psychiatry 39:161–166, 1982

Rounsaville BJ, Glazer W, Wilber CH, et al: Short-term interpersonal psychotherapy in methadone-maintained opiate addicts. Arch Gen Psychiatry 40:629–636, 1983

Rounsaville BJ, Gawin F, Kleber H: Interpersonal psychotherapy adapted for ambulatory cocaine abusers. Am J Drug Alcohol Abuse 11:171–191, 1985

Rounsaville BJ, Foley S, Carroll KM, et al: Psychiatric diagnoses of treatment-seeking cocaine abusers. Arch Gen Psychiatry 48:43–51, 1991

Shoptaw S, Frosch D: Substance abuse treatment as HIV prevention for men who have sex with men. AIDS and Behavior 4:193–203, 2000

Shoptaw S, Frosch D, Rawson RA, et al: Cocaine abuse counseling as HIV prevention. AIDS Educ Prev 9:511–520, 1997

Silverman K, Higgins ST, Brooner RK, et al: Sustained cocaine abstinence in methadone maintenance patients through voucher-based reinforcement therapy. Arch Gen Psychiatry 53:409–415, 1996

Stanton MD, Todd TC: The Family Therapy of Drug Addiction. New York, Guilford, 1982

Stephens RS, Roffman RA, Simpson EE: Treating adult marijuana dependence: a test of the relapse prevention model. J Consult Clin Psychol 62:92–99, 1994

Washton A, Stone-Washton N: Abstinence and relapse in cocaine addicts. J Psychoactive Drugs 22:135–147, 1990

Weiss RD, Mirin SM, Michael JL, et al: Psychopathology in chronic cocaine abusers. Am J Drug Alcohol Abuse 12:17–29, 1986

Weiss RD, Griffin ML, Najavits LM, et al: Self-help activities in cocaine dependent patients entering treatment: results from the NIDA Collaborative Cocaine Treatment Study. Drug Alcohol Depend 43:79–86, 1996

Woody GE, Luborsky L, McLellan AT, et al: Psychotherapy for opiate addicts: does it help? Arch Gen Psychiatry 40:639–645, 1983

Woody GE, McLellan AT, Luborsky L, et al: Psychiatric severity as a predictor of benefits from psychotherapy. Am J Psychiatry 141:1172–1177, 1985

Woody GE, McLellan AT, Luborsky L, et al: Psychotherapy and counseling for methadone maintained opiate addicts: results of research studies, in Psychotherapy and Counseling in the Treatment of Drug Abuse (NIDA Research Monograph 104). Edited by Onken LS, Blaine JD. Rockville, MD, National Institute on Drug Abuse, 1990a, pp 9–23

Woody GE, McLellan AT, O'Brien CP: Research on psychopathology and addiction: treatment implications. Drug Alcohol Depend 25:121–123, 1990b

Woody GE, McLellan AT, Luborsky L, et al: Psychotherapy in community methadone programs: a validation study. Am J Psychiatry 152:1302–1308, 1995

Woody GE, McLellan AT, Luborsky L, et al: Psychotherapy with opioid-dependent patients. Psychiatric Times, November 1998

Woody GE, Gallop R, Luborsky L, et al, and the Cocaine Psychotherapy Study Group: HIV risk reduction in the National Institute on Drug Abuse Cocaine Collaborative Treatment Study [sic]. J Acquir Defic Syndr 33:82–87, 2003

Yahne CE, Miller WR, Irvin-Vitela L, et al: Magdalena Pilot Project: motivational outreach to substance abusing women street sex workers. J Subst Abuse Treat 23:49–53, 2002

Group Therapy

Edward J. Khantzian, M.D.
Sarah J. Golden-Schulman, Ph.D.
William E. McAuliffe, Ph.D.

Group therapy has traditionally been the most popular treatment for addictive disorders and is currently the treatment of choice as addictions are increasingly recognized and addressed. The suffering and life disruptions caused by substance abuse and dependence, the heightened awareness of "hidden" addictive disorders, such as gambling and addictions related to eating and sex, and the recognition of comorbidity and of substitution of one addiction for another (Flores 1988, 2001) have all trained attention on the question of what is to be done. Although the controversy over the etiology and conceptualizations of addiction continues unabated, there appears to be an often unacknowledged consensus about the advantages of group treatment over individual treatment in addressing this problem. Thus, while the origins of addiction to substances may be diversely viewed as physiological, intrapsychic, social, and environmental, or as moral and volitional, the group approach has generally been advocated as a remedy.

Group approaches are as wide-ranging in form as the theories that give rise to them. Self-help "fellow-ships" of Alcoholics Anonymous (AA), time-limited psychoeducational and cognitive-behavioral models, and open-ended, psychodynamic group therapies adhere not only to different assumptions about the nature of addiction but also to different practices in the management of and recovery from addiction.

All group approaches share an appreciation of the healing power of connection with others—what Herman (1992) called "the restoration of social bonds" that "begins with the discovery that one is not alone" (p. 215). Individuals with substance use disorders benefit from group psychotherapy because of their disrupted capacity to establish and maintain attachment to others (Flores 2001). Groups serve as a corrective to these persons' self-absorption, counterdependence, and inability to regulate their emotions, self-esteem, and behaviors, especially self-care (Khantzian 2001; Khantzian et al. 1990). Yalom (1983), an existential group theorist, held that in a group, the "disconfirmation of the feeling of uniqueness offers considerable relief and a 'welcome to the human race' experience" (p. 41). Orford (1985) saw the self-help group and therapeutic community as using public testimony, social support, and social coercion to guide the individual through a "moral passage" to forge a new social identity. In the respite from the shame, isolation, and loneliness of addiction that the group offers (Khantzian 1986), and in the possibilities for both support and confrontation that it provides, the group approach holds its own as a force for managing and changing addictive behavior. More recently, Khantzian (2001) elaborated on how and why groups help individuals with addiction contain the impulse to use substances; help them grow, change, and feel better; and thus help make the pull toward addictive behaviors less strong.

Groups and Addiction

The most widely accepted treatment approach for addiction is the group, with the kind of group reflecting a particular view of addiction. Orford (1985) attributed the popularity and success of the self-help group, epitomized by AA, to its ability to "fuse the disease and the moral perspectives" (p. 309)—that is, to offer both a practical explanation and a corrective spiritual and moral approach to the problem of addiction. AA was founded in 1935 by two men, Bill Wilson and Dr. Bob, in an attempt by each to help the other. Their fledgling organization derived from the model of a Christian fellowship, with its "ideas of self-examination, acknowledgment of character defects, restitution for harm done to others, and working with others" (Orford 1985, p. 309).

In the self-help group, change takes place in a public forum. Orford (1985) emphasized that beyond providing support, this forum promotes the expectation that one conform to certain values: the group provides this "new set of attitudes and values, and it is to the group's ideology or 'will' that the novice must submit if he or she is to become a successful member" (p. 303). A wider range of group processes was described by Khantzian and Mack (1989, 1994) as accomplishing change in the group: these authors saw support, surrender, spirituality, and altruism as therapeutic and transformational elements. After five decades of growth, AA has more recently served as a model for 12-step programs addressing many other addictive behaviors, such as drug taking and gambling.

The concept of the individual's submission to the group's ideology has perhaps found its fullest expres-

sion in therapeutic communities for the treatment of addiction. Synanon, which was established in the 1960s to address heroin addiction, aggressively used the group to change attitudes through confinement, structure, daily work assignments, and often demanding interpersonal confrontation (Cherkas 1965). This "total" group approach, in which every aspect of daily life is regimented, continues to thrive in programs such as Daytop and Phoenix House. The therapeutic community model, with group therapy as its mainstay, is also found in shorter-term detoxification and intensive inpatient treatments for a wide range of addictive behaviors, including cocaine addiction, narcotic addiction, eating disorders, and gambling.

Other major group approaches in the treatment of addiction have developed from the cognitive-behavioral and psychoanalytic, psychodynamic clinical traditions. From these schools of thought have emerged both individual and group therapies for addiction. We focus here on the group models.

Cognitive-Behavioral Group Approaches

Cognitive-behavioral theory holds that addiction is learned behavior that is reinforced by contingencies such as the pleasurable effects of drugs (McAuliffe and Ch'ien 1986). The addictive behavior is conditioned and then generalized to a range of stimuli in the environment that perpetuate it. The treatment of addiction thus involves learning to recognize and avoid these stimuli and to suppress conditioned responses to these stimuli. The aim of cognitive-behavioral therapy is to develop alternative thoughts and behaviors to the conditioned, "addictive" responses.

The psychoeducational group is one form of cognitive-behavioral group therapy. This model uses the group format to inform and teach addicted individuals about the behavioral, medical, and psychological consequences of their addictions. Such groups are a staple of most rehabilitation programs (Nace 1987) and are often seen as the first step of a more comprehensive treatment program. By raising awareness of the consequences of addictive behavior through informational materials, didactic presentations, and group discussions, this method educates group members and attempts to show them how the addiction complicates their lives (Drake et al. 1991). Thus, the psychoeducational group intends to prepare the group members to make a commitment to further treatment.

McAuliffe and Ch'ien (1986) developed a cognitive-behavioral group treatment for substance abuse (called *recovery training and self-help*) that uses a curriculum in a highly structured, didactic group format to teach group members about the cognitive and behavioral factors involved in drug use (e.g., to enable group members to recognize the social and environmental cues that can lead to relapse). Restructuring lifestyles that have been associated with the addictive use of substances, anticipating obstacles to recovery, and finding alternative ways to manage problems that have triggered drug use are systematically addressed in the group. Although the focus of this method is on managing and modifying one's own behavior, the group setting emphasizes the commonality of certain situations and responses in lifestyles of addiction and of recovery. This group model was studied experimentally in the Harvard Cocaine Recovery Project (Khantzian et al. 1990).

An outpatient cessation model for early recovery from cocaine addiction, also developed in the Harvard Cocaine Recovery Project, was described by McAuliffe and Albert (1992) in *Clean Start:* "From the initiation of recovery, the model is a group one in which chemical rewards are replaced with social ones" (McAuliffe and Albert 1992, p. 27). The group serves as an arena for social learning and social backing: "Seeing others make changes gives clients a clear picture of how change is accomplished, and provides motivation to try a little harder" (p. 28). Group members experience nonexploitative friendships, perhaps for the first time, and are prepared by this "prosocial abstinent culture" (p. 28) for participation in the larger recovering community.

Psychoanalytic, Psychodynamic Group Approaches

Several group models have emerged from the psychoanalytic, psychodynamic tradition. Most relevant to the treatment of addiction have been groups with a psychodynamic, interpersonal focus that address the addicted individual's particular needs for safety and structure in the group setting (Brown and Yalom 1977; Khantzian et al. 1990; Matano and Yalom 1991; Vannicelli 1982, 1988; Yalom 1974).

In the psychoanalytic, psychodynamic tradition, addiction is understood as the individual's "solution" to the problem of psychological vulnerability. Contemporary psychoanalytic theory has elaborated on these vulnerabilities as defects of self, both intrapsychic and characterological, that can lead to addiction in an attempt to regulate and medicate the distress caused by the defect (Kohut 1977; Meissner 1986; Wurmser 1978). Flores (2001) linked this need to "self-medicate" to inadequate self structures. Khantzian (1974, 1978, 1985, 1995, 1997, 1999) addressed the particular psychological and narcissistic vulnerabilities of the potential addicted person: his self-medication hypothesis holds that addictions result when an individual seeks to relieve the suffering and distress resulting from deficits in ego or self capacities to regulate affects, self-esteem, self-care, and relationships with others as they play themselves out in everyday life. Heightening awareness of self and changing characteristic patterns of handling these vulnerabilities in everyday situations are both addressed in the psychodynamic group treatment of addiction.

Perhaps the most important aspect of Khantzian's model is that it is modified dynamic group therapy (MDGT) (Khantzian et al. 1990, 2001). The modifications mean that the vulnerabilities and difficulties of the addicted individual define and shape the format of the treatment: the group model establishes maximum safety for addicted individuals in requiring and helping to maintain abstinence, in providing outreach and support, in using an active style of leadership, and in always addressing the potential for drug and psychological relapse. Structure and containment rather than confrontation are emphasized. This group model was also studied experimentally as part of the Harvard Cocaine Recovery Project (Khantzian et al. 1990).

Efficacy

The literature on the efficacy of group therapy for addiction is notably sparse, and controlled studies of treatment outcome are needed. The Harvard Cocaine Recovery Project, a National Institute on Drug Abuse–funded study carried out at Harvard Medical School at the Cambridge Hospital from 1987 to 1990, compared two group treatments (cognitive-behavioral and psychodynamic) and a no-group treatment in a controlled clinical trial involving cocaine-addicted individuals. Findings indicated high retention rates for patients receiving group treatment, and these patients benefited from treatment (Khantzian et al. 1990). Other recent studies, although less comprehensive in their conception, shed light on the efficacy issues of abstinence, retention in treatment, matching of patient and treatment, group type, and maintenance of improvement (Carroll et al. 1998; Getter et al. 1992; Martin et al. 1996; Shaffer et al. 1997).

In a study comparing individual therapy, family therapy, and group treatment for cocaine use disorders, Kang et al. (1991) found that improvement was most strongly related to abstinence, and they also concluded that an intense level of therapy is needed to sustain this abstinence. Bowers and al-Redha (1990) studied alcoholic individuals and their spouses and found that group therapy for couples was superior to individual therapy for the couple in decreasing alcohol consumption by the alcoholic partner. They also found a trend for the conjointly treated couples to report better marital adjustment and higher relationship ratings than the individually treated couples. Hellerstein and Meehan (1987) reported that group treatment in substance-abusing patients with schizophrenia resulted in a marked decrease in the number of days of hospitalization over 1 year. These studies provide evidence for the group modality's need to address particular addictive behaviors and other life issues and problems beyond the addiction.

Greene (2002) reviewed evidence of the efficacy of group therapy in the treatment of substance use disorders. In his report, he repeatedly critiqued the methodological shortcomings in the extant literature on group therapy. Although Greene allowed for the limitations imposed by the "insurmountable restrictions" of the clinical setting, his review highlights the difficulty of comparing studies when those studies lack precision in identifying therapeutic factors and in differentiating approaches. Also addressed in the review is the problem of distinguishing group therapeutic factors from other therapeutic elements in the treatment of substance use disorders. Interestingly, Greene (2002) suggested that the schism between dynamic and cognitive-behavioral approaches is unwarranted and is limiting for both approaches, hindering development of clinically meaningful studies that integrate psychodynamic expertise.

Although more definitive studies of outcomes and the efficacy of group treatment of addiction are needed, diverse group treatments have conceptually and practically gained prominence in recent years.

Group Therapy as Treatment of Choice

Group psychotherapy has been described as "the definitive treatment for producing character change" (Alonso 1989, p. 1) because in a group setting, the "cost of character defenses is illuminated and presents a conflict which can render the same traits dystonic and thus available to interpretation and change" (Alonso 1989, p. 8). Similarly, group therapy has been described as "the treatment of choice for chemical dependency" (Matano and Yalom 1991, p. 269). Matano and Yalom (1991) attributed this choice to the "power of groups—the power to counter prevailing cultural pressures to drink, to provide effective support to those suffering from the alienation of addiction, to offer role modeling, and to harness the power of peer pressure, an important force against denial and resistance" (pp. 269–270).

The rapidly growing focus of mental health professionals on the patient with a dual diagnosis (i.e., a diagnosis of a major mental illness and an addiction, usually a substance use disorder) has opened up new possibilities in the treatment of these disorders (Minkoff and Drake 1991). With the acknowledgment that addicted individuals often also have a range of psychological and characterological problems, and that both the addiction and the psychological difficulties need to be actively addressed for improvement to occur in either domain, access to adequate treatment becomes available for the first time. Paradoxically, the acceptance of a dual diagnosis may mean that an individual's treatment can be unified, coherent, and integrated rather than fragmented or divided between care systems—systems that have often worked at cross-purposes.

In this context, *dual diagnosis* does not apply only to the individual with severe, chronic mental illness. Klein et al. (1991) asserted that individuals who have severe personality disorders—disorders diagnosed on Axis II of DSM-III-R (American Psychiatric Association 1987)—and who are also actively abusing substances are most accurately considered to have dual diagnoses. Klein and colleagues' conceptualization of Axis II therapy groups addressed the special problems of providing group therapy to patients with these severe personality disorders and substance abuse. Such patients pose recurrent danger to themselves and others; they can be demanding and act out anxiety and depression, causing splits and powerful countertransference in treating clinicians (Klein et al. 1991; Vannicelli 2001). The supportive holding environment of the group facilitates treatment of the addiction. At the same time, the group is tailored to manage the characterological difficulties of these patients. In the same manner, the MDGT model developed for cocaine-addicted patients by Khantzian et al. (1990) actively addresses both the substance abuse and the psychological and characterological problems of the group members. Group therapies for substance-abusing patients based on the interpersonal model, variants of this same conceptualization, were described by Vannicelli (1988) and by Matano and Yalom (1991). Here the attempt is to make available to substance-abusing patients in groups "a very powerful therapeutic element: the interactive group process" (Matano and Yalom 1991, p. 270). The group is seen as an adaptation of "regular" interactive group therapy, in which a focus on the here-and-now interpersonal relationships in the therapy group as a "social microcosm" offers a rich source of learning and change.

Special Needs of Addicted Individuals in Group Therapy

Addicted individuals face particular difficulties in the therapeutic process. They may be seen as vulnerable to addiction because they are narcissistically compromised through early experiences of deprivation and damage, with the persistent feelings of shame, loneliness, depression, defectiveness, and emptiness described by Kohut (1977), Wurmser (1978), and Meissner (1986); they may be understood to be narcissistically vulnerable and impaired *secondary* to the addiction (Vaillant 1983); they may be thought to have an attachment disorder (Flores 2001); or some factor may be responsible for both addiction and characterological problems (Flores 1988). A narcissistically vulnerable individual may crave empathy and contact with others and yet fear and reject such attention (Liebenberg 1990). The characteristically uneven and inconsistent way in which cocaine-addicted patients relate suggests their dilemma on entering therapy. As Khantzian et al. (1990) reported,

> [T]hey may be alternately charming, seductive, and passively expectant, or they may act aloof, as if they do not need other people. Their supersensitivity may be evident in deferential attitudes and attempts to gain approval and acceptance, but they may rapidly shift and become ruthless and demanding in their dealings with others. (p. 40)

Action, rather than talking about things or silently enduring negative affect or anxiety, is the preferred ex-

pressive mode, and the acting out may well involve relapsing to the addictive behavior (drinking, using drugs, or gambling). Other characteristic acting-out behaviors involve splitting, violations of boundaries, and violations of the group contract (e.g., attempting to do group business outside the group, either with therapists or with other group members).

In a report on group treatment of alcohol-abusing patients, Matano and Yalom (1991) noted these patients' tendency to externalize, to "see themselves as being influenced or controlled primarily by external events," and to compensate by employing the defenses of "defiance, grandiosity, and counterdependency" (pp. 288–289). Because the patients do not see themselves as being effective or in control, they rebel against control experienced as coming from outside. These defenses, or characteristic ways of coping, must be taken into account in tailoring group therapy to the needs of the addicted patient.

Flores (2001) turned to attachment theory (Bowlby 1973) to explain the force and benefit of group approaches and therapies in the treatment of substance use disorders. Flores stated that addictive behavior results from an attachment disorder. He affirmed a biological basis for interpersonal closeness: humans and other species are driven to "secure assistance for survival," and this closeness has "important emotional regulatory functions" (Flores 2001, p. 65). Walant (1995) viewed addiction as a means of substituting addictive behaviors for needs unmet developmentally. Like Flores, she criticized cultural tendencies to extol separation and individuation and instead argued for human needs that are more relational and intimate, especially in patients with addictive vulnerability. Flores suggested that self-structure, and thus the ability to self-regulate, develops as a function of *optimal* frustration, and group therapy provides a context for spontaneous repair of the inevitable rupture of bonds that occurs in social situations. Therapeutic structure formation becomes a desired by-product of group interaction.

Khantzian (1985, 1995) identified four areas of psychological vulnerability in the addicted individual: 1) regulation of affects, 2) self-care (the capacity to protect oneself from undue risk or danger), 3) relationships with others, and 4) self-esteem. Disturbances or deficits in these areas of ego functioning potentiate characterological problems. Difficulty in regulating affect manifests in an intensity of unmodulated feeling, often dysphoric, or in an inability to identify one's own emotions. Self-care deficits find their expression in poor attention to health, engagement in risky behaviors such as unsafe sex, and a general lack of concern for emotional and physical self-preservation. Relationships with others can be problematic in many ways—tumultuous, dependent, or lacking because of the individual's isolation and withdrawal. Finally, self-esteem is compromised or shaky and may manifest as idealization or devaluation of others, feelings of shame and inadequacy, or bravado and grandiosity.

When group treatment is modified for the special needs of the addicted individual, these four dimensions of everyday intrapsychic and social life become the organizing foci for understanding the individual's distress, behavioral difficulties, characteristic ways of handling problems, and possibilities for change. The dimensions provide clarity and structure for handling complex issues with action-oriented, crisis-prone, and affectively constricted or volatile group members.

The Tradition of Exclusion

Although group therapy has advantages in the treatment of addiction in patients with character disorders, the addicted individual is often excluded from group therapy through being too unstable, disruptive, or unmotivated. Often he or she is unwelcome as a group candidate because of difficulty in tolerating affect and managing anxiety; characteristic postures of self-sufficiency, disavowed need, and bravado (Khantzian 1986); a tendency toward use of more primitive defenses (splitting, denial); and a propensity for action rather than reflection. The addicted individual as candidate for therapy can easily be seen as one of the "difficult" patients who can make the therapist feel "puzzled, overwhelmed, depressed, angry, [and] confused" and on whom "all our skill and knowledge has little impact" (Rice and Rutan 1987, p. 131).

Negative countertransference responses, often unacknowledged and resulting in a reluctance to work with addicted individuals, have been a problem in providing adequate individual or group treatment to addicted individuals (Levy 1987). Levy (1987, p. 786) reported, for example, that the therapist may "not be able to tolerate the alcoholic's repeated 'falls off the wagon' and might, in subtle ways, castigate the patient, adding to the alcoholic's already low self-esteem and

causing the alcoholic to continue drinking as a way to cope with such feelings." The ongoing possibility of relapse—relapse to the addictive behavior and psychological relapse to the unadaptive, problematic emotional state—must be tolerated and actively addressed. The characteristic "difficult" postures, attitudes, and behaviors of addicted patients must be understood and worked with. The propensity for impulsive action leads to crisis, instability, and lack of safety, a situation that continually tests the therapist's empathy, objectivity, and steadiness. As Klein et al. (1991) pointed out, these difficulties are geometrically increased in a group. The group, like its individual members, can change rapidly, verge on dissolution, and regroup just in the nick of time.

The exclusion from treatment can be rationalized from either the addiction treatment or the mental health perspective. A situation develops in which an individual is either excluded from both systems, shuttled back and forth from one to the other, or administered parallel yet potentially uncoordinated treatments.

Sciacca (1991) distinguished between the characteristics of traditional addiction treatment and those of traditional mental health treatment approaches. Programs to treat addictions stress willingness and motivation (with the exception of hospitalization for detoxification) and often involve highly confrontational encounters that aim to break down denial of the problematic consequences of addiction and denial about one's own behavior. In a similar vein, addiction treatment may emphasize the necessity of "hitting bottom." Sciacca (1991) reported that "patients must experience severe losses or deterioration in order to perceive that they need help for addiction" (p. 72). Otherwise, addicted individuals are seen as not ready for treatment. The addicted patient must be willing and motivated by dint of having hit bottom, thereby becoming ripe for confrontation.

On the other hand, mental health or psychotherapeutic approaches, according to Sciacca, characteristically require first that the patient have a diagnosable mental illness. If addiction is the most salient presenting feature of the individual coming for treatment, the care provider might refer the patient for addiction treatment rather than consider the larger, more comprehensive, psychological picture. Mental health approaches, however, are less likely than addiction treatment programs to emphasize motivation or even awareness or acceptance of the addiction as a prerequisite for treatment. This emphasis is seen as the work of the therapy itself, and the approach is more likely to be supportive than confrontational, with less interest in breaking down defenses than in shoring them up (Sciacca 1991, p. 73). Finally, the mental health professional may be unaccepting of addictive problems, either being unaware of and unable to easily identify them or being judgmental and critical in response to recognizing them.

Thus, the traditional mental health approach to the addicted individual with a character disorder may emphasize outreach and engagement, understanding and tolerance of defensive structures, and support during treatment. However, because of a lack of awareness of the psychological aspects of addictive suffering—the way in which the addiction expresses the vulnerable, compromised ego or self—addiction may be seen as the only problem, and there may be an unwillingness to provide therapy. Negative prejudices toward the addicted individual may result in exclusion from mental health or psychotherapeutic services. Therapy programs specializing in addiction, on the other hand, welcome the most desperate of addicted patients, but there is a tendency to desire a degree of preparation and readiness in the patient at the time of treatment, to underplay the importance of psychological factors and defenses, and to confront rather than support. The addicted individual is assumed to have certain strengths to sustain the treatment and a capacity for individual responsibility; otherwise, he or she is considered "not ready." The stages of change model (Prochaska and DiClemente 1985), which more realistically identifies the process of getting ready to change, and the articulation of motivational interviewing techniques (Miller and Rollnick 1991) serve as refreshing antidotes to these pessimistic and fatalistic attitudes about motivation for treatment among patients with substance use disorders.

Failure to appreciate the whole of the addicted individual's experience leads to fragmented, exclusionary, and ineffective treatments. Getting caught between two systems is a real possibility. Taking into account the strengths and shortcomings of both traditional addiction treatment and mental health treatment approaches, as in Sciacca's schema, can aid in the development of an integrated treatment. Conceptually and practically, these two traditions can then inform the treatment of choice for the addicted patient with a character disorder—the specially modified group therapy.

Features of the Group

Specific features of group therapy for the addicted individual derive from the consideration of the addicted person's special needs and have been discussed by several authors in the literature on addiction and group psychotherapy (Brown and Yalom 1977; Flores 1988; Golden et al. 1993; Khantzian 1995; Khantzian et al. 1990, 1992; Matano and Yalom 1991; McAuliffe and Albert 1992; Vannicelli 1982, 1988; Yalom 1974). In addition, the emerging literature on group psychotherapy for the difficult patient, one whose character defenses and acting-out behavior challenge the traditional group therapy format, contributes to an understanding of what is needed (Fenchel and Flapan 1985; Klein et al. 1991; Leszcz 1989; Rice and Rutan 1987; Roth et al. 1990; Stone and Gustafson 1982). Finally, the literature on the dual diagnosis of major mental illness and substance use disorder offers guidance in modifying group therapy for this population (Levy and Mann 1988; Minkoff and Drake 1991).

Pregroup Preparation

Group therapy in the treatment of addiction begins pregroup with outreach and preparation. The goal of this preparation is to provide a welcome that will increase motivation for the treatment, reduce premature dropping out, ease fears of and resistance to the group modality, and increase self-awareness. Sciacca (1991) emphasized the supportive, collaborative nature of the pregroup contacts: the potential group member's level of motivation and readiness is assessed and accepted, and he or she is encouraged to keep an open mind regarding self and others. Assessing the potential member's specific stage in the change process according to the scheme presented by Prochaska and DiClemente (1985) will assist the group leader in determining the best way to help the individual join the group. A clear therapeutic contract is presented, including guidelines for boundaries between group members and between therapist and group member, and a statement about "the necessity for therapist communication and collaboration with other treaters" (Klein et al. 1991, p. 99).

Khantzian et al. (1990) stated that the therapist "can play a critical role at this point in establishing optimistic and realistic member expectations regarding the efficacy" of the group. The therapist (in this case, for a psychodynamic group treating cocaine addiction) not only "acquaints the new members with the established ground rules, which include strict confidentiality, attendance and promptness, and abstinence from drugs and alcohol," but also discusses the benefits of group therapy, explains the focus of the group, acknowledges the difficulty of joining groups, "explains the work of therapy," and identifies the new members' personal goals (Khantzian et al. 1990, pp. 46–48). Reaching out to the prospective group member, anticipating what will follow, and concretely outlining the expectations provide necessary structure to allay overwhelming anxiety.

Structure

Structure in the group for addicted patients is provided in several ways. The group contract serves as an organizing feature initially and as the group progresses. It is a given that the contract will be tested and perhaps hotly debated; this is part of the work of the group. Matano and Yalom (1991) cautioned against an overly authoritarian stance and advised that the group therapist be sensitive to the addicted patient's feeling of loss of personal control, which evokes defiant and counterdependent reactions.

Shared norms, explicitly stated and reiterated, also provide structure. Abstinence from the problematic, addictive behavior, commitment to talking about feelings and problems rather than acting on them in the group, and agreement about the goals of the treatment are important. In describing a group for alcoholic patients, Vannicelli (1988) emphasized that a shared understanding about "what it means to be working on one's drinking problem" and "what it means to be getting better" is necessary to the integrity of the group (p. 349). These norms are essential for dealing with the regression to the addictive behavior (relapse and "slips") and for providing a vision of progress, improvement, and recovery. Khantzian (2001) stated that healthy play, laughter, and humor are important elements of a friendly supportive group.

Didactic and psychoeducational groups, self-help and 12-step programs, and cognitive-behavioral groups are all models with a high degree of structure. This chapter's focus is on the less structured, psychodynamic and interpersonal groups and how they can be modified to provide adequate containment and comfort for the addicted group member. Enhanced structure in a psychodynamically oriented group

means explicitly endorsing certain group norms, an active leadership style for the therapist, and, as in Khantzian's MDGT model, a focus on specific characterological and self-regulation problems.

Safety

Safety considerations in the group setting include ensuring immediate physical safety during group meetings, ensuring safety for therapeutic exploration and change by establishing the norm of abstinence, and promoting an atmosphere of enough interpersonal comfort and psychological security for the interactive work of the group to proceed. Physical safety is a consideration in selection of the meeting place, the group leadership, and the strongly upheld norm of putting things into words instead of actions.

In the treatment of addiction, especially in the beginning stages, "nothing takes precedence over recovery—it is a life or death issue" (Matano and Yalom 1991, p. 273). In their interpersonal group model for alcoholic patients, Matano and Yalom (1991) advocated active facilitation of achieving and maintaining sobriety. Thus, early on in the group, any interpersonal interaction is "gentle, supportive, and directly supportive of sobriety" (p. 274). Vigilance for any threats to the recovery process is counseled.

Safety is also of paramount importance in MDGT (Khantzian et al. 1992). One of the four foci of MDGT—self-care—addresses the self-defeating, destructive, and dangerous nature of activities associated with addictive behavior: the addicted individual's poor capacity for self-preservation plays itself out through the addiction. Cognitive-behavioral and psychoeducational groups emphasize the risks that are external to the individual, such as dangerous companions who actively engage in addictive behavior, or environments that can stimulate cravings or actual relapse. In the group, the individual learns to recognize and avoid these dangers and to find new, safe friends and activities to replace them.

McAuliffe and Albert (1992) emphasized building "walls" and a "foundation" through a "system of steps that creates a life space that is free of drugs and that ensures support for recovery" (p. 33). Attention to the real dangers of the addiction and relapse in everyday life and the strengthening of the motivation for abstinence are necessary from the inception of group therapy.

Discovering what increases safety for individual group members may lead to directing members to other, concomitant treatments. Some individuals, for example, may need support between weekly group meetings and may find the accessibility of AA meetings vitally important. As one group member who attends a weekly Cocaine Anonymous meeting and a psychodynamic group meeting for cocaine-addicted individuals each week put it, "I need to keep seeing guys who are right at the beginning so I don't forget, and some who have a lot of recovery, but I want to talk about *all* the problems in my life." Some may need concurrent individual and group treatment. Others may need to use emergency or crisis intervention services. Developing an individualized combination of services to increase safety is an ongoing aspect of the work of the group therapist for addicted patients.

Within the group, safety is maintained by attending to the ever-possible psychological relapse or relapse to the addictive behavior. In a group for pathological gamblers, for example, the ongoing stress of overwhelming debt, often compounded by the unfamiliar tension of paying back slowly, puts the abstinent gambler at continued risk that must be monitored in the group. It may be common to find the group struggling with the question of what constitutes gambling (running a game at a carnival, buying a raffle ticket for a good cause, investing in stock for the children's college education) long after "the last bet." The question of openness versus keeping secret the extent of the ongoing debt also persists and may add to the risk. Even as self-awareness grows in the group, new stressors appear (e.g., long-term debt, the family's anger), and the risk of relapse remains high.

The atmosphere of the group also must be maintained as one safe for listening and disclosure—that is, the group must be accepting, empathic, and respectful of varying amounts of awareness and motivation; encourage participation; and be understanding of resistance. Modeling this accepting stance, the group leader maintains safety by protecting members from attack, shame, or premature self-disclosure, such as of traumatic material (Khantzian et al. 1990). Acknowledging the possible discomfort and anxiety of being in a group, the group leader assists the group in managing these feelings and in persisting with abstinence and psychological recovery.

Confrontation Versus Support

Matano and Yalom (1991) pointed to the dangers of an overly confrontational approach in the group. Al-

though increasing the addicted patient's honesty with self and others is necessary, the attempt to break down denial can backfire, causing the patient to leave the treatment program or to "dissemble compliance while inwardly retreating" (Matano and Yalom 1991, p. 291). Addicted patients should be treated like other patients—that is, they should be related to in an empathic, supportive, and understanding manner. A central task of the group leader is thus to manage the anxiety that the group process, particularly confrontation, inevitably stimulates in the group members and to keep this anxiety to a tolerable level.

Leszcz (1989), in writing about group treatment of the characterologically difficult patient, saw the group as first providing a holding environment—a place that is reliable, constant, and accepting, a place where group members can "relate in a nonrelated way, until they are able to ascertain that it is safe" (p. 326). The confrontation itself is spelled out as "a forceful, but supportive pressure on the patient to acknowledge something that is conscious or preconscious, but avoided because of the distress that it involves" (p. 327).

The group model of Khantzian et al. (1990) encourages an understanding of addictive behavior as an attempt to deal with feelings and experiences and an adaptation that has outlived its usefulness. The model encourages an understanding of resistance to change: group members are guided "to appreciate how their ways of coping and the crises they precipitate are linked to the past; they need to acknowledge their painful feelings from the past and in the present, and to support each other in finding alternative ways to cope with their painful feeling states and problems in living" (p. 76). In other words, group members, although held responsible for their choices and actions and asked to look squarely at themselves, are not blamed and judged.

The group modality offers a particular advantage when it comes to confrontation: group members are more likely to respond to confrontation by their peers. As Leszcz (1989) put it, "group members are less restricted in their range of responses and may be better able to use humor, cajole, or shock one another to force attention to a disavowed issue" (p. 327). The following case example is from a psychodynamic group led by one of the authors (S.J.G.):

> For many months, Bob, a group member who kept his distance from others and refused to "come clean" with his family about the extent of his addictive behavior, never removed his coat during the group

meetings, stating that he was "too cold." After other group members had "worked" on him for a while, he not only began to consider the problem of his secretiveness but also actually shed his coat for the first time, which was greeted by pleased laughter and a fellow group member's remark: "We *must* be hot tonight if Bob is taking off his coat!" Bob's joining in was acknowledged, gladly but lightly, without making him unduly self-conscious.

Perhaps the question of responsibility lies at the heart of balancing confrontation and support. Matano and Yalom (1991) distinguished between the *addictive process* (called the *disease* in AA terms) and the *recovery process*. Although they did not hold the alcoholic patient responsible for the addiction itself, for the "psychological loss of control," or for his or her culturally learned beliefs about drinking, they did "demand that patients assume responsibility for their recovery" (pp. 277–278). Clarity about responsibility is crucial in group therapy for addiction, especially because this treatment may represent the confluence of the mental health and the addiction treatment traditions that have so widely diverged on the question.

Cohesion and "Addict Identification"

The importance of cohesiveness in group therapy has been likened to the importance of the relationship or therapeutic alliance in individual therapy (Yalom 1985). Cohesiveness, or the attraction of the members to the group and their sense of belonging, has been correlated with tenure in the group (prevention of early dropout) and with the stability necessary for any kind of long-term therapeutic work to occur (Yalom 1985). Cohesiveness has also been cited as the central mediator of outcome (Budman et al. 1989). Matano and Yalom (1991), in their work specifically addressing group therapy for the alcoholic patient, linked the individual's identification as an "alcoholic," as well as the emphasis on sameness among group members, with feeling connected to the group and with the growth of group cohesion and safety. Vannicelli (1988) warned against overdoing the bonding that occurs through talking about the addiction. War stories about the glory days of drinking and how bad things finally got, for example, can also serve as a defense against further development of the group—a way to avoid other emotionally charged issues. Group members, even while seeking mutuality and safety in their identification as "addicts," can withdraw in this way from other contact with fellow group members.

Khantzian et al. (1990) described the group process in MDGT for substance-abusing individuals as moving toward the discovery of common ground. Initially, the group bonds around the identity as an addicted person. Many patients with dual diagnoses see their addicted status as preferable and more socially acceptable than other labels. Calling oneself an alcoholic or a drug addict and belonging to a group for addicted individuals translates to a less stigmatized identity than that of psychiatric patient, borderline personality disorder patient, or narcissist. The "outlaw" life of the addicted individual and the desperate extremities of addiction bring the group together and are idealized even as they are disavowed. Self-esteem is maintained, and cohesion is established.

However, the group must progress to find common bonds in some larger, universal human experience if the members are to grow and begin to see themselves as part of the human mainstream. For addicted individuals in group therapy, the common ground to seek is the middle ground about which they may be ambivalent, "as if the price of ordinary life were one of unremitting drudgery and joyless obligation" (Khantzian et al. 1990, p. 95). Personal material shared after the initial identification as an addicted person may be equally extreme or grandiose, or it may be withheld as not worthy of exposure in the group. Here is where the work of the group on awareness of self and others and on addressing problems of living can proceed.

The very nature of the psychodynamic or interpersonal group, with its emphasis on interpersonal interactions in the here and now and on the understanding of individual characterological patterns as they emerge within the group, provides a way to talk about ordinary life. For instance, a member of a group for cocaine-addicted individuals offered her group members a chance for greater involvement with one another when she remarked that she felt closer to them than to her family. This remark led to a discussion of alienation from neglectful or intrusive parents, instead of the usual accounts of past ruthless quests for cocaine and the enumeration of the pitfalls of addiction. Ordinary problems, part of everyday life beyond the addiction, offer the group members a way into the ordinary world.

The Group Therapist

The therapist administering group therapy for addiction has an active, demanding role to play. Concerns for safety and structure require an alert presence—a readiness to manage and help modulate anxiety, to address acting-out behavior, and to intervene if necessary by setting limits and upholding the group contract, even as the building of cohesion and the developing of the work of the group proceed. This active mode of leadership is important because, as reported by Khantzian et al. (1990), addicted individuals with histories of neglect and trauma "do not respond well to the traditions of therapeutic passivity…instead they need therapists who can actively and empathically help to engage them and each other around their vulnerabilities and the self-defeating defenses and behaviors they adopt to avoid their distress and suffering" (p. 162).

The therapist may become the focus of anger and dependence, the mediator of struggles, and the unintentional voice of the superego. Co-therapists are split into good and evil. Countertransference feelings may be difficult, especially when helplessness and fear are evoked, as they often are in these groups (Klein et al. 1991). Supervision, opportunities to share the work, concurrent therapies, and supports for group members—working as part of a team or a program—all help to make group therapy for addiction possible and effective.

Conclusion

Current group approaches to addiction have emerged from several traditions: self-help fellowships; the psychoeducational, cognitive-behavioral modality; and the psychodynamic, interpersonal tradition. Although the group approach has evolved from these diverse theoretical and ideological viewpoints, there is a dearth of controlled studies of efficacy and outcome that could support a particular school of thought. Conceptually and pragmatically, practitioners working with addicted individuals have reached similar conclusions regarding their special needs in a group setting. If addicted individuals are to receive the full benefit of treatment, their characterological and psychological vulnerabilities must be recognized and addressed. Traditional treatments are then modified, particularly if they do not already provide the high degree of structure and safety necessary for engaging and retaining the addicted individual. The group approach—in its powerful capacity to support and confront, to comfort and to challenge, and to involve its members in en-

counters that vividly heighten awareness of interpersonal and characterological problems and provide a safe place for change—is now viewed as the treatment of choice for addiction. Special features of group therapy for the treatment of addiction are an emphasis on outreach and preparation for involvement in the group; a high degree of structure and active leadership; a concern for safety (particularly an awareness of the risk of relapse to the addictive behavior); a balance between confrontation and support; and a goal of moving beyond the initial cohesiveness of the group members' identification as addicted individuals to helping them discover common bonds in living ordinary lives.

References

Alonso A: Character change in group therapy. Paper presented at Psychiatric Grand Rounds, the Cambridge Hospital, Cambridge, MA, September 1989

American Psychiatric Association: Diagnostic and Statistical Manual of Mental Disorders, 3rd Edition, Revised. Washington, DC, American Psychiatric Association, 1987

Bowers TG, al-Redha MR: A comparison of outcome with group/marital and standard/individual therapies with alcoholics. J Stud Alcohol 51:301–309, 1990

Bowlby J: Attachment and Loss, Vol 2: Separation: Anxiety and Anger. New York, Basic Books, 1973

Brown S, Yalom ID: Interactional group therapy with alcoholics. J Stud Alcohol 38:426–456, 1977

Budman SH, Soldz S, Demby A, et al: Cohesion, alliance and outcome in group psychotherapy. Psychiatry 52:339–350, 1989

Carroll KM, Nich C, Ball SA, et al: Treatment of cocaine and alcohol dependence with psychotherapy and disulfiram. Addiction 93:713–727, 1998

Cherkas MS: Synanon Foundation: a radical approach to the problem of addiction (editorial). Am J Psychiatry 121:1065, 1965

Drake RE, Antosca LM, Noordsy DL, et al: New Hampshire's specialized services for the dually diagnosed, in Dual Diagnosis of Major Mental Illness and Substance Disorder. Edited by Minkoff K, Drake RE. San Francisco, CA, Jossey-Bass, 1991, pp 57–67

Fenchel GH, Flapan D: Resistance in group psychotherapy. Group 9:35–47, 1985

Flores PJ: Group Psychotherapy With Addicted Populations. New York, Haworth, 1988

Flores PJ: Addiction as an attachment disorder: implications for group therapy. Int J Group Psychother 51:63–81, 2001

Getter H, Litt MD, Kadden RM, et al: Measuring treatment process in coping skills and interactional group therapies for alcoholism. Int J Group Psychother 42:419–430, 1992

Golden S, Halliday K, Khantzian EJ, et al: Dynamic group therapy for substance abuse patients: a reconceptualization, in Group Therapy in Clinical Practice. Edited by Alonso AA, Swiller HI. Washington, DC, American Psychiatric Press, 1993, pp 271–287

Greene LR: Research in group psychotherapy for substance abuse: fiction, fact and future, in Group Psychotherapy of Substance Abuse. Edited by Brook DW, Spitz HI. New York, Haworth Medical, 2002, pp 391–410

Hellerstein DJ, Meehan B: Outpatient group therapy for schizophrenic substance abusers. Am J Psychiatry 144:1337–1339, 1987

Herman JL: Trauma and Recovery. New York, Basic Books, 1992

Kang SY, Kleinman PH, Woody GE, et al: Outcomes for cocaine abusers after once-a-week psychosocial therapy. Am J Psychiatry 148:630–635, 1991

Khantzian EJ: Opiate addiction: a critique of theory and some implications for treatment. Am J Psychother 131:160–164, 1974

Khantzian EJ: The ego, the self, and opiate addiction: theoretical and treatment considerations. Int Rev Psychoanal 5:189–198, 1978

Khantzian EJ: The self-medication hypothesis of addictive disorders: focus on heroin and cocaine dependence. Am J Psychiatry 142:1259–1264, 1985

Khantzian EJ: A contemporary psychodynamic approach to drug abuse treatment. Am J Drug Alcohol Abuse 12:213–222, 1986

Khantzian EJ: Self-regulation vulnerabilities in substance abusers: treatment implications, in The Psychology and Treatment of Addictive Behavior. Edited by Dowling S. New York, International Universities Press, 1995, pp 17–41

Khantzian EJ: The self-medication hypothesis of substance use disorders: a reconsideration and recent applications. Harv Rev Psychiatry 4:231–244, 1997

Khantzian EJ: Treating Addiction as a Human Process. Northvale, NJ, Jason Aronson, 1999

Khantzian EJ: Reflections on group treatments as corrective experiences for addictive vulnerability. Int J Group Psychother 51:11–20, 2001

Khantzian EJ, Mack JE: Alcoholics Anonymous and contemporary psychodynamic theory, in Recent Developments in Alcoholism, Vol 7: Treatment Research. Edited by Galanter M. New York, Plenum, 1989, pp 67–89

Khantzian EJ, Mack JE: How AA works and why it's important for clinicians to understand. J Subst Abuse Treat 11:77–92, 1994

Khantzian EJ, Halliday K, McAuliffe WE: Addiction and the Vulnerable Self. New York, Guilford, 1990

Khantzian EJ, Halliday KS, Golden S, et al: Modified group therapy for substance abusers: a psychodynamic approach to relapse prevention. Am J Addict 1:67–76, 1992

Khantzian EJ, Golden SJ, McAuliffe WE: Group therapy for psychoactive substance use disorders, in Treatments of Psychiatric Disorders, 3rd Edition, Vol 1. Edited by Gabbard GO. Washington, DC, American Psychiatric Publishing, 2001, pp 891–900

Klein RH, Orleans JF, Soule CR: The Axis II group: treating severely characterologically disturbed patients. Int J Group Psychother 41:97–115, 1991

Kohut H: Preface, in Psychodynamics of Drug Dependence (NIDA Research Monograph 12; DHEW Publ No ADM-77-470). Edited by Blaine JD, Julius DA. Rockville, MD, National Institute on Drug Abuse, 1977, pp vii–ix

Leszcz M: Group psychotherapy of the characterologically difficult patient. Int J Group Psychother 39:311–335, 1989

Levy MS: A change in orientation: therapeutic strategies for the treatment of alcoholism. Psychotherapy: Research and Practice 24:786–793, 1987

Levy MS, Mann DW: The special treatment team: an inpatient approach to the mentally ill alcoholic patient. J Subst Abuse Treat 5:219–227, 1988

Liebenberg B: The unwanted and unwanting patient: problems in group psychotherapy of the narcissistic patient, in The Difficult Patient in Group: Group Psychotherapy With Borderline and Narcissistic Disorders. Edited by Roth BE, Stone WN, Kibel HD. Madison, CT, International Universities Press, 1990, pp 311–322

Martin K, Giannandrea P, Rogers B, et al: Group intervention with pre-recovery patients. J Subst Abuse Treat 13:33–41, 1996

Matano RA, Yalom ID: Approaches to chemical dependency: chemical dependency and interactive group therapy: a synthesis. Int J Group Psychother 41:269–293, 1991

McAuliffe WE, Albert J: Clean Start: An Outpatient Program for Initiating Cocaine Recovery. New York, Guilford, 1992

McAuliffe WE, Ch'ien JM: Recovery training and self help: a relapse-prevention program for treated opiate addicts. J Subst Abuse Treat 3:9–20, 1986

Meissner WW: Psychotherapy and the Paranoid Process. New York, Jason Aronson, 1986

Miller WR, Rollnick S: Motivational Interviewing: Preparing People to Change Addictive Behavior. New York, Guilford, 1991

Minkoff K, Drake RE (eds): Dual Diagnosis of Major Mental Illness and Substance Disorder. San Francisco, CA, Jossey-Bass, 1991

Nace EP: The Treatment of Alcoholism. New York, Brunner/Mazel, 1987

Orford J: Excessive Appetites: A Psychological View of Addictions. New York, Wiley, 1985

Prochaska O, DiClemente CC: Common processes of change in smoking, weight control, and psychological distress, in Coping and Substance Abuse. Edited by Schiffman S, Willis TA. San Diego, CA, Academic Press, 1985, pp 345–363

Rice CA, Rutan JS: Inpatient Group Psychotherapy. New York, Macmillan, 1987

Roth BE, Stone WN, Kibel HD (eds): The Difficult Patient in Group: Group Psychotherapy With Borderline and Narcissistic Disorders. Edited by Roth BE, Stone WN, Kibel HD. Madison, CT, International Universities Press, 1990

Sciacca K: An integrated treatment approach for severely mentally ill individuals with substance disorders, in Dual Diagnosis of Major Mental Illness and Substance Disorder. Edited by Minkoff K, Drake RE. San Francisco, CA, Jossey-Bass, 1991, pp 69–84

Shaffer HU, LaSalvia TA, Stein JP: Comparing hatha yoga with dynamic group psychotherapy for enhancing methadone maintenance treatment: a randomized clinical trial. Altern Ther Health Med 3:57–66, 1997

Stone WN, Gustafson JP: Technique in group psychotherapy of narcissistic and borderline patients. Int J Group Psychother 32:29–56, 1982

Vaillant GE: The Natural History of Alcoholism. Cambridge, MA, Harvard University Press, 1983

Vannicelli M: Group psychotherapy with alcoholics. J Stud Alcohol 43:17–37, 1982

Vannicelli M: Group therapy aftercare for alcoholic patients. Int J Group Psychother 38:337–353, 1988

Vannicelli M: Leader dilemmas and countertransference considerations in group psychotherapy with substance abusers. Int J Group Psychother 51:43–62, 2001

Walant KB: Creating the Capacity for Attachment: Treating Addiction and the Alienated Self. Northvale, NJ, Jason Aronson, 1995

Wurmser L: The Hidden Dimension: Psychodynamics in Compulsive Drug Use. New York, Jason Aronson, 1978

Yalom ID: Group psychotherapy and alcoholism. Ann N Y Acad Sci 233:85–103, 1974

Yalom ID: Inpatient Group Psychotherapy. New York, Basic Books, 1983

Yalom ID: The Theory and Practice of Group Psychotherapy. New York, Basic Books, 1985

Family Therapy

Alcohol

Peter Steinglass, M.D.
Sari Kutch, M.S.W.

In the past three decades, a growing body of research literature and clinical experience has established that alcoholism is a family problem as well as an individual problem; that alcoholism runs in families; that families are devastated by the secondary consequences of alcoholism; and that inclusion of the family as a central partner in the therapy process significantly improves treatment outcome. The following statistics serve as reminders of the importance of including a family perspective in the design and implementation of treatment and public health approaches to alcoholism:

- Of the approximately 18 million individuals in the United States who abuse alcohol, 3 in 4 live in families.
- Three in 10 adults report that drinking has been a cause of trouble in their families.
- Alcoholism has been linked to marital and family discord, job loss, divorce, inadequate parenting, child abuse, and other forms of family violence.

- Alcohol abuse and drug abuse are factors in the placement of 75% of children who enter foster care.
- Separated and divorced adults are three times more likely than their married counterparts to have been married to or to have lived with an alcoholic individual or problem drinker.
- More than 75% of female victims of nonfatal domestic violence report that their assailants were drinking or using drugs immediately before the assault.
- Among adult drinkers (defined as adults who have consumed 12 or more alcoholic drinks in the past year), 56% report a blood relative with alcoholism.

Given these compelling statistics, one would imagine that families have long been seen as important targets for alcoholism treatment programs. Instead, well into the 1980s, clinicians treating alcoholism by and large ignored families. A number of factors may have contributed to this marginalization of a family perspective in the treatment of alcoholism, including a health care system built around diagnosis and treatment of individuals; an absence of clinicians with training in both addiction psychiatry and family therapy; and a belief widely held by clinicians and the lay public that family members are often part of the problem rather than part of the cure.

This last issue has been a particularly pervasive and corrosive one for families trying to get help for alcohol problems. For many years, clinicians promulgated a pathologizing view of their patients' family members, who were not infrequently seen as directly or indirectly contributing to the patients' drinking. For example, in literature published in the 1970s and 1980s on the "alcoholic marriage," it was argued that alcoholism is often the product of pathological personality traits in the nonalcoholic spouse (usually the wife) that either cause or maintain the alcoholic partner's misuse of alcohol (Rotunda et al. 1995). As another example, the popular literature on recovery long depicted the "alcoholic family" as dysfunctional. These stigmatizing labels, combined with long-standing public and professional perceptions of alcoholism as a reflection of moral weakness or lack of willpower, have increased the reluctance of families to seek help. In addition, the view frequently expressed in this literature that an alcoholic individual must "hit bottom" before he or she can stop drinking, or that loved ones are powerless to influence the alcoholic's drinking, seems to argue against active involvement of families in the treatment process.

Yet there is little empirical evidence to support any of these views. Although current thinking about factors influencing the onset of alcoholism includes an emphasis on the familial nature of alcoholism, and although there are genetic factors that predispose individuals to alcoholism, few would currently argue that there is either a unique individual personality structure or a specific family behavioral style that contributes to alcoholism. Aspects of family interactional style clearly influence the clinical course of alcoholism, but these family characteristics seem to be associated with a wide range of chronic psychiatric conditions rather than only with alcohol or drug abuse disorders.

Put another way, the current research literature supports a view that families with alcoholic members are highly heterogeneous in their structural and behavioral characteristics (Lipps 1999; Rotunda and O'Farrell 1997). Furthermore, there is reason to believe that many of the seemingly dysfunctional behavioral patterns seen in families with alcoholic members are stress-related reactions secondary to the traumas frequently associated with chronic alcoholism (e.g., family violence, sexual abuse of children, financial crises) (Rotunda and O'Farrell 1997; Rotunda et al. 1995). This view also supports a position that effective treatment for alcoholism should target the needs of all family members because the effects of alcoholism on family life are profound.

The argument for a family-focused approach to alcoholism treatment has been further strengthened by emerging research literature indicating that active participation of family members in alcoholism treatment both significantly increases engagement and retention of the alcoholic individual in treatment and improves treatment outcomes for all involved (Baucom et al. 1998; Edwards and Steinglass 1995; Miller et al. 1999a; C. Thomas and Corcoran 2001). As this evidence continues to accumulate, an earlier view that family therapy interventions are appropriate only for alcoholic patients with attendant severe marital and/or family problems has given way to the view that active involvement of the spouse and the family is warranted across the full spectrum of patients (Rotunda and O'Farrell 1997). If these impressions continue to be supported by the wealth of data emerging from the current round of treatment outcome studies, this would strongly suggest that some form of family therapy should be routinely included in alcoholism treatment protocols.

This trend toward active inclusion of families in alcoholism treatment programs is already evident in many clinical settings. Whereas 30 years ago, clinicians treating alcoholic patients at best tolerated families, one is now hard-pressed to find a credible alcoholism treatment program that does not at least give lip service to the importance of including family members in the treatment plan. Nevertheless, despite this growing interest in the family on the part of alcoholism specialists, and despite the widespread perception that family therapy is being offered as a standard component of most treatment programs, considerable confusion remains regarding how this family component should be implemented. For example, one commonly implemented strategy used in many inpatient and residential programs is to establish a separate program for family members but to prohibit or significantly limit patient-family contact during the early phases of treatment. This approach is predicated on the belief that these relationships may be toxic to the individual in treatment and might therefore serve as triggers for resumption of alcohol use.

At the same time, a growing number of programs now include extensive use of family therapy approaches that bring family and patient together to participate conjointly in the rehabilitation program and to plan for the aftercare/relapse prevention phase of treatment. By and large, these programs rely on elements from one or more of the three models of family therapy for alcoholism most frequently mentioned in the clinical literature: 1) family systems therapy (Steinglass et al. 1987), a model that applies principles of general system theory to family behavior and focuses on how family reorganization around alcohol use alters patterns of behavior and distorts long-term family growth; 2) behavioral family therapy (Baucom et al. 1998; Edwards and Steinglass 1995; Lipps 1999; Miller et al. 1999a; Rotunda and O'Farrell 1997; C. Thomas and Corcoran 2001), a model that extends classical conditioning principles to interactional behavior, with particular emphasis on the interactional contingencies that contribute to alcohol use; and 3) social network therapy (Galanter 1999), a model that uses constructs such as social support, social networks, and stressful life events to help identify the factors that either assist or hinder families in solving problems in the face of stressful events. These, therefore, are the approaches we will be describing in greater detail.

Family Therapy Approaches to Alcoholism

Overview

Although family systems therapy, behavioral family therapy, and social network therapy differ significantly both in concept and in technique, when applied to alcoholism treatment they also have many overlapping features. Most important are three central ideas, all of which have strong research support:

1. Active inclusion of family members during the assessment/diagnostic phase of treatment substantially increases the clarity of the clinical picture (i.e., the quantity and frequency of drinking behavior and its impact on family, work, social relationships, and physical health).

2. Early family involvement increases subsequent engagement of both the patient and the family in ongoing treatment (including rehabilitation and aftercare).

3. All three of these treatment approaches substantially improve long-term outcomes not only for the alcoholic family member (e.g., increased sobriety rates) but for others in the family as well (e.g., increased marital satisfaction and stability).

These different family therapy models also share a reliance on a therapeutic stance that emphasizes therapist neutrality, use of nonpathologizing language with patients and families, and family-therapist collaboration (rather than a hierarchical approach in which the therapist takes the position of expert and unilaterally defines the treatment goals for the family). This collaborative stance bears strong resemblance to that of the motivational interviewing approach advocated by Miller and Rollnick (2002), which has become central to the treatment protocols developed for use with alcoholic individuals in many of the major controlled clinical trials carried out in recent decades.

Another feature shared by all three models is the belief that to be effective, therapy must remain focused on the drinking behavior itself and on developing a credible action plan for addressing this issue. Family therapists working in this area are of mixed opinion about whether a reduction in alcohol consumption levels is a credible treatment goal (the "harm reduction" approach) or whether total abstinence is the only viable goal. But regardless of where they fall on this continuum, family therapists share the belief that if the therapist can contextualize drinking behavior within family relationships, family members can then be mobilized to work with the therapist to design and implement a more effective action plan for addressing problematic drinking behavior.

Lastly, in these different family therapy approaches, alcoholism treatment is seen as existing on a continuum, meaning that different techniques are called for depending on what stage of change the family is in (precontemplation, contemplation, preparation, action, or maintenance) (Prochaska and DiClemente 1984) and which phase of treatment is occurring (initiation/engagement, primary treatment/rehabilitation, or aftercare/relapse prevention).

Initiation/engagement. During the initiation/engagement stage of treatment, family members are often the ones requesting help, and a history of significant alcohol abuse emerges, either directly or indirectly, during history taking. By not waiting for the problem drinker to find his or her own motivation for change, family-oriented therapists can work with the rest of the family and effect a substantial alteration in the problem drinker's motivation to seek help (Miller et al. 1999b). Typically, this is accomplished by working with the family to change interactional patterns around alcohol use. Examples might include refusing to allow important family rituals to be disrupted because of alcohol use, removing inadvertent reinforcers of drinking behavior, and increasing coping skills that result in more effective ways to address the drinking problem. These techniques have the direct consequence of making family life more positive and the secondary effect of empowering the family to lobby the alcoholic member to enter treatment.

Put another way, motivation for change on the part of nonalcoholic family members is directly correlated with potential family supportiveness of the problem drinker, which in turn is a key factor in the success of initiation of treatment. Furthermore, inclusion of nonalcoholic family members in the initial assessment phase is invaluable to the clinician, not only because a more complete history of drinking and its consequences can be obtained but also because a treatment plan can be developed that is consistent with the needs of all family members (Edwards and Steinglass 1995; Miller et al. 1999b).

Strategies for subsequent engagement of alcoholic family members in treatment vary from the collaborative, motivational interviewing style advocated by Miller and Rollnick (2002) to the hierarchical strategies associated with what have been called family interventions. The various engagement strategies can also be classified on the basis of whether they involve family members only or the larger social or community network of the identified patient.

Interventions that focus on the family or spouse alone are typically referred to as unilateral family therapy by their designers (namely, Barber and Gilbertson [1996] and E.J. Thomas et al. [1987]). Studies undertaken by these two sets of investigators demonstrated that this approach is effective not only in motivating alcoholic individuals to enter treatment but also in reducing their drinking behavior before entering treatment. Participation in unilateral family therapy is also associated with a decrease in spousal psychopathology and life distress (Edwards and Steinglass 1995; C. Thomas and Corcoran 2001).

A variant of unilateral family therapy is community reinforcement and family training (CRAFT) (Meyers and Smith 1997), an outgrowth of the community reinforcement approach first described by Hunt and Azrin (1973). In a clinical trial, CRAFT proved substantially more effective in engaging initially unmotivated problem drinkers in treatment (64%), compared with Al-Anon (13%) and a standard family intervention (30%) (Miller et al. 1999a).

At the other end of the continuum is perhaps the best-known family intervention used to motivate problem drinkers unwilling to stop—the family intervention model developed by the Johnson Institute (Johnson 1980). The confrontational Johnson approach, although proved to be an effective method for inducing treatment engagement, appears to be an unacceptable strategy for many families. Empirical studies consistently find that a substantial majority of families do not go through with the intervention (Edwards and Steinglass 1995; Miller et al. 1999a).

Primary treatment/rehabilitation.   During the primary treatment/rehabilitation phase, a focus on general family processes and relationship issues (at the same time that the primary focus is on cessation or significant reduction of alcohol consumption) takes what might otherwise be seen as a task for the problem drinker alone and places it instead in a relational context. This is not to say that the family is responsible for getting the problem drinker to stop drinking; rather, significant relationships (both within the family and in the larger social network) become resources for change. That such a relational approach to primary treatment and rehabilitation is warranted has been amply demonstrated by treatment outcome studies comparing individual counseling with a variety of treatment models that include family members in this phase of therapy (Edwards and Steinglass 1995; Rotunda and O'Farrell 1997; Rotunda et al. 1995). Findings of these studies include a significant reduction in drinking behavior, longer stays in treatment, and improved marital satisfaction and stability.

Aftercare/relapse prevention.   In contrast to the growing research-based evidence of the value of including families in the initiation and primary treatment phases of therapy for alcoholism, much less is known about factors contributing to better outcomes during the aftercare/relapse prevention phase of treatment. However, early findings again support the view that families are a positive influence during this phase as well and that family involvement seems to promote both more consistent attendance and higher rates of long-term abstinence (Edwards and Steinglass 1995; C. Thomas and Corcoran 2001).

With this overview in mind, we will now outline the main tenets of the three family-oriented treatment models for alcoholism that have received the most clinical and research attention to date: family systems therapy, behavioral family therapy, and social network therapy. We will also discuss Al-Anon, the most widely used of the lay self-help groups offering help to family members in alcoholic families.

Family Systems Therapy

The family systems model of treatment for alcoholism centers around the concept of the *alcoholic system,* defined as a behavioral system in which alcohol acquisition and/or consumption is a major organizing principle for patterns of interactional behavior. This process of reorganization around alcoholism is most apparent in 1) a reordering of family priorities and routines of daily living to accommodate alcoholism-generated demands and 2) a skewing of the course of family development, attendant on an emphasis on short-term stability at the expense of long-term growth (as a way of coping with the challenges posed by alcoholism), a process that gives the family the appearance of rigidity or narrowness, as frequently mentioned in the clinical literature.

Three areas of family life have been suggested as foci for assessment: family problem-solving strategies; daily routines; and family rituals (e.g., holidays, vacations, family dinners). For each area, the central question is the extent to which family behavior patterns have been invaded (i.e., substantively changed) to accommodate the unique demands generated by the family's alcoholic member, and with what consequences for the family. The importance of this "invasion" process for family life has been supported by a series of empirical studies, which demonstrated 1) striking differences between interactional behavior in the presence of alcohol and in its absence (Jacob and Seilhammer 1987)—often referred to as the contrast between *wet* and *dry* family behavior patterns; 2) the link between a family's daily routines and clinical course issues related to alcoholism (Steinglass 1981); and 3) correlations between alcoholic family rituals and intergenerational transmission of alcoholism (Wolin et al. 1980).

Because this model posits that over time, the entire family reorganizes itself around alcohol issues, treatment is also directed at the entire family, instead of treatment of family members being seen as adjunctive to treatment of the alcoholic member. Thus, the assessment phase of treatment is typically carried out through conjoint interviews of the whole family and/or important subunits (especially the marital dyad), with an eye toward obtaining the multiple perspectives of all family members on the history of alcohol use and the effect of such use on individuals and relationships within the family. Because this approach allows for immediate comparisons of the perspectives of all family members about drinking behavior and family life, it typically generates a clinical database that tends to be both richer and more reliable than is the case with assessment of the alcoholic individual alone.

This ability to obtain multiple perspectives is especially valuable in assessing the effect of intoxicated behavior on family regulatory mechanisms. (As discussed earlier in this section, these mechanisms include family problem-solving styles, daily routines, and family rituals.) In that a key aspect of family systems therapy posits that understanding differences between patterns of interactional behavior in the presence versus the absence of active drinking is critical to the ultimate success of treatment, obtaining this history from the entire family is vastly preferable to interviewing the alcoholic family member alone. Failure to appreciate and understand the complex ways in which alcohol-related behaviors have become incorporated into family life may lead to inadvertent destabilization rather than improvement of family life after the removal of alcohol secondary to participation in an alcoholism treatment program.

Consequently, interest has been generated in the development of assessment techniques for addressing these differences. In some instances, an opportunity to assess behavior under so-called wet conditions is afforded by the alcoholic family member's appearing for a treatment session in an intoxicated state. The therapist can use this opportunity to observe differences in interaction patterns regarding variables such as activity and passivity of various family members, interaction rates, range of affective expression, levels of direct conflict, verbal content (especially related to problems not previously raised), interactional distance, prevailing mood, and degree of interpersonal engagement. For example, an observation that a married couple seems more emotionally engaged during such a session might lead to speculations that the couple is inadvertently using this engagement to carry out problem solving during periods of intoxication, a factor that might become a reinforcer of subsequent episodes of drinking.

A second aspect of the family systems model of alcoholism treatment that differentiates this model from other treatment approaches is its approach to detoxification. In family systems therapy, the primary goal of detoxification is not only cessation of drinking on the part of the alcoholic patient but the establishment of an alcohol-free family environment as well. Thus, the term *family-level detoxification* has been introduced to describe this phase of treatment. To accomplish this aim, a multiphase process is instituted, made up of six integrated components:

1. Development of a written contract (the family detoxification contract) by the family and the therapist
2. Use of a core set of metaphors around which the detoxification contract is framed
3. Use of a multistage strategy for implementing the terms of the detoxification contract
4. Use of public disclosure to reinforce the meaning and importance of the detoxification contract
5. Use of a prospective, anticipatory stance to identify potential challenges to abstinence
6. Ample rehearsal of strategies to effectively meet these potential challenges to abstinence

The family detoxification component is the most distinctive aspect of the family systems treatment model. By asking the couple (or the patient and the family) to work together on framing the contract, and by establishing as a treatment goal an alcohol-free family environment, the therapist is automatically reframing the entire alcoholism issue in family terms. Although not disputing that the patient has been consuming the alcohol, the therapist is dramatically reinforcing the concept that alcoholism has in important ways taken over family life. Thus, at the same time that this phase of treatment is aimed at the important goal of cessation of drinking as a necessary prerequisite for further treatment, the therapist is also carrying out essential reframing work to enable the couple (or the patient and the family) to reorganize family life so that the necessary relapse prevention tools and structures are in place.

The most detailed discussion of the family systems model of alcoholism, including the empirical research on which it is based, is that by Steinglass and colleagues (1987). A manual-based version of a family systems treatment approach, developed by Shoham and colleagues (Rohrbaugh et al. 1995), is also available. The manual was developed in conjunction with the only controlled clinical trial to date of a family systems approach for alcoholism (Beutler et al. 1997; Shoham et al. 1998).

Behavioral Family Therapy

Behaviorally oriented marital and family therapy is an extension of the basic constructs of learning theory to behavior in families. In the alcoholism field, behaviorally oriented treatment approaches have been based primarily on social learning theory, a variant of behavior theory that starts with the basic stimulus-response models of operant and classical conditioning but also incorporates the role of cognitive processes. As outlined by McCrady (1986) (one of the major proponents of the use of behavior therapy techniques for the treatment of alcoholism), reinforcement patterns involving families struggling with alcoholism issues take three major forms (i.e., types of responses or consequences that families establish for drinking behavior): 1) reinforcing drinking behavior through giving attention or caretaking; 2) shielding the alcoholic individual from the negative consequences; and 3) punishing drinking behavior.

To combat this intertwining of drinking behavior and family response patterns, a behavioral family therapist attempts to 1) identify specific sequences of behavior in order to uncover the stimulus-response patterns associated with repetitive drinking episodes, 2) categorize these response patterns (consequences) as either positively or negatively reinforcing drinking behavior, and 3) introduce interventions to increase and reinforce positive behavioral interactions at the spousal or family level and concomitantly decrease negative behavioral response patterns related to drinking. The terms *positive* and *negative* here denote consequences that seem to increase drinking behavior (negative reinforcers) or those that reinforce or reward decreased drinking (positive reinforcers).

Toward these goals, the assessment phase of treatment focuses on identification of specific behaviors that can be targeted for subsequent interventions. Treatment approaches involve the same types of techniques used in cognitive-behavioral therapy with individuals: monitoring behavior, establishing and rehearsing alternative behavioral sequences, and establishing specific behavioral goals regarding positive reinforcement patterns (O'Farrell and Cutter 1984).

The study by Beutler et al. (1997) mentioned above in the "Family Systems Therapy" section also included a cognitive-behavioral, couples treatment as one of its comparison treatments. A detailed manual describing this approach was prepared as part of the study (Wakefield et al. 1996) and is the clearest explication to date of behavioral principles applied to couples therapy for alcoholism.

Also important to mention here is a particularly promising multicomponent treatment program developed by O'Farrell and colleagues (O'Farrell et al. 1998; Rotunda and O'Farrell 1997) called Counseling for Alcoholic Marriages (Project CALM). This program has been extensively researched in controlled clinical trials comparing it with individually oriented alcoholism treatment programs. It has four major components: initial engagement; couple sessions; a multicouple group session; and relapse prevention. Although it relies on many of the behavioral marital therapy principles outlined by McCrady (1986), it also shares many features with the family systems treatment approach, including the use of motivational interviewing to help build the marital couple's commitment to treatment, contracting around cessation of alcohol use (although not around family-level detoxification), and a focus on enhancing couple-level problem solving, considered a key to building stronger relationship skills.

Central to the Project CALM treatment approach is the hypothesis that increased marital relationship stability will amplify the couple's commitment to treatment in general and long-term sobriety in particular. Toward that end, techniques are used that include training the couple to recognize and reinforce positive behavior, teaching communication skills (e.g., reflective listening, direct expression of feelings, negotiation as part of effective problem solving), and guiding partner-assisted contracting around compliance with disulfiram therapy. Furthermore, the couple is taught specific skills (through role-playing, covert rehearsal, and homework) to help reduce sources of family stress, which presumably in turn reduces the risk of relapse.

Social Network Therapy

Social network therapy, based on a social systems model (Colletti and Brownell 1982; Galanter 1999;

Moos et al. 1988–1989), uses a variety of family interventions in support of a treatment plan targeted at the alcoholic individual as the primary patient. Here, the family's involvement is undertaken with one or more of the following goals in mind:

- To obtain more accurate and complete historical data regarding the identified patient's alcoholism history
- To increase the likelihood of engaging the patient in the treatment process
- To increase compliance rates, especially for disulfiram therapy and detoxification strategies
- To increase the social supports available to the alcoholic individual, especially during the postdetoxification period
- To provide independent counseling to family members regarding their own coping strategies and psychological sequelae related to the effect of chronic alcoholism on family life

Typically, these goals are achieved by establishing a concurrent program for family members parallel to and integrated with the treatment program for the identified patient. For example, family sessions (often without the alcoholic family member present) might occur on a regular basis during the time when the alcoholic patient is engaged in a residential detoxification program. Another popular approach has been the use of multiple-family group therapy—groups that focus on issues presumably relevant to the nonalcoholic members of the family, including supportive approaches geared to help families deal with common difficulties they face as a result of having an alcoholic member. In some instances, groups for spouses and/or children meet concurrently with groups for the alcoholic family members. In other instances, the alcoholic members are included in the group, but the focus remains a social systems one.

A detailed description of the social network therapy approach to alcohol and drug abuse treatment can be found in Chapter 28 ("Network Therapy") in this volume.

Al-Anon Groups

It is important to include a word here about the use of self-help groups designed for family members as part of treatment planning. The models of family therapy for alcoholism discussed earlier in this chapter have all been proposed by family therapy specialists. For the most part, they are also designed to be implemented by family therapy clinicians.

However, by far the most active family-oriented program for alcoholism is a self-help one: the Al-Anon family group. Al-Anon is an indigenous self-help movement that arose spontaneously as a movement parallel to but separate from Alcoholics Anonymous (AA) in the 1940s. Al-Anon family groups are modeled after AA (i.e., a group fellowship of peers sharing a common problem), but in the case of Al-Anon, the peers are spouses, children, and close relatives of alcoholic individuals who are usually, but not necessarily, part of an AA group.

Ablon (1977), who studied the Al-Anon movement extensively, suggested that to be successful, Al-Anon members must accept one basic didactic lesson and three principles for operating in the groups themselves. The didactic lesson is the acceptance of the AA concept of alcoholism as an obsession of the mind and an allergy of the body, implying that the alcoholic individual has a disease that is totally outside his or her control. The three operating principles are 1) a loving detachment from the alcoholic individual, in which family members accept as a given that they are powerless to intervene constructively in the behavior of the alcoholic family member; 2) the reestablishment of the individual's self-esteem and independence; and 3) a reliance on a higher power—a spiritual emphasis that, of course, also closely parallels the spiritual emphasis in AA.

Family therapists are divided about combining traditional family therapy approaches with concurrent involvement in AA or Al-Anon groups. Some therapists have argued that the two approaches work at cross purposes in that AA and Al-Anon clearly see the alcoholic individual, not the family, as the patient. However, the prevailing view is that for many families, participation in self-help groups is a useful adjunct to family therapy, especially as a component of the rehabilitation and relapse prevention phases of treatment.

Efficacy

Although there are still far fewer controlled clinical trials of family therapy approaches to alcoholism and drug abuse treatment than of individual therapy, studies carried out to date have consistently indicated that family therapy approaches are at least as effective

in reducing the patient's alcohol consumption but also have the advantage of improving relationships between family members and with the extended social network (for reviews of this literature, see Baucom et al. 1998; Collins 1990; Edwards and Steinglass 1995; Lipps 1999; and C. Thomas and Corcoran 2001). Furthermore, involvement of family members substantially increases patient engagement in both detoxification and rehabilitation phases of treatment (Miller et al. 1999a; Rotunda and O'Farrell 1997; Stark 1992). Thus, the importance of family involvement in substance abuse treatment has solid empirical support.

Reviews of the family therapy literature make it clear that a wide array of family treatment techniques (e.g., family systems therapy, behavioral family therapy, multiple-couples therapy, multiple-family group therapy) have been used with this population of families, and all techniques have their strong advocates. Thus far, these family therapy approaches have not been tested against one another; hence, it is unknown whether, for example, systems-oriented approaches are superior to behavioral family therapy. Nor can one make any statements about the relative effectiveness of the different family therapy approaches for different patient populations (patient-to-therapy-match designs). Given the heterogeneity not only of alcoholic patients but also of their families, clinical wisdom would suggest that no single approach could be best for all patients and families. However, efforts to validate the patient–therapy-match approach have thus far been unsuccessful (Project MATCH Research Group 1997). Hence, an empirical approach that uses clinical judgment not only to combine the different family therapy models but also to integrate individual and family components within the treatment program seems the most reasonable one at this point.

Treatment Outcome Literature

A modest literature now exists on the efficacy of a variety of family therapy approaches for the treatment of alcoholism. The following generalizations about this literature seem warranted:

- *Efficacy of family therapy.* Both clinical reports and findings of controlled studies are overwhelmingly favorable with regard to the use of family therapy for the treatment of alcoholism. Put another way, no reports in the literature suggest either that family therapy is less effective than an alternative treatment approach to which it has been compared or that inclusion of family members in a treatment program has had detrimental effects. Furthermore, various family treatment approaches have been tried, including conjoint family therapy, behavioral marital therapy, concurrent group therapy, multiple-couples therapy, and multiple-family group therapy. All approaches have been reported to be efficacious; none has occupied a dominant position in the field.

With rare exceptions, however, all studies published to date must be characterized as pilot in nature. Yet, even though in most studies sample sizes are small, random assignment of patients is infrequent, and details regarding treatment programs and qualifications of therapists are scanty, Edwards and Steinglass (1995) identified 21 studies adequate in design quality to be included in a meta-analysis of treatment effect.

- *Involvement of nonalcoholic spouse.* On the basis of their meta-analysis, Edwards and Steinglass (1995) concluded both that compelling evidence indicates that involvement of a nonalcoholic spouse in a treatment program significantly improves the participation rate of an alcoholic family member in treatment and that such involvement also has a positive effect on the likelihood that the individual will alter his or her drinking behavior after treatment. This conclusion was based on an examination of three family-oriented treatment approaches: 1) a family intervention method (Liepman et al. 1989), 2) unilateral family therapy (E.J. Thomas and Ager 1993), and 3) community reinforcement training (Sisson and Azrin 1986). The meta-analysis by Edwards and Steinglass (1995) demonstrated that alcoholic individuals whose spouses participate in treatment engage in treatment at rates almost two standard deviations higher than rates for alcoholic individuals whose spouses do not participate in treatment. Alcoholic individuals whose family members were involved in some form of treatment entered treatment at rates ranging from 57% to 86% across the studies reviewed, compared with rates ranging from 0% to 31% in the control groups.

- *Relevance to overall compliance.* A related theme is overall compliance with ongoing treatment, even biomedically oriented treatment. For example,

Keane et al. (1984) demonstrated an unusually high rate of compliance with disulfiram therapy (88%) when the treatment regimen included a contract to take the disulfiram in the presence of the spouse, as well as subsequent positive reinforcement for taking disulfiram. The idea that compliance should improve if spouses are appropriately involved in treatment planning and implementation has considerable face validity. It is thus encouraging to see the emergence of data supportive of this notion.

- *Need for more study of long-range outcomes.* Although family therapy approaches have clear-cut effects on engagement of alcoholic individuals in treatment and also seem to have short-term effects on drinking behavior, remarkably few studies have examined long-range outcomes for these approaches. Given that alcoholism is a chronic disorder, much more attention will need to be paid to these long-range issues before clinicians can be satisfied that they know how to evaluate the true effect of family-oriented treatment approaches on alcoholism.

- *Need for clinical understanding of family dynamics.* Although most clinicians acknowledge that family issues are relevant to the comprehensive treatment of alcoholism, they often approach alcoholism without a sophisticated sense of family dynamics or family systems principles. Furthermore, little evidence indicates that clinicians fully appreciate the heterogeneity of alcoholic individuals' families. Instead, the dominant model in clinical practice remains heavily influenced by the AA/Al-Anon philosophy of separate but equal treatment. For example, it would be unusual to find an alcoholism treatment program in which a sophisticated family assessment was considered a mandatory part of a patient workup and in which a treatment program was designed on the basis of the findings of such a workup. Much more likely, a standard program exists and the alcoholic individual and his or her family are pushed and squeezed to fit the preconceived notions, treatment schedule, and goals of this already-established program.

- *Need to determine the role of family intervention.* Overall, professionals in the alcoholism field are receptive to the notion that family intervention has an appropriate place in the treatment process, but they are still struggling to determine what the scope of such intervention should be and what form it should take.

References

Ablon J: Perspectives on Al-Anon family groups, in Alcoholism: Development, Consequences, and Interventions. Edited by Estes NJ, Heinemann ME. St Louis, MO, CV Mosby, 1977

Barber JG, Gilbertson R: An experimental study of brief unilateral intervention for the partners of heavy drinkers. Research on Social Work Practice 6:325–336, 1996

Baucom DH, Shoham V, Mueser KT, et al: Empirically supported couple and family interventions for marital distress and adult mental health problems. J Consult Clin Psychol 66:53–58, 1998

Beutler LE, Shoham V, Jacob T, et al: Family Versus Behavioral Treatment of Alcoholism: A Final Report on Grant No 1-RO-11108486. Rockville, MD, National Institute on Alcoholism and Alcohol Abuse, 1997

Colletti G, Brownell KD: The physical and emotional benefits of social support: application to obesity, smoking, and alcoholism, in Progress in Behavior Modification. Edited by Hersen M, Eisler RM, Miller PM. New York, Academic Press, 1982, pp 109–178

Collins RL: Family treatment of alcohol abuse: behavioral and systems perspectives, in Alcohol and the Family: Research and Clinical Perspectives. Edited by Collins RL, Leonard KE, Searles JS. New York, Guilford, 1990, pp 285–308

Edwards ME, Steinglass P: Family therapy treatment outcomes for alcoholism. J Marital Fam Ther 21:475–509, 1995

Galanter M: Network Therapy for Alcohol and Drug Abuse. New York, Guilford, 1999

Hunt GM, Azrin NH: A community-reinforcement approach to alcoholism. Behav Res Ther 11:91–104, 1973

Jacob T, Seilhammer R: Alcoholism and family interaction, in Family Interaction and Psychopathology: Theories, Methods and Findings. Edited by Jacob T. New York, Plenum, 1987, pp 535–580

Johnson VE: I'll Quit Tomorrow. San Francisco, CA, Harper & Row, 1980

Keane TM, Foy DW, Nunn B, et al: Spouse contracting to increase Antabuse compliance in alcoholic veterans. J Clin Psychol 40:340–344, 1984

Liepman MR, Nirenberg TD, Begin AM: Evaluation of a program designed to help families and significant others to motivate resistant alcoholics into recovery. Am J Drug Alcohol Abuse 15:209–221, 1989

Lipps AJ: Family therapy in the treatment of alcohol related problems: a review of behavioral family therapy, family systems therapy and treatment matching research. Alcoholism Treatment Quarterly 17:13–23, 1999

McCrady BS: The family in the change process, in Treating Addictive Behaviors: Processes of Change. Edited by Miller WR, Heather NH. New York, Plenum, 1986, pp 305–318

Meyers RJ, Smith JE: Getting off the fence: procedures to engage treatment resistant drinkers. J Subst Abuse Treat 14:467–472, 1997

Miller WR, Rollnick S: Motivational Interviewing: Preparing People for Change, 2nd Edition. New York, Guilford, 2002

Miller WR, Meyers RJ, Tonigan JS: Engaging the unmotivated in treatment for alcohol problems: a comparison of three strategies for intervention through family members. J Consult Clin Psychol 67:688–697, 1999a

Miller WR, Zweben A, DiClemente CC, et al: Motivational Enhancement Therapy Manual: A Clinical Guide for Therapists Treating Individuals With Alcohol Abuse and Dependence. Rockville, MD, National Institute on Alcoholism and Alcohol Abuse, 1999b

Moos RH, Fenn CB, Billings AG, et al: Assessing life stressors and social resources: applications to alcoholic patients. J Subst Abuse 1:135–152, 1988–1989

O'Farrell TJ, Cutter HSG: Behavioral marital therapy couples groups for male alcoholics and their wives. J Subst Abuse Treat 1:191–204, 1984

O'Farrell TJ, Choquette KA, Cutter HSG: Couples relapse prevention sessions after behavioral marital therapy for male alcoholics: outcomes during the three years after starting treatment. J Stud Alcohol 59:357–370, 1998

Prochaska JO, DiClemente CC: The Transtheoretical Approach: Crossing Traditional Boundaries of Therapy. Homewood, IL, Dow Jones/Irwin, 1984

Project MATCH Research Group: Matching alcoholism treatments to client heterogeneity: Project MATCH posttreatment drinking outcomes. J Stud Alcohol 58:7–29, 1997

Rohrbaugh MJ, Shoham V, Spungen C, et al: Family systems therapy in practice: a systemic couples therapy for problem drinking, in Comprehensive Textbook of Psychotherapy: Theory and Practice. Edited by Bongar B, Beutler LE. New York, Oxford University Press, 1995, pp 228–253

Rotunda RJ, O'Farrell TJ: Marital and family therapy of alcohol use disorders: bridging the gap between research and practice. Professional Psychology: Research and Practice 28:246–252, 1997

Rotunda RJ, Scherer DG, Imm PS: Family systems and alcohol misuse: research on the effects of alcoholism on family functioning and effective family interventions. Professional Psychology: Research and Practice 26:95–104, 1995

Shoham V, Rohrbaugh MJ, Stickle TR, et al: Demand-withdraw couple interaction moderates retention in cognitive-behavioral versus family-systems treatments for alcoholism. J Fam Psychol 12:557–577, 1998

Sisson RW, Azrin NH: Family member involvement to initiate and promote treatment of problem drinkers. J Behav Ther Exp Psychiatry 17:15–21, 1986

Stark MJ: Dropping out of substance abuse treatment: a clinically oriented review. Clin Psychol Rev 12:93–116, 1992

Steinglass P: The alcoholic family at home: patterns of interaction in dry, wet, and transitional stages of alcoholism. Arch Gen Psychiatry 38:578–584, 1981

Steinglass P, Bennett L, Wolin SJ, et al: The Alcoholic Family. New York, Basic Books, 1987

Thomas C, Corcoran J: Empirically based marital and family interventions for alcohol abuse: a review. Research on Social Work Practice 11:549–575, 2001

Thomas EJ, Ager RD: Unilateral family therapy with spouses of uncooperative alcohol abusers. Journal of Social Service Research 10:145–162, 1993

Thomas EJ, Santa C, Bronson D, et al: Unilateral-family therapy with the spouses of alcoholics. Journal of Social Service Research 10 (special issue):145–162, 1987

Wakefield P, Williams RE, Yost E, et al: Couples Therapy for Alcoholism: A Cognitive-Behavioral Treatment Manual. New York, Guilford, 1996

Wolin SJ, Bennett LA, Noonan DL, et al: Disrupted family rituals: a factor in the intergenerational transmission of alcoholism. J Stud Alcohol 41:199–214, 1980

Family Therapy

Other Drugs

Edward Kaufman, M.D.
David W. Brook, M.D.

Drug abuse has a profound effect on the family, and the family plays a crucial role in the treatment of drug abuse. In this chapter, we address the role of the family in drug abuse treatment. It is important for therapists to understand the necessity for changing adverse interactions in the family that may lead to drug abuse. Therapists must especially attend to risk factors for and protective factors against the onset and maintenance of drug abuse. Treating the family necessitates further involvement with the patient's ecosystem, which also includes the treatment team, 12-step groups, sponsors, employers, employee assistance program counselors, managed care workers, parole officers, and other representatives of the legal system. At the time of treatment initiation, the family is generally the most critical part of this ecosystem.

In family therapy, there are three basic phases of the family's involvement in treatment: 1) developing a system that is acceptable to the patient and the family for establishing and maintaining a drug-free state,

2) establishing a workable method of family therapy, and 3) guiding the family's readjustment after the cessation of drug abuse. These three phases are discussed in detail, with an emphasis on variations in treatment techniques to meet the needs of different types of drug-abusing individuals. The variations are based on the following factors: substance(s) abused, family reactivity, risk factors and protective factors, stage of disease, and gender of the individual. Before presenting this material, we review the efficacy of family treatment of drug abuse.

Efficacy of Family Therapy in Drug Abuse Treatment

A number of family therapies have undergone rigorous empirical testing over the past decade. Both the quantity and quality of empirical testing have been greatly enhanced during that time. Although space limitations prohibit a complete review of all the work done, we will examine some of the studies that have focused on the family treatment of dependence on and abuse of substances other than alcohol.

Although a number of systems of family therapy have emerged more distinctly over the past decade, the clinical and theoretical work on which they are based has been in development for many years. These systems are also based in part on understanding gained from earlier family therapists. The development of these systems has also been marked by a great increase in the amount of research on family therapy, including process research and outcome research. Specific systems that have emerged include multidimensional family therapy (MDFT) (Dakof et al. 2001; Liddle and Hogue 2000; Liddle et al. 2001), family systems therapy (Szapocznik and Kurtines 1989; Szapocznik et al. 1990), and multisystemic therapy (MST) (Henggeler et al. 1998, 1999, 2002). Many of these systems of family treatment have developed from the work of researchers investigating the processes occurring in interactions and in families, including the work of Brook et al. (1990, 2002) on family interactional theory. Research on the bases of family interactions has found that changes in family interactions have effects on problem behaviors and adolescent development, including adolescent involvement with drug use and abuse.

Although early attempts to evaluate treatment outcome tended to be anecdote based or to take the form of nonquantifiable studies, some studies more than 20 years ago did use more precise methods. Stanton and Todd (1982) evaluated a model of family therapy that may be regarded as a form of family systems therapy. Male opioid-addicted individuals and their families were randomly assigned to one of the three treatments under study (two treatments were family treatments). The control group (53 families) received only methadone and individual counseling, not family treatment. After 1 year of treatment, patients in the two family treatment groups were engaging in less drug use and showed more improvement on measures of drug use compared with subjects in the two non–family therapy groups.

A study in the Netherlands (Romijn et al. 1992) attempted to replicate the work of Stanton and Todd (1982). Family therapy sessions using the techniques of Stanton and Todd (1982) were conducted about once every 4 or 5 weeks over 12–15 months. Subjects in the family therapy group achieved better results in terms of frequency of drug use compared with the control group, as well as better social functioning and improvement in communication with parents.

MDFT has been tested in controlled studies. In one randomized controlled study, MDFT was compared with multifamily educational intervention and adolescent group therapy (Liddle et al. 2001). The subjects were 95 drug-using adolescents and their families. Assessments were performed at intake and 6 and 12 months after termination of treatment, and outcome measures included drug use (reported by adolescents), adolescent acting-out behavior (reported by parents), family competence (observed by the therapist), and adolescent grade point averages. Adolescents in all three treatment programs showed improvement, but those who received MDFT showed more improvement in a wider range of areas, particularly in reduction of adolescent drug use. Significant improvement in family competence and grade point averages was shown only by subjects in the MDFT group, and more subjects in that group completed treatment (Liddle and Hogue 2000; Liddle et al. 2001).

In another study, MDFT was compared with individual cognitive-behavioral therapy (Turner 1992, 1993). Two hundred twenty-four drug-using adolescents and their families were randomly assigned to treatment. All adolescents met the criteria for substance abuse or dependence, and 78% had at least one comorbid diagnosis. Although both treatments resulted in significantly lessened drug use, only subjects who had received MDFT maintained the gain in reduction of symptoms after termination of treatment. MDFT was also tested in a multisite field effectiveness trial involving cannabis-using youth. Here, too, MDFT had a positive effect on drug use and other problem behaviors.

Another approach was used to study substance-abusing men ($N=40$) receiving behavioral couples therapy as well as individual therapy. In a series of studies done over a number of years, the investigators found that behavioral couples therapy was associated with a greater reduction in substance use and improvement in the marital relationship (Fals-Stewart et al. 2000, 2002; O'Farrell and Fals-Stewart 2002).

Over the past 25 years, Szapocznik and colleagues have studied an approach called brief strategic family therapy (BSFT). BSFT was developed when a structural-strategic systems approach was used to apply the principles of family therapy in the treatment of Hispanic youth with drug use and behavioral problems. BSFT was designed to have an effect on intergenerational and cultural differences in the family. In a study comparing BSFT with a community comparison intervention, 104 families were randomly assigned to either treatment method. BSFT was associated with more engagement and greater retention in treatment, especially retention of individuals with more severe problems (Coatsworth et al. 1997; Szapocznik and Kurtines 1989; Szapocznik et al. 1990).

Multisystemic therapy is another method of family treatment that has been studied empirically. Henggeler and colleagues (1999) studied 118 juvenile offenders with substance abuse or substance dependence. Subjects were randomly assigned to MST or community services. MST was found to have reduced substance use at an assessment immediately after treatment, and such a reduction was noted in 50% of subjects 6 months after treatment. After 4 years of participation in MST, the 80 subjects participating in the follow-up showed significant long-term treatment effects on aggressive criminal activity and a reduction in marijuana use.

Functional family therapy uses an integrative approach to address dysfunction in the family as a system and in family members. Treatment is based on altering interactions to help family members learn more adaptive ways of responding. Functional family therapy has been examined in controlled studies, and the findings have indicated positive change compared with other treatment methods and control conditions, with an alteration of delinquent behavior among youth (Alexander et al. 1994; Waldron et al. 2001).

Other approaches have been used to engage the family and significant others in treatment. The two approaches next described combine some of the principles of both family therapy and group therapy.

Network therapy was devised by and has been studied by Galanter and colleagues (1997). In this time-limited, standardized treatment approach, a training manual is used and individual treatment is combined with sessions in which family members and peers—used as a therapeutic network—join the patient and therapist. In a study supported by the National Institute on Drug Abuse, patients were evaluated during a short-term treatment program (average program length, 15.4 weeks). The results indicated the effectiveness of this form of treatment in reducing ongoing drug use, as measured by random urine testing involving observation (Galanter et al. 1997). In addition,

network therapy patients remained in treatment longer than did control subjects (Keller and Galanter 1999).

Multiple-family group therapy is another treatment method that involves techniques from both group and family therapy (Kaufman and Kaufmann 1977). A number of families meet in a group therapy session, the idea being that people perceive and discuss issues more easily when they are manifested in families other than their own. Early results indicated the potential clinical utility of such an approach (Kymissis et al. 1995).

Development of a System for Achieving and Maintaining Abstinence

Family treatment of drug abuse begins with development of a system to achieve and maintain abstinence. This system, together with specific family therapeutic techniques and knowledge of family patterns commonly seen in families with a drug-abusing member—also known as the *identified patient* (IP)—provides a workable, therapeutic approach to drug abuse.

Family treatment of drug abuse must begin with an assessment of the extent of drug abuse or dependence and the difficulties it presents for the individual and the family. Quantification of the individual's drug abuse can take place with the entire family present; the IP often will be honest in this setting, and "confession" is a helpful way to begin communication. Moreover, other family members can often provide more accurate information than the IP can. However, some IPs will give an accurate history only when interviewed alone. In taking a drug abuse history, the clinician should determine the IP's current and past use of every type of abusable drug, including alcohol. IPs also should be asked about the quantity and quality of the substances they have used, the duration of use, the expense, the methods used to support and prevent their drug intake, and the presence of physical effects, tolerance, withdrawal, and medical complications. Other past or present drug-abusing family members may be identified, and their drug use and its consequences should be quantified without the family's being put on the defensive. It is also essential to document the family's patterns of reactivity, codependence, and enabling of drug use and abuse, as well as the interactions of risk factors and protective factors in the IP and the family. The specific method necessary to achieve abstinence can be decided on only after the extent and nature of drug abuse are determined.

Establishing a System for Achieving Abstinence

It is critical to first establish a system for enabling the IP to become drug free, so that family therapy can take place effectively. The specific methods used to achieve abstinence vary according to the extent of use, abuse, and dependence; achieving abstinence should be regarded as a process as well as a goal and may take some time to accomplish. Mild to moderate abuse in adolescents can often be controlled if both parents agree on clear limits and expectations and on how to enforce them. Older individuals may stop abusing drugs if they are aware of the medical or psychological consequences to themselves or the effects on their family.

If drug abuse is moderately severe or intermittent and is not associated with physical dependence (e.g., intermittent use of hallucinogens, weekend cocaine abuse), the family can be offered a variety of measures, such as regular attendance by the IP at Narcotics Anonymous (NA) or Cocaine Anonymous (CA) meetings and by family members at Al-Anon meetings. Outpatient detoxification can be used for selected patients.

If the pattern of abuse or dependence is severe, if symptoms of physical dependence are present, or if there is an increase in symptoms, loss of control, or a history of treatment failures, hospitalization should be set as a requirement early in therapy.

Establishing a System for Maintaining Abstinence

The family is urged to adopt some system that will enable the IP to stay drug free. This system is part of the therapeutic contract made early in treatment. A lifetime commitment to abstinence is not required. Rather, the "one day at a time" approach of Alcoholics Anonymous is recommended. The patient is asked to establish a system for abstinence, which is committed to for only one day at a time but which is renewed daily using the basic principles of NA and CA. In a patient with a history of drug dependence, therapy is most successful when total abstinence is advocated and achieved; the longer the patient remains in treatment, the greater is the likelihood that treatment will be successful.

Many individuals need to shop around for a CA or NA group in which they feel comfortable. Every recovering patient is strongly encouraged to participate in small study groups (which work on the 12 steps) and attend larger meetings (which often have speakers and are open to anyone, including family members). Abstinence can also be achieved in heroin-addicted individuals through drug-aided measures such as methadone maintenance or naltrexone blockade or through the use of buprenorphine in office treatment. These medications work quite well in conjunction with family therapy, because work with the family enhances compliance and the blocking effects on the primary drug of abuse helps calm the family system so that family and individual therapy can take place. Hospitalization also calms an overreactive family system. Another advantage of hospitalization is that it provides an intensive 24-hour-a-day orientation to treatment.

Individuals who have been dependent on illicit drugs for more than a few years generally do not do well in short-term programs, although these programs may buy time so that effective individual and family therapy can occur. For drug-dependent patients who fail to improve in outpatient and short-term hospital programs, long-term residential treatment is the only workable alternative. Most families, however, will not accept this approach until other methods have failed. Therefore, a therapist must be willing to maintain long-term ties with the family, through multiple treatment failures, because drug dependence is a chronic, relapsing disease of the brain, with biopsychosocial and physiological concomitants and consequences (Leshner 1997). However, it may be more helpful to terminate treatment if the patient continues to abuse drugs, because continuation of family treatment implies that change is occurring when it is not. One way to continue therapist-family ties while not condoning drug abuse is to work with the family without the patient present. In other cases, it is more effective to terminate treatment until all family members are willing and able to adopt a workable program for reinforcing abstinence. Families that believe that therapy is being terminated in their best interest often return a few months or years later, ready and willing to commit to abstinence from drugs of abuse (Kaufman 1985).

Working With Families in Which Drug Abuse Continues

The family therapist is in a unique position in regard to continued drug abuse and other manifestations of the IP's resistance to treatment, including total non-participation. The family therapist still has a workable and highly motivated patient: the family. A technique that can be used to reach out to resistant patients is *contingency contracting,* which involves using a "level system" in which the IP's abstinence from drugs and his or her prosocial behavior are linked to parental rewards. With this technique, both family members and the IP have a mutual understanding of each domain of behavior that needs improvement and the therapist helps the parents establish standards of daily monitoring of the IP's drug use. Therapist feedback is an essential part of this technique, in which the therapist can act as a mediator between the IP and family members (Donohue and Azrin 2001).

Another technique, developed by Johnson, is the *intervention,* which involves working with patients and their families to focus on the IP's resistance to treatment ("How to Use Intervention in Your Professional Practice" 1987).

If the drug-abusing patient continues to use drugs despite active therapeutic intervention, one is faced with the problem of dealing with a drug-abusing family. Berenson (1979) offered a workable, three-step therapeutic strategy for dealing with spouses or other family members of individuals who continue to abuse drugs or are drug dependent. The three steps are as follows:

1. Calm down the family system by explaining problems, solutions, and coping mechanisms.
2. Create an external supportive network for family members so that the emotional intensity is not concentrated in the relationship with the IP or redirected to the therapist. Two types of support systems are available: a self-help group in the Al-Anon model and a significant-others group led by a trained therapist. In the first type, the group and sponsor provide emotional support, reinforce detachment, and help calm down the family. A significant-others group may provide more insight and less support for remaining with a drug-abusing spouse.
3. Give the spouse or other overinvolved family member three choices: a) keep doing exactly what you are doing, b) detach or emotionally distance yourself from the patient, or c) separate or physically distance yourself.

As part of the initial contract with a family, the therapist suggests that the patient's spouse, partner, or parents continue individual treatment or participation in Al-Anon, Co-Anon, or a group for spouses, partners, or parents, even if the patient drops out. Other family members are also encouraged to continue in family therapy and support groups. It should be reemphasized that whenever the therapist maintains therapy with a family in which serious drug abuse continues, he or she has the responsibility not to maintain the illusion that a family is resolving problems when the family is in fact reinforcing them. In contrast, even when the IP does not participate in treatment, the therapist may be quite helpful to the rest of the family.

Motivating the Entire Family to Participate

Although treatment works best when the entire family is available for therapy, once the family therapist has knowledge of the risk and protective characteristics of the drug-abusing family, a program for dealing with drug abuse, and a workable personal method of family therapy, it becomes remarkably easy to get the entire family to come in for therapy. The individual who calls for an initial appointment is generally the one who is best able to get the entire household to participate. However, in some cases, the therapist may have to contact one or more family members directly. It then becomes imperative for the therapist to establish a contract with the family that all members believe will relieve the pain that they and the IP are experiencing.

The concept of the family as a multigenerational system necessitates that the entire family be involved in treatment. The family members necessary for optimum treatment include the entire household and any relatives who maintain regular contact with the family. Relatively emancipated family members who have less-than-weekly contact may be helpful to these families; sessions that include them should be scheduled around their visits home.

It is advisable to use a multigenerational approach involving grandparents, parents, spouse, and children at the beginning of family therapy and at certain key points throughout the therapy. Research has demonstrated the multigenerational transmission of risk factors and protective factors for substance abuse (Brook et al. 1999). For IPs younger than about age 24, however, the critical family unit is often the IP and his or her siblings and parents, although many adolescents become emancipated from their families by age 18. The critical family unit for married IPs older than 24 years is the IP and his or her spouse. However, the more dependent the IP is on his or her parents, the more critical is work with the parents. Most sessions should be held with these family units; participation of other family members is essential for a more thorough understanding and permanent change in the family.

The most effective drug abuse treatment programs for women with young children are those that house the children jointly, provide child care, and attend directly to parenting and child care issues.

An Integrated Approach to a Workable System of Family Treatment

Family Diagnosis

Accurate diagnosis is as important a cornerstone in family therapy as it is in individual therapy. In family diagnosis, family interactional and communication patterns and relationships are examined. In assessing a family, it is helpful to construct a map of its basic alliances and roles (Minuchin 1975). Family rules and boundaries are also examined, as are child-rearing practices and the nature of the child-parent bond. Coalitions (particularly transgenerational ones), shifting alliances, splits, cutoffs, and triangulation are observed, as well as communication patterns, confirmation and disconfirmation, unclear messages, and conflict resolution. The family's stage in the family life cycle is also noted. Mind reading (i.e., predicting reactions and reacting to them before they happen, or knowing what someone thinks or wants), double binds, and types of conflicts are also observed. It is helpful to obtain an abbreviated three-generation genogram that focuses on the IP, his or her parents and progeny, and the parents of the IP's spouse.

Overview of Family Treatment Techniques

In this chapter, family therapy systems are summarized, with an emphasis on the application of these techniques to IPs. These systems are classified into several systems of treatment (although recent research has focused on the development of integrated models of family interventions). These approaches include structural-strategic family therapy, psychodynamic family therapy, multisystemic family therapy, and multidimensional family therapy. The work of Bowen (1971) will also be described briefly, as will a number of behavioral techniques. Any of these types of family therapy can be applied to IPs if the IPs' common family patterns are kept in mind and if a method to handle drug abuse is used.

Structural-Strategic Family Therapy

In structural-strategic family therapy, the structural and strategic types of family therapy are combined (they were developed by many of the same practitioners) and shifts between the two types are frequently made, depending on the family's needs. The thrust of structural family therapy is to restructure the system by creating interactional change within the session. The therapist actively becomes a part of the family yet retains sufficient autonomy to restructure the family (Stanton 1981; Stanton and Todd 1992).

According to strategic therapists, symptoms are maladaptive attempts to deal with difficulties that develop a homeostatic life of their own and continue to regulate family transactions. The strategic therapist works to substitute new behavior patterns for the destructive repetitive cycles. The therapist is responsible for planning a strategy to solve the family's problems. Techniques used by strategic therapists include the following (Stanton 1981):

- Putting the problem in solvable form
- Placing considerable emphasis on change outside sessions
- Learning to take the path of least resistance so that the family's existing behaviors are used positively
- Using the paradox (described later in this chapter [see "The Paradox"]), including restraining change and exaggerating family roles
- Allowing the change to occur in stages (The therapist may create a new problem so that solving it leads to solving the original problem. The family hierarchy may be shifted to a different, abnormal one before it is reorganized into a new functional hierarchy.)
- Using metaphorical directives in which the family members do not know they have received a directive

Stanton and Todd (1982) successfully used an integrated structural-strategic approach with heroin-addicted patients who were receiving methadone maintenance.

Psychodynamic Family Therapy

A psychodynamic family therapy approach has rarely been applied to IPs because such patients usually require a more active, limit-setting emphasis on the here and now than is usually associated with psychodynamic techniques. However, if certain basic limitations are kept in mind, psychodynamic principles can be extremely helpful in the family therapy of drug abuse (Kaufman 1992).

Important elements of psychodynamic family therapy include the following:

Countertransference. A fundamental difference in work with families is that the therapist may have a countertransference problem toward the entire family or any individual subsystem or member of the family. The therapist may particularly rally to the defense of his or her IP against "oppressive" family members; this can set up power struggles between the therapist and the family. Judicious expression of countertransference feelings may be helpful in breaking fixed family patterns. For example, sharing anger at a controlling patient may give the family enough support to express its anger at that patient in a manner that finally has an effect.

Family therapists view their emotional reactions to families in a systems framework and in a countertransference context. Thus, they must be aware of how families will replay their problems in therapy by attempting to detour or triangulate their problems onto the therapist. The therapist must be particularly sensitive about becoming an enabler who, like the family, protects or rejects the IP.

Therapist's role in interpretation. Interpretations can be extremely helpful if they are made in a complementary way, without blaming, guilt induction, or dwelling on the hopelessness of long-standing, fixed patterns. The therapist can point out to each family member repetitive patterns and their maladaptive aspects and can give tasks to these individuals to help them change these patterns. An emphasis on mutual responsibility when making any interpretation is an example of a beneficial fusion of structural and psychodynamic therapy (Kaufman 1985).

Overcoming resistance. *Resistance* is defined as behaviors, feelings, patterns, or styles that prevent change (Anderson and Stewart 1983) and enable the abuser to continue drug use. Every drug-abusing family has characteristic patterns of resistant behavior in addition to individual resistances. Some families may need to deny all conflict and emotion and are almost totally unable to tolerate any displays of anger or sadness; others may overreact to the slightest disagreement.

The treatment contract can focus on resistance by having each family member agree to cooperate in overcoming resistance, by performing assigned tasks. The therapist can directly discourage resistances such as blaming, dwelling on past injustices, and scapegoating. He or she may overcome resistance using joining techniques (see "Joining," later in this chapter), including minimizing demands on the family to change so that the family moves more slowly but in the desired direction.

Working through. Derived from psychoanalysis, the important concept of working through underscores the need to work repeatedly on many overt issues, all of which have the same dysfunctional core, to produce long-lasting change. Thus, to produce real change, a family must deal with a problem over and over until it has been worked through. If the family's behavior returns—if the family is back to old maladaptive ways—it becomes necessary to work through the conflicts in many different transactions until stable change takes place.

Multisystemic Therapy

MST focuses on variables in the IP's life that are connected to problem behaviors, including drug use (Henggeler et al. 1998). Psychosocial treatment and psychopharmacological treatment are delivered in an integrated manner.

One goal of MST is to help family members and the IP monitor at-risk behavior and to provide positive reinforcements for responsible behavior and negative restrictions for irresponsible behavior. The therapist tries to help the family develop an increasingly functional family structure and identifies barriers to positive change in the IP. Another goal of MST is to help the IP decrease associations with drug-using peers and increase associations with prosocial peers. Strategies to improve school or job performance are also presented. Improved communication between all family members and nonfamily significant others is emphasized. MST is conducted in community settings and is generally time limited (lasting 4–6 months). Use of a home-based method of treatment helps overcome barriers to treatment.

MST incorporates the work of a number of previous family therapists and includes structural-strategic and cognitive-behavioral therapy methods.

Multidimensional Family Therapy

MDFT was developed on the basis of research findings concerning adolescent development and the risk factors and protective factors for drug use or abuse; it also incorporates findings from treatment research. MDFT targets multiple problem behaviors in an integrative way and may incorporate parts of other empirically based approaches. A tenet of MDFT is that positive change can take place through multiple mechanisms and in many contexts. In addition to family sessions, MDFT also involves individual sessions, with both the IP and family members, as well as sessions with significant others in the life of the IP. In MDFT, conflict between parents and adolescents is often used to develop therapeutic interventions. The importance of engaging the adolescent and the family in treatment is stressed. The initial process of engagement is called joining (see "Joining," later in this chapter). MDFT strategies to engage families early in treatment include a focus on the presenting problem, evaluation of stressors, preparation for crises from therapy, and mobilization of community resources. The use of individual sessions enhances the process of family therapy, particularly in building rapport in the therapeutic relationship (the adolescent-therapist alliance) (Diamond and Liddle 1993). Building the therapeutic alliance with the IP takes place at the same time as sessions with the parents and family sessions. Techniques used in therapy include working with negative affect and building a constructive dialogue, and the therapist also acts as a mediator to help create satisfactory emotional relationships in the family.

Bowen's Systems Family Therapy

In Bowen's (1971) approach, the cognitive is emphasized and the use of affect is minimized. Systems theory focuses on triangulation, which implies that whenever emotional distance or conflict occurs between two individuals, tensions will be displaced onto a third party, issue, or drug. Drugs are frequently the subject of triangulation.

Cognitive-Behavioral Family Therapy

Cognitive-behavioral family therapy is commonly used with drug-abusing adolescents. Its popularity may be attributed to the fact that it can be elaborated in clear, easily learned steps. The following steps using cognitive-behavioral techniques can be applied in family therapy (Winters et al. 1999):

1. *Functional analysis.* Families are taught to understand the interactions that maintain drug abuse, and stressors and coping skill strengths and weaknesses are identified.

2. *Stimulus control.* Coping skills are taught so that stress and irrational beliefs can be dealt with. Drug use is viewed as a habit triggered by certain antecedents and maintained by certain consequences. The family is taught to avoid or change these triggers.

3. *Rearrangement of contingencies.* The family is taught techniques to provide reinforcement for efforts at achieving a drug-free state. These techniques involve frequent reviewing of positive and negative consequences of drug use and self-contracting for goals and specific rewards for achieving these goals.

4. *Cognitive restructuring.* IPs are taught to modify their self-derogatory, retaliatory, or guilt-related thoughts and to replace them with more rational ideation. The learning techniques used include instruction, modeling, peer guidance, and homework assignments.

5. *Planning of alternatives to drug use.* IPs are taught techniques for refusing drugs through role-playing and covert reinforcement.

6. *Problem solving and assertion.* IPs and their families are helped to decide if a situation calls for an assertive response and then, through role-playing, to develop effective assertive techniques.

7. *Maintenance planning.* The entire course of therapy is reviewed, and the new armamentarium of skills is emphasized. IPs are encouraged to practice these skills regularly.

8. *Communication.* Families can also be taught through behavioral techniques to become aware of their nonverbal communications, to make the nonverbal message concordant with the verbal, and to express interpersonal warmth nonverbally and verbally (Stuart 1980).

Specific Structural Techniques

In this section, useful family therapy techniques are discussed. Many of these techniques evolved from the structural family therapy work of Minuchin (1975, 1992) and Haley (1977). The approach described here also borrows from systems and psychoanalytic techniques. The reader is advised to choose those methods that are compatible with his or her personality, to learn and practice these techniques with precision at first, and eventually to use them in a spontaneous manner. These techniques are described individually, although most techniques are a fusion of several others as they are implemented in clinical practice. These techniques include the contract, joining, actualization, boundary marking, assignment of tasks, reframing, the paradox, balancing and unbalancing, and creation of intensity.

The Contract

The contract is an agreement to work on mutually agreed on, workable issues. The contract should always promise help with the IP's problem before being expanded to other issues.

The primary contract is drafted with the family at the end of the first interview. In subsequent sessions, the concept of a contract is always maintained so that family assignments and tasks are agreed on and their implementation is contracted by the family. The likelihood that the family will return after the first session is greatly enhanced by a contract that includes measures for problem resolution. In establishing a contract, the family must choose a system to achieve abstinence and must agree to pursue that system after it has been agreed on as part of the initial evaluation.

The family should be provided with the beginnings of a system of shifting overreactivity to drug abuse in the initial contract. Family members may be coached to disengage from the IP, using strength gained from support groups and the therapist. At times, this disengagement can be accomplished only by powerful restructuring or paradoxical interventions. Later in therapy, contingency contracting principles can be used to facilitate mutual trust, particularly in areas such as adolescent individuation (e.g., a child agrees to be more respectful if his or her curfew is extended).

Joining

In joining, the therapist adjusts himself or herself in a number of ways to affiliate with the family system and to engage the family early in treatment. Joining enhances the therapist's leverage to change the system. The therapist alternates between joining that supports and joining that challenges the family system and family members. Joining with only one part of a family may severely stress or change the rest of the family. The therapist must make contact with all family members so that they will comply with the therapist even when they feel that the therapist is being unfair (Kaufman 1985). The therapist should join by respecting and not challenging the initial defensiveness so common in these families.

Joining begins in the first moment of the session, when the therapist makes the family comfortable through social amenities and by chatting with each member. The three types of joining techniques are maintenance, tracking, and mimesis (Minuchin 1975).

In *maintenance,* the therapist supports the family structures and behaves according to the family rules. In its most extreme form, maintenance includes accepting the family scapegoats as the problem when another family member is much more problematic. Maintenance operations include supporting areas of family strength, rewarding, affiliating with a family member, complimenting or supporting a threatened member, and explaining a problem. The therapist uses the family's metaphors, expressions, and language.

In *tracking,* the therapist follows the content of the family's interactions by listening carefully to what everyone has to say and by providing comments and expressions that help each member know he or she has been heard and understood.

In *mimesis,* the therapist adopts the family's style and affect. If a family uses humor, so should the therapist. If a family communicates through touching, the therapist can also touch. The therapist supports family members or the entire family by means of nonverbal identification.

Actualization

Patients usually direct their communications to the therapist. They should be trained to talk to one another rather than to the therapist. They should be asked to enact transactional patterns rather than describe them.

Drug-abusing families frequently gravitate to a rehash of past fights, hoping to trap the therapist into deciding who started the fight, who is wrong and who is right, and what decision is the proper one. The therapist should not be triangulated into such a position but rather should have the family choose an unresolved conflict and actualize its problem-solving methods or lack of them in the session. If a family arrives with an intoxicated member, the family should not be dismissed. Instead, the family's interactions should be observed, because it will be seen how family members interact during a good portion of their time together. If intoxication recurs, the family must develop a system to end the drug abuse before therapy can continue.

Boundary Marking

All individuals and subsystems are encouraged to preserve their appropriate boundaries. Each individual should be spoken to, not about, and no one should talk, feel, think, answer, or act for anyone else. Each family member is encouraged to tell his or her own story and to listen to and acknowledge the communications of others. Nonverbal checking and blocking of communications should also be observed and, when appropriate, pointed out and halted. Mind reading is common but should be strongly discouraged, because even if the mind reader is correct, this behavior almost always starts an argument. No one likes his or her reactions to be anticipated.

The most important boundary shift in family therapy is a weakening of ties between an overinvolved parent and a child and a strengthening of the boundary that protects the parents as a unit and supports them in dealing with their own parents, in-laws, potential or actual lovers, and the rest of the world (external to the nuclear family).

If a role or tie is removed from a family member, this relationship should be replaced by ties with other family members or individuals outside the family. When boundaries are strengthened around a system, the system's functioning invariably improves.

Assignment of Tasks

Tasks are used to gather information, intensify the relationship with the therapist, and continue the therapy outside sessions, and tasks also give family members

the opportunity to behave differently (Haley 1977). Tasks should be chosen that work in the framework of family goals, particularly those involving changing the IP's behaviors. Tasks should involve everyone in the family and bring gains to each member. A task should be completed successfully in a session before being assigned as homework.

Tasks should be specific, clear, and concise. If tasks are performed successfully, they will restructure the family toward optimal functioning. Tasks that family members fail to complete are used as learning experiences that reveal family dysfunction. Still, the family should not be let off easily, and the reasons for the failure to complete a task should be explored.

Reframing

In reframing (Minuchin and Fishman 1981), the therapist takes information received from the family and transforms it into a format that will be most helpful to changing the family. Reframing, or relabeling, begins at the start of the first session, when the therapist receives information from the family and molds it so that family members feel their problems are clear and solvable. Reframing is achieved by focusing material as it is received, selecting the elements that will facilitate change, and organizing the information to give it new meaning. Perhaps the most common use of reframing occurs when an IP's behaviors are broadened to include the entire family system.

The Paradox

Paradoxical techniques work best with chronically rigid, repetitive, circular, highly resistant family systems, particularly ones that have had many therapeutic failures (Papp 1981).

The paradox is often used 1) to slow progress so that a family is chafing at the bit to move faster or 2) to exaggerate a behavior in order to emphasize the family's need to eliminate it. A behavior that is an externalized acting-out of family conflicts (e.g., stealing, secret drug-taking) can be prescribed to be performed within the family (i.e., family members are told to behave as they are already behaving) so that the family can deal with it. An individual's behavior is not prescribed without its being related to its function in the family system. At times, psychodynamic interpretations can be made in a paradoxical way that gives greater impact in order to reach and change the family.

Balancing and Unbalancing

Balancing techniques, which tend to support a family, are conceptually similar to Minuchin and Fishman's (1981) complementary technique. They challenge the family's views of behaviors as part of a linear hierarchy and emphasize the reciprocal involvement of behavior formation while supporting the family. When balancing is used, mutual responsibility is emphasized, and tasks that involve change in all parties should be given.

Unbalancing involves changing or stressing the existing hierarchy in a family. The therapist unbalances by affiliating with a family member of low power (so that this individual can challenge his or her prescribed family role) or by escalating a crisis, emphasizing differences, blocking typical transactional patterns, developing implicit conflict, and rearranging the hierarchy (Minuchin and Fishman 1981).

Creation of Intensity

Techniques for creating intensity are verbal devices used to ensure that the family hears and incorporates the therapist's message. One simple way to be heard is to either repeat the same phrase or say different phrases that convey the same concept. Another way to create intensity is through isomorphic transactions that use many interventions to attack the same underlying dysfunctional pattern.

Variations in Family Treatment for Different Types of Drug-Abusing Patients

In this section, we consider modifications of treatment that are necessary for optimal results with abusers of various types of drugs and their families. In family treatment, the needs of at least one other individual (in most cases, many others) must be considered as the therapist adapts his or her treatment techniques to each family. It may not be the drug of abuse that demands modification in techniques but other variables, such as the extent and severity of drug abuse, psychopathology, ethnicity, family reactivity, the stage of disease, and gender (Kaufman 1985). Other variables, such as parental warmth and the quality of the parent-child relationship, also play a role in drug abuse

(Brook et al. 1990) and can be modified in the course of family therapy.

By Drug Type

Most modifications in family treatment that are based on drug type occur in the first phase of treatment, when a system is developed for establishing and maintaining a drug-free state. Family self-help groups are extremely helpful adjuncts to family therapy. Co-Anon is extremely helpful in dealing with the specific problems of relatives of cocaine-abusing individuals. Some relatives of abusers of minor tranquilizers participate well in Al-Anon, whereas relatives of abusers of other types of drugs may find it difficult to relate to relatives of alcoholic individuals and would work best in a specialized group. In most geographic areas, groups such as Co-Anon and Nar-Anon do not exist, and it is helpful to use significant-others groups that are organized according to the drug of abuse and according to other factors such as social class and ethnicity.

By Type of Family Reactivity

Drug-abusing families have been categorized into four types—functional, enmeshed, disintegrated, and absent—each with different needs for family therapy (Kaufman and Pattison 1981).

Functional Families

Functional families have minimal overt conflict and a limited capacity for insight as they protect their working homeostasis. Thus, the therapist should not be too ambitious about cracking the defensive structure of the family, which is likely to be resistant. The initial use of family education is often well received. Explanation of the medical effects of drugs provides a concrete way for the family to face up to the consequences of drug abuse (Kaufman and Pattison 1981). These families can usually be taught appropriate family rules and roles. Cognitive modes of interaction are usually acceptable; more uncovering and emotional interactions may be resisted. If abstinence and equilibrium are achieved, the therapist should be content, even if the family members continue to use a great deal of denial and emotional isolation.

Short-term hospitalization may be required. Drug-abusing patients from functional families are often resistant to long-term residential treatment because they are protected by the family homeostasis.

Enmeshed Families

The therapeutic approach used with enmeshed families is much more difficult and prolonged than that used with functional families. Educational and behavioral methods may provide some initial relief but are not likely to have much effect on enmeshed neurotic relationships. Often these families are resistant to ending drug abuse, and the therapist is faced with working with the family while drug abuse continues. The more hostile the enmeshed family's interactions, the poorer the prognosis.

Although initial hospitalization or detoxification may achieve temporary abstinence, the IP is highly vulnerable to relapse. Therefore, long-term family therapy with substantial restructuring is required for development of an affiliated-family system that is free of drug abuse. An integrated synthesis of several schools of family therapy techniques may be required.

Because of the enmeshment and explosiveness of these families, the therapist usually must reinforce boundaries, define personal roles, and diminish reactivity. The therapist must be active and directive to keep the emotional tensions within workable limits. Disengagement can be assisted by getting family members involved in external support groups.

Disintegrated Families

Disintegrated families have a history of reasonable vocational function and family life but also a history of deterioration of family function and, finally, separation from the family. Use of family intervention might seem irrelevant in such a case; however, many of these marriages and families fell apart only after severe drug-related behavior. Furthermore, there is often only pseudoindividuation (i.e., false individuation by rebellion, which keeps children close to their family of origin through failure) of the patient from marital, family, and kinship ties.

These families cannot and will not reconstitute during the early phases of rehabilitation. Early therapeutic sessions are usually characterized by apathy or by intense hostility toward the IP; thus, the early stages of treatment should focus primarily on the IP. Potential ties to a spouse, immediate family, more distant relatives, and friends should be explored early in treatment, and some contact should be initiated. When abstinence and personal stability have been achieved over several months, the therapist can work with the family to reestablish family ties, but reconstitution of the family unit should not be a required goal.

Absent Families

In absent-family systems, there is a total loss of the family of origin, as well as a lack of other permanent relationships. Nevertheless, two types of social network intervention are possible. The first is the elaboration of existing friend and relative contacts. Often these social relationships can be revitalized and provide meaningful social support. Second, younger patients have a positive response to peer-group approaches, such as long-term therapeutic communities, NA, church fellowships, and recreational and avocational clubs, which draw them into social relationships and vocational rehabilitation. These patients can develop new skills and the ability to engage in satisfactory married and family life.

By Gender

Historically, drug abuse treatment in the United States has been male oriented. In countering this one-sided approach, family therapists must be aware that families of chemically dependent women demonstrate much greater disturbance than those of male patients seeking treatment: there is a greater incidence of chemical dependence among other family members, as well as a greater incidence of mental illness, suicide, violence, and physical and sexual abuse. Family-related issues also bring far more women than men into treatment; potential loss of custody of minor children heads the list (Sutker 1981).

Because of the differences between families of drug-abusing men and those of drug-abusing women, family intervention strategies for women must differ from those for men. Family therapy may be more essential for drug-abusing women because of symbolic or often actual losses of spouse and children. The therapist should not impose a stereotyped view of femininity on female patients; this could intensify the conflicts that may have precipitated the drug use (Sandmaier 1980). The therapist should be sensitive to the specific problems of women and drug-abusing women in this society and should address these issues in treatment.

Drug-abusing women have special concerns about their children and child care. Family therapy may help them see how the parenting role fits into their lives and how to develop parenting skills, perhaps for the first time. Many women have been victimized (e.g., through incest, battering, or rape). Catharsis and understanding of these feelings may be essential before a woman can build new relationships or improve her current ties (Kaufman 1985). Several studies have demonstrated that drug abuse treatment programs that address women's needs and accommodate children have better program retention and treatment outcomes.

In the case of male patients, special issues such as pride and acceptance of their own dependence needs often have to be addressed (Metsch et al. 1995).

Family Readjustment After Cessation of Drug Abuse

Once the drug abuse has stopped, the family may enter a honeymoon phase in which major conflicts are denied. The family may maintain a superficial harmony based on relief and suppression of negative feelings. Alternatively, when the IP stops using drugs, other family problems may be uncovered, particularly in the parent's marriage or in other siblings. These problems, which were present all along but were obscured by the IP's drug use, will be "resolved" by the IP's return to symptomatic behavior if not dealt with in family therapy. If symptomatic behavior recommences, the family will reunite around its problem person, according to its familiar pathological style.

Too many treatment programs in the drug abuse field focus their efforts on an intensive inpatient or partial hospital program, neglecting aftercare. Many of these programs include a brief but intensive family educational and therapeutic experience but include even less focus on the family in aftercare. These intensive short-term programs have great impact on the family system, but only temporarily. The pull of the family homeostatic system will draw the IP and/or other family members back to symptomatic behavior. The family must be worked with for months and often years after drug abuse first abates, in order to create a new homeostasis without drugs and a meaningful affective relationship among family members. Because drug abuse is a chronic, relapsing illness, ongoing family therapy is also necessary for the emotional well-being of the IP and other family members. If ongoing family therapy cannot be achieved, the therapist's door should remain open, because IPs and their families may return to treatment a number of times, even after prolonged absences. In some cases, recurrent episodes of family therapy may produce better results over the long term than ongoing family therapy.

Conclusion

Family therapy can reduce the incidence of premature withdrawal from treatment, act as a preventive measure for other family members, and create structural family changes that protect the IP from relapse and a return to drug abuse.

References

Alexander JF, Holtzworth-Monroe A, Jameson PB: The process and outcome of marital and family therapy research: review and evaluation, in Handbook of Psychotherapy and Behavior Change, 4th Edition. Edited by Bergin AE, Garfield SL. New York, Wiley, 1994, pp 595–630

Anderson CM, Stewart S: Mastering Resistance: A Practical Guide to Family Therapy. New York, Guilford, 1983

Berenson D: The therapist's relationship with couples with an alcoholic member, in Family Therapy of Drug and Alcohol Abuse. Edited by Kaufman E, Kaufmann P. New York, Gardner, 1979, pp 233–242

Bowen M: Family therapy and family group therapy, in Comprehensive Group Psychotherapy. Edited by Kaplan H, Sadock B. Baltimore, MD, Williams & Wilkins, 1971, pp 181–189

Brook JS, Brook DW, Gordon AS, et al: The psychosocial etiology of adolescent drug use: a family interactional approach. Genet Soc Gen Psychol Monogr 116:111–267, 1990

Brook JS, Whiteman M, Brook DW: Transmission of risk factors across three generations. Psychol Rep 85:227–241, 1999

Brook JS, Whiteman M, Zheng L: Intergenerational transmission of risks for problem behavior. J Abnorm Child Psychol 30:65–76, 2002

Coatsworth JD, Szapocznik J, Kurtines W, et al: Culturally competent psychosocial interventions with antisocial problem behavior in Hispanic youth, in Handbook of Antisocial Behavior. Edited by Stoff DM, Breiling J, Maser JD. New York, Wiley, 1997, pp 395–404

Dakof GA, Tejeda M, Liddle HA: Predictors of engagement in adolescent drug abuse treatment. J Am Acad Child Adolesc Psychiatry 40:274–281, 2001

Diamond GM, Liddle HA: Improving a negative therapist-adolescent alliance in family therapy, in 101 Interventions in Family Therapy, 2nd Edition. Edited by Trepper T, Nelson T. Binghamton, NY, Haworth, 1993, pp 87–95

Donohue B, Azrin NH: Family behavior therapy, in Innovations in Adolescent Substance Abuse Interventions. Edited by Wagner EF, Waldron HB. Amsterdam, Pergamon/Elsevier Science, 2001, pp 205–227

Fals-Stewart W, O'Farrell TJ, Feehan M, et al: Behavioral couples therapy versus individual-based treatment for male substance-abusing patients. An evaluation of significant individual change and comparison of improvement rates. J Subst Abuse Treat 18:249–254, 2000

Fals-Stewart W, Kashdan TB, O'Farrell TJ, et al: Behavioral couples therapy for drug-abusing patients: effects on partner violence. J Subst Abuse Treat 22:87–96, 2002

Galanter M, Keller DS, Dermatis H: Network therapy for addiction: assessment of the clinical outcome of training. Am J Drug Alcohol Abuse 23:355–367, 1997

Haley J: Problem Solving Therapy. San Francisco, CA, Jossey-Bass, 1977

Henggeler SW, Schoenwald SK, Borduin CM, et al: Multisystemic Treatment of Antisocial Behavior in Children and Adolescents. New York, Guilford, 1998

Henggeler SW, Pickrel SG, Brondino MJ: Multisystemic treatment of substance-abusing and dependent delinquents: outcomes, treatment fidelity, and transportability. Ment Health Serv Res 1:171–184, 1999

Henggeler SW, Clingempeel WG, Brondino MJ, et al: Four-year follow-up of multisystemic therapy with substance-abusing and substance-dependent juvenile offenders. J Am Acad Child Adolesc Psychiatry 41:868–874, 2002

How to Use Intervention in Your Professional Practice: A Guide for Helping-Professionals Who Work With Chemical Dependents and Their Families. Minneapolis, MN, Johnson Institute Books, 1987

Kaufman E: Substance Abuse and Family Therapy. New York, Grune & Stratton, 1985

Kaufman E: The application of the basic principles of family therapy to the treatment of drug and alcohol abusers, in Family Therapy of Drug and Alcohol Abuse, 2nd Edition. Edited by Kaufman E, Kaufmann P. Boston, MA, Allyn & Bacon, 1992, pp 287–314

Kaufman E, Kaufmann P: Multiple family therapy: a new direction in the treatment of drug abusers. Am J Drug Alcohol Abuse 4:467–468, 1977

Kaufman E, Pattison EM: Different methods of family therapy in the treatment of alcoholism. J Stud Alcohol 42:951–971, 1981

Keller DS, Galanter M: Technology transfer of network therapy to community-based addiction counselors. J Subst Abuse Treat 16:183–189, 1999

Kymissis P, Bevacqua A, Morales N: Multifamily group therapy with dually diagnosed adolescents. Journal of Child and Adolescent Group Therapy 5:107–113, 1995

Leshner AI: Drug abuse and addiction treatment research: the next generation. Arch Gen Psychiatry 54:105–107, 1997

Liddle HA, Hogue A: A developmental, family based, ecological preventive intervention for antisocial behavior in high-risk adolescents. J Marital Fam Ther 26:265–279, 2000

Liddle HA, Dakof GA, Parker K, et al: Multidimensional family therapy for adolescent drug abuse: results of a randomized, clinical trial. Am J Drug Alcohol Abuse 27:651–688, 2001

Metsch L, Rivers J, Miller M, et al: Implementation of a family centered treatment program for substance abusing women and their children: barriers and resolutions. J Psychoactive Drugs 27:73–83, 1995

Minuchin S: Families and Family Therapy. Cambridge, MA, Harvard University Press, 1975

Minuchin S: Constructing a therapeutic reality, in Family Therapy of Drug and Alcohol Abuse, 2nd Edition. Edited by Kaufman E, Kaufmann P. Boston, MA, Allyn & Bacon, 1992, pp 1–14

Minuchin S, Fishman HC: Family Therapy Techniques. Cambridge, MA, Harvard University Press, 1981

O'Farrell TJ, Fals-Stewart W: Behavioral couples and family therapy for substance abusers. Curr Psychiatry Rep 4:371–376, 2002

Papp P: Paradoxical strategies and countertransference, in Questions and Answers in the Practice of Family Therapy. Edited by Gurman AS. New York, Brunner/Mazel, 1981, pp 38–44

Romijn CM, Platt JJ, Schippers GM, et al: Family therapy for Dutch drug users: the relationship between family functioning and success. Int J Addict 27:1–14, 1992

Sandmaier M: The Invisible Alcoholics: Women and Alcohol Abuse in America. New York, McGraw-Hill, 1980

Stanton MD: An integrated structural/strategic approach to family therapy. J Marital Fam Ther 7:427–439, 1981

Stanton MD, Todd TC: The Family Therapy of Drug Abuse and Addiction. New York, Guilford, 1982

Stanton MD, Todd TC: Structural-strategic family therapy with drug addicts, in Family Therapy of Drug and Alcohol Abuse, 2nd Edition. Edited by Kaufman E, Kaufmann P. Boston, MA, Allyn & Bacon, 1992, pp 46–62

Stuart RB: Helping Couples Change. New York, Guilford, 1980

Sutker PB: Drug dependent women: an overview of the literature, in Treatment Services for Drug Dependent Women, Vol 1 (NIDA Publ No ADM-81-1177). Edited by Beschner GM, Reed B, Mondanaro J, et al. Rockville, MD, National Institute on Drug Abuse, 1981, pp 25–51

Szapocznik J, Kurtines WN: Breakthroughs in Family Therapy With Drug Abusing and Problem Youth. New York, Springer, 1989

Szapocznik J, Kurtines W, Santisteban DA, et al: Interplay of advances between theory, research, and application in treatment interventions aimed at behavior problem children and adolescents. J Consult Clin Psychol 58:696–703, 1990

Turner RM: Launching cognitive-behavioral therapy for adolescent depression and drug abuse, in Case Book of Brief Therapy. Edited by Budman S, Hoyt M, Friedman S. New York, Guilford, 1992, pp 135–156

Turner RM: Dynamic cognitive-behavioral therapy, in Handbook of Effective Psychotherapy. Edited by Giles P. New York, Plenum, 1993, pp 437–454

Waldron HB, Slesnick N, Brody JL, et al: Treatment outcomes for adolescent substance abuse at 4- and 7-month assessments. J Consult Clin Psychol 69:802–813, 2001

Winters KC, Latimer WL, Stinchfield RD: Adolescent treatment, in Sourcebook on Substance Abuse: Etiology, Epidemiology, Assessment, and Treatment. Edited by Ott PJ, Tarter RE, Hammerman RT. Boston, MA, Allyn & Bacon, 1999, pp 350–361

Alcoholics Anonymous and Other 12-Step Groups

Chad D. Emrick, Ph.D.
J. Scott Tonigan, Ph.D.

Since its founding in 1935, Alcoholics Anonymous (AA) has grown into a worldwide organization with an estimated 2.2 million members in more than 100,000 groups in about 150 countries (Alcoholics Anonymous 1976; Alcoholics Anonymous World Services 2002). Its success as a social movement is indisputable, with the organization exercising considerable influence on the professional community, government agencies and programs, and the general public. The shape of public policy and opinion has been substantially determined by the depiction in film, on television, and in the print media of AA's primacy and potency in helping "alcoholics" "recover" from "alcoholism." The primary purpose of this chapter is to inform health care providers about pertinent findings from recent quantitative research on AA and other 12-step groups and to amplify these findings with observations from contemporary clinical writings concerning the organization. On the basis of these findings, suggestions are given for how caregivers can maximize the use of AA and other 12-step groups. The term *12-step group* refers to any group whose structure and function are guided by the Twelve Steps and Twelve Traditions of AA (see Appendix).

AA's Philosophy, Structure, and Therapeutic Processes

AA's philosophy, though rooted in the Judeo-Christian tradition, contains thought elements that are consonant with a variety of religious and philosophical traditions. Thus, this organization accommodates a wide spectrum of beliefs. The organization itself is structured around the Twelve Steps and the Twelve Traditions (see Appendix). Therapeutic processes are embedded in "working" the steps and having (for some members) one-to-one guidance and support from a senior member (a "sponsor"), and AA meetings involve therapeutic processes akin to those found in professionally led psychotherapy groups (Emrick et al. 1977).

Demographics of Current AA Membership

In general, a majority of problem drinkers will self-select some AA exposure. Timko et al. (2000) found that during an 8-year period, about 67% of problem drinkers sought assistance from AA: 14% used AA alone, and 53% used AA in combination with formal treatment (N=466). Findings from the most recent triennial survey of AA members in North America reveal the demographics of the current membership (Alcoholics Anonymous World Services 1999). Because only active members were surveyed, the findings may not accurately reflect the characteristics of individuals who sample AA but discontinue AA affiliation. The average age of AA members is 46 years; 11% of members are age 30 years or younger, and 14% are age 61 years or older. Sixty-seven percent of members are men, and 33% of members are women. Married persons make up 37% of the membership, 31% of members are single, 24% are divorced, 5% are widowed, and 3% are separated. Eighty-eight percent of members are white, 5% are black, 4% are Hispanic, and 2% are Native American. Only 7% of the membership is unemployed. Twenty-nine percent hold professional/technical, managerial/administrative, or health professional positions.

When given the chance to identify the two factors most responsible for their joining AA, 33% of members reported that they had sought the support of AA on their own, whereas 32% were influenced to begin participation by an AA member, 32% were influenced by a treatment facility (a dramatically lower percentage than that reported by Timko et al. [2000]), 23% by a family member, 8% by a counseling agency, and 7% by an individual health care provider. Twelve percent of the members indicated that a court order was most responsible for their joining AA. After beginning participation in AA, 64% of members received some type of treatment or counseling, with 85% of those members indicating that this treatment or counseling played an important part in their recovery.

Who Attends 12-Step Group Meetings?

Individual and social factors have an effect on who does and who does not attend 12-step group meetings.

Severity of alcohol-related problems is by far the strongest predictor of AA meeting attendance. Analyses of data from the widely known Project MATCH (Connors et al. 2001a), for example, showed that greater intake symptomatology (a composite measure of severity of psychiatric symptoms, alcohol dependence and involvement, and readiness to change) was predictive of AA participation in both an outpatient sample and a sample of patients who were in aftercare following inpatient or day hospital treatment. Studies using single measures of alcohol-related severity have likewise demonstrated that frequency of alcohol-related consequences and heavy alcohol use were modestly predictive of subsequent AA affiliation.

Tonigan and colleagues (1996) demonstrated that study quality is an important consideration when drawing conclusions about AA affiliation. Poorly executed studies concluded, for example, that drinking severity was not predictive of AA affiliation (r=0.04, 10 studies) and that improved psychosocial functioning and AA meeting attendance were, at most, mildly related (r=0.16, 14 studies). In contrast, better executed studies tended to show that drinking severity was positively and modestly related to AA affiliation (r=0.20, 5 studies) and that improved psychosocial functioning and AA meeting attendance were significantly and positively related (r=0.33, 3 studies).

Findings are inconsistent with respect to the role played by the patient's support system in seeking the resources of AA. Generally, research findings indicate that an individual with a drinking problem is more likely to join and become involved in AA if family and friends provide weak or inconsistent support for overcoming the problem or if familial and friendship networks are impoverished. This relationship appears to be more robust for outpatients than for inpatients.

A complex picture emerges when one considers whether ethnicity, gender, and religious involvement are predictive of 12-step group membership. On the one hand, Caetano (1993) reported that a majority of Hispanics regarded AA as a useful resource. In contrast, work in the Southwest has consistently found that Hispanics receiving formal treatment are significantly less likely to become AA members after treatment (Arroyo et al. 1998, 1999, 2003). Although AA is regarded by many to be male-oriented in philosophy and practice, there is scant evidence that gender is a predictor of AA membership. In particular, no gender differences in rates or patterns of AA meeting attendance were found between male and female clients receiving outpatient or aftercare treatment in Project MATCH (Project MATCH Research Group 1997, 1998). Whether men or women are more likely to affiliate with AA without the encouragement of formal treatment is unclear. In general, religious involvement has been a poor predictor of AA affiliation, in spite of the explicitly spiritual nature of 12-step programs (Connors et al. 2001b; Emrick et al. 1993; Winzelberg and Humphreys 1999). Although there is some evidence that individuals endorsing strong atheistic beliefs are less likely to attend AA meetings (Tonigan et al. 2002c), the evidence is not strong enough at this time to contraindicate referring atheists to AA.

The relationships among personal and pretreatment/intake contextual variables and AA membership provide the health care professional with few, if any, clear guidelines for determining who will be a good match for AA or a similar 12-step group. For now, health care practitioners should keep in mind that any given individual patient may or may not be a suitable candidate for AA or another 12-step group. Generally, the more severe the individual's drinking or other identified problem and the fewer the individual's interpersonal supports among family and friends (particularly in the case of an outpatient), the more likely the person is to join AA or another 12-step group.

Attitudes of Health Care Practitioners Toward 12-Step Programs

Most physicians consider participation in AA an effective treatment for alcoholism, yet physicians often lack belief in the benefits of other forms of alcoholism treatment, despite scientific proof that other treatments can be beneficial (Miller et al. 1995). Such lack of belief may result in the underuse of effective professionally delivered treatments for individuals with substance abuse disorders.

Mental health treatment providers and substance abuse counselors vary in their endorsement of 12-step groups, although many believe in the effectiveness of these programs. Depending on their theoretical orientation, mental health treatment providers vary in the importance they place on 12-step groups. Similarly, substance abuse treatment providers vary in the degree to which they endorse the spiritual thinking found in the philosophy of AA, their level of endorse-

ment varying according to such factors as their own involvement in 12-step groups, their religious affiliation, and their educational background.

Effectiveness of AA

Ample research data document the effectiveness of AA (and, by extension, other 12-step groups) in helping individuals maintain a substance-free lifestyle. In effect, this evidence substantiates the intuitive knowledge held by 12-step group members, their families and friends, and large numbers of health care providers concerning the effectiveness of 12-step programs.

Outcome Studies

An impressive amount of data, summarized and analyzed in large-scale reviews, point to a positive relationship between AA membership and improvement in both drinking and nondrinking outcome measures. A meta-analysis of AA studies suggested that "professionally treated patients who attend AA during or after treatment are more likely to improve in drinking behavior than are patients who do not attend AA, although the chances of drinking improvement are not overall a great deal higher" (Emrick et al. 1993, p. 57). And in another meta-analysis of AA studies, Tonigan et al. (1996) found that "better designed studies report moderate and positive relationships between AA attendance and improved psychosocial functioning" (p. 68).

The most salient research reports that have been published since the aforementioned reviews have come from the Center for Health Care Evaluation (CHCE) in Menlo Park, California, and from Project MATCH. In one CHCE study, 515 subjects from an original sample of 631 individuals with previously untreated drinking problems were followed up at 1 year (Humphreys et al. 1997). Among subjects who attended AA meetings but did not receive inpatient or outpatient professional treatment, significant improvement was found on all measures of drinking problems as well as on several other measures of functioning. A total of 395 subjects in this sample were followed up at 8 years, at which time it was found that the number of AA meetings attended during the first 3 years of follow-up was positively related to remission from alcohol problems 8 years after the beginning of the project. AA meeting attendance in the first 3 years of the study also predicted, at 8-year follow-up, lower levels of depression as well as higher-quality relationships with friends and partners or spouses. Of particular note is that inpatient professional treatment services, which some in the sample received, failed to predict any outcome measure at the 8-year follow-up. Although outpatient professional treatment was found to predict drinking outcome at 8-year follow-up, no other benefits of such treatment were observed. This comparison of AA and outpatient professional treatment leads to the obvious conclusion that, at least in this sample with previously untreated drinking problems, AA's therapeutic benefits had a broader effect on alcoholic individuals' lives than did outpatient professional treatment. Humphreys et al. (1997) concluded that compared with professionally delivered inpatient or outpatient treatment, "AA probably helped more people more substantially in this sample" (p. 237).

This same research group evaluated the effects of different types of aftercare treatment 1 year after inpatient treatment in a large sample of veterans (Finney et al. 1999; Moos et al. 1999; Ouimette et al. 1998, 1999). Followed up were 3,018 veterans who had been treated for substance abuse in an inpatient setting. The majority of patients, all of whom were male, were non-Caucasian. Eighty-three percent of the sample was dependent on alcohol, and about 52% of those with alcohol problems were also dependent on other substances. Subjects were evaluated with regard to outcome status approximately 1 year after discharge from the inpatient program. Participation in AA or Narcotics Anonymous in the 3 months before the 1-year follow-up was associated with a greater likelihood of being abstinent, being free of substance use problems, being free of significant distress and psychiatric symptoms, and being employed. These findings still held when the influence of aftercare treatment was controlled for, and they applied to patients with dual diagnoses as much as to patients with only substance use disorders (for the latter, see Ouimette et al. 1999). Statistical analyses suggested that 12-step group involvement after inpatient treatment helped maintain the gains made during inpatient treatment (Finney et al. 1999). These results led the researchers to conclude: "Overall, 12-step attendance and involvement were more strongly related to positive outcomes than was outpatient treatment attendance" (Ouimette et al. 1998, p. 519).

In yet another CHCE study, Moos et al. (2001) examined the 1-year substance use and social functioning outcomes of 2,376 outpatient veterans who were staying in community residential facilities while receiving outpatient treatment. The amount of outpatient mental health care was not predictive of outcome (although regularity of such care was predictive of better outcomes), whereas the amount of attendance at self-help-group meetings *was* predictive of better outcomes.

Project MATCH findings (Project MATCH Research Group 1997, 1998) are in agreement with those of the CHCE group and, in general, offer a more detailed description of the nature of AA participation. Tonigan et al. (2000), for instance, analyzed data from both outpatients and aftercare patients using a composite measure of the AA experience (a construct entailing subjective and objective measures of involvement) and found that this construct accounted for 28% of the variance in drinking outcome in the outpatient sample and 12% of the drinking outcome variance in the aftercare sample. The 12% figure may seem modest, but the AA experience construct was "four times the size of the largest matching effect reported in Project MATCH" and was "substantially larger than the effect of client motivation, the largest prognostic indicator of client treatment response" (Tonigan et al. 2000, p. 37).

In the context of recent research, the AA variable retains its hegemony among predictors of good drinking and nondrinking outcomes.

Treatment Cost

Humphreys and Moos (1996) compared the per-person treatment costs for professionally treated outpatients who had alcohol problems with the costs of treatment for individuals who initially chose to go to AA. Costs were assessed for 3 years. Over the course of the study, some individuals in both groups required detoxification and inpatient or residential treatment. Furthermore, some persons who initially went to AA meetings also received outpatient treatment and vice versa. When all cost factors were calculated, those individuals who initially attended AA meetings were found to have incurred per-person treatment costs that were 45% lower than the costs incurred by those individuals who initially sought outpatient treatment.

A more recent report from the CHCE fortifies these findings (Humphreys and Moos 2001). Twelve-step-group-oriented inpatient treatment was compared with cognitive-behavioral inpatient treatment. In the 1-year follow-up of 1,774 patients, those in 12-step-group-oriented programs used considerably fewer mental health services than did patients in cognitive-behavioral treatment programs, with the result that overall mental health care costs were 64% higher for patients in cognitive-behavioral programs than for those in 12-step-group-oriented programs. Of note is that psychiatric and substance abuse outcomes were comparable across program types, with the exception that the 12-step-group-oriented programs yielded higher rates of abstinence.

If the goal is to get more bang for bucks spent on substance abuse rehabilitation, facilitation of involvement in AA (and, by extension, other 12-step groups) should be among the options exercised by health care providers.

Mechanisms of Effectiveness

It is asserted in clinical writings that AA and, by extension, other 12-step groups are effective because these groups (particularly AA) are readily and widely available, provide a philosophy for living, and present a structured community of individuals who are living life without alcohol. Although there is substantial evidence that AA social group dynamics vary widely (Montgomery et al. 1993; Tonigan et al. 1995), prescribed AA-related behaviors are relatively constant across AA groups. In this context, 12-step groups are normative organizations that help individuals experience, express, and manage feelings, in part through giving members the opportunity to express feelings in group meetings without fear of negative feedback from others. The groups also help members develop the capacity for self-regulation, increase their sense of self-efficacy, perceive the continuity of time, improve a sense of relationship to others, discover their purpose in life or meaning of life, find a way to connect with the unknown reality that exists outside themselves, engage in self-examination and self-expression, increase their ability to listen to others, and repair vulnerabilities in self-care.

Twelve-step groups teach members healthy strategies for interpreting stressful events and experiences and for behaving in response to those events and experiences. For example, participants are taught to distinguish between controllable and uncontrollable events. Active cognitive coping strategies are provided for dealing with uncontrollable events (e.g., members are instructed to think "This too shall pass" when they are faced with a situation they cannot change). For events that are controllable, use of active behavioral coping

strategies is encouraged (e.g., members are taught to deal immediately and actively with interpersonal conflict). No matter what the controllability of the event, members are urged to reduce their use of avoidant and destructive coping strategies, such as turning to alcohol or drugs.

Data from several research efforts have highlighted some mediators that link AA-related behaviors to outcome (Connors et al. 2001a; Humphreys and Noke 1997; Humphreys et al. 1994, 1999b; Kaskutas et al. 2002; Morgenstern and Bates 1999; Morgenstern et al. 1996, 1997; Snow et al. 1994; Vaillant 1995; Zywiak et al. 2002). These data indicate that current, actively involved AA members are more likely to use a variety of therapeutic or adaptive processes, including behavioral change processes such as avoidance of high-risk situations, greater use of active cognitive and behavioral coping strategies, and less reliance on avoidant coping responses (e.g., drinking and using drugs to escape psychological discomfort). Also, active members tend to have larger and higher-quality social networks, with those networks containing a larger proportion of individuals who do not use substances and who are in recovery. Active AA members also report increased self-efficacy to avoid drinking, and this increase predicted higher abstinence rates at early (Morgenstern et al. 1997) and late (Connors et al. 2001a) follow-up in some studies. An important caveat regarding this finding is that although self-efficacy to avoid drinking is generally regarded as a global measure of efficacy in the research literature, confidence to avoid drinking probably varies across different situations and emotional states. Clinicians should be sensitive to the uneven nature of self-efficacy in preparing treatment plans.

Kelly et al. (2000) introduced an intriguing qualification to the above summary: adolescents and adults appear to benefit differently from 12-step groups. In these investigators' sample of adolescents, attendance of 12-step group meetings was not related to enhanced self-efficacy or increased abstinence-focused coping skills. Rather, the beneficial effects were traced to how 12-step group membership maintained and enhanced the motivation to remain drug free. These researchers concluded that "unlike adults, the acquisition of specific abstinence-focused coping skills for youth, although a consequence of attendance at 12-step meetings, is not as crucial in effective substance use behavior change for youth, at least in the early postdischarge months" (Kelly et al. 2000, p. 388).

Health Care Providers and 12-Step Groups

Facilitating Affiliation and Involvement

Because AA and, by extension, other 12-step groups can play a vital part in recovery from chemical dependence, health care practitioners need to prepare their patients for active participation in these groups. Empirical support for this suggestion comes from two major research efforts, both of which show that 12-step-group-oriented treatment results in a higher percentage of patients involving themselves in 12-step groups, and this involvement, in turn, produces higher abstinence rates (Humphreys et al. 1999a; Project MATCH Research Group 1998).

To be successful in their efforts, professionals must have an accurate understanding of the nature of 12-step groups. Practitioners need to understand, for example, that AA does *not* assert that "1) there is only one form of alcoholism or alcohol problem; 2) moderate drinking is impossible for everyone with alcohol problems; 3) alcoholics should be labeled, confronted aggressively or coerced into treatment; 4) alcoholics are riddled with denial and other defense mechanisms; 5) alcoholism is purely a physical disorder; 6) alcoholism is hereditary; 7) there is only one way to recover; or 8) alcoholics are not responsible for their condition or actions" (Miller and Kurtz 1994, p. 165). Also, clinicians must educate their patients about the difference between religion and spirituality, because AA is often perceived to be a form of religion. AA is essentially a "spiritual program of living" (Miller and Kurtz 1994, p. 165) or "a way of life" (Gold 1994, p. 97). This is the case because "there is no dogma, theology, or creed to be learned" in AA (Chappel 1993, p. 181). Knowledgeable clinicians would do well to keep this understanding in mind as they assist their patients in preparing for AA participation. Finally, research supports clinical impressions that AA groups are not all alike. AA groups do differ in perceived cohesiveness, aggressiveness, and expressiveness among AA members, and clinicians should recommend that prospective affiliates sample a number of different AA meetings to determine whether AA is helpful (Horstmann and Tonigan 2000; Montgomery et al. 1993; Tonigan et al. 1995).

Practitioners can also assist their patients in becoming beneficially involved in 12-step groups by offering basic instruction about the meaning and purpose of each of the Twelve Steps and Twelve Traditions of AA. Furthermore, professionals may facilitate involvement by having contact with their patients' sponsors, encouraging their patients to choose home groups and to attend 12-step group meetings frequently (particularly at the beginning of participation), and offering their patients guidance in becoming actively involved in the 12-step group community.

Findings from the meta-analysis by Emrick et al. (1993) can inform clinicians about what this guidance might look like. Members are likely to achieve the greatest benefit from 12-step group membership if they obtain a sponsor; engage in 12-step work; lead a meeting; increase their degree of participation in the organization if they are returning to it after a period of absence; sponsor other members; and "work" the last 7 of the 12 steps.

A further incentive to encourage patients to engage actively in 12-step practices is that the relative benefits of such practices, compared with mere attendance at meetings, appear to be durable. In a 10-year follow-up of 88 Project MATCH subjects, Tonigan et al. (2002a, 2002b) found that frequency of AA meeting attendance did not predict the percentage of abstinent days during the 6 months preceding the 10-year follow-up, but that measurement scores related to the reliance on a higher power and to the taking of a personal inventory were predictive of abstinence.

A recent report by Crape et al. (2002), however, served as a warning against unrestrained assertions concerning the positive effects of 12-step-community practices. Although Crape et al. (2002) observed a strong association between being a sponsor and having sustained abstinence during a 1-year evaluation of former and current injection drug users, having a sponsor was not related to sustained abstinence during the year of evaluation.

This finding notwithstanding, clinicians should operate from the perspective that more active involvement in the fellowship and practices of 12-step groups will, if anything, enhance improvement, which means that attempting to increase a patient's involvement in the 12-step community is an essential component of evidence-based chemical dependence treatment.

Learning How to Integrate 12-Step Programs and Professional Treatment

Health care professionals can further enhance the effective use of AA and other 12-step programs by acquiring knowledge about how best to integrate these programs with professional treatment (see, for example, Zweben 1995). Integration is advised because persons with substance abuse disorders who combine these two systems of care appear to have better outcomes (at least with respect to substance abuse) than do those who avail themselves of only one form of help (see, for example, Fiorentine and Hillhouse 2000).

A common theme in writings about integrating 12-step programs and professional treatment is the need for professionals to learn the language and culture of such programs in order to understand in what ways the two systems differ and where the commonalities in concepts and processes exist. For example, both systems facilitate development of cognitive and behavioral change processes; only the language used to foster this development differs. By having a working knowledge of both systems' languages and cultures, health care providers can more skillfully assist their patients in obtaining both forms of help—simultaneously, alternately, or sequentially. As recent research data suggest, the most effective way to promote use of both types of care is to fashion a professional treatment approach that is consonant with that found in the 12-step environment (Humphreys et al. 1999a).

Tailoring Facilitation Efforts to Specific Groups

Professionals need to tailor their facilitation efforts to the unique characteristics of the particular 12-step groups in which their patients are to become involved. Given the fact that heterogeneity has been found to exist among different AA groups, a patient may find one particular group in his or her community to be compatible with individual needs and may find other groups to be inappropriate. Health care providers are encouraged to help patients understand the heterogeneity of groups and therefore the need to attend meetings of several groups before deciding which group (or groups) is most suitable.

Becoming Knowledgeable About Special-Population Considerations

Reports have identified points of consideration (as well as guidelines, in some cases) for facilitating AA involvement by individuals with special characteristics. These reports focused on the following special populations: veterans with posttraumatic stress disorder (Satel et al. 1993), lesbians (Hall 1994), adolescents (Kennedy and Minami 1993), persons with dual disorders (Kurtz et al. 1995), alcoholic individuals who take medication (Rychtarik et al. 2000), women (Sandoz 1995), persons with substance use disorders who do not have a high degree of need to affiliate with others in a group (Smith 1993), and individuals within particular ethnic groups (Caetano 1993). In general, work with these special populations demonstrates that having these characteristics should not be regarded as a barrier to AA affiliation and benefit. Thus, the health care provider needs to become knowledgeable about, and sensitive to, these special-population issues to be maximally effective in facilitating 12-step group involvement by his or her patients.

Matching Patients to 12-Step Groups

An intuitively appealing, though practically difficult, approach to facilitating use and increasing effectiveness of 12-step programs is to find appropriate matches for these programs. Findings from the Project MATCH study (Project MATCH Research Group 1998) suggest three matching strategies that health care providers should keep in mind when considering a referral to AA or another 12-step group:

1. For drinkers with a social support system that is supportive of drinking (particularly through frequent contact with frequent drinkers), facilitating participation in AA (through 12-step facilitation therapy) appears to result in better drinking outcome than does trying to motivate the individual to give up drinking (through motivational enhancement therapy) or providing treatment based on cognitive-behavioral theory (i.e., cognitive-behavioral coping skills therapy) (Longabaugh et al. 1998; Project MATCH Research Group 1998; Zywiak et al. 2002).

2. Alcohol-dependent individuals who are angry at the start of treatment may benefit more from a nonconfrontational approach to changing their drinking behavior (i.e., motivational enhancement therapy) than from cognitive-behavioral treatment or treatment in which they are encouraged to attend AA meetings (i.e., 12-step facilitation therapy).

3. Inpatients who have relatively high dependence on alcohol may benefit more from 12-step-group-oriented aftercare than from treatment based on cognitive-behavioral theory (Project Match Research Group 1997).

Although not of the stature of a proposed matching strategy, another Project MATCH finding merits noting. Problem drinkers treated in residential settings who sought meaning in life had better drinking outcomes, at least for a time, when they were given aftercare that was oriented toward AA participation rather than comparison aftercare treatments (Tonigan et al. 1997). Because this finding is tentative, further research needs to be undertaken before the variable of seeking meaning in life can serve as a guide in making clinical decisions. Nonetheless, clinicians are encouraged to be sensitive to the interplay between a patient's search for meaning in life and the treatment the patient receives.

12-Step Programs Are Not Always Helpful

Health care practitioners need to keep in mind that any intervention possessing the power to help some people has the potential to harm others. If a health care provider assumes that 12-step group participation "can't hurt," he or she may fail to intervene appropriately when a patient claims to be worsening through his or her involvement in a 12-step community. Quite often, such a complaint is an expression of resistance to a beneficial membership, in which case helping the patient overcome resistance to active membership is appropriate. On the other hand, the organization may truly be having a negative effect on the patient, as evidenced by increased drug use; exacerbation of depressive symptoms such as helplessness, guilt, or inadequacy perceptions; or lack of improvement in family or social relationships.

If the health care practitioner determines that 12-step group involvement is having negative effects on his or her patient, the practitioner needs to work with the patient to reverse such effects. One obvious course of action is to assist the patient in finding alternative treatments. Insisting a patient continue attending 12-step group meetings when he or she is being harmed by such attendance is equivalent to instructing a patient to continue taking medication that not only is failing to improve his or her condition but also is causing harmful side effects. Good medical practice and other professional practice proscribe such behavior.

Alternatives to 12-Step Groups

Given that AA and other 12-step groups are not always effective and may even be harmful to certain individuals, what community group alternatives do persons with substance abuse disorders have for dealing with their disorders? Rational Recovery is one such alternative to 12-step groups (see Galanter et al. 1993), as are Women for Sobriety (see Kaskutas 1996) and Secular Organizations for Sobriety (also called Save Our Selves) (see Connors and Dermen 1996).

Certainly, Rational Recovery and other alternatives to AA are worthy of the health care provider's attention and are organizations to which the practitioner needs to consider making referrals.

Conclusion

In this chapter, a wide spectrum of issues has been surveyed concerning AA and other 12-step groups. Information has been presented regarding the philosophy, structure, and therapeutic processes of AA; the demographics of the current North American membership of AA; the degree to which AA and other 12-step programs are being used; the beliefs and attitudes held by health care providers concerning AA and other 12-step groups; the effectiveness of AA and the mechanisms of effect; ways to enhance the use of 12-step programs; matching patients to 12-step groups; the limits of 12-step groups; and alternatives to 12-step groups.

However, significant areas of 12-step research were not reviewed. For example, researchers are investigating how changes in self-efficacy associated with AA participation may be mediated by cognitive impairment and spirituality (Morgenstern and Bates 1999; Tonigan et al. 2002a), and initial efforts are under way to examine how self-efficacy to abstain from addictive behaviors may vary across different situations (Gwaltney et al. 2002). Interested readers are encouraged to examine professional, peer-reviewed journals to monitor the rapid progress in understanding how and under what circumstances 12-step programs are beneficial.

Our understanding of AA and other 12-step groups continues to deepen as a result of the dedicated efforts of the bright minds responsible for the research reviewed in this chapter. Armed with this understanding, health care providers can now, more than ever, work effectively with their substance-abusing patients.

References

Alcoholics Anonymous: The Story of How Many Thousands of Men and Women Have Recovered From Alcoholism, 3rd Edition. New York, Alcoholics Anonymous World Services, 1976

Alcoholics Anonymous World Services: Alcoholics Anonymous 2001 Membership Survey. New York, Alcoholics Anonymous World Services, 1999

Alcoholics Anonymous World Services: Estimates of A.A. Groups and Members as of January 1, 2002. New York, Alcoholics Anonymous World Services, 2002

Arroyo JA, Westerberg VS, Tonigan JS: Comparison of treatment utilization and outcome for Hispanics and non-Hispanic whites. J Stud Alcohol 59:286–291, 1998

Arroyo JA, Miller WR, Tonigan J: The influence of ethnic identification on long term outcome in three treatment modalities (abstract #426). Alcohol Clin Exp Res 23 (5 suppl):76A, 1999

Arroyo JA, Miller WR, Tonigan JS: The influence of Hispanic ethnicity on long-term outcome in three alcohol-treatment modalities. J Stud Alcohol 64:98–104, 2003

Caetano R: Ethnic minority groups and Alcoholics Anonymous: a review, in Research on Alcoholics Anonymous: Opportunities and Alternatives. Edited by McCrady BS, Miller WR. New Brunswick, NJ, Rutgers Center of Alcohol Studies, 1993, pp 209–231

Chappel JN: Long-term recovery from alcoholism. Psychiatr Clin North Am 16:177–187, 1993

Connors GJ, Dermen KH: Characteristics of participants in Secular Organizations for Sobriety (SOS). Am J Drug Alcohol Abuse 22:281–295, 1996

Connors GJ, Tonigan JS, Miller WR, et al: A longitudinal model of intake symptomatology, AA participation, and outcome: retrospective study of the Project MATCH outpatient and aftercare samples. J Stud Alcohol 62:817–825, 2001a

Connors GJ, Tonigan JS, Miller WR: Religiosity and responsiveness to alcoholism treatments, in Project MATCH Hypotheses: Results and Causal Chain Analyses (National Institute on Alcohol Abuse and Alcoholism, Project MATCH Monograph Series, Vol 8 [NIH Publ No 01-4238]). Edited by Longabaugh R, Wirtz PW. Rockville, MD, National Institute on Alcohol Abuse and Alcoholism, 2001b, pp 166–175

Crape BL, Latkin CA, Laris AS, et al: The effects of sponsorship in 12-step treatment of injection drug users. Drug Alcohol Depend 65:291–301, 2002

Emrick CD, Lassen CL, Edwards MT: Nonprofessional peers as therapeutic agents, in Effective Psychotherapy: A Handbook of Research. Edited by Gurman AS, Razin AM. Oxford, UK, Pergamon, 1977, pp 120–161

Emrick CD, Tonigan JS, Montgomery H, et al: Alcoholics Anonymous: what is currently known? In Research on Alcoholics Anonymous: Opportunities and Alternatives. Edited by McCrady BS, Miller WR. New Brunswick, NJ, Rutgers Center of Alcohol Studies, 1993, pp 41–76

Finney JW, Moos RH, Humphreys K: A comparative evaluation of substance abuse treatment, II: linking proximal outcomes of 12-step and cognitive-behavioral treatment to substance use outcomes. Alcohol Clin Exp Res 23:537–544, 1999

Fiorentine R, Hillhouse MP: Drug treatment and 12-step program participation: the additive effects of integrated recovery activities. J Subst Abuse Treat 18:65–74, 2000

Galanter M, Egelko S, Edwards H: Rational Recovery: alternative to AA for addiction? Am J Drug Alcohol Abuse 19:499–510, 1993

Gold MS: Neurobiology of addiction and recovery: the brain, the drive for the drug, and the 12-step fellowship. J Subst Abuse Treat 11:93–97, 1994

Gwaltney CJ, Shiffman S, Paty JA, et al: Using self-efficacy judgments to predict characteristics of lapses to smoking. J Consult Clin Psychol 70:1140–1149, 2002

Hall JM: The experiences of lesbians in Alcoholics Anonymous. West J Nurs Res 16:556–576, 1994

Horstmann MJ, Tonigan JS: Faith development in Alcoholics Anonymous (AA): a study of two AA groups. Alcoholism Treatment Quarterly 18:75–84, 2000

Humphreys K, Moos RH: Reduced substance-abuse-related health care costs among voluntary participants in Alcoholics Anonymous. Psychiatric Serv 47:709–713, 1996

Humphreys K, Moos R: Can encouraging substance abuse patients to participate in self-help groups reduce demand for health care? A quasi-experimental study. Alcohol Clin Exp Res 25:711–716, 2001

Humphreys K, Noke JM: The influence of posttreatment mutual help group participation on the friendship networks of substance abuse patients. Am J Community Psychol 25:1–16, 1997

Humphreys K, Finney JW, Moos RH: Applying a stress and coping framework to research on mutual help organizations. Am J Community Psychol 22:312–327, 1994

Humphreys K, Moos RH, Cohen C: Social and community resources and long-term recovery from treated and untreated alcoholism. J Stud Alcohol 58:231–238, 1997

Humphreys K, Huebsch PD, Finney JW, et al: A comparative evaluation of substance abuse treatment, V: substance abuse treatment can enhance the effectiveness of self-help groups. Alcohol Clin Exp Res 23:558–563, 1999a

Humphreys K, Mankowski ES, Moos RH, et al: Do enhanced friendship networks and active coping mediate the effect of self-help groups on substance abuse? Ann Behav Med 21:54–60, 1999b

Kaskutas LA: Pathways to self-help among Women for Sobriety. Am J Drug Alcohol Abuse 22:259–280, 1996

Kaskutas LA, Bond J, Humphreys K: Social networks as mediators of the effect of Alcoholics Anonymous. Addiction 97:891–900, 2002

Kelly JF, Myers MG, Brown SA: A multivariate process model of adolescent 12-step attendance and substance use outcome following inpatient treatment. Psychol Addict Behav 14:376–389, 2000

Kennedy BP, Minami M: The Beech Hill Hospital/Outward Bound Adolescent Chemical Dependency Treatment Program. J Subst Abuse Treat 10:395–406, 1993

Kurtz LF, Garvin CD, Hill EM, et al: Involvement in Alcoholics Anonymous by persons with dual disorders. Alcoholism Treatment Quarterly 12:1–18, 1995

Longabaugh R, Wirtz PW, Zweben A, et al: Network support for drinking, Alcoholics Anonymous and long-term matching effects. Addiction 93:1313–1333, 1998

Miller WR, Kurtz E: Models of alcoholism used in treatment: contrasting AA and other perspectives with which it is often confused. J Stud Alcohol 55:159–166, 1994

Miller WR, Brown JM, Simpson TS, et al: What works? A methodological analysis of the alcohol treatment outcome literature, in Handbook of Alcoholism Treatment Approaches: Effective Alternatives, 2nd Edition. Edited by Hester RK, Miller WR. Needham Heights, MA, Allyn & Bacon, 1995, pp 12–44

Montgomery HA, Miller WR, Tonigan JS: Differences among AA groups: implications for research. J Stud Alcohol 54:502–504, 1993

Moos RH, Finney JW, Ouimette PC, et al: A comparative evaluation of substance abuse treatment, I: treatment orientation, amount of care, and 1-year outcomes. Alcohol Clin Exp Res 23:529–536, 1999

Moos R[H], Schaefer J, Andrassy J, et al: Outpatient mental health care, self-help groups, and patients' one-year treatment outcomes. J Clin Psychol 57:273–287, 2001

Morgenstern J, Bates ME: Effects of executive function impairment on change processes and substance use outcomes in 12-step treatment. J Stud Alcohol 60:846–855, 1999

Morgenstern J, Kahler CW, Frey RM, et al: Modeling therapeutic response to 12-step treatment: optimal responders, nonresponders, and partial responders. J Subst Abuse 8:45–59, 1996

Morgenstern J, Labouvie E, McCrady BS, et al: Affiliation with Alcoholics Anonymous following treatment: a study of its therapeutic effects and mechanisms of action. J Consult Clin Psychol 65:768–777, 1997

Ouimette PC, Moos RH, Finney JW: Influence of outpatient treatment and 12-step group involvement on one-year substance abuse treatment outcomes. J Stud Alcohol 59:513–522, 1998

Ouimette PC, Gima K, Moos RH, et al: A comparative evaluation of substance abuse treatment, IV: the effect of comorbid psychiatric diagnoses on amount of treatment, continuing care, and 1-year outcomes. Alcohol Clin Exp Res 23:552–557, 1999

Project MATCH Research Group: Project MATCH secondary a priori hypotheses. Addiction 92:1671–1698, 1997

Project MATCH Research Group: Matching alcoholism treatments to client heterogeneity: Project MATCH three-year drinking outcomes. Alcohol Clin Exp Res 22:1300–1311, 1998

Rychtarik RG, Connors GJ, Dermen KH, et al: Alcoholics Anonymous and the use of medications to prevent relapse: an anonymous survey of member attitudes. J Stud Alcohol 61:134–138, 2000

Sandoz CJ: Gender issues in recovery from alcoholism. Alcoholism Treatment Quarterly 12:61–69, 1995

Satel SL, Becker BR, Dan E: Reducing obstacles to affiliation with Alcoholics Anonymous among veterans with PTSD and alcoholism. Hosp Community Psychiatry 44:1061–1065, 1993

Smith AR: The social construction of group dependency in Alcoholics Anonymous. Journal of Drug Issues 23:689–704, 1993

Snow MG, Prochaska JO, Rossi JS: Processes of change in Alcoholics Anonymous: maintenance factors in long-term sobriety. J Stud Alcohol 55:362–371, 1994

Timko C, Moos RH, Finney JW, et al: Long-term outcomes of alcohol use disorders: comparing untreated individuals with those in Alcoholics Anonymous and formal treatment. J Stud Alcohol 61:529–540, 2000

Tonigan JS, Ashcroft F, Miller WR: AA group dynamics and 12 step activity. J Stud Alcohol 56:616–621, 1995

Tonigan JS, Toscova R, Miller WR: Meta-analysis of the literature on Alcoholics Anonymous: sample and study characteristics moderate findings. J Stud Alcohol 57:65–72, 1996

Tonigan JS, Miller WR, Connors GJ: The Search for Meaning in Life as a Predictor of Treatment Outcome (Project MATCH Monograph Series, Vol 8). Rockville, MD, National Institute on Alcohol Abuse and Alcoholism, 1997

Tonigan JS, Miller WR, Connors GJ: Project MATCH client impressions about Alcoholics Anonymous: measurement issues and relationship to treatment outcome. Alcoholism Treatment Quarterly 18:25–41, 2000

Tonigan JS, Miller WR, Carroll L: Internalization of AA practices 10 years after treatment: Project MATCH preliminary findings (abstract #219). Alcohol Clin Exp Res 26 (5 suppl):42A, 2002a

Tonigan JS, Miller WR, Chavez R, et al: AA participation 10 years after Project MATCH treatment: preliminary findings (abstract #218). Alcohol Clin Exp Res 26 (5 suppl): 42A, 2002b

Tonigan JS, Miller WR, Schermer C: Atheists, agnostics and Alcoholics Anonymous. J Stud Alcohol 63:534–541, 2002c

Vaillant GE: The Natural History of Alcoholism Revisited. Cambridge, MA, Harvard University Press, 1995

Winzelberg A, Humphreys K: Should patients' religiosity influence clinicians' referral to 12-step self-help groups? Evidence from a study of 3,018 male substance abuse patients. J Consult Clin Psychol 67:790–794, 1999

Zweben JE: Integrating psychotherapy and 12-step approaches, in Psychotherapy and Substance Abuse: A Practitioner's Handbook. Edited by Washton AM. New York, Guilford, 1995, pp 124–140

Zywiak WH, Longabaugh R, Wirtz PW: Decomposing the relationships between pretreatment social network characteristics and alcohol treatment outcome. J Stud Alcohol 63:114–121, 2002

Appendix

The Twelve Steps of Alcoholics Anonymous

1. We admitted we were powerless over alcohol—that our lives had become unmanageable.
2. Came to believe that a Power greater than ourselves could restore us to sanity.
3. Made a decision to turn our will and our lives over to the care of God *as we understood Him.*
4. Made a searching and fearless moral inventory of ourselves.
5. Admitted to God, to ourselves and to another human being the exact nature of our wrongs.
6. Were entirely ready to have God remove all these defects of character.
7. Humbly asked Him to remove our shortcomings.
8. Made a list of all persons we had harmed, and became willing to make amends to them all.
9. Made direct amends to such people wherever possible, except when to do so would injure them or others.
10. Continued to take personal inventory and when we were wrong promptly admitted it.
11. Sought through prayer and meditation to improve our conscious contact with God, *as we understood Him,* praying only for knowledge of His will for us and the power to carry that out.
12. Having had a spiritual awakening as the result of these steps, we tried to carry this message to alcoholics, and to practice these principles in all our affairs.

The Twelve Traditions of Alcoholics Anonymous

1. Our common welfare should come first; personal recovery depends up A.A. unity.
2. For our group purpose, there is but one ultimate authority—a loving God as He may express Himself in our group conscience. Our leaders are but trusted servants; they do not govern.
3. The only requirement for A.A. membership is a desire to stop drinking.
4. Each group should be autonomous except in matters affecting other groups or A.A. as a whole.
5. Each group has but one primary purpose—to carry its message to the alcoholic who still suffers.
6. An A.A. group ought never endorse, finance, or lend the A.A. name to any related facility or outside enterprise, lest problems of money, property, and prestige divert us from our primary purpose.
7. Every A.A. group ought to be fully self-supporting, declining outside contributions.
8. Alcoholics Anonymous should remain forever non-professional, but our service centers may employ special workers.
9. A.A., as such, ought never be organized; but we may create service boards or committees directly responsible to those they serve.
10. Alcoholics Anonymous has no opinion on outside issues; hence the A.A. name ought never be drawn into public controversy.
11. Our public relations policy is based on attraction rather than promotion; we need always maintain personal anonymity at the level of press, radio and films.
12. Anonymity is the spiritual foundation of all our traditions, ever reminding us to place principles before personalities.

Source. The Twelve Steps and Twelve Traditions are reprinted with permission of Alcoholics Anonymous World Services, Inc. Permission to reprint the Twelve Steps and Twelve Traditions does not mean that A.A. has reviewed or approved the contents of this publication, nor that A.A. agrees with the views expressed herein. A.A. is a program of recovery for alcoholism *only*—use of the Twelve Steps and Twelve Traditions in connection with programs and activities which are patterned after A.A., but which address other problems, or in any other non-A.A. context, does not imply otherwise.

Inpatient Treatment

Roger D. Weiss, M.D.
Jennifer Sharpe Potter, Ph.D., M.P.H.

In recent years, few subjects in the field of addiction research have generated as much debate as the role of inpatient treatment for patients with substance use disorders. This controversy has been fueled in part by the enormous cost of substance abuse treatment in the United States. In 1992, the cost of specialized services for treating substance-related problems and the medical consequences of addiction was estimated to be $28 billion, of which $10 billion was devoted to the treatment of substance use disorders themselves (Harwood et al. 1999). The annual cost to society of alcohol- and drug-related problems has been estimated to be more than $200 billion (Holland and Mushinski 1999; U.S. Department of Health and Human Services 1998). Therefore, establishing effective treatment methods for patients with substance use disorders is both a public health and a financial priority. Because the resources available to tackle this issue are finite, treatment should be not only effective but also cost-effective. Because the cost differential between in-

patient and outpatient treatment is substantial, and because there is wide variation in per diem costs even among inpatient facilities, determining the proper role of hospital treatment is critical.

Unfortunately, discussions regarding inpatient treatment have often been fueled by political and financial considerations rather than by clinical research data. This has sometimes led to the promulgation of extremist positions. As a result, arguments have been presented that support either the extraordinary effectiveness of (McElrath 1988) or the virtual lack of need for (Miller and Hester 1986) inpatient treatment. This debate has been intensified by the fact that in the late 1970s and early 1980s, private sector (much of it for-profit) hospital treatment of substance-dependent individuals increased dramatically at the same time that the number of public hospital units decreased. By the mid-1980s, however, inpatient treatment of substance use disorders had become the focus of cost-containment efforts (Steenrod et al. 2001). As clini-

Supported by National Institute on Drug Abuse grants DA00326, DA09400, DA15831, and DA15968; National Institute on Alcohol Abuse and Alcoholism grant AA11756; and a grant from the Dr. Ralph and Marian C. Falk Medical Research Trust.

cians, researchers, government officials, and entrepreneurs attempted to develop less costly alternatives to hospitalization, the rationale for inpatient treatment was questioned, and this treatment has remained a subject of considerable controversy. As a result, in 2000, only 2% of individuals receiving treatment for substance use disorders received that treatment in a conventional inpatient setting (Substance Abuse and Mental Health Services Administration 2002).

In this chapter, we present an overview of inpatient treatment, discuss current thinking about the indications for hospital care, and review research on the effectiveness of treatment in this setting.

What Is Inpatient Treatment?

The term *inpatient treatment* actually refers to a variety of forms of treatment that take place in many different settings. Inpatient treatment may involve detoxification, rehabilitation, a combination of the two, or one followed by the other. The treatment may take place either in a medical or general psychiatric setting or on a specialized substance dependence unit, in a general hospital, a psychiatric hospital, or a freestanding substance dependence treatment facility. The level and nature of staffing may vary as well, depending on the facility and the patient population. For example, an inpatient substance abuse treatment facility that treats patients with complex medical comorbidity has more medical staff than does a facility that primarily treats patients who have both substance use disorders and psychiatric illnesses; the latter setting, conversely, requires more psychiatric staff. The American Society of Addiction Medicine Patient Placement Criteria (Mee-Lee et al. 2001) distinguish between "medically managed" and "residential" intensive inpatient treatment; in some facilities, the latter is referred to as "acute residential" treatment. This form of treatment offers the psychosocial intensity of an inpatient program, with less need for physician and nursing services. Many clinicians who work with substance-dependent patients recommend that these patients be treated in a specialized setting because of the availability of peer support and confrontation, the presence of a knowledgeable and dedicated clinical staff, and the fact that substance-dependent patients and patients with other psychiatric disorders may feel uncomfortable around each other. Although little empirical research has

been conducted to test this idea, one study found that heroin-dependent patients treated on a specialized unit had better long-term outcomes than did heroin-dependent patients who underwent detoxification on a general psychiatric unit (Strang et al. 1997).

The recognition during the past two decades of the frequent comorbidity of addictive disorders and other psychiatric illness (Brooner et al. 1997; Kessler et al. 1997; Mirin et al. 1991; Regier et al. 1990; Ross et al. 1988) has led to the creation of numerous *dual diagnosis* inpatient units, which are devoted to the treatment of patients with coexisting mental illness and substance use disorders. One problem with the use of the term *dual diagnosis patients* is that it connotes more similarities among this population than actually exist (Weiss et al. 1992). Patients with coexisting mental illness and substance use disorders are heterogeneous. Thus, although such patients may be grouped together for the purpose of creating greater cohesion on an inpatient unit, this desired result might not occur. For example, a young, bulimic, cocaine-dependent patient will not necessarily feel commonality with an elderly, depressed alcoholic patient merely because they each have two disorders. Thus, although treating patients with dual diagnoses together may make programmatic sense in a particular institution, it is important to recognize the potential pitfalls of this approach.

Dual diagnosis treatment may occur on a unit with a primarily psychiatric focus, on a substance abuse unit with a psychiatric consultant (who may be either peripherally involved or well integrated), or on a unit that attempts to integrate principles of psychiatric and substance use disorder treatment. Minkoff (2001), for example, has argued that substance-dependent patients, psychiatric patients, and individuals with both types of disorders are best treated together in an integrated therapeutic model. He has posited that many of the concepts that have traditionally been associated with substance dependence treatment (e.g., acceptance of and recovery from a chronic illness, the need to overcome denial and shame, the importance of asking for help, active use of treatment, development of new coping skills) are equally useful in the treatment of patients with other primary psychiatric disorders. The rationale behind an integrated treatment approach is that the likelihood of recovery in an individual with a substance use disorder and a co-occurring psychiatric disorder will be enhanced if the treatment addresses both problems concurrently (Swindle et al.

1995; Weiss and Najavits 1998). Kofoed (1993) has suggested that for patients with coexisting psychiatric illness and substance use disorders, the choice of setting should be based on the stage of illness, level of motivation, and current symptom picture (e.g., acute withdrawal, substance-induced psychiatric symptoms). Not surprisingly, on formal dual diagnosis units there is a tendency toward more frequent use of psychotropic medications, longer stays, and greater emphasis on psychiatric aftercare compared with other substance abuse treatment programs (Swindle et al. 1995).

Relatively few controlled studies have examined the effectiveness of integrated inpatient treatment of substance use disorders. Swindle et al. (1995) examined readmission rates among 7,177 patients treated within the Veterans Affairs (VA) dual diagnosis treatment system. Readmission rate variability was studied as a function of program type (specialized dual diagnosis unit, substance abuse unit with dual diagnosis groups, or general substance abuse treatment program). The large sample size allowed the researchers to control for patient factors (e.g., complexity of substance use disorder), permitting a more rigorous investigation of programmatic factors. Overall, after controlling for case mix, there was no significant association between program type and readmission rate. However, it is important to note that outcome in this study was defined only as readmission to a VA substance abuse unit. Across treatment program types, two programmatic factors were associated with lower readmission rates: 1) tolerance of problem behaviors (e.g., poor hygiene, other behavioral issues) during hospitalization and 2) the presence of 12-step groups during hospitalization. Although the results of this study suggest that the effect of programmatic factors on readmission rates may be small relative to the effect of patient case mix factors, the area warrants additional research.

In virtually all inpatient substance abuse treatment programs in the United States, abstinence from all drugs of abuse, including alcohol, is considered the cornerstone of successful treatment. The most common form of inpatient treatment in this country is the *Minnesota Model* (Cook 1988a), so named because of its development in that state in the 1950s. A Minnesota Model treatment program often features a standardized, fixed length of stay, commonly 4 weeks (although in recent years, there has been more flexibility in this regard). After initial detoxification, patients attend educational lectures based on the disease concept of chemical dependence. In addition to learning about the harmful psychological and medical consequences of drug and alcohol use, patients are typically taught about the natural history of alcoholism; the effects of substance abuse on the family; conditioned cues and relapse prevention techniques; the importance of making lifestyle changes; and alternative coping mechanisms. Patients are often asked to recount their drug and alcohol histories in front of other patients and staff members in a forum similar to Alcoholics Anonymous (AA) meetings. The purpose of this exercise is to help patients confront and accept the adverse effects of their substance use; minimization or denial of the severity of their problems is common among patients admitted to inpatient units. Minnesota Model programs rely strongly on group therapy and peer confrontation and heavily employ recovering alcoholic individuals as primary counselors. Systems interventions, including involvement of employers and family members, are also frequently used in these programs.

Many therapy groups in Minnesota Model programs are based on principles of AA and Narcotics Anonymous. Indeed, orienting patients to AA and establishing their continued AA and group therapy involvement after discharge are major goals of such programs.

Psychiatrists may be involved to a variable extent in Minnesota Model treatment programs, often playing a consultative role in dealing with patients who have clear coexisting psychiatric disorders. The degree of integration between the psychiatric and counseling staff is variable, ranging from cooperation and integration to mutual distrust.

Minnesota Model programs provide immersion in an environment that is dedicated to challenging addictive thoughts and beliefs through group therapy, peer evaluation, and meetings with counselors who themselves are recovering from substance use disorders. One of the most powerful tools in these programs is the instillation of hope, helpful for many individuals who have felt trapped in their addiction. To this end, these programs generally emphasize the importance of spirituality in the recovery process.

Cook (1988b) referred to the "comprehensive and dogmatic ideology" of Minnesota Model programs as one of their most powerful therapeutic tools. This aspect of these programs, however, has also been a target of criticism. For example, some patients who have objected to the spiritual aspects of these programs or who have found AA distasteful (for whatever reason) have believed that treatment staff members have given up on them. Some of these patients are accused of being resistant to treatment, when in fact they are merely resistant to AA. Alternative self-help groups such as SMART Recovery and Secular Organizations for Sobriety have arisen partly in response to this complaint. Despite these criticisms, however, Minnesota Model programs remain popular in the United States.

Rationale for Inpatient Treatment

Inpatient treatment offers several advantages over less intensive programs. First, a hospital setting permits a high level of medical supervision and safety for individuals who require intensive physical and/or psychiatric monitoring. Thus, inpatient treatment in a hospital setting is indicated for patients with medically dangerous conditions or for those who represent an acute danger to themselves or others. The intensity of inpatient treatment may also be helpful for patients who, for whatever reason, do not respond to lesser measures. For example, hospital treatment may benefit patients who are too discouraged or unmotivated to regularly undergo outpatient treatment on their own. Moreover, inpatient treatment may benefit some individuals by increasing their awareness of the internal triggers that place them at risk for returning to substance abuse. For example, the intensity and degree of discomfort that some patients feel in a 24-hour-a-day treatment setting may precipitate drug urges. Experiencing these urges in a protected setting, where patients are not in danger of acting on them, may help patients learn enough about their vulnerability to either avoid such situations in the future or learn to cope with them. Moreover, inpatient treatment can help to interrupt a cycle of drug use, even in the absence of medically dangerous withdrawal symptoms. The safety of an inpatient environment and a period of respite from a barrage of conditioned cues may help some patients in their attempts to make life decisions that are in their best interests.

The protectiveness of an inpatient unit can also be a disadvantage. Because one of the major determinants of craving is drug availability (Meyer and Mirin 1979), patients admitted to inpatient units may not experience drug urges simply because they are living in a drug-free environment. Thus, they may not be fully prepared to handle the drug urges that they will surely have after discharge, when they return to a setting in which drugs are once again available. Therefore, some inpatient programs gradually expose patients to such triggers by granting them brief passes during their hospital stay.

The other disadvantages of inpatient treatment are obvious. First, hospital treatment is expensive, typically costing more than several hundred dollars per day. Second, patients who enter a hospital are unable to work, care for their families, study, or conduct their normal daily activities. Finally, patients may be stigmatized as a result of being hospitalized. Thus, inpatient treatment should not be recommended lightly and should generally be used only when less intensive treatment methods have failed or are considered too risky.

When Should Patients Be Hospitalized?

Cost-containment efforts, when combined with data challenging the effectiveness of inpatient treatment, have led clinicians to hospitalize substance-dependent patients less often than previously (Galanter et al. 2000; Steenrod et al. 2001). Lists of indications for inpatient treatment have been developed by a variety of health care insurers, managed care companies, hospitals, and professional groups. For example, Mee-Lee et al. (2001) have listed six areas that should be assessed when determining whether a patient requires inpatient treatment, partial hospital care, or less intensive ambulatory treatment. These areas are 1) acute intoxication and/or withdrawal potential, 2) biomedical conditions and complications, 3) emotional, behavioral, or cognitive conditions and complications, 4) readiness to change, 5) the potential for relapse, continued use, or continued problems, and 6) the recovery environment or living environment. Although one may argue with the emphasis placed on specific criteria in this or any other document, it is important to recognize the importance of a multidimensional assessment in determining the optimal treatment plan for a substance-dependent patient.

When this assessment has been completed, the clinician must ultimately consider two major issues in deciding whether to hospitalize a patient: 1) the danger that the patient might imminently be harmful to himself or herself or others and 2) the likelihood that the patient would achieve treatment success in a less restrictive environment. These issues can sometimes be extremely difficult to evaluate in patients abusing substances. For example, although patients who engage in active homicidal ideation and/or those who have made a recent suicide attempt might be considered clear candidates for hospitalization, substance-abusing patients may be a danger to themselves or to others in the absence of overt threats or self-destructive or violent acts. Patients who regularly drive while intoxicated, share needles with others, or commit violent crimes to finance their drug habits may also represent a substantial risk to themselves and to society. Because one of the functions of inpatient treatment is to protect the substance-dependent patient and/or the people around him or her during a period of acute danger, decisions regarding the timing of hospitalizing individuals who represent a chronic recurrent danger are complicated.

An inpatient setting may also provide safety during detoxification. This is particularly true for patients who are being detoxified from alcohol and/or sedative-hypnotic drugs, because withdrawal from these agents may have serious medical consequences, including grand mal seizures, delirium, and death. A number of studies have shown that alcohol detoxification can be accomplished safely and effectively in selected outpatient settings (Collins et al. 1990; Hayashida et al. 1989). However, inpatient detoxification is still commonly used because of the risk of potentially serious medical sequelae of withdrawal and the potential unreliability of this patient population. For example, some patients undergoing outpatient alcohol detoxification may concomitantly use other drugs, such as cocaine, which lowers the seizure threshold.

Although detoxification from therapeutic doses of benzodiazepines is frequently done on an outpatient basis, patients with mixed benzodiazepine and alcohol dependence and patients who have been abusing benzodiazepines are often detoxified as inpatients. Moreover, although opioid withdrawal is generally less medically dangerous than sedative-hypnotic or alcohol withdrawal, the discomfort that many opioid-dependent patients experience in attempting detoxification may lead to frequent relapses, which may diminish the effectiveness of outpatient treatment. Some patients who are unable to be successfully detoxified from opioids on an outpatient basis may thus be admitted as inpatients to complete the withdrawal process. Complicated detoxification regimens such as those prescribed

for patients who are dependent on two or more classes of drugs should generally be administered in a hospital because of the need for frequent reevaluation and adjustment of such regimens. Similarly, patients with significant organ (e.g., cardiac, cerebral, hepatic) dysfunction should generally be detoxified in a hospital.

As can be seen in the latter examples of indications for hospitalization, there is frequently an overlap between use of the hospital as a protective environment and use of the hospital to reap the benefits of a maximally intensive treatment program. Some individuals are treated as inpatients because of their actual or perceived inability to benefit from less intensive forms of treatment. Although hospitalization was frequently recommended as an initial treatment modality in the 1980s (Steenrod et al. 2001), patients currently are recommended for hospital care either in the case of imminent danger (as described earlier in this section) or after outpatient or partial hospital treatment efforts have failed. For patients who need to be in a structured and safe environment while undergoing rehabilitation, residential treatment programs may be appropriate, whereas patients who represent a more acute danger to themselves or others, who require intensive medical supervision to achieve detoxification, or who need psychiatric stabilization during detoxification require medically managed, hospital-based treatment.

Studies comparing inpatients and outpatients typically show that the former have more severe substance use histories and a greater prevalence of medical, psychosocial, and vocational difficulties, including less social stability, more unemployment, and a greater preponderance of medical and psychiatric disorders (Harrison and Asche 1999, 2001; Harrison et al. 1988; Hser et al. 1998; Skinner 1981). Of course, these data in part reflect referral patterns and do not necessarily indicate which populations fare best in which settings. A number of studies have been undertaken in which alcohol- or drug-dependent patients were randomly assigned to inpatient treatment or a less intensive alternative. Although these studies have generally shown little difference between inpatient treatment and other modalities (Longabaugh 1988; Miller and Hester 1986; Schneider et al. 1996), methodological flaws in some of these studies may have affected results (Craig et al. 1996; Nace 1990; Pettinati et al. 1993; Sell 1995). For example, in one frequently cited study, it was concluded that individuals treated as inpatients or in a partial hospital setting had similar outcomes (Longabaugh et al. 1983). However, the patients in each of the two groups in this study were initially treated as inpatients. In another well-known study, it was concluded that a session of outpatient "advice" was as effective as inpatient treatment (Edwards et al. 1977). However, later analysis of the data from this study showed that patients with more severe alcohol dependence responded better to inpatient treatment than to outpatient treatment (Nace 1990).

One of the difficulties with studies that compare inpatient and outpatient treatment for substance use disorders is related to the framing of the question that is frequently asked—namely, "Which is better: inpatient or outpatient treatment?" This type of head-to-head competition has been called "nonsensical" (Weddington and McLellan 1994) because the goals and structure of and overall approach to treatment of substance dependence problems are different in inpatient and outpatient settings. Asking about the place of inpatient treatment for substance use disorders is similar to asking about the use of inpatient treatment for other chronic illnesses such as diabetes or asthma. These are all lifelong, chronic relapsing illnesses, for which inpatient treatment is required for certain complications and to support long-term outpatient management of the conditions.

Even in studies in which patients were randomly assigned to inpatient treatment or to intensive outpatient or partial hospital treatment, patients were systematically excluded if they had serious medical, psychiatric, or social comorbidity that might make random assignment to anything other than inpatient treatment hazardous (Weddington and McLellan 1994). For example, McKay et al. (1997) found that the *psychosocial* dimensions of the original American Society of Addiction Medicine Patient Placement Criteria (Hoffman et al. 1991) did not predict who would do well in inpatient compared with intensive outpatient substance abuse rehabilitation. However, these researchers did not study the two *medical* problem areas (acute intoxication/withdrawal and physical complications) in these patient placement criteria because random treatment assignment of patients meeting those criteria would not have been possible.

Results of studies of randomized treatment have been conflicting with regard to the role of inpatient treatment. Walsh et al. (1991) showed inpatient treatment to be more effective than assignment to AA meetings for alcohol-dependent individuals referred for treatment by their employee assistance programs. However, intermediate-level options (e.g., partial hos-

pitalization or intensive outpatient treatment) were not offered in this study. Alterman et al. (1994) found day hospital treatment of cocaine-dependent patients to be as effective as inpatient treatment at 7-month follow-up, although the treatment completion rate among the inpatients was higher. Schneider et al. (1996) studied cocaine-dependent patients who, after completing a 5-day inpatient detoxification, were randomly assigned to 2 weeks of partial hospital day treatment or inpatient treatment. Although treatment outcome at 3-month follow-up favored the inpatient participants, the difference between the two groups was not statistically significant at 6-month follow-up. Pettinati et al. (1993) examined the role of psychiatric severity and level of social support in predicting the rate of early attrition from inpatient or intensive outpatient treatment. These investigators found that outpatients were more likely to experience early treatment failure, regardless of psychiatric severity.

More recent research indicates that inpatient hospitalization may be preferable to outpatient treatment for subsets of patients with substance use disorders. Under the auspices of the Minnesota Department of Human Services, Harrison and Asche (1999, 2001) examined treatment outcomes of 2,300 inpatient and outpatient substance use disorder patients throughout the state; level of care was determined clinically rather than by random assignment. In their first study, Harrison and Asche (1999) used admission data in examining abstinence rates. Among patients with suicidal ideation at the time of initiation of treatment, subsequent abstinence rates were higher among those who participated in an inpatient treatment program than among those who received outpatient treatment. In a follow-up analysis, patients with greater severity of pretreatment problems (e.g., alcohol or drug problems, psychological distress, social isolation, unemployment) were more likely to complete treatment and to remain abstinent if they received inpatient treatment rather than outpatient treatment (Harrison and Asche 2001). In contrast, there was no difference in abstinence rates between inpatient and outpatient treatment among individuals with less severe problems at the time of treatment initiation.

Moos et al. (2000) examined the effect of inpatient treatment as a precursor of community residential treatment. In this naturalistic study, 257 patients who underwent inpatient treatment immediately before admission to one of 44 community residential facilities were compared with 257 matched patients who underwent no inpatient treatment before receiving community residential treatment. The study results indicated that patients with co-occurring psychiatric disorders were more likely to continue their substance use and withdraw from residential treatment prematurely if they entered the community treatment program directly rather than after inpatient treatment. However, patients with substance use disorders only were more likely to complete residential treatment if they entered it directly from the community rather than after inpatient treatment. These results suggest the importance of identifying clinically meaningful subgroups in order to examine the effects of inpatient treatment on outcome among patients with substance use disorders.

Outcome of Inpatient Treatment

General Findings

A number of follow-up studies involving patients treated in hospital programs have yielded impressive success rates. For example, Gilmore et al. (1986) conducted 6-month and 12-month follow-up questionnaire assessments of patients who had been treated at the Hazelden Foundation (a well-known Minnesota Model treatment center) and two other facilities. These researchers found that 73% of patients who completed the questionnaires (approximately one-half the total sample) were abstinent from alcohol at the time of the 6-month assessment, and 58% of respondents were abstinent 1 year after discharge. Wallace et al. (1988) presented similarly favorable results among patients treated at Edgehill Newport, an analogous facility that has since closed. They found that 57% of patients interviewed had been continuously abstinent from alcohol and drugs for 6 months after discharge. However, in both treatment samples, patients who were discharged prematurely were excluded from the follow-up study, as were unmarried patients in the study by Wallace et al. (1988). In a 4-year follow-up of inpatients treated at the Carrier Foundation, approximately half the study sample had favorable outcomes (Pettinati et al. 1982). However, fluctuations in outcome status were common, and only one-fourth of patients were continuously abstinent for all 4 years.

In a study involving nearly 75,000 alcoholic men identified through the VA's computerized database, Bunn et al. (1994) found that patients who completed extended formal inpatient alcoholism treatment had lower mortality rates in the 3 years after discharge than did patients who had shorter inpatient stays (either because they entered a short-term detoxification program or because they did not complete a longer-term program) or patients who were hospitalized without receiving any formal alcoholism treatment.

Unfortunately, all of the studies mentioned here were uncontrolled and were therefore subject to the biases inherent in uncontrolled research. It is because of these concerns that an increasing number of controlled studies have recently been undertaken. However, as explained earlier, controlled studies are also not immune to methodological flaws. Thus, continued research on this topic is needed.

Patient Characteristics in Inpatient Treatment Outcome Research

Although some authors have written that inpatient treatment of substance-dependent individuals is often not superior to less intensive treatment, some subgroups of patients do appear to respond better than others to hospitalization. Most studies of inpatient treatment have found that the following groups have a better prognosis: patients who are older, patients who are married, patients who abuse alcohol rather than other drugs, and patients whose families participate in treatment (Harrison et al. 1991). Individuals with histories of intravenous drug use or antisocial behavior tend to fare less well in inpatient treatment outcome studies (Harrison et al. 1991). However, these same patient characteristics are associated with a favorable prognosis in other forms of substance dependence treatment. Patients with greater psychosocial stressors and those with more severe substance use disorders may receive greater benefit from inpatient treatment than from outpatient treatment (Harrison and Asche 2001).

Program Characteristics in Inpatient Treatment Outcome Research

Although a number of studies have focused on the contribution of patient factors to substance abuse treatment outcome, there has been a relative paucity of research on inpatient treatment program characteristics that affect prognosis. Some authors have argued that programmatic variables are less important than patient characteristics in determining treatment outcome (Armor et al. 1976), but Cronkite and Moos (1978), who conducted a path analysis of treatment outcome among 429 alcoholic patients treated in five programs, concluded that program-related characteristics did influence treatment outcome substantially.

Several characteristics of inpatient substance abuse treatment have been examined to determine their effect on treatment outcome (Adelman and Weiss 1989), but many of these studies either were uncontrolled or did not include a carefully matched control group. Moreover, these studies were generally performed in the 1970s and 1980s, when hospitalization was often a first-line treatment for patients with substance use disorders.

In a study of the effect of the referral process on outcome, employed alcoholic individuals who were forced by their employers to enter treatment fared better than individuals who volunteered for treatment (Chopra et al. 1979). Moberg et al. (1982) also found that involving a patient's employer during hospitalization had a beneficial effect on treatment outcome.

Case management augmentation, dual diagnosis groups, and motivational interviewing have also been studied and appear to be useful. Traditionally, inpatient case management has involved identifying referral sources and working with family members and aftercare providers. Some evidence suggests that augmenting these traditional case management services with additional services may enhance treatment outcome. These additional services include identifying adjunctive services for patients, encouraging patients to take the initiative for their own treatment and aftercare, and providing additional structure to the aftercare referral process (see, for example, Franco et al. 1995 and Siegal et al. 1995). In one strategy that has been shown to be effective, the patient becomes familiar with the aftercare treatment by attending at least one meeting before discharge (Verinis and Taylor 1994), meeting a member of the outpatient team before discharge (Lash 1998), or being escorted from the inpatient unit to the outpatient facility (Chutuape et al. 2001). Another promising approach is motivational interviewing. This brief treatment approach, which is designed to foster internal motivation to change addictive behaviors, lends itself to the short length of stays typical in an inpatient setting (Miller and Rollnick 2002). Van Horn and Bux (2001) conducted a pilot study of group motivational interviewing among patients with dual diagnoses and reported

that the intervention is feasible for implementation in an inpatient setting.

Some evidence indicates that the level of emphasis on peer group interaction in a treatment center may affect treatment efficacy (Barnett and Swindle 1997). Stinson et al. (1979) randomly assigned 466 patients to two alcoholism treatment programs: one with an emphasis on intensive individualized treatment and a high staff-to-patient ratio and the other with a lower staff-to-patient ratio and an emphasis on peer group interaction. Patients who entered the latter program had better treatment outcomes, which suggests the potential importance of peer support in alcoholism treatment programs.

Characteristics of staff members have been examined in several studies. Valle (1981) found that the interpersonal skills of alcoholism counselors in an inpatient treatment facility had a marked effect on treatment outcome. McLellan et al. (1988) obtained similar results in a study involving counselors working in an outpatient methadone maintenance treatment program. These findings add weight to the argument that characteristics of specific counselors may substantially affect treatment outcome within a given treatment setting.

Psychiatric assessment has also been shown to be an important part of treatment. For example, in a well-known series of studies, McLellan et al. (1986) demonstrated the importance of severity of psychopathology as a predictor of outcome in patients with substance use disorders. These researchers found that patients with moderate levels of psychiatric severity, as measured by the Addiction Severity Index, had the best response to inpatient treatment. The recent development of psychological and pharmacological treatment approaches for specific subgroups of patients with coexisting substance use disorders and psychiatric illness (Weiss and Najavits 1998) points to the importance of performing careful psychiatric evaluations in substance-dependent patients.

One of the major components of virtually all inpatient treatment programs is the emphasis on group therapy and attendance at AA meetings. Because of the near ubiquity of these aspects of inpatient treatment, little research has been done on their relative contribution to treatment outcome. However, some specific types of groups have been examined, and positive results have been reported for groups teaching social skills (Eriksen et al. 1986) or coping skills (Vogel et al. 1997). Other specific interventions that have been reported to be beneficial include thermal and electromyographic biofeedback (Denney et al. 1991) and the use of patient-written treatment contracts (as opposed to staff-written or mutually written contracts) in treatment planning (Vannicelli 1979). Physical exercise was shown in one study to reduce state and trait anxiety and depression in substance-dependent inpatients, although the long-term effects of exercise on outcome are not clear (Palmer et al. 1988).

Aftercare has long been considered an essential part of inpatient treatment; several studies have shown the positive effect of aftercare on treatment outcome. Some researchers have questioned whether the aftercare program itself improves treatment outcome or whether the patients who are likely to have good treatment outcomes are the ones who also participate in aftercare more often. Two studies using cross-lagged analyses have supported the former hypothesis (Costello 1980; Vannicelli 1978). However, McLatchie and Lomp (1988) disputed this theory. These investigators randomly assigned 155 patients who had completed a 4-week inpatient alcoholism treatment program to one of three aftercare groups: 1) a mandated aftercare group; 2) a voluntary aftercare group, in which patients could decide on their own whether to participate; and 3) a group in which patients were dissuaded from participating in aftercare. No differences were found among groups with respect to relapse to drinking, lifestyle, satisfaction, or level of anxiety. However, 66% of patients in the voluntary aftercare group did request aftercare.

Finally, the correlation between length of stay and inpatient treatment outcome has long been controversial. Although some research has found that inpatient treatment offered no more benefit than a session of outpatient advice (Edwards et al. 1977), other studies have found a positive correlation between length of stay and treatment response (Barnett and Swindle 1997; Finney et al. 1981; McLellan et al. 1982). However, many of these results are difficult to evaluate because of lack of randomization or poor comparability of study groups. Gottheil et al. (1992) examined 131 alcoholic male veterans who received inpatient treatment for the recommended period of 90 days. The authors found that patients with less severe impairment, as measured by the Addiction Severity Index, fared best. Moreover, in these patients, a longer hospital stay resulted in better treatment outcome. Patients with the most severe problems, on the other hand, did not benefit from an increase in length of stay. The results

of this study are similar to those of Simpson (1979), who found that drug-dependent patients who received less than 90 days of treatment in either inpatient or outpatient programs did less well than patients who received 90 or more days of treatment. Gottheil et al. (1992) posited that the more severely psychiatrically ill patients may have failed to benefit from treatment because even 90 days of hospitalization was insufficient for their needs.

Future Implications

The role of inpatient treatment for patients with substance use disorders remains a complex and controversial issue, with public health, political, philosophical, financial, and moral implications attached to its discussion. It is clear, however, that attempting to formulate simplistic guidelines about the use of this treatment modality serves no one's best interest. Thus, the question should not be "Is inpatient treatment effective?" but rather "For which patients is inpatient treatment effective, at what time or times, and for how long?" To that end, the emphasis of current research in this area is on discerning which aspects of inpatient treatment are effective for which groups of patients. As future research helps to clarify these issues, it is hoped that inpatient treatment will have a more stable and defined place in the therapeutic approach to patients with substance use disorders.

References

Adelman SA, Weiss RD: What is therapeutic about inpatient alcoholism treatment? Hosp Community Psychiatry 40:515–519, 1989

Alterman AI, O'Brien CP, McLellan AT, et al: Effectiveness and costs of inpatient versus day hospital cocaine rehabilitation. J Nerv Ment Dis 182:157–163, 1994

Armor DJ, Polich JM, Stambul H: Alcoholism and Treatment. Santa Monica, CA, Rand Corporation, 1976

Barnett PG, Swindle RW: Cost-effectiveness of inpatient substance abuse treatment. Health Serv Res 32:615–629, 1997

Brooner RK, King VL, Kidorf M, et al: Psychiatric and substance use comorbidity among treatment-seeking opioid abusers. Arch Gen Psychiatry 54:71–80, 1997

Bunn JY, Booth BM, Cook CAL, et al: The relationship between mortality and intensity of inpatient alcoholism treatment. Am J Public Health 84:211–214, 1994

Chopra KS, Preston DA, Gerson LW: The effect of constructive coercion on the rehabilitative process: a study of the employed alcoholics in an alcoholism treatment program. J Occup Med 21:749–752, 1979

Chutuape MA, Katz EC, Stitzer ML: Methods for enhancing transition of substance dependent patients from inpatient to outpatient treatment. Drug Alcohol Depend 61:137–143, 2001

Collins MN, Burns T, van den Berk PAH, et al: A structured programme for out-patient alcohol detoxification. Br J Psychiatry 156:871–874, 1990

Cook CCH: The Minnesota Model in the management of drug and alcohol dependency: miracle, method or myth? part I: the philosophy and the programme. Br J Addict 83:625–634, 1988a

Cook CCH: The Minnesota Model in the management of drug and alcohol dependency: miracle, method or myth? part II: evidence and conclusions. Br J Addict 83:735–748, 1988b

Costello RM: Alcoholism aftercare and outcome: cross-lagged panel and path analyses. Br J Addict 75:49–53, 1980

Craig TJ, Branchey M, Buydens-Branchey L, et al: Admission criteria for inpatient substance abuse/dependence rehabilitation: implications for managed care. Ann Clin Psychiatry 8:11–17, 1996

Cronkite RC, Moos RH: Evaluating alcoholism treatment programs: an integrated approach. J Consult Clin Psychol 46:1105–1119, 1978

Denney MR, Baugh JL, Hardt HD: Sobriety outcome after alcoholism treatment with biofeedback participation: a pilot inpatient study. Int J Addict 26:335–341, 1991

Edwards G, Orford J, Egert S, et al: Alcoholism: a controlled trial of "treatment" and "advice." J Stud Alcohol 38:1004–1031, 1977

Eriksen L, Bjornstad S, Gotestam KG: Social skills training in groups for alcoholics: one-year treatment outcome for groups and individuals. Addict Behav 11:309–330, 1986

Finney JW, Moos RH, Chan DA: Length of stay and program component effects in the treatment of alcoholism: a comparison of two techniques for process analyses. J Consult Clin Psychol 49:120–131, 1981

Franco H, Galanter M, Castaneda R, et al: Combining behavioral and self-help approaches in the inpatient management of dually diagnosed patients. J Subst Abuse Treat 12:227–232, 1995

Galanter M, Keller DS, Dermatis H, et al: The impact of managed care on substance abuse treatment: a report of the American Society of Addiction Medicine. J Addict Dis 19:13–34, 2000

Gilmore K, Jones D, Tamble L: Treatment Benchmarks. Center City, MN, Hazelden, 1986

Gottheil E, McLellan AT, Druley KA: Length of stay, patient severity and treatment outcome: sample data from the field of alcoholism. J Stud Alcohol 53:69–75, 1992

Harrison PA, Asche SE: Comparison of substance abuse treatment outcomes for inpatients and outpatients. J Subst Abuse Treat 17:207–220, 1999

Harrison PA, Asche SE: Outcomes monitoring in Minnesota: treatment implications, practical limitations. J Subst Abuse Treat 21:173–183, 2001

Harrison PA, Hoffman NG, Gibb L, et al: Determinants of chemical dependency treatment placement: clinical, economic, and logistic factors. Psychotherapy 25:356–364, 1988

Harrison PA, Hoffman NG, Streed SG: Drug and alcohol addiction treatment outcome, in The Comprehensive Handbook of Drug and Alcohol Addiction. Edited by Miller NS. New York, Marcel Dekker, 1991, pp 1163–1197

Harwood HJ, Fountain D, Fountain G: Cost estimates for alcohol and drug abuse. Addiction 94:631–635, 1999

Hayashida M, Alterman AI, McLellan AT, et al: Comparative effectiveness and costs of inpatient and outpatient detoxification of patients with mild-to-moderate alcohol withdrawal syndrome. N Engl J Med 320:358–365, 1989

Hoffman NG, Halikas JA, Mee-Lee D, et al: ASAM Patient Placement Criteria for the Treatment of Psychoactive Substance Use Disorders. Washington, DC, American Society of Addiction Medicine; Irvine, CA, National Association of Addiction Treatment Providers, 1991

Holland P, Mushinski M: Costs of alcohol and drug abuse in the United States, 1992: Alcohol/Drugs COI Study Team. Stat Bull Metrop Insur Co 80(4):2–9, 1999

Hser YI, Anglin MD, Fletcher B: Comparative treatment effectiveness: effects of program modality and client drug dependence history on drug use reduction. J Subst Abuse Treat 15:513–523, 1998

Kessler RC, Crum RC, Warner LA, et al: Lifetime co-occurrence of DSM-III-R alcohol abuse and dependence with other psychiatric disorders in the National Comorbidity Survey. Arch Gen Psychiatry 54:313–321, 1997

Kofoed L: Outpatient vs. inpatient treatment for the chronically mentally ill with substance use disorders. J Addict Dis 12:123–137, 1993

Lash SJ: Increasing participation in substance abuse aftercare treatment. Am J Drug Alcohol Abuse 24:31–36, 1998

Longabaugh R: Longitudinal outcome studies, in Alcoholism: Origins and Outcome. Edited by Rose RM, Barrett J. New York, Raven, 1988, pp 267–280

Longabaugh R, McGrady B, Fink E, et al: Cost effectiveness of alcoholism treatment in partial vs inpatient settings: six-month outcomes. J Stud Alcohol 44:1049–1071, 1983

McElrath D: The Hazelden treatment model. Testimony before the U.S. Senate Committee on Governmental Affairs, Washington, DC, June 16, 1988

McKay JR, Cacciola JS, McLellan AT, et al: An initial evaluation of the psychosocial dimensions of the American Society of Addiction Medicine criteria for inpatient versus intensive outpatient substance abuse rehabilitation. J Stud Alcohol 58:239–252, 1997

McLatchie BH, Lomp KGE: An experimental investigation of the influence of aftercare on alcoholic relapse. Br J Addict 83:1045–1054, 1988

McLellan AT, Luborsky L, O'Brien CP, et al: Is treatment for substance abuse effective? JAMA 247:1423–1428, 1982

McLellan AT, Luborsky L, O'Brien CP: Alcohol and drug abuse treatment in three different populations: is there improvement and is it predictable? Am J Drug Alcohol Abuse 12:101–120, 1986

McLellan AT, Woody GE, Luborsky L, et al: Is the counselor an "active ingredient" in substance abuse rehabilitation? an examination of treatment success among four counselors. J Nerv Ment Dis 176:423–430, 1988

Mee-Lee D, Shulman GD, Fishman M, et al (eds): ASAM Patient Placement Criteria for the Treatment of Substance-Related Disorders, 2nd Edition, Revised. Chevy Chase, MD, American Society of Addiction Medicine, 2001

Meyer RE, Mirin SM: The Heroin Stimulus: Implications for a Theory of Addiction. New York, Plenum, 1979

Miller WR, Hester R: Inpatient alcoholism treatment: who benefits? Am Psychol 41:794–805, 1986

Miller WR, Rollnick S: Motivational Interviewing: Preparing People for Change, 2nd Edition. New York, Guilford, 2002

Minkoff K: Program components of a comprehensive integrated care system for seriously mentally ill patients with substance disorders. New Dir Ment Health Serv 91:17–30, 2001

Mirin SM, Weiss RD, Griffin ML, et al: Psychopathology in drug abusers and their families. Compr Psychiatry 32:36–51, 1991

Moberg DP, Krause WK, Klein PE: Posttreatment drinking behavior among inpatients from an industrial alcoholism program. Int J Addict 17:549–567, 1982

Moos RH, Finney JW, Moos BS: Inpatient substance abuse care and the outcome of subsequent community residential and outpatient care. Addiction 95:833–846, 2000

Nace EP: Inpatient treatment of alcoholism: a necessary part of the therapeutic armamentarium. Psychiatr Hosp 21:9–12, 1990

Palmer J, Vacc N, Epstein J: Adult inpatient alcoholics: physical exercise as a treatment intervention. J Stud Alcohol 49:418–421, 1988

Pettinati HM, Sugerman AA, DiDonato N, et al: The natural history of alcoholism over four years after treatment. J Stud Alcohol 43:201–215, 1982

Pettinati HM, Meyers K, Jensen JM, et al: Inpatient vs outpatient treatment for substance dependence revisited. Psychiatr Q 64:173–182, 1993

Regier DA, Farmer ME, Rae DS, et al: Comorbidity of mental disorders with alcohol and other drug abuse: results from the Epidemiologic Catchment Area (ECA) Study. JAMA 264:2511–2518, 1990

Ross HE, Glaser FB, Germanson T: The prevalence of psychiatric disorders in patients with alcohol and other drug problems. Arch Gen Psychiatry 45:1023–1031, 1988

Schneider R, Mittelmeier C, Gadish D: Day versus inpatient treatment for cocaine dependence: an experimental comparison. J Ment Health Adm 23:234–245, 1996

Sell J: Academic outcome studies: the research and its misapplication to managed care of alcoholism. Alcoholism Treatment Quarterly 13:17–31, 1995

Siegal HA, Rapp RC, Kelliher CW, et al: The strengths perspective of case management: a promising inpatient substance abuse treatment enhancement. J Psychoactive Drugs 27:67–72, 1995

Simpson DD: The relation of time spent in drug abuse treatment to posttreatment outcome. Am J Psychiatry 136:1449–1453, 1979

Skinner HA: Comparison of clients assigned to inpatient and outpatient treatment for alcoholism and drug addiction. Br J Psychiatry 138:312–320, 1981

Steenrod S, Brisson A, McCarty D, et al: Effects of managed care on programs and practices for the treatment of alcohol and drug dependence. Recent Dev Alcohol 15:51–71, 2001

Stinson DS, Smith WG, Amidjaya I, et al: Systems of care and treatment outcomes for alcoholic patients. Arch Gen Psychiatry 36:535–539, 1979

Strang J, Marks I, Dawe S, et al: Type of hospital setting and treatment outcome with heroin addicts: results from a randomised trial. Br J Psychiatry 171:335–339, 1997

Substance Abuse and Mental Health Services Administration: Results From the 2001 National Household Survey on Drug Abuse: Volume 1. Rockville, MD, Office of Applied Studies, Substance Abuse and Mental Health Services Administration, 2002

Swindle RW, Phibbs CS, Paradise MJ, et al: Inpatient treatment for substance abuse patients with psychiatric disorders: a national study of determinants of readmission. J Subst Abuse 7:79–97, 1995

U.S. Department of Health and Human Services: The Economic Costs of Alcohol and Drug Abuse in the United States 1992. Washington, DC, U.S. Government Printing Office, 1998

Valle SK: Interpersonal functioning of alcoholism counselors and treatment outcome. J Stud Alcohol 42:783–790, 1981

Van Horn DH, Bux DA: A pilot test of motivational interviewing groups for dually diagnosed inpatients. J Subst Abuse Treat 20:191–195, 2001

Vannicelli M: Impact of aftercare in the treatment of alcoholics: a cross-lagged panel analysis. J Stud Alcohol 39:1875–1886, 1978

Vannicelli M: Treatment contracts in an inpatient alcoholism treatment setting. J Stud Alcohol 40:457–471, 1979

Verinis JS, Taylor J: Increasing alcoholic patients' aftercare attendance. Int J Addict 29:1487–1494, 1994

Vogel PA, Eriksen L, Bjornelv S: Skills training and prediction of follow-up status for chronic alcohol dependent inpatients. European Journal of Psychiatry 11:51–63, 1997

Wallace J, McNeill D, Gilfillan D, et al: Six-month treatment outcomes in socially stable alcoholics: abstinence rates. J Subst Abuse Treat 5:247–252, 1988

Walsh DC, Hingson RW, Merrigan DM, et al: A randomized trial of treatment options for alcohol-abusing workers. N Engl J Med 325:775–782, 1991

Weddington WW, McLellan AT: Substance abuse treatment (letter). Hosp Community Psychiatry 45:80, 1994

Weiss RD, Najavits LM: Overview of treatment modalities for dual diagnosis patients: pharmacotherapy, psychotherapy, and twelve-step programs, in Dual Diagnosis: Substance Abuse and Comorbid Medical and Psychiatric Disorders. Edited by Kranzler HR, Rounsaville BJ. New York, Marcel Dekker, 1998, pp 87–105

Weiss RD, Mirin SM, Frances RJ: The myth of the typical dual diagnosis patient. Hosp Community Psychiatry 43:107–108, 1992

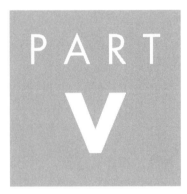

PART

V

Special
Approaches and
Treatment
Programs

Employee Assistance Programs and Other Workplace Interventions

Paul M. Roman, Ph.D.
Terry C. Blum, Ph.D.

Employed people constitute the majority of those with substance abuse problems (Roman 2002). The significant presence of alcohol problems in the workforce was most recently documented in a 1997 national survey indicating that about 7.6% of the full-time employed workforce are heavy drinkers (Zhang et al. 1999). According to this study, about one-third of the heavy drinkers are also illegal drug users. Substance abuse problems among working people can produce substantial economic and social impacts if they are not addressed in a timely and effective manner. Because most workers are employees of organizations, workplaces are critical venues for addressing substance abuse problems. Yet, as we describe in this chapter, there are numerous barriers to making full use of these intervention opportunities.

Employee assistance programs (EAPs) are currently the principal means used by work organizations to provide services to employees with substance abuse

problems. These programs have proliferated widely in the United States and are becoming established internationally. The broad focus of EAPs deflects them from fully attending to workplace substance abuse problems. Furthermore, they are not the only workplace strategy focused on substance abuse; therefore, following an in-depth discussion of EAPs, this chapter includes a section on alternative and complementary strategies for preventing workplace substance abuse problems.

As platforms for addressing substance abuse problems, workplaces have several unique features that are easily overlooked but that must be understood if effective programs are to be implemented. Workplace concern about substance abuse is two-pronged. First, the organization and its members must be *protected from adverse impacts* of co-workers' substance abuse. Second, the organization must *protect its investment in employees* and its relationships with them. Therefore it is typically in the organization's interest to correct employees' impairments and provide for treatment of illnesses that undermine job performance. These two concerns often represent opposite reactions by the organization: one leading to the segregation or exclusion of substance abusers and the other suggesting the value of undertaking efforts to sustain membership in the organization despite evidence of an inability to perform at full capacity (Roman and Blum 1999). These potentially conflicting concerns are represented in many organizations by the presence of both employee drug screening and employee assistance programs.

Other important features of workplace intervention are also unique. First, nearly all substance abuse interventions in other settings involve *short-term* relationships with the affected individuals. Caseloads undergo constant turnover in all types of treatment and also in other interventions such as education courses for those who have been arrested for driving while intoxicated. Likewise, educational settings that are commonly used as prevention and intervention platforms are characterized by a steady turnover of students as they graduate or drop out. By contrast, employees who receive workplace-sponsored intervention are provided with these services on the assumption that their organizational membership will be *long-term*. There is no limit set on the period of "recovery." This suggests that particular tensions are likely to arise if there is an expectation that treated employees should never have a "slip," because relapse is in fact an expected and normal feature of the long-term recovery process.

Second, whether private or public, workplaces are centered on making products or providing services. Success in meeting these goals rests on the coordinated performance of the workforce. Thus the salient definition of adequately functioning employees is based on *job performance,* not health status. Therefore, although most treatment systems are focused on abstinence from alcohol and drug use as the outcome of successful treatment, a return to adequate job performance is the appropriate criterion for judging the success of an intervention sponsored by the workplace. Abstinence from substance use is neither a necessary nor a sufficient condition for adequate job performance, and attempted enforcement of abstinence is clearly outside the employer-employee relationship.

Finally, workplace programming for employee substance abuse issues is typically viewed as though all workplaces were structured along similar lines, in the same way that schools or treatment programs are iso-

morphic in their structures and activities. In fact, however, a vast *diversity* in structures and occupational mixes characterizes populations of work organizations in the United States and throughout the world. Therefore, flexibility and creativity are necessary in adapting substance abuse interventions to multiple types of workplaces.

Variations Across EAPs

Within a workplace, an EAP should have two main components: 1) *access to qualified personnel* who can implement the employee assistance technology (i.e., identification, intervention, motivation, referral, and follow-up) and 2) *written policies and procedures* whereby the core techniques of employee assistance work are integrated with the bureaucratic features of the workplace. The provision of such services varies considerably. In many work sites, access to professional assistance may be fairly remote, with services provided by an external contracted organization. Such contracts vary greatly in their scope of services and in the supervision that the contracting work site exercises over the provider. In other (but increasingly rarer) instances, fully staffed EAP units are incorporated into the work site's human resource management function.

Variations in EAPs are functions of workplace size and of the physical or geographic distribution of employees. Typical in many large multisite organizations is an internal EAP staffed by corporate employees, whose duties include providing services to employees at corporate headquarters as well as selecting and monitoring contractors to provide these services at other corporate sites. In such settings, despite the EAP administration's being internally staffed, the majority of corporate employees actually receive EAP services from external providers.

EAPs are found in nearly 60% of American workplaces, and their presence is directly correlated with workplace size (Hartwell et al. 1996; Roman 2002). Although the widespread presence of EAPs suggests extensive opportunities for substance abuse interventions, there are a number of reasons to doubt the validity of this assumption. Recent data reported by McFarland and colleagues (2003) indicate that even where EAPs are present, benefits managers rank alcohol and drug treatment programs as a bottom-level priority and indicate little interest in improving such benefits. In another study (Rost et al. 2000), it was found that large employers are primarily concerned with the costs of substance abuse and mental health services and are minimally interested in evaluating providers' track record of clinical outcomes. Other research (Roman 2002) reveals that substance abuse treatment centers have shown a sharp decline in referral relationships with EAPs, and national survey data suggest that utilization of EAPs for substance abuse problems is declining. An understanding of this dilemma may begin with discussion of how EAPs evolved in the United States.

The Discovery of Substance-Abusing Individuals in the Workplace

Use of the workplace for intervention was an established idea in the early 1940s, when industrial alcoholism programs were launched in a number of prominent workplaces as a direct spin-off of the influence of Alcoholics Anonymous (AA) (Trice and Schonbrunn 1981). However, this early programming model had a number of limitations that prevented its widespread dissemination. This situation changed during the 1970s, beginning with the American alcoholism movement's symbolic construction of the "hidden alcoholic" as the central target of intervention (Roman 1991; Roman and Blum 1987). This shift substantially altered the political base of the alcoholism movement and set the stage for using workplaces as venues for the identification of alcohol problems.

The transformation followed this pattern: a residue of the temperance movement that accompanied the repeal of Prohibition in 1933 was the pervasive characterization of the American alcoholic as a "skid row bum." Through the 1950s and 1960s, a concerted effort centered on the decriminalization of alcohol problems, replacing criminalization with medicalization by substituting treatment for incarceration (J. Schneider 1978). This movement never attracted strong public attention; custody of public inebriates, decriminalized or not, was a weak basis for attracting public interest, involvement, and support.

To gain treatment parity with other diseases, alcoholism needed to be brought into the mainstream of the health care system. Bringing the public inebriate into the middle-class health care system was clearly not

the key to success in such an effort. With the concerted support of the National Institute on Alcohol Abuse and Alcoholism (NIAAA), founded in 1970, the social construction of the socially integrated "hidden alcoholic" began in earnest and has more or less succeeded (Roman 1991). Prominent today across multiple media is the characterization of the typical American alcoholic individual as being employed, with a stable residence and family. This image has implications for intervention. Unlike the homeless inebriate panhandling in public view, hidden alcoholics are socially integrated, are embedded in active social roles, and are surrounded by systems of enabling that make identification and referral particularly difficult. The theme that most hidden alcoholic persons were employed set the stage for the emergence of substance abuse programming centered in the workplace.

EAPs and the Mainstreaming of Substance Abuse Treatment

Through its control over continued employment and the expectation of adequate job performance, the workplace possesses unique leverage to motivate behavioral change (Roman and Trice 1968; Trice and Roman 1972). A key assumption for implementing this leverage is that in the early middle stage (Jellinek 1960) of serious dependence, an individual developing alcohol dependence manifests measurable job performance deterioration that can be used by supervisors as a basis for motivating behavioral change (Sonnenstuhl and Trice 1986).

Such an intervention is responsive to the two-pronged concern of the workplace described above. On the one hand, the intervention generates savings for employers by curbing alcoholic behavior before such behavior results in serious losses from poor quality or quantity of job output. At the same time, the intervention may allow for conservation of the jobs of employees in whom there may be substantial investment. Through prompt implementation of these interventions, employers may substantially reduce on-the-job safety risks and reduce the effects of alcoholic behavior on fellow employees and supervisors.

These concepts and benefits were embedded in workplace programs from the early 1940s; however, as attractive as they may seem, they were not adopted by workplaces during the 1950s and 1960s despite considerable effort by specialists based in the National Council on Alcoholism. In retrospect, two clear barriers to workplace adoption are evident. First, employers' acceptance of such a program was tacit admission that alcohol problems existed in their workplace, a stigma that could affect both customer and stockholder relations. Second, despite knowledge of the success of AA in many quarters, few employers had been convinced of the viability and feasibility of the rehabilitation of workers with alcohol problems.

Less evident was a potentially fatal flaw in program design. The procedures were based on the assumption that supervisors and managers would be able to accurately target employees whose job performance problems were linked with alcohol abuse and would be able to distinguish them from those whose work was deteriorating for other reasons. Educating supervisors in such diagnostic skills is clearly not feasible, to say nothing of the potential legal and moral ramifications of supervisors' exercise of such arbitrary judgments.

Once it became clear that the industrial alcoholism model had very limited prospects for wider adoption, the NIAAA supported refinement of a new strategy that became embellished as the EAP (Roman 1975, 1981, 1988; Roman and Trice 1976; Wrich 1973). Instead of focusing on the substance-abusing employee per se, this strategy moved directly to the expected outcome of alcohol misuse—poor job performance—and emphasized the clear mandate of the employer to address job performance issues. By necessity, program focus was broadened to the wide variety of behavioral-medical problems that are known to affect employees' job performance. Substance abuse is only one category of these problems, albeit an important category. These problems would be caught in the broad net cast by the emphasis on identifying performance problems. A program specialist would perform the diagnostic role and would direct those in different problem categories to the appropriate treatment. On receiving a referral from a supervisor, the employee assistance coordinator would assess, motivate, and direct referred employees to the treatment resources in the community that were most appropriate for their needs. Thus the new strategy effectively eliminated the diagnostic and moralistic barriers of the old model.

As long as the NIAAA used its resources to promote attention to alcohol problems by EAPs, such attention was largely sustained. However, those resource investments have gradually disappeared over the past 20 years. As is now evident, it cannot be assumed that employee alcohol and drug problems will receive adequate attention through a broad EAP approach that focuses solely on performance issues. First among the barriers to such attention is the stigma associated with substance abuse and the many ways in which this stigma impedes identification and referral behaviors. Second is the sheer amount of time and energy required to effectively deal with the alcohol-dependent employee who denies a problem and eludes attempts at confrontation. Furthermore, an assumption that alcohol and drug problems will be adequately addressed overlooks the potential service demand that can be created by a program that offers assistance for virtually any problem, particularly when the program is specifically designed to encourage self-referrals (Wrich 1973). Finally, unless the employer sponsoring the program is specifically committed to addressing substance abuse, evaluation of the EAP model is likely to be based on its level of activity and overall caseload size. Thus, minimal attention to employee substance abuse can be easily overlooked and the program judged to be a success.

In retrospect, the apparent success of the EAP model in the 1970s and 1980s in identifying and providing services to employees with alcohol problems was in many ways an artifact of educational and promotional resources provided by the NIAAA. Although addressing substance abuse issues does not require re-engineering or redesigning an EAP, it does require special efforts and emphases by medical and human resource specialists to overcome the barriers that are built into the processes by which employee problems are channeled to EAP services.

The EAP Process

As illustrated above, an EAP is a broad-based employee problem-identification policy with a clear potential for addressing employee substance abuse problems. However, this potential may not be achieved without a concerted effort to overcome the natural barriers to managing substance abuse when there are abundant opportunities to focus attention elsewhere. Identification and referral to an EAP can occur through a supervisor's documentation of deteriorated job performance or through self-referral. Evidence from many sources indicates that self-referrals dominate caseloads, accounting for up to 90% of those who use EAP services (Cagney 1999).

After an employee's entry into the program, it is the task of the designated EAP coordinator to identify the nature of the presenting problem. Especially important are the coordinator's skills in determining whether 1) the employee's performance difficulties reflect an underlying *behavior problem* that fits or approximates a diagnostic category, 2) the performance difficulties are an outcome of a *poor fit* between abilities and job demands, or 3) the referral is a consequence of underlying *interpersonal conflicts* or workgroup politics. Thus, along with clinical expertise, familiarity with the workplace and knowledge of organizational behavior are critical for the effective performance of EAP coordinator roles.

As EAPs were originally designed, after the problem was identified the EAP coordinator would link the individual with the community resource most appropriate for managing the problem. The EAP coordinator would then function as a case manager from that point on. Such an approach is used in a minority of instances today. Under norms that have emerged in response to managed care, EAP counselors refrain from making external referrals but instead offer a limited number of counseling sessions with the expectation that these will result in a resolution of the problem. This approach may be a reasonable adaptation in the face of limits imposed by managed care and may be a cost-effective component of an external EAP contract. However, offering such counseling through an internal program or through an external program contracted by the employer creates potential conflicts of interest. Provision of such counseling raises the question of what occurs if the counseling does not produce the desired results.

There are no published research data on the efficacy of short-term counseling provided directly by employee assistance counselors. Several questions are of interest. First is the extent to which such counseling addresses substance abuse problems and under what conditions it leads to problem resolution. The notable impact of such brief interventions in other settings (Fleming et al. 2002) suggests potential efficacy for work-based brief interventions, but no published data address this question. A second issue concerns external referrals. At what point in the brief counseling process is a decision made to seek external assistance, and what is the role of the EAP counselor once such a referral is made? Again, no available research data address these questions.

The reliance on direct counseling clearly alters the essence of the contract between the employer and the employee that was part of the original conceptualization of EAPs. This contract took the following form: The employer is responsible for providing the employee with opportunities to engage in treatment and must not stigmatize or penalize the employee after treatment is completed—that is, the problem is to be handled like any other employee health issue. The employee is not forced to undergo treatment but must work to resolve the job performance problems that precipitated the referral, and thus probably he or she would be wise to cooperate with the prescribed treatment regimen.

The existence and utility of this contract have been altered in several ways by changes that have come about in the EAP process. First, the contract assumes a supervisory referral based on performance problems, but today the vast majority of EAP utilization comes via self-referral. Without an evidence base regarding performance, there is no contract and there is no leverage. Second, with the provision of counseling directly by the EAP, the employer is potentially in the role of both judge and jury. It would seem unfair for an employer to discipline a poorly performing employee if the counseling provided directly by the employer is not effective in solving the employee's problem.

Potential Contributions by EAPs to Effective Workplace Functioning

Recognizing the barriers that need to be overcome in keeping an EAP focused on employee substance abuse, it is important to address the broader benefits that these programs can offer in the employment setting when they sustain such a focus. Review of these benefits should serve as encouragement to maximize the potential for EAPs to address employee substance abuse.

The first potential contribution is the *retention of employees* who have developed substance abuse problems but in whom the organization has a substantial training investment. The intervention strategies embedded in EAPs can be used to reduce or eliminate the job performance problems of substance-abusing employees by motivating these employees to change their behavior with the assistance of counseling or treatment. Employee turnover is generally considered by management to be expensive and undesirable. Especially when dismissals occur, turnover is disruptive to the morale and efficiency of work groups. Therefore, turnover prevention or employment conservation is valuable for the work organization.

The second area where EAPs can make a potential contribution is in the *reduction of managerial responsibility* for and involvement in counseling of employees with substance abuse problems (Roman 1988). It is typically believed that without supportive assistance from an EAP, supervisors and managers facing a substance-abusing employee will engage in denial and will try their best to cover up and ignore the problem. The EAP community has long promoted this self-serving belief. However, data show that there is a marked degree of co-worker and supervisory activity relative to the problem as it progresses (Roman et al. 1992; cf. Trice and Beyer 1984). It should be emphasized that in the absence of an EAP and the supportive resources that it offers to supervisors and managers, there is an implicit policy that delegates the responsibilities for troubled employees to these supervisors and managers.

In undertaking these counseling responsibilities by default, some managers might be effective in leading an employee to rehabilitation, but there is little reason to expect such an outcome. Without knowing the right thing to do, others in the workplace will be hesitant and often inconsistent in their efforts to deal with such problems, which typically become increasingly visible over time. EAP implementation policies should mandate that supervisors and managers seek consultative assistance from an EAP specialist when it is evident that they are faced with such a problem. Such a policy would not exclude supervisors from the process but would give them the necessary support to ensure that policy guidelines are followed.

A third potential contribution by EAPs in managing substance-abusing employees is the *provision for due process* for employees whose substance abuse is affecting their work performance. The value of this contribution centers on several features of the contemporary environment within which work organizations operate:

- A multitude of legal protections that have developed around the employment relationship
- Labor-management relationships that are governed by collective bargaining agreements
- The organization's own guidelines regarding employees' rights, benefits, and responsibilities and the steps in the implementation of progressive discipline

Offering assistance to employees with substance abuse problems may protect the employer against subsequent legal action. Court decisions have tended to be based on this logic: because a health-based technology exists for managing substance abuse and mental health problems, employees should be given the opportunity to use such technology before their employment is terminated because of substandard job performance. Such litigation typically arises when employees charge their employers with discriminatory behavior vis-à-vis a substance abuse issue (Sonnenstuhl and Trice 1986). Here is where the principle of employee responsibility is critical (as contrasted to the mistake of requiring participation in treatment as a condition of continued employment). EAP policy should ensure that through the offer of assistance through an EAP, an employer is not committed to ensuring employees' recovery or their permanent employment.

More recently, EAPs have demonstrated their value as a referral outlet for employees who produce positive results on random or for-cause urine screening for the use of illegal drugs (Roman and Blum 1992). Firing such employees is not always a reasonable alternative and invites litigation that may serve no one's interest (Blum 1989). The presence of an EAP encourages approaches in which assistance is offered but responsibility for adequate job performance (and for continuing negative results when drug screens are administered randomly) after receiving assistance is placed on the substance-abusing employee. When the EAP is part of written human resource management policy, the likelihood of equitable implementation is enhanced.

A fourth potential EAP contribution is *health care cost containment* through encouragement of substance abuse treatment by employees and their dependents. As a group, untreated alcoholic individuals show levels of health care use that markedly exceed the levels of their nonalcoholic peers. This heavy use pattern extends to their families as well (Fein 1984; Holder 1987; Holder and Hallan 1986). These high levels of health care use, by both substance-abusing individuals and their family members, decrease substantially after successful interventions to deal with substance abuse problems.

These reductions in service use do not occur immediately; in fact, they usually require several years. Therefore, although the initial investment involved in providing treatment for substance abuse problems may appear high, follow-up studies indicate that these investments have the ultimate effect of health care cost containment (Smith and Mahoney 1989). Unfortunately, managed care firms have not yet recognized these benefits of intensive substance abuse treatment at the point when motivated clients are first identified.

A fifth potential function served by EAPs is the *gatekeeping and channeling* of employees' use of substance abuse treatment services. Choosing the right service to match an employee's problem is a critical employee assistance function; this function is sometimes missing today when employee assistance specialists do not have an adequate training background in substance abuse. EAP experts' evaluative knowledge of the quality and cost-efficiency of community-based substance abuse treatment alternatives is often superior to that of managed care contractors. In some instances, employees and their dependents have lower co-payments if their use of substance abuse or mental health services is channeled through the EAP.

Involvement of the EAP in the managed care loop varies from setting to setting, and cost-containment procedures do not always include the EAP in key gatekeeping decisions. Such inclusion varies with the extent to which the EAP is integrated into human resources management (particularly benefits management). Sometimes, rather than being empowered in the gatekeeping process, the EAP itself can be the subject of gatekeeping review. EAP staff members can sometimes be considered outsiders in conflicts over access to care that result from the use of managed care and utilization-review devices. Clear lines of communication and coordination, reasonable outcome-oriented databases, and mutual professional respect are all necessary if EAPs and managed care devices are to produce the desired outcomes of the more effective use of care, particularly in the case of substance abuse. There is a need for proactive efforts to educate workplace leaders about the value of full-scale treatments for substance abuse problems, including structured posttreatment follow-up that can be effectively managed by the EAP.

A sixth potential contribution of EAPs is in *transforming the image of substance abuse* within the organizational cultures of workplaces. Specifically, the effective use of an EAP with substance-abusing employees can promote cultural norms that treatment rather than punishment is the appropriate approach to these problems. Furthermore, through the presence of employees who are recovering from substance abuse problems, the reality of effective rehabilitation

is communicated to those who are skeptical about recovery.

The Dynamics of EAP Implementation

How effectively can EAPs fulfill the expectations of the six potential contributions outlined above? Evidence indicates that EAPs are effective in resolving problems of employee substance abuse (Blum and Roman 1995). Several key ingredients should be present for these results to be realized. These components are outlined below.

Policy Statements

The development and promulgation of a written policy statement is the initial step in the implementation of an EAP. The policy serves four purposes:

1. It introduces the program, explains its goals and philosophy, and generates support for the EAP at all levels of the work organization.
2. It spells out roles and expectations. Self-referrals are typically encouraged. The policy should direct supervisors and managers to contact the EAP for assistance rather than attempt a referral on their own.
3. It promotes equal access and fairness. In addition, it should assure employees that their confidentiality will be protected and that disciplinary procedures will be suspended when applicable.
4. It provides a vehicle for top management to indicate both symbolically and tangibly its support for the new program. Furthermore, it can signal a shift in organizational culture to the acceptance of substance abuse as a health problem to be dealt with in the same manner as other health issues.

Policy Dissemination and Training

Dissemination of the policy is essential for an EAP to be effective. Since the early days of industrial alcoholism programs, specific training of supervisors and managers has been deemed essential for effective program implementation. It is especially important if an emphasis on substance abuse issues is to be maintained (Colan and Schneider 1992). Training can demonstrate to supervisors how the EAP can solve difficult and time-consuming problems and can reduce the occurrence of complaints, grievances, or threats of legal action.

Training is ideally conducted by EAP staff. Training can serve to acquaint company personnel with the staff and reduce "social distance." Interaction between trainers and trainees helps to ferret out and eliminate barriers to program use. Conducting training is time-consuming for EAP staff, who must also continue to perform their direct service functions. Support for EAP-related training must emanate from top management levels.

EAP Referral Routes

There are many barriers that hinder supervisors from taking definitive actions toward subordinates whose behavior and demeanor do not meet organizational standards (Roman et al. 1992). A variety of beliefs may be embedded in workplace subcultures:

- The employee's problem will eventually diminish or disappear.
- A referral to another part of the organization might harm the subordinate's well-being.
- The supervisor is uncertain whether this is the kind of problem covered by EAP policy.
- The referral may reflect badly on supervisors' abilities to manage their responsibilities.
- It is easier to put up with the troublesome situation than to get involved in embarrassing and unpredictable referral actions.

These beliefs can lead supervisors to try to "go it alone" in resolving the problem. The risk is that the supervisor and subordinate may become enmeshed in a cycle of enabling and denial with regard to the employee's substance abuse. The self-referral is much more easily facilitated, even though it compromises the leverage that the employer may have in ultimately resolving the employee's performance deficits. In any event, referral delays are inevitable. Accumulated knowledge about substance abuse suggests that cases of substantial alcohol and drug dependence are well known to supervisors and co-workers as well as to the affected individual long before any kind of referral occurs.

Furthermore, what appear as self-referrals are not always private decisions to seek help. Data from a large-scale study of EAP referral routes indicate that most cases involving employee substance abuse that are recorded as self-referrals are indeed the result of informal "nudges" by supervisors and other significant others (Blum and Roman 1992; Blum et al. 1995). Rather than initiate a formal referral of the employee, a supervisor might threaten such a referral unless the employee undertakes a self-referral. This minimizes the likelihood of the supervisor's becoming enmeshed in red tape or interpersonal complications. Furthermore, from the supervisor's perspective, self-referral accomplishes the same result as a supervisory referral. However, from the perspective of the potential of the EAP process, there is less motivation for the employee to change his or her behavior when the supervisor is not formally involved.

Despite these barriers to referral and the use of EAP leverage, research has made it clear that a sound EAP can greatly curtail the delays that would occur in the natural course of events and thus can reduce the hidden costs associated with the substance-abusing employee. Over time, the existence of the EAP becomes well known throughout the workplace and to employees' family members, and data indicate that both family members and work peers play important roles in motivating self-referrals (Blum and Roman 1992; Blum et al. 1995).

Diagnosis and Use of Treatment

Although some EAPs include staff members with professional-level diagnostic skills, other EAPs may use central diagnostic and referral agencies. Use of a central agency frees the employer of the critical and potent diagnostic role and prevents the potential conflicts of one organizational employee diagnosing the problems of another. Furthermore, use of a central diagnostic agency frees the EAP for organizational development activities rather than clinical duties. On the other hand, conducting diagnoses within the work organization allows short steps in the processing of employees and avoids the potential loss of motivation.

After diagnosis, suggestions are made to the employee with regard to the type of counseling or treatment that may be necessary. According to EAP principles, these must be suggestions rather than directives and should never be a condition for avoiding discipline or continuing employment. Any coercion should be implicit, and indeed it should be repeatedly clear that individuals must be able to perform their jobs if they expect to keep them. But entry into a treatment regimen should be an individual choice, because treatment success is heavily dependent on individuals' acceptance of responsibility for working on their recovery. Any statement that the employee must undergo treatment in order to keep his or her job can create an implied contract that such treatment will solve the employee's problems.

An effective workplace referral should be a complex matching of the employee's treatment needs, the employee's job and family situation, the kinds of third-party coverage available to pay for treatment, the availability of appropriate facilities, and the accessibility of facilities. The complexity of these considerations lends support to the importance of having an EAP specialist who genuinely knows the particular workplace. These considerations also underline the inadequacy of relying on contracted service agents who have knowledge only of the employee's clinical status.

Thus, in making a referral decision, EAP staff members need to be highly informed about the effectiveness of service providers and also need to keep up with changing provisions in employee insurance and benefits coverage. EAP specialists must be able to work closely and, if necessary, aggressively with managed care gatekeepers. Finally, EAP staff members should monitor the employee's passage through the substance abuse treatment process.

Posttreatment Follow-up

Although follow-up associated with substance abuse treatment programs is critical in sustaining treatment gains, such efforts are notably weak. It is obviously difficult to track those who have completed care into the community, and it is even more difficult to be reimbursed for such efforts. Despite the built-in opportunities in workplace-based programs, effective posttreatment follow-up is an area of weakness in the operation of most EAPs (Blum and Roman 1992; Blum et al. 1995).

One of the greatest advantages of EAP policies is their intention to maintain the substance-abusing worker's employment throughout the course of treatment and recovery. The workplace also provides opportunities for relapse prevention. Follow-up in the form of participation in self-help groups or brief follow-up counseling sessions can be crucial during the first year after treatment and beyond. Follow-up counseling may reveal the need for change in work role assignments, and such changes are often a key step in relapse prevention.

Lack of attention to follow-up is a consequence of some combination of a lack of time on the part of EAP staff and adherence to the norms of the clinical community. Given the obvious value of follow-up as insurance on the multiple investments that have been made to return the employee to adequate performance, this is regrettable. The neglect stems in part from the tendency of human resource managers to focus on utilization rates to monitor EAP effectiveness. Such rates are obviously important relative to what EAPs are supposed to accomplish, but placing undue emphasis on them has the unfortunate consequence of minimizing emphasis on long-term outcomes, thus undermining the value of follow-up.

Efficacy of EAPs

EAPs have about a 70% success rate, based on reports of coordinators of 317 internal programs and the contract monitors of 126 external programs (Blum and Roman 1989; Blum et al. 1992), as well as a range of other summaries of discrete studies of program functioning (Blum and Roman 1995; Roman and Blum 1996; Sonnenstuhl and Trice 1986). Another way to look at outcome is to examine components of EAPs. Trice and Beyer (1984) established that constructive confrontation—as described by a sample of supervisors from several locations of a large corporation—was highly efficacious for alcoholic subordinates, and more recent work has confirmed the value of the confrontational approach (R.J. Schneider et al. 2000). Data from several different sources confirm the cost-effectiveness of EAPs (Blum and Roman 1995; Foote et al. 1978; French et al. 1997; Smith and Mahoney 1989; Zarkin et al. 2000).

However, the question of efficacy needs to be framed carefully. There is no answer to the questions of how efficacious EAPs are under the multitude of different circumstances in which they operate. Furthermore, the efficacy question poses the EAP as a treatment modality, which it is not. The outcomes of most substance abuse referrals to EAPs are tied to the treatments that are provided, which should be completely independent of the EAP. Therefore, outcomes associated with EAPs reflect the consequences of multiple inputs wherein it is impossible to disentangle the positive or negative influences of EAP inputs, treatment inputs, and aftercare or follow-up inputs.

An outcome focus is at least partially misplaced because it presumes that EAPs are primarily focused on patient outcomes. Research indicates that EAP personnel spend substantial amounts of their time in resolving problems between supervisors and subordinates that do not lead to referral, in giving advice to individuals that is not recorded in case records, in providing education to employees that may have primary preventive impacts, and in attempting to motivate providers to upgrade the quality of treatment services so that treatment efficacy is improved, to cite only a few examples (Blum and Roman 1989; Blum et al. 1992; Roman and Blum 1987).

EAPs are human resource management practices based in the workplace, not freestanding human service programs. These practices do not lend themselves to typical evaluations of efficacy because there is such a broad range of outcomes of interest to different constituency groups and because there is great variation in their structure and design.

Finally, EAPs are not publicly funded but rather are funded by their sponsoring workplace. Therefore, effectiveness is relative to their workplace settings, their integration within these settings, and the extent to which the EAPs attract the investment of organizational resources. It is impossible to determine EAP efficacy in managing employee substance abuse or other employee problems without considering the relatively complex context within which given EAPs function.

Complements and Alternatives to EAPs

Given the dominance of the EAPs as a strategy for addressing employee substance abuse, it is easy to overlook complementary or alternative interventions, several of which are well established. Nearly half of the workforce does not have access to EAPs. Some proportion of this group likely has access to these alternative services. Furthermore, these interventions may have important (but largely undocumented) effects on employee substance abuse.

Workplace Prohibition of Psychoactive Substance Use

Prohibition is a passive primary prevention strategy. Employers do not mandate that their employees actively do anything; rather, employers require that their employees not perform certain acts that in themselves are not directly linked to work. In nearly all cases, these rules proscribe the use of alcohol or drugs during work hours and before arriving for work.

Prohibition of alcohol and drug use is found in nearly all workplaces, and workplace prohibition rules predate nationwide Prohibition (Staudenmeier 1989). With the emergence of attention to illegal drugs, these substances were included in the general list of intoxicating substances and were recognized and addressed in prohibition policy statements in most workplaces, beginning about 35 years ago.

Alcohol and work have not always been segregated. Drinking breaks and on-the-job drinking were historically part of many occupational settings (Ames 1989). Industrialists' interests and capitalist economic growth in the nineteenth and early twentieth centuries in America brought about changes in the links between alcohol and work (Rumbarger 1989).

Workplace prohibition cannot be easily evaluated because settings without prohibition are essentially nonexistent. Even without data, however, it is reasonable to conclude that many accidents and injuries would occur if alcohol and drugs were intermingled with the work technologies of today.

Workplace Drug and Alcohol Testing

With its use increasing widely during the past two decades, workplace drug testing has been the subject of much debate (Macdonald and Roman 1995). At issue is whether preemployment screening identifies persons with drug problems and whether it is an accurate predictor of job performance. It has been found that drug use does not necessarily connote the existence of a drug problem and that evidence of drug use does not necessarily mean that a person cannot perform a job; furthermore, it is possible that preemployment drug testing facilitates discrimination in hiring (Normand et al. 1994). There is also no evidence that preemployment drug screening reduces the rate of drug problems that are subsequently identified in workplaces (Blum 1989; Roman 1989). Nonetheless, it appears that preemployment drug testing may become universally adopted, perhaps in large part for its symbolic value in demonstrating managerial authority and workplaces' support for the War on Drugs (Roman and Blum 1999).

Parallel tests for alcohol are considerably less feasible, but such testing is being adopted in safety-sensitive industries. This is not a new concept; as part of their rules of conduct or fitness-for-duty regulations, many workplaces have reserved the right to test employees for the presence of alcohol either on suspicion of intoxication or after an accident or other disruptive incident.

Random drug screening of current employees might be seen as a follow-up to preemployment screening or possibly as a means of screening employees who were hired before the practice of preemployment screening was instituted. Random drug screening is associated with the same problems as preemployment screening, in terms of identification of drug abuse and prediction of job performance. For-cause screening (i.e., screening after the occurrence of a major job performance problem) fits more closely with traditional workplace intervention approaches and, like random screening, is sometimes accompanied by referral to an EAP for assistance—but often with the condition that such an offer of help will not be repeated. Because for-cause screening is linked to a performance problem, which may involve accidents or injury, this form of screening comes closer to the assumptions underlying EAPs.

In some instances, random drug screening protocols are developed for individuals who have undergone treatment for drug problems under the auspices of an EAP. These cases may also provide only a single opportunity for an observed slip, although EAP policies vary in the extent to which they regard relapse as one of the common or even expected features of recovery from a substance dependence problem. There is anecdotal evidence that the use of random testing can be a strong motivator for treated employees who desire to keep their jobs, and therefore this form of testing can be an important complement to EAPs.

Health Promotion and Stress Management

Recent research suggests that health promotion and wellness programs may be effective in preventing substance abuse problems, and educational programs have been shown to have a measurable impact on self-reported drinking behavior (Stolzfus and Benson

1994; Trudeau et al. 2002). As yet, there is no evidence that health risk appraisals have a widespread impact on employee drinking. It is possible, but undocumented, that employees participating in exercise programs or other health-oriented leisure activities may change their drinking behavior because excessive drinking does not fit in with their new healthy regimen. Likewise, although stress management is a widely used intervention in the workplace, its effect on employee substance abuse has not been studied. In a recently reported study in which several of these concepts were combined and alcohol use reduction education was embedded into a cardiovascular wellness program, significant reductions in participants' drinking were demonstrated (Heirich and Sieck 2000).

Peer Intervention Programs and Member Assistance Programs

Since the 1970s, in the fields of medicine, law, dentistry, psychology, and nursing, there have been reports of activities oriented toward resolving problems of alcohol abuse and alcoholism through peer intervention programs (Hughes et al. 1999; Mansky 1999). Two intertwined concepts underlie such programs.

First, professionals often have autonomy in determining work hours and other aspects of work styles. Indeed, independence of performance often marks highly creative or heroic accomplishments among professionals. Second, there exists a strong sense of community in these professions, with members of a professional group tending to protect one another from external confrontations, interventions, or criticism. This concept relates to the first: to the extent that supervision of professionals occurs at all, it is typically one member of a profession who is supervising other members.

With these characteristics of work, typical organizationally based interventions directed toward substance abuse problems would have a low likelihood of utilization. It would be expected that professionals' problematic performance would be minimally visible, that professionals would readily cover up for one another, and that because of their power and autonomy, professionals would be highly resistant to any form of confrontation.

It is likely that the person who is aware of a professional's drinking or drug problem is another professional. Furthermore, because of professionals' shared interest and shared fate, the deviance, misbehavior, or malpractice of one professional may put at risk the reputation and status of professional peers and might jeopardize the credibility of the organization employing them. Finally, because most professions are certified or licensed through boards composed of professional peers, the profession itself may be in the position to threaten sanctions against members with substance use problems.

Peer intervention programs reportedly exist in numerous locations, generally within the local or state-wide association of a particular professional group (Flowers 1999). These programs are operated and governed by members of the profession, sometimes by members who have recovered from their own substance abuse problems.

Although private surveys of some "impaired professionals" programs have been conducted, detailed evidence about how these programs work and how effective they are is almost nonexistent. As might be expected, outsiders are not readily admitted to carry out objective research studies on professions, particularly studies of potentially threatening behaviors such as patterns of substance abuse. Given the nature of professional power and how it is maintained, this is not surprising. Although there are a number of partially circulated reports on the success of these programs, they were prepared by the program administrators or by others with a clear vested interest in sustaining good public relations for the professional group.

Another complement to EAPs are member assistance programs. A research group at Cornell University has been examining member assistance programs in labor unions for more than a decade. In a first set of studies (summarized in Sonnenstuhl 1996), the focus was on a small, independent union with an intense drinking culture that included on-the-job drinking. With the slow introduction of a union-based program providing recovery assistance to alcoholic union members (a program staffed by a union member who was a recovering alcoholic individual), the workplace drinking culture gradually changed. Recovery and abstinence became accepted as chosen lifestyles, and nearly universal pressure to drink with work peers both on and off the job diminished. This was a dramatic example of a change in what appeared to be deeply entrenched drinking norms, and the study findings suggest that it may be possible to prevent worker disability associated with substance abuse through workplace interventions directed toward cultural change.

A second set of studies by the Cornell group (Bacharach et al. 1994, 2001) focused on member assistance programs with broader ranges of coverage. The researchers examined programs in the railroad industry and in a broad-based transportation union and a program organized by flight attendants. The effect of these programs was found to be almost uniformly positive. There were no means for comparing the efficacy of these member assistance programs with that of management-based EAPs. However, the programs did have an effect on substance abuse among union members across these wide-ranging settings within the transportation industry.

The American workplace is said to be moving away from hierarchical management and toward a model of peer organization, one involving participative management and collective responsibility. Should these predictions prove correct, peer intervention and member assistance programs may be particularly appropriate means for managing employee substance abuse. Perhaps the most attractive feature of these programs is their lack of association with authority, power, and accompanying opportunities for coercion and threat.

On the other hand, peer intervention is not without problems. Defining and implementing actions toward deviant behavior within an informal and undocumented framework may lead to abuses that are greater than in a bureaucratic hierarchy. A bureaucratic system offers opportunities for obtaining equitable treatment and for lodging grievances when authority, procedure, and rules are breached.

Conclusion

The workplace is a platform of great potential value for intervention with employees who have substance abuse problems. Voluntary adoption of EAPs over the past 30 years—to the point where their coverage extends to more than 60% of the American workforce—is testimony to their value as perceived by workplace managers and labor unions. If EAPs are better than another alternative is impossible to address because EAPs are essentially value-added human resource management practices in the workplace rather than substitutes or replacements for preexisting structures or programs.

Because EAPs are widely involved in the mainstreaming of substance abuse treatment and tend to identify with this behavioral health mainstream, the community of EAP workers lies outside the community of substance abuse interventionists. EAPs are not well understood by this broader community, and the fact that they are perceived as work-based treatment programs leads to frustrations for those who demand simple analyses of program efficacy. As human resource management practices that are adapted to particular workplace settings, EAPs require a different frame of reference if their value in managing substance abuse issues is to be understood. However, EAPs are unique in their access to the employed population, which includes the vast majority of recovering, active, and potential substance-abusing individuals. A better understanding of the roles of EAPs by substance abuse interventionists and by interventionists whose primary focus is on psychiatric and family problems is critical if treatment interventions are to have a substantial effect on the consequences of behaviors linked to substance abuse. Such understanding should be accompanied by more research on the complements and alternatives to EAPs, especially strategies that can be successfully embedded in other types of health service delivery and peer intervention programs.

As external support for attention to alcohol and drug problems within broadly focused EAPs has diminished, development of this intervention potential in workplaces has slowed considerably in recent years and is in need of revitalization. The apparent diminution of workplace attention to substance problems through EAPs highlights the important elements of infrastructure necessary to sustain such interventions in institutional settings that do not have a primary mission to address substance abuse. Until there is a level playing field with other human problems and disorders, it is essential that supportive infrastructure be developed and maintained to ensure continuing attention to alcohol and drug problems in settings where the opportunities to do so are present.

References

Ames G: Alcohol related movements and their effects on drinking policies in American workplaces: an historical review. J Drug Issues 19:489–510, 1989

Bacharach SB, Bamberger P, Sonnenstuhl WJ: Member Assistance Programs in the Workplace. Ithaca, NY, ILR Press, 1994

Bacharach SB, Bamberger P, Sonnenstuhl WJ: Mutual Aid and Union Renewal: Cycles of Logics of Action. Ithaca, NY, Cornell University Press, 2001

Blum TC: The presence and integration of drug abuse intervention in human resource management, in Drugs in the Workplace: Research and Evaluation Data (NIDA Research Monograph No 91). Edited by Gust S. Rockville, MD, National Institute on Drug Abuse, 1989, pp 271–286

Blum TC, Roman PM: Employee assistance and human resources management, in Research in Personnel and Human Resources Management, Vol 7. Edited by Rowland K, Ferris G. Greenwich, CT, JAI Press, 1989, pp 258–312

Blum TC, Roman PM: Identifying alcoholics and persons with alcohol-related problems in the workplace: a description of EAP clients. Alcohol Health Res World 16:120–128, 1992

Blum TC, Roman PM: Cost Effectiveness and Preventive Impact of Employee Assistance Programs (Center for Substance Abuse Prevention Monograph 5). Washington, DC, Department of Health and Human Services, 1995

Blum TC, Martin JK, Roman PM: A research note on EAP prevalence, components and utilization. Journal of Employee Assistance Research 1:209–229, 1992

Blum TC, Roman PM, Harwood E: Employed women with alcohol problems who seek help from employee assistance programs: description and comparisons, in Recent Developments in Alcoholism, Vol 12. Edited by Galanter M. New York, Plenum, 1995, pp 126–161

Cagney T: Models of service delivery, in The Employee Assistance Handbook. Edited by Oher J. New York, Wiley, 1999, pp 59–70

Colan NB, Schneider R: The effectiveness of supervisor training: one-year follow-up. Journal of Employee Assistance Research 1:83–95, 1992

Fein R: Alcohol in America: The Price We Pay. Minneapolis, MN, Care Institute, 1984

Fleming MF, Mundt MP, French MT, et al: Brief physician advice for problem drinkers: long-term efficacy and cost-benefit analysis. Alcohol Clin Exp Res 26:36–43, 2002

Flowers WM: Sometimes doctors need help too: the Mississippi recovering physicians program. J Miss State Med Assoc 40:252–255, 1999

Foote A, Erfurt J, Strauch P, et al: Cost Effectiveness of Occupational Employee Assistance Programs. Ann Arbor, MI, Institute of Labor and Industrial Relations of the University of Michigan, 1978

French MT, Zarkin GA, Bray JW, et al: Costs of employee assistance programs: findings from a national survey. Am J Health Promot 11:219–222, 1997

Hartwell TD, Steele PD, French MT, et al: Aiding troubled employees: the prevalence, cost and characteristics of employee assistance programs in the United States. Am J Public Health 86:804–808, 1996

Heirich M, Sieck CJ: Worksite cardiovascular wellness programs as a route to substance abuse prevention. J Occup Environ Med 42:47–56, 2000

Holder HD: Alcoholism treatment and potential health care cost savings. Med Care 25:52–71, 1987

Holder HD, Hallan JB: Impact of alcoholism treatment on total health care costs: a six-year study. Adv Alcohol Subst Abuse 6:1–15, 1986

Hughes PH, Storr CL, Brandenburg NA, et al: Physician substance use by medical specialty. J Addict Dis 18(2):23–37, 1999

Jellinek EM: The Disease Concept of Alcoholism. New Brunswick, NJ, Publications Division of the Rutgers Center of Alcohol Studies, 1960

Macdonald S, Roman P (eds): Drug Testing in the Workplace. New York, Plenum, 1995

Mansky PA: Issues in the recovery of physicians from addictive illnesses. Psychiatr Q 70:107–122, 1999

McFarland BH, Lierman WK, Penner NR, et al: Employee benefits managers' opinions about addiction treatment. J Addict Dis 22(2):15–29, 2003

Normand J, Lempert RO, O'Brien CP (eds): Under the Influence? Drugs and the American Workforce. Washington, DC, National Academy Press, 1994

Roman PM: Secondary prevention of alcoholism: problems and prospects in occupational programming. J Drug Issues 5:327–343, 1975

Roman PM: From employee alcoholism to employee assistance: an analysis of the de-emphasis on prevention and on alcoholism problems in work-based programs. J Stud Alcohol 42:244–272, 1981

Roman PM: Growth and transformation in workplace alcoholism programming, in Recent Developments in Alcoholism, Vol 6. Edited by Galanter M. New York, Plenum, 1988, pp 131–158

Roman PM: The use of employee assistance programs to deal with drug abuse in the workplace, in Drugs in the Workplace: Research and Evaluation Data (NIDA Research Monograph 91). Edited by Guste S. Rockville, MD, National Institute on Drug Abuse, 1989, pp 245–270

Roman PM: Problem definitions and social movement strategies: the disease concept and the hidden alcoholic revisited, in Alcohol: The Development of Sociological Perspectives on Use and Abuse. Edited by Roman PM. New Brunswick, NJ, Center of Alcohol Studies, Rutgers University, 1991, pp 235–254

Roman PM: Missing work: the decline in infrastructure and support for workplace alcohol intervention in the United States, with implications for developments in other nations, in Changing Substance Abuse Through Health and Social Systems. Edited by Miller W, Weisner C. New York, Kluwer/Plenum, 2002, pp 197–210

Roman PM, Blum TC: Notes on the new epidemiology of alcoholism in the USA. J Drug Issues 11:321–332, 1987

Roman PM, Blum TC: Employee assistance and drug screening programs, in Treating Drug Problems, Vol 2. Edited by Gerstein DR. Washington, DC, National Academy of Sciences Press, 1992, pp 221–262

Roman PM, Blum TC: Effectiveness of workplace alcohol problem interventions. Am J Health Promot 11:112–128, 1996

Roman PM, Blum TC: Internalization and externalization as frames for understanding workplace deviance. Research in the Sociology of Work 8:139–164, 1999

Roman PM, Trice HM: The sick role, labeling theory and the deviant drinker. Int J Soc Psychiatry 12:245–251, 1968

Roman PM, Trice HM: Alcohol abuse in work organizations, in The Biology of Alcoholism, Vol 4: Social Aspects of Alcoholism. Edited by Kissin B, Begleiter H. New York, Plenum, 1976, pp 445–518

Roman PM, Blum TC, Martin JK: "Enabling" of male problem drinkers in work groups. Br J Addict 87:275–289, 1992

Rost K, Smith J, Fortney J: Large employers' selection criteria in purchasing behavioral health benefits. J Behav Health Serv Res 27:334–338, 2000

Rumbarger JJ: Power, Profits and Prohibition: Alcohol Reform and the Industrializing of America, 1800–1930. Albany, NY, State University of New York, 1989

Schneider J: Deviant drinking as disease: alcoholism as a social accomplishment. Soc Probl 25:361–372, 1978

Schneider RJ, Casey J, Kohn R: Motivational versus confrontational interviewing: a comparison of substance abuse assessment practices at employee assistance programs. J Behav Health Serv Res 27:60–74, 2000

Smith D, Mahoney J: McDonnell Douglas Corporation's EAP produces. The ALMACAN 19:18–26, 1989

Sonnenstuhl WJ: Working Sober. Ithaca, NY, ILR Press, 1996

Sonnenstuhl W, Trice HM: Strategies for Employee Assistance Programs: The Crucial Balance (Key Issues 30). Ithaca, NY, ILR Press, 1986

Staudenmeier WJ: Contrasting organizational responses to alcohol and illegal drug abuse among employees. J Drug Issues 19:451–472, 1989

Stolzfus JA, Benson PA: The 3M alcohol and other drug prevention program. J Prim Prev 15:147–159, 1994

Trice HM, Beyer J: Work-related outcomes of constructive confrontation strategies in a job-based alcoholism program. J Stud Alcohol 45:393–404, 1984

Trice HM, Roman PM: Spirits and Demons at Work: Alcohol and Other Drugs on the Job. Ithaca, NY, Publications Divisions of the New York State School of Industrial and Labor Relations at Cornell University, 1972

Trice HM, Schonbrunn M: A history of job-based alcoholism programs, 1900–1955. J Drug Issues 11:171–198, 1981

Trudeau JV, Deitz DK, Cook RF: Utilization and cost of behavioral health services: employee characteristics and workplace health promotion. J Behav Health Serv 29:61–74, 2002

Wrich J: The Employee Assistance Program. Center City, MN, Hazelden Foundation, 1973

Zarkin GA, Bray JW, Qi J: Effect of employee assistance programs use on healthcare utilization. Health Serv Res 35:77–100, 2000

Zhang Z, Huang L, Brittingham AM: Worker Drug Use and Workplace Policies and Programs: Results from the 1994 and 1997 NHSDA. Rockville, MD, Office of Applied Studies, Substance Abuse and Mental Health Services Administration, 1999

Community-Based Treatment

Jonathan I. Ritvo, M.D.
Gregory L. Kirk, M.D.

In this chapter we discuss community-based substance abuse treatment from two perspectives. The first perspective, the community's role in treatment, encompasses substance abuse identification and intervention ranging from noncoercive brief interventions in primary care settings to coercive interventions through social service agencies and criminal courts. The second perspective, specific non-hospital-based treatment services, encompasses outpatient treatment programs, outpatient detoxification, community residential facilities, and case management approaches.

Community Intervention

Brief Interventions in Primary Care Settings

Several studies have demonstrated that brief intervention by primary care providers reduces heavy drinking and its health consequences (Fleming and Manwell 1999). A typical brief intervention process consists of screening to identify at-risk alcohol use, expression of concern by the provider, advice on moderate drinking levels, brief application of motivational and cognitive-behavioral techniques, provision of informational materials, and three or four follow-up visits or phone calls (Fleming and Manwell 1999).

Fleming et al. (1997) and Manwell et al. (2000) studied 774 heavy drinkers screened in 10 primary care practices in southern Wisconsin. The brief intervention group received two 15-minute physician advice sessions and a telephone follow-up by a nurse. At 1-year follow-up, men in the brief intervention group showed significant ($P<0.001$) reductions in comparison with control subjects in number of drinks, episodes of binge drinking, and frequency of excessive drinking in the previous month (Fleming et al. 1997). Women of childbearing age showed significant intervention effects in number of drinks and episodes of binge drinking, with the most dramatic decreases in those who became pregnant during the follow-up year (Manwell et al. 2000).

The minimum threshold for heavy drinking as defined in studies demonstrating the effectiveness of brief intervention has ranged from 12 to 25 drinks per week for men and 9 to 16 drinks per week for women (Fleming and Manwell 1999). The studies typically exclude individuals who have been treated for alcoholism or meet criteria for abuse or dependence. The heavy drinkers targeted for brief intervention are at risk both for excess alcohol-related morbidity and for developing an alcohol use disorder. For the Wisconsin study, Fleming et al. (2000) calculated an average benefit of $1,151 versus an average cost of $205 for each individual receiving the intervention, resulting in a benefit–cost ratio of 5.6:1. These heavy drinkers represent a much larger population than drinkers who meet criteria for alcohol abuse or dependence, who would be candidates for more specialized intervention and treatment. Clearly, brief intervention research has profound implications for many health care fields, including public health, prenatal care, general medical practice, and the education of health professionals.

Brief Interventions in Colleges

The brief intervention approach is also appropriate for problem drinking among college students. A report from the Institute of Medicine (1990) recommended a harm-reduction approach designed to foster moderate and safe drinking practices through the use of personalized feedback "containing non-judgmental normative information." The report postulated that this approach would speed up the normal maturational process of increasing personal responsibility for drinking practices.

Marlatt et al. (1998) described programs at the University of Washington for accomplishing this goal with college students who drink heavily. These programs do not involve diagnosis of alcoholism, labeling of problem drinking, or prescribing of abstinence. They present risks, benefits, choices, normative data, and personalized feedback as well as strategies and standards for moderate and safe drinking. Outcome analysis showed that first-year students identified as heavy drinkers who received a brief motivational intervention of this type demonstrated greater reductions in their drinking rates and drinking problems than did control subjects. Both the intervention and the control groups, as well as their peers who did not drink heavily, showed reduction in drinking over the study period, consistent with the postulated maturational effect.

Social Service Agency Interventions

Child Protective Services

MacMahon (1997) reviewed the cases of 53 infants in San Mateo County, California, who were reported to child protective services because of urine screens positive for illicit substances in the newborn nursery. As a result of the hospital report, all mothers were court-ordered to participate in a drug rehabilitation program and to undergo urine monitoring. The 44% who complied with treatment had repeatedly drug-free urine tests. All mothers with repeatedly drug-free urine regained custody of their infants. Forty-six percent of infants were returned to their mothers within a week of birth, and 76% were living with a relative within the first month. Seventeen percent were eventually adopted, and another 17% entered long-term guardianships with relatives. Failure of family reunification was most strongly predicted by a history of unsuccessful drug treatment, previous involvement with child protective services, or previous removal of a child because of substance abuse and was highly correlated with noncompliance with current treatment and positive urine test results. For a few mothers, the threat of losing custody of their child in the final disposition hearing at 18 months was critical in motivating treatment. In this county with progressive services, the process of identifying maternal substance abuse in the newborn nursery, with intervention and follow-up by child protective services and the courts and referral to substance abuse treatment, appears to work as intended in the best interests of the child.

Nishimoto and Roberts (2001) studied treatment retention of postpartum women in two types of 6-month outpatient programs located in inner-city Los Angeles: a traditional coed outpatient program requiring 1.5 hours of participation each week and an intensive gender-specific program that required 5.5 hours of participation a day, 7 days a week. The intensive program offered family therapy, child care, transportation, and infant assessment and tracking. Eighty-three percent of subjects were referred by child protective services, 84% abused cocaine, and 49% had current custody of the newborn. The intensive program had superior treatment retention and completion figures. Custody of the newborn correlated with treatment retention in the intensive program but not in the traditional program.

Disability and Public Support

Recent legislative action has reflected societal concern regarding substance abuse by recipients of public support. Shaner et al. (1995) documented increased cocaine use, psychiatric symptoms, and hospitalization among cocaine-dependent individuals with schizophrenia around the first of the month, when they received their support payments. In contrast, Frisman and Rosenheck (1997) found no increased drug and alcohol use among homeless mentally ill veterans who received disability payments. Other reports have linked the receipt of large lump-sum retroactive disability payments with negative treatment events such as premature, abrupt termination of long-term residential substance abuse treatment (Satel et al. 1997) and missed visits and positive urine tests during methadone maintenance treatment (Herbst et al. 1996).

Herbst et al. (1996) also found that the use of a representative payee (an agency or individual appointed to receive and manage disability payments for the use and benefit of the disabled individual) protected against the negative effect on treatment of large lump-sum retroactive payments. Rosenheck et al. (1997) found that the use of representative payees had a positive effect on homelessness but not on substance abuse in homeless mentally ill individuals. Neither report presented data on the practices of the payees or whether the payees were agencies or individuals. Ries and Comtois (1997) described a successful community mental health center program that managed benefits for some of its chronically mentally ill, substance-abusing patients as part of their treatment. Case managers served as representative payees. The form and frequency of disbursement depended on the patient's functional stability, sobriety, and treatment participation. Compared with a control group of patients in the same program who were not on payee status, the payee-managed patients were more likely to be male and were more likely to have a diagnosis of schizophrenia, a history of high utilization of inpatient services, greater severity of psychiatric and substance abuse symptoms, and lower functional stability. However, during the time they were payee-managed, this group showed no difference from the control group in hospitalization, homelessness, or incarceration rates and attended outpatient services twice as frequently.

Until 1997, Social Security regulations required a representative payee whenever substance abuse contributed to a beneficiary's disability. The Contract With America Administration Act of 1996 disqualified beneficiaries for whom substance abuse contributed to disability. As an unintended consequence, this provision made it more difficult to appoint payees for beneficiaries with substance use disorders (Rosen and Rosenheck 1999). An additional obstacle is the Department of Veterans Affairs (VA) policy prohibiting its programs and clinicians from serving as representative payees (Satel 1995). Considering the role of money in access to substances and in relapses, greater coordination of policy and practice between entitlement and support programs and local treatment services regarding the representative payee mechanism could add considerable leverage to substance abuse treatment.

For the substance-abusing individual, disability benefits may be a mixed blessing. Before supporting an application for disability benefits, the clinician needs to consider potential negative aspects: disincentive to work, ineligibility for many rehabilitation programs, loss of the structuring of time and the rewards for sobriety provided by work, and availability of money for addictive substances. For the substance-abusing patient receiving disability payments, the clinician should weigh the benefits of including a representative-payee arrangement as part of the treatment plan.

Adult Protective Services

Adult protective services seldom use their guardianship capacity to address the problem of substance abuse among payees. In addition, judges are reluctant to appoint conservators for financial incompetence attributable solely to substance use (Satel 1995). For example, in Denver, even when the substance-abusing individual has dementia, understaffed and underfunded adult protective services may choose not to become involved unless the patient is elderly (J.I. Ritvo, personal observations, 1989–2002). The nonelderly alcoholic patient with dementia who needs ongoing custodial care but is long estranged from family and is unwelcome in nursing homes—and who is also unwanted by adult protective services, the public mental health system, and state hospitals—poses a difficult problem and is often left to receive care through emergency and acute hospital services.

Interventions Through the Criminal Justice System

The criminal justice system should be an ideal community setting for substance abuse identification and intervention. The National Center on Addiction and Substance Abuse at Columbia University (1998) estimated that 1.2 million prisoners (70% of America's prison population) are alcohol and drug abusers and addicts, as are another 2 million probationers (Tauber 1998). Among probationers, 64% report driving while under the influence of drugs and alcohol and 35% report a history of violence while drinking (Mumola and Bonczar 1998).

Drug Courts

Beginning in Miami, Florida, in 1989, drug treatment courts have demonstrated that coerced treatment can be effective and have provided a model for cooperation between the criminal justice system and addiction treatment services. By 2001 there were almost 700 drug courts in the United States, including adult, family, juvenile, and combination courts; it was estimated that these courts had enrolled 226,000 clients and that 67% of clients had graduated with considerable overall savings on correctional expenses (American University 2001). The drug-court model depends on the collaboration of judges, prosecutors, public defenders, and community treatment programs to apply the leverage of the criminal justice system to the treatment of the drug-abusing offender (Table 37–1).

Table 37–1. Standard features of the drug-court model

---

1. Judicial supervision of structured community-based treatment
2. Timely identification of defendants in need of treatment and referral to treatment as soon as possible after arrest
3. Regular status hearings before the judicial officer to monitor treatment progress and program compliance
4. Increased defendant accountability through a series of graduated sanctions and rewards
5. Mandatory periodic drug testing
6. Dismissal of charges or reduction of sentence on successful treatment completion
7. Provision of aftercare and support services following treatment to facilitate reentry into the community

---

Source. Adapted from Belenko 1998 and National Center on Addiction and Substance Abuse at Columbia University 1998.

The judge plays a key role by administering sanctions—which often consist of brief jail stays—for positive urine screens or missed treatment appointments. Two drug-court judges have called this "smart punishment" (Hora et al. 1999). Satel (1998) pointed out that these sanctions conform to basic principles of behavioral therapy by being "swift and sure but not necessarily severe." The drug court's use of sanctions can also be conceptualized as shoring up the offender's weakened ego with firm, consistent limits that better promote emotional growth and mature accountability than do traditional court sanctions, which more closely follow the model of the offender's rigid, harsh, and unpredictable primitive superego. Reviewing the emerging research literature on drug courts, Belenko (1998) concluded that these courts engaged and retained felony offenders in treatment, saved money for the criminal justice system, and were associated with reduced recidivism and drug use both during and after the drug-court program.

Most drug-court programs target the least serious felonies (typically crack or cocaine possession). An exception is the Drug Treatment Alternative to Prison program in Brooklyn, New York, which offers the option of deferred prosecution and admission to long-term (15–24 months) residential treatment to defendants arrested for felony drug sales who have prior nonviolent felony convictions and a drug abuse problem. Those who have completed the program have lower rearrest rates than do program noncompleters or control subjects (National Center on Addiction and Substance Abuse at Columbia University 1998). Recently, some courts have reported successful engagement of a broader spectrum of the offender population through the use of multitrack systems. In these courts, the more serious offenders begin with jail time and then enter the traditional drug-court model under the supervision of probation (Tauber 1998). Realizing the potential of probation and parole to offer surveillance, monitoring, and contingencies for treatment will require investment in substance abuse training for probation and parole officers and immediate access to comprehensive treatment services that can also address issues of poverty, employment, health, and drug-free housing (National Center on Addiction and Substance Abuse at Columbia University 1998).

Drunk Driving

Alcohol use patterns among drunk drivers range from social drinking to incipient problem drinking to alcohol dependence. In the late 1960s and early 1970s, the Alcohol Safety Action Programs of the National Highway Traffic Safety Administration expanded the interventions for drunk driving from jail and license actions to education and rehabilitation. Evaluation revealed that social drinkers might benefit from alcohol-safety schools, that education and rehabilitation programs had a small effect on recidivism (compared with no intervention) and had no effect on the frequency of subsequent accidents, and that license sanctions were superior to rehabilitation alone in reducing accidents and convictions (Hagen 1985).

In the 1970s and 1980s, many states adopted statutes called *administrative per se laws* or *administrative license revocation* that permit swift license suspension for drivers who fail sobriety tests. Retrospective studies have shown decreases in recidivism and subsequent accidents involving offenders after initiation of these laws (McArthur and Kraus 1999). For drunk drivers, education and rehabilitation serve as adjuncts to, but not replacements for, community intervention in the form of license sanctions. (Preventive community interventions in drunk driving are discussed in Chapter 49, "Prevention of Alcohol-Related Problems," in this volume.)

Non-Hospital-Based Treatment Services

The 1990s saw a major change in the substance abuse treatment paradigm. In the 1980s, the Minnesota Model of 28-day residential treatment followed by aftercare and participation in Alcoholics Anonymous was the treatment standard and was supported by generous insurance coverage of inpatient treatment. The pressure to provide less costly, less restrictive treatment increased interest in community-based treatment (as opposed to hospital-based treatment) and led to limiting inpatient and intensive residential (Minnesota Model) treatment to cases involving more severe complications or in which "life is in danger or other forms of treatment have failed" (Book et al. 1995). The standard of care now emerging involves individualized treatment determined through the matching of a patient's biopsychosocial needs to a continuum of levels of care and a spectrum of specific services (Gastfriend and McLellan 1997). In this section we discuss the portion of the continuum of care that is based in the com-

munity. (Other community-based treatment services are discussed in Chapter 34, "Alcoholics Anonymous and Other 12-Step Groups," and Chapter 38, "Therapeutic Communities," in this volume.)

Day Hospital and Intensive Outpatient Services

Day or partial hospital programs evolved from inpatient programs through the subtraction of the costly overnight residential component. In the 1980s, comparisons of day and inpatient programs for alcoholic patients who were physically and psychiatrically stable demonstrated equivalent outcomes and a 50% cost savings for day programs (Longabaugh et al. 1983; McLachlan and Stein 1982). With cocaine-dependent patients, day programs have had more difficulty with retention in early treatment and inpatient programs have had more difficulty with the transition to aftercare. The net result is equivalent outcomes at 6–7 months (Alterman et al. 1994; Schneider et al. 1996). Two factors, the intense cue reactivity associated with cocaine use and the lack of an aversive pharmacotherapy such as disulfiram, may explain why community-based settings are more problematic for the cocaine-dependent patient than for the alcohol-dependent patient.

McKay et al. (1994) described and evaluated a 4-week (27 hours/week) day hospital rehabilitation program at the Philadelphia VA Medical Center, with most of the features of Minnesota Model programs, for individuals who abused alcohol or cocaine. Continuity of care, with up to 5 months of twice-weekly aftercare, and an emphasis on participation in a 12-step group were important features of the program. Alterman et al. (1994) compared the outcomes of 56 cocaine-dependent patients in this day program with the outcomes of 55 patients undergoing 28-day inpatient treatment at another Pennsylvania VA hospital located 35 miles away in Coatesville. After 28 days of inpatient treatment at Coatesville, patients returned to the twice-weekly aftercare program of the Philadelphia VA day program. Although the inpatient program had better treatment retention than the day hospital in the first 28 days, the difference between the groups largely disappeared when the inpatients returned to Philadelphia for aftercare. At 7 months, there was no difference in outcome. Obviously, the goal of facilitating the transition to ongoing involvement in self-help groups is more practical for community-based programs than for residential programs at a distance from the patient's community.

The distinction between intensive outpatient and day or partial hospital programs is not always precise. McKay et al. (1997) used the term *intensive outpatient* to refer to the 27 hours/week Philadelphia VA day program (described in the previous paragraph as a day hospital). Guidelines published by the American Society of Addiction Medicine (2001) require 9 hours/week of structured programming for intensive outpatient programs and 20 hours/week for partial hospital programs, which are described as having more immediate access to medical and psychiatric services. McLellan et al. (1997) used a similar minimum criterion of 9 hours/week (three sessions a week) to define 10 intensive outpatient programs. They then compared these programs with 6 "traditional" outpatient programs that offered no more than two 2-hour sessions a week. All programs were non-hospital-based and were oriented toward abstinence. Patients in the intensive outpatient programs engaged in more severe substance use and had more social and health problems. They received more addiction-focused treatment but not more comprehensive services related to medical, employment, family, or social problems. At 6 months, patients in both kinds of programs showed notable improvement in substance use, personal health, and social functioning. These research findings should prompt referring clinicians to examine individual intensive outpatient programs before assuming that they are intensive in terms of providing comprehensive services. Day or partial hospital programs may better serve patients who have a substantial need for comprehensive services. Intensive outpatient programs, which often have evening schedules, may better serve patients for whom continued employment or attendance at school is indicated during treatment.

Community Residential Treatment Facilities

Community residential facilities (CRFs), often called halfway houses, typically receive patients, from inpatient treatment or detoxification services, who are not yet ready for independent living and who need the supervision and support of a living environment committed to sobriety. Moos et al. (1995) studied the 127 CRFs receiving the most VA referrals in 1991. Facilities generally had a 12-step orientation and averaged 30 residents and a 42-day length of stay. Greater lengths of stay were associated with lower rates of readmission to

inpatient facilities. Study patients were severely and chronically ill and were more ill than were patients in CRFs in 1987. Moos et al. (1999) reported that CRFs offering structured, coherent treatment approaches had better retention and substance abuse outcomes than CRFs with an undifferentiated approach. No differences in retention or outcome were found among three types of treatment approach (therapeutic community, psychosocial rehabilitation, or 12-step program). For one VA hospital, CRF placement improved involvement in aftercare for patients returning from out-of-town inpatient treatment (Hitchcock et al. 1995). In general, halfway houses or CRFs can address both the residential and treatment needs of many substance-abusing individuals with limited sober social supports or limited sober housing resources.

Detoxification Services

Detoxification Centers

The Uniform Alcoholism and Intoxication Treatment Act promulgated by the National Conference of Commissioners on Uniform State Laws in 1971 sought to replace the criminal justice solution to public drunkenness with medical alternatives. Persons incapacitated by alcohol were to be taken home or to health care or treatment facilities instead of being arrested and held in "drunk tanks." By 1980, more than half of the states had implemented major provisions of the act (Finn 1985). This legislation led to the development of detoxification centers as the medical alternative to the drunk tank.

Detoxification centers developed according to two major models, medical and nonmedical/social; the latter relies on rest, comfort, and support, with minimal use of medication or medical examination and supervision (Whitfield et al. 1978). The social model initially predominated because of its low cost and the refusal of some hospitals to provide detoxification services (Finn 1985). Over time, the distinctions between the two models became blurred. As benzodiazepine therapy became the standard treatment for alcohol withdrawal, some nonmedical detoxification centers were medicalized, adopting protocols whereby nurses could administer benzodiazepines. Although the Uniform Alcoholism and Intoxication Treatment Act encouraged voluntary, community-based treatment through a continuum of services, Finn (1985) concluded that it did little to rehabilitate the so-called skid row alcoholic and that it replaced one revolving door with another. The detoxification center is certainly more hospitable and humane than the drunk tank; however, decriminalization does nothing to address the conditions that perpetuate the problem, such as inadequate shelter, poverty, and vocational and social handicaps. In the 1990s the demography of patients treated in detoxification centers shifted away from older white male alcoholics in the direction of minorities, women, and heroin and cocaine addicts (McCarty et al. 2000).

Outpatient Detoxification

Mild to moderate alcohol withdrawal can be managed on an outpatient basis with safety and efficacy, although the dropout rate is higher than for inpatient detoxification (Hayashida et al. 1989). Wiseman and colleagues (1997) reported that providing housing and starting psychosocial treatment during detoxification resulted in improved retention. In their study, 5% of patients undergoing outpatient detoxification required transfer to inpatient facilities. Outpatient cost can be as little as 10% of inpatient cost (Hayashida et al. 1989).

Case Management

The goals of case management are to ensure continuity of care and to integrate other functions of the treatment system (Institute of Medicine 1990). Case management activities can include performing patient advocacy, shepherding patients through bureaucratic red tape, improvising to fill gaps in services, conducting outreach to engage and retain patients in treatment, providing basic services such as transportation, and developing an individualized supportive, therapeutic relationship. A wide variety of persons can perform case management functions: psychiatrists, primary care physicians, social workers, caseworkers, probation officers, college counselors, substance abuse counselors and other therapists, Alcoholics Anonymous sponsors, trained laypersons, or even the patient himself or herself (Institute of Medicine 1990). Community institutions that perform case management functions include employee assistance programs, physician health programs, and similar programs for dentists, nurses, and other health professionals (see Chapter 36, "Employee Assistance Programs and Other Workplace Interventions," and Chapter 46, "Impaired Physicians," in this volume). Programs for

health care professionals perform these functions by integrating community identification, patient advocacy, relations with licensing boards, assessment and referral for professional treatment, and ongoing monitoring.

Multiple factors help determine whether patients will require case management to achieve optimal therapeutic results. On the patient's side, these factors include motivation or resistance, experience, knowledge, intelligence, and other internal and external resources or deficits. On the system's side, relevant variables include the complexity of the system, the accessibility of the relevant components, and how well the components are integrated with one another and match the patient's needs. Perhaps the most important factor is the need for individualized, caring, long-term relationships that may not be met elsewhere in treatment. Given the variations in the types of case management and in the settings, populations, and systems in which they are applied, it is not surprising that the literature on the efficacy of case management for substance-abusing patients is inconsistent.

The most intensive case management approaches have been used in the treatment of substance abusers with severe and chronic mental illness (i.e., the dually diagnosed). The term *assertive community treatment* (ACT) describes outpatient programs that combine assertive outreach, medication management, integration of treatment, rehabilitation and support, a multidisciplinary team approach, low client-to-staff ratios (in the range of 12:1 or 8:1), extended or around-the-clock service hours, and a long-term commitment to clients (Drake et al. 1998). ACT and other intensive case management programs that also use stepwise motivational approaches to substance abuse and that integrate mental health and substance abuse counseling and services through the same staff have shown better treatment retention and better long-term outcomes than have short-term intensive dual-diagnosis programs or programs that provide mental health and substance abuse treatment and services separately (Drake et al. 1998).

Case management approaches less intensive than ACT have been effective in engaging and helping substance-abusing individuals who are not seeking treatment. Rhodes and Gross (1997) found that noncoerced case management offered to arrestees who were using illicit drugs other than marijuana decreased drug use and recidivism and increased use of substance abuse treatment. It is noteworthy that this study attributed its case management effect more to personalized, supportive relationships than to referral activity.

Other evaluations of case management for substance-abusing patients have shown mixed results, with some indication that case management services may be most valuable for indigent substance-abusing patients who need housing. A survey of a nationally representative sample of drug treatment programs found that case management services did correlate with utilization of housing assistance and financial services (Friedmann et al. 2000). However, in this survey, transportation and on-site location of ancillary services were more important than case management as correlates of ancillary service utilization. A positive outcome was found in a study of the "chronic public inebriates" who were the most frequent users of the King County (Seattle, Washington) Detoxification Center. In this study, intensive outreach-oriented case management improved financial and residential stability and reduced alcohol and detoxification center admissions in this "revolving door" population (Cox et al. 1998). However, for homeless substance-abusing persons seeking treatment, less intensive case management approaches that are more office-based, more time-limited, and more directed toward arranging rather than directly providing services have not demonstrated a differential effect on substance abuse outcome (Braucht et al. 1995; Stahler 1995; Stahler et al. 1995).

Conclusion

In this chapter, we reviewed substance abuse identification and intervention in a variety of community settings and examined both the community-based portion of the continuum of levels of care and the case management approaches that serve to integrate the complex treatment system for the individual patient. We described instances, such as in drug courts and child protective services, in which the relationship between community institutions and treatment services has been fruitful. We highlighted promising community interventions in primary care settings and colleges that we hope will be disseminated, and we identified community institutions, such as the criminal justice system and public support programs, in which much of the potential for community-based substance abuse treatment remains to be realized.

References

Alterman AI, O'Brien CP, McLellan AT: Effectiveness and costs of inpatient versus day hospital rehabilitation. J Nerv Ment Dis 182:157–163, 1994

American Society of Addiction Medicine: Patient Placement Criteria for the Treatment of Substance-Related Disorders, 2nd Edition, Revised. Chevy Chase, MD, American Society of Addiction Medicine, 2001

American University: OJP Drug Court Clearinghouse and Technical Assistance Project: Drug court activity update: summary information on all programs and detailed information on adult drug courts, June 25, 2001. Available at: http://www.american.edu/spa/justice/publications/allcourtactivity.pdf. Accessed October 1, 2002

Belenko S: Research on drug courts: a critical review. National Drug Court Institute Review 1:1–42, 1998

Book J, Harbin H, Marques C, et al: The ASAM and Green Spring alcohol and drug detoxification and rehabilitation criteria for utilization review. Am J Addict 4:187–192, 1995

Braucht GN, Reichardt CS, Geissler LJ, et al: Effective services for homeless substance abusers. J Addict Dis 14(4):87–109, 1995

Cox GB, Walker RD, Freng SA, et al: Outcome of a controlled trial of the effectiveness of intensive case management for chronic public inebriates. J Stud Alcohol 59:523–532, 1998

Drake RE, Mercer-McFadden C, Mueser KT, et al: Review of integrated mental health and substance abuse treatment for patients with dual disorders. Schizophr Bull 24:589–608, 1998

Finn P: Decriminalization of public drunkenness: response of the health care system. J Stud Alcohol 46:7–23, 1985

Fleming M, Manwell LB: Brief intervention in primary care settings. Alcohol Res Health 23:128-137, 1999. Available at: http://www.niaaa.nih.gov/publications/arh23-2/128-137.pdf. Accessed October 31, 2003

Fleming MF, Barry KL, Manwell LB, et al: Brief physician advice for problem alcohol drinkers: a randomized controlled trial in community-based primary care practices. JAMA 277:1039–1045, 1997

Fleming MF, Mundt MP, French MT, et al: Benefit-cost analysis of brief physician advice with problem drinkers in primary care settings. Med Care 38:7–18, 2000

Friedmann PD, D'Aunno TA, Jin L, et al: Medical and psychosocial services in drug abuse treatment: do stronger linkages promote client utilization? Health Serv Res 35:443–465, 2000

Frisman LK, Rosenheck R: The relationship of public support payments to substance abuse among homeless veterans with mental illness. Psychiatr Serv 48:792–795, 1997

Gastfriend DR, McLellan AT: Treatment matching: theoretical basis and practical implications. Med Clin North Am 81:945–966, 1997

Hagen RE: Evaluation of the effectiveness of educational and rehabilitation efforts: opportunities for research. J Stud Alcohol 46 (suppl 10):179–183, 1985

Hayashida M, Alterman A, McLellan AT, et al: Comparative effectiveness and cost of inpatient and outpatient detoxification of patients with mild to moderate alcohol withdrawal syndrome. N Engl J Med 320:358–365, 1989

Herbst MD, Batki SL, Manfredi LB, et al: Treatment outcomes for methadone clients receiving lump-sum payments at initiation of disability benefits. Psychiatr Serv 47:119–120, 142, 1996

Hitchcock HC, Stainback RD, Roque GM: Effects of halfway house placement on retention of patients in substance abuse aftercare. Am J Drug Alcohol Abuse 21:379–390, 1995

Hora PF, Schma WG, Rosenthal JTA: Therapeutic jurisprudence and the drug treatment court movement: revolutionizing the criminal justice system's response to drug abuse and crime in America. Notre Dame Law Rev 74:439–537, 1999

Institute of Medicine: Broadening the Base of Treatment for Alcohol Problems. Washington, DC, National Academy Press, 1990

Longabaugh R, McCrady B, Fink E, et al: Cost effectiveness of alcoholism treatment in partial vs inpatient settings: six-month outcomes. J Stud Alcohol 44:1049–1071, 1983

MacMahon JR: Perinatal substance abuse: the impact of reporting infants to child protective services. Pediatrics 100:E1, 1997. Available at: http://www.pediatrics.org/cgi/content/full/100/5/e1. Accessed October 1, 2002

Manwell LB, Fleming MF, Mundt MP, et al: Treatment of problem alcohol use in women of childbearing age: results of a brief intervention trial. Alcohol Clin Exp Res 24:1517–1524, 2000

Marlatt GA, Baer JS, Kivlahan DR, et al: Screening and brief intervention for high-risk college student drinkers: results from a 2-year follow-up assessment. J Consult Clin Psychol 66:604–615, 1998

McArthur DL, Kraus JF: The specific deterrence of administrative per se laws in reducing drunk driving recidivism. Am J Prev Med 16 (1 suppl):68–75, 1999

McCarty L, Caspi Y, Panas L, et al: Detoxification centers: who's in the revolving door? J Behav Health Serv Res 27:245–256, 2000

McKay JR, Alterman AI, McLellan AT, et al: Treatment goals, continuity of care and outcome in a day hospital substance abuse rehabilitation program. Am J Psychiatry 151:254–259, 1994

McKay JR, Cacciola JS, McLellan AT: An initial evaluation of the psychosocial dimensions of the American Society of Addiction Medicine criteria for inpatient versus intensive outpatient substance abuse rehabilitation. J Stud Alcohol 58:239–252, 1997

McLachlan JFC, Stein RL: Evaluation of a day clinic for alcoholics. J Stud Alcohol 43:261–272, 1982

McLellan AT, Hagan TA, Meyers K, et al: "Intensive" outpatient substance abuse treatment: comparison with "traditional" outpatient treatment. J Addict Dis 16(2):57–84, 1997

Moos RH, Pettit B, Gruber VA: Characteristics and outcomes of three models of community residential care for substance abuse patients. J Subst Abuse 7:99–116, 1995

Moos RH, Moos BS, Andrassy JM: Outcomes of four treatment approaches in community residential programs for patients with substance abuse disorders. Psychiatr Serv 50:1577–1583, 1999

Mumola CJ, Bonczar TP: Substance abuse and treatment of adults on probation, 1995. U.S. Department of Justice, Bureau of Justice Statistics, 1998. Available at: http://www.ojp.usdoj.gov/bjs/pub/ascii/satap95.txt.

National Center on Addiction and Substance Abuse at Columbia University: Behind Bars: Substance Abuse and America's Prison Population. New York, National Center on Addiction and Substance Abuse at Columbia University, 1998

Nishimoto RH, Roberts AC: Coercion and drug treatment for postpartum women. Am J Drug Alcohol Abuse 27:161–181, 2001

Rhodes W, Gross M: Case management reduces drug use and criminality among drug-involved arrestees: an experimental study of an HIV prevention intervention (National Institute of Justice Research Report). Washington, DC, U.S. Department of Justice, Office of Justice Programs, 1997. Available at: http://www.ncjrs.org/txtfiles/155281.txt. Accessed October 1, 2002

Ries RK, Comtois KA: Managing disability benefits as part of treatment for persons with severe mental illness and comorbid drug/alcohol disorders: a comparative study of payee and non-payee participants. Am J Addict 6:330–338, 1997

Rosen MI, Rosenheck R: Substance use and assignment of representative payees. Psychiatr Serv 50:95–98, 1999

Rosenheck R, Lam J, Randolph F: Impact of representative payees on substance use by homeless persons with serious mental illness. Psychiatr Serv 48:800–806, 1997

Satel SL: When disability benefits make patients sicker. N Engl J Med 333:794–796, 1995

Satel SL: Observational study of courtroom dynamics in selected drug courts. National Drug Court Institute Review 1:43–72, 1998

Satel S, Reuter P, Hartley D, et al: Influence of retroactive disability payments on recipients' compliance with substance abuse treatment. Psychiatr Serv 48:796–799, 1997

Schneider R, Mittelmeier C, Gadish D: Day versus inpatient treatment for cocaine dependence: an experimental comparison. J Ment Health Adm 23:234–245, 1996

Shaner A, Eckman TA, Roberts LJ, et al: Disability income, cocaine use and repeated hospitalization among schizophrenic cocaine abusers. N Engl J Med 333:777–783, 1995

Stahler GJ: Social interventions for homeless substance abusers: evaluating treatment outcomes (editorial). J Addict Dis 14(4):xv–xxvi, 1995

Stahler GJ, Shipley TF Jr, Bartelt D, et al: Evaluating alternative treatments for homeless substance-abusing men: outcomes and predictors of success. J Addict Dis 14(4):151–167, 1995

Tauber J: The future of drug courts: comprehensive drug court systems. National Drug Court Institute Review 1:86–97, 1998

Whitfield CL, Thompson G, Lamb A, et al: Detoxification of 1,024 alcoholic patients without psychoactive drugs. JAMA 239:1409–1410, 1978

Wiseman EJ, Henderson KL, Briggs MJ: Outcomes of patients in a VA ambulatory detoxification program. Psychiatr Serv 48:200–203, 1997

Therapeutic Communities

George De Leon, Ph.D.

Drug-free residential programs for substance abuse appeared a decade later than did therapeutic communities (TCs) in psychiatric hospitals pioneered by Jones (1953) and others in the United Kingdom. The term *therapeutic community* evolved in these hospital settings, although the two models arose independently. The TC for substance abuse emerged in the 1960s as a self-help alternative to existing conventional treatments. Recovering alcoholic and drug-addicted individuals were its first participant-developers. Although its modern antecedents can be traced to Alcoholics Anonymous and Synanon, the TC prototype is ancient, existing in all forms of communal healing and support.

Contemporary TCs for addictions are sophisticated human services institutions. Today, the term *therapeutic community* is generic, describing a variety of short-term and long-term residential programs, as well as day treatment and ambulatory programs that serve a wide spectrum of drug-abusing and alcohol-abusing patients. Although the TC model has been widely adapted, it is the traditional long-term residential prototype that has documented effectiveness in rehabilitating substance-abusing individuals.

The Traditional TC

Traditional TCs are similar to each other in planned duration of stay (15–24 months), structure, staffing pattern, perspective, and rehabilitative regimen, although they differ in size (30 to several hundred beds in a facility) and patient demography. Staffs are composed of TC-trained clinicians, with and without recovery experiences, and other human service professionals who provide medical, mental health, vocational,

---

This chapter is abstracted from a comprehensive account of the therapeutic community theory, model, and method provided elsewhere (De Leon 2000). Descriptive accounts of the therapeutic community for substance-abusing patients, which are less formal than the description presented here, are contained in the literature (e.g., Casriel 1966; Deitch 1972; Yablonsky 1965), as are formal accounts of the therapeutic community from sociological (Sugarman 1986), anthropological (Frankel 1989), and psychodynamic (Kooyman 1993) perspectives.

educational, family counseling, fiscal, administrative, and legal services.

TCs accommodate a diversity of drug-abusing patients. Although TCs originally attracted individuals addicted to narcotics, most of the current TC patient populations are non-opioid-abusing persons with different lifestyles; various social, economic, and ethnic or cultural backgrounds; and drug problems of varying severity.

In TCs, drug abuse is viewed as a deviant behavior, reflecting impeded personality development or chronic deficits in social, educational, and economic skills. Such behavior is a result of socioeconomic disadvantage, poor family effectiveness, and psychological factors. Therefore, the principal aim of the TC is a global change in lifestyle, involving abstinence from illicit substances, elimination of antisocial activity, development of employability, and development of prosocial attitudes and values. The rehabilitative approach requires multidimensional influence and training, which for most can occur only in a 24-hour residential setting.

The traditional TC can be distinguished from other major drug treatment modalities in three general ways. First, the TC coordinates a comprehensive range of interventions and services in a single treatment setting. Vocational counseling; work therapy; recreation, group, and individual therapy; and educational, medical, family, legal, and social services are all offered within the TC. Second, the primary "therapist" and teacher in the TC is the community itself, consisting of peers and staff members who serve as role models of successful personal change. Staff members also serve as rational authorities and guides in the recovery process. Thus, the community as a whole provides a crucial 24-hour context for continued learning in which individual changes in conduct, attitudes, and emotions are monitored and mutually reinforced in the daily regimen. Third, the TC approach to rehabilitation is based on an explicit perspective of the substance use disorder, the patient, the recovery process, and healthy living. It is this perspective that shapes its organizational structure, staffing, and treatment process.

The TC Perspective

The TC perspective consists of four interrelated views, each of which is briefly outlined here.

View of the Disorder

Drug abuse is viewed as a disorder of the whole person, affecting some or all areas of functioning. Cognitive and behavioral problems are evident, as are mood disturbances. Thinking may be unrealistic or disorganized; values are confused, nonexistent, or antisocial. Frequently there are deficits in verbal, reading, writing, and marketable skills. Moral or even spiritual issues, whether expressed in existential or psychological terms, are apparent.

The problem is the individual, not the drug. Addiction is a symptom, not the essence of the disorder. In the TC, chemical detoxification is a condition of entry, not a goal of treatment. The focus of rehabilitation is on maintaining a drug-free existence.

View of the Person

In TCs, individuals are distinguished along dimensions of psychological dysfunction and social deficits rather than according to drug use patterns. In many TC residents, vocational and educational problems are marked; middle-class, mainstream values are either missing or not sought. Usually these residents emerge from a socially disadvantaged sector, where drug abuse is more a social response than a psychological disturbance. Their TC experience is better termed *habilitation*, development of a socially productive, conventional lifestyle for the first time.

Among patients from more advantaged backgrounds, drug abuse is more directly expressive of psychological disorder or existential malaise. For these, the word *rehabilitation* is more suitable, because the term emphasizes a return to a lifestyle previously lived, known, and perhaps rejected.

Notwithstanding these social differences, substance-abusing individuals in TCs have important similarities. Either as a cause or as a consequence of their drug abuse, all such persons exhibit features of personality disturbance and impeded social function (see "Clinical Characteristics" section below). Therefore, all residents in the TC follow the same regimen. Individual differences are recognized in specific treatment plans that modify the emphasis, not the course, of their experience in the TC.

View of Recovery

In the view of recovery employed in the TC, the aim of rehabilitation is global, involving both a change in lifestyle and a change in personal identity. The primary psychological goal is to change the negative patterns of behavior, thinking, and feeling that predispose the individual to drug use; the main social goal is to develop the skills, attitudes, and values of a responsible drug-free lifestyle. Stable recovery, however, depends on a successful integration of these social and psychological goals. Behavioral change is unstable without insight, and insight is insufficient without felt experience. Therefore, to ensure enduring change, conduct, emotions, skills, attitudes, and values must all be addressed.

Motivation

Recovery depends on pressures to change, positive and negative. Some patients seek help, driven by stressful external pressures; others are moved by more intrinsic factors. For all, however, remaining in treatment requires continued motivation to change. Therefore, elements of the rehabilitation approach are designed to sustain motivation or to enable detection of early signs of premature termination.

Self-Help and Mutual Self-Help

Strictly speaking, treatment is not provided; rather, it is made available to the individual in the TC through its staff and peers and the daily regimen of work, groups, meetings, seminars, and recreation. However, the effectiveness of these elements depends on the individual, who must constantly and fully engage in the treatment regimen. In self-help recovery, the individual makes the main contribution to the change process. In mutual self-help, the principal messages of recovery, personal growth, and "right living" are mediated by peers through confrontation and sharing in groups, by example as role models, and as supportive, encouraging friends in daily interactions.

Social Learning

A lifestyle change occurs in a social context. Negative patterns, attitudes, and roles were not acquired in isolation, nor can they be altered in isolation. Thus, recovery depends not only on what has been learned but also on how and where learning occurs. This assumption is the basis for the community's serving collectively as teacher. Learning is active, involving doing and participating. A socially responsible role is acquired by acting the role. What is learned is identified with the individuals involved in the learning process—

supportive peers and staff members serving as credible role models.

Sustained recovery requires a perspective on self, society, and life that must be continually affirmed by a positive social network of others within and beyond the TC.

Treatment as an Episode

Residence in the TC is a relatively brief period in an individual's life, and the influence of this period must compete with the influences of the years before and after treatment. For this reason, unhealthy outside influences are minimized until the individual is better prepared to deal with them on his or her own. As a result, life in the TC is necessarily intense, the daily regimen is demanding, and the therapeutic confrontations are unmoderated.

View of Right Living

TCs adhere to certain precepts that constitute a view of healthy personal and social living. These precepts concern moral behavior, values, and a social perspective that are intimately related to the TC view of the individual and of recovery. For example, in TCs, unambiguous moral positions are held regarding social and sexual conduct. Explicit right and wrong behaviors are identified for which there are appropriate rewards and sanctions. These include antisocial behaviors and attitudes; the negative values of the street, jails, or negative peers; and irresponsible or exploitative sexual conduct.

Guilts relating to self, significant others, and the larger community outside the TC are central issues in the recovery process. Although they are associated with moral matters, guilts are special psychological experiences that if not addressed maintain the individual's disaffiliation from peers and block the self-acceptance that is necessary for authentic personal change.

Certain values are emphasized as being essential to social learning and personal growth. These values include truth and honesty (in word and deed), a work ethic, self-reliance, earned rewards and achievement, personal accountability, responsible concern (being one's brother's or sister's keeper), social manners, and community involvement.

Treatment helps the individual to focus on the personal present (here and now) versus the historical past (then and when). Past behavior and circumstances are explored only to illustrate the current patterns of dysfunctional behavior, negative attitudes, and outlook. Residents are encouraged and trained to assume personal responsibility for their present reality and destiny.

Who Comes for Treatment

Most patients who enter TCs have histories of multiple drug use, including use of marijuana, opioids, alcohol, and prescription medications (although in recent years most residents report cocaine or crack as their primary drug of abuse). However, research has documented that persons admitted to TCs have a considerable degree of psychosocial dysfunction in addition to their substance abuse.

Social Profiles

Patients in traditional programs are usually men (70%–75%), but the number of admissions of women is increasing. Most community-based TCs are integrated across gender, race or ethnicity, and age, although the demographic proportions differ according to geographic regions and specific programs. In general, Hispanics, Native Americans, and patients younger than 21 years represent smaller proportions of admissions to TCs.

Most patients admitted are from broken homes or have ineffective families, have poor work histories, and have engaged in criminal activities. Among adults who are admitted to TCs, fewer than one-third have been employed full-time in the year before treatment, more than two-thirds have been arrested, and 30%–40% have drug treatment histories (e.g., De Leon 1984; Hubbard et al. 1997; Simpson and Sells 1982).

Psychological Profiles

Patients differ in demographics, socioeconomic background, and drug use patterns, but psychological profiles obtained with the use of standard instruments appear uniform, as has been shown in a number of TC studies (e.g., Biase et al. 1986; Brook and Whitehead 1980; De Leon 1984; De Leon et al. 1973; Holland 1986; Kennard and Wilson 1979; Zuckerman et al. 1975).

Typically, symptom measures on depression and anxiety are deviantly high, socialization scores are poor, and IQ is in the dull-to-normal range. Self-esteem is markedly low and Minnesota Multiphasic Personality Inventory scores are deviant, reflecting confusion (high F), character disorder (high Pd), and disturbed thinking and affect (high Sc). Smaller but still deviant peaks are seen on depression (D) and hypomania (Ma).

The psychological profiles mirror features of both psychiatric and criminal populations. For example, the character disorder elements and poor self-concept of delinquent and repeat offenders are present, as are the elements of dysphoria and confused thinking seen in emotionally unstable or psychiatric populations. Therefore, in addition to their substance abuse, patients in TCs have considerable degrees of psychological disability.

Clinical Characteristics

Regardless of drug preference or severity, most individuals admitted to TCs have shared clinical features that are directly addressed in the TC treatment. These characteristics center around immaturity or antisocial dimensions. For example, they include low tolerance for all forms of discomfort and delay of gratification; problems with authority; inability to manage feelings (particularly hostility, guilt, and anxiety); poor impulse control (particularly sexual or aggressive impulse control); poor judgment and reality testing concerning consequences of actions; unrealistic self-appraisal regarding discrepancies between personal resources and aspirations; prominence of lying, manipulation, and deception as coping behaviors; and personal and social irresponsibility (e.g., inconsistency or failures in meeting obligations). In addition, many TC residents have marked deficits in learning and in marketable and communication skills.

These clinical characteristics are not necessarily indicative of an addictive personality, although many of these features are typical of conduct disorder in younger substance-abusing individuals, which later evolves into adult character disorder. Nevertheless, whether they are antecedent or consequent to serious involvement with drugs, these characteristics are commonly observed to be correlated with chemical dependency. More important, in TCs, a positive change in these characteristics is considered to be essential for stable recovery.

Psychiatric Diagnoses

In diagnostic studies in which the Diagnostic Interview Schedule was used, nearly three-fourths of patients admitted to TCs had a lifetime (i.e., beginning before the last 30 days) non-drug-related psychiatric disorder in addition to substance-related problems. One-third had a current (beginning within the last 30 days) mental disorder in addition to substance-related problems. The most frequent non-drug-related diagnoses were phobias, generalized anxiety, psychosexual dysfunction, and antisocial personality. There were few cases of schizophrenia, but lifetime affective disorders occurred in more than one-third of those studied (De Leon 1993; Jainchill 1994).

That the psychological and psychiatric profiles reveal few psychotic features and relatively low variability in symptoms or personality characteristics reflects several factors: the TC exclusionary criteria, the common characteristics among all substance-abusing individuals, and to some degree the self-selection among those who seek admission to residential treatment programs. Nevertheless, patients do differ, as attested by the differences in patient dropout and success rates (discussed below).

Contact and Referral

Voluntary contacts with TCs occur through self-referral, social agencies, treatment providers, and active recruitment by TCs. Outreach teams (usually trained graduates of TCs and selected human services staff members) recruit in hospitals, jails, courtrooms, and social agencies and on the street, conducting brief orientations or face-to-face interviews to determine receptivity to the TC. Among adolescents, 40%–50% have been legally referred for treatment, compared with 25%–30% of adults; in some programs, considerably higher percentages of patients have been legally referred (e.g., Pompi and Resnick 1987).

Although most admissions to TCs are voluntary, many of these patients come to treatment programs under various forms of perceived pressures originating from conflicts with family members or significant others, employment difficulties, or anticipated legal consequences (De Leon 1988).

Detoxification Status

With few exceptions, admission to residential treatment does not require medically supervised detoxification. Therefore, traditional TCs do not usually provide this service on the premises. Most individuals whose primary drugs of abuse are opioids, cocaine, alcohol, barbiturates, or amphetamines have undergone self-administered or medical detoxification before seeking admission to the TC. A small proportion require detoxification during the admission evaluation, and these persons are offered the option of detoxification at a nearby hospital. Individuals who use barbiturates are routinely referred for medically supervised detoxification, after which they are assessed for admission. A minor percentage of patients admitted to TCs have been primarily involved with hallucinogens or phencyclidine (PCP). In the case of those who appear compromised, a referral is made for psychiatric service, after which the individuals can return for residential treatment.

Criteria for Residential Treatment

Traditional TCs maintain an open-door policy with respect to admission for residential treatment. This understandably results in a wide range of treatment candidates, not all of whom are equally ready for, suited for, or motivated to face the demands of the residential regimen. Relatively few are excluded, because the TC policy is to accept individuals who elect residential treatment, regardless of the reasons influencing their choice.

One factor that is useful to consider during the process of deciding whether to admit a patient to a TC is community risk. *Risk* refers to the extent to which patients present a management burden to the staff or pose a threat to the security and health of the community. Specific exclusionary criteria most often include histories of arson, suicide attempts, and serious psychiatric disorder. Psychiatric exclusion is usually based on documented history of psychiatric hospitalizations or evidence of psychotic symptoms on interview (e.g., frank delusions, thought disorder, hallucinations, confused orientation, signs of serious affect disorder). An important differential diagnostic issue concerns drug-related mood or mental states. For example, disorientation, dysphoria, and thought or sensory disorders clearly associated with use of hallucinogens, PCP, and sometimes cocaine may not exclude an otherwise suitable individual from the TC. When diagnosis remains in question, most TCs will use a psychiatric consultation after admission. Referral, however, is based on the patient's suitability or risk rather than on diagnosis alone.

Generally, patients on regular regimens of psychotropic medication are excluded because these regimens are usually correlated with chronic or severe psychiatric disorders. Patients taking medication for medical conditions can be admitted, as can disabled individuals or persons who require prosthetics, providing these patients can participate fully in the program. Physical examinations and laboratory workups (blood and urine profiles) are performed after admission. Because of concern about communicable disease in a residential setting, some TCs require tests for conditions such as hepatitis to be performed before patients enter the facility or at least within the first weeks of admission.

Policies and practices concerning testing for human immunodeficiency virus (HIV) and management of acquired immune deficiency syndrome (AIDS) and hepatitis C emphasize voluntary testing with counseling, special education seminars on health management and sexual practices, and special support groups for residents who are HIV positive or who have a clinical diagnosis of AIDS or hepatitis C (e.g., Barton 1994; De Leon 1996b; McCusker and Sorensen 1994).

Suitability for the TC

A number of those seeking admission to a TC may not be ready for treatment in general or may not be suited for the demands of a long-term residential regimen. Assessment of these factors at admission provides a basis for treatment planning in the TC or sometimes appropriate referral. Some indicators of motivation, readiness, and suitability for TC treatment are acceptance of the severity of the drug problem; acceptance of the need for treatment (the patient thinks he or she "can't do it alone"); willingness to sever ties with family and friends and halt current lifestyle while in treatment; and willingness to surrender a private life and meet the expectations of a structured community. Although motivation, readiness, and suitability are not criteria for admission to the TC, the importance of these factors often emerges after entry to treatment, and these factors, if not identified and addressed, are related to early dropout (De Leon et al. 1994).

The TC Approach

The TC approach can be summarized in the phrase "community as method" (De Leon 1997). The TC uses the diverse elements and activities of community to foster rehabilitative change. These can be organized in terms of the TC structure or social organization and the TC process in terms of the individual's passage through stages of change within the context of community life.

TC Structure

The relatively small staff of the TC is complemented by resident peers at junior, intermediate, and senior levels. These groups constitute the community or family in the residence. This peer-to-community structure strengthens the individual's identification with a perceived ordered network of others. More important, it arranges relationships of mutual responsibility to others at various levels in the program.

The daily operation of the community itself is the task of the residents, who work together under staff supervision. The broad range of resident job assignments illustrates the extent of the self-help process. Residents perform all house services (e.g., cooking, cleaning, kitchen service, minor repair); serve as apprentices; run all departments; and conduct house meetings, certain seminars, and peer encounter groups.

The TC is managed by the staff, whose members monitor and evaluate patient status, supervise resident groups, assign and supervise resident jobs, and oversee house operations. The staff conduct therapeutic groups (other than peer encounter groups), provide individual counseling, organize social and recreational projects, and confer with significant others. They make decisions about resident status, discipline, promotion, transfers, discharges, furloughs, and treatment planning.

The new patient enters a setting of upward mobility. The resident job assignments are arranged in a hierarchy, according to seniority, clinical progress, and productivity. Residents are first assigned the most menial tasks (e.g., mopping the floor) and then work their way up to levels of coordination and management. In fact, individuals come in as patients and can leave as staff members. This social organization of the TC reflects the fundamental aspects of its rehabilitative approach: work as education and therapy, mutual self-help, peers as role models, and staff members as rational authorities.

Work as Education and Therapy

Work and job changes have clinical relevance for substance-abusing patients in TCs, most of whom have not successfully negotiated the social and occupational world of the larger society. Vertical job movements carry the obvious rewards of status and privilege. However, lateral job changes are more frequent and permit exposure to all aspects of the community.

Job changes in the TC are singularly effective therapeutic tools, providing both measures of and incentives for behavioral and attitudinal changes. In the vertical structure of the TC, ascendancy marks how well the patient has assimilated what the community teaches and expects; hence, job promotion is an explicit measure of the resident's improvement and growth. Lateral or downward job movements also create situations that require demonstrations of personal growth. These movements are designed to teach new ways of coping with reversals and change that appear to be unfair or arbitrary.

Mutual Self-Help

The essential dynamic in the TC is mutual self-help. In their jobs, groups, meetings, recreation, and personal and social time, residents continually transmit to one another the main messages and expectations of the community.

Peers as Role Models

Peers, serving as role models, and staff members, serving as role models and rational authorities, are the primary mediators of the recovery process. TC members who demonstrate the expected behaviors and reflect the values and teachings of the community are viewed as role models. Thus, all members of the community—roommates, older and younger residents, and junior, senior, and directorial staff—are expected to be role models. TCs require these multiple role models in order to maintain the integrity of the community and ensure the spread of social learning effects. Two main examples of how role models function in the community are given below:

1. *Resident role models "act as if."*   The resident behaves as the person that he or she should be, rather than as the person that he or she has been. Despite resistances, perceptions, or feelings to the contrary, residents engage in the expected behaviors and consistently maintain the attitudes and values of the community. These include self-motivation, commitment to work and striving, positive regard for staff as authority, and an optimistic outlook toward the future. In the TC's view, acting as if is not merely an

exercise in conformity; it is an essential mechanism for more complete psychological change. Feelings, insights, and altered self-perceptions often follow rather than precede behavioral change.

2. *Role models display responsible concern.*   This concept is closely akin to the notion of being one's brother's or sister's keeper. Showing responsible concern involves willingness to confront others whose behavior is not in keeping with the rules of the TC, the spirit of the community, or the community expectations of growth and rehabilitation. Role models are obligated to be aware of the appearance, attitude, moods, and performance of their peers and to confront negative signs in these areas. In particular, role models are aware of their own behavior in the overall community and the process prescribed for personal growth.

Staff Members as Rational Authorities

Staff members foster the self-help learning process through performance of the managerial and clinical functions described above and through maintenance of psychological relationships with the residents as role models, parental surrogates, and rational authorities. TC residents often had difficulties with authorities who have not been trusted or who have been perceived as guides and teachers. Therefore, residents need a positive experience with an authority figure that is viewed as credible (recovered), supportive, corrective, and protective so that they may gain authority over themselves (personal autonomy). As rational authorities, staff members provide the *reasons* for their decisions and explain the *meaning* of consequences. They exercise their powers to teach, guide, facilitate, and correct rather than to punish, control, or exploit.

The TC Process: Basic Program Elements

The recovery process may be defined as the interaction between treatment interventions and patient change. Unlike other treatment approaches, however, the TC treatment intervention is the daily regimen of structured and unstructured activities and social intercourse occurring in formal and informal settings.

The typical day in a TC is highly structured. It begins at 7:00 A.M. and ends at 11:00 P.M. During this time, residents participate in a variety of meetings, encounter and other therapeutic groups, and recreational activities; perform job functions (work therapy); and receive individual counseling. The interplay of these activities is part of the TC process. As interventions these activities may be divided into three main groups: therapeutic-educative activities, community enhancement activities, and community and clinical management.

Therapeutic-Educative Activities

Therapeutic-educative activities consist of various group processes and individual counseling. These activities provide residents with opportunities to express feelings, divert negative acting-out, and resolve personal and social issues. They increase communication and interpersonal skills, bring about examination and confrontation of behavior and attitudes, and offer instruction in alternative modes of behavior.

The four main forms of group activity in the TC are encounters, probes, marathons, and tutorials. These differ somewhat in format, objectives, and method, but all have the goal of fostering trust, personal disclosure, intimacy, and peer solidarity to facilitate therapeutic change. The focus of the encounter is behavioral. Its approach is supportive confrontation, and its objective is to modify negative behavior and attitudes directly. Probes and marathons have as their primary objective substantial emotional change and psychological insight. In tutorials, the learning of concepts and specific skills is emphasized.

Encounters are the cornerstone of group process in the TC. The term *encounter* is generic, describing a variety of forms that use supportive confrontational procedures as their main approach. The basic encounter group is a peer-led group composed of 12–20 residents in the community; it meets at least three times weekly, usually for 2 hours in the evening, and an additional 30-minute period follows for snacking and socializing. The basic objective of each encounter is to heighten individual awareness of specific attitudes or behavioral patterns that should be modified. The weekly or biweekly "static" group, a variant of the encounter, is composed of the same peer members to address continuing issues and sustain relationships as residents move through the stages of the program.

Probes are staff-led group sessions, involving 10–15 residents, that are conducted to obtain in-depth clinical information on patients early in their residence (in the first 2–6 months). They are scheduled when needed and usually last from 4 to 8 hours. Their main objectives are to increase staff understanding of individuals' backgrounds for the purposes of treatment planning and to increase openness, trust, and mutual identification. Unlike the encounter, in which confrontation is emphasized, the probe involves the use of support, understanding, and the empathy of the other group members. Probes go beyond the here-and-now behavioral incident, which is the material of the encounter, to past events and experiences.

Marathons are extended group sessions whose objective is to initiate resolution of life experiences that have impeded individuals' development. During his or her 18 months of residence, every patient participates in several marathons. All staff members conduct these sessions and are assisted by senior residents with marathon experience. Marathons usually include large groups of selected residents and last for 18–36 hours. Considerable experience, both personal and professional, is required to ensure safe and effective marathons.

The intimacy, safety, and bonding in the marathon setting facilitate emotional processing ("working through") of a significant life event and encourage the individual to continue to deal with certain life-altering issues of the past. These issues are identified in counseling, probes, or other group sessions and may include violence, sexual abuse, abandonment, illness, and deaths of significant others. A wide variety of techniques—including psychodrama, primal therapy, and pure theater—are employed to produce impact.

Tutorials are primarily directed toward training or teaching. Tutorial groups, usually staff led, consist of 10–20 residents. Tutorials are scheduled as needed and focus on certain themes, including personal growth, recovery, and right-living concepts (e.g., self-reliance, maturity, relationships); job skills training (e.g., training in management of the department or the reception desk); and clinical skills training (e.g., training in the use of encounter tools).

Other groups that convene as needed supplement the four main groups. These vary in focus, format, and composition. For example, gender, ethnic, or age-specific theme groups may use encounter or tutorial formats. Dormitory, room, or departmental encounters may address issues of daily community living. In addition, sensitivity training, psychodrama, and conventional gestalt and emotionality groups are used to varying extents.

One-to-one counseling balances the needs of the individual with those of the community. Peer exchange is ongoing and is the most consistent form of informal counseling in TCs. Staff counseling sessions may be formal or informal and are usually conducted as needed. The staff counseling method in the TC is not conventional, as is evident in its main features: transpersonal sharing, direct support, minimal interpretation, didactic instructions, and concerned confrontation.

Community Enhancement Activities

Community enhancement activities, which facilitate assimilation into the community, include the four main facility-wide meetings: the morning meeting, the seminar, the house meeting (these three meetings are held each day), and the general meeting (which is called when needed).

All residents of the facility and the staff on the premises attend the morning meeting, which takes place after breakfast and usually lasts 30 minutes. The purpose of the meeting is to instill a positive attitude at the beginning of the day, motivate residents, and strengthen unity. This meeting is particularly relevant because most residents of TCs have never adapted to the routine of an ordinary day.

Seminars take place every afternoon and usually last 1 hour. Because it brings all residents together, the seminar in the afternoon complements the daily morning meeting and the house meeting in the evening. A clinical aim of the seminar is to balance the individual's emotional and cognitive experience. Residents lead most seminars, although some are led by staff members or outside speakers. The seminar is unique among the various meetings and group processes in the TC in its emphasis on listening, speaking, and conceptual behavior.

House meetings take place nightly after dinner, usually last 1 hour, and are coordinated by a senior resident. The main aim of these meetings is to transact community business, although they also have a clinical objective. In this forum, social pressure through public acknowledgment of positive or negative behaviors is judiciously applied to facilitate individual change.

General meetings take place only when needed and are usually called so that negative behavior, attitudes, or incidents in the facility can be addressed. All residents and staff members (including those not on duty) are assembled at any time and for an indefinite duration. These meetings, conducted by multiple staff members, are designed to identify problem individuals or conditions or to reaffirm motivation and reinforce positive behavior and attitudes in the community.

Community enhancement occurs in a variety of nonscheduled informal activities as well. These include activities related to rituals and traditions, celebrations (e.g., celebrations of birthdays, graduations, phase changes), ceremonies (e.g., those relating to general and cultural holidays), and memorial observances for deceased residents, family members of residents, and staff members. These activities reflect humanistic reactions of the membership and increase cohesiveness of the community.

Community and Clinical Management Elements

Community and clinical management elements maintain the physical and psychological safety of the environment and ensure that resident life is orderly and productive. They protect the community as a whole and strengthen it as a context for social learning. The main elements are privileges, disciplinary sanctions, surveillance, and urine testing.

Privileges. In the TC, privileges are explicit rewards that reinforce the value of achievement. Privileges are accorded with overall clinical progress in the program. Displays of inappropriate behavior or negative attitude can result in loss of privileges, which can be regained through demonstrated improvement.

Staff members deliver all privileges, which may range from telephone use and letter writing early in treatment to overnight furloughs later in treatment. Successful movement through each stage earns privileges that grant wider personal latitude and increased self-responsibility.

Privileges acquire importance because they are earned through investment of time, investment of energy, and self-modification and because residents seeking them risk failure and face disappointment. Thus, the earning process establishes the value of privileges and gives them potency as social reinforcements. Although the privileges offered in the TC are quite ordinary, it is their social and psychological relevance to the patient that enhances their importance.

Moreover, because substance-abusing patients often cannot distinguish between privilege and entitlement, the privilege system in the TC teaches that productive participation or membership in a family or community is based on an earning process.

Finally, privileges are tangible rewards that are contingent on individual change. This concrete feature of privilege is particularly suitable for those with histories of performance failure or incompletion.

Disciplinary sanctions. TCs have their own specific rules and regulations that guide the behavior of residents and the management of facilities. The explicit purpose of these rules is to ensure the safety and health of the community. However, their implicit aim is to train and teach residents through the use of discipline.

In the TC, social and physical safety is a prerequisite for psychological trust. Therefore, sanctions are invoked against any behavior that threatens the physical safety of the therapeutic environment. For example, breaking one of the TC's cardinal rules (such as that of no violence or threat of violence) or a house rule (such as the unapproved borrowing of a book) is a threat that must be addressed. Loss of privileges or a speaking ban may be applied for less severe infractions. Job demotion or loss of accrued time may be invoked for more serious infractions. Expulsion may be appropriate for behavior that is incorrigible or dangerous to others.

All sanctions are implemented by staff members as contracts with the resident. Although sanctions are often perceived as punitive, the basic purpose of contracts is to create a learning experience by compelling residents to attend to their own conduct, to reflect on their own motivation, to feel some consequence of their behavior, and to consider alternative forms of acting under similar situations.

The entire facility is made aware of all disciplinary actions. This helps to deter contract violations. Contracts thus create vicarious learning experiences for others, and as symbols of safety and integrity, they strengthen community cohesiveness.

Surveillance: the house run. The TC's most comprehensive method for assessing the overall physical and psychological status of the residential community is the house run. Several times a day, staff members and senior residents walk through the entire facility, examining its overall condition. This single procedure has clinical implications as well as management goals. House runs provide global snapshot impressions of the facility: its cleanliness, planned routines, safety procedures, morale, and psychological tone. They also illuminate the psychological and social functioning of individual residents and peer groups.

Urine testing. Most TCs use unannounced random urine testing or incident-related urine-testing procedures. Residents who deny the use of drugs or refuse to undergo urine testing on request are rejecting a fundamental expectation in the TC, which is to trust staff and peers enough to disclose undesirable behavior. The voluntary admission of drug use initiates a learning experience, which includes exploration of conditions precipitating the infraction. Denial of actual drug use, either before or after urine testing, can block the learning process and may lead to termination or dropout.

When urine tests positive for drugs, the action taken depends on the drug used, the resident's time and status in the program, the resident's history of drug and other infractions, and the locus and condition of use. Actions may involve expulsion, loss of accrued time, radical job demotion, or rescinding of privileges for specific periods. Review of the triggers or reasons for drug use is also essential.

The TC Treatment Process: Program Stages and Phases

Rehabilitation and recovery in the TC are a developmental process, one that occurs in a social learning setting. The developmental process itself can be understood as a passage through stages of learning. The learning that occurs at each stage facilitates change at the next, and each change reflects movement toward the goals of recovery.

Three major program stages characterize change in long-term residential TCs: orientation-induction, primary treatment, and reentry. Additional substages or phases are also discussed.

Stage 1: Orientation-Induction (0–60 Days)

The main goals of the orientation-induction phase of residence are further assessment and orientation to the TC. The aim of orientation in the initial phase of residence is for the individual to be assimilated into the community through full participation and involvement in all of its activities. Rapid assimilation is crucial at this point, when patients are most concerned about the amount of time they are required to spend in the TC.

Formal seminars and informal peer instruction focus on reducing anxiety and uncertainty, which is accomplished through dissemination of information and instruction concerning cardinal rules (i.e., no use of drugs, no violence or threat of physical violence); house regulations (e.g., no leaving the facility, stealing, borrowing, or lending; the maintenance of manners) or expected conduct (e.g., punctuality, attendance, conduct relating to speaking and dressing); the program itself (e.g., TC structure, job functions, the privilege system, TC process stages, TC philosophy and perspective); and TC tools (e.g., encounter and other groups).

Successful passage through the initial stage is reflected mainly in retention. The fact that patients have remained for 30–60 days indicates that they have adhered to the rules of the program well enough to meet the orientation objectives of this stage and have passed through the period of time when they are most vulnerable to drop out.

Stage 2: Primary Treatment (2–12 Months)

The three phases of primary treatment roughly correlate with time spent in the program (2–4, 5–8, and 9–12 months). These phases are marked by plateaus of stable behavior that signal the need for further change. The daily therapeutic-educational regimen of meetings, groups, job assignments, and peer and staff counseling remains the same throughout the year of primary treatment. However, progress is reflected at the end of each phase in terms of three interrelated dimensions of change: community status, development or maturity, and overall psychological adjustment. The following brief profile of a resident who has completed 9–12 months of primary treatment serves to illustrate this concept.

Twelve-month residents are established role models in the program. Privileges reflect the increasing degree of personal autonomy. These residents enjoy more privacy and can obtain regular furloughs. Although they cannot hold jobs outside the facility, their positions within the TC indicate that they effectively run the house. As senior coordinators, for example, they are responsible for arranging resident schedules, trips, and seminars—tasks they perform under staff supervision. Similarly, their status in terms of earning power is also increased; they are eligible to be staff-in-training in executive management offices, in special ancillary services, or as junior counselors. They are expected to assist the staff in monitoring the facility overnight and on weekends. Those beginning vocational-educational programs experience the pressures and challenges of academics or training. They accept responsibility for themselves and for other members in the community.

The maturity of 12-month residents is most evident in their emotional self-management and increased autonomy. Job performance is consistent, and self-assessment is realistic, as is goal setting. Their social interactions with staff are more spontaneous and re-laxed, and they socialize with positive peers during recreational activities and on furlough. Their movement past conformity is evident in their ability to adapt to new situations and teach others TC values.

Twelve-month residents show some insight into their drug problems and personalities. These residents also display paradoxical signs of positive change. Although they are confident and eager to move forward, a certain degree of anxiety and insecurity emerges, associated with their uncertainty about the future. Their openness about anticipated problems is considered a positive psychological sign. After a year, residents are fully trained participants in the group process and often serve as facilitators. A high level of personal disclosure is evident in groups, in peer exchange, and in their increased use of staff counseling.

Stage 3: Reentry (13–24 Months)

Reentry is the stage at which the patient must strengthen skills for autonomous decision making and the capacity for self-management and must rely less on rational authorities or a well-formed peer network. The two phases of the reentry process are early reentry and later reentry.

Early reentry phase (13–18 months). The main objective of the early reentry phase, during which patients continue to live in the facility, is to prepare patients for separation from the community. Emphasis on rational authority decreases, the assumption being that patients in this phase are sufficiently capable of self-management. This capability is reflected in more individual decision making about privileges, social plans, and life design. Particular emphasis is placed on life-skills seminars, which provide training for life outside the community. Attendance is mandated for sessions on budgeting, job seeking, use of alcohol, sexuality, parenting, use of leisure time, and so on.

During this phase, the development of plans for the individual is a collective task of the patient, a key staff member, and peers. These plans are comprehensive blueprints for long-term psychological, educational, and vocational efforts, which include goal attainment schedules, methods of improving interpersonal and family relationships, and counseling on social and sexual behavior. Patients may be attending school or holding full-time jobs, either within or outside the TC. Still, they are expected to participate in house activities when possible and to have some community responsibilities (e.g., monitoring of the facility at night).

Later reentry phase (18–24 months). The objective of the later reentry phase is successful separation from the community. Patients have a "live-out" status; they hold full-time jobs or attend school full-time, and they maintain their own households, usually with live-out peers. They may participate in Alcoholics Anonymous or Narcotics Anonymous or attend family or individual therapy sessions. Contact with the TC is frequent at first and is gradually reduced to weekly telephone calls and monthly visits with a primary counselor.

Graduation

Completion marks the end of active program involvement. Graduation itself, however, is an annual event conducted in the facility for individuals who have completed the program, usually 1 year after their residence is over. Thus, the TC experience is preparation rather than a cure. Residence in the program facilitates a process of change that must continue throughout life, and what is gained in treatment are tools to guide the individual on a path of continued change. Completion, or graduation, therefore, is not an end but a beginning.

Aftercare

Until recently, an aftercare period was not formally acknowledged in long-term TC programs as a definable period after program involvement. Nevertheless, in TCs, patients' efforts to maintain sobriety and a positive lifestyle beyond graduation have always been appreciated. In most TCs, key clinical and life adjustment issues of aftercare are addressed during the reentry stages of the 2-year program. However, as discussed in the later section on modifications, many contemporary TCs now have explicit aftercare components within their systems or through linkages with outside agencies.

Research: Effectiveness and Retention

Success Rates

A substantial amount of evaluation literature documents the effectiveness of the TC approach in rehabilitating drug-abusing individuals (see reviews in Anglin and Hser 1990; Condelli and Hubbard 1994; De Leon 1984, 1985; Gerstein and Harwood 1990; National Institute on Drug Abuse 2002; Simpson 1997; Simpson and Curry 1997; Simpson and Sells 1982; Tims and Ludford 1984; Tims et al. 1994). The findings of single-program and multiprogram studies regarding short- and long-term posttreatment outcome are summarized in this section.

Substantial improvements are noted on separate outcome variables (i.e., drug use, criminality, and employment) and on composite indices for measuring individual success. Maximally to moderately favorable outcomes (in terms of opioid, nonopioid, and alcohol use; arrest rates; retreatment; and employment) occur in more than half of the sample of patients who have completed programs and dropouts.

There is a consistent positive relationship between time spent in residential treatment and posttreatment outcome. For example, in long-term TC programs, success rates (on composite indices of no drug use and no criminality) determined 2 years after completion of treatment are approximately 90% for graduates or completers, 50% for dropouts who remain in residential treatment for more than 1 year, and 25% for dropouts who remain in residential treatment for less than 1 year (e.g., De Leon et al. 1982).

In a few studies that investigated psychological outcomes, results uniformly showed marked improvement at follow-up (e.g., Biase et al. 1986; De Leon 1984; Holland 1983). A direct relationship has been demonstrated between posttreatment behavioral success and psychological adjustment (De Leon 1984; De Leon and Jainchill 1981–1982).

Since the early 1980s, most patients admitted to residential TCs have been multiple-drug-abusing individuals—primarily abusing cocaine, crack, and alcohol—and there have been relatively few patients admitted whose primary drug of abuse is heroin (e.g., De Leon 1993). Several large-scale federally funded evaluation efforts have documented the effectiveness of TCs for the changing population of substance-abusing individuals. These studies include the Drug Abuse Treatment Outcome Study (Hubbard et al. 1997; Simpson and Curry 1997) and the multisite program of research carried out in the Center for Therapeutic Community Research (De Leon 1997).

Retention

Dropout is the general rule for all drug treatment modalities. For TCs, retention is of particular importance because research has established a firm relationship between time spent in treatment and successful outcome. However, most patients admitted to TCs leave the programs, with many leaving before treatment influences are presumed to be effectively rendered.

Research on retention in TCs has been increasing. Reviews of the TC retention research are contained in the literature (e.g., De Leon 1985, 1991; Lewis and Ross 1994; Simpson and Curry 1997). The key findings from these are summarized here.

Retention Rates

Dropout rates are highest (30%–40%) for the first 30 days of residence but decrease sharply thereafter (De Leon and Schwartz 1984). This temporal pattern of dropout is uniform across TC programs (and other modalities). In long-term residential TC programs, completion rates range from 10% to 25% of all admissions. One-year retention rates range from 20% to 35%, although more recent findings suggest gradual increases in annual retention compared with the period before 1980 (De Leon 1991). Retention rates vary considerably across programs, implicating differences in organizational sophistication and fidelity of treatment delivery (Simpson and Curry 1997).

Predictors of Dropout

No reliable patient characteristics predict retention, with the exceptions of severe criminality and severe psychopathology, which are correlated with earlier dropout. Studies point to the importance of dynamic factors in predicting retention in treatment, such as perceived legal pressure, motivation, and readiness for treatment (e.g., Broome et al. 1997; Condelli and De Leon 1993; Condelli and Dunteman 1993; De Leon 1988; De Leon et al. 1994; Hubbard et al. 1988).

Enhancing Retention in TCs

Some attempts to enhance retention in TCs have involved supportive individual counseling, improved orientation to treatment by experienced staff members as "senior professors" (De Leon et al. 2000a), and family alliance strategies to reduce early dropout (e.g., De Leon 1991). Other efforts involve providing special facilities and programming for mothers and children (e.g., Coletti et al. 1997; Stevens et al. 1997) and teaching curriculum-based relapse-prevention methods (Lewis and Ross 1994) to sustain retention throughout residential treatment. Although results are promising, these efforts require replication in multiple sites.

Although it is a legitimate concern, retention should not be confused with treatment effectiveness. TCs are effective for those who remain long enough for treatment influences to occur. Obviously, however, a critical issue for TCs is maximizing holding power to benefit more patients.

Treatment Process

Recent developments have facilitated empirical studies into the hitherto underinvestigated area of treatment process. These developments include formulations of the essential elements of the TC approach and of the stages of recovery in the TC (e.g., De Leon 1995, 1996a, 2000). Preliminary findings based on these formulations illuminate some of the essential program elements, which may serve as the active ingredients in the treatment process (Melnick and De Leon 1999; Melnick et al. 2001b).

The Evolution of the TC: Modifications and Applications

The traditional TC model described in this chapter is actually the prototype of a variety of TC-oriented programs. Today, the TC modality consists of a wide range of programs serving a diversity of patients who use a variety of drugs and present with complex social and psychological problems in addition to their chemical abuse. Patient differences as well as clinical requirements and funding realities have encouraged the development of modified residential TC programs with shorter planned durations of stay (3, 6, and 12 months) as well as TC-oriented day-treatment and outpatient ambulatory models. Having become overwhelmed with alcohol and drug abuse problems, correctional facilities, medical and mental hospitals, and community residences and shelters have implemented TC programs within their institutions. Highlighted in the following sections are some of the key modifications and applications of the TC approach for different patient populations in different settings.

Current Modifications of the TC Model

Most community-based traditional TCs have expanded their social services or have incorporated new interventions to address the needs of their diverse residents. These changes and additions include family services; primary health care specifically geared toward HIV-positive patients and individuals with AIDS (e.g., Barton 1994; De Leon 1996b; McCusker and Sorensen 1994); aftercare, particularly for special populations such as substance-abusing inmates (e.g., Lockwood and Inciardi 1993); relapse-prevention training (e.g., Lewis and Ross 1994); components of 12-step groups (De Leon 1990–1991); and mental health services (e.g., Carroll and Sobel 1986). Mostly these various modifications are additions to the program activities and enhance but do not alter the basic TC regimen. In some cases, these modifications substantially change the TC model itself.

The Multimodal TC and Patient-Treatment Matching

Traditional TCs are highly effective for a certain segment of the drug-abusing population. However, those who seek assistance in TCs represent a broad spectrum of patients, many of whom may not be suited for a long-term residential stay. Improved diagnostic capability and assessment of individual differences have clarified the need for options other than long-term residential treatment.

Many TC agencies are multimodality treatment centers that offer services in their residential and nonresidential programs depending on the clinical status and situational needs of the individual. The modalities include short-term (less than 90 days), medium-term (6–12 months), and long-term (1–2 years) residential components and drug-free outpatient services (6–12 months). Some TC agencies have drug-free day-treatment and methadone maintenance programs. Attempts are made to match the patient to the appropriate modality within the agency. For example, the spread of drug abuse, particularly cocaine use, in the workplace has prompted the development of short-term residential and ambulatory TC models for more socialized patients. Also, initial studies indicate better retention rates in patients matched to TC-oriented residential and outpatient settings, based on multiple domains of drug use severity and social and psychological functioning (Melnick et al. 2000; Melnick et al. 2001a).

To date, the effectiveness of TC-oriented multimodality programs has not been systematically evaluated. Several relevant studies indicate that positive outcomes are obtained in various shorter-term residential, day-treatment, and outpatient programs (e.g., Bu-

cardo et al. 1997; Karson and Gesumaria 1997; McCusker and Sorensen 1994). However, given what is known about the complexity of the recovery process in addiction and the importance of length of stay in treatment, there is little likelihood that shorter-term treatment alone will be sufficient to produce stable positive outcomes for individuals with serious substance-abuse and related lifestyle problems. This conclusion is supported by evidence in the national Drug Abuse Treatment Outcome Study showing that clients with the highest problem severity have better outcomes in long-term TCs than in other settings (Simpson and Curry 1997). Therefore, for serious substance abusers entering multimodality TC agencies, combinations of residential and outpatient services are needed for long-term treatment involvement and effectiveness.

Current Applications to Special Populations

An important sign of the evolution of the TC is its application to special populations and special settings. It is beyond the purview of this chapter to detail the modifications of these adapted TC models. In the main examples of these models, the focus on mutual self-help is retained, along with basic elements of the community approach, meetings, groups, work structure, and perspective on recovery and right living. Examples of these adaptations are more fully described elsewhere (De Leon 1997).

Recent research provides evidence for the effectiveness of modified TCs for special populations. These study populations include adolescents in various adaptations of the community-based TC (Hubbard et al. 1988; Jainchill 1997), inmates in prison TCs (Inciardi et al. 1997; Simpson et al. 1997; Wexler et al. 1999a, 1999b), mentally ill chemical-abusing individuals (De Leon et al. 2000b; Sacks et al. 1997), addicted mothers and their children (Coletti et al. 1997; Winick and Evans 1997), and (although not described here) patients receiving methadone in a day-treatment TC (De Leon et al. 1995).

The TC in Human Services

The modifications of the traditional model and its adaptation for special populations and settings are redefining the TC modality within mainstream human services and mental health services. Most contemporary

TC programs adhere to the perspective and approach described in this chapter. However, the basic peer/social-learning framework has been enlarged to include additional social, psychological, and health services. Staffing compositions have been altered, reflecting the fact that traditional professionals—correctional, mental health, medical and educational, family, and child care specialists; social workers; and case managers—serve along with experientially trained TC professionals.

These changes in patients, services, and staffing have also brought to the surface complex issues, particularly concerning divergence of the program from the proven TC model as well as staff divergence and integration. Program diversity has led to problems of maintaining treatment fidelity and effectiveness. The response to this issue has been the development of national standards of TC programming (Commission on Accreditation of Rehabilitative Facilities 2000 [cited in De Leon 2000, p. 390]; Therapeutic Communities of America 1999) and quality assurance models (Kressel et al. 2002) based on theory and clinical practice.

Staff issues are related to the TC's philosophy of drug-free living and the TC's self-help perspective; other issues are related to differences in therapeutic concepts and terms, staff members' academic education, staff members' experience with addiction, and their roles and functions within the context of a peer-community model. The issues of staff integration have been addressed through the development of TC training curricula based on theory and standards (Therapeutic Communities of America 1999). Vigorous training and orientation efforts are guided by a common perspective of recovery (Carroll and Sobel 1986; Deitch and Solit 1993; De Leon 1985; Galanter et al. 1991; Talboy 1998). Indeed, the cross-fertilization of personnel and methods between traditional TCs and mental health and human services portends the evolution of a new TC: a general treatment model applicable to a broad range of populations for whom affiliation with a self-help community is the foundation for effecting the process of individual change.

References

Anglin MD, Hser YI: Treatment of drug abuse, in Crime and Justice: An Annual Review of Research, Vol 13. Edited by Tonry M, Wilson JQ. Chicago, IL, University of Chicago Press, 1990, pp 393–460

Barton E: The adaptation of the therapeutic community to HIV/AIDS. Proceedings of the Therapeutic Communities of America 1992 Planning Conference. Providence, RI, Manisses Communications Group, 1994, pp 66–70

Biase DV, Sullivan AP, Wheeler B: Daytop miniversity—phase 2—college training in a therapeutic community: development of self concept among drug free addict/abusers, in Therapeutic Communities for Addictions: Readings in Theory, Research, and Practice. Edited by De Leon G, Ziegenfuss JT. Springfield, IL, Charles C Thomas, 1986, pp 121–130

Brook RC, Whitehead IC: Drug-Free Therapeutic Community. New York, Human Sciences Press, 1980

Broome KM, Knight DK, Knight R, et al: Peer, family, and motivational influence on drug treatment process and recidivism for probationers. J Clin Psychol 53:387–397, 1997

Bucardo J, Guydish J, Acampora A, et al: The therapeutic community model applied to day treatment of substance abuse, in Community as Method: Therapeutic Communities for Special Populations and Special Settings. Edited by De Leon G. Westport, CT, Greenwood, 1997, pp 213–224

Carroll JFX, Sobel BS: Integrating mental health personnel and practices into a therapeutic community, in Therapeutic Communities for Addictions: Readings in Theory, Research, and Practice. Edited by De Leon G, Ziegenfuss JT. Springfield, IL, Charles C Thomas, 1986, pp 209–226

Casriel D: So Fair a House: The Story of Synanon. New York, Prentice-Hall, 1966

Coletti SD, Schinka JA, Hughs PH, et al: Specialized therapeutic community treatment for chemically dependent women and their children, in Community as Method: Therapeutic Communities for Special Populations and Special Settings. Edited by De Leon G. Westport, CT, Greenwood, 1997, pp 115–128

Commission on Accreditation of Rehabilitative Facilities: The 2000 Behavioral Health Standards Manual. Tucson, AZ, Commission on Accreditation of Rehabilitative Facilities, 2000. Available from: CARF, 4891 East Grant Rd. Tucson, AZ 85712

Condelli WS, De Leon G: Fixed and dynamic predictors of retention in therapeutic communities. J Subst Abuse Treat 10:11–16, 1993

Condelli WS, Dunteman GH: Issues to consider when predicting retention in therapeutic communities. J Psychoactive Drugs 25:239–244, 1993

Condelli WS, Hubbard RL: Client outcomes from therapeutic communities, in Therapeutic Community: Advances in Research and Application, (NIH Publ No 94-3633). Edited by Tims FM, De Leon G, Jainchill N. Rockville, MD, National Institute on Drug Abuse, 1994, pp 80–98

Deitch DA: Treatment of Drug Abuse in the Therapeutic Community: Historical Influences, Current Considerations, and Future Outlooks, Vol 4. Washington, DC, National Commission on Marihuana and Drug Abuse, 1972, pp 158–175

Deitch DA, Solit R: Training drug abuse treatment personnel in therapeutic community methodologies. Psychotherapy 30 (special issue):305–316, 1993

De Leon G: The Therapeutic Community: Study of Effectiveness (NIDA Treatment Research Monograph ADM-84-1286). Rockville, MD, National Institute on Drug Abuse, 1984

De Leon G: Legal pressure in therapeutic communities. NIDA Res Monogr 86:160–177, 1988

De Leon G: Aftercare in therapeutic communities. Int J Addict 25:1225–1237, 1990–1991

De Leon G: Retention in drug free therapeutic communities. NIDA Res Monogr 106:218–244, 1991

De Leon G: Cocaine abusers in therapeutic community treatment. NIDA Res Monogr 135:163–189, 1993

De Leon G: Therapeutic communities for addictions: a theoretical framework. Int J Addict 30:1603–1645, 1995

De Leon G: Integrative recovery: a stage paradigm. Subst Abuse 17:51–63, 1996a

De Leon G: Therapeutic communities: AIDS/HIV risk and harm reduction. J Subst Abuse Treat 13:411–420, 1996b

De Leon G (ed): Community as Method: Therapeutic Communities for Special Populations and Special Settings. Westport, CT, Greenwood, 1997

De Leon G: The Therapeutic Community: Theory, Model, and Method. New York, Springer, 2000

De Leon G, Jainchill N: Male and female drug abusers: social and psychological status 2 years after treatment in a therapeutic community. Am J Drug Alcohol Abuse 8:465–497, 1981–1982

De Leon G, Schwartz S: The therapeutic community: what are the retention rates? Am J Drug Alcohol Abuse 10:267–284, 1984

De Leon G, Skodol A, Rosenthal MS: Phoenix House: changes in psychopathological signs of resident drug addicts. Arch Gen Psychiatry 23:131–135, 1973

De Leon G, Wexler HK, Jainchill N: Success and improvement rates 5 years after treatment in a therapeutic community. Int J Addict 17:703–742, 1982

De Leon G, Melnick G, Kressel D, et al: Circumstances, motivation, readiness and suitability (the CMRS scales): predicting retention in therapeutic community treatment. Am J Drug Alcohol Abuse 20:495–515, 1994

De Leon G, Staines G, Perlis PE, et al: Therapeutic community methods in methadone maintenance (Passages): an open clinical trial. Drug Alcohol Depend 37:45–57, 1995

De Leon G, Hawke J, Jainchill N, et al: Therapeutic communities: enhancing retention in treatment using "senior professor" staff. J Subst Abuse Treat 19:375–382, 2000a

De Leon G, Sacks S, Staines G, et al: Modified therapeutic community for homeless mentally ill chemical abusers: treatment outcomes. Am J Drug Alcohol Abuse 26:461–480, 2000b

Frankel B: Transforming Identities, Context, Power, and Ideology in a Therapeutic Community. New York, Peter Lang, 1989

Galanter M, Egelko S, De Leon G, et al: Crack/cocaine abusers in the general hospital: assessment and initiation of care. Am J Psychiatry 149:810–815, 1991

Gerstein DR, Harwood HJ (eds): Treating Drug Problems, Vol 1: A Study of the Evaluation, Effectiveness, and Financing of Public and Private Drug Treatment Systems. Institute of Medicine. Washington, DC, National Academy Press, 1990

Holland S: Evaluating community based treatment programs: a model for strengthening inferences about effectiveness. International Journal of Therapeutic Communities 4:285–306, 1983

Holland S: Measuring process in drug abuse treatment research, in Therapeutic Communities for Addictions: Readings in Theory, Research, and Practice. Edited by De Leon G, Ziegenfuss JT. Springfield, IL, Charles C Thomas, 1986, pp 169–181

Hubbard RL, Collins JJ, Rachal JV, et al: The criminal justice client in drug abuse treatment. NIDA Res Monogr 86:57–80, 1988

Hubbard RL, Marsden ME, Valley Rachal J, et al: Drug Abuse Treatment: A National Study of Effectiveness. Chapel Hill, NC, University of North Carolina Press, 1989

Hubbard RL, Craddock SG, Flynn PM, et al: Overview of 1-year follow-up outcomes in the Drug Abuse Treatment Outcome Study (DATOS). Psychol Addict Behav 11 (special issue):261–278, 1997

Inciardi JA, Martin SS, Butzin CA, et al: An effective model of prison-based treatment for drug-involved offenders. J Drug Issues 27:261–278, 1997

Jainchill N: Co-morbidity and therapeutic community treatment. NIDA Res Monogr 144:209–231, 1994

Jainchill N: Therapeutic communities for adolescents: the same and not the same, in Community as Method: Therapeutic Communities for Special Populations and Special Settings. Edited by De Leon G. Westport, CT, Greenwood, 1997, pp 161–178

Jones M: Therapeutic Community: A New Treatment Method in Psychiatry. New York, Basic Books, 1953

Karson JS, Gesumaria RV: Program description and outcome of an enhanced, six-month residential therapeutic community, in Community as Method: Therapeutic Communities for Special Populations and Special Settings. Edited by De Leon G. Westport, CT, Greenwood, 1997, pp 199–212

Kennard D, Wilson S: The modification of personality disturbance in a therapeutic community for drug abusers. Br J Med Psychol 52:215–221, 1979

Kooyman M: The Therapeutic Community for Addicts: Intimacy, Parent Involvement, and Treatment Success. Rotterdam, The Netherlands, Erasmus University, 1993

Kressel D, Zompa D, De Leon G: A statewide integrated quality assurance model for correctional-based therapeutic community programs. Offender Substance Abuse Report 2(4):49–64, 2002

Lewis BF, Ross R: Retention in therapeutic communities: challenges for the nineties. NIDA Res Monogr 144:99–116, 1994

Lockwood D, Inciardi JA: CREST outreach center: a work release iteration of the TC model, in Innovative Approaches in the Treatment of Drug Abuse: Program Models and Strategies. Edited by Inciardi J, Tims FM, Fletcher BW. Westport, CT, Greenwood, 1993, pp 61–69

McCusker J, Sorensen JL: HIV and therapeutic communities. NIDA Res Monogr 144:232–258, 1994

Melnick G, De Leon G: Clarifying the nature of therapeutic community treatment: a survey of essential elements. J Subst Abuse Treat 16:307–313, 1999

Melnick G, De Leon G, Hiller ML, et al: Therapeutic communities: diversity in treatment elements. Subst Use Misuse 35:1819–1847, 2000

Melnick G, De Leon G, Thomas G, et al: A client-treatment matching protocol for therapeutic communities: first report. J Subst Abuse Treat 21:119–128, 2001a

Melnick G, De Leon G, Thomas G, et al: Treatment process in therapeutic communities: motivation, progress and outcomes. Am J Drug Alcohol Abuse 27:633–650, 2001b

National Institute on Drug Abuse (NIDA) Research Report Series: Therapeutic Community. What Is a Therapeutic Community? Rockville, MD, National Institute on Drug Abuse, 2002

Pompi KF, Resnick J: Retention in a therapeutic community for court-referred adolescents and young adults. Am J Drug Alcohol Abuse 13:309–325, 1987

Sacks S, Sacks J, De Leon G, et al: Modified therapeutic community for mentally ill chemical "abusers": background; influences; program description; preliminary findings. Subst Use Misuse 32:1217–1259, 1997

Simpson DD: Effectiveness of drug abuse treatment: a review of research from field settings, in Treating Drug Abusers Effectively. Edited by Egertson JA, Fox DM, Leshner AI. Cambridge, MA, Blackwell, 1997, pp 41–73

Simpson DD, Curry SJ (eds): Drug Abuse Treatment Outcome Studies (DATOS). Psychol Addict Behav 11 (special issue) 4:211–337, 1997

Simpson DD, Sells SB: Effectiveness of treatment for drug abuse: an overview of the DARP research program. Adv Alcohol Subst Abuse 2:7–29, 1982

Simpson DD, Joe GW, Brown BS: Treatment retention and follow-up outcomes in DATOS. Psychol Addict Behav 11 (special issue):294–307, 1997

Stevens SJ, Arbiter N, McGrath R: Women and children: therapeutic community substance abuse treatment, in Community as Method: Therapeutic Communities for Special Populations and Special Settings. Edited by De Leon G. Westport, CT, Greenwood, 1997, pp 129–142

Sugarman B: Structure, variations, and context: a sociological view of the therapeutic community, in Therapeutic Communities for Addictions: Readings in Theory, Research, and Practice. Edited by De Leon G, Ziegenfuss JT. Springfield, IL, Charles C Thomas, 1986, pp 65–82

Talboy ES: Therapeutic Community Experiential Training: Facilitator Guide. Kansas City, MO, University of Missouri–Kansas City, Mid-America Addiction Technology Transfer Center, 1998

Therapeutic Communities of America: Therapeutic Communities in Correctional Settings: The Prison-Based TC Standards Development Project. Final report of phase II. Washington, DC, White House Office of National Drug Control Policy, 1999

Tims FM, Ludford JP (eds): Drug Abuse Treatment Evaluation: Strategies, Progress, and Prospects (NIDA Research Monograph No 51). Special Issue on Research Analysis and Utilization System. Rockville, MD, National Institute on Drug Abuse, 1984

Tims FM, De Leon G, Jainchill N (eds): Therapeutic Community: Advances in Research and Application. Proceedings of a meeting. May 16–17, 1991. NIDA Res Monogr 144:1–286, 1994

Wexler HK, De Leon G, Thomas G, et al: The Amity Prison TC evaluation: reincarceration outcomes. Crim Justice Behav 26:147–167, 1999a

Wexler HK, Melnick J, Lowe L, et al: Three-year reincarceration outcomes for Amity in-prison therapeutic community and aftercare in California. The Prison Journal 79:321–336, 1999b

Winick C, Evans JT: A therapeutic community for mothers and their children, in Community as Method: Therapeutic Communities for Special Populations and Special Settings. Edited by De Leon G. Westport, CT, Greenwood, 1997, pp 143–160

Yablonsky L: Synanon: The Tunnel Back. New York, Macmillan, 1965

Zuckerman M, Sola S, Masterson J, et al: MMPI patterns in drug abusers before and after treatment in therapeutic communities. J Consult Clin Psychol 43:286–296, 1975

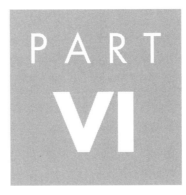

PART VI

Special Populations

Adolescent Substance Abuse

Yifrah Kaminer, M.D.
Ralph E. Tarter, Ph.D.

Childhood and adolescence are not only critical phases for normal development but are also periods when various pathological behaviors or disorders—including substance use disorders—are first recognized. Substance use among American youths dropped to a low point in the 1980s and early 1990s. It then rose continuously between 1992 and 1997 and since then has leveled off (Johnston et al. 2001). Although recent reports suggest that the drug epidemic may be leveling off in older adolescents, secular trends suggest that the magnitude of the problem will not change dramatically until at least the year 2010 (Kaminer 2001a). The upward trend in the 1990s was primarily due to a rate of marijuana use that almost tripled among eighth graders and doubled among twelfth graders. Lifetime diagnoses of alcohol and drug abuse among adolescents in different states in the United States range from 3% to 10% (Harrison et al. 1998; Lewinsohn et al. 1996; Ungemack et al. 1997). Consequently, there is mounting concern regarding the short- and long-term physical and mental health outcomes of adolescents who use psychoactive drugs. This includes observations that use of alcohol and other drugs is a leading cause among adolescents of morbidity and death from motor vehicle accidents, suicidal behavior, violence, drowning, and unprotected sexual activity (Kaminer 1994). Because of limited resources, inadequate age-appropriate programs, and lack of a broad consensus on preferred treatment strategies, only a small proportion of all adolescents in need of treatment—including those with high severity of substance use disorders, comorbid psychiatric disorders, and legal problems—actually receive services.

In this chapter, we review the literature on the development of adolescent substance use, placing particular emphasis on the transition from substance use to substance abuse or dependence. We discuss the difference between substance use and substance use disorders and then review the natural history of substance use disorders among adolescents and the pattern of psychiatric comorbidity. We conclude with an evaluation of the efficacy of prevention and treatment of substance use disorders in adolescents.

Nosology

Normative Behavior

Although any nonmedical use of drugs (including tobacco and alcohol) by adolescents is illegal and can therefore be viewed as a form of abuse, this perspective ignores some key epidemiological findings. Specifically, the high prevalence of alcohol and tobacco use underscores the fact that use of alcohol and tobacco can be viewed as normative, or at least not exceptionally deviant. By age 18 years, approximately 80% of youths in the United States have drunk alcohol, 4% drink alcohol regularly, 66% have smoked cigarettes, and 13% smoke half a pack daily (Johnston et al. 2001). Approximately 8% have used cocaine and 15% have been exposed to the use of inhalants, stimulants, or hallucinogens. These figures illustrate the extent of drug use in the population of 18-year-old high school students in the United States.

Most adolescents who engage in substance use do not develop substance use disorders as defined by criteria in DSM-IV and DSM-IV-TR (American Psychiatric Association 1994, 2000). It is therefore imperative to understand adolescent substance use in the context of changeable patterns of normative behavior and to distinguish this behavior from substance use disorder.

Adolescence has long been recognized as a phase of transition (Erikson 1968). During this period of life, biological and psychological maturation is completed. The social roles of adulthood are increasingly assumed during the final stage of sexual, physical, and psychological maturation. Working, driving, engaging in sexual activity, and using psychoactive substances (particularly alcohol and tobacco) are adult-like activities and behaviors that become increasingly common in persons ages 13–18 years. Alcohol and drug use (particularly tobacco use) can therefore be viewed as one facet of adolescent socialization (Newcomb 1995). In one study, adolescents who experimented with psychoactive substances had better psychological outcomes than did adolescents who used substances frequently or who abstained (Shedler and Block 1990). It should not be concluded from the presentation of this finding that experimentation with psychoactive substances is recommended. However, the finding is evidence that some substance use during adolescence does not necessarily portend an adverse outcome.

Pathological Behavior

Approximately 8% of the United States population will fulfill the criteria for a diagnosis of a substance use disorder during their lifetimes. The cutoff point for a diagnosis of substance use disorder or dependence is somewhat arbitrary, however, particularly in adolescents (Rohde et al. 1996). In clinical psychiatry, a categorical paradigm (e.g., normal versus abnormal) has traditionally been used, even though this theoretical perspective has limitations in terms of understanding pathogenesis and improving treatment (Bukstein and Kaminer 1994). In addition, serious negative effects of drugs in adolescents at the subdiagnostic levels have been recognized, although they have not yet been addressed in DSM (Lewinsohn et al. 1996).

The notion that it is important to differentiate between substance abuse and dependence before beginning treatment was supported by empirical evidence obtained by Hasin and associates (1990). These researchers concluded that most adults with a diagnosis of substance abuse had never progressed to dependence. Abuse and dependence are therefore distinct, and abuse is not always a prodrome and may be developmentally limited in many adolescents. DSM-IV-TR diagnostic criteria for substance abuse and dependence are the same for adolescents and adults. Empirical data generally support the validity of the DSM-IV-TR criteria for adolescents (Lewinsohn et al. 1996; Martin et al. 1995). Pollock and Martin (1999) demonstrated the importance of a new nosological entity for youths called orphan diagnoses that includes subthreshold symptoms of alcohol dependence (i.e., only one or two symptoms). A 3-year follow-up study demonstrated that this entity has a unique trajectory that is similar to neither abuse nor dependence (Martin 2002).

Temperament deviations have also been shown to be associated with psychopathology and substance abuse (Reich et al. 1993). Children who have a "difficult" temperament commonly manifest externalizing and internalizing behavior problems by middle childhood (Earls and Jung 1987) and in adolescence (Maziade et al. 1990). High levels of behavioral activity have been noted in youths at high risk for substance abuse as well as in those with substance use disorder. High levels of activity also correlate with severity of the disorder (Tarter et al. 1990a, 1990b). Other temperamental trait deviations found in youths at high risk include reduced attention span (Schaffer et al. 1984), high impulsivity (Noll et al. 1992) and negative affect states such as irritability (Brook et al. 1990) and emotional reactivity (Blackson 1994). Tarter and colleagues (1994) used the difficult-temperament index to classify adolescent alcoholic patients. The obtained clusters were similar to the adult subtypes reported by Cloninger (1987) and Babor et al. (1992). The smaller subset of adolescents manifesting behavioral dyscontrol and hypophoria were included in Cluster 2, whereas those with primarily negative affect were included in Cluster 1. Compared with Cluster 1 subjects, Cluster 2 patients were younger at the time of first substance use, first diagnosis of substance abuse, and first psychiatric diagnosis. Moreover, adolescents with a difficult temperament had a high probability of developing psychiatric disorders such as conduct disorder, attention-deficit/hyperactivity disorder (ADHD), anxiety disorders, and mood disorders (Tarter et al. 1994). Tarter et al. (1997) also reported that Cluster 1 and Cluster 2 were identified in both male and female adolescents.

Initiation, Maintenance, and Transitions of Substance Use

A number of behavioral dispositions and environmental influences are predictive of age at initiation of drug use, intensity of drug use, and the experience of negative consequences during adolescence (Hawkins et al. 1992; Petraitis et al. 1995). Behavioral characteristics most commonly include impulsivity, aggression, sensation seeking, low levels of harm avoidance, inability to delay gratification, low levels of striving to achieve, lack of religiosity, and psychopathology, especially conduct disorder. Contextual or environmental factors that are most common include stressful life events, lack of support from parents, absence of normative peers, perception of high availability of drugs, social norms that facilitate drug use, and relaxed laws and regulatory policies. Clearly, manifold risk factors, each having different salience, determine overall risk for each person. In aggregate, these risk factors determine the slope and momentum of the developmental trajectory into adulthood, culminating in substance use, abuse, or dependence (Bates and Labouvie 1995). Although adolescence is a time of heightened risk, heavy use is often limited to the period of adolescence. That is, substance use does not invariably increase and lead to dependence. Indeed, moderation or even cessation may occur during or after adolescence (Labouvie 1996).

Kandel (1982), the initial proponent of the "gateway" theory, argued that there are at least four distinct developmental stages of drug use: 1) beer or wine consumption, 2) cigarette smoking or hard liquor consumption, 3) marijuana use, and 4) use of other illicit drugs.

According to Kandel (1982), 26% of adolescents who use illicit drugs progress to the next of the four stages, compared with only 4% who have never used marijuana. A recent study by Golub and Johnson (1994) indicated that alcohol is losing its importance as a prerequisite for progression to marijuana, but marijuana's role as a gateway drug appears to have increased, and marijuana use nearly always precedes use of substances that have less general acceptance (e.g., heroin).

Kandel et al. (1986) studied the 10-year outcome of adolescent substance use at age 15–16 years. They found that the strongest predictor of drug use is prior drug use. However, the consequences of drug use affect every aspect of life in early adulthood. Illicit drug use begun at an early age has also been found to increase the risk of drug problems during late adolescence. According to the results of a retrospective analysis of the Epidemiologic Catchment Area data (Anthony and Petronis 1995), prior drug use predicts future drug use. However, in a prospective study of adolescents (Bates and Labouvie 1997), age at first use of illicit drugs did not emerge as an independent risk factor for either persistence or severity of drug use in adulthood.

When substance use behaviors at age 18 years are controlled for, there is no significant relationship between adolescent risk and the intensity and consequences of adult substance use (Teichman et al. 1989). This suggests that the effect of child and adolescent risk factors on adult substance use may be mediated by the intensity of substance use in late adolescence (Bates and Labouvie 1997).

Temperament precursors such as impulsivity, novelty seeking, and sensation seeking tend to peak in late adolescence or early adulthood (Zuckerman 1994) and to decrease toward the fourth decade of life, with the decrease being accompanied by an increase in cognitive structure. These changes may be partly responsible for the low predictive utility of differences in these and other variables of adolescent risk at age 18 years, as reported by Bates and Labouvie (1997). More study is needed to link changes over the long term in both interpersonal and environmental risk and protective factors to long-term use patterns.

The available results suggest that programs aimed at reducing risk factors during adolescence may have more beneficial long-term effects if they can limit drug use during the peak lifetime period, at ages 18–21 years. Programs that focus on postadolescence therefore need to concentrate on the concurrent risk factors, which are not necessarily the same as those during adolescence. In early adolescence, prevention efforts should be directed at delaying the onset and increase of drug use, because (although not in an invariant fashion) drug use predicts future drug use.

Psychiatric Comorbidity

Psychiatric disorders in childhood, particularly the disruptive behavior disorders, confer an increased risk for the development of substance use disorders (Bukstein et al. 1989; Christie et al. 1988; Loeber 1988). However, the etiological mechanisms have not been systematically researched. A number of possible relationships exist between substance use disorders and psychopathology. Psychopathology may precede substance use disorders, may develop as a consequence of preexisting substance use disorders, may moderate the severity of substance use disorders, or may originate from a common vulnerability (Hovens et al. 1994).

A number of psychiatric disorders are commonly associated with substance use disorders in youth. Conduct disorder is commonly associated with adolescent substance use disorders, and if it occurs, it usually precedes the substance use disorder (Loeber 1988; Milin et al. 1991). Rates of conduct disorder range from 50% to 80% in adolescent patients with substance use disorders. Although ADHD is frequently observed in substance-using and substance-abusing youths, such an association is likely the result of the high level of comorbidity between conduct disorder and ADHD (Alterman and Tarter 1986; Wilens et al. 1994). An earlier onset of conduct problems and aggressive behavior, in addition to ADHD, increases the risk for substance abuse (Loeber 1988). In a prospective follow-up study, Biederman et al. (1997) found that adolescents with and adolescents without ADHD had similar magnitudes of risk for substance use disorders. Conduct disorder and bipolar disorder mediated the association between childhood ADHD and substance use disorder outcome.

In addition, mood disorders, especially depression, frequently precede substance use and substance use disorders in adolescents (Bukstein et al. 1992; Deykin et al. 1992). The prevalence of depressive disorders ranges from 24% to more than 50%.

The empirical literature also supports an association between substance use disorders and suicidal behavior in adolescents (Kaminer 1996). Adolescents who commit suicide are frequently under the influence of alcohol or other drugs at the time of suicide (Brent et al. 1987). Possible mechanisms underlying this relationship include the direct acute pharmacological and chronic neurological effects of psychoactive substances. Acute intoxication may be experienced as a transient but intense dysphoric state, with behavioral disinhibition and impaired judgment. Substance use may also exacerbate preexisting psychopathology, especially impulse dyscontrol, depression, and anxiety.

Several studies of clinical populations have found a high rate of anxiety disorder among youths with substance use disorders (Clark and Sayette 1993; Clark et al. 1995). In adolescent patients with substance use disorders, the prevalence of anxiety disorder ranged from 7% to more than 40% (Clark et al. 1995; Stowell 1991). The order of appearance of anxiety and substance use disorders is variable, depending on the specific anxiety disorder. Social phobia usually precedes substance abuse, whereas panic and generalized anxiety disorder more often follow the onset of substance use disorders (Kushner et al. 1990). Adolescents with substance use disorders often have a history of posttraumatic stress disorder from physical or sexual abuse (Clark et al. 1995; Van Hasselt et al. 1993). Bulimia nervosa (Bulik 1987) and personality disorders, particularly those in Cluster B (Grilo et al. 1995), are also commonly found in adolescents with substance use disorders. Griffiths (1995) reported that pathological gambling in British youths preceded substance abuse. However, Kaminer and colleagues (2002b) did not find elevated rates of pathological gambling among adolescent substance abusers.

There are no reports of research regarding the stability of psychiatric disorders in adolescents with dual diagnoses. A study of the stability of comorbid psychiatric disorders in alcoholic men after 1 year of follow-up revealed that the symptoms are stable over time and therefore constitute a potential target for treatment (Penick et al. 1988). On the other hand, Rounsaville and Kleber (1986) reported good stability of comorbid psychiatric disorders at 6-month follow-up among opiate-addicted individuals, and this stability deteriorated by 2.5-year follow-up, resulting in a low rate of stability. Penick and colleagues (1988) attributed these differences to a threshold effect.

Treatment of dual diagnoses should be addressed simultaneously and not sequentially. Integrative psychosocial interventions or a combination of psychopharmacological and psychosocial interventions are the rule rather than the exception (Kaminer 2001a; Riggs and Davies 2002).

Prevention

Efforts to curtail substance abuse have historically concentrated on modifying the supply-to-demand ratio. However, reduction of supply cannot succeed as long as a demand exists. Hence, *reducing demand* is an integral component of prevention. Laws and regulations can reduce demand. For example, Coate and Grossman (1987) found that alcohol consumption decreased in youths when the cost of alcoholic beverages or the legal drinking age was increased. O'Malley and Wagenaar (1991) reported a reduction in automobile accidents among youths after the legal drinking age was increased to 21 years.

An overarching goal of prevention is to delay initiation of the use of *gateway substances* such as cigarettes, alcohol, and marijuana. Research findings over the past two decades have provided foundation for the development of effective approaches to substance abuse prevention. The traditional prevention strategy involves an educational program designed to increase knowledge of the consequences of drug use. However, the notion that increased knowledge alone prevents drug use is not supported by available evidence (Schinke et al. 1991). Alternative activities programs and affective education, which is designed to increase self-esteem and responsible decision making, have also been found to be ineffective in preventing drug use (Bangert-Drowns 1988; Tobler 1986). More promising prevention strategies are aimed at enhancing social skills and drug-refusal skills. Botvin developed a curriculum involving teaching of general life skills and of skills for resisting social influences to use drugs. This Life Skills Training (LST) program was initially developed as a smoking prevention program led effectively by older peer leaders or classroom teachers (Botvin and Griffin 2001). Botvin et al. (1995) implemented

the LST curriculum in the seventh grade ($N=3,597$) in 56 schools and booster sessions during the 2 years after completion of the intervention. The investigators reported evidence of long-term effectiveness and lasting reduction in drug use 6 years later among the twelfth graders in the experimental condition compared with those in the control condition. The generalizability of the LST prevention approach for African American and Hispanic youths has been supported (Botvin and Griffin 2001).

The challenge confronting health care providers is to identify high-risk individuals before or shortly after initiation of substance use. One of the largest high-risk populations is children who have a biological parent with a diagnosis of substance dependence. The risk of substance use disorders is 4–10 times greater in these children (Goodwin 1985). Children of parents with opioid dependence also have a high rate of psychopathology and more frequently have academic, family, and legal problems (Kolar et al. 1994; Wilens et al. 1995). A balanced view is needed regarding the development and outcomes of children of alcoholic individuals, since most children raised by an alcoholic parent do not develop alcoholism (Wilson and Crowe 1991). Moreover, the labeling of children of alcoholic individuals as such is potentially harmful (Burk and Sher 1990). Thus, although children of substance-abusing persons are at an increased risk for developing substance use disorders themselves, prevention efforts need to take into account the adverse effect of labeling and recognize that most children do not experience the negative outcome. The interaction between risk and protective factors may influence the development or arrest of substance abuse in the vulnerable child. The study of resilience among youths growing up in substance-abusing families is continuing (Wolin and Wolin 1996).

Obtaining the most favorable outcome requires an understanding of the heterogeneity of the adolescent population. In addition, prevention efforts should take into account the developmental staging of substance use behavior. In this regard, prevention must address the needs of adolescents in multiple domains of life. Prevention programs that are sensitive to ethnic differences also need to be continuously devised (Catalano et al. 1993). Finally, dissemination is important because prevention programs proven to be successful, such as LST, are unlikely to have any real public health impact unless they are used in a large number of schools.

Assessment and Treatment

In an excellent review of issues in the assessment of adolescent substance use, Winters and colleagues (2001) emphasize the importance of meaningful assessment of a wide range of variables. Two major sets of assessment variables are considered here. One set of measures has been traditionally included in standardized screening and comprehensive assessment tools and is viewed as being essential to the identification, referral, and treatment of problems associated with adolescent drug involvement. The measures in this set include severity of the drug abuse problem (e.g., preferred drugs, past and present use, age at onset, frequency, quantity, consequences, treatment experience, and treatment response), risk factors, and protective factors. The second set of variables is important for the understanding of its mediating and moderating effects on treatment outcome. The variables in this set include reasons for drug use and drug preference, expectancies, readiness to change behavior, and self-efficacy. Self-reporting of substance use among adolescents is generally valid and detects more use than do laboratory tests and collateral reports (Buchan et al. 2002; Godley et al. 2002). Parental or collateral reporting of internalizing disorders has traditionally been much lower than that of externalizing disorders. Collateral reporting of alcohol and drug abuse has been low to moderate compared with self-reporting or drug urinalysis (Burleson and Kaminer 2002; Cantwell et al. 1997).

The use of screening instruments is essential as a brief first step for assessment of drug use before moving if necessary to the assessment of problem severity. Examples of reliable and valid screening tests include the Personal Experience Screening Questionnaire (Winters 1992), the Substance Abuse Subtle Screening Inventory (Miller 1990), the Drug Use Screening Inventory—Revised (Tarter 1990), and the Problem Oriented Screening Instrument for Teenagers (Rahdert 1991). Measures for the assessment of severity include the Teen Addiction Severity Index (Kaminer et al. 1991, 1993), the Adolescent Drug Abuse Diagnosis (Friedman and Utada 1989), and the Personal Experience Inventory (Winters and Henly 1988). For an updated, comprehensive list of domains of measurement and respective instruments, please refer to Winters et al. (2001).

The limited literature on treatment outcome studies is characterized by significant methodological limitations (Kaminer 2000). These include small sample size, lack of placebo-controlled condition, varying selection criteria, inadequate measurement of psychosocial and comorbid psychiatric conditions, failure to indicate compliance and attrition rates, little description of actual treatment involved or measures to maintain treatment fidelity by counselors, unmanualized interventions (making replication difficult), variability of therapists, lack of or deficiency in objective measurement such as drug urinalysis for treatment outcome, and inadequate follow-up of treatment completers as well as noncompleters. These shortcomings in the studies conducted to date limit the capacity to draw definitive conclusions (Kaminer 2001a).

After reviewing studies conducted in the last 25 years on the treatment outcome of adolescents with substance use disorders, we concluded that some treatment is better than no treatment. However, the effects of treatment are not uniform, and a substantial variability is observed in posttreatment outcome (Catalano et al. 1990–1991; Deas and Thomas 2001; Kaminer 1994; Winters 1999).

In most studies in which prediction of outcome was a goal, there was a focus on patient characteristics determined at the time of treatment initiation. Factors such as age, race, socioeconomic status, severity of drug use, and mental health status have been postulated to be associated with prognosis. Although some studies provide evidence of a relationship between pretreatment patient characteristics and outcome, the findings are not consistent. Variables such as severity of alcohol problems and of other drug use, severity of internalizing symptoms, and level of self-esteem are prognostic of treatment completion in American, Canadian, and Irish adolescents (Blood and Cornwall 1994; Doyle et al. 1994; Kaminer et al. 1992). Psychopathology, particularly conduct disorder, is negatively correlated with treatment completion and posttreatment abstinence (Myers et al. 1995).

Most studies on treatment outcome of adolescents with substance use disorders have focused on completion of treatment rather than follow-up status. Reports of follow-up studies indicate that relapse rates are high, ranging between 35% and 85% (Brown et al. 1989; Catalano et al. 1990–1991; Doyle et al. 1994). The high relapse rate is associated with social pressures. Abstinent teens experience decreased interpersonal conflict, improve academically, and demonstrate increased involvement in normative social and occupational activities (Brown et al. 1994; Vik et al. 1992).

Treatment research on adolescents in the 1980s focused on three general areas: length of time in treatment, staff characteristics, and program environment and treatment services. The most important findings are discussed below.

Length of time in treatment has been shown to be less predictive of treatment outcome than staff characteristics, program environment, and treatment services. However, a comprehensive review of studies has shown that the longer the adolescent remains in treatment, the better the prognosis is (Catalano et al. 1990–1991). It was suggested that longer time in treatment means more opportunities for improvement.

Staff characteristics that affect treatment success include amount of professional experience, competence in taking a problem-solving approach, and availability of volunteers in the program who interact with patients (Friedman et al. 1989). Staff members who themselves have recurring addiction problems do not have a positive effect on treatment outcome (Catalano et al. 1990–1991).

Finally, treatment setting (e.g., inpatient, residential, or outpatient) was found to be less important to treatment outcome than the menu and dosage of treatment provided (Kaminer 1994).

Psychosocial treatment strategies studied in the 1990s that have shown promise in reducing substance use disorders among adolescents include family therapies such as multisystemic therapy (Henggeler et al. 1996), functional family therapy (Waldron et al. 2001), and multidimensional family therapy (Liddle et al. 2001); behavioral therapy (Azrin et al. 1994); cognitive-behavioral therapy (CBT) (Kaminer et al. 1998a, 2002a; Waldron and Kaminer, in press); motivational interviewing (Wagner et al. 1999); the Minnesota 12-step model (Winters et al. 2000); contingency management reinforcement (Corby et al. 2000); community reinforcement (Godley et al. 2002); and integrative models of treatment (Cannabis Youth Treatment Group 2000; Waldron et al. 2001).

The two interventions most commonly studied in recent decades are family therapy and CBT. The involvement of the family increases the likelihood that the patient will complete treatment and reduces problem behavior during treatment (Barrett et al. 1988). Several investigators have demonstrated the benefits of family-based approaches in treating substance use disorders in adolescents (Friedman and Utada 1989; Liddle and Dakof 1995; Szapocznik et al. 1988). The multisystemic therapy model is a successful family-based

ecological systems approach in which interventions simultaneously target family functioning and communication, school and peer functioning, and adjustment in the community (Henggeler et al. 1992, 1996).

Behavioral treatment has been reported to be superior to supportive counseling (Azrin et al. 1994). Manual-guided therapy has been shown to be helpful in improving drug-refusal, problem-solving, and social skills (Kaminer et al. 1998a). Comparison of the effectiveness of two 12-week psychosocial interventions revealed that adolescents enrolled in a CBT program fared better than those who participated in an interactional therapy program. Those assigned to CBT demonstrated a statistically significant reduction in severity of substance use—as determined through use of the Teen Addiction Severity Index (Kaminer et al. 1991, 1993) and controlled by the Teen Treatment Services Review (Kaminer et al. 1998b)—compared with those assigned to interactional therapy (Kaminer et al. 1998c). Improvements were also observed in the areas of family function, school adjustment, peer or social relationships, legal problems, and psychiatric disturbance in patients receiving CBT (Kaminer et al. 1998c).

Kaminer and colleagues (2002a) compared the efficacy of CBT versus psychoeducational therapies for adolescent substance abusers. This study was designed to replicate the findings from the earlier investigation, establishing the efficacy of the CBT intervention in a larger-scale, controlled, randomized trial. The 88 predominantly dually diagnosed adolescents were randomized to one of the two 8-week group interventions. Youths in the CBT group exhibited significantly lower rates of positive urinalysis than did subjects receiving psychoeducational therapies for older youths at 3-month follow-up. Moreover, Teen Addiction Severity Index subscales (Kaminer et al. 1991) indicated sound improvement from baseline to 3-month and to 9-month follow-up across conditions.

The Cannabis Youth Treatment (2000) study has been the largest (N=600), most influential collaborative project designed to address the differential efficacy of the treatments implemented and the contribution of treatment dose to outcome. A total of five interventions were evaluated across the four study sites. Two group CBT interventions were offered. Both began with two individual motivational-enhancement therapy (MET) sessions, followed by either three CBT sessions (MET/CBT-5) (Sampl and Kadden 2001) or 10 CBT sessions (MET/CBT-12) (Webb et al. 2002). A third intervention represented a family-based add-on intervention involving MET/CBT-12 plus a 6-week family psychoeducational intervention. In addition, a 12-session individual adolescent community reinforcement approach and a 12-week family therapy condition were included. The five treatment models were evaluated in two arms, in a community-based program and an academic medical center. Although all five models were not implemented within treatment sites, the replication of the MET/CBT-5 intervention across all four sites made it possible to study site differences and conduct quasi-experimental comparisons of the interventions across study arms.

Dennis and his colleagues (in press) reported that all five interventions produced significant reductions in cannabis use and negative consequences of use from pretreatment to the 3-month follow-up, and that these reductions were sustained through the 12-month follow-up. In addition, changes in marijuana use were accompanied by reductions in behavioral problems, family problems, school problems, school absences, argumentativeness, violence, and illegal activity.

Although they were not entirely expected, some initial differences were found across conditions. For example, the 12-session CBT produced initially poorer outcomes, whereas the CBT plus support produced initially better outcomes, relative to the briefer CBT intervention—findings that are inconsistent with a simple dose-response relationship. Also, despite considerable support for family interventions in the literature, the individual (community reinforcement approach) and individual/group (MET/CBT-5) behavioral interventions produced better outcomes than the family approach (multidimensional family therapy) in terms of days of substance use at 3 months. Nevertheless, these initial differences were not sustained, and the best predictor of long-term outcomes was initial level of change.

Recognition of the heterogeneity of individuals with substance use disorders led to increasing interest in the issue of patient-treatment matching, or the identification of variables that predict differential responses to various interventions (Litt et al. 1992; Mattson et al. 1994). However, no evidence for matching was found in Project MATCH, a large multicenter study on the treatment of alcoholism that employed CBT, MET, and 12-step treatment strategies (Project MATCH Research Group 1997). No matching effects specific for adolescents have been found in a study in which a potential matching between psychopathology (e.g., internalizing and externalizing disorders) and

therapeutic interventions (e.g., CBT, interactional therapy) was hypothesized (Kaminer et al. 1998a). Most recently, however, Kaminer and colleagues (2002a) reported that older as well as male adolescent substance abusers responded better to CBT than to a psychoeducational approach. Babor and colleagues (2002) noted that there was evidence for treatment matching in the Cannabis Youth Treatment study. Adolescents with internalizing disorders and those with difficult temperament did best in family therapy, whereas those without difficult temperament did better in the MET/CBT-5 condition. It is noteworthy that these results do not preclude the possibility that there may be a differential response to other treatment modalities that were not included in these studies.

Another effort to establish a matching effect is the development by the American Society of Addiction Medicine of placement criteria for adults and adolescents. The purpose of these criteria is to enhance objective matching decisions for different severity levels to various settings of care. There has been little research on placement criteria despite their extensive use in clinical settings. Results indicate that the validity of these criteria and their clinical utility is rather limited (Steinberg and Babor 1997). Matching a substance-abusing patient with the right type of treatment program is a much discussed but elusive goal in the real world. A patient may not have the option of referring or switching to a more appropriate treatment program. Opportunities may be limited by geographical, slot availability, insurance, psychiatric comorbidity, legal, or other considerations.

It is suggested that following a comprehensive multidimensional functional assessment of a patient's needs, efforts should be redirected from matching patients with programs to matching patients' problems with targeted services meeting their needs within the program. This model could be tailored to be complementary or an alternative to future revised and tested American Society of Addiction Medicine placement criteria.

A comorbid psychiatric disorder may be the primary reason adolescents with substance use disorder seek treatment. Indeed, Friedman and Glickman (1987) reported that 28% of adolescents sought treatment because of an emotional or psychiatric problem. The effect of psychiatric comorbidity on treatment outcome in adolescents with comorbid disorders has been addressed by Kaminer and colleagues (1992, 2002a), who reported that subjects who were noncompleters and those who failed to show for follow-up were more likely to have a diagnosis of conduct disorder.

Relative to research evaluating the efficacy of psychosocial interventions for adolescent substance use problems, research evaluating the efficacy of pharmacotherapeutic interventions for substance abuse in teenagers has been neglected. Yet the largest subgroup of adolescents with substance use disorders presenting in clinical settings are those with both substance use and other psychiatric disorders. This particular subgroup may stand to benefit the most from effective pharmacotherapies. Studies of pharmacotherapies specific to a substance of abuse or a comorbid psychiatric disorder in youths have usually been in the form of single case reports or of small open-label studies. Only recently have several controlled studies been initiated. It is still premature to report any findings. However, preliminary guidelines for the use of integrated pharmacotherapy and psychosocial interventions in dually diagnosed youths were published by Riggs and Davies (2002). For a comprehensive review of specific pharmacotherapies, the interested reader is referred to Kaminer (2001b).

Conclusion

The recent controlled clinical trials evaluating treatments for adolescent substance use disorders have contributed substantial new empirical evidence supporting the efficacy of treatment for substance use disorders. Research focused on improving short-term and long-term outcomes, improving engagement techniques (especially for individuals with conduct disorder and other severe disturbances), and identifying youths for whom different treatment modalities or integrative interventions are likely to be beneficial is urgently needed. Moreover, the problems of relapse and lack of maintenance of treatment gains make research on continuing care or aftercare an important focus of investigation.

References

Alterman AI, Tarter RE: An Examination of Selected Topologies: Hyperactivity, Familial and Antisocial Alcoholism: Recent Developments in Alcoholism, Vol 4. New York, Plenum, 1986

American Psychiatric Association: Diagnostic and Statistical Manual of Mental Disorders, 4th Edition. Washington, DC, American Psychiatric Association, 1994

American Psychiatric Association: Diagnostic and Statistical Manual of Mental Disorders, 4th Edition, Text Revision. Washington, DC, American Psychiatric Association, 2000

Anthony JC, Petronis KR: Early-onset drug use and risk of later drug problems. Drug Alcohol Depend 40:9–15, 1995

Azrin NH, Donohue B, Besalel VA: Youth drug abuse treatment: a controlled outcome study. Journal of Child and Adolescent Substance Abuse 3:1–16, 1994

Babor TF, Dolinsky ZS, Meyer RE, et al: Types of alcoholics: concurrent and predictive validity of some common classification schemes. Br J Addict 87:1415–1431, 1992

Babor TF, Webb C, Burleson JA, et al: Subtypes for classifying adolescents with marijuana use disorders: construct validity and clinical implications. Addiction 97 (suppl 1):58–69, 2002

Bangert-Drowns RL: The effects of school-based substance abuse education: a meta-analysis. J Drug Educ 18:243–264, 1988

Barrett ME, Simpson DD, Lehman WE: Behavioral changes of adolescents in drug abuse intervention programs. J Clin Psychol 44:461–473, 1988

Bates ME, Labouvie EW: Personality-environment constellations and alcohol use: a process-oriented study of intraindividual change during adolescence. Psychology of Addiction Behavior 9:23–35, 1995

Bates ME, Labouvie EW: Adolescent risk factors and the prediction of persistent alcohol and drug use into adulthood. Alcohol Clin Exp Res 21:944–950, 1997

Biederman J, Wilens T, Mick E, et al: Is ADHD a risk factor for psychoactive substance use disorders? Findings from a four-year prospective follow-up study. J Am Acad Child Adolesc Psychiatry 36:21–29, 1997

Blackson TC: Temperament: a salient correlate of risk factors for alcohol and drug abuse. Drug Alcohol Depend 36:205–214, 1994

Blood L, Cornwall A: Pretreatment variables that predict completion of an adolescent substance abuse treatment program. J Nerv Ment Dis 182:14–19, 1994

Botvin GJ, Griffin KW: Life skills training: theory, methods, and effectiveness of a drug abuse prevention approach, in Innovations in Adolescent Substance Abuse Interventions. Edited by Wagner EF, Waldron HB. Amsterdam, Elsevier Science, 2001, pp 31–50

Botvin GJ, Baker E, Dusenbury I, et al: Long-term follow-up results of a randomized drug abuse prevention trial in a white middle-class population. JAMA 273:1106–1112, 1995

Brent DA, Perper JA, Allman C: Alcohol, firearms and suicide among youth: temporal trends in Allegheny County, Pennsylvania, 1960 to 1983. JAMA 257:3369–3372, 1987

Brook JS, Whiteman M, Gordon AS, et al: The psychosocial etiology of adolescent drug use: a family interactional approach. Genet Soc Gen Psychol Monogr 116:113–267, 1990

Brown SA, Vik PN, Creamer V: Characteristics of relapse following adolescent substance abuse treatment. Addict Behav 14:291–300, 1989

Brown SA, Myers MG, Mott MA, et al: Correlates of success following treatment for adolescent substance abuse. Appl Prev Psychol 3:61–73, 1994

Buchan BJ, Dennis ML, Tims FM, et al: Cannabis use: consistency and validity of self-report, on-site urine testing and laboratory testing. Addiction 97 (suppl 1):98–108, 2002

Bukstein OG, Kaminer Y: The nosology of adolescent substance abuse. Am J Addict 3:1–13, 1994

Bukstein OG, Brent DA, Kaminer Y: Comorbidity of substance abuse and other psychiatric disorders in adolescents. Am J Psychiatry 146:1131–1141, 1989

Bukstein OG, Glancy LJ, Kaminer Y: Patterns of affective comorbidity in a clinical population of dually diagnosed substance abusers. J Am Acad Child Adolesc Psychiatry 31:1041–1045, 1992

Bulik CM: Drug and alcohol abuse by bulimic women and their families. Am J Psychiatry 144:1604–1606, 1987

Burk JP, Sher KJ: Labeling the child of an alcoholic: negative stereotyping by mental health professionals and peers. J Stud Alcohol 51:156–163, 1990

Burleson J, Kaminer Y: Adolescent alcohol and marijuana use: concordance among objective-, self-, and collateral reports of use. Paper presented at the 25th annual meeting of the Research Society on Alcoholism, San Francisco, CA, June 28, 2002

Cannabis Youth Treatment Group: Cannabis Youth Treatment (CYT) Experiment: Preliminary Findings. A Report to the Center for Substance Abuse Treatment (CSAT). Rockville, MD, Substance Abuse and Mental Health Services Administration, U.S. Department of Health and Human Services, 2000

Cantwell DP, Lewinsohn PM, Rohde P, et al: Correspondence between adolescent report and parent report of psychiatric diagnostic data. J Am Acad Child Adolesc Psychiatry 36:610–619, 1997

Catalano RF, Hawkins JD, Wells EA, et al: Evaluation of the effectiveness of adolescent drug abuse treatment, assessment of risks for relapse, and promising approaches for relapse prevention. Int J Addict 25:1085–1140, 1990–1991

Catalano RF, Hawkins JD, Krenz C, et al: Using research to guide culturally appropriate drug abuse prevention. J Consult Clin Psychol 61:804–811, 1993

Christie KA, Burke JD, Regier DA, et al: Epidemiologic evidence for early onset of mental disorders and higher risk of drug abuse in young adults. Am J Psychiatry 145:971–975, 1988

Clark DB, Sayette MA: Anxiety and the development of alcoholism. Am J Addict 2:56–76, 1993

Clark DB, Bukstein OG, Smith MG, et al: Identifying anxiety disorders in adolescents hospitalized for alcohol abuse or dependence. Psychiatr Serv 46:618–620, 1995

Cloninger CR: Neurogenetic adaptive mechanisms in alcoholism. Science 236:410–415, 1987

Coate D, Grossman N: Change in alcoholic beverage prices and legal drinking age. Alcohol Health Res World Fall: 22–25, 1987

Corby EA, Roll JM, Ledgerwood DM, et al: Contingency management interventions for treating the substance abuse of adolescents: a feasibility study. Exp Clin Psychopharmacol 8:371–376, 2000

Deas D, Thomas SE: An overview of controlled studies of adolescent substance abuse treatment. Am J Addict 10:178–189, 2001

Dennis ML, Godley SH, Diamond G, et al: Main findings of the Cannabis Youth Treatment randomized field experiment. J Subst Abuse Treatment (in press)

Deykin EY, Buka SL, Zeena TH: Depressive illness among chemically dependent adolescents. Am J Psychiatry 149:1341–1347, 1992

Doyle H, Delaney W, Trobin J: Follow-up study of young attendees at an alcohol unit. Addiction 89:183–189, 1994

Earls F, Jung K: Temperament and home environment characteristics in the early development of child psychopathology. J Am Acad Child Adolesc Psychiatry 26:491–498, 1987

Erikson EH: Identity: Youth and Crisis. New York, WW Norton, 1968

Friedman AS, Glickman NW: Program characteristics for successful treatment of adolescent drug abuse. J Nerv Ment Dis 174:669–679, 1987

Friedman AS, Utada A: A method for diagnosing and planning the treatment of adolescent drug abusers (the Adolescent Drug Abuse Diagnosis [ADAD] instrument). J Drug Educ 19:285–312, 1989

Friedman AS, Schwartz R, Utada A: Outcome of a unique youth drug abuse program: a follow-up study of clients of Straight, Inc. J Subst Abuse Treat 6:259–268, 1989

Godley MD, Godley SH, Dennis ML, et al: Preliminary outcomes from the assertive continuing care experiment for adolescents discharged from residential treatment. J Subst Abuse Treat 23:21–32, 2002

Golub A, Johnson BD: The shifting importance of alcohol and marijuana as gateway substances among serious drug abusers. J Stud Alcohol 55:607–614, 1994

Goodwin DW: Alcoholism and genetics: the sins of the fathers. Arch Gen Psychiatry 42:171–174, 1985

Griffiths M: Adolescent Gambling. London, Routledge, 1995

Grilo CM, Becker DF, Walker ML, et al: Psychiatric comorbidity in adolescent inpatients with substance use disorders. J Am Acad Child Adolesc Psychiatry 34:1085–1091, 1995

Harrison PA, Fulkerson JA, Beebe TJ: DSM-IV substance use disorder criteria for adolescents: a critical examination based on a statewide school survey. Am J Psychiatry 155:486–492, 1998

Hasin DS, Grant B, Endicott J: The natural history of alcohol abuse: implications for definitions of alcohol use disorders. Am J Psychiatry 147:337–341, 1990

Hawkins JD, Catalano RF, Miller JY: Risk and protective factors for alcohol and other drug problems in adolescence and early adulthood: implications for substance abuse prevention. Psychol Bull 112:64–105, 1992

Henggeler SW, Melton GB, Smith LA: Family preservation using multi-systemic therapy: an effective alternative to incarcerating serious juvenile offenders. J Consult Clin Psychol 66:953–961, 1992

Henggeler SW, Pickrel SG, Brondino MJ, et al: Eliminating treatment dropout of substance abusing or dependent delinquents through home-based multisystemic therapy. Am J Psychiatry 153:427–428, 1996

Hovens J, Cantwell DP, Kiriakos R: Psychiatric comorbidity in hospitalized adolescent substance abusers. J Am Acad Child Adolesc Psychiatry 33:476–483, 1994

Johnston LD, O'Malley IM, Bachman JG: Results of the 26th national "Monitoring the Future" survey (press release). Ann Arbor, MI, University of Michigan, 2001

Kaminer Y: Adolescent Substance Abuse: A Comprehensive Guide to Theory and Practice. New York, Plenum, 1994

Kaminer Y: Adolescent substance abuse and suicidal behavior, in Adolescent Substance Abuse and Dual Disorders. Child Adolescent Psychiatric Clinics in North America Series. Edited by Jaffe SL. Philadelphia, PA, WB Saunders, 1996, pp 59–71

Kaminer Y: Contingency management reinforcement procedures for adolescent substance abuse. J Am Acad Child Adolesc Psychiatry 39:1324–1326, 2000

Kaminer Y: Alcohol and drug abuse: adolescent substance abuse treatment; where do we go from here? Psychiatr Serv 52:147–149, 2001a

Kaminer Y: Psychopharmacological therapy, in Innovations in Adolescent Substance Abuse Interventions. Edited by Wagner EF, Waldron HB. Amsterdam, Elsevier Science, 2001b, pp 285–311

Kaminer Y, Bukstein OG, Tarter TE: The Teen Addiction Severity Index: rationale and reliability. Int J Addict 26:219–226, 1991

Kaminer Y, Tarter RE, Bukstein OG, et al: Comparison between treatment completers and noncompleters among dual-diagnosed substance-abusing adolescents. J Am Acad Child Adolesc Psychiatry 31:1046–1049, 1992

Kaminer Y, Wagner E, Plummer B, et al: Validation of the Teen Addiction Severity Index: preliminary findings. Am J Addict 2:221–224, 1993

Kaminer Y, Blitz C, Burleson JA, et al: Measuring treatment process in cognitive-behavioral and interactional group therapies for adolescent substance abusers. J Nerv Ment Dis 186:407–413, 1998a

Kaminer Y, Blitz C, Burleson JA, et al: The Teen Treatment Services Review (T-TSR). J Subst Abuse Treat 15:291–300, 1998b

Kaminer Y, Burleson JA, Blitz C, et al: Psychotherapies for adolescent substance abusers: a pilot study. J Nerv Ment Dis 186:684–690, 1998c

Kaminer Y, Burleson JA, Goldberger R: Cognitive-behavioral coping skills and psychoeducation therapies for adolescent substance abuse. J Nerv Ment Dis 190:737–745, 2002a

Kaminer Y, Burleson J, Jadamec A: Gambling behavior in adolescent substance abusers. Subst Abus 23:191–198, 2002b

Kandel DB: Epidemiological and psychosocial perspective on adolescent drug use. J Am Acad Child Adolesc Psychiatry 20:328–347, 1982

Kandel DB, Davies M, Karus D, et al: The consequences in young adulthood of adolescent drug involvement. Arch Gen Psychiatry 43:746–754, 1986

Kolar AF, Brown BS, Haertzen CA, et al: Children of substance abusers: the life experiences of children of opiate addicts in methadone maintenance. Am J Drug Alcohol Abuse 20:159–171, 1994

Kushner MG, Sher KJ, Beitman BD: The relation between alcohol problems and anxiety disorders. Am J Psychiatry 147:685–695, 1990

Labouvie E: Maturing out of substance use: selection and self-correction. J Drug Issues 26:455–474, 1996

Lewinsohn PM, Rohde P, Seeley J: Alcohol consumption in high school adolescents: frequency of use and dimensional structure of associated problems. Addiction 91:375–390, 1996

Liddle HA, Dakof GA: Family based treatment for adolescent drug use: state of the science, in Adolescent Drug Abuse: Clinical Assessment and Therapeutic Interventions (NIH Publ No 95-3908). Edited by Rahdert E, Czechowicz D. Rockville, MD, National Institute on Drug Abuse, 1995, pp 218–254

Liddle HA, Dakof GA, Diamond G, et al: Multidimensional family therapy for adolescent substance abuse: results of a randomized clinical trial. Am J Drug Alcohol Abuse 27:651–687, 2001

Litt MD, Babor TF, DelBoca FK, et al: Types of alcoholics, II: application of an empirically derived typology to treatment matching. Arch Gen Psychiatry 49:609–614, 1992

Loeber R: Natural histories of conduct problems, delinquency and associated substance use, in Advances in Clinical Child Psychology. Edited by Lahey BB, Kazdin AE. New York, Plenum, 1988, pp 73–124

Martin CS: Presented at the annual meeting of the Research Society on Alcohol, San Francisco, CA, June 27, 2002

Martin CS, Kaczynski NA, Maisto SA, et al: Patterns of DSM-IV alcohol abuse and dependence symptoms in adolescent drinkers. J Stud Alcohol 56:672–680, 1995

Mattson ME, Allen JP, Longabaugh R, et al: A chronological review of empirical studies matching alcoholic clients to treatment. J Stud Alcohol Suppl 12:16–29, 1994

Maziade M, Caron C, Cote P, et al: Extreme temperament and diagnosis: a study in a psychiatric sample of consecutive children. Arch Gen Psychiatry 47:477–484, 1990

Milin R, Halikas JA, Meller JE, et al: Psychopathology among substance abusing juvenile offenders. J Am Acad Child Adolesc Psychiatry 30:569–574, 1991

Miller G: The Substance Abuse Subtle Screening Inventory—Adolescent Version. Bloomington, IN, SASSI Institute, 1990

Myers MG, Brown SA, Mott MA: Preadolescent conduct disorder behaviors predict relapse and progression of addiction for adolescent alcohol and drug abusers. Alcohol Clin Exp Res 19:1528–1536, 1995

Newcomb MD: Identifying high-risk youth: prevalence and patterns of adolescent drug abuse, in Adolescent Drug Abuse: Clinical Assessment and Therapeutic Interventions (NIH Publ No 95-3908). Edited by Rahdert E, Czechowicz D. Rockville, MD, National Institute on Drug Abuse, 1995, pp 7–38

Noll RB, Zucker RA, Fitzgerald HE, et al: Cognitive and motoric functioning of sons of alcoholic fathers and controls: the early childhood years. Dev Psychol 28:665–675, 1992

O'Malley PM, Wagenaar AC: Effects of minimum drinking age laws on alcohol use, related behaviors and traffic crash involvement among American youth: 1976–1987. J Stud Alcohol 52:478–491, 1991

Penick EC, Powell BJ, Liskow BI, et al: The stability of coexisting psychiatric syndromes in alcoholic men after one year. J Stud Alcohol 49:395–405, 1988

Petraitis J, Flay BR, Miller TQ: Reviewing theories of adolescent substance use: organizing pieces of the puzzle. Psychol Bull 117:67–86, 1995

Pollock NK, Martin CS: Diagnostic orphans: adolescents with alcohol symptoms who do not qualify for DSM-IV abuse or dependence diagnoses. Am J Psychiatry 156:897–901, 1999

Project MATCH Research Group: Matching alcoholism treatments to client heterogeneity: Project MATCH post-treatment drinking outcomes. J Stud Alcohol 58:7–29, 1997

Rahdert E: The Adolescent Assessment and Referral System Manual (DHHS Publ No ADM 91-1735). Rockville, MD, National Institute on Drug Abuse, 1991

Reich W, Earls F, Frankel O, et al: Psychopathology in children of alcoholics. J Am Acad Child Adolesc Psychiatry 32:995–1002, 1993

Riggs PD, Davies RD: A clinical approach to integrating treatment for adolescent depression and substance abuse. J Am Acad Child Adolesc Psychiatry 41:1253–1255, 2002

Rohde P, Lewinsohn PM, Seeley JR: Psychiatric comorbidity with problematic alcohol use in high school students. J Am Acad Child Adolesc Psychiatry 35:101–109, 1996

Rounsaville BJ, Kleber HD: Psychiatric disorders in opiate addicts: preliminary findings on course and interaction with program type, in Psychopathology and Addictive Disorders. Edited by Meyer RE. New York, Guilford, 1986, pp 140–168

Sampl S, Kadden R: Motivational Enhancement Therapy and Cognitive Behavioral Therapy for Adolescent Cannabis Users: Five Sessions. Cannabis Youth Treatment Series, Vol 1. Rockville, MD, Center for Substance Abuse Treatment, 2001

Schaffer K, Parson O, Yohman J: Neuropsychological differences between male familial alcoholics and nonalcoholics. Alcohol Clin Exp Res 8:347–351, 1984

Schinke SP, Botvin GJ, Orlani MA: Substance Abuse in Children and Adolescents: Evaluation and Intervention. Newbury Park, CA, Sage, 1991

Shedler J, Block J: Adolescent drug use and psychological health: a longitudinal inquiry. Am Psychol 45:612–630, 1990

Steinberg KL, Babor TF: Patient-treatment matching using the ASAM criteria. Paper presented at the American Society of Addiction Medicine Medical-Scientific Conference, San Diego, CA, April 18–20, 1997

Stowell RJ: Dual diagnosis issues. Psychiatr Ann 21:98–104, 1991

Szapocznik J, Perez-Vidal A, Briskman AL, et al: Engaging adolescent drug abusers and their families in treatment. J Consult Clin Psychol 56:552–557, 1988

Tarter RE: Evaluation and treatment of adolescent substance abuse: a decision tree method. Am J Drug Alcohol Abuse 16:1–46, 1990

Tarter RE, Laird SB, Moss HB: Neuropsychological and neurophysiological characteristics of children of alcoholics, in Children of Alcoholics: Critical Perspectives. Edited by Windel M, Searles JS. New York, Guilford, 1990a, pp 73–98

Tarter RE, Laird SB, Mostefa K, et al: Drug abuse severity in adolescents is associated with magnitude of deviation in temperamental traits. Br J Addict 85:1501–1504, 1990b

Tarter RE, Kirisci L, Hegedus A, et al: Heterogeneity of adolescent alcoholism. Ann NY Acad Sci 708:172–180, 1994

Tarter RE, Kirisci L, Mezzich A: Multivariate typology of adolescents with alcohol use disorder. Am J Addict 6:150–158, 1997

Teichman M, Barnea Z, Ravav G: Personality and substance use among adolescents: a longitudinal study. Br J Addict 84:181–190, 1989

Tobler NS: Meta-analysis of 143 adolescent drug prevention programs: quantitative outcome results of program participants compared to a control or comparison group. J Drug Issues 16:537–567, 1986

Ungemack JA, Hartwell SW, Babor TF: Alcohol and drug abuse among Connecticut youth: implications for adolescent medicine and public health. Conn Med 61:577–585, 1997

Van Hasselt VB, Null JA, Kempton T: Social skills and depression in adolescent substance abusers. Addict Behav 18:9–18, 1993

Vik PW, Grisel K, Brown SA: Social resource characteristics and adolescent substance abuse relapse. Journal of Adolescent Chemical Dependency 2:59–74, 1992

Wagner EF, Brown SA, Monti PM, et al: Innovations in adolescent substance abuse intervention. Alcohol Clin Exp Res 23:236–249, 1999

Waldron HR, Kaminer Y: On the learning curve: the emerging evidence supporting cognitive-behavioral therapies for adolescent substance abuse. Addiction (in press)

Waldron HR, Slesnick N, Brody JL, et al: Treatment outcomes for adolescent substance abuse at 4- and 7-month assessments. J Consult Clin Psychol 69:802–813, 2001

Webb C, Scudder M, Kaminer Y, et al: Motivational Enhancement Therapy and Cognitive Behavioral Therapy for Adolescent Cannabis Users: Seven Sessions. Cannabis Youth Treatment Series, Vol 1. Rockville, MD, Center for Substance Abuse Treatment, 2002

Wilens TE, Biederman J, Spencer TJ: Comorbidity of attention-deficit disorder and psychoactive substance use disorders. Hosp Community Psychiatry 45:421–435, 1994

Wilens TE, Biederman J, Kiely K: Pilot study of behavioral and emotional disturbances in the high-risk children of parents with opioid dependence. J Am Acad Child Adolesc Psychiatry 34:779–785, 1995

Wilson JR, Crowe L: Genetics of alcoholism: can and should youth at risk be identified? Alcohol Health Res World 15:11–17, 1991

Winters KC: Development of an adolescent alcohol and drug abuse screening scale: Personal Experience Screening Questionnaire. Addict Behav 17:479–490, 1992

Winters KC: Treating adolescents with substance use disorders: an overview of practice issues and treatment outcome. Subst Abus 20:203–225, 1999

Winters KC, Henly G: Personal Experience Inventory (PEI). Los Angeles, CA, Western Psychological Services, 1988

Winters KC, Stinchfield RD, Opland E: The effectiveness of the Minnesota Model approach in the treatment of adolescent drug abusers. Addiction 95:601–612, 2000

Winters KC, Latimer WW, Stinchfield R: Assessing adolescent substance use, in Innovations in Adolescent Substance Abuse Interventions. Edited by Wagner EF, Waldron HB. Amsterdam, Elsevier Science, 2001, pp 1–29

Wolin S, Wolin SJ: The challenge model: working with strengths in children of substance-abusing parents, in Adolescent Substance Abuse and Dual Disorders. Child Adolescent Psychiatric Clinics in North America Series. Edited by Jaffe SL. Philadelphia, PA, WB Saunders, 1996, pp 243–255

Zuckerman M: Behavioral Expressions and Biosocial Bases of Sensation Seeking. New York, Cambridge University Press, 1994

Ethnic Minorities and the Elderly

Edith S. Lisansky Gomberg, Ph.D.

Study of ethnic minorities has increased in recent years, and more attention has been paid to special populations. Treatment and research on addictions in these populations is a subject for *Alcohol Alert,* a publication of the National Institute on Alcohol Abuse and Alcoholism (2002). Even nonprofessional publications have occasional stories on such topics, particularly on elderly people. In April 2002, an article entitled "Hidden Plague of Alcohol Abuse by the Elderly" by medical reporter Jane Brody (2002) appeared in the *New York Times.* In its magazine *Modern Maturity,* the American Association of Retired Persons (2002) published a story entitled "Too Much Time in a Bottle?" The article concerns an elderly father "who chooses to spend his last years in an alcoholic haze."

Minorities, of course, are not only characteristic of the United States. For example, as a result of population shifts that have taken place in the European Union, political issues have arisen about dealing with immigrant populations and limiting further immigration in several European countries where there are large groups of North Africans, Arabs from various countries, Turks, and Gypsies. The minorities discussed in this chapter are the four federally mandated

minority groups in the United States: African Americans; American Indians and Alaska Natives; Hispanics; and Asian Americans and Pacific Islanders. None of these groups are homogeneous. African Americans are of varied racial origin (admixtures of Caucasian and American Indian as well as African backgrounds); Hispanics, who constitute a language group, come from Central and South America, Mexico, Puerto Rico, and Cuba and the other Caribbean islands with all their different subcultures; Asian Americans include those from China, Japan, Korea, and other Asian countries; and American Indians are divided by tribal groupings, such as Hopi, Plains Indians, Apache, and Navaho, with variations in customs and language.

The epidemiology of substance use and abuse has been well studied and documented in two areas: the use and abuse of alcohol and the use and misuse of prescription drugs. In the year 2000, rates of heavy alcohol use were highest in the age group 21–25. Underage (ages 12–20) past-month alcohol use was highest among whites, followed by American Indians and Alaska Natives.

Although drinking in general drops off among older adults, it should be noted that alcohol was the primary substance of abuse among individuals age 55 and older who were admitted to publicly funded substance abuse treatment (Substance Abuse and Mental Health Services Administration 2001a). Older persons tend to be more frequent users of prescribed drugs. The 2000 National Household Survey on Drug Abuse (Substance Abuse and Mental Health Services Administration 2001b) indicated that about 1% of older adults in the United States had used an illicit drug in the past month, usually psychotherapeutic drugs used nonmedically or marijuana; among older adults, use of illicit drugs was highest in the age group 55–59 and declined with increasing age. Whites had higher rates of past-month illicit drug use (possibly because of more access to health systems and hence to medications). It is estimated that illicit drug use among the elderly will increase in the coming decades because the "baby boom" generation is aging.

National surveys show that current and heavy drinking are most prevalent among American Indians and Alaska Natives. Alcohol intake is lowest among Asian Americans. Among adolescents, the heaviest alcohol intake occurs among Hispanic youths, followed by whites (Johnston et al. 2001). African American adolescents show a very low rate of alcohol intake and the lowest frequency of being drunk. Insofar as effects of alcohol intake go, most medical research has focused on cirrhosis. Related to drinking levels and problems, deaths from liver disease and cirrhosis are four times more prevalent among American Indians and Alaska Natives. Hispanics are twice as likely as whites to die from liver cirrhosis. (It is estimated that they consume more alcohol per drinking occasion than do whites.) Reported percentages for drinking and driving were 19% for American Indians and Alaska Natives, 11% for whites and Hispanics, 7% for African Americans, and below 6% for Asian Americans (Beauvais 1998; Stinson et al. 1998).

Studies of ethnic groups' attitudes toward drinking and drinking behaviors in the 1940s and the 1950s involved several immigrant groups: the Irish, the Jews, the Italians, and the Chinese. In the 1960s, national survey research developed, and ethnic identification increased. The perception of the "drunken Indians" was reexamined (MacAndrew and Edgerton 1969). Stivers's (1976) report on drinking among Irish Americans called attention to the changes that could occur with new circumstances; for example, drinking among Irish Americans was not the same as premigration drinking in Ireland.

African Americans

Herd (1985) concluded that ambivalence about alcohol is universal and is particularly high among African Americans. Two different subcultures emerged during the twentieth century. The first is the result of Southern African Americans migrating northward and developing urban attitudes of tolerance and a nightclub culture (e.g., in Harlem during Prohibition); this subculture produced the Black Renaissance in literature and the other arts during the 1920s. The second subculture is that comprising churchgoers and the temperance movement. Members of this subculture were often involved in the struggle to attain political and social equality. Even though there were segregated black chapters, many African American women joined the Women's Christian Temperance Union. During the Prohibition years, hospital admissions rose and there were disproportionate alcohol-related deaths among African Americans; rates of mortality from cirrhosis increased steeply in the 1950s. Some theorists have advanced views about "stress" and response to oppression; however, the evidence offers little support. Herd offers an alternative view—that is, that African American attitudes toward alcoholic beverages are affected by changes in the larger society and by major demographic changes among African Americans.

Gaines (1985) distinguished between "respectable drinking" (sipping, moderate weekend drinking) and problem drinking. Among adults (ages 30–50), prevailing attitudes about alcohol use by men and by women differed sharply; for example, "it was considered totally unacceptable for any woman to be drunk in public." (It would be useful to study whether this difference in attitude still exists; African Americans have, to a limited extent, joined the feminist movement.)

Reporting on a survey done in the mid-1980s, Herd (1989) noted that black and white men had similar drinking patterns. Black and white women's patterns were different, however. For example, half of the black women were abstainers, whereas only one-third of the white women abstained. The age differences identified in the same survey were that less drinking occurred among black adolescents than among white adolescents and more heavy and problem drinking occurred among middle-aged blacks than among middle-aged whites. Cirrhosis appeared to be a problem, but, interestingly enough, this was not the case among the blacks who did not migrate north.

Gaines also pointed out that African American culture is "familistic" and tends to resist accepting treatment from strangers. Lack of trust and fear of criminalization and oppression, a commonly held theory of the etiology of problem drinking, is based on attitudes and behaviors encountered in the problem drinker's social world, relatives, lovers, and work companions. Drinking heavily is seen as a response to frustration—the "blues." Another area of concern is confidentiality and the possibility of gossip being spread about those receiving treatment. It is important to note that in Malcolm X's autobiography (X 1965) his description of the preferred Black Muslim treatment for those having problems with drugs or alcohol closely parallels the 12 steps of Alcoholics Anonymous (AA).

Black culture is not unitary. For example, a growing number of African Americans can be described as middle class. Whether social class definition and point of origin (e.g., Africa, the southern United States, the Caribbean) may be added to age and gender differences as variables remains to be seen, but treatment will have to deal with all of these—to say nothing of the lightness or darkness of the patient, occupation, drinking history, and other factors. Early ethnographic studies were of "street corner men" (currently referred to as "the homeless"), but more recent studies have focused on working black men and women and on middle-class respondents.

American Indians/Alaska Natives

There is a long history of alcohol-related problems—and, more recently, problems with drugs in general—among American Indians and Alaska Natives. A study of the Navaho by Venner and Miller (2001) suggests that the symptomatic progression of problem drinking differs from that seen in Jellinek's (1960) original sample of AA members. Gender differences are quite marked; women show more comorbidity (e.g., depression), more cocaine dependence, less marijuana dependence, and more medication use. Such differences must obviously be considered in treatment planning.

Two recent publications by the National Institute on Alcohol Abuse and Alcoholism are relevant. In 1998, *Alcohol Health and Research World* published a special edition on minorities. Beauvais (1998) reviewed the work on Native American subgroups and noted that the inclusion of their belief systems about alcohol

and their approaches to problem drinking would be useful in treatment and prevention.

There are more than 200 tribes of Native Americans, each with its own customs and belief systems. Some tribes vigorously enforce abstinence, and some tribes have major problems with alcohol abuse and abuse of other drugs. The use of traditional treatment methods by professional counselors and therapists has not met with much success. It is probably true that traditional Native American forms of treatment and healing combined with orthodox treatment techniques would be most effective. It does seem clear that the most effective therapists for this population are probably Native Americans who are recovering alcoholics.

In a recent comparison of beverage choices of Native American and black women, Graves and Kaskutas (2002) concluded that alcohol research concerning urban subjects should inquire not only about consumption of beer, wine, and spirits but also about stronger beer products. These authors note that urban minorities, particularly the African American and Hispanic communities, are the chief target populations for marketing of alcoholic beverages.

Weibel-Orlando (1985) describes many treatment modalities that are in use with Native Americans:

1. *Medical model:* alcoholism as a disease (AA)
2. *Abusive drinking as symptoms:* sociopsychoanalytic orientation
3. *Assimilative model:* Indian-run, using standard modalities
4. *Culture-sensitive model:* group therapy using Indian themes and counselors
5. *Syncretic model:* use of Indian ceremonial practices and standard interventions
6. *Traditional model:* use of Indian spirituality

The programs that are most successful are those that integrate spiritual elements into treatment strategies. The American Indian Movement strongly advocates abstinence from all intoxicants.

Hispanics

The Substance Abuse and Mental Health Services Administration (1998) issued a report on substance abuse among racial and ethnic subgroups during the early 1990s. The highest percentage of heavy alcohol use was by Mexican Americans, followed by Caucasians and some other Hispanic groups (e.g., Puerto Ricans). Still other Hispanic groups (Cubans, Central Americans, Caribbean Islanders, and South Americans) ranked lower. Alcohol dependence was highest among Native Americans, followed by Mexican Americans.

There are many subgroups of Hispanics: Mexican Americans, Puerto Ricans, Dominicans, Guatemalans, Salvadorians, and others. Caetano (1989) reported from an interview survey that the Hispanics from Mexico drank larger quantities of alcoholic beverages and reported more alcohol-related problems. Quantity and frequency of drinking varied within the Hispanic population by gender, age, income, and education. Drinking problems among the general American male population peak in the 20s and begin to decline in the 30s, but Hispanic men tend to maintain alcohol-related problems longer and to show a decline in such problems in their 40s. All Hispanic males (from different Hispanic subgroups) responded that in their 30s, men had more freedom to drink than younger men.

Three Hispanic groups in the northeastern United States have been studied: Dominicans, Guatemalans, and Puerto Ricans. Dominicans tend to migrate with their families, and they drink in moderate amounts on Saturday nights with families at social clubs. Guatemalans drink beer heavily through extended weekends. Puerto Ricans have assimilated the drinking customs of the mainland United States, and when problem drinking occurs, they are likely to seek treatment in a Pentecostal church group, whereas other Hispanic groups tend to reject the Pentecostals. Puerto Ricans vary in their attitudes toward and acceptance of AA; in New York City they were active in AA, but in other northeastern cities they did not participate. It is of interest that AA is a more accepted cultural tradition in Guatemala than in other Central American states. Another source of treatment for alcohol and drug addiction among Puerto Ricans has been the *centros espiritismos* (spiritual centers).

The perception that Hispanics do not seek help with alcohol and drug problems reflects their tendency not to use formal clinical settings. These formal settings tend to treat alcoholism as a disease (i.e., medically), and indigenous treatments do not. Dominicans view heavy drinking as irresponsible; Pentecostals see the use of drugs and alcohol as sinful (other sins include smoking, dancing, and accepting welfare). Alcohol and drugs are not the basic problem; the problem is one of lifestyle and the rejection of Jesus. The efficacy of Pentecostal treatment has not been studied.

Cherpitel (2001) reported the differences in service utilization between Caucasian and Mexican Americans who had been arrested for driving under the influence; the Mexican Americans were less likely to use the services offered (such arrests being a potential source for treatment referrals.)

A recent analysis of liver cirrhosis mortality data (Stinson et al. 2001) shows the highest rate among white Hispanic men, followed by African American men and Caucasian men. Among Hispanics, the largest group was of Mexican origin; large numbers had been born outside the United States and had low educational achievement levels.

Asian Americans

Kitano et al. (1985) and Kitano and Chi (1989) wrote about the "strong family system" among Japanese Americans. Japanese Americans appear in very low numbers in drug and alcohol treatment programs. In Japan, although drinking is frequently linked to social problems it is believed that it is fundamentally a private matter. Although Japanese Americans drink less than Caucasian Americans, whether this is due to Asians' heightened flushing response to alcohol is a question that has not been answered. Alcohol is perceived as the social cement in groups; however, overt motives for drinking include alienation and culture conflict. Of an estimated 157 Japanese Americans with alcohol-related problems, only about 3% entered treatment programs. In Japan, the All Nippon Sobriety Association (patterned after AA) is available.

Asian Americans have lower rates of alcohol consumption and alcohol-related problems than other groups, but it should be noted that Japanese Americans have significantly higher drinking rates than Chinese Americans. It is of interest that among Japanese in Japan and in America, the percentage of drinkers was highest among the most educated and those of the highest income. In Korea, heavy drinking by males is more or less accepted, but Korean Americans (in California) drink less.

Alcohol consumption in traditional Chinese society is sanctioned for ceremonial or medicinal purposes. According to Chinese classical literature, there are two groups of drinkers: the literati or gentry, and the elderly, for whom drinking is tolerated ostensibly for health reasons.

Issues Concerning Substance Abuse Treatment in Minorities

1. It is likely that more African Americans and Hispanics will find their way to treatment in addition to whites. Studies have shown larger numbers of liquor stores in minority neighborhoods, and the availability of alcohol and drugs is probably greater in some neighborhoods with predominantly minority populations.

2. Some authors have identified a phenomenon they call "acculturation stress." Experiences vary, but some individuals and groups have a harder time adapting to a new culture. The therapist would do well to be aware of the issue.

3. There is a community reinforcement intervention that seeks information from and utilizes family and community networks. This approach has demonstrated some success with alcoholic Navahos in New Mexico when Native American spiritual traditions that encourage abstinence have been included. The approach could be extended beyond the Navaho to include Hispanic and African American subcultures. Weibel-Orlando (1985) described an assimilative model of treatment that is staffed and run by Native Americans; a culture-sensitive model with Native American counselors; a model that integrates Native American values and ceremonial curing practices with standard interventions; and a traditional model that excludes therapies other than traditional Native American approaches.

4. When treating African Americans, the therapist may combine his or her skills with church contacts. The therapist may also discuss confidentiality with the client to allay possible concerns.

5. Cherpitel (2001) studied the differences in service utilization between whites and Mexican Americans. Because social service is one of the points of contact with Mexican Americans, outreach techniques should be tried and studied.

Older Adults

The proportion of older people in the general population has been increasing, not only in the industrialized Western nations but in developing nations as well. For the purposes of this discussion, ages 65 and up will be considered "elderly." It is clear that the different forms of aging—biological, psychological, and social—occur at varying intraindividual and interindividual rates. In gerontology, the question of "normal" aging is critical; the assumption that aging equals loss is open to new thinking and research. The older population is heterogeneous by age (65–100+ years) and gender (women tend to live longer), by economic status (older women have less money than older men), by marital status (more older men are married), and by cultural background and religion.

Some psychosocial issues relevant to older adults (Gomberg 1990) are the following:

- Role and status changes
- Increase in chronic illnesses
- Cognitive change
- Retirement and work
- Widowhood
- Losses; affect and life satisfaction
- Social networks and social supports
- Substance use (from prescribed medications to "street" drugs)

Several factors are associated with the use of substances by the elderly. First are pharmacokinetics (absorption, tissue distribution, metabolism and excretion, and relationship of drug intake to intensity and duration of effects) and pharmacodynamics (physiological and psychological responses to drugs taken; e.g., enhanced response to benzodiazepines). Second, there is evidence that adverse drug reactions occur more frequently among older people than among younger ones; this is evident in the records of emergency rooms. Third, the issue of noncompliance, usually attributed to cognitive loss, appears to be a more complex matter than simple memory loss (Gomberg 1990).

Prescribed and Over-the-Counter Medications

Although persons age 65 and over constitute approximately 13% of the population, they account for a third of prescription drugs used and about half of over-the-counter drugs purchased. The American Association of Retired Persons (AARP), which is involved in the politics of prescribed drugs for the elderly, has launched a campaign encouraging elderly consumers to learn more about their prescriptions and to question their physicians about prescriptions. (The term used by the AARP for noncompliance by the elderly is *misuse* and includes not having a prescription filled, stopping medication before the course of treatment has terminated, and changing the timing or dosage recommended by the physician.)

The most commonly prescribed drugs among older patients include diuretics, cardiovascular drugs, and sedative-hypnotics (Gomberg 2000). The most commonly purchased over-the-counter drugs are nonnarcotic analgesics, vitamins, and laxatives. Psychoactive drugs such as antidepressants and sedatives are prescribed more often for elderly patients, particularly elderly women.

The advancement of psychopharmacology in medical treatment and the increase in advertising by drug companies have markedly expanded the range of use of prescription drugs in the past few decades. Because of the increase of chronic disease in the aging population and the growing proportion of the elderly in the general population, older people will probably continue to consume disproportionate amounts of both prescription and over-the-counter medications.

Nicotine

The use of nicotine among older people has dropped during the past several decades. Men are more likely to be smokers than women, but the gender gap has narrowed in all age groups studied. In 1993, 13.5% of older men and 10.5% of older women were smokers. A Massachusetts study revealed that 23% of respondents over age 65 were smokers; those least likely to be smokers were older people living alone or with their children, those who reported their health as being poor or fair, and the frail elderly. Studies of smoking cessation in the elderly are rarely done.

Illegal Drugs

Illegal drugs are used very little by older adults (except possibly by the homeless elderly or street people). This has less to do with the illegality or the effects of the drug and more to do with the lifestyle that is part of heroin or cocaine addiction. A group of heroin-addicted older persons have been studied (DesJarlais et al. 1985) for the bases of their survival. Earlier in the twentieth century, persons who were addicted to heroin usually died prematurely, often violently, or it was believed that they "matured out." Virtually nothing is known about street drug usage among the elderly in

poor minority populations, although it is a safe guess that such drugs are more readily available in poorer neighborhoods.

Although alcohol-related problems are more likely to be found among older adults than are street drug–related problems, this may change: with the aging of the baby boom generation, it is likely that the use of marijuana or hashish will be greater in people over age 65 in the coming decades.

Alcohol

Generally, the consumption of alcoholic beverages drops during the later years of life. However, it should be noted that this conclusion is based largely on cross-sectional studies; data derived from longitudinal surveys are not necessarily supportive of this reduction. Older women are as likely to consume alcoholic beverages as older men, but the latter outnumber older women in the proportion of heavy drinkers. For the present older generation, alcohol abuse is probably the most frequently seen substance abuse. In a column in the *New York Times*, medical reporter Jane Brody (2002) pointed to heavy drinking as "a growing and hidden problem" that poses health risks for older adults.

The diagnosis of drinking-related problems among older people has not yet been standardized. For example, because so many elderly people are retired, lost time from work is not a relevant cue. The elderly are less likely to be picked up for driving under the influence of alcohol. This population subgroup is often sheltered by family; a large proportion (particularly of widowed women) live alone. Older women are more likely than older men to begin problem drinking at a later age and are more likely to have a spouse who drinks heavily. Older women also manifest more depression and use other psychoactive drugs more than older men.

Although it is generally agreed that older persons drink less and manifest less problem drinking than younger persons, several reports have suggested that the problems are greater than was originally thought. Alexander and Duff (1988) interviewed residents of a retirement community. This study revealed more social drinking and problem drinking than had earlier studies.

Despite reports that older problem drinkers are identified in hospital settings (e.g., inpatient admissions and emergency room cases), relatively few older problem drinkers enter treatment. It has been suggested that age-specific criteria for problem drinking (e.g., housing problems, falls, poor nutrition, poor activities of daily living, inadequate exercise, and social isolation) should be added to screening instruments because such instruments have been inadequate in detecting problems related to alcohol use by elders (Dupree and Schonfeld 1998). Dupree and Schonfeld (1998) caution against the use of confrontational interviewing; although they indicate that supportive interviewing is preferable, they recommend the use of motivational interviewing. These authors further recommend a structural behavioral interview in which triggers to drinking and the consequences of drinking are asked about. This information is useful in predicting relapse.

Considering that most therapists agree that group treatment is central to elderly problem drinkers, the question arises whether such drinkers are best treated in a group of age peers or in a mixed-age group (Atkinson 1998). Evidence is limited, but the programs designed for a specific group of elderly problem drinkers have shown greater compliance than occurs in the mixed-age groups (Atkinson 1995). The few available studies emphasize compliance rather than outcome, and there are other elder-related issues that need to be addressed, including risk factors for relapse and dropout; the management of comorbidities; and requirements for staffing, case management, and psychosocial programs.

Whatever the numbers and the demography, the therapist of an elderly problem drinker faces problems of lifestyle, loneliness, aging-related illness, sex, and family attitudes. Also of relevance is social attitude toward older people—the view of the elderly as unproductive, cognitively impaired, and a general burden on the community. The first step in treatment may well be reassurance and a positive view of the patient. The second step is recognition by the therapist that there are age-related differences in alcohol withdrawal (Brower 1998). In an inpatient setting, elderly patients undergoing detoxification developed more symptoms that lasted longer than those observed in a group of comparable younger patients. Brower's review of alcohol withdrawal studies in older populations consistently found symptoms of greater intensity and duration than occurred in younger groups. It is generally agreed that group treatment, whether it is patterned after AA or another social support model, is essential. The other aspects of treatment (denial, abstinence as a goal, diagnostic features other than drinking, evaluation of treatment outcome, etc.) are the same for all age groups. It should also be noted that elderly persons with recent-onset drinking problems appear to have better prognoses than those with early-onset problems.

Treatment modalities for older adults. Some of the many relevant treatment modalities for older adults are listed below. Among these are individual-focused cognitive-behavioral therapy; outpatient and inpatient treatment; supportive group therapy with or without family therapy; and specific treatments for older women, aging homosexuals, and elderly ethnic minorities. There is also the matter of related mental health conditions (e.g., cognitive impairment and depression) and of chronic medical conditions.

1. *Cognitive therapy.* Glantz (1995) discussed screening and the selection of patients, the initial sessions, the establishment of goals, problem solving and skills training, tapering off the sessions, and relapse prevention. Cognitive-behavioral therapies are currently popular with counselors and psychologists.
2. *Outpatient versus inpatient treatment.* The choice between outpatient and inpatient treatment will depend on the intensity of the problem and the patient's living conditions and health status.
3. *Supportive group therapy with or without family therapy.* It is generally believed that group intervention is essential and that resocialization, directed toward depression and isolation, is critical.
4. *Therapies that are not helpful with older patients.* Confrontation, aversion therapy, and chemotherapy (e.g., disulfiram) have not demonstrated any benefit in elderly patients.
5. *Family therapies.* If there is a family (a spouse, children, siblings), family members may be functioning as enablers. Older problem drinkers report more family difficulties and interpersonal conflict and less support—social or material—than comparison age groups. The coping mechanisms of older problem drinkers are frequently resignation and avoidance of family problems.
6. *Adjunctive services.* Working with the elderly, it is necessary for the therapist to maintain contact with a variety of community agencies, medical and dental resources, senior centers, home health services, meals-on-wheels, and others.

In treatment planning and information gathering, the therapist should get some idea of the situations and feelings that precede a drinking bout. The role of stress is not clear, although significant loss (such as widowhood or retirement) is clearly a factor. There does not seem to be a major role for acute stress; there is a stronger relationship between chronic stress and elderly problem drinking.

Older alcohol abusers are more likely to have medical comorbidities (e.g., anemia, dementia, diabetes, hypertension, osteoporosis, liver pathology or pancreatitis). Even with comorbidity factored in, recovery rates for older and younger alcohol abusers under treatment are reasonably similar.

Theories about the etiology of alcohol abuse in older persons include developmental, biopsychosocial, genetic, neurophysiological, psychopharmacological, psychological, classical conditioning, and social learning theories (Gomberg 2000). An interesting research question presents itself: Are the theoretical foundations of alcohol abuse the same for younger and older alcoholics? It is helpful for the therapist to select the modality with which he or she is most comfortable and to offer treatment on the basis of his or her views about the etiology of alcohol abuse.

A note about treatment for older adults. There is general agreement in the published literature that elder-specific groups are more effective than "mainstreaming" or mixed-age groups. One possible explanation is that in a group of age peers, the older individual feels more accepted. What is the societal status of older people? Obviously, it varies in different cultures. Some societies grant high status to elders, but as the world becomes globalized and industrialized, older people, seen as nonproductive, are not likely to gain greater respect and status. It is clear also that increases in the number and proportion of older persons in the population will put strains on the Social Security system and health care institutions, and increased media attention has focused on societal problems that the elderly pose (such as the need for care). At the same time, there is some feeling that people have earned the right to retirement, and there are negative sanctions on "ageism." Over all, the impression is one of ambivalence toward the elderly. In treatment of this population, it is likely that the clinician will be younger—possibly considerably younger—than the patient. Clinicians need to examine their attitudes, fears, and perceptions of aging. The elderly are a reminder that we are all mortal.

Older substance abusers may present with comorbid illnesses and psychological symptoms. They are likely to present with depression and feelings of unworthiness; they are more likely to have memory losses than younger patients; and they are likely to be somewhat slower in responding to the treatment modality. It behooves the clinician working with elderly patients (whose numbers are increasing) to respect the dignity of the older patient (Gomberg 2000). Elderly substance abusers are, in every sense, a new group, and the appropriate social attitudes to adopt are still being worked out. An awareness of these issues will be very useful to the clinician who is available for geriatric work.

References

Alexander FM, Duff RW: Drinking in retirement communities. Generations 12:58, 1988

American Association of Retired Persons: Too much time in a bottle? Modern Maturity July/August 2002

Atkinson RM: Treatment programs for aging alcoholics, in Alcohol and Aging. Edited by Beresford TP, Gomberg E. New York, Oxford University Press, 1995, pp 186–210

Atkinson RM: Age-specific treatment programs for older adult alcoholics, in Alcohol Use Among U.S. Minorities. Edited by Gomberg ESL, Hegedus AM, Zucker RA. Rockville, MD, National Institute on Alcohol Abuse and Alcoholism, 1998, pp 425–435

Beauvais P: American Indians and alcohol. Alcohol Health Res World 22:253–259, 1998

Brody J: Hidden plague of alcohol abuse by the elderly. New York Times, April 2, 2002, F7

Brower KJ: Alcohol withdrawal and aging, in Alcohol Problems and Aging. NIAAA Research Monograph 33. Edited by Gomberg ESL, Hegedus AM, Zucker RA. Rockville, MD, National Institute on Alcohol Abuse and Alcoholism, 1998, pp 359–372

Caetano R: Drinking patterns and alcohol problems in a national sample of U.S. Hispanics, in Alcohol Use Among U.S. Ethnic Minorities (NIAAA Research Monograph 18). Rockville, MD, National Institute on Alcohol Abuse and Alcoholism, 1989, pp 147–162

Cherpitel CJ: Differences in service utilization between white and Mexican American DUI arrestees. Alcohol Clin Exp Res 25:122–127, 2001

DesJarlais DC, Joseph H, Courtwright DE: Old age and addiction: a study of elderly patients in methadone maintenance treatment, in The Combined Problems of Alcoholism, Drug Abuse and Aging. Springfield, IL, Charles C Thomas, 1985, pp 339–358

Dupree LW, Schonfeld L: Older alcohol abusers: recurring treatment issues, in Alcohol Problems and Aging (NIAAA Research Monograph 33). Edited by Gomberg ESL, Hededus AM, Zucker RA. Rockville, MD, National Institute on Alcohol Abuse and Alcoholism, 1998, pp 339–358

Gaines AD: Alcohol cultural conceptions and social behavior among urban Blacks, in The American Experience With Alcohol. Edited by Bennett LA, Ames GM. New York, Plenum, 1985, pp 171–197

Glantz M: Cognitive therapy with elderly alcoholics, in Alcohol and Aging. Edited by Beresford TP, Gomberg E. New York, Oxford University Press, 1995, pp 211–229

Gomberg ESL: Drugs, alcohol and aging, in Advances in Alcohol and Drug Problems, Vol 10. Edited by Kozlowski LT, Annis HM, Cappell HD, et al. New York, Plenum, 1990, pp 171–213

Gomberg ESL: Substance abuse disorders, in Psychopathology in Later Adulthood. Edited by Whitbourne SK. New York, Wiley, 2000, pp 277–298

Graves K, Kaskutas LA: Beverage choice among Native American and African American urban women. Alcohol Clin Exp Res 26(2):218–222, 2002

Herd D: Ambiguity in Black drinking norms: an ethnohistorical interpretation, in The American Experience With Alcohol. Edited by Bennett LA, Ames GM. New York, Plenum, 1985, pp 149–170

Herd D: The epidemiology of drinking patterns and alcohol-related problems among U.S. Blacks, in Alcohol Use Among U.S. Ethnic Minorities (NIAAA Research Monograph 18). Rockville, MD, National Institute on Alcohol Abuse and Alcoholism, 1989, pp 3–50

Jellinek EM: The Disease Concept of Alcoholism. Highland Park, NJ, Hillhouse Press, 1960

Johnston LD, O'Malley PM, Bachman JG: Monitoring the Future National Survey Results on Drug Use, 1975–2000, Vol 1: Secondary School Students (NIH Publ No 01-4924). Rockville, MD, National Institute on Drug Abuse, 2001

Kitano HHL, Chi I: Asian Americans and alcohol: The Chinese, Japanese, Koreans and Filipinos in Los Angeles, in Alcohol Use Among U.S. Ethnic Minorities (NIAAA Research Monograph 18). Rockville, MD, National Institute on Alcohol Abuse and Alcoholism, 1989, pp 375–382

Kitano HHL, Hatanake HM, Young W, et al: Japanese-American drinking patterns, in The American Experience With Alcohol. Edited by Bennett LA, Ames GM. New York, Plenum, 1985, pp 335–358

MacAndrew C, Edgerton RB: Drunken Comportment: A Social Explanation. New York, Aldine, 1969

National Institute on Alcohol Abuse and Alcoholism: Alcohol Alert/National Institute on Alcohol Abuse and Alcoholism. Alcohol and Minorities: An Update. No 55. Rockville, MD, National Institute on Alcohol Abuse and Alcoholism, 2002

Substance Abuse and Mental Health Services Administration: Analytic Series A-6: Prevalence of Substance Abuse Among Racial and Ethnic Subgroups in the United States 1991–1993 (DHHS Publ No SMA 98-3202). Rockville, MD, Substance Abuse and Mental Health Services Administration, Office of Applied Studies, 1998

Substance Abuse and Mental Health Services Administration: Alcohol Use. Rockville, MD, Substance Abuse and Mental Health Services Administration, Office of Applied Studies, 2001a

Substance Abuse and Mental Health Services Administration: 2000 National Household Survey on Drug Abuse. Rockville, MD, Substance Abuse and Mental Health Services Administration, Office of Applied Studies, 2001b

Stinson FS, Grant BF, Dufour MC: The critical dimension of ethnicity in liver cirrhosis morality statistics. Alcohol Clin Exp Res 25:1181–1187, 2001

Stivers R: Hair of the Dog: Irish Drinking and American Stereotype. University Park, PA, Pennsylvania State University Press, 1976

Venner KL, Miller WR: Progression of alcohol problems in a Navaho sample. J Stud Alcohol 62(2):158–165, 2001

Weibel-Orlando J: Indians, ethnicity and alcohol: contrasting perceptions of the ethnic self and alcohol use, in The American Experience With Alcohol. Edited by Bennett LA, Ames GM. New York, Plenum, 1985, pp 201–226

X M: The Autobiography of Malcolm X; with the assistance of Alex Haley. New York, Grove, 1965

Substance Use Disorders and Co-occurring Axis I Psychiatric Disorders

Kathleen T. Brady, M.D., Ph.D.
Robert J. Malcolm, M.D.

The relationship between substance use and psychiatric disorders is a complex one, and co-occurrence may manifest itself in several ways: 1) substance use and psychiatric disorders may co-occur by coincidence; 2) substance use may cause psychiatric conditions or increase the severity of psychiatric symptoms; 3) psychiatric disorders may cause or increase the severity of substance use disorders; 4) both disorders may be caused by a third condition; and 5) substance use and withdrawal may produce symptoms that mimic those of a psychiatric disorder (Meyer 1989). In any individual case, different aspects of this complex relationship may be involved. This complexity can lead to difficulties in diagnosis and management of comorbid conditions.

Two epidemiological surveys emphasized the prevalence of comorbid psychiatric and substance use disorders in community samples: the Epidemiologic Catchment Area (ECA) study sponsored by the National Institute of Mental Health (Reiger et al. 1990) and the National Comorbidity Survey (NCS) (Kessler et al. 1994). In the ECA study, an estimated 45% of individuals with an alcohol use disorder and 72% of individuals with a drug use disorder had at least one co-occurring psychiatric disorder (Reiger et al. 1990). In the NCS, approximately 78% of alcohol-dependent men and 86% of alcohol-dependent women met lifetime criteria for another psychiatric disorder, including drug dependence (Kessler et al. 1994).

General Diagnostic Considerations

One of the most difficult challenges in the area of comorbidity is diagnosis. Manifestations of substance use and withdrawal can mimic nearly every psychiatric disorder. Substances of abuse have profound effects on neurotransmitter systems involved in the pathophysiology of most psychiatric disorders; long-term use of these substances may unmask a vulnerability or lead to organic changes that manifest as a psychiatric disorder. The best way to differentiate substance-induced, transient psychiatric symptoms from psychiatric disorders that warrant treatment is through observation of symptoms during a period of abstinence. It is likely that the minimum amount of time necessary for diagnosis will vary depending on the comorbid condition being diagnosed and the expected residual effects of the substance in question. In the case of depression and many anxiety symptoms, there appears to be symptom resolution for 2–4 weeks after last use. This probably partly reflects the fact that many of the symptoms of depression and anxiety disorders overlap with common symptoms associated with substance withdrawal. Other psychiatric disorders are less well studied in this regard. A family history of psychiatric illness, clear onset of psychiatric symptoms before onset of the substance use disorder, and sustained psychiatric symptoms during lengthy periods of abstinence in the past can all weigh in favor of making a psychiatric diagnosis in cases that are unclear.

General Treatment Considerations

In general, treatment efforts addressing psychiatric and substance use disorders have developed in parallel. To design treatments specifically tailored for patients with comorbidity, it is necessary to determine the appropriate integration of treatment modalities from both the psychiatric and the substance abuse fields. Psychosocial treatments are powerful interventions for both substance use and psychiatric disorders. There are common themes in the psychosocial treatments from both fields, and these themes can be built on to optimize outcome.

Research in pharmacotherapies for both substance use and psychiatric disorders is progressing rapidly. Integration of information from both the psychiatric and the substance abuse fields has led to the testing of strategies targeting individuals with both disorders. Specific comorbid disorders are discussed in detail below, but general principles involved in

choosing a pharmacological agent include paying particular attention to potential toxic interactions of the agent with drugs and alcohol (should relapse occur) and assessing the abuse potential of the agent being used.

This chapter contains an overview of the most common and clinically relevant comorbidities of Axis I psychiatric disorders and substance use disorders. For every category of psychiatric diagnosis discussed, prevalence rates, differential diagnosis, and information on pharmacotherapeutic and psychotherapeutic treatment options are briefly reviewed.

Psychotic Disorders

Prevalence

Psychotic symptoms may occur with substance use disorders as a direct result of chemical intoxication or withdrawal or because of a primary underlying psychotic disorder. As many as 50% of treatment-seeking schizophrenic patients have alcohol or illicit drug dependence, and more than 70% are nicotine dependent (Ziedonis et al. 2000). Epidemiological surveys indicate that individuals with schizophrenia are at substantial risk (odds ratio, 4–5) for having a substance use disorder, compared with the general population (Kessler et al. 1994; Reiger et al. 1990). The relationship between psychosis and substance use is complex. Individuals with schizophrenia may use substances to decrease the negative symptoms of schizophrenia (depression, apathy, anhedonia, passivity, social withdrawal), to combat the overwhelming positive symptoms of schizophrenia (typically auditory hallucinations and paranoid delusions), or as an attempt to ameliorate the adverse effects of neuroleptic medications (dysphoria, akathisia, and sedation).

Diagnosis

Differential diagnosis frequently involves differentiating a substance-induced psychotic disorder from a primary psychotic disorder. Findings that might support a diagnosis of substance-induced psychotic disorder rather than primary psychotic disorder are younger age at onset of psychosis, family history of drug use, male gender, and good premorbid adjustment (Ziedonis et al. 2000). Obtaining a thorough history regarding symptoms during abstinent periods and observing the patient during monitored abstinence are essential to accurate diagnosis.

Treatment

The optimal management of patients with comorbid schizophrenia and substance use involves both pharmacotherapy and psychotherapy. There are few empirical data concerning specific pharmacotherapeutic strategies, but atypical antipsychotic agents are an excellent choice for a number of reasons. Compared with typical antipsychotics, these agents have fewer side effects that might compromise compliance, are more efficacious in treating negative symptoms of schizophrenia, and may decrease craving for substances. Management of dysphoric affect in substance abuse in patients may be an important step in successful treatment. One group of investigators studying adjunctive desipramine treatment in a small group of cocaine-abusing schizophrenic individuals found that the desipramine-treated group stayed in treatment longer and had fewer cocaine-positive urine drug screens (Ziedonis et al. 2000). Disulfiram must be used with caution in this comorbid population because it may increase central levels of dopamine by blocking dopamine β-hydroxylase and thereby exacerbate psychosis (Wilkins 1997). The use of naltrexone to decrease alcohol consumption in individuals with schizophrenia is an intriguing idea that has not been explored in a systematic manner. The use of medications demonstrated to be effective in the treatment of nicotine dependence (bupropion hydrochloride and nicotine replacement therapies) in schizophrenic patients has been underexplored, but preliminary studies have shown promise (Ziedonis et al. 2000).

The psychotherapeutic management of comorbid schizophrenia and substance abuse is critical. Patients must be closely monitored with urinalysis and Breathalyzer, and clear limits must be set. Feedback should be given in an empathic and nonjudgmental manner. The confrontational group process approach often used for substance-abusing persons has little value in the treatment of the substance-abusing schizophrenic individual (Ziedonis et al. 2000) and may exacerbate psychosis. A dual-diagnosis, treatment-matching strategy based on motivation levels, substance of abuse, and illness severity has been suggested (Ziedonis et al. 2000).

Affective Disorders

Prevalence

Symptoms of mood instability and depression are among the most common psychiatric symptoms seen in individuals with substance use disorders. In the ECA study, 32% of individuals with an affective disorder also had a comorbid substance use disorder (Reiger et al. 1990). Of the individuals with major depression, 16.5% had an alcohol use disorder and 18% had a drug use disorder, and 56.1% of individuals with bipolar disorder had a substance use disorder. In both the ECA study and the NCS, bipolar disorder was the Axis I condition most likely to occur with a substance use disorder.

Studies in treatment-seeking samples have resulted in variable estimates of the comorbidity of affective illness with substance use disorders. One reason for this is that diagnostic issues at the interface of affective illness and substance use disorders are particularly complex. Estimates of the prevalence of depressive disorders in treatment-seeking alcoholic individuals range from 15% to 67% (W.E. Brown and Schuckit 1988). In studies of cocaine-dependent individuals, estimates of affective comorbidity range from 33% to 53% (Brady and Sonne 1999). Bipolar disorders appear to be more prevalent (20%–30%) among cocaine-dependent individuals than among alcoholic individuals. In opiate-dependent samples, the rates of lifetime affective disorder (primarily depressive disorders) range from 16% to 75% (Brooner et al. 1997).

Diagnosis

Up to 98% of individuals presenting for substance abuse treatment have some symptom of depression. Many of these symptoms resolve with abstinence alone. Obviously, assessment done too early in recovery may lead to overdiagnosis and unnecessary treatment. Underdiagnosis also presents a risk because evidence indicates that appropriate treatment of depression can improve substance-related outcomes. Clinical features that should influence treatment decisions are affective symptoms that predate the onset of substance use, a strong family history of affective disorder, and symptoms that have persisted during abstinent periods in the past.

Treatment

Pharmacotherapy for Depression

Studies of treatment of major depressive episodes and alcoholism with tricyclic antidepressants (TCAs) indicate that such treatment modestly decreases alcohol use and the symptoms of depression (Mason et al. 1996; McGrath et al. 1996). Serotonin has been implicated in the control of alcohol intake. A number of serotonin reuptake inhibitors (SRIs) have been shown to modestly decrease alcohol consumption in persons with problem drinking as well as in alcoholic individuals (Gorelick 1989). In a study investigating the use of fluoxetine in a group of alcoholic persons with major depression (Cornelius et al. 1997), individuals who received fluoxetine had significantly greater reduction in both depressive symptoms and alcohol consumption compared with the placebo group. This study is particularly important because the clinical improvement was more substantial than that seen in the studies involving TCAs, and SRIs have less potential for toxicity and interaction with drugs of abuse than do TCAs.

Several trials of TCAs have been performed with opioid-dependent patients. Nunes and colleagues (1998) found that imipramine significantly decreased depression in a group of depressed patients receiving methadone maintenance treatment. The effect of imipramine on drug use was not remarkable. Although self-report measures indicated significantly less craving and drug use, there were no differences in positive urine drug screens.

The primary focus of the use of TCAs in cocaine-dependent patients has been on treatment of cocaine dependence, rather than on treatment of depression. Several studies involving desipramine have shown improvement in anhedonia and cocaine craving and increased initial abstinence in nondepressed patients, and one small study showed improvement in depressed patients (Rao et al. 1995). Clinicians should be aware, however, that desipramine may have an activating effect in cocaine-dependent individuals, which can precipitate relapse; furthermore, should relapse occur, desipramine may have additive cardiotoxicity in combination with cocaine. Unlike the promising data gathered from investigating the use of SRIs in comorbid alcohol dependence and major depression, recent placebo-controlled trials investigating the use of fluoxetine in depressed cocaine-dependent (Schmitz et al. 2001) and methadone-maintained (Petrakis et al.

1998) individuals have shown no effect of medication on drug use or symptoms of depression.

In summary, for the pharmacotherapeutic treatment of comorbid alcohol dependence and major depression, available data support the use of SRI agents. For cocaine-dependent and opiate-dependent individuals with major depressive episodes, there are limited data supporting the use of TCAs, but studies thus far testing the efficacy of SRIs have shown no benefit. It is possible that the different pharmacological properties of these substances of abuse are involved in determining pharmacological specificity in treatment responsivity. Trials of some of the newer antidepressants with mixed serotonin and norepinephrine activity (venlafaxine or duloxetine) in alcohol-, cocaine-, and opiate-dependent individuals with major depressive episodes would be of interest in this regard.

Pharmacotherapy for Bipolar Disorder

There are few published data on the treatment of bipolar disorder complicated by substance abuse. Lithium has been the standard treatment for bipolar disorder for several decades; however, substance abuse may be a predictor of poor response to lithium (Bowden 1995). Patients with mixed manic episodes or rapid-cycling disorder have a better response to anticonvulsant drugs than to lithium. Patients with bipolar disorder and concomitant substance use disorders appear to have more mixed and rapid-cycling episodes and therefore may have a better treatment response with anticonvulsant mood-stabilizing medications. Controlled studies testing this hypothesis need to be performed. Weiss and colleagues (1998) reported better medication compliance with valproate, compared with lithium, in a group of substance-abusing patients with bipolar disorder. Brady and colleagues (2002) recently reported on results from a placebo-controlled, double-blind trial in which carbamazepine showed preferential efficacy in decreasing cocaine use in cocaine-dependent subjects with affective disorder compared with those without affective disorders.

Psychotherapeutic Treatment

The psychotherapeutic and psychosocial strategies used in the treatment of comorbid conditions should be specifically tailored and should contain elements of effective treatment from the areas of both substance abuse and affective disorders. Many of the principles of cognitive-behavioral therapy are common to the treatment of affective disorder and substance use disorders. There are several recently published pilot studies demonstrating efficacy for psychotherapeutic strategies specifically designed for dually diagnosed populations. R.A. Brown and colleagues (1997) demonstrated that alcoholic individuals with depressive symptoms had improved outcomes at 3- and 6-month follow-up visits after treatment with cognitive-behavioral treatment for depression, compared with a control group that received relaxation training. Weiss and colleagues (2000) compared a manual-based group therapy for patients with bipolar disorder and substance dependence to treatment as usual and found that subjects receiving the group treatment had significantly better outcomes in a number of domains.

Alcoholics Anonymous and Narcotics Anonymous are found in most communities, and active participation can be a major factor in an individual's recovery. It is important that dually diagnosed individuals choose 12-step recovery groups in which they are not likely to receive mixed or negative messages about the use of psychotropic medications under the direction of a physician. Further work is needed in developing therapies specifically geared toward comorbid affective and substance use disorders, in which therapeutic techniques for each type of disorder are combined.

Anxiety Disorders

Prevalence

Data from the NCS indicate that approximately 36% of individuals with anxiety disorders also have a substance use disorder (Kessler et al. 1994). Because the anxiety disorders are heterogeneous and the issues concerning diagnosis, treatment, and prevalence differ substantially between disorders, each disorder is discussed in a separate subsection.

Panic Disorder

In the ECA survey, 36% of individuals with panic disorder had lifetime substance use disorder (Reiger et al. 1990). In the NCS, the odds ratio for co-occurrence of drug and alcohol dependence with panic disorder was 2.0 (Kessler et al. 1994). The estimated prevalence of panic disorder and agoraphobia in treatment-seeking samples of alcoholic persons is variable, with estimates ranging from 5% to 42% (Kushner et al. 1990). This variability is, in part, related to diagnostic difficulties. Anxiety symptoms in general and panic attacks in particular are commonly seen during withdrawal periods. Alcohol, sedative-hypnotic, and opiate withdrawal are all marked by hyperexcitability of the noradrenergic systems, which also occurs with panic attacks. Other drugs of abuse (cocaine, marijuana, other stimulants) may induce panic attacks during acute intoxication.

The most widely used classes of pharmacotherapeutic agents for the treatment of panic disorder are the SRIs, although TCAs, monoamine oxidase inhibitors (MAOIs), and benzodiazepines have demonstrated efficacy in non-substance-using patients (Lydiard et al. 1988). As mentioned above (see "Pharmacotherapy for Depression"), some investigators have shown that SRIs can modestly decrease alcohol consumption. SRIs are therefore a logical choice for the patient with comorbid panic disorder and alcoholism, but controlled clinical trials in substance-using populations have not been conducted. Benzodiazepines are generally contraindicated in substance-using populations because of their abuse potential. This is a controversial issue, however, and a recent review of the literature questions the empirical justification for this and suggests that benzodiazepines may be indicated in certain patients with a history of a substance use disorder (Posternak and Mueller 2001). When a benzodiazepine is being prescribed to a patient with comorbid substance use, limited amounts of medication should be given and the patient should be closely monitored for relapse.

MAOIs are also difficult to use in patients with comorbid substance use disorders. Dietary restrictions are necessary because of the interaction with tyramine in the diet, which may result in a hypertensive crisis. Moreover, MAOIs in combination with stimulant drugs may precipitate a hypertensive crisis.

Panic disorder is responsive to nonpharmacological treatment. Cognitive-behavioral techniques, such as exposure and systematic desensitization, have been shown to be particularly effective in the treatment of panic disorder (Barlow and Lehman 1996). It is important to maximize nonpharmacological treatments in patients with substance use disorders. The ability to self-regulate subjective states and the confidence that can result from successful mastery through therapy can be helpful to individuals in recovery. Many of the techniques used in anxiety disorders overlap with therapies known to be successful in the treatment of substance use disorders. Therefore, combination therapy is feasible. Finally, by learning therapeutic anxiety-reducing strategies, patients may be able to acquire alternative coping strategies and break out of the mindset of using external agents to combat intolerable subjective states.

Generalized Anxiety Disorder

For generalized anxiety disorder (GAD) and substance use disorders, diagnostic issues are particularly complex. The DSM-IV-TR (American Psychiatric Association 2000) criteria for GAD specify that symptoms must occur for 6 months without being directly related to physiological effects of a substance. Symptoms of GAD substantially overlap with symptoms of acute intoxication with stimulants and withdrawal from alcohol, sedative-hypnotics, and opiates, and the 6-month period of abstinence may be difficult to ascertain. Although many substance-using individuals report anxiety symptoms consistent with GAD, they may not meet diagnostic criteria for GAD because of difficulty in distinguishing symptoms of anxiety from substance-related symptoms.

The treatment of GAD complicated by a substance use disorder is challenging. Benzodiazepines are effective in the treatment of GAD; however, as discussed above, their abuse potential limits utility in the substance-abusing population. Buspirone is a nonbenzodiazepine anxiolytic with no abuse potential that has been shown in several studies of alcoholic individuals with anxiety to decrease alcohol consumption and to improve symptoms of anxiety (Kranzler et al. 1994). Because of the low abuse potential and reports of success in well-controlled studies, buspirone remains a good choice in individuals with comorbid GAD and substance use disorders. Although there have been no reported systematic trials of TCAs or SRIs in the treatment of GAD in individuals with substance use disorders, these agents have been useful in non-substance-abusing populations (Lydiard et al. 1988).

As mentioned above under "Panic Disorder," nonpharmacological treatments for anxiety disorders can be useful. GAD can be effectively managed with the use of relaxation, coping, and cognitive-behavioral therapy techniques (Barlow and Lehman 1996). Pharmacotherapy and psychotherapy are likely to complement each other in maximizing patient outcomes.

Social Phobia

Studies examining the interface of alcohol abuse and dependence with social phobia have found rates of co-

morbidity ranging from 8% to 56% (Kushner et al. 1990). Social phobia in drug dependence has not been well studied, but in one study (Myrick and Brady 1996), the lifetime prevalence of social phobia in a cocaine-dependent population was approximately 14%.

Because social phobia may interfere with an individual's ability to engage in treatment effectively, early recognition is paramount. Social phobia can be recognized without a lengthy period of abstinence because fear of interaction in a social situation is not a specific feature of substance use or withdrawal. However, social fears that arise only during periods of intoxication with marijuana or stimulants should not be considered sufficient for diagnosis of social phobia.

MAOIs (reversible inhibitors of monoamine oxidase), SRIs, and benzodiazepines have documented efficacy (Lydiard et al. 1988) for the treatment of uncomplicated social phobia. There was one placebo-controlled pilot study in comorbid alcohol dependence and social phobia in which paroxetine was significantly more efficacious than placebo in decreasing symptoms of social anxiety and improving global severity ratings for alcohol consumption (Randall et al. 2001). Gabapentin, an anticonvulsant agent, has also demonstrated efficacy in the treatment of social phobia in a placebo-controlled trial (Pande et al. 1999). Although there are no studies of gabapentin treatment in comorbid populations, because of the utility of anticonvulsants in treating alcohol withdrawal, a controlled trial in a comorbid population would be of interest.

Psychotherapeutic treatment is important. It may be difficult for socially phobic patients to participate in group therapy or 12-step programs. Although there are no published studies that have systematically examined psychotherapeutic treatments in patients with comorbid social phobia and substance use, several types of nonpharmacological treatments—such as systematic desensitization, imaginal flooding, graduated exposure, social skills training, and cognitive approaches—have proved effective in non-substance-using individuals with social phobia.

Posttraumatic Stress Disorder

The prevalence of comorbid posttraumatic stress disorder (PTSD) and substance use disorders is high. In the NCS study, approximately 30%–50% of men and 25%–30% of women with lifetime PTSD had a co-occurring substance use disorder (Kessler et al. 1994).

In studies conducted in substance abuse treatment settings, the lifetime prevalence of PTSD is between 36% and 50% and the current prevalence is between 25% and 42% (Dansky et al. 1994).

TCAs, MAOIs, and SRIs have been shown in double-blind, placebo-controlled trials to improve symptoms of PTSD (Davidson 1992). Unfortunately, none of the trials included individuals with substance use disorders. There is one report of an open trial of sertraline treatment in a small group of individuals with comorbid PTSD and alcohol dependence that resulted in decreased alcohol consumption and decreased symptoms of PTSD (Brady et al. 1995), and a double-blind, placebo-controlled trial is under way.

The appropriate psychotherapeutic approach to comorbid PTSD and substance use disorders remains unclear. Cognitive-behavioral therapies have shown efficacy in the treatment of PTSD but have been under-explored in comorbid populations. There have been several preliminary studies reporting promising results for manual-guided cognitive-behavioral treatment in comorbid populations (Brady et al. 2001; Najavits et al. 1996). This area warrants further investigation.

Attention-Deficit/Hyperactivity Disorder

The co-occurrence of attention-deficit/hyperactivity disorder (ADHD) and psychoactive substance use disorders has received much recent attention. In an analysis summarizing data from several studies of adults and adolescents with substance use disorders, the mean percentage of subjects with a comorbid diagnosis of ADHD was determined to be 23%. In investigations of substance use disorders in adults with ADHD, rates of alcohol use disorders have been estimated to be between 17% and 45%, and rates of drug use disorders have been estimated to be between 9% and 50% (Wilens et al. 1994).

As with many comorbid conditions, diagnostic issues with ADHD in substance use disorders are problematic. Because attentional problems are common during withdrawal and acute intoxication, symptoms must be assessed during abstinence. Because the symptoms of ADHD must first occur in childhood and then persist over time, careful screening for childhood symptoms may be of help in differentiating substance withdrawal from ADHD.

Pharmacotherapy plays an important role in the treatment of ADHD. Stimulants are ordinarily the first-line drug of choice for uncomplicated ADHD in children and adults. Because of the abuse potential of the stimulants, there has been concern about their use in the population. However, in one pilot treatment study, cocaine-dependent patients with ADHD receiving methylphenidate under carefully controlled conditions reported a reduction in ADHD symptoms and had reduced cocaine use documented by urine drug screening (Levin et al. 1999). Desipramine, bupropion, and tomoxetine (not available in the United States) have all been studied in placebo-controlled trials and have been found to be efficacious in the treatment of ADHD in non-substance-using patients. Because these agents have no abuse potential, they should be considered the first line of treatment in substance-using patients. Pemoline, a stimulant drug with a longer half-life than methylphenidate, might have less abuse potential. However, recent evidence concerning the hepatotoxicity of pemoline may limit its usefulness in substance-using patients.

Psychotherapy for patients and families should address psychoeducation about ADHD, substance use disorders, interpersonal difficulties, low self-esteem, impulsivity, and time management. Behavioral treatments to improve focus and attention can be helpful in the treatment of childhood ADHD but have not been adequately studied in the treatment of ADHD in adults. As with other comorbid conditions, it is important to maximize nonpharmacological treatment approaches. Because inattention and impulsivity can interfere with successful substance abuse treatment, careful attention to diagnosis and effective treatment may be important in improving treatment outcome.

Conclusion

Converging evidence from multiple lines of investigation indicates that substance use disorders and psychiatric disorders commonly co-occur. This comorbidity presents challenges for diagnosis and for optimal patient management. For diagnosis, strategies focused on the features most likely to facilitate early diagnosis will be helpful. Regarding treatment, psychotherapeutic techniques used in the psychiatric and substance use fields can be combined to design specifically tailored strategies for comorbid populations. In addition, the development of scientific techniques capable of elucidating the common neurobiological pathways in comorbid disorders is promising for the development of specifically targeted pharmacotherapeutic strategies. Recent studies have provided helpful information concerning diagnostic, psychotherapeutic, and pharmacotherapeutic strategies tailored for this population, but much work remains to be done in developing the optimal treatment for this prevalent group of disorders.

References

American Psychiatric Association: Diagnostic and Statistical Manual of Mental Disorders, 4th Edition, Text Revision. Washington, DC, American Psychiatric Association, 2000

Barlow DH, Lehman CL: Advances in the psychosocial treatment of anxiety disorders: implications for national health care. Arch Gen Psychiatry 53:727–735, 1996

Bowden CL: Predictors of response to divalproex and lithium. J Clin Psychiatry 56:25–30, 1995

Brady KT, Sonne SC: The role of stress in alcohol use, alcoholism treatment, and relapse. Alcohol Res Health 23:263–271, 1999

Brady KT, Sonne SC, Roberts JM: Sertraline treatment of comorbid posttraumatic stress disorder and alcohol dependence. J Clin Psychiatry 56:502–505, 1995

Brady KT, Dansky BS, Back SE, et al: Exposure therapy in the treatment of PTSD among cocaine-dependent individuals: preliminary findings. J Subst Abuse Treat 21:47–54, 2001

Brady KT, Myrick H, Henderson S, et al: The use of divalproex in alcohol relapse prevention: a pilot study. Drug Alcohol Depend 67:323–330, 2002

Brooner RK, King VL, Kidorf M, et al: Psychiatric and substance comorbidity among treatment-seeking opioid abusers. Arch Gen Psychiatry 54:71–80, 1997

Brown RA, Evans DM, Miller IW, et al: Cognitive-behavioral treatment for depression in alcoholism. J Consult Clin Psychol 65:715–726, 1997

Brown WE, Schuckit M: Changes in depression among abstinent alcoholics. J Stud Alcohol 49:412–417, 1988

Cornelius JR, Salloum IM, Ehler JG, et al: Fluoxetine in depressed alcoholics: a double-blind, placebo-controlled trial. Arch Gen Psychiatry 54:700–705, 1997

Dansky BS, Brady KT, Roberts JT: Post-traumatic stress disorder and substance abuse: empirical findings and clinical issues. Subst Abus 15:247–257, 1994

Davidson J: Drug therapy of post-traumatic stress disorder. Br J Psychiatry 160:309–314, 1992

Gorelick DA: Serotonin uptake blockers and the treatment of alcoholism. Recent Dev Alcohol 7:267–281, 1989

Kessler RC, McGonagle KA, Zhao S, et al: Lifetime and 12-month prevalence of DSM-III-R psychiatric disorders in the United States: results from the National Comorbidity Survey. Arch Gen Psychiatry 51:8–19, 1994

Kranzler HR, Burleson JA, DelBoca FK, et al: Buspirone treatment of anxious alcoholics: a placebo-controlled trial. Arch Gen Psychiatry 51:720–731, 1994

Kushner MG, Sher KJ, Beitman BD: The relation between alcohol problems and the anxiety disorders. Am J Psychiatry 147:685–695, 1990

Levin FR, Evans SM, Kleber HD: Practical guidelines for the treatment of substance abusers with adult attention-deficit hyperactivity disorder. Psychiatr Serv 50:1001–1003, 1999

Lydiard RB, Roy-Byrne PP, Ballenger JC: Recent advances in the psychopharmacological treatment of anxiety disorders. Hosp Community Psychiatry 39:1157–1165, 1988

Mason BJ, Kocsis JH, Ritvo EC, et al: A double-blind, placebo-controlled trial of desipramine for primary alcohol dependence stratified on the presence or absence of major depression. JAMA 275:761–767, 1996

McGrath PJ, Nunes EV, Stewart JW, et al: Imipramine treatment of alcoholics with primary depression: a placebo-controlled clinical trial. Arch Gen Psychiatry 53:232–240, 1996

Meyer RE: Prospects for a rational pharmacotherapy of alcoholism. J Clin Psychiatry 50:403–412, 1989

Myrick DH, Brady KT: Social phobia in cocaine-dependent individuals. Am J Addict 6:99–104, 1996

Najavits LM, Weiss RD, Liese BS: Group cognitive-behavioral therapy for women with PTSD and substance use disorder. J Subst Abuse Treat 13:13–22, 1996

Nunes EV, Quitkin FM, Donoval SJ, et al: Imipramine treatment of opiate-dependent patients with depressive disorders. Arch Gen Psychiatry 55:153–160, 1998

Pande AC, Davidson JR, Jefferson JW, et al: Treatment of social phobia with gabapentin: a placebo-controlled study. J Clin Psychopharmacol 19:341–348, 1999

Petrakis I, Carroll KM, Nich C, et al: Fluoxetine treatment of depressive disorders in methadone-maintained opioid addicts. Drug Alcohol Depend 50:221–226, 1998

Posternak MA, Mueller TI: Assessing the risks and benefits of benzodiazepines for anxiety disorders in patients with a history of substance abuse or dependence. Am J Addict 10:48–68, 2001

Randall CL, Johnson MR, Thevos AK, et al: Paroxetine for social anxiety and alcohol use in dual-diagnosed patients. Depress Anxiety 14:255–262, 2001

Rao S, Ziedonis D, Kosten T: The pharmacotherapy of cocaine dependence. Psychiatr Ann 25:363–368, 1995

Reiger DA, Farmer ME, Rae DS, et al: Comorbidity of mental disorders with alcohol and other drug abuse: results from the Epidemiologic Catchment Area (ECA) Study. JAMA 264:2511–2518, 1990

Schmitz JM, Averill P, Stotts AL, et al: Fluoxetine treatment of cocaine-dependent patients with major depressive disorder. Drug Alcohol Depend 63:207–214, 2001

Weiss RD, Greenfield SF, Najavits LM, et al: Medication compliance among patients with bipolar disorder and substance use disorder. J Clin Psychiatry 59:172–174, 1998

Weiss RD, Griffin ML, Greenfield SF, et al: Group therapy for patients with bipolar disorder and substance dependence: results of a pilot study. J Clin Psychiatry 61:361–367, 2000

Wilens TE, Biederman J, Spencer TJ, et al: Comorbidity of attention-deficit hyperactivity and substance use disorders. Hosp Community Psychiatry 45:421–435, 1994

Wilkins JN: Pharmacotherapy of schizophrenia patients with comorbid substance abuse. Schizophr Bull 23:215–228, 1997

Ziedonis D, Williams J, Corrigan P, et al: Management of substance abuse in schizophrenia. Psychiatr Ann 30:67–75, 2000

Addiction in Women

Sheila B. Blume, M.D.
Monica L. Zilberman, M.D., Ph.D.

Why Study Addiction in Women?

Addiction has traditionally been considered a disease of men. Although it is true that the lifetime prevalence of substance use disorders remains higher in men than in women, evidence shows convergence of these rates, especially among younger individuals. Women have increasingly entered the job market, particularly in formerly male-dominated professions, increasing their opportunities to drink and to use drugs. This convergence is also associated with a lowering of the age at onset of substance use. Early use of substances is associated with a higher risk of developing dependence, an effect more pronounced in women than in men. Addictive disorders remain a major source of mortality and morbidity in women, who are more sensitive to the physiological effects of some substances than men are and have a higher incidence of comorbid sexually transmitted and psychiatric disorders. Women of childbearing age are at risk for perinatal complications and for bearing offspring with fetal alcohol and/or drug ef-

fects (covered in Chapter 43, "Perinatal Substance Abuse," in this volume). Thus, addiction in women requires a special emphasis on prevention, case finding, treatment, and research (Zilberman et al. 2002).

Physiological Factors

Alcohol

A given amount of alcohol will lead to a higher blood alcohol concentration in a woman than in a man, even adjusting for body weight. In part, this is because women have lower levels of alcohol dehydrogenase in the gastric mucosa, leading to lower rates of first-pass metabolism, higher alcohol absorption, and therefore higher blood alcohol concentrations. Also, women have a higher proportion of fat and a lower proportion of water in their bodies. Because the absorbed alcohol is distributed in total body water, less water produces higher blood concentration (Lieber 2000). Higher rates of alcohol metabolism by the liver could contribute to the higher prevalence of liver damage in women, and estrogen can produce an additive effect in the alcohol-related liver damage. Gender variations in the action of neurosteroids in the brain are also reported to influence gender differences in response to alcohol (Brady and Randall 1999). Women's greater sensitivity to alcohol might explain, at least in part, why alcohol dependence and the physical damage caused by alcohol progress more rapidly in women ("telescoping" of the disease). Physical effects of alcohol and metabolic differences, however, might not be the sole explanations; recent studies on pathological gambling, a nonchemical dependence, have also found a telescoped (shortened) course among female pathological gamblers (Tavares et al. 2001). Both alcohol-related symptoms and physical complications such as fatty liver, cirrhosis, hypertension, anemia, malnutrition, gastrointestinal hemorrhage, peptic ulcer, peripheral myopathy, cardiomyopathy, and cognitive impairment advance more rapidly in women (Greenfield and O'Leary 2002), meaning that the window for therapeutic interventions is shorter in women than in men.

Although alcohol is perceived by the public to be a sexual stimulant for women, it actually depresses female sexual arousal and orgasm. The mistaken notion that alcohol has improved their sexual responsiveness causes many alcoholic women to fear sexual intercourse in early recovery. In fact, most alcoholic women report improved responsiveness and pleasure in their sexual relationships once alcohol abstinence is established (Blume 1998). Sex-specific effects of alcoholism in women include amenorrhea, anovulation, luteal phase dysfunction, and early menopause (Greenfield and O'Leary 2002).

Evidence of gender differences in the genetics of alcoholism is mixed. Some studies indicate that the genetic influence is higher in men (Sigvardsson et al. 1996). More recent evidence shows that the magnitude of the genetic influence is equally high for men and women, but the genetic sources of vulnerability might not be the same across genders (Prescott et al. 1999).

Other Drugs

Physiological gender differences in the effects and the medical consequences of other drugs have been less studied than those of alcohol. Regarding cocaine, for instance, a greater subjective response in women compared with that in men has been reported (as well as the opposite), linked to an increased cocaine metabo-

lism by cholinesterases in women. In addition, menstrual cycle variations in the plasma levels, though not in the subjective effects, of inhaled cocaine were found among women, attributed to an increased viscosity of the nasal mucosa of women during the luteal phase, with consequent decreased cocaine absorption. The occurrence of a telescoping course of cocaine dependence among women remains a controversial topic.

Similar to that with alcohol, a telescoping of the course of opioid dependence among women has been described, with women presenting more genitourinary and respiratory problems and a higher mortality rate than men. Regarding cannabis use, neuropsychological impairments appear to be more prominent among men who are heavy users, but women display a gender-specific impairment on visuospatial recall memory (Zilberman et al. 2002).

Psychological Factors

Alcohol

Depressive and anxiety symptoms are common in female drinkers (even recreational drinkers), and the accustomed level of alcohol consumption influences the relationship between mood and drinking outcome. Depressed mood predicts more drinking in frequently intoxicated women, whereas in women who consume alcohol moderately, it predicts less drinking (Sexton et al. 1999). In a 27-year follow-up study of college women, the best predictors of later drinking problems were drinking to relieve shyness, drinking to feel high, and drinking to get along better on dates. These patterns differed from predictive factors for men and predicted later problems better than did actual drinking problems while still in college (Fillmore et al. 1979). Other longitudinal studies show that depression is not predictive of increased alcohol use in men, but depressed women are at higher risk of heavy drinking at follow-up (Wang and Patten 2001). Women with major depression face a risk 2.6 to 4.1 times greater of later developing alcohol abuse or dependence than do nondepressed women (Dixit and Crum 2000; Kessler et al. 1997). A history of sexual abuse and posttraumatic stress disorder also increases the risk for substance-related disorders in women (Breslau et al. 1997; Wilsnack et al. 1997).

Data from the National Comorbidity Survey (NCS) have demonstrated a significantly higher lifetime prevalence of psychiatric comorbidity in women than in men with alcohol abuse (72% and 57%, respectively) (Kessler et al. 1994). In addition, the Epidemiologic Catchment Area (ECA) study showed that this was the case for both alcohol abuse and dependence (65% for women versus 44% for men) (Helzer et al. 1991). Furthermore, comorbid diagnoses are more often primary (that is, preceding the addictive disorder or occurring during a prolonged period of abstinence) in women, whereas the opposite occurs with men (Kessler et al. 1997).

Among women with both major depression and alcohol dependence, the major depression is independent or primary approximately two-thirds of the time, whereas in men, the alcohol diagnosis is primary about two-thirds of the time and the depression is predominantly alcohol-related (Prescott et al. 2000). In addition, depression seems to mediate gender differences in the severity of each disorder in comorbid subjects, depression being more severe in women and alcoholism more severe in men. No gender differences in the severity of alcoholism were found in nondepressed alcoholic men and women (Pettinati et al. 1997). Recent evidence points out that comorbidity between alcoholism and depression is linked to gender-specific genetic and environmental risk factors and that the factors underlying it differ between women and men (Prescott et al. 2000).

There is a complex relationship between comorbid alcoholism and depression, and this co-occurrence has differential significance for the outcome of alcoholism treatment between genders. For instance, no gender differences were found in the relapse rate after detoxification in currently depressed alcoholic women and men (Greenfield and O'Leary 2002). However, a lifetime diagnosis of depression among treatment-seeking alcoholic women predicted a better prognosis in terms of drinking outcomes compared with that of nondepressed women, whereas the opposite occurred among men (McGrath et al. 2000).

Other psychiatric disorders significantly comorbid with alcohol use disorders in women include bulimia, but not anorexia (Schuckit et al. 1996). Moreover, this comorbidity is more likely to occur in the presence of other psychiatric disorders, particularly depression and posttraumatic stress disorder (Dansky et al. 2000; Sinha and O'Malley 2000). Alcoholic women also have increased risk of a drug use disorder, especially that of tranquilizing drugs, compared with that risk for alcoholic men (Graham and Wilsnack 2000; Kessler et al.

1997). The comorbidity between alcoholism and social phobia is associated with higher severity of the anxiety disorder in women than in men, despite similar alcoholism severity (Randall et al. 2000).

Other Drugs

Among individuals dependent on drugs other than alcohol, there is contradictory evidence regarding gender differences in the occurrence of psychiatric comorbidity, possibly related to greater heterogeneity of the populations surveyed. Data from the ECA study showed a significantly higher lifetime prevalence of psychiatric comorbidity (excluding alcohol abuse and dependence) among women with other drug abuse and dependence than that among men, phobic and depressive disorders being more frequent among women and antisocial personality disorder being more frequent among men (Anthony and Helzer 1991). A recent study with treatment-seeking individuals with other drug dependence showed no significant gender differences in the overall rate of psychiatric comorbidity. Nevertheless, women present greater rates of depression, mania, and anxiety disorders, as well as a higher mean number of non–substance use disorders. Men have more alcohol dependence and antisocial personality disorder (Compton et al. 2000). Furthermore, the association of substance use disorders and posttraumatic stress disorder is especially salient for female adolescents, in comparison with male adolescents (Lipschitz et al. 2000).

Sociocultural Factors

Whether or not addictive disorders turn out to be determined less by nature and more by nurture in women, the importance of sociocultural factors in shaping their etiology and course is clearly established. The traditional expectations that women will drink less than men and will drink only on special occasions protect women from developing alcohol problems, whereas societal changes in women's roles have been associated with increasing drinking and alcohol problems among women. Cross-cultural analyses of drinking behavior show that women with higher education tend to consume more alcohol than less educated women, a pattern not observed among men. Also, unemployment is more strongly associated to women's drinking than to that of men (Ahlstrom et al. 2001). Additionally, evidence shows that women may be affected more than men are by family history of alcoholism and violence (Chermack et al. 2000) as well as by the drinking patterns of their spouses or significant others (Blume 1998).

Although societal norms protect women to some degree, they can also be destructive. The social stigma attached to heavy drinking and to drug use in women (a stigma that is associated with the incorrect expectation of sexual arousal and promiscuity) brands such individuals as "fallen women." When alcoholic women do not fit the societal stereotype, their disease is not recognized. Thus, the stigma reinforces denial in the affected women as well as in their families and among professionals, who might otherwise diagnose and treat the disease earlier. The probability that a diagnosis of alcoholism will be missed in a general medical and surgical hospital population is highest when the patient is better educated, of higher socioeconomic status, privately insured, and female (Moore et al. 1989).

This societal stereotyping also encourages sexual assault, including date rape, against women who drink. A woman who is drinking is assumed to be sexually available. Society considers a rapist who is intoxicated to be less responsible for his behavior, whereas a victim who is intoxicated is blamed for the assault (Blume 1991).

A recent trend in many states is to prosecute pregnant or postpartum women for alcohol or other drug use during their pregnancy. In some jurisdictions, a positive urine toxicology result in a newborn leads to automatic removal of the child, without any effort to diagnose or treat the mother or to help the family unit. In others, criminal charges of "prenatal child abuse" or delivering a controlled substance to a minor (via the umbilical cord) have been pressed, even when the accused woman had tried to obtain treatment during her pregnancy and had been unsuccessful because of a lack of facilities (Blume 1997). Such policies are widely publicized and tend to further erode the addicted woman's tenuous trust in the public medical system. By deterring pregnant addicts from seeking either addiction treatment or prenatal care, these policies have the potential to increase the numbers of alcohol- and drug-affected newborns rather than improve infant health. At the same time, growing evidence shows that brief intervention is associated with sustained reductions in substance use in pregnant women (Manwell et al. 2000).

Treatment

The continuum of treatment modalities and settings that has evolved over the past half century was initially developed to help alcoholic and addicted men. Common sense dictates that professionals and programs tailor their treatment to women's needs. However, this is not always done. For example, the so-called boot camp model of military-style discipline and physical challenge for convicted drug-addicted men has been applied, unchanged (even with regard to male-style clothing and haircuts), to young women. The Twelve Steps of Alcoholics Anonymous (AA), also used in some form by other mutual-help groups for addicted individuals and their families, were originally written as a distillation of the recovery experience of the first hundred or so AA members, most of them middle-class white men (White and Chaney 1993). Although many women have recovered through participation in 12-step programs, and at present, fully one-third of AA members are women, an understanding of gender differences can enhance the ability of health professionals to recommend these steps to and interpret these steps for women. For example, admitting powerlessness over alcohol (the first step in AA) often represents a spiritual crisis for a culturally empowered man who is accustomed to running his own life. In contrast, a single mother who lives in urban poverty and has been sexually abused might think that to admit she is powerless and that her life is unmanageable is merely to describe her situation. For such women, learning to take control rather than give it up will be a major goal of treatment.

National data reveal that women are currently underrepresented in addiction treatment, particularly in alcoholism treatment facilities. In addition to the role played by stigma and denial, other barriers experienced by women needing treatment include a lack of child care (virtually no residential programs accommodate both women and their children), the reluctance of many addiction programs to accept pregnant patients (Blume 1997), and lack of health insurance (more women than men are employed in low-paying and/or part-time jobs that do not provide health insurance). Furthermore, the most common organized referral programs (employee assistance programs in the workplace and drinking driver or other criminal justice–based programs) are much more effective at identifying addicted men than addicted women. For example, among convicted drunk drivers, men outnumber women by about nine to one.

What case-finding methods would work better for women? When male and female patients in alcoholism facilities are asked to identify the problems that brought them into treatment, they reply differently. Among men, the problems most frequently cited are problems related to work and those involving the justice system, reflecting current intervention techniques. Among women, the most frequently mentioned problems relate to health and family. Age differences are likely to influence these responses, with younger women more often reporting job and legal problems and alcohol-related symptoms such as blackout, and middle-aged women frequently citing problems with children or an "empty nest" after children have grown and left home (Gomberg 1993).

Simple screening programs in health facilities would identify a large number of women with addictive disorders. Five studies in different sites by different researchers, using simple screening tests for alcohol abuse and dependence in women receiving medical services, found serious problems at rates well above the general population prevalence. Among ambulatory primary care and gynecological patients, the rates ranged from 11% to 17%, and 12% to 14% of medical and surgical inpatients screened positive (Blume 1998). However, such screening is rarely done. Likewise, screening among the clients of divorce lawyers and family service agencies could uncover addictive disorders at earlier stages than are now generally recognized.

Once a female patient enters treatment, she should be carefully evaluated for additional psychiatric and substance use disorders. Many alcoholic and other drug-addicted women develop iatrogenic dependence on sedatives, benzodiazepines, and/or opiates, prescribed for a variety of reported symptoms by clinicians who have failed to recognize the underlying addictive disorder. Such dependencies must be treated along with the primary alcohol or other drug dependence.

Because suicidal behavior is especially common among women with substance use disorders (Pirkola et al. 1999), particular attention should be given to this issue when assessing psychiatric status at treatment entry.

When comorbid psychiatric disorders are discovered, it is helpful to determine whether the disorder preceded the addiction or had its onset during a prolonged period of abstinence and therefore might be regarded as primary. In these cases particularly, the patient should be prepared to recognize early indications of recurrence of the disorder during her recovery from addiction. Prompt treatment—of recurrent major depression, for example—can relieve symptoms and avert a relapse of addiction. Primary psychiatric disorders are less likely than secondary ones (such as depression with onset during active addiction) to be relieved without specific treatment during early recovery. Whether primary or secondary, however, some disorders, such as anorexia nervosa, bulimia, severe depression, or psychosis, will require treatment along with the addictive disorder. Substance use may be a weight control measure for many women, pointing the need for careful evaluation of comorbid eating disorders (Cochrane et al. 1998).

Female substance abusers are more likely than male substance abusers to report unsafe sexual practices and unsafe injection drug use (Pugatch et al. 2000). Much research has shown that successful treatment of drug-dependent women is associated with improved health-related behaviors, including safer sexual practices and more appropriate treatment seeking. Therefore, a review of physical health status, with special attention to human immunodeficiency virus (HIV) risk factors, is warranted, along with the appropriate referrals.

In evaluating an addicted woman, it is important to obtain an adequate history of physical and/or sexual abuse. Women in a currently abusive relationship might need help in obtaining safe shelter before treatment can be successfully undertaken. Additional effort should be made to assess the female patient's children for problems related to intrauterine exposure or to living with an addicted parent. Such children can often profit from programs designed for school-age children of alcoholic and addicted individuals. Parenting programs and programs that offer assistance for single parents are particularly helpful in the long-term rehabilitation of addicted women. Often from families made dysfunctional by the substance dependence of their own parents, these women commonly feel overwhelmed by the parental role. Family members should be involved in the female patient's treatment whenever possible and should be encouraged to participate in mutual-help groups such as Al-Anon, Nar-Anon, Alateen, and Adult Children of Alcoholics. Because having a substance-using partner is frequent among these women, it is useful to suggest the appropriate treatment referrals for the partner as well because this may have an impact on the woman's treatment.

Vocational rehabilitation is also a useful adjunct in women's treatment. Often unemployed or underemployed and restricted in outlook by narrow gender-stereotyped role choices, recovering women can gain a feeling of competence and control through job training and adequately paid employment. Care must be taken to avoid maintenance of sexist attitudes within the treatment program itself. In mixed-gender programs, women should not be role-stereotyped, assigned only "women's work," or allowed to defer to male group members without challenge. On the other hand, women's stereotyping of men (e.g., all men are batterers) should also be challenged to enlarge such women's understanding of the world and the opportunities that are open to them in recovery.

To avoid the problem of gender stereotyping, a number of all-female treatment programs have been developed, both as residential and outpatient models, with some preliminary evidence showing improved retention in comparison with mixed-gender models (Grella 1999). The all-female programs tend to employ female staff members and apply feminist principles to their treatment. Other programs that serve both genders have developed woman-led women's groups of various types, either as primary therapy groups or as supplements to mixed-gender groups. It is often easier for women to discuss sexual and abuse problems in all-female settings. Though preliminary evidence does not show meaningful advantages of therapist/client gender matching for treatment outcome (Sterling et al. 2001), female staff members provide role models for patients, as do recovering women encountered in mutual-help groups. An all-women mutual-help group, Women for Sobriety, meets in some parts of North America, as do some all-women AA and Narcotics Anonymous groups (check http://www.womenforsobriety.org and http://www.aa.org). Women-only programs seem to be attractive particularly for women with young children, women with a history of abuse, and lesbians (Hodgins et al. 1997).

Special populations of addicted women—including lesbians; Native American, African American, and Hispanic women; women in the military; and female health professionals—require special approaches that recognize the specific cultural context in which their addictive disorder developed (and in which their recovery will be played out) (Smith and Weisner 2000).

Research aiming at pharmacotherapy for substance-related problems should break down results by gender because recent evidence shows gender differential responses, with men benefiting more than women from citalopram in the treatment of alcohol dependence, for instance (Naranjo et al. 2000).

Prevention

Little effort has been devoted to the development of prevention methods that are specifically geared toward women. Because of society's double standard that accepts intoxication in men while condemning it in women, young women's perceptions regarding drinking are somewhat more conflicted than men's, suggesting that preventive efforts might have more impact if directed at either men or women independently (Ricciardelli et al. 2001). Most preventive programs for women have concentrated on the effects associated with substance use during the perinatal period. In addition, campaigns should target women in other age brackets, particularly adolescents. Recent studies have found that smoking is in danger of becoming a predominantly female drug usage because among adolescents ages 14–15 years, female daily smokers are less likely than male daily smokers to cease smoking (Patton et al. 1998). Primary prevention efforts geared toward girls might successfully include measures to combat sex-stereotyping, raise self-esteem, and decrease emphasis on thinness (many girls begin to smoke as a way to lose weight) and offer help to girls who have been abused. For adult women, primary prevention can be accomplished through group support for women involved in separation, divorce, or widowhood and through support for single mothers, caregivers of elderly or chronically ill persons, battered women, and other women in stressful situations. Helping these women to cope with their problems without the use of alcohol or other drugs will prevent abuse and dependence. Helping society to see addicted women as people with treatable illnesses will bring about an end to the prejudice that now keeps those in need from receiving help.

References

Ahlstrom S, Bloomfield K, Knibbe R: Gender differences in drinking patterns in nine European countries: descriptive findings. Subst Abus 22:69–85, 2001

Anthony JC, Helzer JE: Syndromes of drug abuse and dependence, in Psychiatric Disorders in America. Edited by Robins LN, Regier DA. New York, Free Press, 1991, pp 116–155

Blume SB: Sexuality and stigma: the alcoholic woman. Alcohol Health Res World 15:139–146, 1991

Blume SB: Women and alcohol: issues in social policy, in Gender and Alcohol: Individual and Social Perspectives. Edited by Wilsnack RW, Wilsnack SC. New Brunswick, NJ, Rutgers Center of Alcohol Studies, 1997, pp 462–489

Blume SB: Women and addictive disorders, in Principles of Addiction Medicine, 2nd Edition. Edited by Graham A, Schultz P. Chevy Chase, MD, American Society of Addiction Medicine, 1998, pp 15.1.1–15.1.30

Brady KT, Randall CL: Gender differences in substance use disorders. Psychiatr Clin North Am 22:241–252, 1999

Breslau N, Davis GC, Peterson EL, et al: Psychiatric sequelae of posttraumatic stress disorder in women. Arch Gen Psychiatry 54:81–87, 1997

Chermack ST, Stoltenberg SF, Fuller BE, et al: Gender differences in the development of substance-related problems: the impact of family history of alcoholism, family history of violence and childhood conduct problems. J Stud Alcohol 61:845–852, 2000

Cochrane C, Malcolm R, Brewerton T: The role of weight control as a motivation for cocaine abuse. Addict Behav 23:201–207, 1998

Compton WM 3rd, Cottler LB, Ben Abdallah A, et al: Substance dependence and other psychiatric disorders among drug dependent subjects: race and gender correlates. Am J Addict 9:113–125, 2000

Dansky BS, Brewerton TD, Kilpatrick DG: Comorbidity of bulimia nervosa and alcohol use disorders: results from the National Women's Study. Int J Eat Disord 27:180–190, 2000

Dixit AR, Crum RM: Prospective study of depression and the risk of heavy alcohol use in women. Am J Psychiatry 157:751–758, 2000

Fillmore KM, Bacon SD, Hyman M: The 27-year longitudinal panel study of drinking by students in college: final report, 1979 (Contract No ADM 281-76-0015). Rockville, MD, National Institute on Alcoholism and Alcohol Abuse, 1979

Gomberg ESL: Women and alcohol: use and abuse. J Nerv Ment Dis 181:211–219, 1993

Graham K, Wilsnack SS: The relationship between alcohol problems and use of tranquilizing drugs: longitudinal patterns among American women. Addict Behav 25:13–28, 2000

Greenfield SF, O'Leary G: Sex differences in substance use disorders, in Psychiatric Illness in Women: Emerging Treatments and Research. Edited by Lewis-Hall F, Williams TS, Panetta JA, et al. Washington, DC, American Psychiatric Publishing, 2002, pp 467–533

Grella CE: Women in residential drug treatment: differences by program type and pregnancy. J Health Care Poor Underserved 10:216–229, 1999

Helzer JE, Burnam A, McEvoy LT: Alcohol abuse and dependence, in Psychiatric Disorders in America. Edited by Robins LN, Regier DA. New York, Free Press, 1991, pp 81–115

Hodgins DC, El-Guebaly N, Addington J : Treatment of substance abusers: single or mixed gender programs? Addiction 92:805–812, 1997

Kessler RC, McGonagle KA, Zhao S, et al: Lifetime and 12-month prevalence of DSM-III-R psychiatric disorders in the United States: results from the National Comorbidity Survey. Arch Gen Psychiatry 51:8–19, 1994

Kessler RC, Crum RM, Warner LA, et al: Lifetime co-occurrence of DSM-III-R alcohol abuse and dependence with other psychiatric disorders in the National Comorbidity Survey. Arch Gen Psychiatry 54:313–321, 1997

Lieber CS: Ethnic and gender differences in ethanol metabolism. Alcohol Clin Exp Res 24:417–418, 2000

Lipschitz DS, Grilo CM, Fehon D, et al: Gender differences in the associations between posttraumatic stress symptoms and problematic substance use in psychiatric inpatient adolescents. J Nerv Ment Dis 188:349–356, 2000

Manwell LB, Fleming MF, Mundt MP, et al: Treatment of problem alcohol use in women of childbearing age: results of a brief intervention trial. Alcohol Clin Exp Res 24:1517–1524, 2000

McGrath PJ, Nunes EV, Quitkin FM: Current concepts in the treatment of depression in alcohol-dependent patients. Psychiatr Clin North Am 23:695–711, 2000

Moore RD, Bone LR, Geller G, et al: Prevalence, detection and treatment of alcoholism in hospitalized patients. JAMA 261:403–408, 1989

Naranjo CA, Knoke DM, Bremner KE: Variations in response to citalopram in men and women with alcohol dependence. J Psychiatry Neurosci 25:269–275, 2000

Patton GC, Carlin JB, Coffey C, et al: The course of early smoking: a population-based cohort study over three years. Addiction 93:1251–1260, 1998

Pettinati HM, Pierce JD Jr, Wolf AL, et al: Gender differences in comorbidly depressed alcohol-dependent outpatients. Alcohol Clin Exp Res 21:1742–1746, 1997

Pirkola SP, Isometsae ET, Heikkinen ME, et al: Female psychoactive substance–dependent suicide victims differ from male: results from a nationwide psychological autopsy study. Compr Psychiatry 40:101–107, 1999

Prescott CA, Aggen SH, Kendler KS: Sex differences in the sources of genetic liability to alcohol abuse and dependence in a population-based sample of U.S. twins. Alcohol Clin Exp Res 23:1136–1144, 1999

Prescott CA, Aggen SH, Kendler KS: Sex-specific genetic influences on the comorbidity of alcoholism and major depression in a population-based sample of U.S. twins. Arch Gen Psychiatry 57:803–811, 2000

Pugatch D, Ramratnam M, Strong L, et al: Gender differences in HIV risk behaviors among young adults and adolescents entering a Massachusetts Detoxification Center. Subst Abus 21:79–86, 2000

Randall CL, Thomas SE, Thevos AK: Gender comparison in alcoholics with concurrent social phobia: implications for alcoholism treatment. Am J Addict 9:202–215, 2000

Ricciardelli LA, Connor JP, Williams RJ, et al: Gender stereotypes and drinking cognitions as indicators of moderate and high risk drinking among young women and men. Drug Alcohol Depend 61:129–136, 2001

Schuckit MA, Tipp JE, Anthenelli RM, et al: Anorexia nervosa and bulimia nervosa in alcohol-dependent men and women and their relatives. Am J Psychiatry 153:74–82, 1996

Sexton H, Lipton RI, Nilssen O: Relating alcohol use and mood: results from the Tromso study. J Stud Alcohol 60:111–119, 1999

Sigvardsson S, Bohman M, Cloninger CR: Replication of the Stockholm Adoption Study of alcoholism: confirmatory cross-fostering analysis. Arch Gen Psychiatry 53:681–687, 1996

Sinha R, O'Malley, SS: Alcohol and eating disorders: implications for alcohol treatment and health services research. Alcohol Clin Exp Res 24:1312–1319, 2000

Smith WB, Weisner C: Women and alcohol problems: a critical analysis of the literature and unanswered questions. Alcohol Clin Exp Res 24:1320–1321, 2000

Sterling RC, Gottheil E, Weinstein SP, et al: The effect of therapist/patient race- and sex-matching in individual treatment. Addiction 96:1015–1022, 2001

Tavares H, Zilberman ML, Beites FJ, et al: Gender differences in gambling progression. J Gambl Stud 17:151–159, 2001

Wang J L, Patten SB: A prospective study of sex-specific effects of major depression on alcohol consumption. Can J Psychiatry 46:422–425, 2001

White W, Chaney R: Metaphors of Transformation: Feminine and Masculine. Bloomington, IL, Lighthouse Training Institute, 1993

Wilsnack SC, Vogeltanz ND, Klassen AD, et al: Childhood sexual abuse and women's substance abuse: national survey findings. J Stud Alcohol 58:264–271, 1997

Zilberman ML, Tavares H, Blume S, et al: Towards best practices in the treatment of women with addictive disorders. Addictive Disorders and Their Treatment 1:39–46, 2002

Perinatal Substance Use

Loretta P. Finnegan, M.D.
Stephen R. Kandall, M.D.

The perinatal period should be regarded as a continuum that extends from the beginning of a woman's pregnancy through delivery and the first 3 months of a child's life. Although in this chapter we discuss discrete drugs, clinicians must be aware that the use of a psychoactive drug during pregnancy may mean that other psychoactive agents are being used concomitantly. Perinatal effects may therefore reflect pharmacological effects of individual agents or the combined effects of multiple drugs. In all cases, substance use during pregnancy must be considered to be "high risk" from general medical, obstetric, neonatal, pediatric, psychosocial, and criminal justice standpoints. It is extremely important, however, to recognize that providing comprehensive, supportive, nonjudgmental care for the pregnant woman and her family in a well-integrated, multidisciplinary setting offers a unique opportunity to restructure the woman's life in a positive direction.

Treatment of the Substance-Using Mother

Epidemiology

Determining the epidemiology of drug use during pregnancy has always been an inexact science (American Academy of Pediatrics 1998; National Institute on Drug Abuse 1996). This imprecision has resulted from factors such as changes in drug use patterns over time, variations in sample populations in individual hospitals and larger geographical areas, differing applications of history-taking techniques and drug-detection technologies, and the varying attention that society has paid over time to this specific subset of female drug users (Kandall 1996).

In 1992–1993, using a cross-sectional analysis in their National Pregnancy and Health Survey, the National Institute on Drug Abuse (1996) estimated the annual totals in the U.S. population. The survey was a two-stage probability sample of hospitals within the United States and women delivering live-born infants. Women reported licit and illicit drug use behavior, obstetric history, prenatal events, and demographic information. Drug use patterns were reported prior to pregnancy and within each trimester for 2,613 women from 52 participating hospitals. Data were weighted to represent 4,023,307 live births in the United States in 1992, and national estimates were calculated.

In the United States in 1992, according to these estimates, approximately 220,000 women (5.5% of pregnant women) used an illicit drug during pregnancy. Marijuana was used most frequently (119,000 women; 2.9%) and was followed by amphetamines, sedatives, tranquilizers, and analgesics in a nonmedical context (61,000 women; 1.5%); cocaine (benzoylmethylecgonine) (45,000 women; 1.1%); and smaller percentages for methamphetamine, heroin, methadone, inhalants, and hallucinogens. These numbers are all considerably less, however, than those for alcohol use (757,000 women; 18.8%) and cigarette smoking (820,000 women; 20.4%) during pregnancy.

Although national epidemiological studies are of interest, each community should determine its own incidence of maternal substance use to best assess the impact on its obstetric, medical, social services, and addiction treatment needs.

Medical Issues in Prenatal Substance Use

Given the chronic relapsing nature of addiction and the chaotic lives of substance-abusing women, coupled with the frequent lack of consistent prenatal care, it is not surprising that many medical problems may arise during pregnancy. Substance-abusing women are at increased risk for anemia, bacteremia and septicemia, bacterial endocarditis, cellulitis, dental caries, endocrinopathies, hepatitis, nutritional deficiencies, phlebitis, pneumonia, tetanus, tuberculosis, and urinary tract infections (Finnegan and Kandall 1997). The pregnant opiate addict may have periods of physical well-being but may also feel the extremes of being "high" or "sick" within a relatively brief period of time. During binges, the cocaine user has an increased risk of hypertensive crises, cardiac and cerebrovascular complications, seizures, and a range of psychiatric disorders such as dysphoric agitation.

Sexually transmitted diseases, particularly human immunodeficiency virus (HIV), have become inextricably linked to illicit drug use because of direct sex-for-drugs activity, prostitution to purchase drugs, and the sharing of infected needles and drug paraphernalia. Current recommendations for the treatment of HIV-infected women with HIV RNA levels greater than 1,000 copies/mL include highly active combination antiretroviral regimens including zidovudine. The use of zidovudine alone is recommended for women with RNA below 1,000 copies/mL. Regardless of treatment regimen, all HIV-infected women should receive zidovudine during labor; zidovudine should be continued for 6 weeks in the newborn infant. A zidovudine regimen has reduced the perinatal HIV transmission rate from 25% to 5%–8%; highly active combination antiretroviral therapy has further reduced the transmission rate below 2%.

Illicit substance use during pregnancy also places the fetus and newborn infant at increased obstetric risk. Abruptio placentae, amnionitis, early pregnancy loss, intrauterine growth retardation, late intrauterine death, placental insufficiency, postpartum hemorrhage, preeclampsia and eclampsia, premature labor, premature rupture of membranes, and septic thrombophlebitis are among the potential complications (Finnegan and Kandall 1997).

Treatment for heroin dependency during pregnancy should be tailored to the woman's individual needs. Highly motivated women or those facing barriers to obtaining methadone maintenance may be considered for medical withdrawal during pregnancy if the process can be undertaken under careful medical supervision (Center for Substance Abuse Treatment 1993b). The pharmacological treatment of choice for heroin-dependent women is methadone maintenance, which offers a unique opportunity for careful supervision of a woman for her addiction, pregnancy, and general medical and psychosocial health (Kandall et al. 1999). Potential barriers such as fear of the loss of her children to protective agencies, insufficient financial means, unsafe living conditions, difficulties in obtaining suitable transportation, lack of support from family and social contacts, and inaccessibility of gender-specific programs must be addressed (Murphy and Rosenbaum 1999). Under the Substance Abuse Prevention and Treatment Block Grant (P.L. 102-321 1992), states are required to grant pregnant women priority for treatment and to provide them with access to health care and child care and assistance with transportation. A source for referral of individuals to relevant state and local services is the Health Resources and Services Administration's National Maternal and Child Health Clearinghouse (1-888-275-4772).

All pregnancies associated with drug abuse should be considered obstetrically high-risk. Medical-obstetric management should be carried out by knowledgeable, supportive health care providers in a program that has experience in handling such pregnancies. In such an environment, methadone maintenance treatment has been shown for three decades to reduce both maternal mortality rate and rates of fetal wastage, fetal morbidity, and pregnancy-associated complications (Blinick et al. 1973; Finnegan et al. 1991). Although suggested regimens of methadone maintenance vary, provision of an adequate dosage of methadone (60–150 mg/day) is associated with a lower incidence of illicit drug use and higher rates of treatment retention. Single daily dosing of methadone still represents the standard of care, but split daily dosing may also be considered in order to maintain a steady-state level of medication.

Psychosocial Issues in Prenatal Substance Use

The complexity of medical management of the pregnant substance abuser is mirrored in the attendant psychosocial problems seen in this population. Drug-dependent women often have anxiety, depression, and low self-esteem (Hagan et al. 1994; Murphy and Rosenbaum 1999). Degrading descriptive terms reflect the disrespect with which women are regarded within the drug culture and should never be used in the treatment setting (Murphy and Rosenbaum 1999).

Many addicted women share a history of past and current physical abuse and sexual assault. A Philadelphia study (Finnegan et al. 1991) revealed that 83% of women entering drug treatment came from households in which parents used drugs, 67% had experienced sexual assault, and 60% had been physically assaulted. Similarly, in a New York study, homelessness, sexual abuse, and drug use by family members were prominent historical facts about their past and current environments elicited from drug-dependent women (Chavkin et al. 1993).

In this stressful psychosocial setting, aggravated by reduced socioeconomic circumstances, it is not surprising that an increasing number of women enter the drug subculture. Society's decision to prosecute

women who use drugs during pregnancy (Kandall 1996, pp. 273–279) and draconian sentences for drug-related offenses have resulted in a large increase in the number of women incarcerated during the past 20 years (National Institute on Justice 1990; Snell 1994). Prosecution of drug-using pregnant women was carried out despite opposition by a wide spectrum of medical, public health, and addiction agencies. In addition, fear of criminal prosecution had been shown to deter women from seeking prenatal care (Chavkin 1991). Gynecological-obstetric care in the penal system has been reported to be substandard, which jeopardizes pregnancy outcome (Wellisch et al. 1993).

The complex matrix of intertwining medical and psychosocial risk factors that usually characterize substance use during pregnancy dictate that a successful outcome can best be obtained within a comprehensive, supportive, nonjudgmental environment that focuses on the multidimensional needs of the woman (Center for Substance Abuse Treatment 1993b, 1994; Finnegan et al. 1984).

The existence and interaction of these complex issues make it clear that effective drug treatment must be based on this comprehensive approach to the woman and her addiction. This approach encompasses a wide range of services (residential, outpatient, home-based, and prison-based); multiple counseling modalities (individual, group, and family); counseling on sexual abuse and domestic violence; services for children (day care, play therapy, parental training); concrete services (transportation, housing, food); comprehensive family-based health care (obstetric, pediatric, general medical); educational training (job training, high school equivalency training); appropriate staffing (including female members and being supportive and culturally and racially sensitive); advocacy services (legal, child protection, welfare); and aftercare. Provision of these services at a single location will enhance compliance and will make accessing the multiple aspects of treatment easier for the pregnant woman.

Treatment of the Substance-Exposed Infant

Neonates born to substance-using mothers should be admitted to units that provide observation, assessment, and treatment by trained personnel. In cases in which a suspicion of maternal drug use is under consideration, confirmation of fetal exposure may be accomplished by testing of urine. Analysis of meconium (Ostrea et al. 1992) and/or hair (Callahan et al. 1991) provides a longer window of fetal drug exposure, but these testing methodologies are generally restricted to research laboratories. Under all circumstances, however, testing should be carried out not for the purpose of punitive referral but to identify both mothers who are in need of medical and addiction services and infants who require special observation for medical complications such as neonatal abstinence syndrome.

Opiates

Many pharmacological agents have been reported to produce signs of neonatal abstinence syndrome. The most notable agents are opiates (including opium, meperidine, methadone, morphine, and controlled-release oxycodone hydrochloride), alcohol, barbiturates, and diazepam. Because signs of abstinence syndrome may overlap among these categories of drugs, documentation of maternal drug-taking patterns is critical. This can be accomplished prenatally with sensitive history taking and at birth by means of urine testing.

In the newborn period, signs of drug abstinence may mimic other serious conditions such as sepsis or meningitis, hypoglycemia, adrenal insufficiency, or cardiorespiratory disease. Because most opiates are short acting, signs of abstinence will develop shortly (generally within 1–3 days) after delivery, when the cord is clamped and the infant is acutely deprived of the drug circulating in the maternal bloodstream. Variations in amounts of maternal drug use, placental drug transfer, neonatal metabolism and excretion, and gestational age may all potentially affect the time to onset of abstinence symptoms. The onset of methadone-associated abstinence symptoms, although usually early, is somewhat more unpredictable because methadone establishes a reservoir in fetal tissue and undergoes more variable metabolism and excretion (Finnegan and Kaltenbach 1992).

Signs of neonatal abstinence syndrome are usually divided into four groups (American Academy of Pediatrics 1998; Center for Substance Abuse Treatment 1993a; Finnegan and Kaltenbach 1992; Kandall 1999):

1. *Central nervous system signs* include irritability, high-pitched crying, tremors, hypertonia, hyperreflexia,
and dysrhythmic sucking and swallowing. Seizures may occur in approximately 5% of opiate-exposed infants.
2. *Gastrointestinal signs* include vomiting and diarrhea, which when combined with poor intake of nutrients and increased insensible water loss, often results in excessive weight loss and suboptimal weight gain in the first few weeks of life.
3. *Respiratory signs* include tachypnea and hyperpnea, which may produce respiratory alkalosis, cyanosis, and apnea if untreated.
4. *Autonomic nervous system signs* include sweating, sneezing, tearing, and hyperthermia.

Infants exposed to drugs prenatally are considered to be at high risk and should be cared for in a structured setting by skilled personnel. Liberal amounts of fluids and calories should be provided to offset the infant's hypermetabolic state. Although it has been traditionally recommended that these infants be spared excessive stimulation, swaddling in a darkened room increases the need for close surveillance, including the detection of abstinence-associated seizures.

Because only about 60%–80% of drug-exposed neonates experience significant abstinence symptoms, routine prophylactic treatment is not recommended. Use of the semi-objective abstinence symptom severity scoring system proposed by Finnegan and Kaltenbach (1992) allows accurate evaluation of signs, avoids unnecessary treatment of mildly affected infants, and provides a methodology for effective tapering of medications. This scoring system rates 21 individual signs, assigning each a relative weight based on a postulated relationship with outcomes of perinatal morbidity and death. Infants are evaluated 2 hours after birth and every 4 hours thereafter, or more frequently if the abstinence symptoms are severe. Specific pharmacological treatment is tailored to the severity score.

Although diazepam and chlorpromazine have been used to treat opiate abstinence symptoms, there are no studies to prove their efficacy. Paregoric (camphorated tincture of opium) or another short-acting opiate preparation has been the treatment of choice for neonatal opiate abstinence syndrome (American Academy of Pediatrics 1998; Center for Substance Abuse Treatment 1993a). This treatment is based on the assumption that opiate exposure is best treated with another opiate and on studies performed on neonates. Paregoric is easily administered orally, has little toxicity, restores sucking reflexes to normal more rapidly than nonspecific therapies such as phenobarbital, and offers some protection against abstinence-associated seizures. Paregoric is given every 3–4 hours with monitoring of the clinical response; the final stabilizing dosage is maintained for 3 to 5 days, followed by a slow tapering regimen (Finnegan and Kaltenbach 1992; Kandall 1999).

However, recent concerns have been raised about the safety of other ingredients found in paregoric, despite its record of efficacy and safety (American Academy of Pediatrics 1998). The Committee on Drugs of the American Academy of Pediatrics cautioned that paregoric contains isoquinoline derivatives (noscapine and papaverine), which are antispasmodics. Paregoric also contains camphor, a potentially dangerous central nervous system stimulant (American Academy of Pediatrics 1994), which is lipid-soluble and requires glucuronidation for excretion. In addition, paregoric contains alcohol, anise oil, and glycerin. Paregoric also contains 4 mg/mL of benzoic acid, which may compete for bilirubin binding sites. Benzyl alcohol (its oxidative product) has been reported to cause a syndrome of severe acidosis, central nervous system depression, hypotension, renal failure, seizures, and death in small premature infants who receive large doses (Gershanik et al. 1982).

As a result of these concerns, the AAP Committee on Drugs has recommended tincture of opium as the treatment of choice for neonatal opiate abstinence (American Academy of Pediatrics 1998). The committee's recommendation is for the use of a 25-fold dilution of tincture of opium, which results in a concentration of morphine equivalent to that in paregoric. Dosage regimens can be used in the same way as with paregoric, using the above regimen and the severity scoring system. Tincture of opium dosages may be tapered in the same way as with paregoric.

Phenobarbital is a nonspecific central nervous system depressant that can also be used to treat neonatal abstinence syndrome; however, ineffectual sucking may occur with this medication (Center for Substance Abuse Treatment 1993a). After cessation of either treatment, the infant should be monitored in the hospital for at least 2 days to observe for rebound withdrawal. The reader should refer to other publications for the regimen cited above for the details of treatment of neonatal abstinence syndrome (Finnegan and Kaltenbach 1992). Careful dosing, continued assessment, and appropriate withdrawal of medications will reduce the chances for added morbidity.

Abstinence-associated seizures should be treated acutely with a loading dose of 10–20 mg/kg of phenobarbital supplemented with oral paregoric. The phenobarbital dose may be lowered sequentially once the seizures are controlled and a diagnostic workup has ruled out other causes of neonatal seizures. Most of the infants will be discharged without anticonvulsant medication, and the prognosis of infants with uncomplicated seizures is excellent.

If the mother is HIV-negative, breast-feeding should be encouraged for its attendant medical and psychosocial benefits. Studies are in progress to determine if antiretroviral drugs given to the infant during this period will make breast-feeding safer. Opiates pass to the nursing infant through the breast milk but do not appear to affect the severity of the neonatal abstinence syndrome, nor are they adequate to serve as treatment for neonatal symptoms (McCarthy and Posey 2000).

Stimulants

Maternal cocaine use is associated with specific obstetric complications, including early pregnancy loss, abruptio placentae, premature onset of labor, chronic fetal hypoxia, intrauterine growth retardation, and an increased incidence of stillbirths (Plessinger and Woods 1991). Cocaine has a low molecular weight, is highly soluble in water and lipid, and passes easily transplacentally from mother to fetus. Although the risk of cocaine-associated teratogenicity has been difficult to establish (Koren et al. 1993), cocaine has been reported to be responsible for a series of congenital anomalies in a pattern of "fetal vascular disruption" (Hoyme et al. 1990). After birth, cocaine-associated vasoconstriction has been reported to be the precipitating factor in necrotizing enterocolitis, bowel perforation, arterial thrombosis, hypertension, and myocardial ischemia (Finnegan and Kandall 1997).

Cocaine-exposed newborns show neurological signs that are quite different from those seen in opiate-exposed neonates. Rather than abstinence symptoms, cocaine-exposed infants show direct neurotoxicity manifested initially by transient hypertonia and hyperreflexia, followed by depressed interactive behavior, lability of state, and poor organizational response to environmental stimuli (Chasnoff et al. 1985; Mayes et al. 1993; Oro and Dixon 1987). Less commonly, these infants may show more dramatic neuropathological signs such as seizures and cerebrovascular accidents. Although most infants do not require treatment, excessive irritability may be treated with short courses of phenobarbital. Because cocaine-exposed infants have been reported to be hyporeactive once the initial irritability subsides, they should be provided with an individualized program of structured physical contact, including gentle handling with body support, soft social talking, and eye contact without overstimulation (Center for Substance Abuse Treatment 1993a). Intervention programs provided by trained personnel should include the parents as much as possible. In contrast to opiates, breast-feeding by a cocaine-using mother poses risks of acute neonatal intoxication and is therefore contraindicated.

Similar to the action of cocaine, amphetamine and methamphetamine block the reuptake of neurotransmitters. Use of these drugs during pregnancy has been associated with a high perinatal mortality rate; reductions in birth weight, length, and head circumference; associated congenital malformations; and abnormal neurological signs, including drowsiness, poor feeding, and seizures (Eriksson et al. 1978, 1981; Oro and Dixon 1987).

Nonopiate Central Nervous System Depressants

Maternal use of phenobarbital at a dosage of at least 90 mg/day for 12 weeks before delivery has been reported to produce a neonatal abstinence syndrome marked by hyperactivity, restlessness, excessive crying, tremulousness, hyperreflexia, vomiting, and diarrhea. This complex of signs is similar to opiate abstinence syndrome (American Academy of Pediatrics 1998). The abstinence syndrome usually develops by 4–8 days of age and should be treated with phenobarbital when symptoms cannot be controlled by conservative measures. A more prolonged abstinence syndrome, similar to the subacute withdrawal described occasionally with heroin exposure, may persist for 2–6 months. Barbiturates pass into breast milk, but breast-feeding need not be discouraged.

Hallucinogens

The effects of marijuana (Δ^9-tetrahydrocannabinol) on the human fetus and neonate are not well understood, and no controlled studies have been reported. Some studies have linked maternal marijuana use with reduced fetal growth and an increase in neonatal tremors and startle responses. The same lack of studies applies to lysergic acid diethylamide (LSD), which has been reported to cause chromosomal breakage, spontaneous abortions, and prematurity. Phencyclidine, or 1-(1-phenylcyclohexyl)piperidine, also known as PCP and "angel dust," has been noted in limited studies to cause hypertonia, hyperreflexia, and tremors.

Alcohol

Alcohol abuse may occur by itself or as part of a larger pattern of polysubstance abuse. Management of the pregnant alcohol abuser should be undertaken in the same comprehensive manner as described above for other substances (Center for Substance Abuse Treatment 1993b). Because the fetus is especially vulnerable to the teratogenic effects of alcohol during the first trimester, a discussion of alcohol consumption should be an integral part of both preconception counseling and ongoing discussions during pregnancy.

Although biological variability dictates that the safe limit for alcohol consumption varies among individual women, the diagnosis of fetal alcohol syndrome has been associated with consumption of more than 3 ounces of absolute alcohol daily, often in combination with binge drinking. The term *fetal alcohol effects* is often used when only some of the signs of fetal alcohol syndrome are seen. Fetal alcohol syndrome (Sokol and Clarren 1989) is characterized by the following triad of symptoms:

1. Prenatal and postnatal growth retardation affecting the parameters of body weight, length, and head circumference.
2. A characteristic facial dysmorphism marked by short palpebral fissures, hypoplastic maxilla, short upturned nose, hypoplastic philtrum, thinned upper vermillion, and micrognathia or retrognathia. Ptosis, strabismus, epicanthal folds, microphthalmia, posterior rotation of the ears, and cleft lip or palate are less common features. Other reported malformations involve the cardiac, genitourinary, and gastrointestinal tracts, the skin, and joints.
3. Central nervous system anomalies, including microcephaly. Neurological dysfunction may present in the newborn period with irritability, tremulousness, poor sucking, increased crying, and tonic-clonic seizures. Long-term follow-up examinations (Streissguth et al. 1994) tend to show cerebellar deficits, hypotonia, speech and hearing problems, and reduced mental capacity with reductions in IQ scores.

Nicotine

Long-term maternal smoking has been linked to increased rates of placenta previa, abruptio placentae, placental infarcts, and placental changes caused by vasoconstriction. Elevated levels of carbon monoxide in smokers may also adversely affect the delivery of oxygen to the fetus transplacentally. Many studies have shown a reduction in birth weight by approximately 150–200 g per pack of cigarettes smoked. Hypertonia has been reported in neonates born to smoking mothers. Children born to mothers who smoke have increased rates of sudden infant death syndrome, hospitalization, and death up to 5 years of age, primarily from respiratory disorders such as bronchiolitis and pneumonia.

Conclusion

Perinatal substance abuse is a problem of major public health importance. The stigma that society attaches to women who abuse substances during pregnancy has often originated in societal moral attitudes and in political opportunism (Kandall 1996). These dehumanizing attitudes have placed barriers in the way of women seeking optimal medical and obstetric care for themselves and their fetuses. The best public health result can be obtained once these barriers have been removed and women are able to find appropriate services in a supportive, multidimensional treatment facility.

References

American Academy of Pediatrics: Camphor revisited: focus on toxicity. American Academy of Pediatrics, Committee on Drugs. Pediatrics 94:127–128, 1994

American Academy of Pediatrics: Neonatal drug withdrawal. Pediatrics 101:1079–1088, 1998

Blinick G, Jerez E, Wallach RC: Methadone maintenance, pregnancy and progeny. JAMA 225:477–479, 1973

Callahan CM, Grant TM, Phipps P, et al: Measurement of gestational cocaine exposure: sensitivity of infants' hair, meconium, and urine. J Pediatr 120:763–768, 1991

Center for Substance Abuse Treatment: Improving Treatment for Drug-Exposed Infants (DHHS Publ No SMA-93-2011). Rockville, MD, Substance Abuse and Mental Health Services Administration, 1993a

Center for Substance Abuse Treatment: Treatment Improvement Protocol for Pregnant Substance-Using Women. Rockville, MD, Substance Abuse and Mental Health Services Administration, 1993b

Center for Substance Abuse Treatment: Practical Approaches in the Treatment of Women Who Abuse Alcohol and Other Drugs. Rockville, MD, Substance Abuse and Mental Health Services Administration, 1994

Chasnoff IJ, Burns WJ, Schnoll SH, et al: Cocaine use in pregnancy. N Engl J Med 313:666–669, 1985

Chavkin W: Mandatory treatment for drug abuse during pregnancy. JAMA 266:1556–1561, 1991

Chavkin W, Paone D, Friedmann P, et al: Psychiatric histories of drug using mothers: treatment implications. J Subst Abuse Treat 10:445–448, 1993

Eriksson M, Larsson G, Winbladh B, et al: The influence of amphetamine addiction on pregnancy and the newborn infant. Acta Paediatr Scand 67:95–99, 1978

Eriksson M, Larsson G, Zetterstrom R: Amphetamine addiction and pregnancy. Acta Obstet Gynecol Scand 60:253–259, 1981

Finnegan LP, Kaltenbach K: Neonatal abstinence syndrome, in Primary Pediatric Care, 2nd Edition. Edited by Hoekelman RA, Friedman SB, Nelson N, et al. St Louis, MO, CV Mosby, 1992, pp 1367–1378

Finnegan LP, Kandall SR: Maternal and neonatal effects of alcohol and drugs, in Substance Abuse: A Comprehensive Textbook, 3rd Edition. Edited by Lowinson JH, Ruiz P, Millman RB, et al. Baltimore, MD, Williams & Wilkins, 1997, pp 513–534

Finnegan LP, Kaltenbach KA, Pasto M, et al: Improving outcome of children born to drug-dependent mothers, in Frontiers of Infant Psychiatry, Vol 2. Edited by Call J, Galenson E, Tyson R. New York, Basic Books, 1984, pp 225–231

Finnegan LP, Hagan T, Kaltenbach KA: Scientific foundation of clinical practice: opiate use in pregnant women. Bull N Y Acad Med 67:223–239, 1991

Gershanik J, Boecler B, Ensley H, et al: The gasping syndrome and benzyl alcohol poisoning. N Engl J Med 307:1384–1388, 1982

Hagan TA, Finnegan LP, Nelson-Zlupko L: Impediments to comprehensive treatment models for substance-dependent: treatment and research questions. J Psychoactive Drugs 26(2):163–171, 1994

Hoyme HE, Jones KL, Dixon SD, et al: Prenatal cocaine exposure and fetal vascular disruption. Pediatrics 85:743–747, 1990

Kandall S: Substance and shadow: women and addiction in the United States. Cambridge, MA, Harvard University Press, 1996

Kandall SR: Treatment strategies for drug-exposed neonates. Clin Perinatol 26:231–243, 1999

Kandall SR, Doberczak TM, Jantunen M, et al: The methadone-maintained pregnancy. Clin Perinatol 26:173–183, 1999

Koren G, Graham K, Feigenbaum A, et al: Evaluation and counseling of teratogenic risk: the Motherisk approach. J Clin Pharmacol 33:405–411, 1993

Mayes LC, Granger RH, Frank MA, et al: Neurobehavioral profiles of neonates exposed to cocaine prenatally. Pediatrics 91:778–783, 1993

McCarthy JJ, Posey BL: Methadone levels in human milk. J Hum Lact 16:115–120, 2000

Murphy S, Rosenbaum M: Pregnant Women on Drugs. New Brunswick, NJ, Rutgers University Press, 1999

National Institute on Drug Abuse: National Pregnancy and Health Survey: Drug Use Among Women Delivering Livebirths: 1992. Rockville, MD, National Institute on Drug Abuse, 1996

National Institute on Justice: Drug Use Forecasting Annual Report 1989. Washington, DC, U.S. Department of Justice, 1990

Oro AS, Dixon SD: Perinatal cocaine and methamphetamine exposure: maternal and neonatal correlates. J Pediatr 111:571–578, 1987

Ostrea EM, Brady M, Gause S, et al: Drug screening of newborns by meconium analysis: a large-scale, prospective, epidemiologic study. Pediatrics 89:107–113, 1992

Plessinger MA, Woods JR: The cardiovascular effects of cocaine use in pregnancy. Reprod Toxicol 5:99–113, 1991

Snell TJ: Women in Prison: Survey of State Prison Inmates. Bureau of Justice Statistics Special Report (Publ No NCJ-145321). Washington, DC, U.S. Department of Justice, 1994

Sokol RJ, Clarren SK: Guidelines for use of terminology describing the impact of prenatal alcohol on the offspring. Alcohol Clin Exp Res 13:597–598, 1989

Streissguth AP, Sampson PD, Olson HC, et al: Maternal drinking during pregnancy: attention and short-term memory in 14-year-old offspring—a longitudinal prospective study. Alcohol Clin Exp Res 18:202–218, 1994

Substance Abuse Prevention and Treatment Block Grant 1992, Pub. L. No. 102-321, sec. 1931–1935; 1941–1954

Wellisch J, Anglin MD, Prendergast ML: Numbers and characteristics of drug-using women in the criminal justice system: implications for treatment. J Drug Issues 23:7–30, 1993

HIV/AIDS and Substance Use Disorders

Steven L. Batki, M.D.

Kalpana I. Nathan, M.D.

The Significance of HIV in Substance Use Disorders

Human immunodeficiency virus (HIV) disease is a defining feature of the landscape of substance use disorders. The connection between HIV and substance use is especially significant in that injection drug use is a major conduit for HIV transmission to women, heterosexual men, minorities, and children. HIV-infected drug users are a growing group of patients whose optimal medical and psychiatric care requires adequate assessment and treatment of HIV and acquired immunodeficiency syndrome (AIDS) as well as substance use disorders. HIV infection complicates the treatment of substance use disorders in a number of ways. HIV-related public health concerns are increasingly influencing substance abuse treatment and are adding to the scope of work expected of programs and providers. The most salient public health issues affecting substance abuse treatment are the need for primary prevention of HIV infection (prevention of transmission) as well as secondary and tertiary prevention (reducing HIV-related morbidity). Substance use disorders may make the medical management of HIV diseases more difficult. The behavioral disturbances that accompany drug dependence complicate adherence to treatment regimens. The triple diagnosis of HIV infection, substance use disorders, and comorbid psychiatric disorders creates diagnostic problems and requires special treatment approaches (Batki 1990b; Treisman et al. 2001).

In this chapter we review the epidemiology of HIV infection among drug users, including a summary of its psychiatric, medical, and substance use–related morbidity. We describe the assessment and treatment of HIV-infected patients with substance use disorders and review various models for integrating the treatments for HIV disease and substance use disorders.

Epidemiology

It is estimated that 40 million people worldwide are living with HIV infection or AIDS; AIDS caused the deaths of 3 million people in 2001 (Centers for Disease Control and Prevention 2002a). AIDS incidence in the United States increased rapidly throughout the 1980s, peaked in the early 1990s, and then started declining in 1996. The Centers for Disease Control and Prevention (2002b) has estimated that 41,311 new AIDS cases in adults and adolescents were diagnosed in the United States in 2001. During 1996–1997, after the implementation of highly active antiretroviral therapy (HAART), the number of deaths among persons with AIDS declined by 42%, but declines since then have been much smaller. The prevalence of AIDS has increased steadily: as of December 31, 2001, 816,149 persons were reported to have contracted AIDS, of whom 467,910 had died; leaving an estimated 348,239 persons living with AIDS in the United States. Ethnic and racial minorities were overrepresented among these patients, of whom 41% were African American and 20% were Hispanic.

Of males living with AIDS, 24% were injection drug users (IDUs) and 8% were men who have sex with men and who were also IDUs. Of women living with AIDS, 39% were IDUs (Centers for Disease Control and Prevention 2002b). Injection drug use as a risk factor for AIDS has particularly affected ethnic and racial minority populations. Of new AIDS cases reported in 2000, AIDS associated with injection drug use accounted for 26% of cases among African American adults and adolescents and 31% among Hispanic adults and adolescents, compared with 19% of all cases among whites. Injection drug use–associated AIDS also accounts for a larger proportion of women than men. Since the epidemic began, 57% of AIDS cases among women have been attributed to injection drug use or sex with partners who inject drugs. Noninjection drugs such as crack cocaine also present a risk when users engage in high-risk sexual behaviors.

Prevention of HIV Transmission in Drug Users

Comprehensive HIV prevention strategies include a variety of components, such as 1) community-based outreach; 2) drug abuse treatment; and 3) sterile syringe access programs, which help members of high-risk groups increase protective behaviors and reduce risk for HIV infection and AIDS, as well as hepatitis B and C (National Institute on Drug Abuse 2002). For example, Des Jarlais et al. (2000) found that HIV testing and counseling, public funding, and expansion of the community-based syringe exchange programs in New York City were associated with large reductions in risky behaviors and incidence of HIV infection among IDUs who used these programs.

Community-Based Outreach

Community-based outreach relies on workers who are familiar with the community and its drug use culture and who are able to influence their peers in reducing HIV risk. Outreach workers distribute educational information and offer referrals for drug treatment, syringe access programs, HIV testing, and condoms. Cumulative research from a 23-site study of more than 18,000 drug users reported that 3–6 months after participating in the intervention, 72% of the IDUs stopped or reduced drug injection. Of the crack cocaine users, 26% had stopped using crack at follow-up. Nearly 25% of the drug users who participated in the study had entered drug abuse treatment at follow-up, many for the first time (National Institute on Drug Abuse 2002).

Substance Abuse Treatment as HIV/AIDS Prevention

Substance abuse treatment in and of itself constitutes an effective HIV/AIDS prevention technique (Sorensen and Copeland 2000). A number of studies of substance abuse treatment demonstrate effectiveness in preventing infection. For example, Metzger et al. (1993) found lower rates of seroconversion associated with methadone maintenance treatment. In that study, drug users who remained out of treatment were six times more likely to become infected with HIV than those who remained in methadone maintenance treatment.

Sterile Syringe Access Programs

Access to sterile syringes is a critical issue. Most HIV transmission among IDUs is thought to occur through multiperson use ("sharing") of the needles and syringes used in drug injection. Certain types of sharing, such as in "shooting galleries" involving many different partners within short time periods, are associated with rapid transmission of HIV among IDUs, with HIV incidence rates as high as 20–50 per 100 person-years at risk (Des Jarlais et al. 2001). Most IDUs who continue to inject may be unable to obtain a sufficient number of sterile syringes to effectively reduce their risk of acquiring and transmitting blood-borne viral infections. Syringe exchange programs provide IDUs with free sterile syringes and a way to safely dispose of used syringes. Many syringe exchange programs also provide other services, such as links to substance abuse treatment, counseling, and health services. Studies of syringe exchange programs have so far shown no increase in illicit drug injection associated with the exchanges and have shown significant decreases in drug-related risk behavior (Paone et al. 1995).

HIV Risk Assessment, Testing, Education, and Counseling

HIV counseling and testing appear to be effective intervention strategies for seropositive persons. The Centers for Disease Control and Prevention (2001) recommends that providers in substance abuse treatment settings should recommend counseling, testing, and referral to all clients. Voluntary and confidential HIV testing is helpful in clarifying differential diagnosis of medical conditions, informing infected persons and their partners about how to prevent HIV transmission, and initiating early medical management of HIV infection (Eichler et al. 2002). HIV testing in drug users does not appear to lead to major psychological or behavioral deterioration (Casadonte et al. 1990), and there appear to be no sustained increases in psychological distress (Davis et al. 1995) or suicide risk (van Haastrecht et al. 1994). Furthermore, informing drug users about their positive HIV serostatus is not associated with worse outcome in drug abuse treatment (Wimbush et al. 1996).

Education aimed at reducing risk of HIV infection is also an important prevention strategy. Instruction regarding condom use, syringe access programs, and the use of clean injection equipment are essential components. Small group interventions are a commonly used method to share information and to build social support for changing both drug use and sexual behavior (Sorensen and Batki 1997). There are various models for psychoeducational HIV counseling,

but it has been difficult to demonstrate the clear superiority of any one approach over others (Gibson et al. 1998).

Harm Reduction

Harm reduction refers to a wide range of activities that aim to reduce the adverse health consequences of drug use (Des Jarlais 1995). The harm reduction perspective is essentially pragmatic and nonjudgmental. Examples of harm reduction approaches include making methadone treatment readily available, teaching drug injectors how to inject drugs more safely, and providing syringe exchange.

Treatment

Treatment of Substance Use Disorders in HIV-Infected Patients

The treatment of substance use disorders is important to the overall care of HIV-infected patients and requires more flexibility than is customary in traditional substance abuse programs (Sorensen and Batki 1997). Current guidelines recommend that substance abuse treatment providers give consideration to HIV disease severity to maximize retention of patients in treatment and thereby reduce public health risks (Center for Substance Abuse Treatment 2000).

Methadone Maintenance Treatment Programs

Providing drug abuse treatment such as methadone maintenance treatment to HIV-infected individuals is crucial because it can prevent HIV transmission by reducing drug injection (Sorensen and Copeland 2000). Treatment programs can also provide a setting to deliver other needed services, including HIV medical care, psychiatric treatment, social services, and HIV education. Methadone maintenance treatment is of particular value because opioid dependence is so common among IDUs (Center for Substance Abuse Treatment 2000). It is particularly effective for HIV-infected IDUs because it affords nearly daily contact with patients and provides a stable setting for the provision of medical and psychiatric care (Sorensen and Batki 1997). Despite concerns about the potential of opioids to depress immune function (Carballo-Dieguez et al. 1994), studies of IDUs have found that methadone maintenance treatment is associated with normalization of the alterations in immune function that are associated with heroin abuse (Kreek 1990; Kreek et al. 1990). Furthermore, methadone treatment may have some efficacy in slowing the progression of HIV disease (Weber et al. 1990).

Methadone treatment dosing may be affected by some important interactions with medications used in HIV disease. The liver enzyme cytochrome P450 3A4 extensively metabolizes methadone, and methadone levels may decrease with the use of P450 3A4 inducers such as rifampin. Conversely, P450 3A4 inhibitors can raise methadone levels. Methadone, in turn, inhibits metabolism of some HIV medications and induces metabolism of others. Although methadone has been shown to increase zidovudine blood levels by 50%, it decreases levels of didanosine by 41% and stavudine by 13%. In turn, methadone blood levels are decreased by about 60% by efavirenz, 53% by lopinavir/ritonavir, between 39% and 47% by nelfinavir, 60% by nevirapine, and 40% by ritonavir (Gourevitch and Friedland 2000). Information about drug-drug interactions is a rapidly evolving area, and practitioners should frequently review the latest listings of these interactions.

Psychiatric Care

Psychiatric Disorders, HIV, and Substance Use Disorders

The more severe their HIV symptoms are, the more likely patients with substance use disorders and HIV infection are to require psychiatric services (Burnam et al. 2001). The triple diagnosis of HIV infection, psychiatric disorder, and drug use poses significant assessment and treatment challenges (Batki 1990b). Lyketsos et al. (1996) studied a series of 222 HIV-infected patients in a medical clinic and found that a comorbid substance use disorder was the best predictor of psychiatric distress. In a study of HIV-infected methadone maintenance treatment patients, 79% were found to have Axis I psychiatric disorders (Batki et al. 1996). Although this high rate is similar to that found in opioid-dependent patients in studies done before the AIDS epidemic, it is higher than the rates documented among HIV-infected homosexual and bisexual men

(Lyketsos and Federman 1995). The majority of these disorders—such as depression, anxiety, and insomnia—may be related to substance use or to medical illness (Batki et al. 1996). A number of studies agree on the importance of drug abuse as a major contributing factor to psychiatric disorders in seropositive drug users. In the early stages of HIV infection, drug use appears to be a more important cause of psychopathology than HIV itself (Lipsitz et al. 1994).

Treatment of Psychiatric Disorders

Both psychological and pharmacological treatments are necessary in treating comorbid psychiatric disorders in drug users with HIV infection. Support groups and self-help groups can reduce isolation and teach patients about the basics of HIV-related health care, and supportive psychotherapy by substance abuse counselors can help to bolster the coping abilities of patients as well (Center for Substance Abuse Treatment 2000).

Psychopharmacology in HIV-Infected Drug Users

There has been little systematic study to assess the safety or efficacy of pharmacological treatment of psychiatric disorders in drug users with HIV infection. Available recommendations rely on studies that involved HIV-infected patients who were not drug users (Center for Substance Abuse Treatment 2000). The treatment of anxiety and insomnia is particularly problematic because of abuse liability associated with benzodiazepines and other sedative-hypnotics (Freedman et al. 1996). One approach has been to attempt to treat anxiety disorders with medications with little or no abuse liability, such as buspirone (Batki 1990a). A stepwise, hierarchical approach to the pharmacological treatment of psychiatric disorders in drug users infected with HIV has been proposed (Center for Substance Abuse Treatment 2000). This approach first utilizes medications with lower abuse liability and lower overdose risk (e.g., trazodone for insomnia or serotonin reuptake inhibitors for anxiety disorders) before proceeding to medications with higher abuse liability (e.g., benzodiazepines) or overdose risk (e.g., lithium or tricyclic antidepressants).

HAART involves treatment of HIV disease with three or more antiretroviral drugs. Regimens typically consist of two nucleoside reverse transcriptase inhibitors and either a nonnucleoside reverse transcriptase inhibitor or a protease inhibitor (AIDSinfo 2002). HAART lends itself to multiple drug interactions. The nonnucleoside reverse transcriptase inhibitors and protease inhibitors are largely cleared through metabolism by the cytochrome P450 systems, which accounts for the potential for interactions (Gourevitch and Friedland 2000). Antiretroviral agents can also produce psychiatric and neurological adverse effects (Treisman and Kaplin 2002). For example, efavirenz, a nonnucleoside reverse transcriptase inhibitor, can produce anxiety, depression, suicidal ideation, confusion, and hallucinations, whereas zidovudine, a nucleoside reverse transcriptase inhibitor, can induce mania and can produce agitation and insomnia.

The possibility of drug interactions of psychiatric medications with the antiretroviral medications should also be taken into account. Information about the interactions of psychotropic drugs with antiretrovirals is constantly changing, and providers should refer to current guidelines and resources to check on this evolving knowledge base.

Medical Care for HIV-Infected Drug Users

Behavioral Problems of Drug Users Affecting Medical Care

Drug users may face greater delays in accessing HIV medical services than nondrug users, and they may have worse adherence to treatment regimens (Broers et al. 1994). HIV-infected drug users may have difficulty in accessing antiretroviral therapy. This has been shown in a study of HIV-infected IDUs in British Columbia, where treatment is offered for free. In this study (Strathdee et al. 1998), 11 months after eligibility only 40% of patients had received antiretroviral medications, and the odds of not receiving treatment were increased threefold for those not currently enrolled in a drug or alcohol treatment program.

Settings for Medical Care

There are different models for providing primary medical care for IDUs (Samet et al. 1995). One model of care for HIV-infected drug users in methadone maintenance treatment consists of referring these patients to an off-site AIDS clinic. This approach may be less appropriate for those with ongoing illicit drug use or psychological disorders who may have minimal or strained relationships with health care providers and whose behavioral problems interfere with utilization of medical services. HIV-infected drug users may have particular problems keeping appointments and may be fearful of or ambivalent about medical care. On-site primary medical care for IDUs in substance abuse treatment is another model. The methadone maintenance treatment setting is useful for providing medical services such as primary medical care, tuberculosis prevention, and other medical services to patients with HIV disease. In a study by Umbricht-Schneiter et al. (1994), 92% of methadone maintenance treatment patients who obtained on-site primary medical care received further medical care, whereas only 35% of patients receiving a referral received such care. In a randomized, controlled trial of tuberculosis chemoprophylaxis provided on-site in methadone maintenance treatment versus usual care, significantly higher rates of completion of tuberculosis preventive therapy were found in the on-site condition (Batki et al. 2002). Other studies have demonstrated high utilization of HIV-related medical services when they were provided on-site in substance abuse treatment programs. O'Connor et al. (1992) reported on access to primary care at a substance abuse treatment program in New Haven, Connecticut. Of those eligible, 89% accepted antiretroviral therapy, and 100% accepted *Pneumocystis carinii* pneumonia prophylaxis. Selwyn et al. (1993) conducted a 16-month prospective study on IDUs at a New York City methadone program with on-site primary care services. These researchers found that 81% of IDUs voluntarily used on-site primary care services, with care being utilized more by HIV-positive patients. HIV-related medical care provided on-site is an especially relevant treatment model for methadone maintenance programs because such care can be effectively provided on-site with a relatively moderate investment of resources (Center for Substance Abuse Treatment 2000).

Conclusion

HIV-infected drug users have complex medical, psychiatric, and drug-related problems that require careful assessment and management. HIV disease and its associated neurocognitive problems do not appear to progress more rapidly in drug users, and these patients' psychiatric disorders are more often due to drug use than to HIV infection. Because of the behavioral problems associated with drug use, provision of medical, psychiatric, and substance abuse treatment services in a common site is a useful model of service delivery. The combined treatment of substance use and psychiatric disorders may improve the likelihood that patients will receive adequate medical treatment of HIV disease.

References

AIDSinfo: Guidelines for the Use of Antiretroviral Agents in HIV-Infected Adults and Adolescents. Rockville, MD, National Institutes of Health, 2002. Available at: http://aidsinfo.nih.gov/guidelines. Accessed September 11, 2003

Batki SL: Buspirone in drug users with AIDS or AIDS-related complex. J Clin Psychopharmacol 10 (3 suppl):111S–115S, 1990a

Batki SL: Drug abuse, psychiatric disorders, and AIDS: dual and triple diagnosis. West J Med 152:547–552, 1990b

Batki SL, Ferrando SJ, Manfredi LB, et al: Psychiatric disorders, drug use, and medical status in injection drug users with HIV disease. Am J Addict 5:249–258, 1996

Batki SL, Gruber V, Moon Bradley J, et al: A controlled trial of methadone treatment combined with directly observed isoniazid for tuberculosis chemoprophylaxis in injection drug users. Drug Alcohol Depend 66:283–293, 2002

Broers B, Morabia A, Hirschel B: A cohort study of drug users' compliance with zidovudine treatment. Arch Intern Med 154:1121–1127, 1994

Burnam MA, Bing EG, Morton SC, et al: Use of mental health and substance abuse services among adults with HIV in the United States. Arch Gen Psychiatry 58:729–736, 2001

Carballo-Dieguez AJ, Goetz R, El Sadr W, et al: The effect of methadone on immunological parameters among HIV-positive and HIV-negative drug users. Am J Drug Alcohol Abuse 20:317–329, 1994

Casadonte PP, Des Jarlais DC, Friedman SR, et al: Psychological and behavioral impact among intravenous drug users learning HIV test results. Int J Addict 25:409–426, 1990

Center for Substance Abuse Treatment: Substance Abuse Treatment for Persons with HIV/AIDS. Treatment Improvement Protocol (TIP) Series 37 (DHHS Publ No [SMA] 00-3410). Rockville, MD, Substance Abuse and Mental Health Services Administration, 2000

Centers for Disease Control and Prevention: Revised guidelines for HIV counseling, testing, and referral. MMWR Recomm Rep 50(RR19):1–58, 2001. Available at: http://www.cdc.gov/mmwr/preview/mmwrhtml/rr5019a1.htm. Accessed September 5, 2003

Centers for Disease Control and Prevention: Drug-Associated HIV Transmission Continues in the United States. Atlanta, GA, Centers for Disease Control and Prevention, 2002a. Available at: http://www.cdc.gov/hiv/pubs/facts/idu.htm. Accessed September 11, 2003

Centers for Disease Control and Prevention: U.S. HIV and AIDS cases reported through December 2001. HIV AIDS Surveill Rep 13(2):1–44, 2002b. Available at: http://www.cdc.gov/hiv/stats/hasr1302.htm. Accessed September 11, 2003

Davis RF, Metzger DS, Meyers K, et al: Long-term changes in psychological symptomatology associated with HIV serostatus among male injecting drug users. AIDS 9:73–79, 1995

Des Jarlais DC: Harm reduction: a framework for incorporating science into drug policy. Am J Public Health 85:10–11, 1995

Des Jarlais DC, Marmor M, Friedmann P, et al: HIV incidence among injection drug users in New York City, 1992–1997: evidence for a declining epidemic. Am J Public Health 90(3):352–359, 2000

Des Jarlais DC, Dehne K, Casabona J: HIV surveillance among injecting drug users. AIDS 15 (suppl 3):S13–S22, 2001

Eichler MR, Ray SM, del Rio C: The effectiveness of HIV post-test counseling in determining healthcare-seeking behavior. AIDS 16:943–945, 2002

Freedman JB, O'Dowd MA, McKegney FP: Managing diazepam abuse in an AIDS-related psychiatric clinic with a high percentage of substance abusers. Psychosomatics 37:43–47, 1996

Gibson DR, McCusker J, Chesney M: Effectiveness of psychosocial interventions in preventing HIV risk behaviour in injection drug users. AIDS 28:919–929, 1998

Gourevitch MN, Friedland GH: Interactions between methadone and medications used to treat HIV infection: a review. Mt Sinai J Med 67:429–436, 2000

Kreek MJ: Immune function in heroin addicts and former heroin addicts in treatment: pre- and post-AIDS epidemic. NIDA Res Monogr 96:192–219, 1990

Kreek MJ, Khuri E, Flomenberg N, et al: Immune status of unselected methadone maintained former heroin addicts. Prog Clin Biol Res 328:445–448, 1990

Lipsitz JD, Williams JB, Rabkin JG, et al: Psychopathology in male and female intravenous drug users with and without HIV infection. Am J Psychiatry 151:1662–1668, 1994

Lyketsos CG, Federman EB: Psychiatric disorders and HIV infection: impact on one another. Epidemiol Rev 17:152–164, 1995

Lyketsos CG, Hutton H, Fishman M, et al: Psychiatric morbidity on entry to an HIV primary care clinic. AIDS 10:1033–1039, 1996

Metzger DS, Woody GE, McLellan AT, et al: Human immunodeficiency virus seroconversion among intravenous drug users in- and out-of-treatment: an 18-month prospective follow-up. J Acquir Immune Defic Syndr 6:1049–1056, 1993

National Institute on Drug Abuse: Principles of HIV Prevention in Drug-Using Populations (NIH Publ No 02-4733). Rockville, MD, National Institute on Drug Abuse, 2002

O'Connor PG, Molde S, Henry S, et al: Human immunodeficiency virus infection in intravenous drug users: a model for primary care. Am J Med 8:382–385, 1992

Paone D, Des Jarlais DC, Gangloff R, et al: Syringe exchange: HIV prevention, key findings, and future directions. Int J Addict 30:1647–1683, 1995

Samet JH, Stein MD, O'Connor PG: Models of medical care for HIV-infected drug users. Subst Abus 16:131–139, 1995

Selwyn PA, Budner NS, Wasserman WC, et al: Utilization of on-site primary care services by HIV-seropositive and seronegative drug users in a methadone maintenance program. Public Health Rep 108:492–500, 1993

Sorensen JL, Batki SL: Management of the psychosocial sequelae of HIV infection among drug abusers, in Substance Abuse: A Comprehensive Textbook, 2nd Edition. Edited by Lowinson JH, Ruiz P, Millman R, et al. Baltimore, MD, Williams & Wilkins, 1997, pp 788–792

Sorensen JL, Copeland AL: Drug abuse treatment as an HIV prevention strategy: a review. Drug Alcohol Depend 59:17–31, 2000

Strathdee S, Palepu A, Cornelisse P, et al: Barriers to use of free antiretroviral therapy in injection drug users. JAMA 280:547–549, 1998

Treisman GJ, Kaplin AI: Neurologic and psychiatric complications of antiretroviral agents. AIDS 16:1201–1215, 2002

Treisman GJ, Angelino AF, Hutton HE: Psychiatric issues in the management of patients with HIV infection. JAMA 286:2857–2864, 2001

Umbricht-Schneiter A, Ginn DH, Pabst KM, et al: Providing medical care to methadone clinic patients: referral vs on-site care. Am J Public Health 84:207–210, 1994

van Haastrecht MJ, Mientjes GH, van den Hoek AJ, et al: Death from suicide and overdose among drug injectors after disclosure of first HIV test result. AIDS 8:1721–1725, 1994

Weber R, Ledergerber B, Opravil M, et al: Progression of HIV infection in misusers of injected drugs who stop injecting or follow a program of maintenance treatment with methadone. BMJ 301:1362–1365, 1990

Wimbush J, Amicarelli A, Stein MD: Does HIV test result influence methadone maintenance treatment retention? J Subst Abuse 8:263–269, 1996

Treatment of Pain in Drug-Addicted Persons

Erik W. Gunderson, M.D.
Barry Stimmel, M.D.

The treatment of pain has always been problematic. Surveys have consistently demonstrated that pain, regardless of cause, is most often inadequately relieved, resulting in needless suffering and loss of function. Although the principles physicians should adhere to in relieving pain have been published in numerous journals and monographs (Carr et al. 1992; Jacox et al. 1994; Stimmel 1997), they are often not followed, and consequently pain management has become a treatment priority. The American Pain Society has promoted the concept of pain as "The Fifth Vital Sign" (Campbell 1995) to increase awareness of pain treatment among health care professionals; in addition, the U.S. Department of Health and Human Services has disseminated clinical practice guidelines for the management of acute pain and cancer pain (Carr et al. 1992; Jacox et al. 1994). In addition, the Joint Commission on Accreditation of Healthcare Organizations (JCAHO), the national board responsible for defining standards of care in the United States, enacted its pain standard in January 2001, recognizing patients' rights to appropriate assessment and management of pain (Phillips 2000).

In this chapter we address some of the barriers that lead to inadequate pain management and then focus on the pharmacological treatment of pain in persons who intermittently or consistently use mood-altering substances—licit, illicit, or prescribed for recognized medical disorders. In addressing this issue, we focus only limited attention on the biology of pain, specific pharmacological doses of available analgesics, and nonpharmacological methods of treatment. These subjects are important; however, so many reviews have been published that to repeat such information would be less than productive. What follows then is a pragmatic approach to pain relief in persons who are concurrently dependent on or addicted to mood-altering substances, with an emphasis on the basic principles to be followed in evaluation and management.

Physician Barriers to Adequate Pain Management

Iatrogenic Addiction

Various explanations have been offered to explain why pain is often undertreated. These explanations include fear of sanctions, inadequate training, and negative attitudes such as concern about promoting addiction (American Academy of Pain Medicine and American Pain Society 1997). Available studies suggest that de novo addiction rarely occurs when opioids are used for pain in patients without a history of drug abuse or addiction. Porter and Jick (1980) found that among 12,000 patients who received opioids for moderate to severe pain, only four cases of psychological dependence were documented in patients who had no history of drug abuse. Similar results were found in studies of diverse patient populations that have included patients on burn units (Perry and Heidrich 1982), patients with cancer pain (Kanner and Foley 1981), and patients with chronic nonmalignant pain (Zenz et al. 1992). In addition, a retrospective study of medical records from 1990 to 1996 in the databases of the Drug Abuse Warning Network (DAWN) and the Automation of Reports and Consolidated Orders System (ARCOS) showed that a recent trend of increasing medical use of opioid analgesics to treat pain does not appear to have increased the health consequences of opioid analgesic abuse (Joranson et al. 2000). Although the DAWN system may underreport the true extent of all drug abuse, because only episodes of drug abuse that result in emergency department admission are recorded, a stable trend in opioid abuse levels over the study period suggests that actual abuse of opioid analgesics is also relatively stable (Joranson et al. 2000).

Despite the suggestion by these studies that there is minimal risk of iatrogenic addiction when patients are treated with opioids for pain, there are no long-term, prospective studies assessing such risk in which a definition of addiction is operationalized and measured. Furthermore, these studies did not determine risk in patients with a history of addiction, a population that might be at greater risk for opioid abuse than the pain patients in these studies. A retrospective study of patients with chronic nonmalignant pain and a history of substance abuse who were treated with long-term opioid therapy for at least a year was conducted to determine factors associated with prescription abuse (Dunbar and Katz 1996). Patients who had a history of alcohol abuse alone rather than polysubstance abuse, and those who were active members of Alcoholics Anonymous and had a stable social support system, were less likely to abuse opioid therapy. In a study of opioid abuse among patients with chronic nonmalignant pain at a pain clinic, long-term opioid users and opiate abusers did not differ by history of drug or alcohol abuse (Chabal et al. 1997).

Regulatory Scrutiny

Fear of investigation or sanction by federal, state, and local regulatory agencies may also result in inappropriate or inadequate treatment of pain (Carr et al. 1992). That this fear is not entirely misplaced has been demonstrated by a survey of state medical board members, many of whom stated that they would recommend investigation of a physician based solely on the prescription of an opioid for malignant pain for longer than 6 months (Joranson et al. 1992). It is to be hoped that the Pain Relief Act, a proposed statute that has been emulated by several states in formatting state pain relief policies (American Society of Law, Medicine and Ethics 2002), will lead to more appropriate policies and fewer physician fears. The primary goal of the act is "to terminate actions against providers engaging in justifiable pain management practices as early as possible in the disciplinary or criminal process to prevent unnecessary investigations, protracted proceedings, and inappropriate legal sanction" (Johnson 1996, p. 322). Medical professionals who are in "substantial compliance with accepted practice guidelines," such as those of the American Pain Society or the Agency for Health Care Policy and Research, will receive the protection of the act, including those treating pain in addicted patients (Johnson 1996, p. 322). Standards of practice identified in the act, including "maintenance of accurate and complete medical records, physical examination of the patient, and documentation of a treatment plan" (Johnson 1996, p. 323), are similar to practice guidelines later adopted by the Federation of State Medical Boards (1998). Because state medical board policies have changed in the recent past (Joranson et al. 2002), medical professionals treating pain should be familiar with the policies of the state in which they practice (American Society of Law, Medicine and Ethics 2002).

Inadequate Physician Training

Most clinicians, including pain specialists, are untrained in addiction medicine, and those involved in treating addiction are often untrained in pain management (Portenoy et al. 1997). These facts illustrate the need for improved training on pain and addiction (Schnoll and Finch 1994). Clinicians who prescribe opioids or other drugs with abuse potential should be familiar with addiction, and greater integration of the two disciplines is necessary to improve care for opioid-addicted pain patients (Portenoy et al. 1997). In fact, part of the mission of the JCAHO is to emphasize a collaborative and interdisciplinary approach to pain management (Phillips 2000). Efforts to increase physician education in these two interrelated fields should begin early, but medical school curriculums provide only minimal focus on pain management (Schnoll and Finch 1994). Medical education also needs improvement with regard to addiction; a recent national survey of residency directors in various fields found that only 56% of all the surveyed programs combined had required training on substance use disorders (Isaacson et al. 2000).

Guidelines for Relieving Pain

The specific approach to relief of pain depends on whether the pain is acute, intermittent, or chronic and, if chronic, whether it is due to a malignant or a nonmalignant disorder. However, in an assessment of a person in pain, certain general principles always apply (Table 45–1). These principles are especially important in dealing with a person who may have a concurrent drug dependence.

Define the Etiology of Pain

It is frequently assumed that a person taking mood-altering drugs, especially opioids, will fabricate symptoms to obtain medication; however, it is equally likely (if not more likely) that a specific cause of pain exists that may have been relieved or hidden by the use of other mood-altering drugs. To elucidate the etiology of the pain syndrome, it is essential to obtain a comprehensive history, perform a physical examination, and obtain appropriate diagnostic testing. Prior medical records and diagnostic studies should be reviewed to

Table 45–1. Initial evaluation of a patient in pain

Define the etiology of pain
Classify the type of pain
Assess the severity of pain
Identify existing modifying psychological and environmental factors
Determine prior successful means of pain relief
Evaluate for signs suggestive of opioid addiction
Determine whether drug treatment is needed

monitor potential changes in function and disease progression and also to corroborate the patient's condition. Failure to recognize the etiology of the pain syndrome may have severe consequences; in persons who use drugs parenterally, underlying afflictions can often go undetected until breakthrough pain occurs, whereas in persons using stimulants, pain may be a concomitant symptom heralding the onset of a cardiac or pulmonary event. Unless a careful medical evaluation is carried out, these conditions may go unrecognized, with the physician assuming that the patient is exhibiting manipulative behavior to obtain additional mood-altering drugs.

In addition to well-defined sources of pain, Savage (1994) described a syndrome of pain facilitation or dissipation in currently dependent persons. This state is characterized by a relatively constant level of pain that can be relieved only by a drug in the same group as the one on which the individual is dependent. Individuals undergoing withdrawal may experience nonspecific pain symptoms as part of the withdrawal process due to either sympathetic stimulation (which may intensify the painful experience) or increased muscle activity (seen in withdrawal from sedatives and opioids). These symptoms may be relieved by the provision of appropriate medication, with a subsequent slow detoxification from the primary drug.

Classify the Type of Pain

The classification of pain as acute, intermittent, or chronic is essential to providing appropriate pain relief. This is discussed in detail in a later section.

Assess the Severity of Pain

Obtaining a comprehensive description of the painful experience is important. Although various standardized questionnaires can be used to assess the intensity of pain, asking the person to assess its severity on a scale of 1–10, establishing its intensity based on previous painful experiences, and determining its impact on the ability to engage in various life activities can help guide therapy and will enable monitoring of treatment efficacy. The Pain Disability Index is a useful instrument to measure the extent to which pain interferes with a person's ability to engage in various life activities (Table 45–2) (Tait et al. 1987). Patients rate their level of disability on a scale from 0 (no disability) to 10 (total disability) in seven areas of activity, yielding a general disability score from 0 to 70 after summing the ratings of the seven categories. More important than the actual number generated, however, is the fact that use of the Pain Disability Index ensures that various areas of activity are considered when assessing the functional impact of pain, and the scale can be administered repeatedly over time to monitor change in status. When analgesic therapy is started, pain severity should be assessed at least every 8 hours, and as frequently as every 2 hours when the pain is acute and severe.

Table 45–2. Pain Disability Index

1. **Family/Home Responsibilities:** chores/duties around the house, errands/favors for family members
2. **Recreation:** hobbies, sports, leisure time activities
3. **Social Activity:** participation with nonfamily friends, such as parties, theater, dining out, social functions
4. **Occupation:** activities part of or related to one's job, including nonpaying jobs
5. **Sexual Behavior:** frequency and quality of sexual activity
6. **Self-Care:** personal maintenance and independent daily living, such as showering, driving, dressing
7. **Life-Support Activity:** basic life supporting behaviors: eating, sleeping, breathing

Note. Each area is rated on a scale from 1 (no disability) to 10 (total disability).
Source. Adapted from Tait et al. 1987.

Identify Psychological and Environmental Factors

Many factors are known to modulate the pain threshold (Table 45–3), particularly in persons using mood-altering drugs. Drug craving and its associated anxiety lower the pain threshold, whereas withdrawal may

Table 45–3. Factors affecting the pain threshold

Threshold-lowering factors	Threshold-increasing factors
Anxiety	Sleep
Depression	Sympathy
Discomfort	Understanding
Fatigue	Mood elevation
Fear	
Isolation	
Recalling of last painful experience	

heighten an individual's awareness of pain and lead to increased sympathetic, muscular, abdominal, and neuropathic pain. Fatigue and depression, common with abuse of many mood-altering drugs, also heighten a painful experience. Finally, fear or anger over the inability to have the pain relieved or the feeling that the pain is not being taken seriously will increase intensity of pain. Identifying these factors is important so that they can be addressed.

Determine Prior Successful Means of Pain Relief

A simple but often forgotten way of maximizing pain relief is to ask the patient what has worked in the past. Although people are more than willing to recount their past painful experiences and to describe ways of providing relief that were effective for them, physicians frequently either do not elicit this information or do not believe it when it is given. Patients should be asked about past medication side effects (Sees and Clark 1993): What were the side effects? Were they tolerable? How were they managed? Although patients receiving long-term opioids typically become tolerant to many opioid side effects, such as sedation or euphoria, constipation may persist. A prime example of the importance of inquiring about prior successful means of pain relief is with patients presenting with the acute, painful crises of sickle cell disease. Persons with recurrent sickle cell crises are well aware of the exact strength of opioid needed to relieve their pain; if they are allowed to use patient-controlled analgesia, they relieve their pain quickly and shorten their hospital stay. However, more often than not physicians do not prescribe the requested medication, which causes increasing anxiety and ultimately increased use of opioids.

Evaluate for Signs Suggestive of Opioid Addiction

Perhaps one of the most difficult challenges for clinicians when addressing pain in a patient with a history of addiction is differentiating a patient with pain from a patient addicted to pain medication. Particularly with chronic pain patients on long-term opioid treatment, physical dependence on opioids is often misla-beled as addiction. Identifying the presence of certain drug-taking behaviors can help recognize addiction, in which there is a maladaptive pattern of substance use leading to clinically significant impairment (American Psychiatric Association 2000). Table 45–4 lists some behaviors that not only might help to identify addiction during the initial evaluation but might also be used during subsequent monitoring of patients after the decision to prescribe opioids has been made.

Table 45–4. Behaviors that suggest addiction in patients receiving opioids for pain

Pain patient	Addicted patient
Stable pattern of medication use	Loss of control with medications
Medications improve overall function	Medications decrease overall function
Is concerned about side effects	Wants medication despite persistence of adverse effects
Will follow treatment plan	Does not follow treatment plan
Has leftover medication	No leftover medication; often loses medication or prescriptions
Is no longer preoccupied with obtaining opioids after pain has been adequately controlled	Is preoccupied with obtaining opioids despite adequate analgesia

Source. Adapted from Heit 2001; Savage 1996; Schnoll and Finch 1994.

The addicted patient often experiences a loss of control with medications, as exhibited by frequently running out of medication, repeatedly reporting lost or stolen prescriptions, or using street sources for opioids (Schnoll and Finch 1994). Preoccupation with opioid use is evidenced by an unwillingness to try nonopioid alternative pain treatments or the perception that no interventions other than opioids will have any impact on pain (Savage 1996). Addicted patients may want to continue taking medications despite adverse consequences, such as persistent sedation or euphoria, or a general decreased level of functioning despite adequate analgesia (Savage 1996).

Patients who exhibit addictive behaviors as described above must be distinguished from those exhibiting *pseudoaddiction,* a term used to describe a pattern of drug-seeking behavior resulting from inadequate pain treatment rather than from compulsive use. Initially, a pseudoaddicted patient may request that opioids be distributed more frequently at higher doses, then engage in pain behaviors (vocalizations, grimacing) to convince the physician that the pain is real and that more medication is needed (Weissman and Haddox 1989). If the pain persists, the patient may become less cooperative and appear to have a behavioral problem, which may lead to a loss of trust between patient and physician (Weissman and Haddox 1989). Pseudoaddictive behav-ior can be distinguished from true addictive behavior by observing that the patient's level of functioning improves with adequate analgesia, whereas the previous pattern of addictive behaviors decreases. It is important to note that there is a paucity of data on pseudoaddiction; little is known about the prevalence of this behavior, diagnostic criteria have not been validated, and evidence on management is anecdotal, consisting of a trial of increased pain medication with close monitoring and assessment of the patient's response.

Determine Whether Drug Therapy Is Needed

In many instances pain may be relieved without any pharmacological intervention. Indeed, for various types of pain, nonpharmacological treatment may be more effective and can usually be easily provided (Table 45–5). The use of a nonpharmacological treatment, when indicated, allows an individual using mood-altering drugs to address the factors related to inappropriate drug use and the issues that may be causing the pain. In fact, as noted below, in individuals with chronic pain both pharmacological and nonpharmacological therapies, including psychotherapy, may be warranted in the attempt to assist an individual to function at maximum capacity.

Table 45–5. Nonpharmacological means of relieving pain

Behavioral	Physical
Biofeedback	Active and passive exercises
Imagery	Acupuncture
Meditation	Application of heat or cold
Relaxation	Transcutaneous nerve stimulation
Psychotherapy	Surgical nerve block

Pharmacological Guidelines for Providing Analgesia

If it is decided that pharmacological therapy is needed, guidelines also exist to enable the physician to choose appropriately (Table 45–6). Determining the etiology of the pain, as described above, will help direct treatment, and if it is determined that a specific state does not exist that can be relieved by drugs specifically targeted to the existing pathophysiology, then general analgesic therapy may be warranted.

Table 45–6. Guidelines for pharmacological treatment of pain

Start with an analgesic that is least likely to cause
   dependence
Understand the concepts of dependence, tolerance, and
   withdrawal
Use equivalent doses when changing an analgesic
Use drug combinations carefully
Consider a patient-physician opioid agreement

Start With an Analgesic That Is Least Likely to Cause Dependence

A person who uses opioids will have a tolerance threshold to other opioids. Also, someone dependent on drugs in the alcohol-sedative-hypnotic group may require, because of stimulation of the hepatic microsomal system, an increased dose of opioids to obtain pain relief. Mild to moderate pain often can be relieved with the use of a nonopioid, such as acetaminophen, aspirin, or a nonsteroidal anti-inflammatory drug (NSAID) (Table 45–7). These drugs have therapeutic ceilings, do not cross-react with opioids, and on an individual basis may enhance opioid analgesia when

Table 45–7. Nonopioid analgesics

Generic name	Trade name
Acetaminophen	(various brands)
Aspirin	(various brands)
Diclofenac	Voltaren, Cataflam
Diflunisal	Dolobid
Etodolac	Lodine
Ibuprofen	Advil, Motrin, Nuprin, Saleto-200–600, Genpril
Ketoprofen	Orudis, Actron
Ketorolac	Toradol
Meclofenamate	Meclomen
Naproxen	Anaprox, Naprosyn, Aleve
Tramadol	Ultram

given concurrently; therefore, for mild to moderate pain these medications should be the first line of therapy. Importantly, NSAIDs purchased over the counter are packaged in the lowest possible dose, so incomplete pain relief with an over-the-counter medication does not mean that the same drug, given in appropriate doses, will be ineffective. As an example, ibuprofen is sold as an over-the-counter medication in 200-mg pills, whereas the effective analgesic dosage may be up to 800 mg four times daily. For neuropathic pain, first-line drugs may be antidepressants found effective for neuropathy, rather than the opioid analgesics. In patients with moderate or severe pain, opioids will frequently be needed to relieve the pain and in such cases should be prescribed appropriately.

Understand the Concepts of Dependence, Tolerance, and Withdrawal as Applied to Analgesia

Understanding dependence, tolerance, and withdrawal (concepts that are reviewed elsewhere) is essential when treating pain in individuals who are already taking dependence-producing drugs. Although virtually any mood-altering drug within a particular class (e.g., benzodiazepines) can be substituted in equivalent doses for another in that class, substitution cannot be made across groups (e.g., between benzodiazepines and opioids). Combining drugs from different groups may enhance analgesia but will increase the risk of central nervous system depression. Individuals who regularly take opioids, regardless of the reason, will have developed a tolerance threshold to the analgesic effects of the opioids and require a greater-than-usual dose for pain relief. Therefore, if opioid analgesia is warranted, it is important to estimate the average opioid dose needed to meet the baseline requirement and then to provide an additional dose for analgesia. For persons taking sedative-hypnotic drugs in addition to opioids, there exists a possibility of withdrawal from this group of drugs that can be life-threatening if untreated. Therefore, a complete drug history must be obtained and appropriate medication prescribed when there is a risk of withdrawal.

Use Equivalent Doses When Changing an Analgesic

When changing from one opioid to another, it is always important to use equivalent doses (Table 45–8). Because of incomplete cross-tolerance, it is safest to begin by dividing the calculated equianalgesic dose in half and then adjusting the dose upward for the first 24 hours to obtain analgesia. This rule must be modified in persons who are dependent on opioids (e.g., methadone maintenance) when changing from a nonopioid to an opioid analgesic to account for the presence of tolerance. When converting to an opioid for analgesia, it is simplest to calculate the total baseline opioid dose taken over 24 hours and then prescribe an opioid analgesic dose in excess of the baseline requirement. To diminish the chances of individual variability, two-thirds of the calculated total dose can initially be administered, with adjustment upward as needed. Partial agonists, such as buprenorphine, and agonist-antagonists, such as nalbuphine and butorphanol, should be avoided in opioid-dependent patients because their use in high doses is at times associated with cognitive side effects, and, more importantly, they may produce withdrawal in these patients.

Table 45–8. Equianalgesic doses of oral and parenteral opioid analgesics

	Oral (mg)	Parenteral (mg)	Interval
Opioid agonists			
Codeine	130	75	q 3–4 hr
Hydrocodone (Lorcet, Lortab, Vicodin, others)	30	N/A	q 3–4 hr
Hydromorphone (Dilaudid)	7.5	1.5	q 3–4 hr
Levorphanol (Levo-Dromoran)	4	2	q 6–8 hr
Meperidine (Demerol)	300	100	q 3 hr
Methadone (Dolophine, others)	20	10	q 6–8 hr
Morphine	30–60	10	q 3–4 hr
Oxycodone (Roxicodone, Percocet, Percodan, Tylox)	30	N/A	q 3–4 hr
Opioid agonist-antagonists and partial agonists			
Buprenorphine (Buprenex, Subutex[a])	1 (SL)[b]	0.3–0.4	q 6–8 hr
Butorphanol (Stadol)	N/A	2	q 3–4 hr
Nalbuphine (Nubain)	N/A	10	q 3–4 hr
Pentazocine (Talwin, others)	150	60	q 3–4 hr

Note. Published tables vary in the suggested doses that are equianalgesic to morphine. Clinical response is the criterion that must be applied for each patient; titration to clinical response is necessary. Because there is incomplete cross-tolerance among these drugs, it is usually necessary to use a lower than equianalgesic dose when changing drugs and to re-titrate to response. N/A=not applicable; SL=sublingual.

Caution. Recommended doses do not apply to patients with renal or hepatic insufficiency or other conditions affecting drug metabolism and kinetics.

[a]A combinaton product of buprenorphine with naloxone (Suboxone) exists for maintenance therapy of opioid dependence.
[b]Approximate dose from Johnson et al. 2003.

Source. Adapted from Carr et al. 1992.

Pharmacokinetics must be considered when prescribing opioids. For example, methadone has a long and unpredictable half-life that may result in a delay in symptoms of overdose as the plasma levels increase over several days (Ripamonti et al. 1997). Also, when changing from other opioids to methadone for pain control, methadone should be started at a dose much lower than the equianalgesic dose, down to one-tenth the calculated dose, and patients should be monitored closely over 3–6 days (Ripamonti et al. 1997). In contrast to methadone, meperidine has an extremely short duration of action, and its metabolite normeperidine in increased plasma concentrations can cause seizures. Because meperidine is excreted by the kidneys, use of this drug in individuals with renal disease can be exceptionally hazardous and should be avoided.

Use Drug Combinations Carefully

Combinations of drugs should be used only when specific effects are desired. Excessive sedation may result from the use of drugs in the sedative-hypnotic group, and these drugs should never be used to enhance analgesia. However, there are drugs that can enhance analgesia when used in combination with opioids (Table 45–9). Antidepressants have been found to be an effective adjunctive therapy in persons with pain who are also depressed; they have also been found to be as effective as a single agent in the relief of neuropathic pain. Effective analgesia can also be obtained through combinations of opioids and anti-inflammatory drugs, amphetamines, hydroxyzine, clonidine, or baclofen.

Table 45–9. Drugs used to enhance opioid analgesia

Acetaminophen	Carbamazepine
Amphetamines	Chlorpromazine
Antidepressants	Fluphenazine
Aspirin	Gabapentin
Baclofen	Hydroxyzine

Consider a Patient-Physician Opioid Agreement

Before prescribing opioids to patients at high risk for medication abuse, physicians may consider having the patient sign a contract on the treatment plan (Gitlin 1999). However, we prefer the term *agreement* to minimize legal connotations, and this is the term used by the Federation of State Medical Boards (1998). Opioid agreements often address expectations and issues that are potential points of contention later in treatment, such as the risks and benefits of treatment, the terms and goals of treatment, issues regarding the termination of treatment, the schedule of consensual urine or serum toxicology testing, exclusions for receiving opioids, patient and clinician responsibilities, and prohibited and discouraged behaviors (Fishman et al. 1999). Opioid agreements can improve care through educating the patient about opioid therapy and may enhance compliance with the treatment protocol. Although the Pain Relief Act does not require such agreements, individual U.S. states may require them (Johnson 1996), and physicians should become familiar with the policy of the state in which they are practicing.

Although they are well intended, opioid agreements may have some negative consequences, such as potentially perpetuating the belief that opioid treatment is bad or dangerous and making the patient feel stigmatized. Critics believe that a formal agreement is unnecessary because most patients use opioids responsibly, and that there are other medications that may pose a greater risk than opioids but do not require a contractual agreement (Gitlin 1999). Also, there could be legal consequences should the physician break the agreement (Gitlin 1999). Therefore, it is recommended that the agreement be worded in a nonbinding manner. Ultimately, ongoing communication, evaluation, and documentation are of the greatest importance for proper patient care.

Pain Management According to Type of Pain

Pain can generally be classified as acute, intermittent, or chronic. Chronic pain can be further subdivided into malignant pain, nonmalignant pain, and pain of undefined etiology. Although the general guidelines to be followed in pain management are the same regardless of the type of pain, specific differences exist based on whether the pain is acute or chronic. Both acute and chronic pain are affected by psychological and environmental factors that must be addressed for optimal relief.

Acute Pain

In managing acute pain in an individual who is concurrently using mood-altering drugs, the general guidelines mentioned above (see Table 45–6) should be followed. The administration of opioids to individuals who are already dependent on these drugs must be done in effective doses in excess of a person's baseline requirement. In addition, the medication should be prescribed on an ongoing basis rather than as needed and should be consistent with the pharmacological action of the particular opioid. Once the acute painful episode is resolved, if the opioid has been prescribed for 48–72 hours, it can be abruptly stopped. In individuals who have a tolerance threshold, however, doses of the opioid should be decreased only to the individual's baseline opioid requirement.

Although meperidine is often used for treatment of acute pain, it has considerable disadvantages, including its short duration of action; its frequent irritation of subcutaneous tissues when it is given intramuscularly; its association with delirium in postoperative patients; and its metabolite, normeperidine, which can also cause irritability, confusion, and convulsions, especially in the presence of compromised renal function. For these reasons the U.S. Public Health Service recommends that meperidine not be used for acute pain unless other opioids cannot be tolerated (Carr et al. 1992).

Use of patient-controlled analgesia (PCA) has become an increasingly acceptable way of relieving acute pain, and the efficacy of PCA has been documented. PCA allows an individual to self-administer intravenous doses of narcotics as needed. Limits can be set on the frequency of dispensing and the amount of drug dispensed, and PCA is associated with a lower total dose of analgesia and a shorter time of hospitalization. Because the person must be alert to administer the analgesic, overdose rarely occurs.

The relief of acute pain in persons receiving methadone maintenance therapy has become problematic. This is not because of the difficulty of relieving pain but because of the lack of physician knowledge regarding the appropriate way to provide analgesia. Persons receiving methadone do not have an impaired perception of pain. In the presence of inflammation, use of an NSAID is appropriate. Opioid agonist-antagonists should be avoided because they will precipitate withdrawal symptoms. A mild opioid will probably be ineffective because of the tolerance accompanying methadone maintenance, although the actual degree of tolerance is dependent on the daily methadone dose.

Parenteral narcotics can be effective in relieving pain in persons on methadone maintenance regimens if they are given in appropriate doses. The tolerance threshold to methadone is based on a single oral dose of methadone given every 24 hours. The administration of parenteral, short-acting opioids in doses slightly greater than those usually recommended may be effective. Depending on the tolerance threshold, however, this dose must be increased until analgesia is obtained. If a person receiving methadone is admitted who is unable to take any medication by mouth, intramuscular methadone may be given in divided doses to maintain baseline requirements. Alternatively, the patient's daily methadone dose may be converted to an equivalent dose of morphine sulfate to provide baseline needs, with the dose then increased to provide analgesia. Although this method will relieve pain and prevent withdrawal, it does disturb the steady-state methadone plasma level. Therefore, administering parenteral methadone intramuscularly every 8–12 hours is preferred by many physicians.

Chronic Pain

Defining the etiology of chronic pain is especially important, because if it is of malignant origin, other therapies may be instituted that might be effective in providing pain relief and perhaps in producing a cure or remission. The constant presence of pain often results in depression, anxiety, and a marked disturbance in interpersonal relationships. The use of opioids to relieve pain of malignant origin is well accepted in medical practice, even in persons with a history of drug abuse. However, treatment of chronic pain of nonmalignant origin with opioids has been somewhat more controversial, despite the belief by many physicians that if an etiology for the pain exists, relief of pain should be the primary goal. Analgesia should not be the only goal, because the presence of a chronic debilitative disease may never allow one to be completely free from discomfort. This has to be realized and addressed not only by the physician and the patient but by family members as well. Available nonpharmacological modalities, both invasive and noninvasive, can be effective in providing pain relief. If an opioid is decided on, it should be one with a long duration of action, because tolerance will develop more slowly (Table 45–10). Opioids do not have a ceiling on their effectiveness, so increasing the dose is usually accompanied by increasing analgesia. Breakthrough pain should be managed with short-acting opioids until the dose of the long-acting opioid can be adjusted upward. Pain relief, however, should be accompanied by an increase in function. Use of sedatives should be avoided. It must be emphasized, however, that caution should accompany the use of long-acting opioids to avoid pharmacological overdose, and that patients should be closely observed for behaviors indicative of abuse.

Table 45–10. Long-acting opioids

Generic name	Trade name
Fentanyl, transdermal	Duragesic
Levorphanol	Levo-Dromoran
Morphine, controlled-release	MS Contin
Methadone	Dolophine
Oxycodone, controlled-release	OxyContin

Because a variety of pharmacological and nonpharmacological modalities may be helpful in relieving chronic pain, referral to a center devoted to pain management can often provide a needed team approach by a staff that is both interested in and knowledgeable about the relief of chronic pain and that is comfortable in dealing with the specific demands of patients with chronic pain. However, if a person wishes to obtain treatment outside a pain center, it is essential that analgesic care be provided by a single physician, with ongoing review and assessment carefully documented in the medical record.

Finally, it must be noted that there will be persons with chronic pain in whom a demonstrative cause cannot be found. This presents a physician with a dilemma: whether it is appropriate to prescribe opioid medications when the reason for prescribing these drugs is not fully defined. In many instances patients may be dependent on multiple substances or medications and, as mentioned earlier (see the section "Evaluate for Signs Suggestive of Opioid Addiction"), one must establish whether a primary addictive disorder exists or the dependence is related to an attempt to provide relief (see Table 45–4). After making certain that an organic etiology has not been overlooked, it is helpful to identify associated factors—such as secondary gain, depression, and insomnia—and then to consider attempting slow detoxification with a change to a nonopioid for chronic mild pain (Savage 1994).

Close monitoring is necessary for all patients taking opioids for chronic pain—regardless of whether there is an identifiable etiology—to ensure that the therapy is providing improvement of pain and daily functioning without abuse or adverse consequences. It is essential that the physician set definite boundaries with respect to the development of a reasonable analgesic regimen and maintain ongoing communication with the patient to ensure that there is a clear understanding of the goals and requirements of treatment. In the end a clear message should be provided that the physician will not merely function as a supplier of drugs but will work with the patient to enable functioning. If it is believed that addictive behavior is present, referral should be made to an appropriate treatment facility.

Conclusion

There is no reason individuals dependent on or using licit or illicit mood-altering substances cannot obtain adequate relief when pain is experienced. The assessment and management of pain in such persons should differ little from methods used in the general population. If the physician can overcome the cultural biases that are frequently present in dealing with those who abuse drugs, adequate relief from pain can be obtained and a solid, long-lasting physician-patient relationship can be developed. It is this relationship that may be the most important factor in addressing the presence of the addictive behaviors that may exist.

References

American Academy of Pain Medicine and American Pain Society: The Use of Opioids for the Treatment of Chronic Pain: A Consensus Statement From the American Academy of Pain Medicine and the American Pain Society. Glenview, IL, American Pain Society, 1997

American Psychiatric Association: Diagnostic and Statistical Manual of Mental Disorders, 4th Edition, Text Revision. Washington, DC, American Psychiatric Association, 2000

American Society of Law, Medicine and Ethics. Pain and the law: state pain relief acts. 2002. Available at: http://www.painandthelaw.org/statutes/state_pain_acts.php. Accessed September 11, 2003

Campbell J: Pain: The Fifth Vital Sign™. Presidential Address at the American Pain Society Meeting, Los Angeles, CA, November 1995. Available at: http://www.ampainsoc.org/advocacy/fifth.htm. Accessed September 11, 2003

Carr DB, Jacox AK, Chapman CR, et al: Acute Pain Management: Operative or Medical Procedures and Trauma (Clinical Practice Guideline, AHCPR Publ No 92-0032). Rockville, MD, Agency for Health Care Policy and Research, 1992

Chabal C, Erjavec MK, Jacobson L, et al: Prescription opiate abuse in chronic pain patients: clinical criteria, incidence, and predictors. Clin J Pain 13:150–155, 1997

Dunbar SA, Katz NP: Chronic opioid therapy for nonmalignant pain in patients with a history of substance abuse: report of 20 cases. J Pain Symptom Manage 11:163–171, 1996

Federation of State Medical Boards: Model Guidelines for the Use of Controlled Substances for Treatment of Pain. May 1998. Available at: http://www.fsmb.org. (Under "Policy Documents"). Accessed September 11, 2003

Fishman SM, Bandman TB, Edwards A: The opioid contract in the management of chronic pain. J Pain Symptom Manage 18:27–37, 1999

Gitlin MC: Contracts for opioid administration for the management of chronic pain: a reappraisal. J Pain Symptom Manage 18:6–8, 1999

Heit HA: The truth about pain management: the difference between a pain patient and an addicted patient. Eur J Pain 5 (suppl A):27–29, 2001

Isaacson JH, Fleming M, Kraus M, et al: A national survey of training in substance use disorders in residency programs. J Stud Alcohol 61:912–915, 2000

Jacox AK, Carr DB, Payne R, et al: Management of Cancer Pain (Clinical Practice Guideline, AHCPR Publ No 94-0592). Rockville, MD, Agency for Health Care Policy and Research, 1994

Johnson RE, Strain EC, Amass L: Buprenorphine: how to use it right. Drug Alcohol Depend 70 (2 suppl):S59–S77, 2003

Johnson SH: Disciplinary actions and pain relief: analysis of the Pain Relief Act. J Law Med Ethics 24:319–327, 1996

Joranson DE, Cleeland CS, Weissman DE, et al: Opioids for chronic cancer and non-cancer pain: a survey of state medical board members. Federal Bulletin 4:415–449, 1992

Joranson DE, Ryan KM, Gilson AM, et al: Trends in medical use and abuse of opioid analgesics. JAMA 283:1710–1714, 2000

Joranson DE, Gilson AM, Dahl JL, et al: Pain management, controlled substances, and state medical board policy: a decade of change. J Pain Symptom Manage 23:138–147, 2002

Kanner RM, Foley KM: Patterns of narcotic drug use in a cancer pain clinic. Ann N Y Acad Sci 362:161–172, 1981

Perry S, Heidrich G: Management of pain during debridement: a survey of U.S. burn units. Pain 13:267–280, 1982

Phillips DM: JCAHO pain management standards are unveiled. Joint Commission on Accreditation of Healthcare Organizations. JAMA 284:428–429, 2000

Portenoy RK, Dole V, Joseph H, et al: Pain management and chemical dependency: evolving perspectives. JAMA 278:592–593, 1997

Porter J, Jick H: Addiction rare in patients treated with narcotics (letter). N Engl J Med 302:123, 1980

Ripamonti C, Zecca E, Bruera E: An update on the clinical use of methadone for cancer pain. Pain 70(2–3):109–115, 1997

Savage SR: Management of acute and chronic pain and cancer pain in the addicted patient, in Principles of Addiction Medicine. Edited by Miller NS, Doot MC. Chevy Chase, MD, American Society of Addiction Medicine, 1994, pp 1–16

Savage SR: Long-term opioid therapy: assessment of consequences and risks. J Pain Symptom Manage 11:274–286, 1996

Schnoll SH, Finch J: Medical education for pain and addiction: making progress toward answering a need. J Law Med Ethics 22:252–256, 1994

Sees KL, Clark HW: Opioid use in the treatment of chronic pain: assessment of addiction. J Pain Symptom Manage 8:257–264, 1993

Stimmel B: Pain and Its Relief Without Addiction: Clinical Issues in the Use of Opioids and Other Analgesics. Binghamton, NY, Haworth, 1997

Tait RC, Pollard CA, Margolis RB, et al: The Pain Disability Index: psychometric and validity data. Arch Phys Med Rehabil 68:438–441, 1987

Weissman DE, Haddox JD: Opioid pseudoaddiction: an iatrogenic syndrome. Pain 36:363–366, 1989

Zenz M, Strumpf M, Tryba M, et al: Long-term oral opioid therapy in patients with chronic nonmalignant pain. J Pain Symptom Manage 7:69–77, 1992

Impaired Physicians

Peter A. Mansky, M.D.

The term *impaired physician* has both a general and a specific connotation. The general connotation refers to a physician with impairment recognized by a decrease in the quality of practice as the result of a psychiatric illness, another medical illness, or an injury. The specific connotation refers to a physician who has a substance use disorder regardless of whether or not the substance use disorder can be directly related to practice impairment (Mansky 1996). This chapter focuses primarily on substance use disorders in physicians and the impact of these disorders on the practice of medicine. Much of the published information concerning impaired physicians is based on clinical observations. Those who work with impaired physicians have a general recognition of the need for collecting uniform data on substance use disorders in physicians, and systematic efforts are under way to explore relevant clinical research issues (Dilts et al. 1999).

Incidence of Substance Use Disorders in Physicians

Literature reviews suggest that physicians are no more likely to have a substance use disorder than socioeco-

nomically matched professionals serving as control subjects; the lifetime incidence of a substance use disorder in physicians has been promulgated as being 8%–15% (Coombs 1997). Hughes et al. (1992) conducted a retrospective study exploring aspects of drug and alcohol consumption. Structured questionnaires were mailed to about 9,600 physicians across the country, with a response rate of 59% after three mailings; 8% of the physicians reported ever experiencing substance abuse or dependence, and 2% indicated experiencing either during the previous year. This study appears to show that physicians have a lower prevalence of substance use disorders compared with two major epidemiological studies, the Epidemiologic Catchment Area (ECA) study and the National Comorbidity Study (NCS), both of which indicate that far more than 8% of the general population have substance use disorders. The difference may well lie in the methodology; the studies of the general population used trained interviewers and questionnaires specifically structured to diagnose psychiatric illnesses, including substance use disorders. In addition, many of the subjects in the general studies who received a substance use disorder diagnosis did not have a self-perception that they had an illness and had not sought treatment (Narrow et al. 2002). There are no studies of physicians with substance use disorders as defined by structured diagnostic instruments and personal interviews.

Substances of Abuse and Dependence

Alcohol is the principal problem drug used by physicians with substance use disorders. Opioids are the second most common class of drugs used by physicians, who tend to be addicted to prescription opioids and rarely to heroin. Cocaine dependence is the third most common substance use disorder in physicians (Galanter et al. 1990; Mansky 1999). Interestingly, anesthesiologists do not follow the same pattern. Alcohol is the second drug of choice among anesthesiologists, whereas the first choice is opioids, usually highly potent injectable opioids such as fentanyl and sufentanil.

Risk Factors for Physicians

Heredity

In the pathogenesis of a substance use disorder, a family history of alcoholism or other addiction is a major risk factor that is considered to be genetically determined (Schuckit and Smith 1997). Being raised in a family in which one or both parents have a substance use disorder may well foster the choice of a medical career. Once the career has been chosen, the pathogenesis of a substance use disorder may continue through genetic inheritance (Mansky 1999). Physicians with a substance use disorder are often motivated by the seemingly altruistic desire to help others but neglect their own needs because of the values, attitudes, and survival behavior engendered by the interactive dynamics of their family of origin (Vaillant et al. 1970).

Health and Self-Care

In general, physicians as they enter their profession are mentally and physically healthier than a matched control population (Frank 1996; Frank et al. 1998). Physicians are certainly able to withstand vigorous training that requires physical, emotional, and intellectual strengths. However, physicians often work with high stress accompanied by the demand for multiple critical decisions. The long work hours, including on-call time, are stressful and tend to isolate physicians from their social support system. In addition, physicians are less likely to seek routine or preventive health care than are other professionals (Vaillant et al. 1970). It has been proposed that even though physicians start with better physical and mental health, the high stress of the profession without the mitigation of adequate social support equalizes their risk for developing a substance use disorder (Frank 1996).

Specialty

In relating specialty to the prevalence of substance use disorders, investigators have first reported the number of physicians in a specialty who have a substance use disorder and who are enrolled in a physician health program (PHP) or other selected group dealing with substance abuse. The number of enrollees is then linked to the likelihood of a physician within that specialty developing a substance use disorder, using the percentage of the specialty in a given program as a prognostic indicator of the risk. However, the percentage of members of the specialty enrolled in the program may not represent a valid risk factor. The risk is better represented by comparing the percentage of the specialty participating in a program such as a PHP to the percentage of the total number of physicians practicing in that specialty. For example, if a specialty accounts for 3% of the total physician population in the state but 6% of physicians taking part in a PHP, this specialty has a risk factor of 2.

Anesthesiologists and emergency room physicians have the highest risk factor, approximately three times that of the general population of physicians (Mansky 1996). This risk may be related to the choice of this field, the medications used in the field, or the attraction of working in situations that deal with intense periodic clinical activity. It should also be noted that the American Society of Anesthesiologists has an increased awareness of substance use disorders and promotes referrals to PHPs. In the early 1990s there were reports indicating that anesthesiologists who self-administered high-potency opioids needed to retrain in another specialty. More recent data demonstrate that about 50% of anesthesiologists can return to the safe and effective practice of anesthesia (Paris and Canavan 1999).

Professional Experiences and Attitudes

Some of the experiences and attitudes of physicians have been proposed as risk factors for developing a substance use disorder. These have been described as pharmacological optimism and knowledge, reliance on intellectual strength, having a strong will, loving challenges, resorting to the instrumental use of medications, and a daily need for denial (Mansky 1999). These factors have been proposed on the basis of clinical experience, and there still remains a need to establish their etiological role in the pathogenesis of substance use disorders in physicians.

Pharmacological Optimism and Knowledge

Pharmacological optimism and knowledge arise from the experiences of treating patients with medications that work well and rapidly. Cases of severe congestive heart failure, ketoacidosis, acute psychosis, fulminant infections, and acute mania often respond quickly to the administration of medications. Physicians learn to respect the utility and value of medications. The rapid responses to medications in clinically severe cases are frequent occurrences in the practice of emergency medicine and anesthesiology. A personality trait that includes an increased appreciation of excitement and satisfaction with rapid response may lead to choosing either of these two specialties. This may be the same trait that predisposes to the evolution or progression of the substance use disorder disease process.

Pharmacological knowledge or clinical understanding of substance use disorders does not confer immunity to the development of the disease. Physicians with the disease often misuse or distort their knowledge to support their use of substances.

> Physician JB was very knowledgeable about medications. He was a board-certified internist who had completed a 2-year fellowship in clinical pharmacology, and after 10 years of practice he was a full professor of medicine at a prestigious medical school. He self-prescribed various benzodiazepines; with his knowledge of pharmacology he knew that major withdrawal symptoms did not occur at doses below the equivalent of 40 mg of diazepam. He was therefore very careful to keep his daily intake below the 40-mg equivalence level. Over several years he developed severe gastric reflux and was prescribed cimetidine. He knew that the cimetidine increased his blood level of diazepam and that he should lower his dosage well below the 40 mg/day equivalence. He did not do this, and after several months he stopped the medication for a period of time and had a withdrawal seizure.

Reliance on Intellectual Abilities

Reliance on intellectual abilities has been the lifelong pattern for most physicians, and they tend to hold this ability in high regard. Physicians are generally among those who did well in grade school, high school, and college. It is their intellectual abilities reflected in their grades and the importance of their grade scores to their career that add perceived value to their intellectual skills. This reinforcement continues as physicians find that their intellectual abilities help them in their daily work when they are faced with complicated clinical decisions. The importance of the physician's clinical acumen is emphasized by the consequences of the decisions in the prevention of mortality, morbidity, and suffering. This use of intellect is considered to have a negative effect on the recognition of and recovery from a substance use disorder because it contributes to denial of the illness.

Strong Will

Strong will at first appears to be a quality one would not expect to find in individuals with a substance use disorder, which seems to be the result of a weak will or poor self-control. Nevertheless, clinical experience indicates that patients with a substance use disorder are actually strong-willed. The contradiction appears to be resolved when it becomes evident that the strength of the compulsion to continue the use of a substance is much stronger than an individual's ability to maintain abstinence. Strong-willed individuals who correctly perceive their strength of will take risks based on their self-awareness. In contrast, they usually deny or are not aware of the strong reinforcement of the addicting drug.

Physicians who train in tertiary care centers are exposed primarily to patients with end-stage and severe substance use disorders. The physical and mental disabilities associated with end-stage or severe substance use disorders mask manifestations of the patient's strong will. The patient has lost the battle with the substance use disorder and appears to have no self-control or ability to stop use, unlike the physician with less severe stages of the illness characterized by periods of abstinence. Physicians see their the ability to stop or to use periodically as proof that they are not like the patients in the severe stages of the illness. This perception fosters a false sense of being able to use addicting substances with impunity and control.

When physicians are in recovery they often report hearing about "self-will run riot" or having a very "strong self-will" in their mutual-support 12-step meetings. They indicate that they rarely hear a discussion concerning a weak will or lack of self-control.

Love of Challenges

Love of challenges may lead to risk-taking behavior, the willingness to take chances, and sensation seeking. These are factors in the pathogenesis of substance use disorders in physicians (McAuliffe et al. 1987) and are often interpreted to be related to self-will. The practice reflected in the old adage "see one, do one, teach one" leads to actions that require courage, initiative, and assertiveness. This pattern of learning early in a physician's career engenders a sense that taking risks may apply to situations outside the practice of medicine. Weissberg (1996) administered questionnaires to medical students at the University of Colorado concerning three types of risk-taking behavior: driving without seat belts, smoking tobacco, and driving while intoxicated. Almost all used seat belts, very few used tobacco, and about one-third admitted to driving while intoxicated. This willingness to use an addicting substance in a dangerous situation is striking and is an impetus for the additional study of risk-taking behavior in medical students and physicians.

Instrumental Use of Drugs

The use of drugs to fulfill a demanding work role, often termed instrumental or implemental use, is a risk factor for developing a substance use disorder among physicians (McAuliffe et al. 1987). At-risk physicians may have started using amphetamines or other stimulants to cram for examinations in college or in medical school.

> A resident physician, Dr. S, suffered from mild headaches during her first postgraduate year. Because her headaches continued and the pain seemed to decrease her ability to concentrate while on call, she took aspirin and occasionally extra strength acetaminophen to relieve the pain. The headaches continued into her second postgraduate year and she decided to add a nonsteroidal anti-inflammatory medication, which provided pain relief up until her third postgraduate year. During this year Dr. S maintained an active follow-up outpatient clinic for her patients. She was treating a young attorney who had a traumatic back injury followed by chronic pain. The attorney was prescribed acetaminophen and a low dose of codeine to take at night so she could sleep. She eventually also used the combination medication throughout the day and reported to Dr.
>
> S that she was able to work well and was able to prepare documents and argue in conference without making errors or losing her concentration.
>
> Dr. S realized that she should not prescribe an opioid for herself, so she persuaded a fellow resident to prescribe the medication for her. Dr. S's use of opioids continued into her first five years of practice. She eventually became addicted to opioids, wrote prescriptions for herself, and stole supplies from her office practice of gastroenterology. She also wrote prescriptions in the names of several patients, some fictitious. She presented the prescriptions at numerous pharmacies and was eventually referred to a PHP by a pharmacist who worked at several different pharmacies and observed Dr. S picking up the prescriptions.

Systematic study of resident physicians revealed that many started to use minor opiates or benzodiazepines during their residency (Hughes et al. 1991). It is also significant that Dr. S did not seek formal evaluation or treatment for her headache. She had several "curbside consultations" but did not seek the care she needed and deserved.

Denial

Denial as used in relation to substance use disorders implies that patients with a substance use disorder very frequently use their intellect and experience to convince themselves that they do not have the illness. It is considered one of the major explanations for patients not seeking treatment for their substance use disorder. Denial, of course, is also an ego defense mechanism that has been thought to indicate prominent regression, even to the level of psychosis. There appears to be a healthy form of denial that helps individuals cope with illness and even with everyday life situations. For example, without denial it would be difficult to drive a car with the constant awareness and fear of having an accident. In clinical settings it has been noted that cardiac patients who express denial but follow their physician's advice tend to do better than patients without denial (Dimsdale and Hackett 1982; Hackett and Cassem 1982).

It is a common experience for medical students to be convinced they have symptoms of a disease they are studying during their introduction to pathology. They are surprised when they find out that many of their classmates have had the same thought but perhaps about a different disease. The students learn early the value of ignoring their own symptoms in an effort to dissociate from the potential danger of having the illness (Vaillant et al. 1970). Throughout medical practice they learn about frightening and destructive illnesses and frequently include these illnesses in their daily differential diagnoses of their patients. It requires some degree of denial to keep out of conscious awareness the possibility that they will develop the illnesses seen daily in their work setting.

Healthy denial, although used as a mechanism of daily coping, delays the possibility of physicians recognizing that they might have a substance use disorder. The denial of illness may become so entrenched over time that it is difficult to convince a physician who drank socially for many years that the drinking is pathological and that the pattern qualifies for the diagnosis of a substance use disorder.

Recognition and Intervention

As a substance use disorder in a physician progresses, marital, financial, social, and legal difficulties are the first to become evident. Usually the last area of a physician's life to be affected by the illness is the practice setting (Centrella 1994). The most important aspect of recognizing the illness is personality change in the physician. The change may be very rapid in opioid and cocaine addiction, but it may be much slower and more difficult to perceive in alcohol dependence because it develops slowly over many years. In the practice setting it may be noticed that the physician is increasingly irritable and moody. Difficulties or arguments may be evident with nurses and other nonphysician health care workers. These attitudes and behaviors may then become evident to patients and to other colleagues as the disease progresses. Absences from work or canceling of office hours, especially on Monday or the day after a major holiday weekend, are not uncommon and are often attributed to other illnesses as well as to financial or social crisis. The physician may conduct rounds at unusual hours, either late in the evening or very early in the morning. The physician's clinical record keeping often suffers, and the hospital staff as well as office personnel may have difficulties reaching the physician at times. The physician frequently explains that financial, legal, and family problems are causing all the difficulties, whereas in reality it is likely that the substance use disorder is the origin of most of the difficulties. Intoxication at social functions and arrests for drinking and driving or for behavior resulting from substance use occur as the disease

progresses. These events often precede the physician's withdrawal from social activities and isolation from colleagues and social support systems. As the illness continues into more severe stages, the physician begins to show obvious impairment at the work site, with the odor of alcohol appearing on his or her breath. Noticeable signs of intoxication may be present at work. Anesthesiologists have been found unconscious on the floor between appointments and sometimes cannot be aroused in the on-call room even during daytime hours.

At various stages in the illness a colleague may want to confront the physician or intervene to urge the physician to get a clinical evaluation. A general rule to follow is never to approach the physician alone. In most cases when this is done the physician simply dismisses the concerns of the colleague who makes the solo approach. Confrontation is best done with a group of concerned family members, colleagues, and friends. It is useful to contact the state PHP or the hospital physician health committee to aid in convincing the physician to seek an evaluation.

Hospital physician health committees are now becoming common as a result of the physician health standard adopted in 2001 by the Joint Commission on Accreditation of Healthcare Organizations (2003). Medical Staff Standard 2.6 requires that hospitals develop a mechanism for handling matters of physician health separately from physician discipline; educate physicians and staff about physician impairment; and implement a procedure to identify impaired physicians who can then be referred for evaluation and treatment. Many hospitals are turning to state PHPs to help in this process.

Treatment

In clinical treatment settings, physicians who are patients are often able to use their knowledge to control or intimidate other patients and treating clinicians. In essence they use their clinical skills to avoid being a patient, and they become the unofficial physician for the group of patients in the treatment setting. This phenomenon can be avoided by sending physicians with substance use disorders to clinicians and clinical centers that specialize in treating physicians. If such treatment is not available to a physician in his or her locality, there are recognized national centers specializing in the evaluation and treatment of physicians. These centers tend to have extensive experience treating physicians and have a substantial patient population of health care professionals. A center that is removed from the physician's home location provides a setting for increased confidentiality and helps avoids the bias and pitfalls related to the physician's local reputation, status, and professional relationships. Alternatively, local outpatient treatment may be appropriate in some cases, especially if the physician is experiencing a mild level of substance abuse.

The treating clinicians and centers are aware of medical workplace issues and are often called on to make recommendations for the physician's return to active practice. When it is deemed that the physician can return to the safe and effective practice of medicine, these centers have the ability to issue reports and case summaries that are clinically accurate and at the same time help preserve the physician's ability to continue to practice medicine within the scrutiny of hospital administrations and managed care organizations, as well as legal and regulatory agencies. These centers are able to complement and support the efforts of state PHPs. Physicians who are returning to practice must be abstinent, and techniques of harm reduction can be used only if a physician is not practicing.

The social and family consequences of substance use disorders in physicians are also addressed. The clinicians and centers support programs for family members and other people of significance in the physician's life with parallel or supportive programs for family issues facing the physician. Occasionally, a physician will not respond to treatment specifically geared for physicians and will respond only when treated in a center with the general population, often with a more diverse socioeconomic stratum.

The physicians are introduced to two mutual support groups: caduceus groups and International Doctors in Alcoholics Anonymous (IDAA) groups. Caduceus groups, first called caduceus clubs in the 1970s, originally encompassed various activities of support and aftercare following inpatient treatment (Angres et al. 1998). Today the caduceus groups provide a confidential support group for recovering physicians to discuss issues pertinent to their careers and recovery. They supplement attendance at other mutual help groups or 12-step meetings. IDAA is an organization of recovering physicians, dentists, and doctoral-level health care professionals. IDAA holds an annual meeting with international attendance for mutual support along with scientific sessions through a relationship with the American Society of Addiction Medicine. Some communities have IDAA meetings instead of caduceus meetings for mutual support.

Clinicians treating physicians need to be skilled in the delivery of care and therapy while at the same time reporting the progress of the physician's response to a PHP or a state medical board. This requires the clinician to have developed expertise in effectively employing techniques of therapy that depend on the strength of the therapeutic relationship while also reporting to an outside program or agency. Such expertise is especially important when treating the physician with long-term insight-oriented psychotherapy during the more advanced stages of recovery (Fayne and Silvan 1999). In addition to reporting progress in therapy, clinicians may be asked to testify for the physician at board hearings regarding issues of licensure. Furthermore, they may also treat the physician under mandates from medical boards.

Physician Health Programs

Statewide PHPs now exist in all 50 U.S. states (American Medical Association 2002), whereas other countries have regionwide programs. The programs are clinically oriented and provide support for physicians with various illnesses. The American Medical Association and the Canadian Medical Association have periodically sponsored international meetings addressing physician health with worldwide attendance.

In the early 1970s it was recognized by medical organizations that there was a need for confidential collegial support of physicians with substance use disorders and that identifying and treating physicians with psychiatric illnesses would improve patient safety (Goldman et al. 2000). Many states developed programs called *physician health committees* that served as confidential peer support. These committees consisted of a network of physicians who were successfully recovering from substance use disorders and were available to help physicians with active substance use disorders. Over time the programs have systematically developed organizations supported by state law, run by professional staffs, and addressing many illnesses.

Most state PHPs have remained affiliated with state medical societies. Many are now established under state laws that protect the confidentiality of the physician and the referral source. A small number are run by state medical boards, which limits the protection of confidentiality. Programs are funded from various sources, mostly by medical societies. Varying by state, they are also financially supported by state medical boards, malpractice carriers, hospitals, and participant fees. About one-quarter are structured as independent corporations that have the affiliations and financial support described above.

Illnesses Addressed and Other Activities

All of the state PHPs enroll physicians with substance use disorders, and 85% of the programs include participants with other Axis I psychiatric disorders, including a percentage having both a substance use disorder and another Axis I illness at the time of the referral. About 60% of the programs also help physicians who have physical illnesses. More than 70% of the programs accept referrals for disruptive behavior and address the issues resulting from the behavior, often using cognitive and directive techniques even in the absence of an Axis I disorder. More than 60% of the programs assist physicians with boundary issues, and 40% provide support to assist with stress, 20% specifically with stress from malpractice litigation.

Functional Aspects

PHPs have several basic functions. These include outreach and education, case identification and referral, intervention, clinical evaluation, monitoring, and advocacy.

Outreach and Educational Functions

Outreach and educational functions inform physicians about PHPs and the illnesses they address, primarily substance use disorders. It is important that physicians learn that they can receive confidential treatment and that despite having an illness they can resume their career while being treated. Outreach and education also provide the basis for preventive measures in educating practicing physicians, medical students, and residents about substance use disorders and the recognition of the illness in themselves and their colleagues.

Case Identification and Referral

Case identification and referral follow from outreach activities but also include referrals from other sources.

Most referrals tend to be from physicians referring either themselves or their colleagues, in the latter case frequently in the capacity of representing a hospital or group practice. Other sources of referrals are pharmacists; patients; family members; physicians or therapists treating the physician being referred; and regulatory agencies, including medical boards. Most of the self-referrals are done under pressure from hospitals, managed care organizations, regulatory agencies, or families.

Intervention

Interventions can be done directly by the PHP, done locally and then referred to the PHP, or done in coordination with the PHP. The interventions may be confrontive and supportive and may use either the confrontive johnsonian approach or that approach modified by the motivational techniques of persuasion (Merrill et al. 2002). Most important is that intervention with the physician can be supported by the pressure of mandate. PHPs are usually permitted by law to interact with the physician confidentially, contingent on the physician's adherence to the clinical guidelines as developed by the PHP along with the clinicians evaluating and treating the physician.

Evaluation and Treatment

Evaluation and treatment are guided by the PHP in conjunction with the treating clinicians approved by the PHP. Evaluations may be either outpatient or inpatient. Inpatient evaluations usually last for 3–5 days and allow for observations of behavior throughout the entire 24 hours of each day. Gathering of collateral information from family members and colleagues with the physician's consent is essential. PHPs often offer the physician the opportunity to remain or to choose a different center for treatment, thus decreasing the physician's perception that the center may be biased toward diagnosing the substance use disorder so that they can treat the physician.

Monitoring

Monitoring is an important aspect of the PHP and includes the monitoring of body fluids, treatment, and practice. Monitoring also has value in treatment in that it substantially increases the chance of a positive outcome (Shore 1987). This is also evident in other programs that monitor professionals, such as the program developed by the Federal Aviation Administration for pilots (Pakull 2002). Many PHPs and the Federal Aviation Administration program can demonstrate a recovery rate above 90%, occasionally with a brief relapse as part of the recovery process. Previously, PHPs customarily monitored physicians for 2 years, but most now require 5 years of monitoring, with less intensity as the time of participation increases. Some PHPs monitor physicians indefinitely, although with substantially decreased frequency.

Advocacy

Advocacy is an important and essential feature of PHPs. These organizations support physicians in their recovery from their illness and in their return to practice. PHPs aid physicians recovering from illness in their dealings with hospitals, employers, group practices, managed care organizations, regulatory and licensing agencies, the community, and the family. Such advocacy is helpful in the physicians' treatment, recovery, and reintegration into social and professional life.

Conclusion

Physicians treating their fellow physicians who are impaired have been trained in a variety of specialties and have become proficient in treating substance use disorders. As this special area of treatment has grown, it has become more evident that impaired physicians frequently include those who have a multitude of psychiatric illnesses. This tendency places the clinician with psychiatric training in a unique position to treat impaired physicians and to work with other, nonpsychiatrist physicians who are trained in addiction medicine in the treatment of their fellow physicians. Psychiatrists have become medical directors of PHPs in increasing numbers in recent years.

References

American Medical Association: State Program Listing, Federation of State Physician Health Programs. Chicago, IL, American Medical Association, 2002. Available at: http://www.ama-assn.org/ama/pub/category/6020.html. Accessed September 11, 2003

Angres DH, Talbott GD, Berttinardi-Angres K: Healing the Healer: The Addicted Physician. Madison, CT, Psychosocial Press, 1998

Centrella MC: Physician addiction and impairment: current thinking: a review. J Addict Dis 13:91–105, 1994

Coombs RH: Drug-Impaired Professionals. Cambridge, MA, Harvard University Press, 1997, pp 27–30

Dilts S, Goldman L, Shore J: Physician Health Research Conference (Estes Park, Colorado, September 15–17, 1996): progress report one year later. Psychiatr Q 70:123–135, 1999

Dimsdale JE, Hackett TP: Effect of denial on cardiac health and psychological assessment. Am J Psychiatry 139:1477–1480, 1982

Fayne M, Silvan M: Treatment issues in the group psychotherapy of addicted physicians. Psychiatr Q 70:123–135, 1999

Frank E: Research issues for physician health programs in prevention and special populations. Paper presented at the Physician Health Research Conference, Estes Park, CO, September 15–17, 1996

Frank E, Brogan DJ, Mokdad AH, et al: Health-related behaviors of women physicians vs other women in the United States. Arch Intern Med 158:342–348, 1998

Galanter M, Talbott D, Gallegos K, et al: Combined Alcoholics Anonymous and professional care for addicted physicians. Am J Psychiatry 147:64–68, 1990

Goldman LS, Myers MF, Dickstein LJ: Evolution of the physician health field, in The Handbook of Physician Health. Edited by Goldman LS, Myers MF, Dickstein LJ. Chicago, IL, American Medical Association, 2000, pp 1–8

Hackett TP, Cassem NH: Coping with cardiac disease. Adv Cardiol 31:212–217, 1982

Hughes PH, Conard SE, Baldwin DC Jr, et al: Resident physician substance use in the United States. JAMA 265:2069–2073, 1991

Hughes PH, Brandenburg N, Baldwin DC Jr, et al: Prevalence of substance use among U.S. physicians. JAMA 267:2333–2339, 1992

Joint Commission on Accreditation of Healthcare Organizations: Hospital Accreditation Standards Manual, Medical Staff Standard 2.6. Oakbrook Terrace, IL, Joint Commission on Accreditation of Healthcare Organizations, 2003

Mansky PA: Physician health programs and the potentially impaired physician with a substance use disorder. Psychiatr Serv 47:465–467, 1996

Mansky PA: Issues in the recovery of physicians from addictive illnesses. Psychiatr Q 70:107–122, 1999

McAuliffe WE, Santangelo S, Magnuson E, et al: Risk factors of drug impairment in random samples of physicians and medical students. Int J Addict 22:825–841, 1987

Merrill JO, Marlatt GA, Verghese A: Health care workers and addiction. N Engl J Med 347:1044–1045, 2002

Narrow WE, Rae DS, Robins LN, et al: Revised prevalence estimates of mental disorders in the United States: using a clinical significance criterion to reconcile 2 surveys' estimates. Arch Gen Psychiatry 59:115–123, 2002

Pakull B: The Federal Aviation Administration's role in evaluation of pilots and others with alcoholism or drug addiction. Occup Med 17:221–226, 2002

Paris RT, Canavan DI: Physician substance abuse impairment: anesthesiologists vs. other specialties. J Addict Dis 18:1–7, 1999

Schuckit MA, Smith TL: Assessing the risk for alcoholism among sons of alcoholics. J Stud Alcohol 58:141–151, 1997

Shore JH: The Oregon experience with impaired physicians on probation: an eight-year follow-up. JAMA 257:2931–2934, 1987

Vaillant GE, Brighton JR, McArthur C: Physicians' use of mood-altering drugs: a 20-year follow-up report. N Engl J Med 282:365–370, 1970

Weissberg MP: Survey of medical students: research issues for physician health programs in prevention and special populations. Presented at the Physician Health Research Conference, Estes Park, CO, September 15–17, 1996

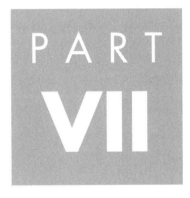

PART

VII

Special Topics

Laboratory and Psychological Diagnostic Testing

Robert L. DuPont, M.D.
Carl M. Selavka, Ph.D.

The diagnosis of substance use disorder, like most other medical diagnoses, is primarily clinical, with the patient's history and the mental status examination playing the central role in the diagnostic process. Laboratory and psychological testing nevertheless are increasingly important in clinical settings in addiction medicine, ranging from the initial diagnosis to treatment management, and from research and epidemiology to health care assessment. Laboratory testing is essential for identifying the recent use of specific abused substances, both for initial evaluation and for monitoring of compliance with treatment. Laboratory testing is also helpful in medical settings as part of the screening process to identify patients for evaluation for substance use disorder. Psychological tests are being used to identify people at high risk for substance use disorders and to assess readiness for and progress during substance abuse treatment.

In this chapter we review the uses of laboratory and psychological testing. We describe some of the tests now in common use, including the science on which they rely, and the information that these tests can provide to clinicians.

Laboratory Testing

Laboratory testing in addiction medicine can be separated into tests that identify recent, repetitive, or ongoing *use* of particular drugs of abuse and tests that identify the common *biological consequences* of the use of alcohol and other drugs, including infectious diseases and abnormal clinical chemistry findings. Laboratory tests cannot detect or measure drug-caused impairment, physical dependence, or addiction to alcohol or other drugs (DuPont 2000). Like the diagnosis of addictive illness itself, those important assessments rely primarily on clinical assessments, with the laboratory findings often providing supportive data.

Identifying Recent Drug Use

Two of the hallmarks of addictive disorders are denial and dishonesty. Addicted people characteristically deny to themselves and to others the negative consequences of their use of alcohol and other drugs, and they characteristically lie about their use of alcohol and other drugs to anyone who might interfere with their continued substance use (DuPont 1998). When it comes to illegal drugs, drug users might not know what drugs they are actually taking, so even if they wanted to tell their doctors what drugs they were taking they could not do so.

Users of alcohol and other drugs consume their substances of choice for the effect these specific substances have on the reward centers of their brains (DuPont and Gold 1995). To achieve this brain-rewarding effect, users consume the drugs by various routes of administration, including oral, intranasal, inhalation (smoking), and intravenous, with the common preference of many experienced drug users being the routes of administration that produce the most rapid increase in blood levels because these are the most intensely rewarding.

Once in the body, the abused drugs are distributed so widely that they can be identified in virtually all parts of the body and in all body fluids. The drugs are typically metabolized by the liver and in the blood, producing characteristic metabolites that are often longer lasting and detectable at higher levels than the parent drug. Although the pharmacokinetics of this process are complex and substance-specific, the general pattern is universal. This common pattern is what makes drug testing for all drugs similar and relatively easily understood. On the other hand, the pharmacokinetics of each drug are important in the linkage of laboratory results to specific drug use.

Although drugs and their metabolites can be identified by using a wide range of techniques, modern drug testing has settled into a pattern that usually involves the use of a relatively inexpensive immunoassay screening test that has high sensitivity but not necessarily high specificity. That means that the immunoassay screen can detect very low levels of drugs and drug metabolites in the tested specimen but that the results occasionally may be confounded by cross-reactivity with nondrug substances.

In the workplace and other settings where the results must be forensically defensible, positive results from screening drug tests are confirmed by using a highly specific confirming test, such as a gas chromatography/mass spectrometry test. Screening tests can be done on site and do not require a clinical laboratory, although confirming drug tests are performed in a laboratory. This picture of an initial screening test followed by a confirming drug test is used to produce optimal reliability for all tested specimens from urine and blood to sweat, saliva, and hair.

In many settings where this forensic standard is unnecessary—including most addiction treatment settings and the criminal justice system—an immunoassay test is typically sufficient without confirmation (DuPont and Selavka 2003). An important exception to this general testing regimen involves the determination of the presence of ethanol. For this volatile substance, breath testing, using relatively automated methods, and oral fluid (saliva) tests provide generally reliable results without the need for laboratory confirmation.

Two decades ago, drug testing technology was relatively primitive and the only commonly used sample for drug testing was urine, in which drugs and drug metabolites are relatively concentrated and easily identified. The exception was breath and blood testing for alcohol, which has been common for several decades. In more recent years, as drug detection technology has improved and as more reliable procedures for collection and sample handling have been developed, it has become practical to test sweat, saliva, and hair for recent drug use.

The sample selected for alcohol and other drug testing reflects many factors, including ease of access, cost of test, and the most appropriate detection window (i.e., the period of time that is sampled to identify drug use). Breath, saliva, and hair samples are the most easily collected, whereas urine can present logistical and reliability issues, and blood and organ samples (such as liver biopsies) are the most difficult to obtain. Costs of analysis, when considered as a part of a total patient assessment, are similar, although hair, saliva, sweat, and blood testing are somewhat more expensive than urine testing. Sweat, saliva, and hair testing are done only at specialized laboratories at present, but urine testing for drugs of abuse is done at most clinical laboratories. More recently, urine testing kits have become available for on-site screening, which produces results within a few minutes of collection. Saliva tests can also be performed on site. If the alcohol and other drug testing relates to the workplace, then legal regulations are important considerations, including secure collection with forensic standards of specimen handling and laboratory confirmation (U.S. Department of Health and Human Services 1988).

Blood has the shortest window of detection because most drugs are cleared to below measurable levels from the blood in 12 hours or less. Urine has a detection window of about 1–3 days because most drugs are cleared within this time after the most recent use of the drug. This is true even for marijuana, unless the tested individual has been a long-term heavy smoker of marijuana, in which case the urine results can remain positive for up to a month after use stops. In the absence of previous heavy long-term marijuana use, after smoking one or two marijuana cigarettes many subjects have urine testing results that are negative within 24 hours, and all results will be negative at the 100-ng/mL cutoff within 3 days. After smoking one or two marijuana cigarettes, all subjects will have urine test results that will be negative at the more sensitive 20-ng/mL cutoff within 5 days of last marijuana use (Schwartz 1988).

Hair grows at the rate of about 0.5 inch (or a bit more than 1 cm) per month. With each day of drug use, a subject's newly created hair cells incorporate drug from the bloodstream on that day. If a patient has only a single day of drug use, the incorporation of drug into hair is predominantly localized to the tiny 0.3-mm length of hair representing that one day. When surrounded by the "ocean of abstinence" represented by hair growing on days without drug use, this single ingestion cannot be detected in a conventional hair drug test. In fact, hair-testing positive results are generally expected only when a patient has used a drug four to six times or more (for single individual recreational doses) per month, when conventional hair test reporting thresholds (cutoffs) are employed. For this reason, hair-testing positive results are generally interpreted as reliable indicators of long-term drug ingestion.

It takes about a week for the hair to grow long enough to be sampled in routine clipping of head hair. Thus, a standard 1.5-inch sample of head hair contains drug residuals from the previous 90 days, minus the week immediately before sample collection. Hair testing is particularly useful and superior to urine testing in various situations in which the longer detection window is important (DuPont and Selavka 2003). Because preemployment urine drug testing is a scheduled test, a drug user has to refrain from nonmedical drug use for only 3–5 days before submitting a urine sample in order to pass a urine test for abused drugs. It is much harder for most long-term drug abusers to refrain from drug use for 90 days before preemployment testing, the period covered by a hair sample. Longer hair, and therefore longer time periods, can also be tested.

In contrast to urine samples, hair samples do not pose problems with sample substitution, adulteration, or dilution. However, hair treatments—such as perming, bleaching, and straightening—can reduce drug levels in hair in a way that can convert borderline positive results to negative results. Research has shown, on the other hand, that conventional hygienic hair treatments have little impact on the detection of drug use involving hair tests. Collection of hair is also less offensive to the subject than collection of urine. However, as noted above, substantial drug use in the 90 days before sample collection is required to create a positive hair-test result. This higher threshold for a positive hair-test result means that eating poppy seeds will not produce a positive hair laboratory test result for opiates, as it commonly does in urine tests. Positive laboratory results for opiates on urine tests are routinely reversed by medical review officers, making an opiate testing of urine samples in the workplace all but worthless because of the poppy seed problem. More importantly, high cutoffs for urine opiate detection make it nearly impossible to detect abusers of heroin—a substance for which hair testing is particularly well suited.

Workplace drug testing conducted under federal guidelines is limited to a small number of drugs (codeine/morphine, amphetamine/methamphetamine, phencyclidine [PCP], marijuana, and cocaine) with urine tests. This means that under federal guidelines the use of any other drug is not detected, including lysergic acid diethylamide (LSD), methylenedioxymethamphetamine (MDMA, Ecstasy) and other stimulants, and synthetic opioids (such as hydromorphone hydrochloride, oxycodone hydrochloride, and methylphenidate hydrochloride). Urine tests, when employed under nonregulated standards, can offer important diagnostic information. Even a single dose of important abuse substances—including inhalants (such as nitrous oxide), solvents (involved in "huffing"), and a myriad of drugs available to medical professionals (e.g., meperidine, fentanyl)—can be detected in urine. But the clinician will need to seek out a reference toxicology laboratory to provide these specialty urine testing services.

Sweat patch testing is a relatively new technique for drug testing. The person wears a patch, similar to a nicotine patch worn by people attempting to quit smoking, that, once removed, cannot be easily replaced without noticeable puckering of the edges of the patch. This feature provides reasonable integrity in the sweat patch collection process. Sweat is continuously absorbed into the patch, with the water in the sweat evaporating through the outer patch membrane while the drug substance is accumulated on the absorbent patch. Because skin normally desquamates, patches can be worn only 2–4 weeks before they fall off. Drug detection sweat patches can be worn for periods of a few hours to a few weeks. During that time, they prospectively collect evidence of drug use that occurs. Once removed, the patches are sent to a laboratory for testing.

Patches are commercially tested for the detection of cocaine, opiates, marijuana, PCP, and amphetamine/methamphetamine. Sweat patches are not routinely marketed for the detection of alcohol use, but alcohol detection patches might find greater application in the future. Sweat patch testing is especially useful for follow-up testing, for example, in a return-to-work setting where daily urine testing for drug use or even more repetitive breath testing for ethanol are impractical.

Hair testing and sweat patches offer important advantages over urine testing for abuse drugs in many settings. Both are far more resistant to cheating, both can offer rough quantitation (enabling the rough separation of heavy users from light users), and both more reliably produce positive test results for opiates after heroin ingestion. See Table 47–1 for summary comparison of blood, urine, hair, and sweat patch testing for abused drugs.

Saliva testing for drugs of abuse is now commonly used by the insurance industry to detect use of nicotine (as cotinine), cocaine, and other drugs. Saliva testing for abused drugs is also gaining popularity in the workplace and other settings. For example, saliva tests of impaired drivers can significantly improve the overall detection of ingested drugs in drivers whether these impaired drivers also drank alcohol or not. Saliva is in equilibrium with blood; therefore, saliva testing, like blood testing, can detect only very recent use of drugs, often within the previous 6–12 hours. Saliva testing for alcohol is also available. Because saliva is easily obtained (unlike urine and blood) and can be screened on site (unlike hair samples), it is especially useful in postaccident and highway testing and in other settings in which immediate results and easy collection are important. The one limitation of saliva testing is that it is much less effective than urine testing in detecting recent marijuana use, whereas saliva and urine testing are similar in positive rates for other drugs of abuse in side-by-side testing (Yacoubian et al. 2001).

Identifying Common Correlates of Alcohol and Other Drug Use

Clinical chemistry tests can be useful in identifying and following alcohol use because of the wide range of adverse biological effects of long-term heavy drinking (Allen and Litten 1994). Laboratory tests are neither as specific nor as sensitive as clinical assessment for diagnosing alcoholism (DuPont 1994). Nevertheless, it is useful to have a clear picture of the common laboratory results seen after heavy drinking. Abnormal laboratory results are more common in older drinkers, reflecting years of negative health effects of alcohol. Clinical chemistry test results are less likely to be abnormal in younger people, even if they heavily use alcohol.

In about two-thirds of long-term heavy drinkers, the γ-glutamyltransferase (GGT) level is elevated. GGT sensitively but nonspecifically reflects damage to the liver caused by alcohol (and, to a lesser extent, that caused by other drugs) as well as infiltrative liver disorders and biliary obstruction. GGT reflects both liver damage and enzyme induction secondary to heavy drinking over extended periods of time. GGT is induced not only by alcohol but also by phenobarbital, phenytoin, and many other drugs. GGT levels return to normal after about 3 weeks of abstinence from alcohol use.

Mean corpuscular volume (MCV) is elevated in about one-quarter of alcoholic patients. Elevation of the MCV is a relatively late manifestation of alcoholism and can result from both direct toxic effects of alcohol on the bone marrow and disruptions in folate metabolism. Unlike GGT elevations, MCV elevations persist for several months after abstinence from alcohol. The specificity of GGT elevation in identifying alcoholism is enhanced when it occurs in conjunction with MCV elevation because the nonalcoholic factors that raise GGT levels do not raise MCV levels.

Alanine aminotransferase (ALT) and aspartate aminotransferase (AST) are elevated in about one-half of long-term heavy drinkers. Elevations of these trans-

Table 47–1. Comparison of blood, urine, hair, saliva, and sweat patch testing for drugs of abuse

Characteristic	Blood	Urine	Hair	Saliva	Sweat patch
Immunoassay screen	Yes	Yes	Yes	Yes	Yes
GC/MS confirmation option (laboratory-based)	Yes	Yes	Yes	Yes	Yes
Chain-of-custody option	Yes	Yes	Yes	Yes	Yes
Retained positives for retest option	Difficult	Possible	Easy	Difficult	Possible
Medical review officer option	Yes	Yes	Yes	Yes	Yes
Common surveillance window	3–12 hours	1–3 days	7–90 days+	3–24 hours	1–21 days
Intrusiveness of collection	Severe	Moderate	None	Slight	Slight
Retest of same sample	Yes	Yes	Yes	Yes	Yes
Compatibility of new sample if original test disputed	No	No	Yes	No	No
Number of drugs screened	Unlimited[a]	Unlimited[b]	Large[c]	5+alcohol	5[d]
Cost/sample (NIDA 5)	About $200	About $15–$30	About $40–$65	About $50	About $35
Can distinguish between light, moderate, and heavy use	Yes (short term)	No	Yes (long term)	No	Yes (ongoing)
Resistance to cheating	High	Low	High	High	High
Best applications	Postaccident and overdose testing for alcohol and other drugs; Blood alcohol concentration level	Reasonable-cause testing; Frequent testing of high-risk groups such as those in posttreatment follow-up and the criminal justice system; Unannounced, random tests with observed collection	Preemployment testing; Random and periodic testing; Testing to determine severity of drug use for referral to treatment; Testing of subjects suspected of seeking to evade urine-test detection; Opiate addicts claiming poppy seed false positive	Postaccident and overdose testing for alcohol and other drugs; Blood alcohol concentration level; Reasonable-cause testing	Posttreatment testing; Maintaining abstinence; Opiate addicts claiming poppy seed false positive; Compliance testing in DOT and criminal justice system applications

Note. DOT = U.S. Department of Transportation; GC/MS = gas chromatography/mass spectrometry; NIDA = National Institute on Drug Abuse.
Blood testing for alcohol is routine, costing about $25/sample, but blood testing for drugs is done by only a few laboratories in the United States. Blood testing for drugs is relatively expensive, costing about $60 for each drug tested for.
[a]Urine tests for nonroutine drugs are available from most reference laboratories, and costs for broad screens are generally less than $200.
[b]Hair testing is commonly performed for the NIDA 5 (cocaine, opiates, marijuana, amphetamines, and phencyclidine). However, a large number of drugs and metabolites can be detected, and routine broad testing is performed in several toxicology reference laboratories. The cost of nonroutine testing of hair is less than $500 in most cases.
[c]Commonly limited to the NIDA 5. Tests can also be performed for alcohol.

aminase levels are nonspecific signs of liver damage. Also, ALT (formerly serum glutamic-pyruvic transaminase [SGPT]) and AST (formerly serum glutamic-oxaloacetic transaminase [SGOT]) are elevated in many conditions, including various liver disorders such as cirrhosis, fatty liver, and alcoholic hepatitis; myocardial infarction; circulatory dysfunction; muscle injury; central nervous system disorders; and other diseases unrelated to the liver. The ratio of mitochondrial AST to total AST is more specific to alcoholic liver damage than is the AST level itself. AST levels can be greater than ALT levels in alcoholism because of the toxicity of alcohol on ALT synthesis. Although ALT is equally sensitive and possibly more specific to liver damage than is AST, it adds little of clinical value to AST levels alone.

Carbohydrate-deficient transferrin (CDT) is elevated in about 80% of people who drink heavily every day for 1 week or longer. During periods of abstinence from alcohol consumption, CDT returns to normal, with values declining by about 50% after every 2 weeks of abstinence. Unlike transaminase levels, CDT level is not commonly elevated in liver diseases unrelated to heavy alcohol consumption. CDT can be elevated in people with severe hepatic failure unrelated to heavy drinking, as well as in individuals with rare genetic variants of transferrin, a beta-globulin in blood that transports iron. Carbohydrate-deficient transferrin can be a useful marker of heavy drinking in follow-up studies and in the clinical management of recovering alcoholic patients.

Other laboratory findings that are associated with heavy drinking include the following:

- Uric acid is elevated in about one-tenth of alcoholic patients because alcohol produces excessive levels of lactic acid, which competes with uric acid in the kidney and can produce elevations in serum uric acid levels.
- Triglycerides are elevated in about one-fourth of alcoholic patients.
- Bilirubin levels are elevated for about one-seventh of alcoholic patients. Bilirubin levels can be elevated for many reasons other than alcoholism; their elevation is common in many chronic and acute liver diseases.
- Alkaline phosphatase is elevated in about one-sixth of alcoholic patients.
- Glucose levels are depressed in many alcoholic patients.

Other common abnormal laboratory findings in alcoholism include lowered potassium, magnesium, calcium, phosphate, and zinc levels; lowered red and white blood cell counts; and lowered platelet levels. Amylase is elevated in alcoholic pancreatitis.

Psychological Testing

Screening Tests

Psychological tests can augment clinical interviews and help clinicians recognize clinically important problems resulting from the use of alcohol and/or other drugs of abuse. Structured psychological testing can screen for the presence of drug and alcohol problems. Testing can also help establish a diagnosis using DSM-IV-TR criteria (American Psychiatric Association 2000) and can help define the severity of the substance use disorder. Tests can identify other medical or psychiatric problems of the patients as well as identify patients in need of pharmacological treatment for withdrawal.

The simplest psychological screening test, and still one of the best, is the CAGE test (Ewing 1984; Mayfield et al. 1974). The interviewer asks patients if they have attempted to **C**ut down on drinking, if they have been **A**nnoyed by people's comments about their drinking, whether they have felt **G**uilty about any aspect of their drinking, and whether they have used alcohol early in the day as an **E**ye-opener to get going. This simple test is remarkably effective in identifying drinking problems. Even a single positive answer is ample reason to explore drinking and its consequences more fully.

Another commonly used psychological test is the Michigan Alcoholism Screening Test (MAST; Selzer 1971), which has several versions. The original MAST test is a 25-item, self-administered questionnaire. The Short MAST (SMAST; Selzer et al. 1975) has 13 items, whereas the Brief MAST (BMAST; Pokorny et al. 1972) has only 10 items. The MAST is not copyrighted, so it can be used and duplicated at no cost. Copies of the MAST test are available for $40 each from Melvin L. Selzer, M.D., 6967 Paseo Laredo, La Jolla, CA 92037. Both CAGE and MAST screen for drinking but not drug use because neither is designed to identify problems related to nonmedical drug use.

Three other screening tests have wide support: the Alcohol Use Disorders Identification Test (AUDIT;

Saunders et al. 1993), the Self-Administered Alcoholism Screening Test (SAAST; Swenson and Morse 1975), and the Adolescent Drinking Inventory (ADI; Allen and Litten 1994; Harrell and Wirtz 1989).

The AUDIT is copyrighted by the World Health Organization. The test is free; the training materials can be purchased for $75 from the WHO Program on Substance Abuse, 20 Avenue Appia, 1211 Geneva, Switzerland, or from Thomas F. Babor, Alcohol Research Center, University of Connecticut, Farmington, CT 06030. The SAAST is copyrighted. For information, contact the Mayo Foundation, 200 First Street, S.W., Rochester, MN 55905 or see their Web site: http://www.mayoclinic.org.

Assessment Tests

Because third-party payors want clinicians to reduce costs and raise health care quality, the 1990s saw a new movement to establish systematic approaches to diagnosis and treatment of addictive disorders. Controversies over the use of inpatient addiction treatment, which were especially intense in the 1980s when such treatment represented one of the most rapidly growing health care costs, have encouraged structured assessment of patients' addiction problems and efforts to match these problems to specific levels of addiction treatment. Psychological instruments can provide standardization and credibility for treatment selection and can facilitate the study of treatment outcomes (Gastfriend et al. 1994).

Patient Placement Criteria, published most recently by the American Society of Addiction Medicine (ASAM) in April 2001 (American Society of Addiction Medicine 2001), was one of the earliest and most influential of the efforts to standardize data collection related to treatment. Since their initial publication (American Society of Addiction Medicine 1991), these criteria have had a major impact on substance abuse treatment decisions. The ASAM criteria divide addiction treatment into four levels of care defined by treatment setting: 1) hospital, 2) nonhospital inpatient, 3) day treatment, and 4) outpatient. The criteria were expanded in 1996 (American Society of Addiction Medicine 1996) to include a broader range of addiction treatments within each of the four major levels of care. ASAM criteria assess six patient-related dimensions: 1) acute intoxication and/or withdrawal, 2) medical diagnoses or complications, 3) emotional/behavioral disorders or complications, 4) treatment

acceptance or resistance, 5) relapse or continuing use, and 6) recovery/living environment.

A good test for psychiatric problems other than substance use disorders is the Brief Symptom Inventory (BSI; Derogatis 1993), a shorter version of the Symptom Checklist—90. The BSI is a 53-item self-administered checklist that takes about 10 minutes to complete and is scored on a five-point scale. It assesses nine symptom dimensions (somatization, obsessive-compulsive, interpersonal sensitivity, depression, anxiety, hostility, phobia, paranoid ideation, and psychotic manifestations).

An excellent way to screen for a wide range of Axis I DSM-IV-TR diagnoses, including psychoses as well as affective and anxiety disorders, is the M.I.N.I. (Mini-International Neuropsychiatric Interview). This 25-page structured clinical interview takes about 30 minutes for an experienced clinician to administer. Copyrighted most recently in 2001, it is widely used in research settings. Copies can be obtained from David Sheehan, M.D., M.B.A., Director, Office of Research, University of South Florida Department of Psychiatry, 3515 E. Fletcher Avenue, Tampa, FL 33613.

A standard test to identify the possible need for pharmacological treatment of alcohol withdrawal is the revised Clinical Institute Withdrawal Assessment (CIWA-Ar; Sullivan et al. 1989). The CIWA-Ar is not copyright protected. It is available from the Marketing Services of the Addiction Research Foundation, 33 Russell Street, Toronto, Ontario, Canada M5S 2S1.

Diagnosis of Substance Use Disorder

The Structured Clinical Interview for DSM-IV (SCID; First et al. 1997a, 1997b) is suitable for both clinical and research use. It is the most highly developed of the assessment instruments currently used to establish the diagnosis of alcohol or drug abuse or dependence. The SCID is designed to be administered by trained clinical evaluators from the master's to the doctorate level. However, it is not easily administered by clinicians. It is labor intensive and is not compatible with the more intuitive, subjective way that clinicians usually approach patients.

Detailing both Axis I and Axis II diagnoses, the entire SCID requires more than 2 hours to administer, whereas the Psychoactive Use Disorders module of the SCID can be administered alone in about 30–60 minutes, depending on the extent of the subject's substance use history and the current intensity of substance use and related problems. This module, like the total SCID, now has questions specifically related to each item in the DSM-IV diagnostic criteria. Data are collected to establish lifetime and current diagnoses, age at onset of first abuse, and first dependence for each category of drug.

SCID diagnoses have shown good interrater reliability for substance use disorders but only moderate reliability for comorbid conditions such as anxiety and depression (Skre et al. 1991). The SCID is systematic and comprehensive in gathering the information required to fit the DSM-IV diagnostic criteria. The SCID—Clinician Version is available through American Psychiatric Publishing, Inc., by calling 1-800-368-5777. The SCID—Research Version is available from the Biometrics Research Department, Unit 60, New York State Psychiatric Institute, 1051 Riverside Drive, New York, NY 10032.

Substance Abuse and Dependence Severity

The Addiction Severity Index (ASI; McLellan et al. 1992) is the most widely used instrument for assessing substance use disorder severity. Through administration of a 30-minute semistructured interview, the ASI assesses seven areas typically affected by substance use: medical problems, employment/support, drug/alcohol use, legal status, family history, family/social relationships, and psychiatric problems. Information is obtained about lifetime drug and alcohol use as well as use in the previous 30 days. The ASI can be administered by a trained technician (not necessarily a licensed clinician, as is required for the SCID) and has been used widely for clinical, administrative, and research purposes. A smaller subset of ASI items has been used in follow-up studies.

The ASI is based on patient report without independent verification or review of collateral material (workplace, criminal justice, or family sources). The rater uses a 10-point scale to assess the severity of the patient's overall substance use disorder and the reliability of the patient's self-reports. Thus, the ASI is not totally dependent on what the patient says about his or her own problem. Although the ASI was developed for and initially used in methadone treatment of heroin addiction, it is now employed in a wide variety of settings, including drug-free treatment, homeless shelters, and inpatient psychiatric hospitals (McLellan et al. 1980). Reflecting its origins, the ASI reliably

identifies severe alcohol- and other drug-related impairments but is not as good at characterizing less severely impaired patients, including those commonly seen in outpatient alcohol treatment programs and in many drug-free outpatient programs. The ASI and related materials can be ordered from A. Thomas McLellan, Ph.D., Building 7, Philadelphia VAMC, University & Woodland Avenues, Philadelphia, PA 19104. There is no cost, but there may be minimal charges for photocopying and mailing.

Motivation for Recovery and Treatment Readiness

The Recovery Attitude and Treatment Evaluator Clinical Evaluation (RAATE-CE; Mee-Lee 1988) is the most promising instrument for assessing treatment readiness. The RAATE-CE systematically and quantifiably assesses the patient's resistance and impediments to addiction treatment. This clinician-rated structured interview (like the SCID) assesses five dimensions related to substance treatment planning: 1) resistance to treatment; 2) resistance to continuing care; 3) severity of medical problems; 4) severity of psychiatric problems; and 5) extent of unsupportive family, social, and environmental factors. The RAATE-CE instrument has 35 items scored from 1 to 4; higher scores indicate greater resistance and impediments to recovery. The RAATE-CE material can be ordered through New Standards, Inc., 1080 Montreal Avenue, #300, St. Paul, MN 55116.

Conclusion

Although clinical judgment remains the foundation of addiction medicine, laboratory testing in recent years has provided important new opportunities to identify use of alcohol and other drugs and to study the effects of the use of alcohol and other drugs on the physiology of alcohol and drug abusers. Psychological testing provides an objective and quantifiable basis for the identification of alcohol and other drug problems and a more systematic way to follow the progress of treated individuals over time. Wise clinicians have learned to use laboratory and psychological tests in ways that enhance the effectiveness of patient care and provide powerful scientific evidence for the efficacy of addiction treatment.

References

Allen JP, Litten RZ: Biochemical and psychometric tests, in Principles of Addiction Medicine. Edited by Miller NS. Chevy Chase, MD, American Society of Addiction Medicine, 1994, Section IV, Chapter 3, pp 1–8

American Psychiatric Association: Diagnostic and Statistical Manual of Mental Disorders, 4th Edition, Text Revision. Washington, DC, American Psychiatric Association, 2000

American Society of Addiction Medicine: Patient Placement Criteria. Chevy Chase, MD, American Society of Addiction Medicine, 1991

American Society of Addiction Medicine: Patient Placement Criteria, 2nd Edition. Chevy Chase, MD, American Society of Addiction Medicine, 1996

American Society of Addiction Medicine: Patient Placement Criteria, 2nd Edition—Revised. Chevy Chase, MD, American Society of Addiction Medicine, 2001

Derogatis LR: BSI Brief Symptom Inventory: Administration, Scoring, and Procedures Manual, 4th Edition. Minneapolis, MN, National Computer Systems, 1993

DuPont RL: Laboratory diagnosis, in Principles of Addiction Medicine. Edited by Miller NS. Chevy Chase, MD, American Society of Addiction Medicine, 1994, Section IV, Chapter 2, pp 1–8

DuPont RL: Addiction: a new paradigm. Bull Menninger Clin 62:231–242, 1998

DuPont RL: The Selfish Brain: Learning From Addiction. Center City, MN, Hazelden, 2000

DuPont RL, Gold MS: Withdrawal and reward: implications for detoxification and relapse prevention. Psychiatr Ann 25:663–668, 1995

DuPont RL, Selavka CM: Drug testing in addiction treatment and criminal justice settings, in Principles of Addiction Medicine, 3rd Edition. Edited by Graham AW, Schultz TK, Mayo-Smith MF, et al. Chevy Chase, MD, American Society of Addiction Medicine, 2003

Ewing JA: Detecting alcoholism: the CAGE questionnaire. JAMA 252:1905–1907, 1984

First MB, Spitzer RL, Gibbon M, et al: Structured Clinical Interview for DSM-IV Axis I Disorders, Clinician Version (SCID-CV). Washington, DC, American Psychiatric Association, 1997a

First MB, Spitzer RL, Gibbon M, et al: Structured Clinical Interview for DSM-IV Axis I Disorders, Research Version. Washington, DC, American Psychiatric Association, 1997b

Gastfriend DR, Najavits LM, Reif S: Assessment instruments, in Principles of Addiction Medicine. Edited by Miller NS. Chevy Chase, MD, American Society of Addiction Medicine, 1994, Section IV, Chapter 4, pp 1–8

Harrell AV, Wirtz PW: Screening for adolescent problem drinking: validation of a multidimensional instrument for case identification. Psychol Assess 1:61–63, 1989

Mayfield D, McLeod G, Hall P: The CAGE questionnaire: validation of a new alcoholism instrument. Am J Psychiatry 131:1121–1123, 1974

McLellan AT, Luborsky L, Woody GE: An improved diagnostic evaluation instrument for substance abuse patients: the Addiction Severity Index. J Nerv Ment Dis 168:26–33, 1980

McLellan AT, Kushner H, Metzger D, et al: The Fifth Edition of the Addiction Severity Index. J Subst Abuse Treat 9:199–213, 1992

Mee-Lee D: An instrument for treatment progress and matching: the Recovery Attitude and Treatment Evaluator (RAATE). J Subst Abuse Treat 5:183–186, 1988

Pokorny AD, Miller BA, Kaplan HB: The brief MAST: a shortened version of the Michigan Alcoholism Screening Test. Am J Psychiatry 129:342–345, 1972

Saunders JB, Aasland OG, Babor TF, et al; Development of the Alcohol Use Disorders Screening Test (AUDIT): WHO collaborative project on early detection of persons with harmful alcohol consumption, II. Addiction 88:791–804, 1993

Schwartz H: Urine testing in the detection of drugs of abuse. Arch Intern Med 148:2407–2412, 1988

Selzer ML: The Michigan Alcoholism Screening Test: the quest for a new diagnostic instrument. Am J Psychiatry 127:1653–1658, 1971

Selzer ML, Vinokur A, van Rooijen L: A self-administered Short Michigan Alcoholism Screening Test (SMAST). J Stud Alcohol 36:117–126, 1975

Skre I, Onstad S, Torgersen S, et al: High interrater reliability for the Structured Clinical Interview for DSM-III-R Axis I (SCID-I). Acta Psychiatr Scand 84:167–173, 1991

Sullivan JT, Sykora K, Schneiderman J, et al: Assessment of alcohol withdrawal: the revised Clinical Institute Withdrawal Instrument for Alcohol Scale (CIWA-Ar). Br J Addict 84:1353–1357, 1989

Swenson WM, Morse RM: The use of a self-administered alcoholism screening test (SAAST) in a medical center. Mayo Clin Proc 50:204–208, 1975

U.S. Department of Health and Human Services: Mandatory guidelines for federal workplace drug testing programs. Fed Regist April 11, 1988, pp 11979–11989

Yacoubian GS, Wish ED, Perez DM: A comparison of saliva testing to urinalysis in an arrestee population. J Psychoactive Drugs 33:289–294, 2001

Medical Education

Frances Rudnick Levin, M.D.
Erik W. Gunderson, M.D.
Petros Levounis, M.D.

During the past five decades there has been an increasing awareness of the need for improvement in substance abuse education for medical students, residents, and practicing physicians. In 1956, the annual report of the American Medical Association emphasized that alcoholism is an illness and that "alcoholism must be regarded within the purview of medical practice." This set the stage for a series of milestones (outlined by Lewis 1990) that include the establishment of the federally funded Career Teacher Program in 1971, the establishment of several specialty organizations (e.g., the American Society of Addiction Medicine [initially known as the American Medical Society on Alcoholism], the Association for Medical Education and Research in Substance Abuse, and the American Academy of Addiction Psychiatrists), and the development of fellowships in alcoholism and substance abuse (Galanter et al. 1993).

Perhaps because of the milestones described above, there has been increased addiction training in both medical schools and residencies throughout the country. Although the number of teaching units in medical schools increased substantially during a 16-year period (1976–1992) (Fleming et al. 1994), training in the management of substance use disorders remains disproportionately low compared with other chronic disorders such as diabetes or hypertension (Klamen 1999).

Part of the problem might stem from a lack of faculty members with expertise to teach about substance use (Fleming et al. 1994). The Career Teacher Program, founded in 1971 by the National Institute on Alcohol Abuse and Alcoholism (NIAAA) and the National Institute on Drug Abuse (NIDA), funded 59 teachers in medical school throughout the country and provided a major impetus to improving medical school addiction training (Ewan and Whaite 1982). This funding mechanism lasted 10 years and was subsequently replaced by Faculty Fellow Training grants. Initially these grants were designed to support three to five members from primary care departments and psychiatry, but they were subsequently expanded to include nursing, social work, and psychology school. As Chappel and Lewis (1997) noted, this program provided modest part-time support, and its scope was dramatically diminished over time. Therefore, the critical need for training faculty in the area of substance abuse remains. Some private and not-for-profit treatment organizations such as the Hazelden Foundation have developed faculty training programs, but the scope of these programs is limited, and the impact that these programs have on improving substance abuse training for medical students and residents has not been assessed.

In this chapter we provide an overview of the knowledge, attitudes, and skills of physicians in various stages of their training and what information should be conveyed. We also describe some of the educational initiatives that have been developed to address physicians' deficits in these areas, and we review studies that have evaluated the impact of these educational initiatives.

Knowledge, Attitudes, and Practice Habits

Despite increased awareness of the importance of substance abuse training in medical education, there remain deficits in knowledge and clinical skills that are compounded by negative attitudes toward substance abusers. A comprehensive survey conducted by Geller et al. (1989) assessed the knowledge, attitudes, beliefs about role responsibility, and perceived skills regarding substance use disorders among medical students and house staff at the Johns Hopkins Medical School and Hospital. Whereas level of knowledge was relatively high across all years of medical school and residency training, attitudes became increasingly more negative as individuals progressed in their training. After the third year of medical school, the percentage of individuals who felt that they had a major responsibility for screening, referral, and follow-up dropped dramatically. Furthermore, perceived skills in screening showed no improvement as medical students progressed into their residencies, and perceived skill at follow-up diminished.

Geller et al. (1989) hypothesized that the lack of adequate curriculum, exposure to end-stage addiction, and lack of faculty expertise may all contribute to these findings. The lack of knowledge or responsibility by physicians for the detection of and intervention in substance use disorders was reflected by the practice habits of house staff and physicians within the same

hospital setting (Moore et al. 1989). All patients newly admitted to adult inpatient services were screened for alcoholism. However, detection rates by house staff and faculty physicians were below 50% for all specialties except psychiatry. For patients diagnosed with nonrecovered alcoholism, the rates of initiating treatment ranged from low (less than 50%) to high (100%), depending on the specialty.

Numerous studies at other institutions have also consistently demonstrated a need for improvement in resident practice habits, finding that residents often fail to appropriately screen for or diagnose alcoholism and other substance use disorders in their clinic and hospital patients (Buchsbaum et al. 1992; Bush et al. 1987; Cleary et al. 1988; Coulehan et al. 1987; Dawson et al. 1992). Although such studies have prompted medical educators to address this problematic practicing behavior, more recent studies of residents reveal that sufficient improvements have not been attained (Cerise et al. 1998; Conigliaro et al. 1998; Stein et al. 1996). It is not surprising that practicing physicians also inadequately address substance use by their patients, according to findings based on physician self-reporting (Bradley et al. 1995), medical record charting (Graves et al. 1992), and patient reporting (National Center on Addiction and Substance Abuse at Columbia University 2000).

In the results of a survey conducted by the National Center on Addiction and Substance Abuse at Columbia University (2000) of 648 primary care physicians and 510 adults receiving treatment for substance use in 10 treatment programs throughout the United States, some troubling findings were highlighted. Among these are the following:

- More than 50% of patients reported that their primary care physician did nothing about their substance abuse, with fewer than half of physicians making the diagnosis.
- Ten percent of patients reported that physicians knew about the substance abuse but did nothing to address the problem.
- Fewer than 20% of primary care physicians considered themselves "very prepared to identify alcohol or drug dependence"; this contrasts with more than 80% feeling very comfortable in diagnosing hypertension and diabetes.
- Approximately 75% of patients reported that their primary care physicians were not involved in their decision to seek treatment.

Correlates of Optimal Practices

Research attempting to determine correlates of optimal practices with regard to substance users has had conflicting results. Studies of medical students and primary care residents suggest that self-efficacy and positive attitudes, such as greater confidence, are associated with favorable self-reported practices (Geller et al. 1989; Schorling et al. 1994). However, another study of medical residents found no relationship to attitudes but did find that having had a supervised clinical experience on alcohol abuse was associated with better practices (Warburg et al. 1987).

Surveys attempting to find practice correlates of practicing physicians have tended to focus on self-assessment and attitudes, rather than asking about prior training. A survey of primary care physicians in Texas revealed that self-efficacy and outcome expectation were positively related to screening and counseling for problems with alcohol, tobacco, and other drugs but were negatively related to outside referral (Gottlieb et al. 1987). In a national survey of 2,000 physicians practicing in several specialties, favorable alcohol screening and intervention practices were associated with greater confidence in alcohol history taking, familiarity with expert guidelines, and less concern that patients will object (Friedmann et al. 2000). Favorable screening and intervention for illicit drug abuse were associated with psychiatry specialty, confidence in drug use history taking, optimism about treatment efficacy, and less concern that patients will object (Friedmann et al. 2001).

Training Initiatives on Substance Use Disorders in Medical School

Previously, the major focus in substance abuse education in medical schools was to change the negative course of students' attitudes during medical school with the hope that this might improve clinical practice. Pursch (1978) emphasized that, rather than didactic training, direct patient contact in substance abuse treatment programs and attendance at Alcoholics Anonymous (AA) meetings were key ingredients to changing negative attitudes of physicians. Unfortunately, this advice has often gone unheeded (Hanlon 1985).

What Information Needs to Be Covered

Burger and Spickard (1991) noted that despite efforts made to train faculty and develop curricula to train medical students, the students still lacked adequate skills in diagnosing and treating substance abuse. These authors argued that to emphasize the importance of the material and to bring it into the mainstream of medical education, substance abuse education needs to be integrated within the medical school curriculum. This sentiment has been echoed by Miller et al. (2001), who eloquently stated that substance abuse teaching should be like the "insertion of beads into the overall necklace of medical school education." Using published guidelines from various sources, Burger and Spickard (1991) developed a list of categories and content areas that they believed should be covered in a medical school curriculum (Table 48–1). Importantly, they focused on creative ways to provide this education within the framework of basic science courses and clinical rotations.

Miller and colleagues (2001) found that a substantial number of barriers impede implementation of a substance abuse curriculum or additional training in substance use disorders into medical education. These include lack of curricular time, lack of coordination of efforts among departments, shortage of treatment sites in which to provide relevant clinical experiences, lack of interested or qualified faculty members, and lack of time for faculty to develop an integrated curriculum. Burger and Spickard (1991) provide some concrete solutions to overcome some of these barriers in order to improve substance abuse medical education (Table 48–2). Not surprisingly, one of the greatest difficulties was identifying expert faculty members, particularly during the medical students' clinical training. Without supportive faculty and a "champion" to help initiate change, enhancements in existing medical school substance abuse curricula are unlikely. Furthermore, Miller et al. (2001) note that medical educators need to support parity for addictive disorders with other medical and psychiatric disorders and should not overlook the need to provide detection and intervention training for substance use disorders to students, residents, and physicians. Clearly progress has been made, but much work remains to be done.

Table 48–1. Basic competencies listed on matrix of basic and specialty-specific competencies prepared for the curriculum project

Category	Content
Basic concepts	Abuse, addiction, dependence, tolerance, withdrawal, denial
Epidemiology	Incidence, prevalence, morbidity, mortality, demographic differences, patterns of drug abuse
Biochemistry and pharmacology	Pharmacology of commonly abused drugs (alcohol, heroin, marijuana, cocaine, barbiturates, benzodiazepines), physiology and biochemistry of dependence, drug interactions (synergism, potentiation), nutritional effects of abused drugs, general knowledge of drug overdose
Natural history and history	Progression of drug use within individuals, outcome (spontaneous remission, relapse)
Risk factors	Biological/genetic factors, sociocultural factors, psychological factors
Physician self-awareness	Attitudes toward drug abuse patients, how own drug abuse affects treatment
Diagnosis and treatment of withdrawal, dependence, overdose	Use of diagnostic criteria, history taking, and diagnostic tests; understanding treatment alternatives; assessment of community treatment resources; motivating patient change (e.g., intervention), recognition and treatment of abstinence syndromes
Medical complications	Effects of acute and chronic abuse on organ systems, infectious complications (e.g., acquired immunodeficiency syndrome)
Prevention	Primary, secondary, and tertiary prevention; risk identification and patient education; prescribing practices with psychoactive drugs
Legal and ethical issues	Informed consent and notification of family; laws and regulations regarding controlled substances and legal limits on intervention with children

Source. Reprinted from Burger MC, Spickard WA: "Integrating Substance Abuse Education in the Medical Student Curriculum (Society of General Internal Medicine Symposium)." *American Journal of the Medical Sciences* 302:181–184, 1991. Copyright 1991 Lippincott Williams & Wilkins. Used with permission.

Description of Substance Abuse Training Initiatives

A series of papers published throughout the 1980s described substance use training initiatives (usually of less than 15 hours total) that consisted of lectures alone (Whitfield 1980) or a combination of didactic and experiential training, often within an ongoing clerkship (Coggan et al. 1981; Confusione et al. 1982; Nocks 1980).

Siegal and Rudisall (1983) described an intensive experience at a weekend intervention program that targeted persons involved in alcohol-related vehicular legal offenses. Under the supervision of professional substance abuse counselors, students were exposed to group counseling sessions and to counseling and education sessions with patients' families; they were also required to attend AA meetings. Korcok (1984) also described a comprehensive training experience that consisted of a 4-week-long elective that incorporated

lectures, participation in group therapy, half-day visits to treatment programs such as halfway houses, attendance at AA meetings, and also direct clinical experiences with patients and families. Student satisfaction with these programs was high. Although attitudinal changes or practice behaviors were not formally assessed, these types of integrative programs are potentially of great consequence. Exposing medical students to patients in substance abuse treatment settings is a striking departure from what they normally see in medical settings (i.e., individuals with end-stage addictive disease who are not interested in treatment or have frequently undergone failed treatment) and therefore may challenge the therapeutic nihilism that medical students develop throughout their medical training. In fact, based on the results of annual surveys of medical students administered while a comprehensive substance use curriculum was being developed, Gopalan et al. (1992) suggest that experiential training and electives during the clinical years of medical

Table 48–2. Recommendations to effect curricular change

- Prepare the educational environment for change by identifying and including key faculty members who will promote substance abuse education in the curriculum
- Secure the endorsement of the medical school administration and department chairperson
- Develop support from student leaders in promoting curriculum change such that the impact of the group is enhanced
- Integrate substance training into the ongoing curriculum such that few new curricular hours are needed
- Integrate evaluation into the course design
- Make the evaluation fit the goals of the curriculum
- Provide support to medical school faculty members who want to independently develop their own course offerings in substance abuse
- Identify and support a staff member dedicated to substance abuse training and research who, through contact or the local media, can continually remind the faculty that this is an important area of study

Source. Reprinted from Burger MC, Spickard WA: "Integrating Substance Abuse Education in the Medical Student Curriculum (Society of General Internal Medicine Symposium)." *American Journal of the Medical Sciences* 302:181–184, 1991. Copyright 1991 Lippincott Williams & Wilkins. Used with permission.

school are an important aspect of training to encourage the development of positive attitudes toward managing substance abuse.

Evaluation of Substance Abuse Curriculum

Studies assessing the impact of medical student training programs on substance use have typically focused on assessment of changes in student knowledge and attitudes (el-Guebaly et al. 2000). For example, Chappel and Veach (1987) found that incorporating a course on substance use in the curriculum of second-year medical students can lead to improved attitudes across several areas (e.g., treatment intervention, treatment optimism, nonmoralism). Their 28-hour course included lectures, small group discussions, clinical problems, and visits to treatment programs and AA meetings.

Given the evidence that brief interventions by primary care physicians can lead to reduction in alcohol consumption among problem drinkers (Bien et al. 1993; Fleming et al. 1997), it is not surprising that new training initiatives have focused on teaching these

skills to medical students and that subsequent studies have examined the impact of such training on skills and practices. Using videotaped interviews with simulated patients after participation in a brief (1–3 hour) didactic training session, Roche et al. (1997) and Walsh et al. (1999) demonstrated that alcohol interventions by medical students were improved, regardless of whether the session included an additional interactive component that included feedback.

In a recent study from Australia, Gaughwin et al. (2000) examined the impact of medical student training on history taking and management of alcohol dependence in the emergency department and on the medical wards by assessing charting practices after the medicine students became interns. In this retrospective study, researchers examined charts from interns who as medical students had been exposed to a new 30-hour substance use curriculum and an inpatient drug and alcohol unit. These charts were compared with those of interns who were not exposed to the new training initiative during medical school. The researchers found that interns who participated in the curriculum and rotated on the inpatient unit were more likely to take an alcohol history (although there was no difference in documentation that they quantified consumption) and to appropriately manage alcohol dependence.

Training Initiatives on Substance Use Disorders in Residency

What Information Needs to Be Covered

With the increased recognition that graduating residents should have certain core competencies in managing substance use disorders, guidelines have been developed to help guide training of primary care house staff and other physicians (Table 48–3). These competencies are simply meant to provide a basic framework and may need to be modified based on the type of residency program. For example, a pediatric residency program should include competency in the recognition of possible risk factors and assessment of adolescents for alcohol and drug abuse.

Description and Evaluation of Residency Training Initiatives

Most of the recent literature that has focused on substance abuse training initiatives has provided an evalu-

Table 48–3.   Recommended physician competencies for managing substance use disorders

1. **Screening patients for alcohol and drug use**
   - Physicians should screen all patients for use of tobacco, alcohol, and other drugs. Recommended screening tests are based on estimates of quantity and frequency of substance abuse.

2. **Assessment for problems related to alcohol and drug use**
   - Persons who screen positive for current tobacco use should be assessed for types of tobacco products used and level of dependence or addiction.
   - Persons who drink above established cutoff limits (more than 7 drinks/week or more than 3 drinks/occasion for women; more than 14 drinks/week or more than 4 drinks/occasion for men) or who have problems related to their alcohol use should be assessed for potential problems related to alcohol use and symptoms of dependence or addiction.
   - Persons who screen positive for the use of addictive prescription drugs should be assessed for symptoms of dependence or addiction.
   - Persons who screen positive for illicit drugs (have used illicit drugs five or more times in their lifetime) should be assessed for current level of use, problems related to use, and symptoms of dependence or addiction.

3. **Office-based treatment**
   - To assist patients who are identified as having potential alcohol and drug disorders, physicians should be able to use a number of treatment strategies, including brief intervention techniques, counseling, and pharmacotherapy.

4. **Pharmacotherapy**
   - Physicians should be skilled in the pharmacological treatment of nicotine, alcohol, and drug dependence. This includes the management of drug withdrawal, postwithdrawal abstinence syndromes, drug maintenance, and comorbid conditions.

5. **Referral to specialized treatment and other community programs**
   - Physicians should be able to consult with and refer patients to addiction specialists, alcohol and drug treatment programs, and self-help groups.

6. **Pain management**
   - Physicians need to be skilled in the management of acute pain in hospital and ambulatory care settings and chronic pain in persons with (and without) a history of alcohol and drug disorders.

7. **Clinical indications for drug testing**
   - Physicians should be able to utilize drug testing for the care of persons adversely affected by alcohol and other drugs.
   - Common indications for drug testing include testing patients in acute care settings, confirming information provided by patients, and monitoring patients' recovery.

8. **Care of affected family members**
   - Physicians should be able to recognize and provide counseling services or referral for family members or close friends of persons who are adversely affected by alcohol and drug disorders.

9. **Physician impairment**
   - Physicians should be able to recognize and assist colleagues who may have an alcohol or drug problem. Prevention is an essential component of this clinical competency.

Source.   Adapted from Fleming M: "Competencies for Substance Abuse Training," in *Training About Alcohol and Substance Abuse for All Primary Care Physicians, Proceedings of a Conference Sponsored by the Josiah Macy Jr. Foundation, Phoenix, Arizona, October 2–5, 1994.* Edited by Sirica C. New York, Josiah Macy Jr. Foundation, 1995. Used with permission.

ation component to determine whether the training led to changes in knowledge or practices. Research examining the effect of substance use education in residency programs has typically been conducted in primary care programs. Most curricula studied have focused on alcohol misuse and have attempted to improve skills on screening and patient intervention, although some have also addressed knowledge and attitudes. In a study of primary care residents, attending physicians, and nurse practitioners, Ockene et al. (1997) found that a 3-hour training program to teach a counseling intervention for high-risk and problem drinkers resulted in improved knowledge, attitudes, and skills as assessed by pretest and posttest surveys and performance evaluation using simulated patients. The training program had a small group and individual tutorial session using role-play with simulated patients who provided feedback to the provider (Ockene et al. 1997).

In a retrospective study of family practice resident charting after a 3–4 week rotation on a chemical dependence unit, it was found that there was a significant increase in diagnoses of alcoholism and chemical dependence during the year after the rotation (Mulry et al. 1987). Another study of family practice resident charting practices examined the impact of feedback from the attending physician on charting by house staff and of incorporation of the CAGE screening questionnaire on a standard patient evaluation form (Lawner et al. 1997). During the 6 months after the intervention, residents were more likely to record CAGE screening questions and to document the quantity and frequency of alcohol consumption. Although there was no difference in documentation by house staff of interventions for patients who had positive CAGE screens, this finding is not surprising because the educational effort focused on screening and documentation rather than on how to intervene.

Using simulated patients, Levin et al. (1999) demonstrated an improvement in interviewing and intervention skills among internal medicine and pediatric residents after participation in a 5-day experiential and didactic training program at the Hazelden Residential Program of New York City. Self-reported ratings also improved after participation in the program. A similar training program that combined experiential and didactic training during four half-day sessions for family medicine residents also showed improvement in self-reported knowledge and attitude (Confusione et al. 1988), although there was no statistical comparison and the study lacked a behavioral outcome.

Wilk and Jensen (2002) tested the impact of a 1-hour intervention in which internal medicine residents interviewed, examined, and then intervened with a known simulated patient who used tobacco and reported excessive alcohol use. After the intervention, the resident received feedback and instruction on NIAAA (1995) guidelines on alcohol screening and brief intervention. The intervention was viewed positively by the residents, and a comparison of residents' performance with an unannounced simulated patient before and 1–2 months after the intervention demon-

strated a dramatic two- to threefold improvement in alcohol screening and intervention (Wilk and Jensen 2002).

Although most studies assessing substance use curricula for residents have been in primary care programs, recent studies have evaluated curricula for psychiatry and emergency medicine residents. A 1-day educational conference on knowledge, diagnosis, and management of alcohol, tobacco, and opiate addiction was offered to all psychiatry residents in Michigan. The conference, led by several addiction specialists, was found to enhance the belief that physicians can motivate their patients to seek treatment and to increase residents' interest in pursuing an addiction psychiatry fellowship (Karam-Hage et al. 2001). However, the follow-up survey administered at the end of the training did not assess impact on skills or practices, and those who completed the survey were highly self-selected.

A nonrandomized, controlled educational trial was conducted at two similar emergency medicine residency programs to examine whether a 4-hour training program—which included a didactic session, demonstration video, and skills-based workshop—would improve the knowledge, attitudes, and practices of house staff as reflected by a survey and medical record charting (D'Onofrio et al. 2002). House staff from control and intervention institutions completed surveys on knowledge, attitudes, and practices at baseline and 1 year after the intervention, and their charts were reviewed at baseline and 6 months after the intervention. Compared with residents in the control program, who received no formal didactic or skills-based training related to addressing alcohol problems, residents in the intervention program demonstrated significant improvement in knowledge scores and in screening and intervention practices based on chart review (D'Onofrio et al. 2002).

In a similarly designed nonrandomized, controlled trial conducted at two pediatric residency programs, Kokotailo et al. (1995) examined the impact of an experiential curriculum on alcohol and other drugs in which the intervention group participated in an adolescent assessment program, interactive didactic sessions, role-play, and a session on interviewing skills. Pretest and posttest assessment was performed using written examination, self-assessment, and simulated patients. Compared with control subjects, house staff in the intervention group demonstrated significantly greater improvement in their knowledge, confidence, and screening and interviewing skills.

Training Initiatives on Substance Use Disorders After Residency

Development of Addiction Psychiatry Fellowships

Physicians who have completed a residency program in general psychiatry can pursue further training in addiction psychiatry through a fellowship program (also sometimes called a residency program in addiction psychiatry). As of September 2003, there were 45 such postresidency training programs in the United States that were accredited by the Accreditation Council for Graduate Medical Education (ACGME) (2003). Data from the Center for Medical Fellowships in Alcoholism and Drug Abuse at New York University (2001), which tracks fellowships in addiction psychiatry, indicate that the earliest reported postresidency programs were established in 1978. As of 2001, a total of 245 psychiatrists had graduated from addiction psychiatry fellowship programs, and there were 78 positions available for the year 2000–2001. Most programs last 1 year, although some last 2 years to allow fellows the opportunity to conduct original research. The salaries offered range from a minimum of $34,000 to a maximum of $87,000, with the majority of programs offering annual salaries in the mid-$40,000 range. On average, the fellows spend about half of their time in direct clinical care and the other half in academic activities (Galanter et al. 2002). Some of these programs accept physicians who have completed residency in other fields (e.g., internal medicine or neurology). However, unlike psychiatrists, these fellows would not be eligible for the addiction psychiatry boards.

ABPN Certification and Recertification in Addiction Psychiatry

The first subspecialty certification examination (for what was then called Added Qualifications in Addiction Psychiatry) was given in 1993. As of November 2002, a total of 1,854 psychiatrists had been certified in addiction psychiatry (see the ABPN Web site, http://www.abpn.com/certification/examinations.html). Today, psychiatrists who complete an ACGME-accredited fellowship and are certified in general psychiatry by the American Board of Psychiatry and Neurology (ABPN) are eligible to sit for a subspecialty certification examination given by ABPN once every 2 years.

This is a 4-hour, multiple-choice computerized examination that covers only addiction psychiatry topics (Table 48–4). Both in 2000 and in 2002, all candidates who took the examination passed (see the ABPN Web site, http://www.abpn.com/certification/statistics).

Table 48–4. Content of American Board of Psychiatry and Neurology certification examination in addiction psychiatry

- Evaluation and consultation (including comorbidity, forensic, and legal issues)
- Pharmacotherapy (including detoxification, rehabilitation, new and alternative medications, and side effects)
- Pharmacology of drugs
- Psychosocial treatment
- Biological and behavioral basis of practice

Source. Adapted from American Board of Psychiatry and Neurology: 2004 Part I Psychiatry Examination: Psychiatry Content Outline. Deerfield, IL, American Board of Psychiatry and Neurology, 2003. Available at: http://www.abpn.com/certification/psych-psych_items.html.

The ABPN certification in the subspecialty of addiction psychiatry is valid for 10 years. To maintain his or her certification beyond 10 years, the addiction psychiatrist has to take a recertification examination that is similar to the certification examination in content and format. The American Board of Medical Specialties now mandates that medical specialties and subspecialties, including addiction psychiatry, adhere to the concept of maintenance of certification, a concept that is broader than that of recertification. Maintenance of certification involves not only examinations but also documentation of commitment to lifelong learning and assessment of practice-based performance (Burke 2002).

Certification and Recertification by the American Society of Addiction Medicine

The American Society of Addiction Medicine (ASAM) offers a certification examination to physicians who have completed residency training in any medical specialty and who have an additional year of clinical experience in treating substance abuse patients. The ASAM examination is a 6-hour multiple-choice test. Like the ABPN examination, it is offered every 2 years, with recertification required every 10 years (American Society of Addiction Medicine 2002). Both ASAM and

ABPN certifications are widely recognized and accepted as evidence of expertise in substance abuse. For example, physicians who are certified by either ASAM or ABPN are exempt from taking a special training course before being approved by the U.S. Drug Enforcement Administration to prescribe buprenorphine to their patients (Substance Abuse and Mental Health Services Administration 2002). In 2002, 88% of the physicians who took the ASAM certification examination passed; currently, there are 3,315 certified physicians and 233 recertified. The breakdown of certified physicians by medical specialties is 40% psychiatrists; 20% internists; 20% family practitioners; 9% addiction medicine specialists; 6% pediatricians, anesthesiologists, emergency medicine practitioners, and preventive medicine practitioners; and 3% surgeons and obstetricians (gynecologists) (American Society of Addiction Medicine 2002).

American Osteopathic Association Certification of Added Qualifications in Addiction Medicine

Osteopathic physicians who are certified in anesthesiology, family practice medicine, internal medicine, or psychiatry and neurology and who have either completed 1 year of American Osteopathic Association (AOA) training in addiction psychiatry or fulfilled extensive work and continuing medical education (CME) requirements in addiction psychiatry or addiction medicine are eligible to take the Certification of Added Qualifications in Addiction Medicine examination (American Osteopathic Association 2002). Members of the AOA who have passed the qualification examination are eligible to join the American Osteopathic Academy of Addiction Medicine. Since the inception of the Certification of Added Qualifications in Addiction Medicine examination in 1996, 25 physicians have been certified: 11 in 1997, 4 in 1999, and 10 in 2001. Osteopathic physicians who are certified in addiction medicine, by practice, include 16 family practitioners, 2 internists, and 7 physicians who specialize in psychiatry and neurology.

Description of Programs Targeting Medical School Faculty

After the success of the Physicians in Residence program, which is primarily targeted toward house staff

from all specialties (Levin et al. 1999), the Hazelden Foundation introduced the Faculty Training Program on Addiction for Primary Care Physicians. Up to eight faculty members from primary medical specialties such as internal medicine, pediatrics, psychiatry, and primary care undergo an intensive 5-day, 30-hour program on site at a Hazelden residential program. Similarly to the Physicians in Residence program, the faculty program provides a lecture series and a strong experiential component. The participants fully engage in the activities of the residence, join the group exercises, and assume a participant-observer role in daily treatment. In addition, the faculty train in motivational interviewing techniques and in planning for integration of their training into the academic training of medical students, residents, and fellows at their home institutions (Hazelden Foundation 2002). The program is jointly sponsored by the University of Wisconsin Medical School, and the participants receive CME credits.

Bigby and Barnes (1993) describe an experiential training program targeting general medicine faculty. A 3-day course sponsored by five medical centers covered various addiction topics, with less than 20% of the program being didactic. The experiential components included role-playing, case discussions, the use of simulated patients, and attendance at self-help groups. The participants describe substantial improvements in their attitudes toward substance abusers and their clinical and referral skills. Other faculty programs have been more limited in scope, with on-site lectures or skills-based training (Fleming et al. 1994, 1997).

Project MAINSTREAM (the Multi-Agency INitiative on Substance abuse TRaining and Education for AMerica) is a new program that funds teams of three fellows from different disciplines (e.g., medicine, social work, nursing) to work on faculty development and community projects (Stuart et al. 2002). MAINSTREAM (http://www.projectmainstream.net), administered by the Association for Medical Education and Research in Substance Abuse, represents the first systematic effort to bring together and train substance abuse educators from different professions.

Description and Evaluation of Programs That Target Physicians in Practice

Apart from these postresidency training initiatives, the majority of practicing physicians who want to further their education and training in substance use disorders attend CME programs (Sandlow and Dos Santos 1997). CME activities are a major means by which practicing physicians stay up-to-date with medical information to improve practices and optimize patient outcome (Davis et al. 1999). El-Guebaly et al. (2000) reviewed 11 studies that assessed the outcome of CME programs devoted to teaching physicians about substance use disorders. Most programs tended to use a combination of didactic and interactive interventions to enhance screening, early intervention, and referral by primary care physicians, although a few included psychiatrists and obstetricians. Many studies found it difficult to recruit physicians for CME programs on substance use. The results of the studies examining the impact of these programs were often equivocal, but they suggested a need for educational reinforcement of training to improve the impact of CME (el-Guebaly et al. 2000). These conclusions were supported by a meta-analysis of randomized controlled trials of formal CME programs not specifically related to substance abuse (although one study assessed CME training on tobacco), which showed that multiple longitudinal CME interventions improved physician performance (Davis et al. 1999). This study also concluded that interactive sessions (e.g., role-play or discussion groups), but not didactic sessions, can effect change in physician practices.

Major textbooks in substance abuse also help the practicing physician who is committed to improving her or his skills through self-learning (Table 48–5). Additional information can be obtained from the Web sites of NIDA (http://www.nida.nih.gov), NIAAA (http://www.niaaa.nih.gov), and ASAM (http://www.asam.org). Unfortunately, because such learning in substance abuse is rarely required, the physicians who have negative attitudes toward addicted patients—and who therefore would benefit the most from postresidency addiction training—are less likely to pursue such training.

Observations Based on Outcome Assessment of Educational Strategies

Based on the findings of the studies described above that assessed the impact of various educational strategies, several observations may be made that could help optimize curriculum development for training physi-

Table 48–5. Major substance abuse textbooks

Clinical Textbook of Addictive Disorders. Edited by Richard J. Frances and Sheldon I. Miller; published by Guilford Press; 2nd Edition, 1998

Drug and Alcohol Abuse: A Clinical Guide to Diagnosis and Treatment. By Marc A. Schuckit; published by Kluwer Academic Publishers; 5th Edition, 2000

Principles of Addiction Medicine. By Bonnie Wilford; published by the American Society of Addiction Medicine; 3rd Edition, 2003

Substance Abuse: A Comprehensive Textbook. Edited by Joyce H. Lowinson, Pedro Ruiz, Robert B. Millman, and John G. Langrod; published by Lippincott Williams & Wilkins; 3rd Edition, 1997

Textbook of Substance Abuse Treatment. Edited by Marc Galanter and Herbert D. Kleber; published by American Psychiatric Publishing, Inc.; 3rd Edition, 2004

cians on substance use. Rather than solely using standard didactic programs, curricula should incorporate interactive sessions that are skills based, such as small group discussions and role-play. Attempts should be made to incorporate an experiential component if possible. Although experiential training ideally should take place in a substance use treatment setting, the use of simulated patients is also an effective way to educate medical personnel on substance use (Wilk and Jensen 2002), and the use of simulated patients has been rated favorably compared with prerecorded videotaped interviews and even the use of real patients in one study of teaching medical students about alcohol misuse (Eagles et al. 2001). Because the selection and duration of strategies to train medical personnel depends on available resources (el-Guebaly et al. 2000), simulated patients or substance use treatment settings may not be available for medical training. In these instances, attempts should be made to incorporate an interactive component into the training. Also, the curriculum should incorporate feedback to help reinforce optimal skills and practices, because this has been shown to be effective in several studies (Ockene et al. 1997; Wilk and Jensen 2002). Lastly, the existence of a ceiling effect, whereby the greatest influence of an intervention is on the most negative areas at pretest (el-Guebaly et al. 2000), suggests the need for curricula on substance abuse to be implemented for broad groups of medical personnel, not only those with a high degree of interest in the field.

Persistent Barriers to the Diagnosis and Referral of Substance-Abusing Patients

Although the emphasis has been on improving knowledge, attitudes, and skills, there remain other factors to explain why physicians often do not adequately address substance use problems with their patients. The National Center on Addiction and Substance Abuse at Columbia University (2000) identified several factors that contribute to this problem. These include patient resistance, time constraints, fear that discussing substance abuse may encourage patients to see another physician, and the fact that insurance does not reimburse physicians' time. Managed care has placed even greater time constraints on physicians, and addiction treatment benefits have decreased substantially over the past decade (Hay Group 1999). This lack of insurance coverage "may discourage physicians from discussing substance abuse with patients and referring them for treatment" (National Center on Addiction and Substance Abuse at Columbia University 2000, p. 30). Both patient and physician advocates will be needed to reverse this troubling trend.

Conclusion

Although progress has been made in improving substance abuse education in medical school, residency, and postresidency and training guidelines have been developed, these directives have not been uniformly applied. Repeatedly, the literature emphasizes the importance of developing physician role models who have expertise in substance abuse. These individuals can help implement curriculum change, provide supervised experiences to medical students and residents, and help reduce the stigmatization experienced by alcohol- and drug-dependent patients, a phenomenon that remains common in medical settings. Clearly, there are barriers that make change difficult. However, these obstacles are not insurmountable. Many innovative approaches to substance abuse training are being implemented and evaluated for their success in producing behavioral change. Providing physicians with interactive and clinically relevant training experiences, exposure to patients who have benefited from treatment, adequate reimbursement for time spent assessing patients for substance use disorders, and a supportive administrative environment will almost certainly lead to substantial improvement in the treatment of patients who abuse substances.

References

Accreditation Council for Graduate Medical Education: ACGME Accreditation Program and Institutional Listing. Chicago, IL, Accreditation Council for Graduate Medical Education, 2003. Available at: http://www.acgme.org/adspublic/program/default.asp?specialtyid=87&stateid=0&go=show+resulting+programs (http://www.acgme.org/adspublic, under Accredited Programs: Psychiatry: Addiction psychiatry). Accessed September 20, 2003

American Osteopathic Association: Requirements for Certification: Neurology and Psychiatry. n.d. Available at: http://www.aoa-net.org/certification/neuropsych.htm. Accessed December 19, 2003

American Society of Addiction Medicine: Certification Information. Chevy Chase, MD, American Society of Addiction Medicine, 2002. Available at: http://www.asam.org/cert/03%20CERTIFICATION%20INFO.htm. Accessed September 16, 2003

Bien TH, Miller WR, Tonigan JS: Brief interventions for alcohol problems: a review. Addiction 88:315–335, 1993

Bigby J, Barnes H: Evaluation of a faculty development program in substance abuse education. J Gen Intern Med 8:301–305, 1993

Bradley KA, Curry SJ, Koepsell TD, et al: Primary and secondary prevention of alcohol problems: U.S. internist attitudes and practices. J Gen Intern Med 10:67–72, 1995

Buchsbaum DG, Buchanan RG, Poses RM, et al: Physician detection of drinking problems in patients attending a general medicine practice. J Gen Intern Med 7:517–521, 1992

Burger MC, Spickard WA: Integrating substance abuse education in the medical student curriculum. Am J Med Sci 302:181–184, 1991

Burke T (ed): Implementation of the ABPN maintenance of Certification program. ABPN Diplomate, Newsletter of the American Board of Psychiatry and Neurology, Inc. 1:1–3, 2002

Bush B, Shaw S, Cleary P, et al: Screening for alcohol abuse using the CAGE questionnaire. Am J Med 82:231–235, 1987

Center for Medical Fellowships in Alcoholism and Drug Abuse at New York University: Postgraduate Medical Fellowships in Alcoholism and Drug Abuse, 2001–2003. New York, New York University School of Medicine, 2001. Available at: http://www.med.nyu.edu/subabuse/felldes.html#d. Accessed October 24, 2002

Cerise FP, Scarinci IC, Thibodaux R, et al: Alcoholism among indigent inpatients: identification and intervention by internal medicine residents. South Med J 91:27–32, 1998

Chappel JN, Lewis DC: Medical education: the acquisition of knowledge, attitudes, and skills, in Substance Abuse: A Comprehensive Textbook, 3rd Edition. Edited by Lowinson JH, Ruiz P, Millman RB, et al. Baltimore, MD, Williams & Wilkins, 1997, pp 787–801

Chappel JN, Veach TL: Effect of a course on students' attitudes toward substance abuse and its treatment. J Med Educ 62:394–400, 1987

Cleary PD, Miller M, Bush BT, et al: Prevalence and recognition of alcohol abuse in a primary care population. Am J Med 85:466–471, 1988

Coggan P, Davis A, Rogers J: Teaching alcoholism to family medicine students. J Fam Pract 13:1025–1028, 1981

Confusione M, Jaffe A, Rosen MG: Drug abuse training as part of a family medicine clerkship. J Med Educ 57:409–411, 1982

Confusione M, Leonard K, Jaffe A: Alcoholism training in a family medicine residency. J Subst Abuse Treat 5:19–22, 1988

Conigliaro J, Lofgren RP, Hanusa BH: Screening for problem drinking: impact on physician behavior and patient drinking habits. J Gen Intern Med 13:251–256, 1998

Coulehan JL, Zettler-Segal M, Block M, et al: Recognition of alcoholism and substance abuse in primary care patients. Arch Intern Med 147:349–352, 1987

Davis D, O'Brien MA, Freemantle N, et al: Impact of formal continuing medical education: do conferences, workshops, rounds, and other traditional continuing education activities change physician behavior or health care outcomes? JAMA 282:867–874, 1999

Dawson NV, Dadheech G, Speroff T, et al: The effect of patient gender on the prevalence and recognition of alcoholism on a general medicine inpatient service. J Gen Intern Med 7:38–45, 1992

D'Onofrio G, Nadel ES, Degutis LC, et al: Improving emergency medicine residents' approach to patients with alcohol problems: a controlled educational trial. Ann Emerg Med 40:50–62, 2002

Eagles JM, Calder SA, Nicoll KS, et al: A comparison of real patients, simulated patients and videotaped interview in teaching medical students about alcohol misuse. Med Teach 23:490–493, 2001

el-Guebaly N, Toews J, Lockyer J, et al: Medical education in substance-related disorders: components and outcome. Addiction 95:949–957, 2000

Ewan CE, Whaite A: Training health professionals in substance abuse: a review. Int J Addict 17:1211–1229, 1982

Fleming M, Barry K, Davis A, et al: Medical education about substance abuse: changes in curriculum and faculty between 1976 and 1992. Acad Med 69:362–369, 1994

Fleming MF, Barry KL, Manwell LB, et al: Brief physician advice for problem alcohol drinkers: a randomized controlled trial in community-based primary care practices. JAMA 277:1039–1045, 1997

Friedmann PD, McCullough D, Chin MH, et al: Screening and intervention for alcohol problems: a national survey of primary care physicians and psychiatrists. J Gen Intern Med 15:84–91, 2000

Friedmann PD, McCullough D, Saitz R: Screening and intervention for illicit drug abuse: a national survey of primary care physicians and psychiatrists. Arch Intern Med 161:248–251, 2001

Galanter M, Burns J: The status of fellowships in addiction psychiatry. Am J Addict 2:4–8, 1993

Galanter M, Dermatis H, Calabrese D: Residencies in addiction psychiatry: 1990 to 2000, a decade of progress. Am J Addict 11:192–199, 2002

Gaughwin M, Dodding J, White JM, et al: Changes in alcohol history taking and management of alcohol dependence by interns at The Royal Adelaide Hospital. Med Educ 34:170–174, 2000

Geller G, Levine DM, Mamon JA, et al: Knowledge, attitudes, and reported practices of medical students and house staff regarding the diagnosis and treatment of alcoholism. JAMA 261:3115–3120, 1989

Gopalan R, Santora P, Stokes EJ, et al: Evaluation of a model curriculum on substance abuse at the Johns Hopkins University School of Medicine. Acad Med 67:260–266, 1992

Gottlieb NH, Mullen PD, McAlister AL: Patients' substance abuse and the primary care physician: patterns of practice. Addict Behav 12:23–32, 1987

Graves TG, Terlep GT, Rudy DR, et al: Hospital charting of substance use. Fam Med 24:613–617, 1992

Hanlon MJ: A review of the recent literature relating to the training of medical students in alcoholism. J Med Educ 60:618–626, 1985

Hay Group: Employer Health Care Dollars Spent on Addiction Treatment. Chevy Chase, MD, American Society of Addiction, 1999

Hazelden Foundation: Faculty Training Program on Addiction for Primary Care Physicians. Center City, MN, Hazelden Foundation, 2002. Available at: http://www.hazelden.org/newsletter_detail.dbm?ID=1118. Accessed October 24, 2002

Karam-Hage M, Nerenberg L, Brower KJ: Modifying residents' professional attitudes about substance abuse treatment and training. Am J Addict 10:40–47, 2001

Klamen DL: Education and training in addictive diseases. Psychiatr Clin North Am 22:471–480, 1999

Kokotailo PK, Langhough R, Neary EJ, et al: Improving pediatric residents' alcohol and other drug use clinical skills: use of an experiential curriculum. Pediatrics 96:99–104, 1995

Korcok M: How can we teach students about alcoholism? Can Med Assoc J 130:305–308, 1984

Lawner K, Doot M, Gausas J, et al: Implementation of CAGE alcohol screening in a primary care practice. Fam Med 29:332–335, 1997

Levin FR, Owen P, Stinchfield R, et al: Use of standardized patients to evaluate the physicians in residence program: a substance abuse training approach. J Addict Dis 18:39–50, 1999

Lewis DC: Medical education for alcohol and other drug abuse in the United States. CMAJ 143:1091–1096, 1990

Miller NS, Sheppard LM, Colenda CC, et al: Why physicians are unprepared to treat patients who have alcohol- and drug-related disorders. Acad Med 76:410–418, 2001

Moore RD, Bone LR, Geller G, et al: Prevalence, detection, and treatment of alcoholism in hospitalized patients. JAMA 261:403–407, 1989

Mulry JT, Brewer ML, Spencer DL: The effect of an inpatient chemical dependency rotation on residents' clinical behavior. Fam Med 19:276–280, 1987

National Center on Addiction and Substance Abuse at Columbia University: Missed Opportunity: National Survey of Primary Care Physicians and Patients on Substance Abuse. New York, National Center on Addiction and Substance Abuse at Columbia University, 2000

National Institute on Alcohol Abuse and Alcoholism: The Physicians' Guide to Helping Patients With Alcohol Problems (NIH Publ No 95-3769). Rockville, MD, National Institute on Alcohol Abuse and Alcoholism, 1995

Nocks JJ: Instructing medical students on alcoholism: what to teach with limited time. J Med Educ 55:858–864, 1980

Ockene JK, Wheeler EV, Adams A, et al: Provider training for patient-centered alcohol counseling in a primary care setting. Arch Intern Med 157:2334–2341, 1997

Pursch JA: Physicians' attitudinal changes in alcoholism. Alcohol Clin Exp Res 2:358–361, 1978

Roche AM, Stubbs JM, Sanson-Fisher RW, et al: A controlled trial of educational strategies to teach medical students brief intervention skills for alcohol problems. Prev Med 26:78–85, 1997

Sandlow LJ, Dos Santos SR: Addiction medicine and continuing medical education. J Psychoactive Drugs 29:275–284, 1997

Schorling JB, Klas PT, Willems JP, et al: Addressing alcohol use among primary care patients: differences between family medicine and internal medicine residents. J Gen Intern Med 9:248–254, 1994

Siegal H, Rudisill JR: Teaching medical students about substance abuse in a weekend intervention program. J Med Educ 58:322–327, 1983

Stein MD, Wilkinson J, Berglas N, et al: Prevalence and detection of illicit drug disorders among hospitalized patients. Am J Drug Alcohol Abuse 22:463–471, 1996

Stuart GW, Burland J, Ganju V, et al: Educational best practices. Adm Policy Ment Health 29:325–333, 2002

Substance Abuse and Mental Health Services Administration: Buprenorphine: Physician Waiver Qualifications. Rockville, MD, Substance Abuse and Mental Health Services Administration, 2002. Available at: http://www.buprenorphine.samhsa.gov/waiver_qualifications.html. Accessed October 24, 2002

Taverner D, Dodding CJ, White JM: Comparison of methods for teaching clinical skills in assessing and managing drug-seeking patients. Med Educ 34:285–291, 2000

Walsh RA, Samson-Fisher RW, Low A, et al: Teaching medical students alcohol intervention skills: results of a controlled trial. Med Educ 33:559–565, 1999

Warburg MM, Cleary PD, Rohman M, et al: Residents' attitudes, knowledge, and behavior regarding diagnosis and treatment of alcoholism. J Med Educ 62:497–503, 1987

Whitfield CL: Medical education and alcoholism. Md State Med J 29:77–83, 1980

Wilk AI, Jensen NM: Investigation of a brief teaching encounter using standardized patients: teaching residents alcohol screening and intervention. J Gen Intern Med 17:356–360, 2002

Prevention of Alcohol-Related Problems

Harold D. Holder, Ph.D.

In this chapter on the prevention of alcohol use among underage youths and prevention of alcohol abuse among all age groups, I summarize the state of knowledge concerning various strategies to prevent alcohol-involved problems. The specific goals of alcohol prevention are 1) to delay or prevent the onset of use and 2) to reduce the likelihood that alcohol-related problems will occur in the future. The first goal is important because early initiation of drinking is often associated with later problems, including alcohol dependence. The second goal, the prevention of alcohol-related problems, includes the prevention of acute problems or those immediately associated with heavy drinking (including traffic crashes, falls, burns, drowning, and violence) and the prevention of chronic effects, that is, the long-term exposure to alcohol and the health problems associated with it, including physical and mental illness and early death.

Prevention Is a Result, Not an Activity

One of the basic challenges in the prevention of alcohol abuse throughout the world is the incorrect assumption that specific activities or programs in themselves constitute prevention. For example, providing health messages about substance use or conducting alcohol education in schools might be considered prevention because this is the intention of these programs. However, the *intent* of prevention programs is to reduce alcohol abuse and associated problems, and by definition the *result* is actual prevention (or reduction) of a specific alcohol problem. There may be more than one alternative strategy to accomplish this effect.

The challenge of prevention research is to identify, develop, test, implement, and evaluate alternative strategies or techniques to determine their efficacy or actual achievement of desired effects. Simply implementing a prevention activity is not an end in itself. For example, the goal of medicine is to aid healing and to assist with good health. Providing medicine or treatment is not the same as healing.

Prevention strategies and evidence of their effectiveness are summarized below.

School-Based Education

Many school-based substance abuse educational programs have been developed and evaluated, although the effect of these programs has generally not been large. Peer and media influence programs are called "social influence" strategies, and they are meant to inform students about peer and media influences to use drugs and the negative consequences of their use. They counter the perception that use is widespread and provide modeling and role-play practice of skills for resisting peer influences to use drugs. Life skills programs include social influence features and teach additional skills such as problem solving, assertiveness, decision making, coping, and goal setting. Life Skills Training, for example, is a school-based program that teaches seventh graders social skills and problem-solving skills that focus on decision making, resisting media influences, coping with negative affect, managing their own behavior, communicating effectively with others, behaving appropriately in situations that require assertiveness, and resisting peer pressure to use alcohol (Botvin 1996). The most frequently used school program in the United States is Drug Abuse Resistance Education (DARE), conducted by police officers in upper elementary classes. Unfortunately, evaluation of the program has shown that it is not very effective. A short-term experimental evaluation of Project DARE in North Carolina found that DARE had no effects on use of a range of substances (Ringwalt et al. 1991). A 5-year longitudinal controlled evaluation of Project DARE in Illinois, with random assignment of 18 pairs of schools (6 pairs each in urban, suburban, and rural school districts) to a DARE or no-DARE condition found small or nonexistent long-term effects, as reported by Ennett et al. (1994) and Rosenbaum et al. (1994). Although the effect of school-based programs has generally been modest, there is definite evidence of their value in reducing initial use of alcohol. More didactic prevention programs that do not involve interactions between teachers and students or among students have generally not been found to prevent alcohol use.

Family Education and Intervention

Family interventions are designed to promote effective parenting practices, to improve family communication and parental involvement with their children, and to provide young people with skills for dealing with peer pressure to drink and use drugs. The Iowa Strengthening Families Program (ISFP) is a 7-session intervention that focuses primarily on improving parental use of consequences and on building better relationship skills in both parents and their children. Parents are taught skills for making their expectations clear, using appropriate discipline practices, managing emotions, and communicating with their children. Youths learn skills that complement the skills parents are learning, and they are also taught skills for dealing with peer pressure and stress. In part or all of each session, parents and young people practice communicating with each other.

ISFP was evaluated in a randomized, controlled trial in which families of sixth-grade students in 33 schools in small Iowa communities were randomly assigned to receive either the Strengthening Families Program, the Preparing for the Drug Free Years program (reviewed below), or no intervention. Most families were dual parent (85%) and white (98%). At 2-year follow-up, alcohol consumption differed significantly among ISFP teenagers versus those in the control condition (Redmond et al. 1999). Whereas 30% of adolescents in the control condition had begun the use of tobacco, alcohol, or other drugs between the 1-year follow-up and the 2-year follow-up, only 15% of the adolescents in the ISFP condition had done so. Spoth et al. (1999) also reported that scores on the Alcohol Initiation Index were significantly lower for ISFP adolescents than for control adolescents at both the 1-year and 2-year posttreatment assessments. Moreover, the proportion of young people who began alcohol use was lower for the ISFP condition at both times.

Preparing for the Drug Free Years (PDFY) is a five-session program designed to help parents and teenagers get through early adolescence without developing drug or other behavioral problems, principally through encouraging parents to use consequences and persuasion effectively and to monitor children's behavior. The program also tries to build teenagers' skills for refusing invitations to use drugs or alcohol. By the 2-year follow-up, 30% of control adolescents and only 12% of PDFY adolescents had initiated some sort of substance use. In addition, 50% of the control adolescents who had been using alcohol and/or tobacco at the 1-year follow-up began to use marijuana, whereas only 23% of those in the PDFY condition who had been using alcohol and/or tobacco at 1-year follow-up had begun marijuana use. By tenth grade, the proportion of adolescents using alcohol in the past month was significantly lower for adolescents in the PDFY condition than for those in the control condition (Spoth et al. 1999). Family programs targeted toward high-risk families include Focus on Families, a multicomponent intervention headed by recipients of methadone maintenance treatment (Gainey et al. 1995). Based on one controlled study of effects over 2 years, families and children reported improvements in parental skills and self-efficacy but reported no changes in drinking levels or drinking initiation (Catalano et al., in press). Few targeted family prevention programs have been evaluated with controlled trials, and their efficacy in preventing alcohol-related problems is unknown.

Brief Intervention

During the past two decades, more than 40 randomized, controlled trials have been conducted to evaluate the efficacy of brief interventions. The results of these trials are summarized in several integrative literature reviews and meta-analyses (Babor 1994; Higgins-Biddle and Babor 1996; Kahan et al. 1995; Poikolainen 1999; Wilk et al. 1997). The cumulative evidence of randomized, controlled trials conducted in a variety of settings shows that clinically significant effects on drinking behavior and related problems can follow from brief interventions. Nevertheless, the results have not always been consistent across studies (Poikolainen 1999). Furthermore, there is little evidence that these interventions are beneficial for alcohol-dependent individuals (Mattick and Jarvis 1994).

Public Education and Mass Media

The mass media have been used in two basic ways for alcohol prevention: media campaigns designed to change information and attitudes about alcohol misuse, and campaigns in support of public policy. Babor

et al. (2003) reviewed research on the effects of media designed to reduce alcohol use or its related problems. The types of media they reviewed included public service announcements, news coverage of alcohol issues, and counteradvertising. They cited a single study of the effects of public service announcements about drinking during pregnancy that showed increased awareness of the dangers of drinking while pregnant. However, the study did not have a control group that did not receive the media. The researchers suggest that news coverage could have an effect on both individual drinking behavior and public policy making, but there seem to be no experimental evaluations of the effects of different types of news coverage. Counteradvertising is designed to directly counter the persuasive appeal of advertising for a product. Lipsey and Derzon (2002) did a meta-analysis of 72 evaluations of media campaigns designed to discourage adolescent substance use. They found small but reliable effects of media campaigns on young people's knowledge, attitudes, and behavior concerning substance use. The researchers estimated that the effects in reducing alcohol use were modest (a reduction from 53% to 51%).

Public Policy as Prevention

Alcohol policy is an environmental or structural response to alcohol-related problems. That is, policy is used to produce structural changes in the drinking or smoking or illicit drugs environment. In turn, changes in the environment effect changes in drinking behavior. Examples of alcohol policy and evidence of their effectiveness follow.

Increasing the Price of Alcohol

Alcohol, like any product sold as a retail commodity, is responsive to price fluctuations. That is, as the retail price increases, demand for the product decreases (on average). There are a number of econometric studies from around the world dealing with alcoholic beverages (Clements and Selvanathan 1991; Edwards et al. 1994; Godfrey 1986; Olsson 1991; Österberg 1995; Yen 1994). Several studies have estimated the relationship of alcohol price to drinking, that is, the elasticity or sensitivity of alcohol consumption to changes in price and income (see, for example, Cook and Tauchen 1982; Levy and Sheflin 1983; Ornstein and Levy 1983; Saffer and Grossman 1987). The elasticity of alcohol consumption is influenced by many other factors. It has been pointed out that the more restricted the availability of alcohol, the smaller the influence of changes in prices and income of consumers will be. (See Huitfeld and Jorner 1972 and Olsson 1991 for analyses of Swedish data, and Gruenewald et al. 1993 for analyses of U.S. data.) There are many studies suggesting that increased alcoholic beverage taxes and prices have direct impacts on reductions in alcohol consumption and on outcomes of related problems. For example, Cook (1981) investigated the short-term effects of changes in liquor tax on automobile accident death rates and found that such fatalities declined as taxes increased (resulting in higher retail prices). Laixuthai and Chaloupka (1993) estimated that if the price of beer (the beverage of choice of youths) was indexed to inflation, then overall drinking by youths over any past year would be reduced by 9% and heavy drinking by youths would be reduced by 20%. Using data from the U.S. National Longitudinal Survey of Youth, Pacula (1998) calculated that doubling the tax on beer would reduce alcohol consumption among young people between 3% and 6%. Estimates from studies based on overall crime rates and other measures of violence among adults conclude that higher alcoholic beverage taxes and prices would lead to significant reductions in violence and other crime (Chaloupka et al. 2002; Markowitz 2000; Sloan et al. 1994). Similarly, higher alcoholic beverage taxes and prices would lower child abuse and other violence toward children (Markowitz and Grossman 1998, 2000).

Increasing the Minimum Age for Alcohol Purchase

The goal of a higher minimum legal drinking age is to reduce alcohol consumption among those below age 21 years. In the 1980s, all 50 U.S. states were required to adopt a uniform minimum age of 21 for purchase and consumption of all alcoholic beverages. Yu et al. (1997) in New York State found a 70% decrease in self-reported alcohol purchases by 19- to 20-year-olds after the implementation of a minimum drinking age of 21 years. O'Malley and Wagenaar (1991) found that the reduction in self-reported alcohol use among individuals below the minimum drinking age and an associated reduction in traffic crashes continued well into young adulthood and did not decay after young people reached the legal drinking age. Voas et al. (1999), using data from all 50 states and the District of Columbia for 1982–1997, determined that the enactment of the uniform age 21 minimum drinking age law was re-

sponsible for a 19% net decrease in fatal crashes involving young drinking drivers after controlling for driving exposure, beer consumption, enactment of zero-tolerance laws, and other relevant changes in the laws during that time period. In the most comprehensive review to date, Wagenaar and Toomey (2000) analyzed all identified published studies on the drinking age from 1960 to 1999 and concluded that compared with a wide range of other programs and efforts to reduce drinking among high-school students, college students, and other teenagers, increasing the legal age for purchase and consumption of alcohol to 21 appears to have been the most successful effort to date. The National Highway Traffic Safety Administration, using an average estimated reduction in traffic fatalities due to the legal drinking age of 13%, calculated that the age-21 policy prevented 846 deaths in 1997 and prevented a total of 17,359 deaths since 1975 (National Highway Traffic Safety Administration 1998).

Restricting Hours and Days for Retail Alcohol Sale

Reducing the days and times of alcohol sales restricts the opportunities for alcohol purchasing and can reduce heavy consumption. This is a common policy strategy for reducing drinking-related problems, although the trend in recent years has been to liberalize such restrictions in many countries (e.g., Drummond 2000). Smith (1988), for example, presented a study in which the introduction of Sunday alcohol sales in Brisbane, Australia, was related to an increase in Sunday traffic accidents with casualty and reported property damage. A number of studies have investigated the effects of changing hours of sale on alcohol consumption and problems. In sum, it appears that changes in licensing provisions that substantially modify hours of service can have a significant impact on drinking and drinking-related problems overall. These studies (summarized in Babor et al. 2003) suggest that reduced hours and days of sale can have net effects in reducing overall alcohol consumption and problems levels, with the reduced-consumption effects concentrated during the time of closure but not matched by counterbalancing increases at other times of the week.

Regulating Density or Concentration of Retail Outlets

As with restrictions of hours and days of sale, structuring the geographical location of outlets and restricting their numbers may have strongly focused effects on particularly problematic drinking patterns (Gruenewald et al. 1993). Densities of bars, restaurants, and off-premise establishments have been observed to reach the level of one outlet for every 75 feet of roadway in many California cities (Gruenewald and Treno 2000). Gruenewald et al. (2000) found that a 10% increase in outlet density at the neighborhood level was associated with a 1.7% increase in drinking prevalence and a 0.7% increase in drinking frequency. Although the findings were not statistically significant, this study first demonstrated positive relationships. Such studies of changes in alcohol availability (see summary in Babor et al. 2003) support a conclusion that increases in the number and concentration of alcohol retail outlets result in increased consumer convenience and thereby increase purchases and consumption by consumers (Gruenewald et al. 1999). These findings about the influence of outlet density on alcohol-related problems suggest the appropriateness and potential of regulation at the local level for the prevention of alcohol-related problems (Gruenewald et al. 1996; Holder et al. 2000). Depending on the division of government responsibilities in a given society, it is often at the local level that planning and zoning laws can be used to regulate densities of outlets.

Regulating Types of Retail Outlets

Retail sales of alcoholic beverages take two general forms: 1) off-premises sales (for drinking elsewhere) by liquor stores or other licensed outlets and 2) on-premises sales (for consumption on the site) by bars, restaurants, and pubs. Regulation of off-premises alcohol sales—including regulation of the time, costs, and places of retail sales—is designed to reduce the availability of alcohol. Regulations designed to affect on-premise alcohol consumption can include specifying sizes of drinks, disallowing discounted drinks (such as during "happy hours"), requiring workers to undergo responsible beverage service training, mandating programs to provide "safe rides" for drinking drivers as well as food service, regulating the availability of entertainment, and regulating aspects of the physical design and layout of bars and restaurants. Cross-sectional studies have shown that drinking and driving is associated with bars and restaurants and in particular (in Australia) with bars serving beverages with high alcohol content (Gruenewald et al. 1999, 2000; Stockwell et al. 1993). Violence is associated with bars in particular, but connections have also been found with off-premises outlets (Graham et al. 2000; Stevenson et al. 1999).

One method of regulating the type of outlet is for the government to monopolize ownership of one or more types of retail alcohol outlet. For example, in North America state-owned liquor stores exist. A summary of seven time series analyses of six U.S. states and New Zealand found a consistent increase in total consumption when government-owned off-premises outlets were replaced with privately owned outlets (Wagenaar and Holder 1996). Typically, the network of stores in such a government-operated system is sparse rather than dense and the opening hours are limited. Elimination of a private profit interest also typically facilitates the enforcement of rules against selling to minors or the already intoxicated (Her et al. 1999).

Restricting Licensing of Retail Outlets

A popular prevention strategy is based on licensing restrictions on retail outlets. Licensing has been used in various ways, including granting (or denying) a license to sell alcohol, restricting hours of sales, restricting the number or density of outlets in a given area, and restricting the types of beverages or container sizes that can be sold. Studies in the United States have investigated the effects of privatization of wine sales and the elimination of a state monopoly on retail sales of distilled spirits (e.g., Holder and Wagenaar 1990; Wagenaar and Holder 1995).

Restricting Service of Alcohol

Responsible beverage service (RBS) consists of the implementation of a combination of outlet policies (e.g., requiring clerks or servers to check identification for all customers appearing to be under age 30 years) and training (e.g., teaching clerks and servers to recognize altered or false identification cards). RBS can be implemented at both on-premises (Saltz and Stanghetta 1997) and off-premises establishments (Grube 1997). Overall, such programs have been shown to be effective in some circumstances. Saltz (1988) and Saltz and Hennessy (1990a, 1990b) demonstrated that server training is most effective when coupled with a change in actual serving policies and practices of a bar or restaurant. (See reviews of the impact of beverage server intervention in Gliksman et al. 1993; McKnight 1988; Russ and Geller 1986; and Saltz 1987, 1989, 1993). RBS has been found to reduce the number of intoxicated patrons leaving a bar (e.g., Gliksman et al. 1993; Saltz

1987, 1989) and the number of car crashes (e.g., Holder and Wagenaar 1994). Voluntary clerk and manager training at off-premises establishments had a negligible effect on sales to minors beyond the effects of increased enforcement (Grube 1997). Similarly, a study in Australia revealed that, even after training, age identification was rarely checked in bars, although decreases in the number of intoxicated patrons were observed (Lang et al. 1996, 1998). Research indicates, for example, that establishments that have firm and clear policies (e.g., checking identification for all patrons who appear to be under age 30) and a system for monitoring staff compliance are less likely to sell alcohol to minors (Wolfson et al. 1996a, 1996b).

Enforcing Drinking and Driving Laws

Driving after drinking produces large numbers of alcohol-involved injuries and deaths and considerable property damage in the United States each year. One form of drinking and driving enforcement is random breath testing (RBT), which undertakes extensive and continuous random stops of drivers who are required to take a breath test to establish their actual blood alcohol concentration (BAC) levels. The use of random roadside checks by police for alcohol-impaired drivers in Australia (Homel 1986, 1993), Canada (Mercer 1985), and Great Britain (Ross 1988a, 1988b) has demonstrated the effectiveness of this type of drinking and driving enforcement. The perceived likelihood of apprehension for drinking and driving increased with exposure to RBT, notably when that exposure was recent. Shults et al. (2001) reviewed 23 studies of RBT and selective testing and found a median decline of 22% (range, 13%–36%) in fatal crashes, with slightly lower decreases for noninjury and other accidents for such enforcement strategies. In a time series analysis for four Australian states, Henstridge et al. (1997) found that RBT was twice as effective as selective checkpoints. They estimated that every increase of 1,000 in the daily testing rate corresponded to a decline of 6% in all serious accidents and 19% in single-vehicle nighttime accidents. However, to produce a sustained effect, increased public expectations of arrest must be reinforced with actual increased enforcement (see reviews by Vingilis and Coultes 1990; Zador et al. 1989).

Sobriety checkpoints and a limited version of RBT are often implemented in individual U.S. states under proscribed circumstances, often involving prenotification about when and where they will be implemented.

Even under these restricted circumstances there is some evidence that these strategies reduce drinking and driving and related traffic crashes. An evaluation of a Tennessee checkpoint program (Lacey et al. 1999), for example, found a 20% decrease in alcohol-related fatal crashes and a 6% reduction in single-vehicle nighttime crashes that were maintained up to 21 months after implementation of the program. Public awareness and publicity, however, have been identified as important mediators of enforcement effectiveness.

Setting BAC Limits for Drunk Driving

Complementary to actual enforcement is the legal limit of BAC that a driver can maintain (generally 0.05%—0.08% or, for young drivers, usually 0.00%–0.02%). This is the legal BAC level at which a driver is presumed to be impaired, that is, the level at which a driver can be arrested and charged with drinking and driving. Therefore, the establishment of a specific and measurable BAC limit is a certainty policy that makes enforcement of impaired driving more effective. Jonah et al. (2000) reviewed the international evidence for the impact of lower BAC laws (which outside the United States involves reductions to 0.05 or, in the case of Sweden, to 0.02) and found that consistently lower BAC limits produced positive results. Shults et al. (2001) reviewed six well-designed studies of the effect of these laws in the United States and Australia and estimated reductions in fatal crashes that ranged from 24% to 9%. As a result of such studies, the BAC legal limit has been declining in North America, Europe, Australia, and New Zealand.

Establishing Low BAC Limits for Young Drivers

Younger drivers (those under age 21) who drink and drive are especially at risk for traffic accidents because of their lack of driving experience in addition to the impairing effects of alcohol. Therefore all states have now set lower BAC limits for younger drivers, which are called zero-tolerance laws. Usually the limit is set at the minimum that can be reliably detected by breath testing equipment (i.e., 0.01%–0.02%). Zero-tolerance laws also commonly invoke other penalties such as automatic revocation of one's driver's license. An analysis of the effect of zero-tolerance laws in the first 12 states enacting them revealed a 20% relative reduction in the proportion of nighttime single-vehicle fatal crashes among drivers under age 21 compared with nearby states that did not pass zero-tolerance laws (Hingson et al. 1994; Martin et al. 1996).

Implementing Administrative License Revocation Laws

Many states permit police officers to remove or suspend the driving privilege with court action of a driver with a BAC over the legal limit (Hingson et al. 1996). These laws were associated with a 5%–9% decline in nighttime fatal crashes in some studies (Hingson 1993; Zador et al. 1989). License revocation is one type of punishment that has been shown to be effective in reducing repeated incidents of drinking and driving and to be a major deterrent to youthful drinkers who drive. The threat of the loss of one's driver's license has been shown to have important effects in deterring drinking and driving by persons previously convicted of driving under the influence (see review by Ross 1991).

Implementing Graduated Driving Licenses

Graduated licensing places limits on new or young drivers (e.g., nighttime driving is restricted). A graduated licensing program in Connecticut led to a 14% net reduction in crash involvement among the youngest drivers (Ulmer et al. 2000). Similarly, in New Zealand, a 23% reduction in car crash injuries among novice drivers was found after implementation of a graduated licensing system (Langley et al. 1996). Differences in the enforcement of zero-tolerance laws have been identified as a key issue in understanding why some programs are less successful than others (Ferguson et al. 2000), as was lack of awareness on the part of young people (Balmforth 1999; Hingson et al. 1994). The use of media campaigns to increase young peoples' awareness of reduced BAC limits and of enforcement efforts can significantly increase the effectiveness of zero-tolerance laws, according to Blomberg (1992).

Using Automobile Ignition Interlocks

Ignition interlocks are devices that can check the blood alcohol level of the driver before he or she can operate the vehicle. The automobile cannot be started if the level is above zero or some other preset limit. These devices have been proposed as a potential means of reducing drinking and driving in the general population, but in the United States they have been used primarily with specific individuals after multiple drinking and driving offenses (Voas 1988).

Restricting Advertising

Survey studies consistently find small but significant relationships between awareness of and positive reactions to alcohol advertising and the drinking beliefs and behaviors of adolescents (e.g., Casswell and Zhang 1998; Connolly et al. 1994; Grube and Wallack 1994; Grube et al. 1996; Wyllie et al. 1998). In contrast, although a few econometric studies have found a positive relationship between advertising expenditures and overall consumption or alcohol-related death (e.g., Saffer 1997), most are negative or mixed in their findings (Duffy 1995; Nelson and Moran 1995). Apparently no studies have investigated the specific effects of advertising restrictions on youth drinking or associated problems.

Placing Warning Labels on Alcoholic Beverages

Warning labels on beverage containers constitute another population-based strategy. An early evaluation of warning labels on alcoholic beverage containers in the United States showed that about one-fifth of respondents to a national survey remembered seeing the warnings 6 months after their introduction (Kaskutas and Greenfield 1992). Although somewhat greater proportions of key target groups (e.g., heavy drinkers and young men at risk for drunk driving) remembered seeing the labels, no changes in knowledge of the targeted health risks could be detected. In a national survey of youths, MacKinnon et al. (1993) found increases in self-reported awareness of, exposure to, and memory of the labels after they were required but no substantial changes in alcohol use or beliefs about the risks targeted by the warning. Overall, then, there is little evidence that alcohol beverage warning labels have any discernible effect on drinking by young people or on their attitudes or knowledge of the risks of drinking.

Implementing Keg Registration

Keg registration laws require the purchaser of a keg of beer to complete a form that links their name to a number on the keg. Keg registration is seen primarily as a tool for prosecuting adults who supply alcohol to young people at parties and even establishments that rent to underage persons. Keg registration laws have become increasingly popular in local communities in the United States. There are currently no studies on the effectiveness of these laws in reducing access to alcohol by underage persons.

Community Interventions

Public policy has had and is likely to continue to have an important role in the prevention of social and health problems, especially in the area of addictions. Comprehensive programs have combined school-based education with community environmental interventions (Biglan et al. 2000; Hingson et al. 1996; Perry et al. 1996; Wagenaar et al. 1999, 2000). However, community interventions undertaken only to support school-based education by involving parents in homework or staging school-related alcohol-free or drug-free activities are not true community interventions in that little is accomplished in terms of actual policy or other environmental change (e.g., Paglia and Room 1999).

Project Northland (Perry et al. 1996), which included components targeting sixth graders with family take-home assignments, has led to substantial reductions (19%–46%) in alcohol use among younger adolescents in rural Minnesota. Although the project reports lower drinking levels for high-school students in the treatment compared with the control condition, the effect of Project Northland cannot be attributed with confidence to the environmental strategies implemented. Because few high school students obtain alcohol in licensed on-premises outlets, this strategy has limited potential as a significant barrier against drinking by middle-school students. No information was reported about the level of actual RBS implementation or level of enforcement (Veblen-Mortenson et al. 1999). Project Northland also reported nothing concerning police enforcement of sales to underage persons, which is essential in reducing alcohol access (Grube 1997).

Communities Mobilizing for Change on Alcohol

Wagenaar et al. (1994, 2000) evaluated a community organizing intervention that was designed to bring about change in policies regarding access to alcohol by those under age 21. Communities Mobilizing for Change on Alcohol (CMCA) was evaluated in a randomized trial in which 15 Minnesota and Wisconsin communities were randomly assigned to receive or not receive the program. The CMCA communities had lower levels of sales of alcohol to minors in their retail outlets and had marginally lower sales to minors at bars and restaurants. Telephone surveys of 18- to 20-year-olds indicated that they were less likely to try to buy alcohol and that they were less likely to provide alcohol to others. The proportion of 18- to 20-year-olds who reported drinking in the past 30 days was lower in intervention communities. However, the prevalence of heavy drinking in this age group was not affected. Furthermore, there were no significant effects on the drinking behavior of twelfth graders (who were surveyed in school). Arrests of 18- to 20-year-olds for driving under the influence of alcohol declined significantly more in CMCA communities than in control communities (Wagenaar et al. 2000).

The Saving Lives Project

The Saving Lives Project in Massachusetts was designed to reduce alcohol-impaired driving and related problems such as speeding (Hingson et al. 1996). Local efforts included media campaigns, business information programs, awareness days on speeding and drunk driving, speed watch telephone hot lines, police training, peer-led education in high schools, establishment of Students Against Drunk Driving chapters, and college prevention programs. Outcomes measured included fatal and injury crashes, seat belt use, automotive speed, traffic citations, and telephone surveys of self-reported drinking and driving. Over the 5 years of the program, participating cities experienced a decline in all of these outcomes compared with the rest of the state. Compared with the 5 years before the intervention, the Saving Lives cities had a 42% reduction in fatal automobile crashes, a 47% reduction in the number of fatally injured drivers who tested positive for alcohol, and an 8% decline in crash injuries among 16- to 25-year-olds. In addition, there was a decline in self-reported driving after drinking among youths and about a 50% reduction in observed speeding. The greatest reductions in fatal and injury crashes occurred in the 15- to 25-year age group.

The Community Trials Project

The Community Trials Project (Holder et al. 1997) tested a five-component community intervention to reduce alcohol-related harm among people of all ages. It sought to reduce the primary sources of acute injury and harm related to alcohol: drunken-driving injuries and fatalities and injuries and deaths related to violence, burns, falls, and drowning. The Community Trials fielded five intervention components: 1) a Media and Mobilization component to develop community organization and support for the goals and strategies of the project and to utilize local news to increase public support of environmental strategies; 2) a Responsible Beverage Service component to reduce service to intoxicated patrons at bars and restaurants; 3) a Sales to Youth component to reduce underage access; 4) a Drinking and Driving component to increase local enforcement of laws regarding driving while intoxicated; and 5) an Access component to reduce the availability of alcohol. A comparison of the experimental and control communities found that the intervention produced significant reductions in nighttime injury crashes (10% lower in experimental than in comparison communities) and in crashes in which the driver was found by police to "have been drinking" (6%). Assault injuries observed in emergency departments declined by 43% in the intervention communities versus the comparison communities, and all hospitalized assault injuries declined by 2%. There was a 49% decline in reports of driving after "having had too much to drink" and 51% in self-reports of driving when "over the legal limit." Surprisingly, although the self-reported drinking population increased slightly in the experimental sites over the course of the study, there was a significant reduction in problematic alcohol use: average drinks per occasion declined by 6% and the variance in drinking patterns (an indirect measure of heavy drinking) declined 21% (Holder et al. 2000).

Effectiveness of Prevention Programs

Community decisions about which prevention strategies should actually be implemented to reduce alcohol-related problems are usually a compromise between political values and scientific evidence. This section summarizes what is known about alternative prevention strategies in four general groupings of the general state of knowledge across scientific evaluations of effectiveness.

Solid Evidence

The strategies listed below have been shown to be consistently effective over time and in two or more countries or cultural settings. If a strategy has shown strong effects in only one country, its cultural robustness is considered to be untested and the strategy was placed in the next category.

- Increasing the retail price of alcohol
- Increasing the minimum drinking age
- Restricting hours and days of alcohol sale
- Deterring driving while under the influence of alcohol and drugs, especially through regular and highly visible enforcement
- Establishing limits on the retail sale of alcohol
- Establishing lower BAC limits for driving

Positive Evidence That Needs Replication

Strategies that have shown clear positive evidence of effectiveness but have either been tested under very controlled conditions (usually controlled by a scientist team) or been shown to be effective in one culture but not tested in other cultures constitute this category. These strategies are listed below.

- Responsible beverage service: policies and training regarding the serving of alcohol
- School-based education
- Family education
- Warning labels on alcoholic beverages
- Suspension of driver's license for drinking and driving
- Regulation of the density of establishments selling alcohol
- Restrictions on alcohol sales to youth

Promising, But Too Early to Tell

Strategies that have demonstrated early evidence of the potential to reduce problems, but for which this potential has not been replicated sufficiently to be considered strong evidence, are listed below.

- Workplace policies to restrict on-the-job drinking and employee impairment
- Health care interventions, including brief interventions
- Genetics and genetics counseling
- Limits on alcohol sales to dependent persons
- Automobile ignition controls to prevent drunk driving
- Parent mobilization for restricting availability of alcohol and tobacco to youth
- Restrictions on drinking locations
- Marketing and selling beverages with low or no alcoholic content
- Training heavy drinkers to moderate consumption

Contradictory Findings With Unclear Implications

Listed below are prevention strategies for which evaluation has produced contradictory results that are difficult to fully assess. Often these are strategies that show as many negative as positive results.

- Mass communication and public education alone
- Information alone
- Fear arousal and stimulation
- Restrictions on alcohol advertising

Conclusion

In summary, the most effective public prevention strategies and policies to reduce alcohol-related problems are

1. Taxation or price increases
2. Increases in the minimum drinking age
3. Zero-tolerance laws or graduated licensing
4. Enforcement of restriction of sales of alcohol to underage persons
5. Random breath testing and sobriety checkpoints (a strategy that appears promising for reducing drinking and driving, based on studies in the general population)

In this chapter, the importance of evidence of effectiveness has been emphasized as a critical condition for the use of a prevention strategy. However, in a time of decreased availability of public and private resources for prevention, the cost of a strategy relative to its demonstrated (or potential) effectiveness should be increasingly considered. For example, a particular strategy may have been shown to be effective in a number of controlled studies, but its potential to yield desired effects when compared with an alternative strategy must be weighed against its cost to design, implement, and sustain. Cost-effectiveness is an additional standard that prevention strategies of the future will have to meet.

References

Babor TF: Avoiding the horrid and beastly sin of drunkenness: does dissuasion make a difference? J Consult Clin Psychol 62:1127–1140, 1994

Babor T, Caetano R, Casswell S: Alcohol: No Ordinary Commodity—Research and Public Policy. Oxford, UK, Oxford University Press, 2003

Balmforth D: National Survey of Drinking and Driving, Attitudes and Behavior: 1997 (DOT HS 808 844). Washington, DC, U.S. Department of Transportation, National Highway Traffic Safety Administration, 1999

Biglan A, Ary DV, Smolkowski K, et al: A randomized control trial of a community intervention to prevent adolescent tobacco use. Tob Control 9:24–32, 2000

Blomberg R: Lower BAC Limits for Youth: Evaluation of the Maryland .02 Law (DOT HS 807 860). Washington, DC, U.S. Department of Transportation, National Highway Traffic Safety Administration, 1992

Botvin G: Substance abuse prevention through life skills training, in Preventing Childhood Disorders, Substance Abuse, and Delinquency. Edited by Peter RD, McMahon RJ. Thousand Oaks, CA, Sage, 1996, pp 215–240

Casswell S, Zang JF: Impact of liking for advertising and brand allegiance on drinking and alcohol-related aggression: a longitudinal study. Addiction 93:1209–1217, 1998

Catalano RF, Haggerty KP, Gainey RR, et al: Effectiveness of primary prevention interventions with high-risk families. NIDA Res Monogr (in press)

Chaloupka FJ, Grossman M, Saffer H: The effects of price on alcohol consumption and alcohol-related problems. Alcohol Res Health 26:23–34, 2002

Clements KW, Selvanathan S: The economic determinants of alcohol consumption. Australian Journal of Agricultural Economics 35:209–231, 1991

Connolly GM, Casswell S, Zhang JF, et al: Alcohol in the mass media and drinking by adolescents: a longitudinal study. Addiction 89:1255–1263, 1994

Cook PJ: The effect of liquor taxes on drinking, cirrhosis, and auto accidents, in Alcohol and Public Policy: Beyond the Shadow of Prohibition. Edited by Moore MH, Gerstein DR. Washington, DC, National Academy Press, 1981, pp 255–285

Cook PJ, Tauchen G: The effect of liquor taxes on heavy drinking. Bell Journal of Economics 13:379–390, 1982

Drummond DC: UK government announces first major relaxation in the alcohol licensing laws for nearly a century: drinking in the UK goes 24–7. Addiction 95:997–998, 2000

Duffy M: Advertising in demand systems for alcoholic drinks and tobacco: a comparative study. Journal of Policy Modeling 17:557–577, 1995

Edwards G, Anderson P, Babor TF, et al (eds): Alcohol Policy and the Public Good. New York, Oxford University Press, 1994

Ennett ST, Rosenbaum DP, Flewelling RL, et al: Long-term evaluation of drug abuse resistance education. Addict Behav 19:113–125, 1994

Ferguson SA, Fields M, Voas RB: Enforcement of zero tolerance laws in the United States. Paper presented at the 15th International Conference on Alcohol, Drugs, and Traffic Safety, Stockholm, Sweden, May 2000

Gainey RR, Catalano RF, Haggerty KP, et al: Participation in a parent training program for methadone clients. Addict Behav 8:117–125, 1995

Gliksman L, McKenzie D, Single E, et al: Role of alcohol providers in prevention: an evaluation of a server intervention programme. Addiction 88:1195–1203, 1993

Godfrey C: Factors Influencing the Consumption of Alcohol and Tobacco: A Review of Demand Models. York, UK, Addiction Research Centre for Health Economics, 1986

Graham K, West P, Wells S: Evaluating theories of alcohol-related aggression using observations of young adults in bars. Addiction 95:847–863, 2000

Grube JW: Preventing sales of alcohol to minors: results from a community trial. Addiction 92 (suppl 2):S251–S260, 1997

Grube JW, Wallack L: Television beer advertising and drinking knowledge, beliefs, and intentions among school children. Am J Public Health 84:254–259, 1994

Grube JW, Madden PA, Friese B: Television alcohol advertising increases adolescent drinking. Poster presented at the annual meeting of the American Psychological Society, San Francisco, CA, June 1996

Gruenewald PJ, Treno AJ: Local and global alcohol supply: economic and geographic models of community systems. Addiction 95 (suppl 4):S537–S549, 2000

Gruenewald PJ, Ponicki WB, Holder HD: The relationship of outlet densities to alcohol consumption: a time series cross-sectional analysis. Alcohol Clin Exp Res 17:38–47, 1993

Gruenewald PJ, Millar AB, Treno AJ, et al: The geography of availability and driving after drinking. Addiction 91:967–983, 1996

Gruenewald PJ, Stockwell T, Beel A, et al: Beverage sales and drinking and driving: the role of on-premise drinking places. J Stud Alcohol 60:47–53, 1999

Gruenewald PJ, Millar A, Ponicki WR, et al: Physical and economic access to alcohol: the application of geostatistical methods to small area analysis in community settings, in The Epidemiology of Alcohol Problems in Small Geographic Areas. Edited by Wilson RA, DuFour MC. Rockville, MD, National Institute on Alcohol Abuse and Alcoholism, 2000, pp 163–212

Henstridge J, Homel R, Mackay P: The long-term effects of random breath testing in four Australian states: a time series analysis. Canberra, Australia, Federal Office of Road Safety, 1997

Her M, Giesbrecht N, Room R, et al: Privatizing alcohol sales and alcohol consumption: evidence and implications. Addiction 94:1125–1139, 1999

Higgins-Biddle JC, Babor TF: Reducing Risky Drinking. A report prepared for the Robert Wood Johnson Foundation. Farmington, CT, University of Connecticut Health Center, 1996

Hingson R: Prevention of alcohol-impaired driving. Alcohol Health Res World 17(1):28–34, 1993

Hingson R, Heeren T, Winter M: Effects of lower legal blood alcohol limits for young and adult drivers. Alcohol Drugs Driving 10:243–252, 1994

Hingson RW, McGovern T, Howland J, et al: Reducing alcohol-impaired driving in Massachusetts: the Saving Lives Program. Am J Public Health 86:791–797, 1996

Holder HD, Wagenaar AC: Effects of the elimination of a state monopoly on distilled spirits' retail sales: a time-series analysis of Iowa. Br J Addict 85:1615–1625, 1990

Holder HD, Wagenaar AC: Mandated server training and reduced alcohol-involved traffic crashes: a time series analysis of the Oregon experience. Accid Anal Prev 26:89–97, 1994

Holder HD, Treno AJ, Saltz RF, et al: Summing up: recommendations and experiences for evaluation of community-level prevention programs. Eval Rev 21:268–277, 1997

Holder HD, Gruenewald PJ, Ponicki W, et al: Effect of community-based interventions on high-risk drinking and alcohol-related injuries. JAMA 284:2341–2347, 2000

Homel R: Policing the Drinking Driver: Random Breath Testing and the Process of Deterrence. Canberra, Federal Office of Road Safety, 1986

Homel R: Random breath testing in Australia: getting it to work according to specifications. Addiction 88 (suppl): 275–335, 1993

Huitfeld B, Jorner U: [Demand for alcoholic beverages in Sweden: an econometric study of the development of consumption following the abolishment of the personal ration book] (Swedish). Report from the Alcohol Policy Commission (APU). Stockholm, Swedish Government Official Reports, 1972

Jonah B, Mann R, Macdonald S, et al: The effects of lowering legal blood alcohol limits: a review, in Alcohol, Drugs and Traffic Safety—T 2000: Proceedings of the 15th International Conference on Alcohol, Drugs, and Traffic Safety, Stockholm, Sweden, May 22–26, 2000. Edited by Laurell H, Schlyter F. Stockholm, International Conference on Alcohol, Drugs and Traffic Safety, 2000

Kahan M, Wilson L, Becker L: Effectiveness of physician-based interventions with problem drinkers: a review. Can Med Assoc J 152:851–859, 1995

Kaskutas L, Greenfield TK: First effects of warning labels on alcoholic beverage containers. Drug Alcohol Depend 31:1–14, 1992

Lacey JH, Jones RK, Smith RG: Evaluation of Checkpoint Tennessee: Tennessee's Statewide Sobriety Checkpoint Program. Washington, DC, National Highway Traffic Safety Administration, 1999

Laixuthai A, Chaloupka FJ: Youth alcohol use and public policy. Contemporary Policy Issues 11:70–81, 2003

Lang E, Stockwell T, Rydon P, et al: Use of pseudo-patrons to assess compliance with laws regarding underage drinking. Aust N Z J Public Health 20:296–300, 1996

Lang E, Stockwell T, Rydon P, et al: Can training bar staff in responsible serving practices reduce alcohol-related harm? Drug Alcohol Rev 17:39–50, 1998

Langley JD, Wagenaar AC, Begg DJ: An evaluation of the New Zealand graduated driver licensing system. Accid Anal Prev 28:139–146, 1996

Levy D, Sheflin N: New evidence on controlling alcohol use through price. J Stud Alcohol 44:920–937, 1983

Lipsey M, Derzon J: Effects of mass media interventions on drug abuse: changes in knowledge, attitude, and behavior, in Mass Media and Drug Prevention Communication. Edited by Crano W, Burgoon M. Mahwah, NJ, Erlbaum, 2002, pp 231–258

MacKinnon DP, Pentz MA, Stacy AW: Alcohol warning labels and adolescents: the first year. Am J Public Health 83:585–587, 1993

Markowitz S: The price of alcohol, wife abuse, and husband abuse. South Econ J 67:279–303, 2000

Markowitz S, Grossman M: Alcohol regulation and violence towards children. Contemp Econ Policy 16:309–320, 1998

Markowitz S, Grossman M: The effects of alcohol regulation on physical child abuse. J Health Econ 19:271–282, 2000

Martin SE, Grube JW, Voas RV, et al: Zero tolerance laws: effective public policy? Alcohol Clin Exp Res 20 (suppl 8):147A–150A, November 1996

Mattick RP, Jarvis T: Brief or minimal intervention for "alcoholics"? The evidence suggests otherwise. Drug Alcohol Rev 13:137–144, 1994

McKnight AJ: Development and Field Test of a Responsible Alcohol Service Program (Final Report on NHTSA Contract No. DTNH22–84-C-07170). Washington, DC, U.S. Department of Transportation, National Highway Traffic Safety Administration, 1988

Mercer GW: The relationships among driving while impaired charges, police drinking-driving roadcheck activity, media coverage and alcohol-related casualty traffic accidents. Accid Anal Prev 17:467–474, 1985

National Highway Traffic Safety Administration: Traffic Safety Facts 1997: Alcohol. Washington, DC, Department of Transportation, National Center for Statistics and Analysis, 1998

Nelson JP, Moran JR: Advertising and U.S. alcoholic beverage demand: system-wide estimates. Appl Econ 27:1225–1236, 1995

Olsson O: [The effect of prices and income on alcohol consumption and related problems] (Swedish). Stockholm, The Swedish Council for Information on Alcohol and Other Drugs (CAN), 1991

O'Malley PM, Wagenaar AC: Effects of minimum drinking age laws on alcohol use, related behaviors and traffic crash involvement among Americans youth: 1976–1987. J Stud Alcohol 52:478–491, 1991

Ornstein SI, Levy D: Price and income elasticities and the demand for alcoholic beverages, in Recent Developments in Alcoholism, Vol 1. Edited by Galanter M. New York, Plenum, 1983, pp 303–345

Österberg E: Do alcohol prices affect consumption and related problems? in Alcohol and Public Policy: Evidence and Issues. Edited by Holder HD, Edwards G. New York, Oxford University Press 1995, pp 145–163

Pacula RL: Does increasing the beer tax decrease marijuana consumption? J Health Econ 17:557–585, 1998

Paglia A, Room R: Preventing substance use problems among youth: a literature review and recommendations. J Prim Prev 20:3–50, 1999

Perry CL, Williams CL, Veblen-Mortenson S, et al: Project Northland: outcomes of a community-wide alcohol use prevention program during early adolescence. Am J Public Health 86:956–965, 1996

Poikolainen K: Effectiveness of brief interventions to reduce alcohol intake in primary health care populations: a meta-analysis. Prev Med 28:503–509, 1999

Redmond C, Spoth R, Shin C, et al: Modeling long-term parent outcomes of two universal family focused preventive interventions: one-year follow-up results. J Consult Clin Psychol 67:975–984, 1999

Ringwalt C, Ennett ST, Holt KD: An outcome evaluation of Project DARE (Drug Abuse Resistance Education). Health Educ Res 6:327–337, 1991

Rosenbaum DP, Flewelling RL, Bailey SL, et al: Cops in the classroom: a longitudinal evaluation of Drug Abuse Resistance Education (DARE). Journal of Research in Crime and Delinquency 31:3–31, 1994

Ross HL: British drink-driving policy. Br J Addict 83:863–865, 1988a

Ross HL: Deterrence-based policies in Britain, Canada and Australia, in The Social Control of Drinking and Driving. Edited by Laurence MD, Zimring JR, Snortum FE. Chicago, IL, University of Chicago Press, 1988b, pp 64–78

Ross HL: Administrative License Revocation for Drunk Drivers. Washington, DC, AAA Foundation for Traffic Safety, 1991

Russ NW, Geller ES: Evaluation of a Server Intervention Program for Preventing Drunk Driving (Final Report No. DD-3). Blacksburg, VA, Virginia Polytechnic Institute and State University, Department of Psychology, 1986

Saffer H: Alcohol advertising and motor vehicle fatalities. Rev Econ Stat 79:431–442, 1997

Saffer H, Grossman M: Drinking age laws and highway mortality rates: cause and effect. Econ Inq 25:403–417, 1987

Saltz RF: The roles of bars and restaurants in preventing alcohol-impaired driving: an evaluation of server intervention. Eval Health Prof 10:5–27, 1987

Saltz RF: Server intervention and responsible beverage service programs. Surgeon General's Workshop on Drunk Driving: Background Papers. Rockville, MD, Office of the Surgeon General, 1988, pp 169–179

Saltz RF: Research needs and opportunities in server intervention programs. Health Educ Q 16:429–438, 1989

Saltz RF: The introduction of dram shop legislation in the United States and the advent of server training. Addiction 88 (suppl):95S–103S, 1993

Saltz RF, Hennessy M: The efficacy of "responsible beverage service" programs in reducing intoxication (working paper). Berkeley, CA, Prevention Research Center, 1990a

Saltz RF, Hennessy M: Reducing intoxication in commercial establishments: an evaluation of responsible beverage service practices (working paper). Berkeley, CA, Prevention Research Center, 1990b

Saltz RF, Stanghetta P: A community-wide responsible beverage service program in three communities: early findings. Addiction 92 (suppl 2):S237–S249, 1997

Shults RA, Elder RW, Sleet DA, et al: Reviews of evidence regarding interventions to reduce alcohol-impaired driving. Am J Prev Med 21 (4 suppl):66–88, 2001

Sloan FA, Reilly BA, Schenzler C: Effects of prices, civil and criminal sanctions, and law enforcement on alcohol-related mortality. J Stud Alcohol 55:454–465, 1994

Smith DI: Extended alcohol trading hours during the 1982 Brisbane Commonwealth Games and traffic accidents. Australian Drug and Alcohol Review 7:363–367, 1988

Spoth R, Redmond C, Lepper HS: Alcohol initiation outcomes of universal family focused preventive interventions: one- and two-year follow-ups of a controlled study. J Stud Alcohol Suppl 13:103–111, 1999

Stevenson RJ, Lind B, Weatherburn D: The relationship between alcohol sales and assault in New South Wales, Australia. Addiction 94:397–410, 1999

Stockwell R, Lang E, Rydon P: High-risk drinking settings: the association of serving and promotional practices with harmful drinking. Addiction 88:1519–1526, 1993

Ulmer RG, Preusser DF, Williams AF, et al: Effects of Florida's graduated licensing program on the crash rate of teenage drivers. Accid Anal Prev 32:527–532, 2000

Veblen-Mortenson S, Rissel C, Perry CL, et al: Lessons learned from Project Northland: community organization in rural communities, in Health Promotion at the Community Level 2: New Advances. Edited by Bracht N. Thousand Oaks, CA, Sage, 1999, pp 105–117

Vingilis E, Coultes B: Mass communications and drinking-driving: theories, practices and results. Alcohol Drugs Driving 6(2):61–81, 1990

Voas RB: Emerging technologies for controlling the drunk driver, in Social Control of the Drinking Driver. Edited by Laurence MD, Snortum JR, Zimring FE. Chicago, IL, University of Chicago Press, 1988, pp 321–371

Voas RB, Tippetts AS, Fell J: United States limits drinking by youth under age 21: does this reduce fatal crash involvements? Paper presented at the annual meeting of the Association for the Advancement of Automotive Medicine, Barcelona, Spain, September 1999

Wagenaar AC, Holder HD: Changes in alcohol consumption resulting from the elimination of retail wine monopolies: results from five U.S. states. J Stud Alcohol 56:566–572, 1995

Wagenaar AC, Holder HD: The scientific process works: seven replications now show significant wine sales increases after privatization (letter). J Stud Alcohol 57:575–576, 1996

Wagenaar AC, Toomey TL: Effects of minimum drinking age laws: review and analyses of the literature from 1960 to 2000. J Stud Alcohol Suppl 14:206–225, 2002

Wagenaar AC, Murray DM, Wolfson M, et al: Communities mobilizing for change on alcohol: design of a randomized community trial. J Community Psychol (special issue):79–101, 1994

Wagenaar AC, Gehan JP, Jones-Webb R, et al: Communities mobilizing for change on alcohol: lessons and results from a 15-community randomized trial. J Community Psychol 27:315–326, 1999

Wagenaar AC, Murray DM, Toomey TL: Communities Mobilizing for Change on Alcohol (CMCA): effects of a randomized trial on arrests and traffic crashes. Addiction 95:209–217, 2000

Wilk AI, Jensen NM, Havighurst TC: Meta-analysis of randomized control trials addressing brief interventions in heavy alcohol drinkers. J Gen Intern Med 12:274–283, 1997

Wolfson M, Toomey TL, Forster JL, et al: Characteristics, policies and practices of alcohol outlets and sales to underage persons. J Stud Alcohol 57:670–674, 1996a

Wolfson M, Toomey TL, Murray DM, et al: Alcohol outlet policies and practices concerning sales to underage people. Addiction 91:589–602, 1996b

Wyllie A, Zhang JF, Casswell S: Positive responses to televised beer advertisements associated with drinking and problems reported by 18 to 29-year-olds. Addiction 93:749–760, 1998

Yen ST: Cross-section estimation of U.S. demand for alcoholic beverage. Appl Econ 26:381–392, 1994

Yu J, Varone R, Shacket RW: Fifteen-year review of drinking age laws: preliminary findings of the 1996 New York State Youth Alcohol Survey. New York, Office of Alcoholism and Substance Abuse, 1997

Zador P, Lund A, Fields M: Fatal crash involvement and laws against alcohol-impaired driving. J Public Health Policy 10:467–485, 1989

Forensic Issues

Edgar P. Nace, M.D.
J. Douglas Crowder, M.D.

Addiction-related behaviors often result in legal problems. Examples include intoxication leading to aggravated assault or driving under the influence (DUI); theft to obtain cash for drug procurement or diversion of drugs from medical supplies; and noncompliance with probation (continued drug use or failure to attend treatment). Although these behaviors are encountered commonly by the clinician, forensic issues related to addiction treatment may be less familiar.

In this chapter we review common forensic issues as they apply to addiction. Included are civil competence and guardianship, the Americans with Disabilities Act, malpractice in substance abuse treatment, crime and substance abuse, drug courts, competence to stand trial, diminished capacity and the insanity defense, and treatment during incarceration.

History

During the past century, concerns about drug and alcohol abuse have prompted significant legislative ac-

tion in the United States. For example, in the 1890s importation of opium for use in medication reached its peak. Opium availability, the development of the hypodermic needle, and the unregulated use of morphine in patent medications produced an estimated 250,000 opiate addicts in the United States by 1900 (Musto 1973). The Pure Food and Drug Act of 1906 was a first attempt at discouraging patent medicine abuse. It required any medicine containing opiates, cocaine, chloral hydrate, or cannabis to be so labeled and the percentage of each given. The Harrison Act of 1914 mandated that dealers in narcotics register with the Bureau of Internal Revenue. Record keeping was required, and legal possession of a drug necessitated a physician's or dentist's prescription (Musto 1997). The Marijuana Tax Act was passed in 1937, and the Opium Poppy Control Act, in 1942 (Musto 1997).

Concern over alcohol use in the nineteenth century was reflected in the formation of temperance societies. Churches and temperance groups joined forces, but the Prohibition Act of 1880 was easily defeated in Congress. However, by 1912, several states had adopted prohibition acts, and the Eighteenth Amendment—banning production, importation, and sale of alcohol on a national level—became law on January 17, 1920. Although hospitalization rates, traffic fatalities, and the incidence of cirrhosis declined, organized crime flourished, and the American public chose to repeal Prohibition in 1933 (Howland and Howland 1978).

In addition to concern about regulation or prohibition of drugs and alcohol, there has been a historical focus on what to do with "inebriates" and addicts. During the first half of the nineteenth century, per-capita alcohol consumption was three times what it is today (White 1998). The drunkard was seen as diseased or evil, or as something in between the two.

As early as 1812 Benjamin Rush advocated involuntary treatment of drunkards. With the establishment of inebriety facilities during the latter half of the nineteenth century (the first being Boston's Washington Hall in 1845), involuntary treatment gained favor. Guardianship was the first tentative approach, but by the end of the nineteenth century 14 states had involuntary substance abuse commitment codes (Hall and Appelbaum 2002). This movement was aborted as Prohibition gained precedence and specialty hospitals for alcoholism closed. It was not until the 1960s that involuntary treatment mechanisms for substance-abusing patients reemerged, and today most states have mechanisms of civil commitment available (Hall and Appelbaum 2002).

More recently, the Anti-Drug Abuse Act of 1988 (P.L. 100-690) provided funding for treatment and law enforcement, stipulated penalties for personal possession of drugs, and required that alcoholic beverages contain a warning label. Furthermore, the act established the Office of National Drug Control Policy, which is an executive-branch function tasked with designing a national strategy to curb drug abuse (Musto 1997).

The historical question of how to respond to the addicted person continues to evolve and is expressed in the inclusion of alcohol- and drug-dependent persons in the Americans With Disabilities Act (Starkman 2000) and in the current growth of "drug courts" (Belenko 1998), both of which are discussed in this chapter.

Civil Competence and Guardianship

Civil law implies special concerns for addiction psychiatrists. Most practitioners associate civil incompetence with dementia, but substance abuse can also cause legally incapacitating impairment. Mental *capacity* is a task-specific functional ability. That is, capacity requires that a person's cognitive and more general psychic apparatus constitutes an adequate substrate for decision making with reference to a particular issue. For example, an individual may lack the capacity to transact business while retaining the capacity to marry. No one can make correct choices in every instance, but a basically intact mind must underlie the decision process to an extent that permits an understanding of the probable consequences that would follow the various choices available. *Competence* is the legal status of a person who possesses capacity in all relevant domains. A psychiatrist may offer opinions about either capacity or competence, but only the courts can adjudicate a person incompetent.

Competence affects practice in the areas of consent to treatment and guardianship assessment. Consent to treatment requires that a patient be given information about the risks, benefits, and alternatives of a proposed therapy; that the patient be able to understand and rationally manipulate the information supplied; and that he or she be acting voluntarily. Intoxication and delirium frequently interfere with competence to consent to treatment in obvious ways. Consent is not required when incompetent patients find themselves in emergency situations, and the patient must immediately be protected in these circumstances regardless of protest. Clinicians should be aware of any specific jurisdictional definition of an emergency that may apply, but the imminent threat of physical death or significant physical damage is almost universally accepted as a minimum criterion. After the patient's immediate welfare is ensured, more formal procedures for substituted judgment may be appropriate depending on local law and the expected length of incapacity.

The need for informed consent and for voluntary action are relatively straightforward considerations, but understanding and rational information manipulation can be more subtle parameters of competence. The mere ability to mechanically repeat clinical information is not sufficient to demonstrate competence, because some patients seem to learn that parroting a dire prognosis without really believing it is the price of hospital discharge. Careful exploration of the underlying thought process and the patience to go beyond superficial rationalizations are needed if more than perfunctory assessment is to be performed. Family and friends may help clarify the patient's long-held values in order to detect any change from baseline. A commonly encountered situation involves an intravenous drug user with bacterial endocarditis who voices an intention to leave the hospital against medical advice. The psychiatric clinician is then asked to determine if the patient is competent to refuse treatment. A compulsion to continue using drugs and the characteristic defense mechanism of denial, as well as possible cognitive deficits from chronic substance abuse, cloud the usual presumption of free will. The evaluation is often further complicated by staff countertransference pitting rescuers against autonomy advocates and perhaps some who lack empathy for what they feel is a self-induced illness. Such a patient who is cognitively intact is usually best regarded as competent, especially if there is personal experience with the medical condition or substance treatment. However, a reasonable case can be made for involuntary retention for treatment in individual instances. Family support for such a course, sudden relapse after an extended remission, or the patient's youth might argue for an involuntary confinement based on an incompetence finding. Again, local legal measures—the specific form of which vary by locale and may include court injunctions, temporary guardianship, or civil commitment—need to be pursued to arrange for involuntary treatment. However, it is always preferable to enlist the help of significant people in the patient's life and to deal with intrapsychic conflicts, control struggles, and the patient's reality concerns (e.g., job or child custody problems) before resorting to involuntary treatment.

Guardianship is granted under a best-interest standard when an individual is incompetent to handle his or her financial or personal affairs. The guardian's specific authority for some actions such as inpatient psychiatric hospitalization of a ward is variable from state to state, and clinicians should be aware of local regulations before acting on a guardian's request. However, the guardian generally has broad power to collect monies, pay obligations, manage investments, consent to medical treatment, limit social contacts, and arrange living conditions for the ward. Substance abuse and dependence are adequate bases for the appointment of a guardian, but the adversarial process that can follow a guardianship application sometimes entails substantial expenses, which may or may not be borne by the estate of the proposed ward. Civil commitment and powers of attorney are less costly but are also less permanent and less effective at protecting a person's interests. Powers of attorney, which allow a

designee to conduct business, must be granted in a competent state and do not preclude independent ill-conceived transactions or behaviors because the granting person has not been adjudicated incompetent. The term *durable preceding power of attorney* means that the instrument survives (literally, endures despite) the granting person's subsequent decline into incompetence. Similarly, law enforcement and protective agencies may act to protect an impaired individual more expeditiously than a guardianship could be arranged, but, again, they do not necessarily provide long-term assistance of the type needed. Guardianship should be considered when substance abuse patients prove unable to reverse a habit that significantly compromises their health, repeatedly involves them in high-risk behaviors, causes sustained severe lifestyle deterioration, risks the loss of extensive monetary assets, or leads to cognitive decline that interferes with function. An understandable desire to preserve the autonomy of, or a relationship with, a substance abuse patient may make family members reluctant to take coercive action, but regaining independence is a powerful incentive for recovery.

The Americans With Disabilities Act

When the Americans With Disabilities Act (ADA) of 1990 (P.L. 101-336) was passed by the U.S. Congress on July 26, 1990, the substance abuse treatment community had reason to be pleased. A broad civil rights mandate had been legislated "for the elimination of discrimination against individuals with disabilities," and alcoholism and drug addiction were included.

Three distinct ways to qualify for a disability were defined:

1. Having a physical or mental impairment that subsequently limits one or more major life activities
2. Having a record of such an impairment
3. Being regarded as having such an impairment (Americans With Disabilities Act of 1990)

The inclusion of alcoholism and drug addiction under the ADA does not preclude the employer's right to require employees to conform to the Drug-Free Workplace Act of 1988 (P.L. 100-690, Title V, Subtitle D), as well as to statutes established by other federal agencies. Therefore, employers may ensure that the workplace is free from illegal alcohol or drug use.

In contrast to the alcoholic individual, the drug abuser has a harder time qualifying for ADA protection. Current drug use, on or off the job, is not protected. Current drug use—that is, drug use that has "occurred recently enough to indicate that the individual is actively engaged in such conduct" (29 CFR sec. 1630, App. 1630.31)—is given no protection under the ADA. Drug use does not need to occur on the day that an employer takes action against an employee, and the concept of current use (still vaguely defined) can extend back at least several months (Starkman 2000).

ADA protection is available if the drug addict

1. Has successfully completed a supervised drug rehabilitation program and is no longer engaging in the illegal use of drugs or has been otherwise successfully rehabilitated and no longer uses drugs
2. Is participating in a supervised rehabilitation program and no longer uses drugs
3. Is mistakenly regarded as using drugs (42 U.S.C. 12114 [c])

Use of alcohol away from the job cannot be the basis for employer action against an employee. If the employee poses a threat to the safety of others or breaks workplace rules against the use of alcohol, ADA protection does not apply. An employer cannot inquire as to whether an applicant is an alcoholic or drug addict or has been in alcohol or drug rehabilitation. The employer can ask if the applicant currently uses illegal drugs or drinks (Americans With Disabilities Act of 1990).

In a review of ADA decisions regarding addicted individuals, Westreich (2002) concluded that "a widespread aversion to extending ADA protection to addicted people seems clear" (p. 9). Westreich documented how case law has shaped the application of the ADA in addiction cases. For example, if an employee's aberrant behavior is considered closely attributable to an addiction, ADA protection could be expected. However, the causality of the faulty behaviors may not be seen as being integral to addiction; for example, in the case of an employee's failure to show up for work, his absence was attributed to his inability to make bail rather than to detention from an alcohol-related offense (Westreich 2002).

Furthermore, job performance standards are the same for disabled and nondisabled individuals when ADA protection is sought. Employees may be removed from security positions on the basis of a history of alcoholism if "no reasonable accommodations" on the part of the employer can be found that would enable the employee to be deemed not a security risk. The employee typically would be accommodated by being put in a job that is perhaps less satisfying but that does not involve security issues (Westreich 2002). Barlow (1999) reported that several courts even have ruled that alcoholism is not a disability per se protected by the ADA because there was insufficient evidence that a major life activity was limited. For example, a recovering alcoholic executive who was fired while in rehabilitation was denied protection of the ADA by a federal court because there was not sufficient evidence that he was substantially limited in any major life activities. His hangovers and dulled reactions were considered temporary impairments.

The hope that addicted individuals will receive ADA protection when appropriate is not consistently being fulfilled (Westreich 2002). Quite possibly this disappointing development is reflective of the judiciary struggle with the role of personal responsibility versus the biopsychosocial forces that propel the development of addiction (Committee on Addictions of the Group for the Advancement of Psychiatry 2002).

Malpractice in Substance Abuse Treatment

Addiction specialists must contemplate treatment in light of the growing threat of malpractice actions. The distraction of litigation anxiety can be the greatest impediment to the clinician's primary defense against malpractice: excellent delivery of care. Continuing education, maintenance of empathy, and adequate personal time guard against deficits in judgment. Beyond this, unusual responsibilities in addiction psychiatry lead to singular or at least accentuated malpractice vulnerabilities.

A strong alliance is both a potent agent of therapeutic transformation and a protection against malpractice litigation. However, the astonishing craving, escape, and instant reinforcement that beckon to those with substance use disorders divide patient loyalty to the goal of remission from a desire for immediate comfort even more than most psychiatric illnesses do. Therapist empathy is highly correlated with positive outcome in psychotherapy and guards against the narcissistic injury that is often at the root of malpractice litigation. Miller and Rollnick (2002) proposed a motivation-enhancing interviewing style that relies on eliciting and affirming "change talk" to develop the desire for recovery. Values supporting change and the ambivalence opposing it are clarified and discussed. According to Miller and Rollnick, preserving the alliance depends on remaining in this motivation-enhancing mode while avoiding the role of an active treater shaping a passive patient. Patient passivity and resistance are evoked by the clinician assuming the stance of an omniscient expert, a partisan participant in debates with the patient about the reality of his or her problem or need for treatment, or taking sides with significant others who—often more desperately than the patient—want relief. Resistance is also mobilized by an insistence that the patient accept the clinician's label for him, even subtly blaming him, and by a premature focus on substance abuse as "the problem" when the patient may have other priorities. On the other hand, both motivational interviewing and more confrontational styles may be effective in facilitating substance abuse treatment (Miller et al. 1993). The essential point is to maintain vigilance toward breakdowns of the therapeutic alliance. Although ongoing attention to the quality of interaction improves the chance for a positive treatment alliance, no method can guarantee that a favorable relationship will develop.

Medical treatment increasingly relies on a cooperative model of physician-patient interaction reflecting declining idealization of the medical profession, societal concerns about autonomy, and rising patient sophistication. Although it is somewhat naive and simplistic, this cooperative view emphasizes the patient's responsibility for treatment choices and implies the need to fully inform patients about risks (of both treatment and continued substance use) and therapeutic options. Substance abuse patients are notoriously noncompliant. Treatment regimens should therefore be tailored to the individual patient, but a departure from the usual interventions should be explained in the patient's record so that there is no question about the patient's role in designing the plan. Documentation about a patient's basic ability to understand the treatment prescribed establishes that he or she is competent to consent and therefore is able to shoulder his or her share of responsibility in pursuing it. Even an implicit demonstration of competence, such as a patient

quote about ambivalence toward the treatment that is ultimately accepted, helps in this regard. Regression of the patient increases the clinician's responsibility because the patient has less ego strength to apply to his or her own care. Involving family members mobilizes support and structure for treatment and also minimizes the sense of exclusion that may lead to guilt and litigation in case of a negative outcome. The practitioner should formulate contingency plans for use by the patient and the family if the patient's condition deteriorates.

The high risk of suicide in substance abuse patients is an ever-present issue for both quality of care and malpractice risk management. Even though patients are usually quite aware of the consequences of continued substance use, the tendency that many abusable drugs have to produce suicidal ideation should be explicitly discussed, because completed suicide is the most common cause of successful malpractice litigation. No-harm contracts have not been demonstrated to be reliable means of preventing suicide, but clinical wisdom and experience suggest that they convey benefit in individual instances. Complete or comprehensive suicide assessments have achieved prominence in the professional literature (Simon 1992). Examples of proposed methodology include an explicit evaluation of static (e.g., age, sex) and dynamic (e.g., current support status, recent losses, substance abuse resumption) risk factors; facilitating (e.g., presence of panic attacks) and inhibiting (e.g., no family history of suicide) factors; consideration of intent, plans, means, and perceived consequences; and characterization of patients as being of high, moderate, or low risk (Manley 2000; Simon 1992). By far, most clinicians perform such assessments at every patient visit as they should, although a detailed record including every risk factor is seldom generated. If a suicide should ensue, plaintiff's experts may assume that no assessment took place because it was not documented. The assumption is probably wrong in most cases, and a truly comprehensive risk assessment is seldom written, even though an assessment was performed. However, the clinician should be aware that some authorities would opine that failure to record a comprehensive risk assessment at each visit falls below the standard of care. Despite disagreements, most would assert that it is safer to record suicide risk assessments at each patient contact when significant ongoing suicide potential has been identified. Simon (1992) suggested the use of a checklist to ensure completeness and convenience. It also can be helpful to educate family members or very close associates about suicidal potential and warning signs.

States vary in their view of a clinician's duty to third parties. For example, California and New Jersey tend to regard treating professionals as being responsible for acts or omissions that result in harm to a nonpatient, whereas other states such as Florida and Texas recognize no clinician liability in these instances. Caregivers should familiarize themselves with local precedent so that they can fulfill legal duties to warn, avoid suggesting false abuse scenarios, or conform to other standards. The most salient duty to a third party that might be imposed on substance abuse specialists has to do with negligent release. The act of discharging a patient from an inpatient substance treatment facility implies a belief that the patient is not foreseeably dangerous to others in the community. However, as in the case of suicide risk assessments, it is advisable to conduct some form of risk assessment before proceeding to discharge. Psychiatric professionals should not be, but sometimes are, held responsible for a discharged patient's acting out of antisocial or other personality-related motives. Documentation of a reasonably intact mental status examination (apropos of the discharge environment), understanding of the treatment and aftercare plan, discussion of special risk factors and situations to avoid, agreement by the patient and family that the patient is ready for discharge, and contingency planning should suffice to show that the patient is responsible enough to be at liberty.

Substance abuse clinicians should be aware that working in residential or inpatient treatment facilities entails special malpractice and even criminal vulnerabilities. Such institutions theoretically provide maximal patient protection, but it is precisely this perception of heightened structure that makes mishaps during confinement appear to constitute a priori negligence when scrutinized by lay people. Addiction specialists often function as part-time consultants in these settings, giving them minimal control over the operation of the facility but, in the eyes of attorneys and perhaps juries, partial liability for accidents, suicide attempts, or other problems that may take place there. More disturbing still, some courts have shown a recent and unfortunate inclination to criminalize what has in the past been perceived as negligent care rendered in residential facilities, especially when adolescents are involved. Although it is still rare, this trend should stimulate a very deliberate approach to professional involvement in residential treatment. Those who pursue

such aggressive action and the triers of fact who find against practitioners in equivocal cases seem to be concerned with sanctioning what they see as uncaring and sloppy treatment in settings where it should be most thoughtful and in-depth, regardless of the accuracy of specific allegations. Even when the impression is misleading, nothing so conveys a casual attitude toward treatment to outside observers as slovenly record keeping and the failure to go beyond routine measures when patients are obviously in trouble or are not responding well. Care should be taken to ensure that records are complete and demonstrate more than superficial understanding of the client. Psychiatric practitioners must also promote the cohesion of multidisciplinary teams in inpatient facilities, without which a pall of assembly line–like impersonality and fragmentation may descend over the care rendered. Clinicians working in institutional settings should not hesitate to bring any problems with safety or delivery of treatment to the attention of administrators or simply to decline involvement with entities that deliver substandard care. Otherwise, the clinicians may be assumed to be responsible for the actions of others or for conditions over which they have little actual influence.

Crime and Substance Abuse

Criminal acts seem to be produced by a complex interaction among varying proportions of free will, genetic predispositions, temperament, personality, and facilitating and inhibiting biological and social influences. Because so many of these factors intersect with substance abuse, it is frequently intertwined with illegal behavior. For example, up to 65% of prison inmates are drug dependent at the time of their arrest (Lightfoot and Hodgins 1988). More than half of convicted murderers were abusing a substance at the time they committed a homicide, with half of this number being intoxicated with alcohol (Yarvis 1994). Cannabis abuse and intravenous heroin abuse have also been linked to criminal behavior (Ball et al. 1983; Dembo et al. 1987). The association between substance abuse and crime appears to result from every possible permutation of the two phenomena (Kermani and Castaneda 1996). That is, substance abuse may cause, contribute to, result from, or merely coincide with crime. Specifically, psychosis or intoxication delirium may directly cause crime by altering perceptions to the point that illegal acts appear necessary or appropriate to the impaired person. The agitation that stimulants induce and the disinhibition and magnification of aggression that alcohol evokes may contribute to the mix of factors eventuating in crime. The high price, the interference with work activity, the dread of withdrawal, and even the evanescent half-life associated with illegal drugs such as cocaine propel some addicts toward crime in order to support their habit. On the other hand, the extravagant income that accompanies some criminal lifestyles allows the purchase of otherwise prohibitively expensive drugs in bulk quantities, not to mention the influence of criminal associates who are often involved in purveying or abusing substances themselves. Finally, many individuals with borderline, narcissistic, antisocial, and psychopathic personality disorders choose to commit crimes in a sober state as a reflection of deviant cognitions, values, or goals. The same dysfunctional internal lives may lead to substance abuse as a simple association, rather than its directly contributing to the crime. Like psychiatric clinicians, those involved in criminal law enforcement have struggled to compassionately integrate an understanding of the impact of substances on those who abuse them while limiting inappropriate behavior.

Diminished Capacity and the Insanity Defense

Crime consists of two concurrent essential components: an actus reus (guilty act) coupled with a mens rea (guilty mind). Voluntary substance abuse and addiction do not exculpate perpetrators from criminal responsibility, as some might expect; that is, substance use disorders do not vitiate mens rea. Thus, insanity defenses are not available to defendants who have committed proscribed acts resulting from their voluntary ingestion of legal or illegal psychoactive substances for recreational purposes. However, the specific intent (the particular level of guilty awareness; e.g., knowing, purposeful, intentional, reckless, or negligent) required to secure a conviction for some crimes may be negated by substance intoxication or, arguably, withdrawal states. In such instances, a criminal defendant is considered to be unable to form the intent (mens rea) necessary to commit the crime in question. State jurisdictions vary considerably in their crime classification schemes, but in many localities the effect of substance abuse on intent may be, for example, to reduce applicable charges from first-degree (e.g., willful, deliberate, premeditated) to second-degree (e.g., heat of passion, voluntary manslaughter) homicide. These policies reflect the general awareness in the justice system that substances—particularly alcohol and stimulants—reduce impulse control and impair executive functioning. The state of mind that is so impaired as to interfere with specific intent is termed *diminished capacity*.

Forensic and addiction specialists as well as treating clinicians are often sought out by prosecutors and defense attorneys who need diminished-capacity determinations. It is important to keep in mind a few basic rules of thumb when functioning as an expert witness in these proceedings. First, treating clinicians may or may not feel equipped by their limited knowledge and perspective to supply an opinion about a patient's capacity to form criminal intent or other relevant matters and should not feel compelled to do so simply because they are asked. On the other hand, when one's patient is accused of a serious crime and the clinician possesses relevant information, it seems inappropriate to deny the patient the benefit of that information if it is requested. Becoming the primary forensic expert who exhaustively investigates the alleged criminal act and draws conclusions about diminished capacity issues is not necessary, however, and may be counterproductive because of actual or perceived compromise of evaluator objectivity. Whether forensic evaluators should also administer treatment is the subject of considerable disagreement. The ethical guidelines of the American Academy of Psychiatry and the Law state that these two functions should be separate except in unusual circumstances. Although there is much to recommend this position, real-world situations are often more complicated, and the inconvenience, discomfort, and expense of evaluation, as well as respect for the autonomy of the patient and attorneys involved, suggest that a more flexible approach is warranted. The involved parties should have an opportunity to consent to any role-mixing but should acknowledge that problematic consequences may ensue.

In conducting diminished-capacity determinations forensic evaluators should consider relevant history, especially criminal history, the patient's known behavior during intoxication in other contexts, the commonality or dissonance of the alleged criminal conduct with the person's usual actions and choices, and the possibility of malingering. Neuropsychological testing, functional brain imaging, toxicological screening, and other appropriate laboratory testing are often useful in making diminished-capacity inquiries. The automatic equation of intoxication with diminished capacity—especially when the criminal acts are embedded in a long criminal career accrued in both intoxicated and nonintoxicated states—is a common mistake in such evaluations. Oversubscription to disease or personal-responsibility models of addiction is another often-encountered error. Both stances are reductionistic and may predispose to either excusing perpetrators wholesale or incorrectly assuming that the diminution of executive functioning and the pull and angst of addictive lifestyles have no effect on volition. Finally, diminished-capacity evaluations should never depend on self-reporting and should never be based on diffuse reasoning about substance abuse. That is, the association of substance abuse with antisocial behavior is not by itself a sufficient basis for concluding that a causative relationship exists between the two in a specific instance. The known effects of the substance in question must be compared with the criminal behavior to help determine whether a relationship exists. When diminished capacity does not apply, substance use disorders may still result in mitigation at sentencing.

As implied above, involuntary intoxication or the unexpected effects of prescription medication do constitute an affirmative defense to criminal charges, defined either as insanity or the specific legal entity of involuntary intoxication. The burgeoning psychotropic armamentarium and its ever more complicated drug interaction and metabolism issues make the phenomenon of involuntary intoxication more and more important as time goes on. However, involuntary intoxication is frequently claimed but seldom true, and evaluators must be wary of malingering and the unconscious projection of responsibility for misbehavior onto substances. Intoxication or withdrawal delirium or previously unknown idiosyncratic intoxication could form the basis for an insanity plea, as could the commission of a criminal act related to the unintended long-term consequences of substance abuse, such as psychotic disorders, dementia, or hallucinosis.

Competence to Stand Trial

As discussed earlier, there are several specific competences that a psychiatrist may be asked to assess, including competence to refuse treatment, competence to care for one's self and property (guardianship), and others. There are various competences of the criminal justice process as well. These competences include competence to confess (i.e., to waive rights of pretrial proceedings) competence to stand trial, competence to be sentenced, and competence to be executed (Grisso 1988).

The competences of the criminal justice system as listed above, particularly competence to stand trial, are the areas most likely to confront the addiction psychiatrist.

In most states, competence to stand trial is based on the U.S. Supreme Court decision in *Dusky v. United States* (1960): "the test must be whether he has sufficient present ability to consult with his attorney with a reasonable degree of rational understanding and a rational as well as a factual understanding of the proceedings against him." Most states add that the deficiencies must be due to a mental disease or defect (Grisso 1988).

Areas to explore when assessing competence, originally formulated by McGarry (1973), have been summarized by Grisso (1988) as follows:

- Appraisal of available legal defense
- Unmanageable behavior
- Quality of relating to attorney
- Planning of legal strategy
- Appraisal of roles of judge, prosecutor, defense counsel, jury, and witnesses
- Understanding of court proceedings
- Appreciation of charges
- Appreciation of range and nature of possible penalties
- Appraisal of likely outcome
- Capacity to disclose to attorney available pertinent facts surrounding the offense
- Capacity to realistically challenge the prosecuting witness
- Capacity to testify relevantly
- Self-defeating versus self-serving motivations

In patients with substance use disorders, the capacities listed above may be compromised by delirium withdrawal states, drug-induced psychosis, or drug-induced dementia. Drug withdrawal or drug-induced delirium would typically be of short duration and would be likely to have resolved by the time determination of competence is requested.

Drug Courts

The current model of a drug court first appeared in 1989 in Dade County, Florida. Throughout the 1990s, drug courts proliferated; 140 were identified by 1997. Drug courts provide pretrial diversion for nonviolent drug-involved offenders. Belenko (1998) outlined the features of drug courts as follows:

- Judicial supervision of structured community-based treatment
- Timely identification of defendants in need of treatment and referral to treatment as soon as possible after arrest
- Regular status hearings before the judicial office to monitor treatment progress and program compliance
- Increasing defendant accountability through a series of graduated sanctions and rewards
- Mandated periodic drug testing

Earlier models existed, but treatment was not strongly emphasized (Belenko 1998).

The impetus for the formation of drug courts as well as other judicially mandated treatment arose from the large increase in numbers of incarcerated drug offenders throughout the 1980s. During the 1990s the rate of referrals from the criminal justice system to substance abuse programs increased at least threefold, but still only a minority of substance abusers received treatment (Polcin 2001).

The outcomes of drug court clients are encouraging. In a 30-month follow-up period from a Florida court, predictors of retention and arrest were studied. Overall, 67% of participants were arrested at least once during the 30-month follow-up period. Graduates of the program were significantly less likely to be rearrested, and participants who were not rearrested averaged a 2.5-month longer stay in the program (average stay of 11.6 months versus 9.0 months). Variables that predicted a favorable outcome from this drug court included full-time employment, living with family or friends (versus living alone or living alone with small children), current charges of drug possession (versus other charges), and a primary substance abuse problem with alcohol or marijuana (versus cocaine) (Peters et al. 1999).

A follow-up study from a Delaware drug court found a 19% rearrest rate for graduates and a 55% re-

arrest rate for those who were terminated from the program (Willhite and O'Connell 1999). A drug court in Riverside County, California, found that a comparison group (offenders who did not receive drug court–mandated treatment) reoffended at a rate of 25% over the 2.5-year follow-up period compared with 34% of drug court dropouts but only 5% of drug court graduates (Sechrest and Shichor 1999).

Another favorable aspect of drug courts is cost savings. Examples include a study from Maine that showed costs for drug court clients were $5,600 per year, compared with $30,000 per year if they had been incarcerated (Anspach and Ferguson 1999). Similarly, it was estimated that $1.5 million was saved in the cases of the 102 clients studied in California (Sechrest and Shichor 1999).

Treatment During Incarceration

The extraordinarily frequent co-occurrence of crime and substance abuse poses daunting challenges to jails and prisons. The success of diversion programs in reducing drug-related crime implies that the frequency of such crime and the cost of incarceration can be reduced by the delivery of effective drug treatment programs in correctional institutions. However, a number of monetary factors seem to prevent substance treatment for inmates from achieving its full promise. The cost of initiating programs, the extensive target population, the scarcity of available dollars, the political dangers of diversion of money from more visible police functions, and budgetary compartmentalization (which negates the overall societal financial incentives for individual components of the law enforcement system to provide such treatment) have limited the availability of treatment. For these and other reasons, only 1%–20% of offenders who have substance abuse problems and who are or have been incarcerated have received treatment for those issues (Peters et al. 1997; U.S. General Accounting Office 1991a, 1991b).

Despite this disheartening paucity of correctional resources, some incarceration-based programs have demonstrated effectiveness. The exemplary Stay'n Out program in New York maximizes the advantages of proximity to conditional release, chance for separation from the general prison population, and peer support and confrontation in a therapeutic community setting (Wexler et al 1990). Stay'n Out reduced recidivism more than did nontherapeutic community and individual counseling treatment, yet it added only $8.00 per day to the usual cost of imprisonment (Ehrlich et al. 1989). An inmate could participate in the program for up to 2 years, and length of participation was correlated with successful postrelease adjustment.

Edens et al. (1977) reviewed a number of other incarceration-based treatment programs that deal with both substance abuse and dual-diagnosis patients. Judging from these operations, the ideal program utilizes extended assessment periods, psychoeducation, cognitive-behavioral interventions, medication when indicated, self-help groups, relapse prevention, and provisions for community transition. Like Stay'n Out, many programs employ a therapeutic community approach. At a minimum, incarceration-based substance abuse treatment should include screening for co-occurring mental illness and access to 12-step or similar group experiences. The modest cost of administering such treatment should make it relatively widely available, but a broader range of interventions is obviously desirable. Unfortunately, some jurisdictions limit treatment to that provided by volunteer counselors from the community (Peters et al. 1997).

Clinicians administering substance abuse treatment in incarceration settings deal with a number of practical problems, which—although they may defy definitive solutions—should be considered when delivering care. In jails, the care delivery system should provide for a screening mechanism to identify arrestees who are aggressive or self-destructive due to intoxication and who are at risk for dangerous types of withdrawal. Questionnaires are useful in this regard, but clinicians should seek the opportunity to educate the law enforcement personnel who make first contact to recognize warning signs. Although it may not be practical to arrange for immediate psychiatric evaluation for these patients, the capacity to transfer them to a more capable facility or some form of consultation, even if by telephone, is needed. Safe and humane isolation should be provided for agitated and suicidal patients. Social services can help prevent rearrest by facilitating transition back into the community. Maintaining continuity of care can be difficult because of court appearances, unpredictable release times, and meager community resources. Although it is often neglected, close cooperation with volunteer organizations and community caregivers helps inmates avoid falling through the cracks after release.

Issues change in prison settings where—perhaps even more than in jails—addicted patients may continue to pursue their habits along with the concomitant ills of robbery, prostitution, and corruption. Even intravenous drug abuse is possible in incarceration and can result in hepatitis and transmission of human immunodeficiency virus. Rarely, other countries have provided bleach and have instituted needle-sharing programs in prisons, but domestic correctional institutions are reluctant to do so because they fear the appearance of acceptance and, more understandably, heightened risk of violence. Incarceration-based treatment programs should be designed with these problems in mind, even though they may be insurmountable. Staff development is easily neglected amid these overwhelming concerns. Treatment coordinators should remember that team-building activities and the maintaining of alliances with educational institutions can help prevent the demoralized indifference that may be the greatest enemy of effective correctional health care.

Providing substance abuse treatment in incarceration settings is a demanding task entailing special limitations but also special opportunities to be of service to both patients and society. Community advocacy and strong working relationships with law enforcement—reinforced by a logical appeal to the value of treatment in terms of optimal resource management, improved security for correctional personnel, and enhanced public safety—can prove decisive in assisting this special population.

References

Americans With Disabilities Act of 1990, Pub. L. No. 101-336

Anspach DF, Ferguson AS: Maine's first drug court: Project Exodus. National Drug Court Institute Review 2:116–119, 1999

Anti-Drug Abuse Act of 1988, Pub. L. No. 100-690

Ball J, Schaeffer J, Nurco D: The day-to-day criminality of heroin addicts in Baltimore: a study in the continuity of offense rates. Drug Alcohol Depend 12:119–142, 1983

Barlow T: Rulings make ADA protection for alcoholic employees more difficult. South Carolina Business Journal 18(3):8–12, 1999

Belenko S: Research on drug courts: a critical review. National Drug Court Institute Review 1:1–42, 1998

Committee on Addictions of the Group for the Advancement of Psychiatry: Responsibility and choice in addiction. Psychiatr Serv 53:707–713, 2002

Dembo R, Washburn M, Wish ED, et al: Heavy marijuana use and crime among youths entering a juvenile detention center. J Psychoactive Drugs 19:47–56, 1987

Drug-Free Workplace Act of 1988, Pub. L. No. 100-690, Title V, Subtitle D

Dusky v United States, 362 U.S. 402 (1960)

Edens JF, Peters RH, Hills HA: Treating prison inmates with co-occurring disorders: an integrative review of existing programs. Behav Sci Law 15:439–457, 1977

Ehrlich E, Driscoll L, Green W, et al: Some winning maneuvers in the war on drugs. Business Week, November 27, 1989, pp 120–130

Grisso T: Competency to Stand Trial Evaluations: A Manual for Practice. Sarasota, FL, Professional Resource Exchange, 1988

Hall KT, Appelbaum PS: The origin of commitment for substance abuse in the United States. J Am Acad Psychiatry Law 30:33–45, 2002

Howland RW, Howland JW: 200 years of drinking in the United States: evolution of the disease concept, in Drinking, Alcohol and American Society: Issues and Current Research. Edited by Ewing JA, Rouse BA. Chicago, IL, Nelson-Half, 1978, pp 39–60

Kermani EJ, Castaneda R: Psychoactive substance use in forensic psychiatry. Am J Drug Alcohol Abuse 22:1–27, 1996

Lightfoot LQ, Hodgins D: A survey of alcohol and drug problems in incarcerated offenders. Int J Addict 23:688–706, 1988

Manley MRS: Diagnosis and psychiatry: examination of the psychiatric patient, in Kaplan & Sadock's Comprehensive Textbook of Psychiatry, 7th Edition. Edited by Sadock BJ, Sadock VA. Philadelphia, PA, Lippincott Williams & Wilkins, 2000, pp 652–664

McGarry A: Competency to stand trial and mental illness (DHEW Publ No ADM 77-103). Rockville, MD, National Institute on Drug Abuse, 1973

Miller WR, Rollnick S: Motivational Interviewing: Preparing for Change, 2nd Edition. New York, Guilford, 2002

Miller W, Benefield R, Tonigan J: Enhancing motivation for change in problem drinking: a controlled comparison of two therapist styles. J Consult Clin Psychol 61:455–461 1993

Musto DF: The American Disease: Origins of Narcotic Control. New Haven, CT, Yale University Press, 1973

Musto DF: Historical perspectives, in Substance Abuse: A Comprehensive Textbook, 3rd Edition. Edited by Lowinson JH, Ruiz P, Millman RB, et al. Baltimore, MD, Williams & Williams, 1997, pp 1–10

Peters RH, May RI, Kearns WD: Drug treatment in jails: results of a nationwide survey. J Crim Justice 20:283–295, 1997

Peters RH, Haas AL, Murrin MR: Predictors of retention and arrests in drug courts. National Drug Court Institute Review 2:33–60, 1999

Polcin DL: Drug and alcohol offenders coerced into treatment: a review of modalities and suggestions for research on social model programs. Subst Use Misuse 36:589–608, 2001

Sechrest DK, Shichor D: Riverside County drug court evaluation. National Drug Court Institute Review 2:114–116, 1999

Simon RI: Clinical Psychiatry and the Law, 2nd Edition. Washington, DC, American Psychiatric Press, 1992

Starkman PE: Answering the tough questions about alcoholism and substance abuse under the ADA and EMLA. Employee Relat Law J 25:43–95, 2000

U.S. General Accounting Office: Drug treatment. Despite new strategy, few federal inmates receive treatment. Report to the Committee on Government Operations, House of Representatives (GAO/HRD-92-116). Washington, DC, U.S. General Accounting Office, 1991a

U.S. General Accounting Office: Drug treatment. State prisons face challenges in providing services. Report to the Committee on Government Operations, House of Representatives (GAO/HRD-91-128). Washington, DC, U.S. General Accounting Office, 1991b

Westreich LM: Addiction and the Americans With Disabilities Act. J Am Acad Psychiatry Law 30:355–363, 2002

Wexler HK, Falkin GP, Lipton DS: Outcome evaluation of a prison therapeutic community for substance abuse treatment. Crim Justice Behav 17:71–90, 1990

White WL: Slaying the Dragon: The History of Addiction Treatment and Recovery in America. Bloomington, IL, Chestnut Health Systems, 1998

Willhite SA, O'Connell JP: The Delaware drug court: a baseline evaluation. National Drug Court Institute Review 2(1):110–111, 1999

Yarvis RM: Patterns of substance abuse and intoxication among murderers. Bull Am Acad Psychiatry Law 22:133–144, 1994

Index

Page numbers printed in **boldface** type refer to figures or tables.

alternatives to, 440, 448
attitudes of health care providers
   toward, 435
continued abstinence related to
   involvement in, 436
definition of, 433
difficulty for persons with social
   phobia, 340, 534
drug counseling and, 379, 382
effectiveness of, 435–437
   for adolescents vs. adults, 437
   mechanisms of, 437
   treatment costs and, 436–437
   twelve-step programs are not
      always helpful, 440
facilitating affiliation and
   involvement in, 438
   tailoring to specific groups, 439
group therapy and, 399
for hallucinogen abuse, 206
health care practitioners' need to be
   knowledgeable about, 438
integrating professional treatment
   with, 438–439
lack of formal evaluation of, 137–138
matching patients to, 439–440
Minnesota Model programs based
   on principles of, 447
network therapy and, 353, 358
partial hospitalization and, 479
philosophy of, 379
psychodynamic psychotherapy and,
   339, 346–347
for relapse prevention, 379
during short-term residential
   treatment, 144
who attends meetings of, 434–435
women in, 434, 542
Twin studies, 60–62, 73–74, 110
of alcoholism, 75, 77, 151
of cannabis use, 74–76, 173
of hallucinogen abuse, 74, 75
of opiate abuse, 74, 75
of opioid dependence, 27
of sedative abuse, 74, 75
of stimulant abuse, 74–76
Tylox. *See* Oxycodone
Tyrosine hydroxylase, 36

Ulcers, 271
Unbalancing techniques, 427
Uniform Alcoholism and Intoxication
   Treatment Act, 480
United Kingdom, 60

University of Rhode Island Change
   Assessment (URICA), 115
Urban substance abuse, 62
Uric acid, **159,** 592
URICA (University of Rhode Island
   Change Assessment), 115
Urinary retention, methadone-
   induced, 295
Urinary tract infection, 548
Urine acidification, 214
Urine toxicology testing, 113, 379–380,
   589, **591**. *See also* Laboratory testing
   for anabolic-androgenic steroids,
      259, **260**
   for cannabinoids, 183, 589
   to confirm fetal drug exposure, 550
   drugs detected by, 589
   for hallucinogens, 203
   for inhalants, 252–253, **253**
   during methadone maintenance, 298
   on-site screening kits for, 588
   for opiates, 271, 589
   for phencyclidine, 213
   preemployment, 589
   psychotherapy and, 379–380
   in therapeutic communities, 494
   window of detection for, 589
U.S. National Longitudinal Survey of
   Youth, 614
Utilization of health care resources,
   related to use of patient placement
   criteria, 124

Vaccine, cocaine, 191, 193
Valium. *See* Diazepam
Valproate
   for alcohol withdrawal, 244
   for benzodiazepine withdrawal,
      244–245
   for comorbid bipolar disorder and
      substance abuse, 532
Values in therapeutic communities, 487
Vasoconstriction in newborn, cocaine-
   induced, 551
Venlafaxine, 532
Ventral tegmental area (VTA)
   alcohol effects in, 8, 11
   drug self-administration and, 22
   glucocorticoid receptors in, 23
   mediation of reinforcing properties
      of drugs in, 20, 32
   opioid effects in, 21, **22,** 24, 26
   in stimulant sensitization, 33–34
   toluene effects in, 249

Versed. *See* Midazolam
Vicodin. *See* Hydrocodone
Victimization, 96, 428, 450, 541, 542,
   543
Videotape self-confrontation, for
   alcoholic patients, 133
Vietnam veterans, 62
Violent behavior. *See also* Aggression
   and agitation; Crime and
   substance abuse
   anabolic-androgenic steroid use
      and, 262
   inpatient treatment of suicidal or
      homicidal patient, 449
   toward women, 428
Visual disturbances, drug-induced
   hallucinogens, 201
   γ-hydroxybutyrate, 329
   ketamine, 213
   phencyclidine, 213
   sedative-hypnotics, 237
"Vitamin K," 211, 326. *See also* Ketamine
Vitamin supplements
   during alcohol detoxification, 161
   during opioid detoxification, 284
   use by older adults, 524
Vocational rehabilitation, 486, 544
Volatile substances. *See* Inhalant use
Voltage-sensitive calcium channels
   (VSCCs)
   alcohol and, 10–11
   cannabinoids and, 49, 50
Voltaren. *See* Diclofenac
Voucher systems. *See* Contingency
   management interventions
VSCCs (voltage-sensitive calcium
   channels)
   alcohol and, 10–11
   cannabinoids and, 49, 50
VTA. *See* Ventral tegmental area
Vulnerabilities to substance abuse,
   27–28, 64–66, 74, 84
   genetic factors, 65, 73–79, 84

WAIS-R (Wechsler Adult Intelligence
   Scale—Revised), 249
Warning labels on alcohol beverage
   containers, 617
Weakness, γ-hydroxybutyrate–induced,
   329
Wechsler Adult Intelligence Scale—
   Revised (WAIS-R), 249
Weight gain, after smoking cessation,
   227–228